Basic Mechanisms of the Epilepsies

Editorial Board

Herbert H. Jasper
CHAIRMAN

J. Kiffin Penry
COORDINATING EDITOR

Reginald G. Bickford

William F. Caveness

James L. O'Leary

Alfred Pope

A. Earl Walker

Arthur A. Ward, Jr.

Dixon M. Woodbury

Staff

Bettie Jean Hessie

Teresina M. Williams

Rebecca R. Wise

PUBLIC HEALTH SERVICE
ADVISORY COMMITTEE ON THE EPILEPSIES

CHAIRMAN
H. Houston Merritt

EXECUTIVE SECRETARY
J. Kiffin Penry

RESEARCH AND RESEARCH TRAINING SUBCOMMITTEE

Arthur A. Ward, Jr. (*Subcommittee Chairman*)

Reginald G. Bickford

Herbert H. Jasper

Alfred Pope

J. Preston Robb

Dixon M. Woodbury

SERVICE AND SERVICE TRAINING SUBCOMMITTEE

David D. Daly (*Subcommittee Chairman*)

Edward Davens

Philip R. Dodge

Francis M. Forster

Thomas R. Johns

Herbert R. Karp

Richmond S. Paine

Joseph E. Snyder

NATIONAL INSTITUTE OF NEUROLOGICAL DISEASES AND STROKE

DIRECTOR
Edward F. MacNichol, Jr.

Basic Mechanisms of the
EPILEPSIES

Editors

HERBERT H. JASPER, M.D., D.Sc., F.R.S.C.
Professor of Neurophysiology
University of Montreal

ARTHUR A. WARD, Jr., M.D.
Professor and Chairman
Department of Neurological Surgery
University of Washington School of Medicine

ALFRED POPE, M.D.
Professor of Neuropathology
Harvard Medical School

Foreword by
H. HOUSTON MERRITT, M.D.
Professor of Neurology and Dean
College of Physicians and Surgeons
Columbia University

Little, Brown and Company
BOSTON

Copyright © 1969 by Little, Brown and Company

All rights reserved. No part of this book may be reproduced in any form or by any electronic or mechanical means, including information storage and retrieval systems, without permission in writing from the publisher, except by a reviewer who may quote brief passages in a review.

Library of Congress catalog card No. 75-82926

First Edition

Published in Great Britain by J. & A. Churchill Ltd., London
British Standard Book No. 7000 0155 7

Printed in the United States of America

Foreword

EPILEPSY, the term used to describe the repeated occurrence of any of the various forms of convulsive seizures, is one of the oldest afflictions known to man. It has been the subject of discussion in medical and lay literature since time immemorial.

Known in ancient literature as the dread disease, it was subject to many superstitions, and popular feeling in regard to the disease has changed very little up to modern times. Afflicted individuals are still shunned and excluded by society, in line with the old belief based on the concept expressed in the term *seizure:* the patient is being seized by the devil.

Ideas with regard to treatment have been similarly mystic until recent times. A little more than a hundred years ago, Sieveking gave a dissertation before the Royal Society of Medicine on the treatment of epilepsy. Among the numerous exotic remedies he discussed was extract of mistletoe. The logic behind this therapy was that mistletoe clung to the tree and did not fall, and therefore the administration of this preparation would prevent the patient from falling down during a seizure. It is interesting to note that in the discussion of Sieveking's presentation, Locock stated that he had good results in the control of convulsions by administering bromides. Locock had given bromides as an anaphrodisiac because he thought the seizures were related to sexual excitement. Apparently he had not thought of the possible depressant action of the bromides on the cortical neurones.

We now know that convulsive seizures are the normal mode of expression of the cortex to an excessive, overwhelming discharge, that they occur or can be precipitated in all forms of life with a rudimentary or well-developed nervous system.

Epilepsy in man is a common disease, estimated to occur in approximately one-half of one percent of the population throughout the world. The form in which the convulsive seizure expresses itself is related to a number of factors, including the site or origin of the abnormal discharge and the rapidity of the spread of the discharge.

In so-called grand mal epilepsy, the site of origin of the discharge is in the neurons of the cerebral cortex, or perhaps in the subcortical structures. The discharge spreads rapidly to all parts of the nervous system, resulting in rapid loss of consciousness. The dramatic features of the attacks, the rigidity and convulsive movements, result from stimulation of the motor cortex. If the focus of origin of the abnormal discharge is in the relatively silent area of the cortex, there may be no external clue for the site of origin. If it is in the motor cortex, however, movement of isolated segments of the body musculature may signalize its onset. Similarly, somatic sensory, olfactory, auditory, visual, or other phenomena may precede development of the generalized convulsion; this gives information with regard to the area of brain that gives rise to the abnormal discharge and therefore is presumably the site of the organic lesion or the locus of action of a metabolic disturbance.

In partial seizures, the abnormal discharge may remain localized to restricted portions of the brain, as a result either of low intensity of the discharge or of predominance of inhibitory factors. This nature of the symptoms that develop in localized forms of seizures, minor epilepsy, is related to the affected portion of the nervous system.

In spite of the devastating, although temporary, effects of convulsions of the organism, their occurrences have been of great value to the physiologist in elucidating the form and function of the nervous system. The study of patients with convulsions resulting from experiments of nature, or as a result of electrical stimulation of an isolated portion of the cortex, has provided invaluable information with regard to the function of various portions of the brain and the mode of action of individual components of the nervous system, as well as their interaction with neighboring and distant centers.

A discussion of many of the facets of epilepsy is not possible here. Two, however, should be touched on: the hereditary factor and the possibility of modifying the factors that may precipitate the abnormal discharge or alter its spread.

It is commonly assumed that epilepsy is inherited, and numerous studies attest to the importance of hereditary factors. At one time (I do not know if it still exists) a law prohibited entry into this country by an individual afflicted with so-called idiopathic epilepsy, but a person subject to convulsive seizures as a result of head injury, for example, was allowed free access.

It is not difficult to see the fallacy of this type of reasoning. All of us inherit a nervous system capable of responding to excessive stimuli by the production of a convulsive seizure. Any inherited metabolic disturbance or disease of the nervous system may predispose the affected individual to convulsive disorders. In such an individual, the metabolic defect or disease is inherited, not the epilepsy.

Other causative factors of seizures are of much greater importance. They include maldevelopment of the nervous system due to adverse factors operating during development of the embryo or fetus in utero: trauma, anoxia, hypoglycemia, or other factors presenting in the perinatal period; infections of the nervous system, head trauma, brain tumors, or degenerative disease in youth and adult life. The familial occurrence of epilepsy may be due in part to faulty reproductive apparatus, a small pelvis, or inadequate prenatal or perinatal care. It is interesting to speculate what light the current perinatal study of the National Institute of Neurological Diseases and Stroke will throw on this subject.

The topic of this monograph, spawned by a preceding symposium with the same title, *Basic Mechanisms of the Epilepsies,* is of far greater importance than any speculations regarding the inheritance of epilepsy. If inherited, epilepsy is difficult to modify and may require study extending over many generations; the results of investigations presented here are of much more immediate and practical significance. Information is sorely needed regarding factors that cause isolated neurons or collections of neurons to become epileptogenic; the nature of physiological or biochemical disturbance in those neurons; the mode of spread of the discharge; and how it can be modified by changes in external or internal environment and by administration of drugs or other forms of therapy.

As one who has long been interested in the medical form of therapy, I am forced to admit that we do not as yet have a rational form of therapy; while the available agents are of great value to patients, they are far from ideal.

The information presented here and the results of work yet to be done that hopefully will be stimulated by this monograph should be of value to basic scientists in understanding the nervous system and of great assistance to clinicians in developing more effective forms of therapy.

H. HOUSTON MERRITT

Preface

WHILE the neurological problem of epilepsy is estimated to involve between one and two million Americans, an adequate understanding of this condition is not yet available. In recognizing an urgent need for action at the national level, the Surgeon General of the Public Health Service, Dr. William H. Stewart, created the Public Health Service Advisory Committee on the Epilepsies in May, 1966. Dr. H. Houston Merritt, Professor of Neurology and Dean, College of Physicians and Surgeons, Columbia University, was named chairman.

Two subcommittees were designated: one for service and the other for research. Dr. David D. Daly of Dallas was appointed chairman of the Service and Service Training Subcommittee, and Dr. Arthur A. Ward, Jr., of Seattle was appointed chairman of the Research and Research Training Subcommittee.

A Basic Research Task Force (one of three task forces attached to the Research Subcommittee) was established under the chairmanship of Dr. Herbert H. Jasper. It was apparent to this Task Force that basic research in the epilepsies needed stimulation. Furthermore, those engaged in various facets of such research are scattered throughout the basic and clinical neurosciences, so that optimal communication is difficult. As a consequence, a critical need was identified for a modern, definitive statement of current knowledge regarding fundamental aspects of the epilepsies in the form of a comprehensive monograph. It was determined that this monograph should cover recent advances in knowledge dealing with basic structural and functional neuronal mechanisms of importance to an understanding of the pathophysiology of epileptic seizures. In addition to presenting a collation and synthesis of modern knowledge in this area, it was hoped that this effort would stimulate increased participation and cross-communication among diverse scientific disciplines, so that all the potential of the relevant neurosciences could be brought to bear on the problem of the epilepsies.

It was decided that it would be appropriate that such an effort be made at this particular time. It is now 21 years since the Association for Research in Nervous and Mental Disease published the proceedings of their symposium, entitled *Epilepsy*. The monograph by Penfield and Jasper, entitled *Epilepsy and the Functional Anatomy of the Human Brain,* was originally published in 1954, and was designed for a somewhat different purpose.

It was judged that an authoritative statement of the basic mechanisms of the epilepsies would require the collaboration of colleagues who are particularly sophisticated in their specialized fields. To implement such a project involving a large group of authors, the Basic Research Task Force developed plans for two preliminary and necessary steps, a workshop to be followed by a symposium. These plans were formulated in September, 1967, presented to the full Advisory Committee on the Epilepsies, and promptly approved. It was established that the effort would be sponsored by the Advisory Committee and the National Institute of Neurological Diseases and Stroke.

The Editorial Board, chaired by Dr. Herbert H. Jasper, includes as members: Drs. Reginald G. Bickford, William F. Caveness, James L. O'Leary, J. Kiffin Penry, Alfred Pope, A. Earl Walker, Arthur A. Ward, Jr., and Dixon M. Woodbury. The same group (except Drs. O'Leary and Walker) comprised the organizers of the symposium, with Dr. J. Kiffin Penry as Secretary.

The workshop held in Colorado Springs in February, 1968, surveyed the clinical problem and developed the areas of relevance in the basic sciences. The content of the monograph was firmly programmed and the publication date set for the fall of 1969. Twenty-nine of the authors were present, and three new chapters were proposed. It was decided that a designated discussant for each chapter should make an additional contribution to the monograph by presenting more than a categorical discussion of the author's material and by providing a further contribution to the subject from his own data in order to enhance the completeness of the monograph. The Organizing Committee, in conjunction with the workshop participants, selected the proposed discussants. The structure of the symposium was completed at the workshop.

The symposium on basic mechanisms of the epilepsies took place in November, 1968, again at Colorado Springs. Each of the 33 authors presented pertinent aspects of his research and summarized the contents of his chapter. This was complemented by the contribution of the respective discussant. Final arrangements for publication of the monograph were completed.

Immediately following the symposium, processing and editing of the manuscripts was begun and coordination of the publication schedule was carried out in the Section on Epilepsy of the National Institute of Neurological Diseases and Stroke. A meeting of the Editorial Board was held late in January, 1969, to clarify any problems that had arisen in connection with the monograph, and final review, discussion, and approval of the manuscripts was achieved at that time.

While it is comprehensive, *Basic Mechanisms of the Epilepsies* does not purport to be an all-inclusive presentation on the present state of the subject. Other material, either directly or indirectly related, might have been included, but the practical limitations of space required that a selection be made of both subjects and authors. The enthusiastic contributions from the authors have been most gratifying, but the omission of many who may have made equally important contributions is regretted.

The National Institutes of Health and the Editorial Board are not responsible for the conceptions expressed by the individual authors. The material included represents the judgments of each author and does not necessarily reflect the views and opinions of the Editorial Board.

The Editors would like to express particular thanks to Dr. J. Kiffin Penry who is Head, Section on Epilepsy of the National Institute of Neurological Diseases and Stroke. The creation of this monograph is, in no small measure, a consequence of his diligence, tact, and organizing ability, coupled with his high competence and motivation in the field of epilepsy. The dedication of Dr. Penry and his staff is documented between these covers and appreciated by all who have participated in this endeavor.

It has been the objective of all concerned with this effort that this volume should bring together the current work considered significant, viable, and provocative in the field of epilepsy. It is hoped that by so doing it will serve as a benchmark which summarizes past scientific accomplishments, against which future progress can be measured. To this end, the monograph has a twofold mission: to make available to clinicians, scientists, and students a body of data and concepts relevant to epilepsy; and to serve as a stimulus for an expanded interdisciplinary research effort in the epilepsies.

H. H. J.
A. A. W., Jr.
A. P.

Contents

Foreword BY H. HOUSTON MERRITT		vii
Preface		ix
Contributors		xvii

1 Clinical and Experimental Challenges of the Epilepsies — 1
ARTHUR A. WARD, JR., HERBERT H. JASPER, AND ALFRED POPE

2 Architecture of the Cerebral Cortex — 13
J. SZENTÁGOTHAI

Discussion: HETEROGENEITY OF THE CEREBRAL CORTEX — 29
Marc Colonnier and Serge Rossignol

3 Biophysics of Nerve Membrane — 41
J. WALTER WOODBURY

Discussion: VOLTAGE CLAMP ANALYSIS OF A REPETITIVELY FIRING NEURON — 76
Charles F. Stevens

4 Cerebral Energy Metabolism and Membrane Phenomena — 83
HENRY MC ILWAIN

Discussion: ENERGY METABOLITES IN EXPERIMENTAL SEIZURES — 98
Janet V. Passonneau

5 Central Synaptic Transmitters — 105
DAVID R. CURTIS

Discussion: TRANSMITTER ACTION AND MULTIPLE DISCHARGE — 130
Motoy Kuno

6 Ultrastructural Neurochemistry — 137
EDUARDO DE ROBERTIS, GEORGINA RODRIGUEZ DE LORES ARNAIZ, AND MARTHA ALBERICI

CONTENTS

Discussion: NEUROTRANSMITTERS IN NORMAL AND ISOLATED CORTEX — 159
K. Krnjević

7 Mechanisms of Action of Convulsants — 167
DON W. ESPLIN AND BARBARA ZABLOCKA-ESPLIN

Discussion: ACTION OF CONVULSANTS: NEUROCHEMICAL ASPECTS — 184
William E. Stone

8 Pharmacology of Synaptic Transmitters — 195
GEORGE B. KOELLE

Discussion: FLUORESCENCE HISTOCHEMISTRY OF MONOAMINES IN THE CNS — 212
A. Dahlström

9 Excitatory and Inhibitory Mechanisms in Brain — 229
J. C. ECCLES

Discussion: STUDIES OF PYRAMIDAL TRACT CELLS — 253
Tomokazu Oshima

10 The Epileptic Neuron: Chronic Foci in Animals and Man — 263
ARTHUR A. WARD, JR.

Discussion: EXPERIMENTAL SEIZURE MECHANISMS — 289
Eli S. Goldensohn

11 Acute Effects of Topical Epileptogenic Agents — 299
COSIMO AJMONE-MARSAN

Discussion: MICROELECTRODE STUDIES OF PENICILLIN FOCI — 320
David A. Prince

12 Isolated and Deafferented Neurons: Disuse Supersensitivity — 329
SETH K. SHARPLESS

Discussion: EFFECT OF STIMULATION ON ISOLATED CORTEX — 349
Lester T. Rutledge

13 Physiology and Histochemistry of the Mirror Focus — 357
FRANK MORRELL

	Discussion: THE MIRROR FOCUS AND LONG-TERM MEMORY STORAGE Samuel H. Barondes	371
14	DC Potential Shifts in Paroxysmal States HEINZ CASPERS AND ERWIN-JOSEF SPECKMANN	375
	Discussion: POLARIZATION OF GENICULATE AND CORTICAL NEURONS James L. O'Leary	389
15	Neuronal Mechanisms Underlying the EEG O. D. CREUTZFELDT	397
	Discussion: ON THE GENERATION OF NEOCORTICAL POTENTIALS Daniel A. Pollen	411
16	Mechanisms of Propagation: Extracellular Studies HERBERT H. JASPER	421
	Discussion: MECHANISMS OF PROPAGATION: INTRACELLULAR STUDIES Dominick P. Purpura	441
17	Sleep Mechanisms OTTAVIO POMPEIANO	453
	Discussion: BASAL FOREBRAIN INHIBITION Carmine D. Clemente	474
18	Stability and Seizure Susceptibility of Immature Brain DOMINICK P. PURPURA	481
	Discussion: ELECTRICAL ACTIVITY OF BRAIN TISSUE DEVELOPING IN CULTURE Stanley M. Crain	506
19	Ontogeny of Focal Seizures WILLIAM F. CAVENESS	517
	Discussion: MATURATIONAL FACTORS IN DEVELOPMENT OF SEIZURES Antonia Vernadakis and Dixon M. Woodbury	535
20	Sensory Precipitation and Reflex Mechanisms REGINALD G. BICKFORD AND DONALD W. KLASS	543

Discussion: PHOTOGENIC SEIZURES IN THE BABOON 565
Robert Naquet

21 Synaptic Inhibition in Seizures 575
W. ALDEN SPENCER AND ERIC R. KANDEL

Discussion: ORGANIZATION AND FREQUENCY DEPENDENCE OF HIPPOCAMPAL INHIBITION 604
P. Andersen and T. Lømo

22 Neurochemical Mechanisms 611
DONALD B. TOWER

Discussion: CEREBRAL BLOOD FLOW AND ENERGY METABOLISM 639
Louis Sokoloff

23 Mechanisms of Action of Anticonvulsants 647
DIXON M. WOODBURY

Discussion: FURTHER OBSERVATIONS ON DIPHENYLHYDANTOIN 682
James E. P. Toman

24 Genetics of Seizure Susceptibility 689
GUY M. MC KHANN AND ERIC M. SHOOTER

Discussion: GENETIC STUDIES IN CLINICAL EPILEPSY 700
Julius D. Metrakos and Katherine Metrakos

25 Systemic Electrolyte and Neuroendocrine Mechanisms 709
J. GORDON MILLICHAP

Discussion: ROLE OF HORMONES IN DEVELOPMENT OF SEIZURES 727
Paola S. Timiras

26 Neuroglial-Neuronal Interactions 737
RICHARD K. ORKAND

Discussion: MORPHOLOGY OF NEUROGLIAL CELLS 747
Sanford L. Palay

27 Theoretical Concepts of Synchrony 755
MARVIN MINSKY

	Discussion: MODELS OF BRAIN FUNCTION Valentino Braitenberg	768
28	Perspectives in Neuropathology ALFRED POPE	773
	Discussion: FEATURES OF CHEMICAL STRUCTURE OF SYNAPTIC MEMBRANES Leonhard S. Wolfe	782
29	Epilepsy, Neurophysiology, and Some Brain Mechanisms Related to Consciousness WILDER PENFIELD	791
30	A Prospectus A. EARL WALKER	807
	Index	815

Contributors

Cosimo Ajmone-Marsan, M.D.
Chief, Electroencephalography and Clinical Neurophysiology Branch
National Institute of Neurological Diseases and Stroke
National Institutes of Health
Bethesda, Maryland 20014

Martha Alberici, Ph.D.
Research Assistant
Instituto de Anatomia General y Embriologia
Facultad de Medicina
Universidad de Buenos Aires
Buenos Aires, Argentina

Per Andersen, dosent, M.D.
Associate Professor
Institute of Neurophysiology
University of Oslo
Oslo, Norway

Samuel H. Barondes, M.D.
Associate Professor of Psychiatry and Molecular Biology
Albert Einstein College of Medicine
Yeshiva University
Bronx, New York 10461

Reginald G. Bickford, M.D.
Professor, Department of Neurosciences
University of California, San Diego, School of Medicine
La Jolla, California 92037

Valentino Braitenberg, M.D.
Direktor at the Max-Planck-Institut für Biologische Kybernetik
Tübingen, Federal Republic of Germany

Prof.Dr.med. Heinz Caspers
Direktor des Physiologischen Instituts der Universität Münster
Münster, Federal Republic of Germany

William F. Caveness, M.D.
Chief, Laboratory of Experimental Neurology
National Institute of Neurological Diseases and Stroke
National Institutes of Health
Bethesda, Maryland 20014

Carmine D. Clemente, Ph.D.
Professor and Chairman
Department of Anatomy and
Member, Brain Research Institute
University of California, Los Angeles, School of Medicine
Los Angeles, California 90024

Marc Colonnier, M.D., Ph.D.
Associate Professor, Department of Physiology
University of Montreal
Montreal, Quebec, Canada

Stanley M. Crain, Ph.D.
Associate Professor of Physiology
Albert Einstein College of Medicine
Yeshiva University
Bronx, New York 10461

Dr.med. Otto D. Creutzfeldt
Privat-Dozent für Neurophysiologie
Universität München
Abteilung für Neurophysiologie
Max-Planck-Institut für Psychiatrie
München, Federal Republic of Germany

David R. Curtis, M.B., Ph.D.
Professor of Neuropharmacology
Department of Physiology
The John Curtin School of Medical Research
The Australian National University
Canberra, Australia

Annica B. Dahlström, Docent
Assistant Professor
Institute of Neurobiology
University of Göteborg
Göteborg, Sweden

Eduardo De Robertis, M.D.
Professor of Histology and Director
Instituto de Anatomia General y Embriologia
Facultad de Medicina
Universidad de Buenos Aires
Buenos Aires, Argentina

John C. Eccles, Ph.D.
Distinguished Professor of Biophysics and Physiology
Laboratory of Neurobiology, Faculty of Health Sciences
Schools of Medicine and Dentistry
State University of New York at Buffalo
Buffalo, New York 14214

Don W. Esplin, Ph.D.
Professor, Department of Pharmacology and Therapeutics
McGill University
Montreal, Quebec, Canada

Eli S. Goldensohn, M.D.
Professor of Neurology
College of Physicians and Surgeons
Columbia University
New York, New York 10032

Herbert H. Jasper, M.D., D.Sc., F.R.S.C.
Professor of Neurophysiology
University of Montreal
Montreal, Quebec, Canada

Eric R. Kandel, M.D.
Professor, Departments of Physiology and Psychiatry
New York University School of Medicine
New York, New York 10016

Donald W. Klass, M.D.
Consultant, Section of Clinical Electroencephalography and Physiology
Mayo Clinic and
Assistant Professor of Neurology
Mayo Graduate School of Medicine
University of Minnesota
Rochester, Minnesota 55901

George B. Koelle, Ph.D., M.D.
Professor and Chairman
Department of Pharmacology
University of Pennsylvania School of Medicine
Philadelphia, Pennsylvania 19104

Krešimir Krnjević, M.B., Ch.B., Ph.D.
Director, Wellcome Department of Research in Anaesthesia
McGill University
Montreal, Quebec, Canada

Motoy Kuno, M.D.
Associate Professor of Physiology
The University of Utah College of Medicine
Salt Lake City, Utah 84112

Terje Lømo, M.D.
Assistant Professor
Institute of Neurophysiology
University of Oslo
Oslo, Norway

Georgina Rodriguez de Lores Arnaiz, Ph.D.
Research Associate
Instituto de Anatomia General y Embriologia
Facultad de Medicina
Universidad de Buenos Aires
Buenos Aires, Argentina

Henry McIlwain, D.Sc., Ph.D.
Professor of Biochemistry
Institute of Psychiatry
British Postgraduate Medical Federation, University of London
London, England

Guy M. McKhann, M.D.
Kennedy Professor of Neurology
The Johns Hopkins University School of Medicine
Baltimore, Maryland 21205

H. Houston Merritt, M.D.
Professor of Neurology
Dean, and Vice President in Charge of Medical Affairs
College of Physicians and Surgeons
Columbia University
New York, New York 10032

Julius D. Metrakos, Ph.D.
Professor of Genetics
McGill University
Montreal, Quebec, Canada

Katherine Metrakos, M.D., C.M.
Director, Department of Electroencephalography
The Montreal Children's Hospital
Montreal, Quebec, Canada

J. Gordon Millichap, M.D.
Professor, Departments of Neurology and Pediatrics
Northwestern University Medical School
Chicago, Illinois 60611

Marvin Minsky, Ph.D.
Professor of Electrical Engineering
Massachusetts Institute of Technology
Cambridge, Massachusetts 02139

Frank Morrell, M.D., M.Sc.
Professor of Neurology
Stanford University School of Medicine
Stanford, California 94305

Robert Naquet, M.D.
Maître de Recherche au C.N.R.S.
Directeur du Département de Neurophysiologie appliquée
Institut de Neurophysiologie et de Psychophysiologie
Centre National de la Recherche Scientifique
Marseille, France

James L. O'Leary, M.D.
Professor and Head
Department of Neurology
Washington University School of Medicine
St. Louis, Missouri 63110

Richard K. Orkand, Ph.D.
Associate Professor of Zoology
University of California, Los Angeles
Los Angeles, California 90024

Tomokazu Oshima, M.D., D.Med.Sc., Ph.D.
Associate Professor
Laboratory of Neurobiology, Faculty of Health Sciences
Schools of Medicine and Dentistry
State University of New York at Buffalo
Buffalo, New York 14214

Sanford L. Palay, M.D.
Bullard Professor of Neuroanatomy
Harvard Medical School
Boston, Massachusetts 02115

Janet V. Passonneau, Ph.D.
Associate Professor of Pharmacology
Washington University School of Medicine
St. Louis, Missouri 63110

Wilder Penfield, M.D.
Honorary Consultant
Montreal Neurological Institute
McGill University
Montreal, Quebec, Canada

Daniel A. Pollen, M.D.
Assistant Neurophysiologist
Neurosurgical Service
Massachusetts General Hospital
Boston, Massachusetts 02114

Ottavio Pompeiano, M.D.
Professor of Physiology
II Chair of Human Physiology
Instituto di Fisiologia
Università di Pisa
Pisa, Italy

xxii CONTRIBUTORS

Alfred Pope, M.D.
Professor of Neuropathology
Harvard Medical School
Boston, Massachusetts 02115

David A. Prince, M.D.
Associate Professor of Medicine (Neurology)
Stanford University School of Medicine
Stanford, California 94305

Dominick P. Purpura, M.D.
Professor and Chairman
Department of Anatomy
Albert Einstein College of Medicine
Yeshiva University
Bronx, New York 10461

Serge Rossignol, M.D.
Department of Physiology
University of Montreal
Montreal, Quebec, Canada

Lester T. Rutledge, Ph.D.
Professor of Physiology
The University of Michigan Medical School
Ann Arbor, Michigan 48104

Seth K. Sharpless, Ph.D.
Associate Professor
Department of Pharmacology
Albert Einstein College of Medicine
Yeshiva University
Bronx, New York 10461

Eric M. Shooter, Ph.D.
Professor of Genetics and Biochemistry
Stanford University School of Medicine
Stanford, California 94305

Louis Sokoloff, M.D.
Chief, Laboratory of Cerebral Metabolism
National Institute of Mental Health
Health Services and Mental Health Administration
Bethesda, Maryland 20014

Dr.med. Erwin-Josef Speckmann
Assistent, Physiologischen Instituts der Universität Münster
Münster, Federal Republic of Germany

W. Alden Spencer, M.D.
Professor of Physiology
New York University School of Medicine
New York, New York 10016

Charles F. Stevens, M.D., Ph.D.
Associate Professor
Department of Physiology and Biophysics
University of Washington School of Medicine
Seattle, Washington 98105

William E. Stone, Ph.D.
Professor of Physiology
The University of Wisconsin Medical School
Madison, Wisconsin 53706

John Szentágothai, M.D.
Professor of Anatomy
University Medical School
Budapest, Hungary

Paola S. Timiras, M.D., Ph.D.
Professor of Physiology
University of California, Berkeley, School of Medicine
Berkeley, California 94720

James E. P. Toman, Ph.D.
Professor and Chairman
Department of Pharmacology and Therapeutics
The Chicago Medical School
Chicago, Illinois 60612

Donald B. Tower, M.D., Ph.D.
Chief, Laboratory of Neurochemistry
National Institute of Neurological Diseases and Stroke
National Institutes of Health
Bethesda, Maryland 20014

Antonia Vernadakis, Ph.D.
Assistant Professor
Departments of Psychiatry and Pharmacology
University of Colorado School of Medicine
Denver, Colorado 80220

A. Earl Walker, M.D.
Professor of Neurological Surgery
The Johns Hopkins University School of Medicine
Baltimore, Maryland 21205

Arthur A. Ward, Jr., M.D.
Professor and Chairman
Department of Neurological Surgery
University of Washington School of Medicine
Seattle, Washington 98105

Leonhard S. Wolfe, M.D., Ph.D.
Associate Professor
Department of Neurology and Neurosurgery
Montreal Neurological Institute
McGill University
Montreal, Quebec, Canada

Dixon M. Woodbury, Ph.D.
Professor of Pharmacology
The University of Utah College of Medicine
Salt Lake City, Utah 84112

J. Walter Woodbury, Ph.D.
Professor of Physiology
University of Washington School of Medicine
Seattle, Washington 98105

Barbara Zablocka-Esplin, M.D.
Assistant Professor
Department of Pharmacology and Therapeutics
McGill University
Montreal, Quebec, Canada

Basic Mechanisms of the Epilepsies

1
Clinical and Experimental Challenges of the Epilepsies

ARTHUR A. WARD, JR., HERBERT H. JASPER, AND ALFRED POPE

EPILEPSY is a relatively common disease, affecting at least 15 million people in the world today. It has probably afflicted the human race from the beginning, since the earliest descriptions found date from 2000 B.C. The word *epilepsy* is derived from the Greek word *epilepsia* or *seizure*. Early definitions include: "Epilepsy is a seizure of the mind and the sense together with a sudden fall, in some with convulsions, in others, however, without convulsions" [25]. Under such a broad definition, many seizures may occur which are not truly epileptiform, nor do they justify a clinical diagnosis of epilepsy, strictly defined.

Epileptic seizures are characterized as being spontaneous, episodic, recurrent, and paroxysmal, that is, "a fit of disease." Consequently convulsive seizures induced by intense electrical stimulation of the brain or by convulsant drugs, as well as those which occur during toxic states such as uremia, are not considered epilepsy as strictly defined. These may provide useful models of seizure mechanisms, but since they do not occur in self-perpetuating recurrent episodes and are, on the contrary, self-limiting, such convulsive reactions are not considered to be clinical epilepsy. Likewise, sudden transient losses of consciousness due to concussion or syncope do not fall within the definition of epilepsy. With regard to epilepsy it may be necessary to introduce concepts of seizure mechanism into the definition and not rely solely upon descriptive clinical criteria.

The most commonly accepted mechanistic definition of epilepsy is that proposed by Hughlings Jackson, stated simply by Penfield and Jasper [21]: "An epileptic seizure is a state produced by an abnormal excessive neuronal discharge within the central nervous system." This descriptive definition has been supported by numerous electrophysiological studies described in this volume. Such a definition without further qualification, however, would include as epileptiform many seizures symptomatic of disease processes not primarily epileptic as such. It would include most of the experimental models of epileptiform attack or process to be described in this monograph. It implies that an epileptic seizure is a symptom of many and varied disease processes and that there may be no true epilepsy as a disease sui generis.

If the different conditions that produce recurring epileptic seizures or abnormal excessive neuronal discharge are grouped together, they may be referred to as *the epilepsies,* a term used by Jackson and later by Wilson [28]. Use of this term in the title of this monograph implies acceptance of the principle of the symptomatic nature of all forms of epileptic seizure and that they may be caused by a variety of different diseases affecting the central nervous system. By probing more deeply into basic mechanisms controlling the excitation and discharge of neurons within the brain, it should be possible to describe factors common to all of these diseases. This should provide a more satisfactory definition based upon fundamental causes of excessive neuronal discharge. Such an increase in understanding should lead to more effective and rational methods of treatment. Understanding of normal control mechanisms is the first step toward an understanding of how they are deranged or defective in the epilepsies.

HISTORICAL DEVELOPMENTS OF CONCEPTS

It is little wonder that mystical forces have for centuries been invoked in an attempt to explain the dramatic events of an epileptic seizure; the unfortunate patient was considered to be possessed by evil spirits. Hippocrates, about 400 B.C., first attacked such conceptions in his classical treatise on epilepsy, *The Sacred Disease,* and offered convincing proof that seizures resulted from trauma or disease of the brain. The early Greek writers, however, distinguished between true or essential epilepsy arising in the head without known trauma or disease (*idiopathic*), as opposed to convulsions arising secondarily to traumatic or other brain diseases and those secondary to other diseases of the body (*sympathetic*). Convulsions preceded by a distinct aura, or by local spasms without loss of consciousness, were thought to be of peripheral origin. Manipulations such as tying a ligature around a limb were introduced, even at this time, to "postpone the attack which announced itself in a limb" [25]. More precise conceptions of the location of onset and physiological mechanisms of seizures had to wait until the intellectual reawakening of the Renaissance and the birth of scientific methods of study of the nervous system in the nineteenth and early twentieth centuries.

With the development of concepts of reflex action during the nineteenth century, certain forms of epilepsy were thought to be of reflex origin [5, 10]. The cause was sought in the periphery, where the aura or onset began, the convulsion being due to increased reflex excitability of nerve centers in spinal cord and brain stem. Many authors of this time believed that the brain stem was responsible for seizures, especially major generalized attacks with loss of consciousness. Kussmaul and Tenner [14], for example, believed that the central origin of seizures should be sought in "excitable districts of the brain lying behind the thalamic optici." A modern version of this view will be presented by Penfield in Chap. 29.

The cerebral cortex was not recognized as a major source of seizures until Fritsch and Hitzig [7] and Ferrier [6] demonstrated the electrical excitability of the cerebral cortex, showing that not only movements but local and generalized convulsive seizures could be produced by local electrical stimulation of certain cortical areas in experimental animals. This marked the beginning of the truly experimental study of the epilepsies. At the same time, Hughlings Jackson provided us with his monumental clinical studies of the epilepsies [12], and William Gowers presented his classical clinical observations [9].

At this time there was strong opposition to Jackson's view that all forms of seizure were symptomatic of a common physiopathological process. Jackson agreed that chronic convulsions could be divided into two groups or classes: "(1) Those in which the spasm affects both sides of the body almost contemporaneously . . . usually called epileptic, and sometimes cases of 'genuine' or 'idiopathic' epilepsy. (2) Those in which the fit begins by deliberate spasm on one side of the body, and in which parts of the body are affected one after the other . . . . I trust I am studying the general subject of convulsion methodically when I work at the simplest varieties of occasional spasm I can find." All forms of epilepsy were considered due to "discharging lesions." Those characterized by initial loss of consciousness (petit mal absence) or those with major "grand mal" convulsions without local onset or both, were thought to begin "in the very highest centres of the cerebral hemispheres, that is to say, in the anatomical substrata of consciousness." However, Gowers maintained a more or less clear distinction (as do many, even today) between "(1) convulsions which are the result of organic disease, such as can be recognized after death, and (2) those which are the expression of a condition of the brain which is not evidenced by any visible alteration." It may be hoped that with more refined methods of observation, many of which are to be presented in this volume, those seizures which apparently occur "without visible alteration" in the pathophysiology of the brain will gradually disappear from necessary consideration.

Since the time of Jackson and Gowers, the challenge posed by the many caricatures of brain function presented by many varied manifestations and causes of seizures, both in man and in experimental animals, has contributed much to an understanding of basic mechanisms and functional organization of the normal brain, as exemplified particularly in the work of Penfield. For example, the great importance of central inhibitory mechanisms was recognized in the work of both Jackson and Gowers in their efforts to explain both the cause and some of the manifestations of seizures. In the *Proceedings of the Association for Research in Nervous and Mental Disease* of 1922. J. Ramsay Hunt drew attention again to the precept: "There is much in the convulsive and other paroxysmal phenomena of epilepsy to suggest a loss of inhibitory function" [11]. He continues, providing some evidence from neuropathological studies, to suggest that central inhibition might be attributed to Golgi II cells, a suggestion of considerable interest in view of recent developments in neurophysiological conceptions of central inhibition.

The most significant development in the history of concepts of epilepsy was the introduction of electroencephalography in the early 1930s. Demonstration that most epileptic seizures are associated with dramatic changes in the electrical activity of the brain, recorded from the scalp surface through the unopened skull, revolutionized diagnostic procedures and made possible the detection of electrical signs of latent epilepsy, even in the absence of manifest seizures [13, 15, 19]. Of equal importance was the impetus given to electrophysiological studies of the brain of man and experimental animals in its normal behavior, awake or asleep, and for the objective study of the clinical epilepsies, as well as experimentally induced seizures. A wealth of new empirical data soon became available to aid in localization of onset and in classification of different forms of seizures and their underlying physiopathology. Understanding of basic mechanisms underlying the electrical manifestations of seizures has developed much more slowly and will be the concern of many contributors to this book.

It may be said that the advent of electroencephalography, beginning with the pioneer work of Hans Berger some 40 years ago [3, 4], marked the beginning of the modern era of research in the epilepsies. The definition of epilepsy as a sudden paroxysmal, excessive neuronal discharge was readily confirmed. To it was added the concept of *paroxysmal dysrhythmia* of the EEG and *hypersynchrony* to indicate not only excessive firing of individual cells, but also massive discharge of many neurons in unison, abolishing the finely organized temperospatial patterning characteristic of the normal integrative activity of the brain.

SEIZURE CLASSIFICATION

If a seizure is the consequence of an abnormal, excessive, neuronal discharge, the clinical manifestations should be determined by the functional properties of those neurons and their interconnections. In a highly developed central nervous system such as that of man, in which any assembly of neurons with different functional specializations may be initially involved in a seizure, it is not surprising that the clinical patterns of epilepsy vary widely. This has complicated the clinical classification of the epilepsies.

The purpose of a classification is to categorize a collection of observations into groups sharing common characteristics. Since the clinical phenomenon can usually only be described, operational definitions have evolved which suffer because two seizure forms may differ widely in appearance, yet have fundamental similarities with regard to causation and response to therapy. Even the attempt to categorize the appearance of the seizure is difficult. One or two words cannot describe a dynamic process consisting of a whole procession of events. Even though seizure patterns differ in almost every individual patient, certain recognizable constellations of seizure manifestations merit their grouping under certain headings which form the bases for the attempt to classify different seizure types. As knowledge and insight have grown, clinical classifications of the epilepsies have also evolved.

Detailed descriptions of various clinical manifestations of the epilepsies are available in the classic reports of Hughlings Jackson [12] and Gowers [9] as well as more modern statements such as those of Lennox [18]. Reference is made to the classic monograph by Penfield and Jasper [21] which represents the most comprehensive attempt to categorize the epilepsies in relation to functional anatomy of the brain. An international classification has recently been proposed [8].

Discussion of basic mechanisms in the epilepsies requires definitions of clinical phenomena of the epilepsies. A language in common is necessary to provide communication between the disciplines; in addition, it is useful to provide a brief survey of the clinical problem for those who have not had direct contact with the phenomenon in the human. Certain characteristics of specific types of seizures are not shared by the rest of the epilepsies; other features may be common to the entire group. In an attempt to categorize some of these properties and to provide an orderly means of communication between clinicians dealing with the epilepsies, various classifications of the epilepsies have been constructed. Such classifications are based in part on the state of knowledge regarding epilepsy at that point in time and in part on the models of the mechanisms as viewed by the authors of the classification. Since knowledge is incomplete, any detailed classification tends to become outdated rapidly. The broad classification originally proposed by Penfield and Jasper is perhaps still the most useful since it is the least restrictive. In this scheme, seizures are divided into three groups: (1) focal cerebral seizures; (2) centrencephalic seizures—formerly called *idiopathic* or *essential* epilepsy; and (3) cerebral seizures (unlocalized or generalized).

Focal Seizures

Focal seizures are those which originate in a local area of gray matter of one cerebral hemisphere. The initial clinical phenomenon in an epileptic seizure is usually the most important clue to the localization of origin of the epileptic discharge and thus is also a reliable guide to the anatomical classification of a particular case. In such cases the EEG often shows local abnormality with sporadic epileptiform discharge even during periods between overt clinical attacks (interictal).

When the initial event does not involve propagation of the discharge to circuits involved in consciousness, the neuronal discharge may produce a sensation or feeling which the patient can describe. Galen (A.D. 130–200) reported that a young man with epilepsy likened the sensation he felt just before an attack to a cold breeze (or *aura*) blowing upon a part of his body. The character of this aura is determined by the function of the neurons at the epileptic focus and thus may provide rather specific information regarding localization of origin of the epileptic discharge. The aura is not strictly a *warning*, but rather is the first event in a seizure. The seizure may not progress beyond involvement of that local aggregate of neurons, or it may propagate widely over the axonal projections to other parts of the brain. Widespread involvement of neuronal circuits is clinically manifested by a major convulsive seizure. Such a terminal convulsion or *grand mal* has no localizing pattern or significance, except to indicate general susceptibility of the brain as a whole to the spread of an epileptic process. Focal seizures which remain sharply localized or "partial" are relatively rare; most are propagated to some extent.

For a variety of practical reasons, focal epilepsy is considered to consist largely of that group of focal cerebral seizures which originate in the cerebral cortex. This is partly because our knowledge of localization of function is much more complete for cortical than for subcortical circuits; and because our diagnostic techniques (including EEG) provide more information about cortical dysfunction and relatively little about the pathophysiology of neuronal aggregates buried within the brain. Cases with focal seizures can be divided into groups based on the initial phenomena they present as shown in Table 1-1.

TABLE 1-1. Distribution of Initial Phenomena in 222 Cases of Focal Cerebral Seizures

Initial Phenomena	Percentage
Initial unconsciousness	14
Motor phenomena	13
Sensory phenomena	36
Autonomic motor or sensory phenomena	12
Psychical phenomena	13
Miscellaneous phenomena	12

Modified from Penfield and Kristiansen, 1951 [22].

These initial phenomena, in turn, provide clues regarding localization of origin of the epileptic discharge. In cases in which the initial event is unconsciousness, localization in the majority of focal cortical cases is to the anterior or intermediate frontal lobes. Where motor phenomena are the initial events, localization depends on the type of motor response. Simple adversive seizures tend to be localized in the intermediate frontal region just above the so-called motor speech area or Broca's convolution. Seizures with local motor phenomena or Jacksonian seizures arise in the sensorimotor cortex. Similarly, sensory phenomena are localized primarily to paracentral cortex, visual sensations to occipital cortex, auditory and vestibular sensations to the first temporal convolution, and the like.

The group with autonomic motor and sensory phenomena include epigastric and abdominal sensations, palpitation, thoracic sensation, and other sensations such as thirst. Some of these have been localized to diencephalic-autonomic centers, but most are roughly localized to the Sylvian region comprising the insula and temporal lobe, including the amygdaloid, hippocampal, and uncinate areas deep in the temporal region. Their manifestations can also include hallucinations which may resemble dreams, perceptual illusions, and emotional aurae such as fear. Such seizures often progress into automatisms in which the patient may engage in automatic motor activity for which he has no recollection. Such automatic activity may consist of relatively simple, stereotyped movements such as slapping his thigh; or it may be quite complex as when the patient continues to drive a car, but may change his destination or pay no attention to traffic lights. Such seizures arising in the temporal lobe have also been classified as *psychomotor epilepsy* [17]. The reason for emphasis on this particular seizure pattern is, in part, the obvious, rather dramatic character of the behavior during the seizure; in part, the emphasis is justified by the fact that this is probably the commonest of all seizure patterns in adult epileptic patients. Of all adults having seizures it has been estimated that about 50 percent are of temporal lobe origin.

Alterations of function occurring as a consequence of paroxysmal activity, arising at some cortical focus, are commonly considered a consequence of activation of circuits appropriate to the origin of the discharge. Thus, seizure discharge in the motor cortex produces motor contractions in appropriate muscles of the contralateral body. However, it should be emphasized that alterations of function due to seizure activity can be either positive or negative, as well as combinations of these. Although seizures involving motor cortex do induce motor activity in contralateral muscles, they are also associated with the abolition of ability to carry out coordinated, voluntary "movement." Even subclinical discharges in such circuits can impair normal function in these complex neural nets. This accounts for the *paradoxical* improvement of motor function that can follow excision of an epileptogenic focus in the motor cortex [27]. Improvement is paradoxical because structural lesions of motor cortex commonly produce a motor deficit; but removal of a discharging focus in the same cortical area may permit normal functioning of adjacent neural nets with an improvement in function. In the same fashion, seizure discharge involving cortical circuits subserving speech does not result in the active production of speech but, on the contrary, in paralysis of speech during the seizure, although unstructured vocalization may also be part of the ictal event. Epileptic activation of the temporal region and limbic structures results in the reproduction of complex imagery or recollections. Functional interpretation of these phenomena represents one of the great challenges of epilepsy, to be discussed by Penfield (Chap. 29).

It is well known that after a seizure is over, depression of function can be manifested in a variety of ways. When the motor cortex has been heavily involved in prolonged seizure activity, the seizure may be followed by brief postictal paralysis. Obviously, it may be most difficult for an observer to determine what part of the patient's behavior is due to active discharge of neuronal circuits disrupting their integrated activity and what part is due to postictal depression of function. A seizure discharge in speech cortex will produce sudden loss of speech; as soon as the seizure is over, there may be continuing aphasia, which represents postictal paralysis of this same function. The ambiguities become most troublesome when circuits subserving complex functions are involved. Involvement of limbic circuits by a seizure discharge produces profound alterations of behavior including automatism with amnesia; but is it legitimate to call this *psychomotor* rather than *psychoparetic,* as Penfield has suggested? Finally, this problem must be carefully considered when seizure discharges involve those circuits which maintain consciousness. Involvement by a seizure is heralded by sudden loss of consciousness, while this may be succeeded by stupor as the seizure ends. This conceptual framework is of particular importance when considering those seizure types in which alterations of consciousness constitute the primary symptom.

Centrencephalic Seizures

The second broad category of seizures is the *highest level* or centrencephalic seizures of Penfield. They have a characteristic EEG, the bilaterally synchronous 3-per-sec rhythmic spike-wave complex which appears suddenly from a normal EEG. In contrast with focal cortical seizures, interictal epileptiform discharge is rare in these cases. These have been classified as *simple absence* or *petit mal* and described in great detail by Lennox [16–18]. Unlike other forms of seizures, petit mal attacks occur characteristically without warning. Impairment or lapse of consciousness is the primary symptom. Consciousness is always lost abruptly and usually regained with equal suddenness. The period of unconsciousness is brief in 90 percent of cases, varying between 5 and 30 sec. Because of their brevity, seizures may be difficult to detect. Objectively, there is sudden immobility and a vacant look in the eyes which, in a child, may be confused with a brief period of daydreaming or inattention.

The majority of patients know that they have had a seizure when it lasts more than 4–5 sec. Muscular movements are not prominent, but there may be slight jerks of both arms or blinking of eyes occurring rhythmically at about 3 per sec. In 30–40 percent of the cases, visible muscular movements do not accompany an absence. It is common for the attacks to recur daily and increase to a peak of 5–50 a day. These seizures occur in childhood and tend to disappear with the onset of puberty and, in the great majority of instances, attacks vanish by the time the patient is adult, sometimes being replaced by other forms of seizure.

The centrencephalic epilepsies, of which *petit mal absence* is the classic example, are characterized by certain unique features not shared by other forms of epilepsy. The initial loss of consciousness can be simulated by focal cortical seizures originating in the anterior mesial or orbital frontal cortex. The complete pattern of such frontal cortical seizures with initial loss of consciousness is different from that of the petit mal attack, and the electroencephalogram is usually not of the classic, bilaterally synchronous spike-wave form. Penfield has suggested the term, centrencephalic, for such seizures when a cortical focus can be excluded, and it would seem that a neuronal system involving the brain stem with projections to both hemispheres may be responsible for the symmetrically bilateral, representation of this attack in the EEG, as well as for its unique, clinical manifestations with initial loss of consciousness and minimal bilateral myoclonic movements about the face. Further elaboration of the centrencephalic system concept will be presented by Jasper (Chap. 16) and by Penfield (Chap. 29).

Such seizure states are also distinguished by sensitivity to a variety of changes in the metabolic environment of the organism, are often easily precipitated by hyperventilation and consequent hypocarbia, as well as by hypoglycemia. Such patients often appear to be precipitated into a major convulsion by fever; attacks are also often precipitated by specific sensory stimuli, especially the interrupted flashing of a bright light at critical frequencies, although other forms of generalized seizures may also be sensitive to photic stimulation as described by Bickford in Chap. 20. Response to medical therapy is also different from that of other forms of seizures; those drugs most effective in simple petit mal absence may not modify other types of seizure, in fact, may increase the frequency of generalized convulsive attacks even in the same patients. Thus the petit mal or centrencephalic form of seizure presents a number of distinctive problems to be resolved in any consideration of seizure mechanisms, problems of a different nature than those of the focal cortical seizure.

Cerebral Seizures Unlocalized or Generalized

The final broad category of the epilepsies, *cerebral seizures unlocalized,* is much less distinctive. It includes many forms of generalized epileptic state due to either a diffuse pathological process in the brain or a generalized biochemical or metabolic disturbance in the brain, causing multiple areas of susceptibility to seizures involving widespread areas of both hemispheres or, in some cases, the entire brain. Diffuse or generalized epileptic states must be clearly distinguished from both the focal cortical epilepsies and those designated as centrencephalic, even though certain aspects of their clinical expression may simulate either one or the other of the previously described categories. For example, bilateral myoclonic movements may characterize progressive degenerative diseases of the brain such as in myoclonus epilepsy; this must not be confused with true centrencephalic seizures or "idiopathic petit mal" of Lennox. These cases may, upon occasion, exhibit an apparent focal onset, either motor or sensory in one seizure while in another the focus of onset may be different; the area of initial discharge varies from time to time over the widely susceptible cortical areas involved in the diffuse seizure process. Seizures secondary to metabolic diseases of other organs, such as the hypoglycemia of a pancreatic adenoma, obviously produce generalized changes in the brain, although in some cases their initial expression may appear as a seizure of focal onset, but seldom with a consistent focus. A great deal of confusion has arisen from failure to differentiate between such generalized epilepsies, with diffuse pathological or metabolic disease, and the centrencephalic seizures, or idiopathic petit mal, in which no such pathological process or lesion can be consistently demonstrated. Lennox was the first to point out that the slow spike-wave or petit mal variant was associated with gross diffuse brain pathology, not to be confused with true petit mal or centrencephalic seizures.

MECHANISMS OF SEIZURE

In any discussion of mechanisms, the phenomena exhibited by focal cerebral seizures are perhaps the most pertinent. When it can be demonstrated that the seizure process arises in a given cluster of cortical neurons, the phenomenon is obviously more susceptible to experimental analysis. This enables discussion of possible mechanisms which might throw light on the process generating the autonomous discharge; to determine some of the factors responsible for precipitation of this inter-ictal activity into a propagating seizure; then to study the mechanisms of spread to other parts of the brain. Such a formulation of mechanisms requires major utilization of knowledge in the fields of neuroanatomy, neurophysiology, neurochemistry, biophysics, neuropharmacology, and neurogenetics. Here is the challenge provided by this exquisite experiment of nature which we call epilepsy. The magnitude of the challenge is intensified because the phenomenon involves the most complex organ in the body and the logical inference that complete insight will require essentially full understanding of the brain.

Challenge to Neurophysiology

The disturbances in central neuronal activity which characterize the various forms of epileptic seizure represent caricatures of normal excitatory, inhibitory, and regulatory mechanisms of the brain, thus providing a particularly potent challenge to neurophysiology. Conversely, the exaggeration of function shown in the epilepsies, when studied by sophisticated neurophysiological techniques, may shed light on the nature of control systems regulating normal brain function.

The electroencephalogram has provided an essential link between clinical and experimental approaches to these problems, while at the same time demonstrating their enormous complexity if there is to be penetration beyond the purely descriptive level of understanding. The EEG and microelectrode studies of individual neurons have confirmed Hughlings Jackson's surmise that abnormal excessive discharge of "explosive" cells are present in discharging lesions of the brain. It is necessary now to explore the problem of why they are explosive; what alterations may be found in their intrinsic metabolism, the molecular structure and ionic transport mechanisms of neuronal membranes, their responsiveness to synaptic transmitter substances, both excitatory or inhibitory, and, in fact, all mechanisms, either intrinsic or extrinsic to particular neurons which may play a role in determining their excessive repetitive discharge.

The most fundamental property of all nerve cells is, of course, their excitability, the explosive nature of their response in generating action potentials, and their tendency to repetitive discharge. Even though intrinsically normal, all neurons are potentially epileptic when subjected to excessive excitatory drive or when normal inhibitory controls are reduced. Synaptic circuitry and the external environment of nerve cells must be most important in determining certain forms of epileptic discharge, particularly their fluid and glial environment, as well as electrical field potentials which may affect large populations of neurons, not all of which may be otherwise intrinsically abnormal.

Epileptic seizures, like action potentials, are transient periodic phenomena. Both may be generated at local synaptic junctions and propagated in local reverberating neuronal nets or transmitted over long axonal conduction pathways to induce excitation, inhibition, or self-sustained epileptic states in distant assemblies of neurons. Powerful inhibitory control systems have been found in central neuronal circuitry serving to suppress regenerative recruitment of large masses of neurons in hypersynchronous epileptic discharge. A delicate balance of excitatory and inhibitory synaptic events must be maintained, distributed differentially on soma and dendrites. The structural basis of these will be discussed in detail in the following chapter by Szentágothai and Colonnier and by other contributors to this volume.

The principal problem is twofold: first, to discover what are the *latent defects* in either the intrinsic or extrinsic control systems which cause abnormal susceptibility to epileptic discharge and its propagation even though these circuits may function in a relatively normal manner between seizures; and second, to discover the mechanisms responsible for translation of latent susceptibility into *overt clinical seizures* at intervals of minutes, weeks, months, or years in epileptic patients. Genetic factors, discussed in Chap. 24, are of obvious importance here.

Chronic, continuous, local epileptic discharge may persist in focal epileptogenic lesions with continuous disturbances in cerebral function, or, rarely, in the form of continuously repetitive convulsive movements, as in *epilepsia partialis continua*. But the important problem remains: why does the relatively restricted sporadic discharge of chronic epileptic neurons become periodically enhanced and propagated to produce overt seizures involving more or less of the entire brain in the process? Mechanisms of spread will be considered in detail in Chaps. 10 and 16. Factors of particular importance in the precipitation of seizures are discussed in Chaps. 20 and 25.

In anticipating much in the presentations to follow, we may suggest, for the purpose of orientation, the following general neurophysiological definition of epilepsy. Summation of all intrinsic and extrinsic factors that determine the excitatory state of a neuron or an interconnected assembly of neurons, including their extension in time, and the fact that all excitatory states are normally opposed by intrinsic or extrinsic (inhibitory and other) factors tending to restore the resting equilibrium of neuronal membranes or the stability of neuronal pools, suggests that redefinition of Sherrington's conception of central excitatory and inhibitory states may be useful [24].

Central excitatory states, it is now known, depend upon many interrelated factors, in addition to the spatial and temporal summation of excitatory and inhibitory impulses in central neuronal pools, as described by Sherrington. Structural and functional or metabolic alterations at specific synaptic sites (presynaptic, dendritic, or somatic), involving a variety of neurochemical transmitters and specific receptor substances in postsynaptic membranes, as well as more general structural and chemical factors affecting excitability and stability of neuronal membranes, must be considered as part of the complex of mechanisms determining central excitatory states. Without specifying which of the these factors may be most important in a given instance, epilepsy may be viewed as the result of gross imbalance in central excitatory and inhibitory states in interconnected assemblies of neurons. It follows that inhibitory arrest of function may be one manifestation of an epileptic seizure, and that excessive neuronal discharge may result from defective inhibitory controls as well as from excessive excitation. Individual epileptic neurons, strategically located in an assembly of otherwise normal cells, might act as pacemakers or amplifiers, serving to synchronize and recruit more and more cells into their orbit of abnormal excessive discharge.

CHALLENGE TO NEUROCHEMISTRY

In spite of the relatively meager development of neurochemistry prior to World War II, a number of investigations had been directed toward elucidation of epilepsy in molecular terms. The dynamic development of this subdiscipline of the neurosciences during the past 20 years has also generated numerous attempts to correlate tissue metabolic events with seizure phenomena [26]. If any generalization may be permitted, it is that by and large, biochemical evidence on this subject provides a predictable reflection of states of excessive neuronal discharge, but that no substantial leads have been established concerning molecular level changes of pathogenetic significance.

Nevertheless, the powerful tools and insights of modern biochemistry should furnish ways and means for significant developments in this sphere. Such theoretical possibilities are enhanced by the relative excellence of experimental models for the biochemical epileptologist, as compared with the student of most neuropsychiatric disorders. These facts enhance both the opportunity and urgency for penetrating explorations concerning the molecular pathology of seizures.

In principle, each of the following areas of contemporary biochemistry and molecular biology should have something to offer regarding the molecular pathology of seizures.

The genetically determined predisposition for certain types of seizure development means that as a distant but challenging goal, *molecular genetics* has a role to play in elucidation of the epileptic state. Indeed, it would be axiomatic in this era to assume that molecular biology, as currently defined, may eventually be decisive in this regard for precise understanding and control of human epilepsy. This must be a compelling challenge for the future molecular neurobiologist and genetic engineer.

More amenable to current biochemical technology would be investigation of the comparative macromolecular structure of neuron membranes in cells with demonstrable epileptic properties, by coordinating the physical chemistry of biopolymers with ultrastructure research of the resolving power adequate for description of *membrane molecular morphology*. Alterations in the tertiary structure or conformational properties of membrane proteins and in the modes of protein-lipid articulations involved in membrane structure should have critical relevance for abnormalities in ion distributions and polarization states of *epileptic neurons*.

Even more immediate applications of biochemistry might be addressed to queries concerning abnormalities in cation transport mechanisms and the way in which these are coupled with *intracellular energy-yielding processes*. Sophisticated techniques in metabolic biochemistry now exist for monitoring the steady state levels of intermediary metabolites and the activities of enzymes governing their metabolic transformations. It is not premature to conceive of the application of such technology to the experimental analyses of epileptic foci in relation to ongoing electrocorticographic activity. Suitable miniaturization of techniques should enable establishment of important correlations between biochemical data and tissue ultrastructure and microphysiology. Analogous considerations apply equally to questions concerning the metabolism of biogenic amines in general and of specifically established central neurotransmitters in particular.

Challenge to Neuromorphology

From the earliest days of cellular pathology, neuropathologists have addressed themselves to searching for the "lesion of epilepsy" [20, 22, 23]. An extensive literature developed which, in essence, showed that at the level of light microscopy in cases of seizures without focal origin, there is no generally accepted identifiable or characteristic cytological or histological change having etiological significance. It is now generally agreed that the pathological anatomy often to be found (especially in the hippocampus) is rather the result of repeated epileptic attacks and attendant hypoxia.

From the foregoing considerations, it is apparent that the focal epilepsies are a constellation of symptom complexes arising in all parts of the cerebrum as a result of many kinds of pathologic processes, especially those resulting in slowly progressive destruction of neurons. Thus, seizure discharges may arise from such divergent reactions to injury as those associated with intracerebral traumatic lesions, chronic sepsis, infarction, neoplasia, and spontaneous, degenerative neuronal disease of many kinds. Again, light microscopy has failed to identify those characteristics of such pathological processes that confer on the resultant lesions their epileptogenicity.

Advances in ultrastructure research and in cytochemistry have now provided a new level for descriptive analysis of the morphology of epileptogenous cortex. In this regard, the challenge is particularly manifest for the student of the fine structure of the nervous system. Can he demonstrate in epileptic foci significant electron microscopic changes in the internal structure of nerve cells or particularly of their surface membranes and synaptic contacts? Does the glial sheath exhibit unusual properties that are consistent with significant modifications in the interstitial milieu of the neurons? These and other questions would be part of the total complex of issues that challenge the contemporary morphologist to furnish comparative definitions of structural relationships in epileptogenic as contrasted with normal cerebral tissue. Partial answers to some of these questions and provocative suggestions concerning avenues for future investigation will be found in the pages that follow.

THE EPILEPSIES IN NEUROBIOLOGY AND BRAIN RESEARCH

In view of factors such as the foregoing, the time is ripe for correlative research, involving the physiologist and the biochemist, in the search for sequential events at the ionic and molecular levels that produce or accompany the hypersynchronous, neuronal firing equivalent to seizure activity. Similarly, combined efforts of the biochemist and ultramorphologist should, in principle, be appropriate for precise definition of alterations in neuronal membrane structure accountable for, or consistent with, altered states of polarization and excessive neuronal discharge.

Complex mechanisms apparently must be operating in the genesis and spread of seizure discharge in the process we call epilepsy. An adequate model cannot be provided by examining the phenomenon of epilepsy from the parochial viewpoint of a single discipline in the neurosciences but requires application of knowledge and principles from them all. To quote Santayana, "The same battle in the clouds will be known to the deaf only as lightning and to the blind only as thunder." Our goal is to view the battle of epilepsy from the broad base of neurobiology.

It is particularly appropriate that our knowledge regarding basic mechanisms underlying the epileptic process be collated and synthesized at this time. The last such effort occurred over 20 years ago [2], and in spite of the increase in knowledge regarding seizures and the increased effectiveness of therapy, the epileptic is still the leper of modern society. Although the epilepsies are the commonest manifestation of disease of the brain, relatively more space is devoted to epilepsy by ancient than by modern authors. As Lennox [18] points out, the Hippocratic writings are 2.6 percent about epilepsy, Aretaeus' 3.4 percent, Cecil's *Medicine* (1959) only 0.5 percent, and Wilson and Bruce's *Neurology* (1955), 0.4 percent.

Lennox goes on to point out that "epilepsy is no longer the Cinderella of medicine. The electroencephalograph is her glass slipper. As if to make up for centuries of neglect, epilepsy is now favored above many other diseases in that its essential malactivity can be recorded and analyzed. We speak disparagingly of magic, but what is greater magic than for the brain to write its own confession of wrongdoing on a sheet of moving paper? In ancient Greece certain actions of the patient identified the god responsible for the seizure. Now the writings of the electrographic pens name the sort of seizure the patient is having, help to assign its therapy and to predict the chances of control."

A really complete understanding of epilepsy might require almost total knowledge of the central nervous system. *This is the challenge, also the excitement of the field.* Epilepsy represents one of the most exquisite experiments of nature, and its study may provide basic insight into fundamental functions of the brain. With the clues provided by nature, it may be possible to generate quantal jumps in our knowledge in the neurosciences. It has been said that physics owes more to the steam engine than than steam engine owes to physics. It may transpire that the neurosciences will owe more to epilepsy than epilepsy owes to the brain sciences.

Although the phenomena of epilepsy might be thought superficially to represent a hierarchy of bizarre, pathological events, we are confident that epilepsy is really a modification of the normal principles of neuronal operations.

With the rapid advances in the neurosciences in the past 20 years, it is relevant to bring together that body of knowledge which may provide insight into the basic mechanisms in the epilepsies. The goal of this volume is to establish a benchmark to which future knowledge can be related. It is hoped that the information collected here will also serve as a major resource of data and concepts dealing with fundamental problems relevant to the epilepsies, to which future workers can turn.

Our goal, then, is to bring fundamental knowledge to bear on the basic mechanisms of the epilepsies, to assure that the exciting potential of sophisticated concepts in the various neurosciences which are germane to problems of epilepsy will be brought to the attention of clinicians, clearly and forcefully. Another hope is to interest basic neurobiologists in the applicability of their work to the clinical problems of epilepsy; a rather unique opportunity may exist in that epilepsy is particularly ripe for these developments. Neuroscientists, we hope, will be stimulated to focus interest on this challenging problem.

REFERENCES

1. A.R.N.M.D. *Epilepsy and the Convulsive State*. Baltimore: Williams & Wilkins, 1931, vol. 7.

2. A.R.N.M.D. *Epilepsy*. Baltimore: Williams & Wilkins, 1947, vol. 26.

3. Berger, H. Über das Elektrenkephalogramm des Menschen. *Arch. Psychiat.* 87: 527, 1929. Ibid. 94:16, 1931; 100:301, 1933; 101:452, 1933; 102:538, 1934; 104:678, 1936.

4. Berger, H. Über die Entstehung der Erscheinungen des grossen epileptischen Anfalls. *Klin. Wschr.* 14:217, 1935.

5. Brown-Sequard, E. Nouvelles recherches sur l'épilepsie due à certaines lésions de la moelle épinière. *Arch. Physiol. Norm. Path.* 2:211, 422, 496, 1869.

6. Ferrier, D. Experimental researches in cerebral physiology and pathology. *West Riding Lunatic Asylum Medical Reports* 3:30, 1873.

7. Fritsch, G., and Hitzig, E. Über die elektrische Erregbarkeit des Grosshirns. *Arch. Anat. Physiol.* 37:300, 1870.

8. Gastaut, H. A proposed international classification of epileptic seizures. *Epilepsia* (Amst.) 5:297, 1964.

9. Gowers, W. R. *Epilepsy and Other Chronic Convulsive Diseases: Their Causes, Symptoms and Treatment* (2d ed.). London: J. and A. Church, 1901.

10. Hall, M. *Synopsis of the Spinal System.* London: J. Mallett, 1850.

11. Hunt, J. R. A theory of the mechanism underlying inhibition in the central nervous system and its relation to convulsive manifestations. *Proc. Ass. Res. Nerv. Ment. Dis.* 7:45, 1931.

12. Jackson, J. H. *Selected Writings of John Hughlings Jackson.* Vol. 1. *On Epilepsy and Epileptiform Convulsions,* Ed. by J. Taylor. London: Hodder and Stoughton, 1931.

13. Jasper, H. H., and Kershman, J. Electroencephalographic classification of the epilepsies. *Arch. Neurol. Psychiat.* 45:903, 1941.

14. Kussmaul, A., and Tenner, A. *On the Nature and Origin of Epileptiform Convulsions Caused by Profuse Bleeding and Also of Those of True Epilepsy.* Trans. by E. Bronner. London: New Sydenham Society, 1859.

15. Lennox, W. G. The physiological pathogenesis of epilepsy. *Brain* 59:113, 1936.

16. Lennox, W. G. The petit mal epilepsies; their treatment with tridione. *J.A.M.A.* 129:1069, 1945.

17. Lennox, W. G. Phenomena and correlates of the psychomotor triad. *Neurology* (Minneap.) 1:357, 1951.

18. Lennox, W. G. *Epilepsy and Related Disorders.* 2 vols. Boston: Little, Brown, 1960.

19. Lennox, W. G., Gibbs, F. A., and Gibbs, E. L. Effect on the electroencephalogram of drugs and conditions which influence seizures. *Arch. Neurol. Psychiat.* 36:1236, 1936.

20. Meyer, A. Epilepsy. In Greenfield's *Neuropathology* (2d ed.). Baltimore: Williams & Wilkins, 1963.

21. Penfield, W., and Jasper, H. H. *Epilepsy and the Functional Anatomy of the Human Brain.* Boston: Little, Brown, 1954, p. 20.

22. Penfield, W., and Kristiansen, K. *Epileptic Seizure Patterns.* Springfield, Ill.: Thomas, 1951.

23. Scholz, W. The contribution of pathoanatomical research to the problem of epilepsy. *Epilepsia* (Amst.) 1:36, 1959, Ser. 4.

24. Sherrington, C. S. *The Integrative Action of the Nervous System.* Cambridge, Eng.: Cambridge University Press, 1947.

25. Temkin, O. *The Falling Sickness.* Baltimore: Johns Hopkins Press, 1945.

26. Tower, D. B. *Neurochemistry of Epilepsy.* Springfield, Ill.: Thomas, 1960.

27. Welch, K., and Penfield, W. Paradoxical improvement in hemiplegia following cortical excisions. *J. Neurosurg.* 7:414, 1950.

28. Wilson, S. A. Kinnier, and Bruce, A. N. *Neurology.* 3 vols. Baltimore: Williams & Wilkins, 1955.

2
Architecture of the Cerebral Cortex

J. SZENTÁGOTHAI

GENERAL STRUCTURE: LAMINATION, CELL TYPES

The cerebral cortex (neocortex) is usually described as a six-layered sheet of gray matter, with laminae numbered from the subpial surface toward the depth. Lamination is more obvious in the Nissl picture and is obscured rather than clarified by staining either the dendrites or axonal ramifications or both. This is due to the fact that dendrites, in particular, but also to some extent the axon ramifications, transgress the lamina boundaries liberally. There is difficulty for detailed structural analysis of the neuron network, which is particularly obvious if compared with the strict confinement of dendritic and axonal ramifications to a certain layer in the cerebellar cortex.

Two main categories of nerve cells can be distinguished at first sight: pyramidal and stellate cells. Only two intermediate types cannot be classified easily into one of the two categories: the star-pyramids of the second lamina and fusiform cells of the fifth and sixth laminae. The first type can almost certainly be considered as essentially a pyramidal type, and the second—if not inverted pyramidal cells—are more likely to be stellate cells. Each of the main categories can be subdivided into a number of types and subtypes, mainly according to the ramification of their axons, but to some extent also to that of dendritic arborization pattern or surface structure. Study of the cerebral-cortex neuron network involves a major difficulty in identification of the various cell types under the electron microscope. Although structural differences between the two main cell categories are obvious, it is unlikely that differences in plasma structure of both cell bodies and dendrites will enable identification of various types in the electron microscope picture on sight.

The most significant types of cells are shown in highly diagrammatic fashion in Fig. 2-7. The best recent account of cell types with a remarkable approach for estimating quantitatively both cell types and dendritic arborizations was given by Sholl [26, 27]; however, some oversimplification in this approach has been criticized [3]. Studies in progress in this laboratory [23], using statistical analysis of the Nissl pictures in the cerebellar cortex show that quantitative data gathered from silver impregnation pictures are highly unrealistic; and a correct quantitative approach to neuron-type population analysis needs a completely new methodical approach.

AFFERENTS

Afferent fibers of the cerebral cortex are subdivided: (1) specific afferents—well defined only in the primary sensory regions (specific sensory afferents)—arising from the specific subcortical source of that region; (2) nonspecific afferents arising from nonspecific subcortical source; (3) callosal afferents; (4) association afferents from cortical source; and (5) association afferents from subcortical source.

Reliable data about the modus of termination of various kinds of afferents are exceedingly scarce; only in the case of the specific sensory afferents do the Golgi pictures [18, 25] and degeneration studies [22] appear to give concordant information on

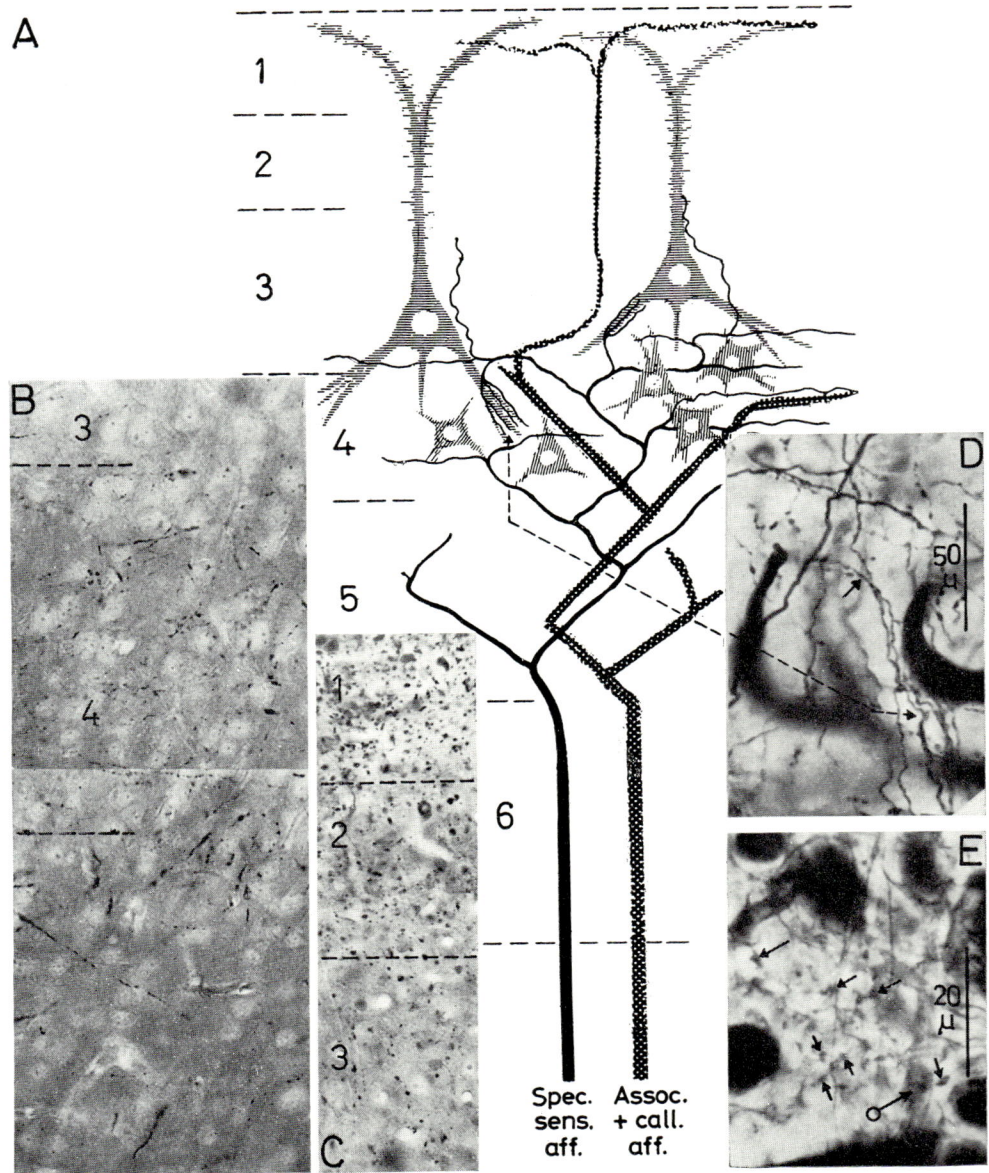

Fig. 2-1. Course and distribution of afferent fibers in the cerebral cortex. (*A*) Arborization of a specific sensory afferent (in full black) and of associative or callosal afferent (crosshatched). Arabic numerals indicate cortical layers. (*B*) Degeneration fragments in striate region (laminae 3, 4, and below) of the cat 5 days after a lesion placed in lateral geniculate body (Nauta-Gygax procedure). (*C*) Degeneration of association afferents in medial cortex surface of rat 5 days after lateral cortical lesion. Predominant localization of terminal fragments in laminae 1 and 2 (Fink-Heimer procedure). (*D*) Curved branch (arrow) of oblique large afferent breaking up in horsetail-type arborization probably for basal dendrite of pyramidal cell as indicated in diagram *A*. (*E*) Bielschowsky degeneration picture in lamina 4 of striate region of cat 5 days after lesion placed in lateral geniculate body. Arrows point to degeneration fragments. Ringed arrow indicates shadow of apical dendrite around which intact ascending terminal axons can be seen.

a very characteristic terminal course of the afferents.

The label *nonspecific* is obviously highly arbitrary. In primary sensory regions or those receiving afferents from some specific source, like the motor cortex afferents arising from the association nuclei of the thalamus (lateralis posterior or pulvinar) might be called nonspecific. But this may not be evident in some other regions. The expression is unequivocal only in the case of the nonspecific (or intralaminar) thalamocortical afferents. The group of association afferents from subcortical source might be separated from the nonspecific group as indicated above, but whether such separation is possible will be seen only on the basis of more detailed study with degeneration methods.

Typical branching pattern of the sensory afferents as deduced from a comparison of degeneration fragments (Fig. 2-1B) and Golgi pictures (Fig. 2-1D) is shown somewhat diagrammatically in Fig. 2-1A. Since an appropriate electron microscope analysis is still lacking, it is not possible as yet to decide about the elements with which contacts are primarily established.

On the basis of light microscope studies using the Bielschowsky stains (Fig. 2-1E), it may be concluded that in the upper part of the fourth layer the degeneration fragments lie so densely that they might have contacts with any part of neurons or dendrites embedded in the neuropil. In the negative sense, it may be concluded from this figure that they do not contribute to the *synaptic cartridges* around the shaft dendrites of pyramidal cells. From the oblique course of the descending or ascending horsetail-shaped terminal arborizations, seen in the Golgi picture, it may be inferred that they contribute to the synaptic terminals surrounding basal dendrites of pyramidal cells, mainly of the third and fourth laminae.

Almost nothing is known about the termination sites of nonspecific subcortical afferents. It has been felt by various authors [22, 28] that callosal fibers are more widely distributed in depth, with some preponderance of termination of the upper layers. But all earlier reasoning has been proven spectacularly wrong by a new staining technique for degenerated terminal fragments by Fink and Heimer [8], who showed that quite a considerable part of first lamina fibers and terminals derive from callosal [14] and association afferents (Fig. 2-1C). This does not invalidate the conclusion reached by cortical isolation experiments [28, 29]; see also figures given by Colonnier [3], that many of the tangential first lamina fibers are of intracortical origin. It shows clearly that all earlier degeneration studies on the cerebral cortex have to be redone using this new light microscope technique and also electron microscope degeneration procedures. Until recently, a difficulty in the study of the cerebral cortex was ambiguity regarding the fine unmyelinated parts of cortical axons, since results of the Nauta-Gygax procedure usually show only the fragments of preterminal parts of most axons. Classical Bielschowsky stains were somewhat better (Fig. 2-1E), but tracing degenerated elements with this method in unknown cortical areas is almost hopeless.

Only now with the Fink-Heimer method can the almost unbelievable wealth of commissural and associative connections be realized. A true appraisal of the new situation emerging from the new degeneration results will be possible in a few years' time, especially if observations are completed by an electron microscope study of the real sites of the synaptic contacts. The same considerations can be applied to both kinds of associative afferents.

Electron Microscope Identification of Pyramidal and Stellate Cells and Synapses

An up-to-date structural analysis of any neuron network has to begin with identification of various cell types under the electron microscope. This is required primarily in order to recognize and identify both structure and origin of their synapses. Most neurohistologists agree that certain information on whether or not any given axonal element is in synaptic contact with any neuronal elements nearby can only be gained by the aid of the electron microscope. Difficulties in identifying neurons in the cerebral cortex, mentioned previously, arise from the fact that it has neither the strict lamination and obvious structural differences of the laminae nor are there the excessive differences in size, location, and arborization nor particularly the low number of cell types of the cerebellar cortex, which made identification under the electron microscope of various cell types relatively easy [6, 9, 12, 13].

PYRAMIDAL CELL CATEGORY. Characteristic form and uniform orientation of pyramidal cells make it relatively easy to identify them mainly on the basis of their apical (or shaft) dendrites (Fig. 2-2 and 2-4). But it is very unlikely that any of the various pyramidal cell types could be distinguished within the pyramidal cell category. It is to be expected that the pyramidal nature of the main cell type of the second lamina (the star-pyramids) and the less certain nature of the more multiform cell types in the fifth and sixth laminae can be established relatively easily in the electron microscope picture; so far, this has not been done. The minute structure of the pyramidal cell will not be discussed here beyond that which is evident from the very low-power electron micrograph of Fig. 2-2A.

It has been long known (Ramón y Cajal [25]) that the cell bodies of some cortical cells, in all probability mainly those of pyramidal cells, are surrounded by a synaptic basket, the fibers of which terminate on the cell surface by means of synaptic boutons. Figure 2-2A shows a classification of synaptic terminals (as far as possible under higher magnification of the same picture) into those that have synaptic contacts including contact specializations with the soma and the initial parts of the dendrites, and into those having none. The latter, being often in direct membrane contact with the soma or initial dendrite surface, have their synaptic membrane specialization on some other parts of their surface that are in contact with some other element of the neuropil, generally with a dendritic spine.

As recently shown, independently by Colonnier [4] and Hámori [11] (Fig. 2-2B and 2-2C), the synaptic terminals having direct specialized contacts with the soma or initial dendrite surface are exclusively of the so-called *flattened vesicular* type of Uchizono [33]. They are believed to be inhibitory; and those having structurally specialized contacts with neuropil elements are of the *spheric vesicular* type, having larger vesicles and considered excitatory. This is of particular interest as the pericellular synaptic baskets, terminating also on the initial smooth parts of the dendrites up to distances of about 10–30 μ, have been considered already by Ramón y Cajal [25] as belonging to a particular kind of horizontal stellate cells. Such a cell from the second lamina is shown in Fig. 2-3D indicating also an interesting feature of this cell type, where the axons of the more superficial *basket*-type cells have a very low tangential spread; their span may be quite considerable—500 μ and perhaps more—in deeper layers.

The intracortical origin of the soma–initial dendrite synapses has been shown by the use of the *persisting elements* method in chronically isolated cortical slabs [29, 30]

FIG. 2-2. The pyramidal cell. (A) A very low-power electron micrograph of small pyramidal neuron in occipital cortex of cat. Axon terminals having direct attachment to soma or initial dendrites with specialized contact region and containing small ovoid vesicles, seen under higher magnification of the same neuron, are stippled with black. Axon terminals having synaptic contacts with spines and containing larger spheric synaptic vesicles are stippled with white. (B) and (C) Synaptic terminals, being in apposition with the same smooth initial part of pyramidal neuron dendrite, D. (B) Specialized synaptic contact is with a spine, Sp, and vesicles are of larger spheroid type. (C) Contact is with initial part of dendrite and synaptic vesicles are of smaller ovoid type. (D) and (E) Details from Golgi pictures of delicate terminal axon branches (arrows) longitudinally attached to apical dendrites of pyramidal cells. (F) Typical vertical axon strand, with indication of relation to apical pyramidal cell dendrite (stippled). (G) Initial collaterals (arrow) of descending pyramidal cell axon may contribute to vertical delicate fiber strands. (D) through (G) Perfusion Golgi-Kopsch procedure.

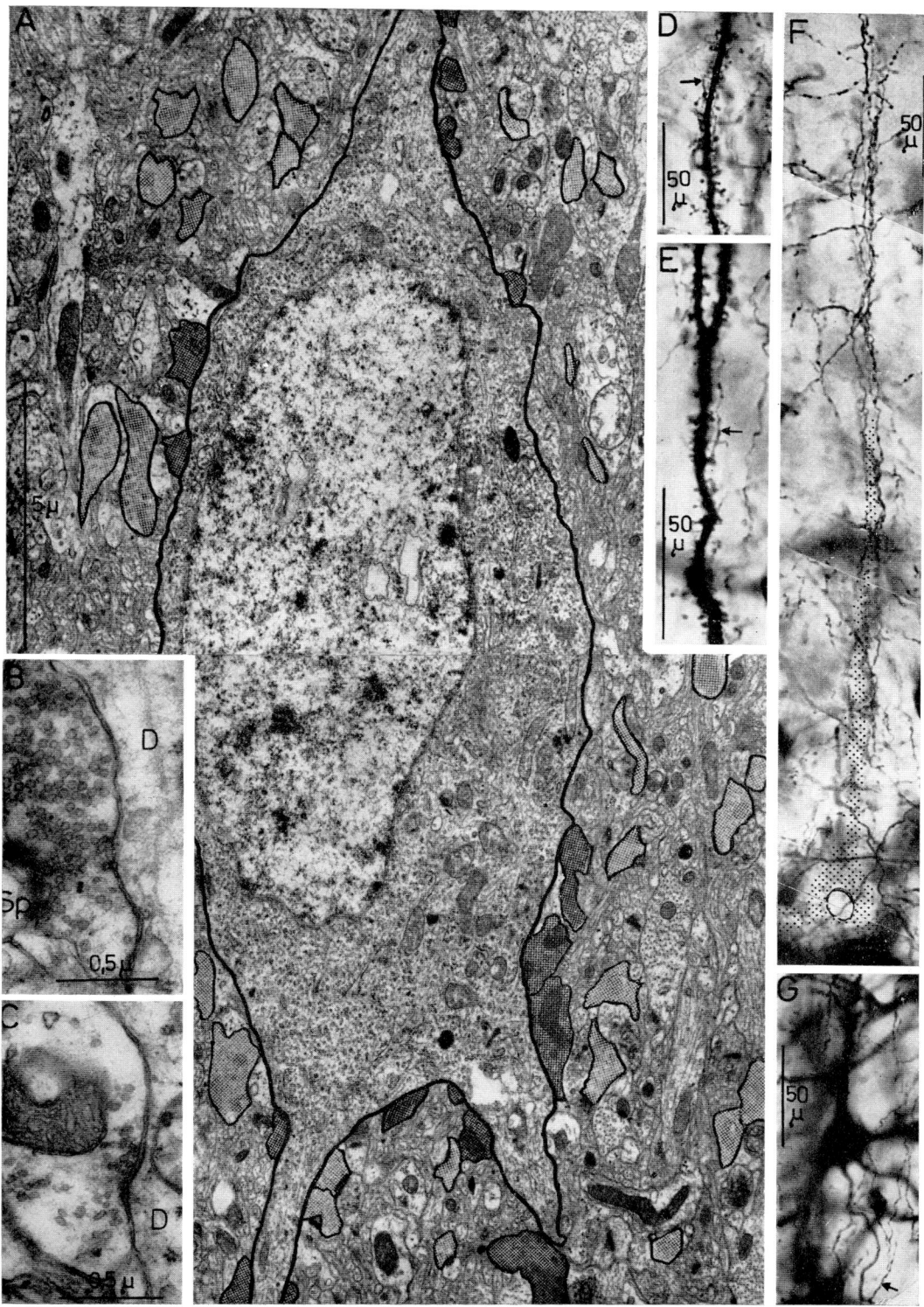

—an additional indirect proof of Ramón y Cajal's conjecture. This problem has been discussed recently by Colonnier [3] including electron microscope evidence but is not treated here further. Only its significance for formation of the integrative unit of the cerebral cortex will be considered. Synaptic apparatus of the dendrites proper will be discussed in the next section, under The Cortical Neuropil.

STELLATE CELL CATEGORY. Irregularity of the dendritic tree, of the stellate cells in most cases, does not permit development of any simple method (of section orientation or the like) for their identification in the electron microscope picture. So far we have been able only to find a cell type, the plasma structure of which—both of the cell body and the dendrites—allows definition that it is no pyramidal cell. A cell type of quite similar plasma and mitochondrial structure can be identified in many thalamic and geniculate nuclear regions as a Golgi type II cell probably of inhibitory nature [20, 32]. In Fig. 2-3A these cells are irregular in shape, the plasma structure very dense, both in the cell body and in the dendrites. The plasma contains wide endoplasmic cisterns, large pale mitochondria, having relatively sparse cristae, that contrast strongly with the darker plasma background. In accordance with the classic Golgi description, the dendrites are beaded and are either devoid of, or have few irregularly arranged spines. Beaded character of the dendrites is also seen well in the electron microscope picture; this is no artifact as might be supposed from the Golgi picture.

Synaptic terminals do occur on the cell body, often deeply impressed into the ruggedly irregular surface, but they are not numerous. Synapses of the dendrites (Fig. 2-3B) are situated on the dendrite surface proper, an arrangement not usual in the pyramidal cells, where most of the distal dendritic synapses are established with the spines.

Only an elementary level of knowledge exists about the several cell types of the cerebral cortex; the road ahead is long before more specific information on the various cell types will be available. Involved is the matter of how far this kind of analysis could be driven, in more easily manageable regions of the central nervous system, as a hopeful key to the situation.

THE CORTICAL NEUROPIL

Axonal arborizations, the finer the more numerous, are arranged predominantly parallel with the general course of the dendrites. The delicate axonal neuropil is tangentially oriented in the first lamina, has obliquely oriented meshes in the second, is predominantly perpendicular in the third, and again tangentially oriented in the fourth lamina. In deeper layers of the cortex, orientation of the delicate synaptic neuropil is obscured by the numerous larger fibers entering or leaving the cortex. Relation between the dendrites and the delicate axonal meshwork is particularly conspicuous in the third lamina, where dendritic shafts of pyramidal neurons are neatly arranged parallel in the perpendicular direction.

In the Golgi picture it is quite common to see a number of very fine terminal axons running for considerable distances closely

FIG. 2-3. The stellate cell. (A) Low-power electron micrograph of cell, presumed a stellate neuron, with characteristic dark plasma structure, Ac = astrocyte. (B) Two synaptic terminals, St, of the spheroid type in contact with dark dendrite, D. Lack or scarcity of spines and beaded character of such dendrites, if cut longitudinally, favors interpretation as stellate dendrites. (C) Two stellate cells from the somatosensory cortex (lamina 4) of cat. Axon, ax, of lower one can be traced clearly to horsetail fiber strand indicated by arrow. Delicate axonal feltwork at left from upper stellate cell cannot be traced to any larger axon but appears to have pericellular contacts with the upper stellate cell body. (D) Small stellate cell in lamina 2 of same area; its axon (arrow) giving basket-type terminal arborization (semicircles) in near neighborhood of cell body. This cell corresponds to S_2 of Fig. 2-7. (C) and (D) Perfusion Golgi-Kopsch procedure.

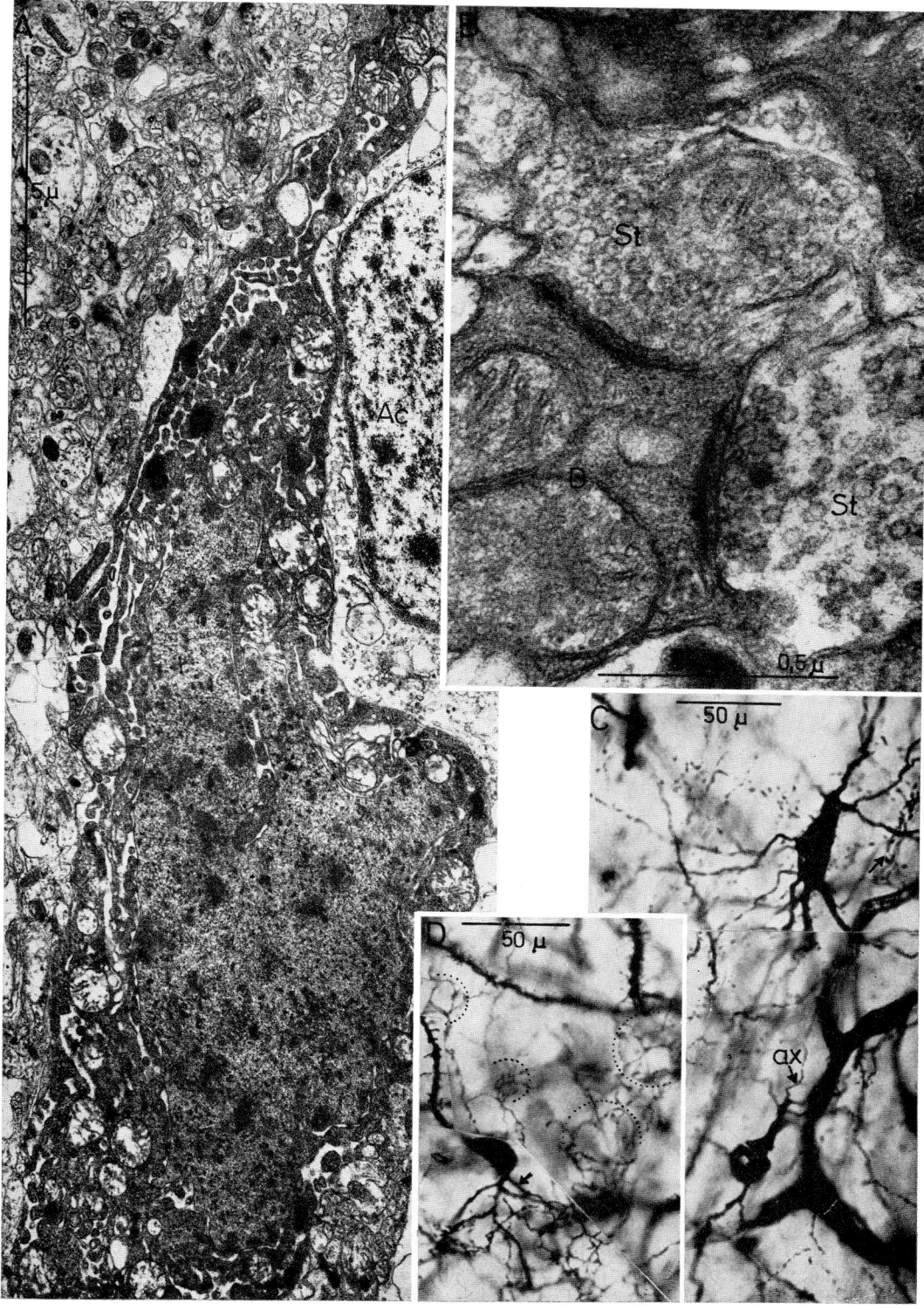

associated into bundles (Fig. 2-2E, 2-2F), which in many cases can be seen to contain a dendritic shaft in their axes (Figs. 2-2D, 2-2E, 2-5C, 2-5D). This arrangement corresponds to the electron microscope picture (Fig. 2-4) of the shaft dendrites, each of which can be clearly seen as surrounded by a dense cylinder of synaptic axonal neuropil containing numerous axon-spine synapses. Visualization of these synaptic *cartridges* of the shaft dendrites and their main branches in a stereodiagram is attempted in Fig. 2-5F. Similar, although less well-organized cartridges may exist also around some of the basal dendrites of the pyramidal cells. This view of the synaptic arrangement around the larger dendrites corresponds to several light-microscope descriptions of the so-called climbing collaterals of dendritic shafts, considered by several authors [3, 24, 31] as the sign of a repeated contact of the same terminal axon with a considerable number of spines of the same dendrite.

Analogous to the similar situation of the climbing fiber in the cerebellum having hundreds of contacts, if not more, between the same single axon and the same Purkinje neuron, and their known powerful action [7], a rather powerful action of the synaptic cartridges upon the dendritic shafts might be assumed. In the frame of this reasoning, parallel orientation of terminal axons with dendrites gains importance. It is worthwhile to compare the two principal kinds of axodendritic synaptic systems, established by means of spines, in the cerebellar and the cerebral cortex. As pointed out [12], axon-spine synapses of the cerebellar molecular layer are, with rare exceptions, synapses of overcrossing (Fig. 2-5E) whereas those of the pyramidal dendritic shaft cartridges are those of parallel arrangement (Fig. 2-5F).

Synaptic action of one parallel fiber on one Purkinje cell is probably negligible and parallel fiber stimulation requires high convergence. Synaptic action would become particularly powerful if terminal axons of the cartridge were branches of the same preterminal fiber. This is often the case with characteristic horsetail-shaped terminal axon ramifications. As shown in Fig. 2-1A (diagrammatically) and in Fig. 2-1D (Golgi picture), such ramifications are given by afferents—probably specific ones—most likely to basal dendrites of pyramidal cells. This is not quite certain, since the horsetail arborizations are too delicate for detection in light microscopy degeneration pictures; however, characteristic downward turns of branches before breaking up in the arborization can be seen in the degeneration picture.

The majority of really dense horsetail arborizations derive undoubtedly from large stellate cells of the fourth lamina; two examples are shown in Fig. 2-3C, a more impressive one in Fig. 2-5A. General significance of the vertically oriented, axonal branchings of a certain kind of Golgi second-type cell, the *cellule à double bouquet dendritique* of Ramón y Cajal [25], has been stressed earlier [3]. But this additional information of specific attachment of several vertical branches of the same axon to one or a few dendritic shafts leads to the conclusion that synaptic linkage in the cerebral cortex might provide means to bring certain cells into action rather specifically.

No similar arrangement has been seen around the dendrites of stellate cells, which is not to be expected, since lack (or scarcity) of dendritic spines would not provide for an appropriate receiving surface of such a dense axonal cartridge. Stellate cells may be embedded, particularly in the fourth lamina (Fig. 2-3C) into extremely dense, terminal axonal meshworks deriving at least partly from other stellate cells. In lamina four of primary sensory regions it is observed that after transection of the sensory radiation, the cells appear literally embedded into numerous degeneration fragments (Fig. 2-1E). This might indicate that stellate cell bodies and probably also dendrites are the main receivers of specific afferent inflow. That shaft dendrite cartridges are rarely affected under such circumstances also supports this assumption. The conclusion that stellate cells are the main receivers of specific afferents is by no means incompatible with the observation by Globus and Scheibel [10] of a spine loss on dendritic shafts of pyramidal cells oc-

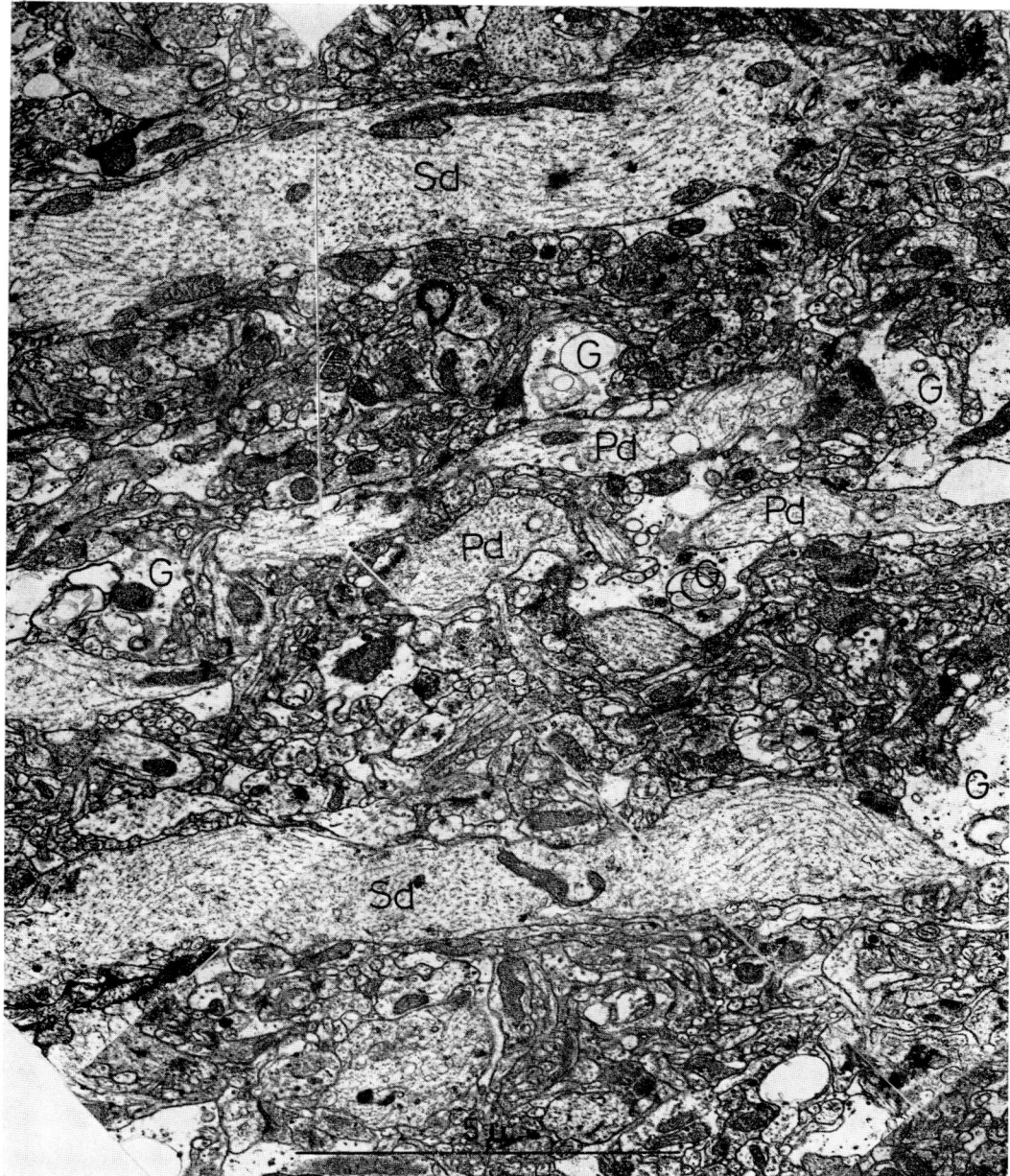

FIG. 2-4. Low-power electron micrograph of neuropil in the upper part of lamina 3, cut perpendicularly. Two dendritic shafts, Sd, can be seen (pial surface is to right) with surrounding darker cylinder of neuropil, the *synaptic cartridge*. Inspection with higher power reveals that cartridge contains mainly delicate axons and spines of apical dendrite. Space between synaptic cylinders is occupied by smaller dendrites, here of pyramidal cells, Pd, with more irregular surrounding neuropil. Residual space between dendrites and attached neuropil is occupied by light glial profiles, G. Little if any glia enters synaptic cartridges of apical dendrites.

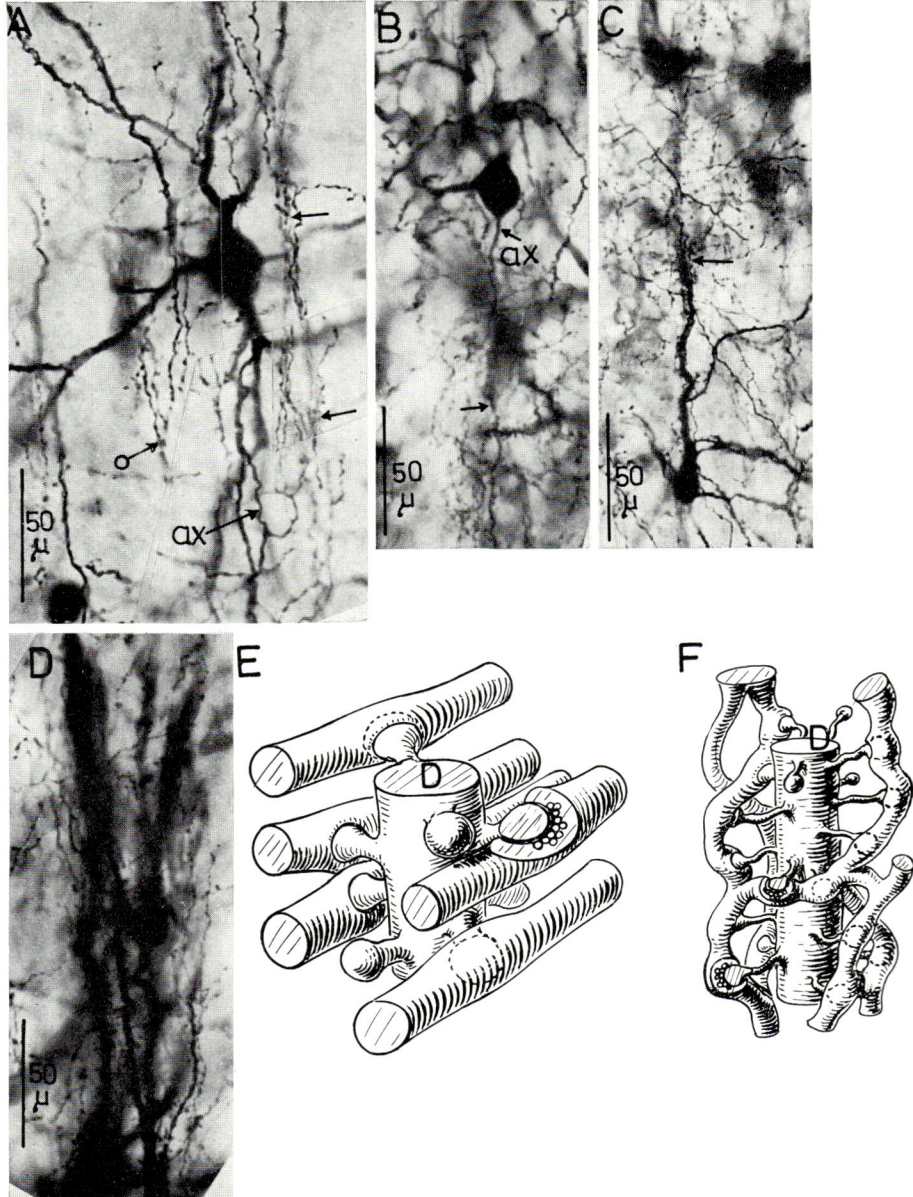

Fig. 2-5. Source and relationships of vertically oriented, delicate axonal neuropil to apical dendrites of pyramidal cells. (*A*) Stellate neuron from lamina 4 of somatosensory cortex of cat. Descending axon, ax, of this cell breaks up into numerous recurrent branches, giving rise to strands of vertically ascending delicate axons (arrows). In axis of right strand, shadow of a pyramidal dendritic shaft can be recognized in preparation (not visible in photograph). Strand at left divides (ringed arrow) in an acute angle corresponding to division of dendritic shafts in this level of the fifth lamina pyramidal cells. This cell corresponds to cell S_1 of Fig. 2-7. (*B*) Stellate cell whose dendritic tree is confined to very small space due to recurring dendrites, giving rise to a descending axon, ax, which breaks up into descending, delicate axon strands (arrow). This cell corresponds to S_4 in Fig. 2-7. (*C*) Pyramidal cell with part of its synaptic cartridge around apical dendrite stained (arrow). (*D*) Apical dendrites of pyramidal cells embedded into vertically oriented axonal

curring after lesions of the lateral geniculate body or after enucleation. The fact itself that enucleation does cause a loss in shaft dendrite spines shows that the effect may be transneuronal, as pointed out correctly by Valverde [34] in the discussion of similar results. (A very considerable transneuronal reduction of spines occurs also in Purkinje cells of the chronically isolated cerebellar cortex, although the majority of the parallel fibers remain intact.) The beautiful figures of Valverde [34] also support the conclusion that dendritic shafts of pyramidal cells are contacted mainly by the axons of local neurons. Some of the cell bodies embedded into the degeneration fragments might, of course, be pyramidal cells, but this is less likely as the axosomatic synaptic knobs of pyramidal neurons persist in chronically isolated cortical slabs [30] and thus are undoubtedly of local origin.

There is also good evidence to assume that pyramidal cell dendrites are directly engaged with specific or other afferents. All these questions are now open for an appropriate degeneration analysis with aid of the electron microscope.

TENTATIVE NEUROPIL GEOMETRY. In regions undisturbed by cell bodies of the neuropil of the third lamina, the dendritic shafts are found fairly regularly at distances of about 10 μ. This would indicate in the case of an ideal distribution that dendritic shafts be arranged in an equilateral triangular pattern. Six units of this pattern would form a hexagonal pattern. However, it is unlikely that such a large area could exist without cell bodies disturbing such a regular arrangement. This would be so in lower mammals; however, decreasing cell density in man, perhaps also in the monkey, might permit even larger spaces of pure neuropil.

As the diameter of apical dendrites is roughly 2 μ and the average length of dendritic spines also around 2 μ, the synaptic cartridge would have a radius of roughly 3 μ. This would leave a minimal distance of 4 μ free between neighboring cartridges for smaller dendritic branches, either those of the dendritic shafts or those of the basal dendrites of more superficially situated pyramidal cells, having their own minor and less regular cylindrical synaptic axonal envelopes. Dark stellate dendrites are found also in spaces between shaft cartridges with more individually arranged direct axodendritic synapses. In contrast to the molecular layer of the cerebellar cortex, where the dendritic surface of Purkinje neurons is specifically isolated by glial processes (Fig. 112 of [16])—with the exception of the synaptic surfaces of the spines—no such arrangement appears to exist in the cerebral cortex. Here the astrocytic processes seem to fill spaces between the cartridges and more specifically to surround the stellate cells and their dendrites which, in the cerebellum (stellate and basket cells), have no glial envelope.

This view of neuropil arrangement is shown tentatively and in oversimplified manner in Fig. 2-6, as are the neuropil of other layers of the cortex. In the first lamina there appears to be no such specific space arrangement between axons and dendrites, except that all are oriented tangentially. Otherwise no order appears in the relatively loose neuropil of this lamina although more specifically aimed electron microscope studies with carefully oriented planes of sectioning and systematic survey, with low magnifications, might well disclose a visible order. Again, this first ap-

---

strands so delicate that few can be resolved at this magnification. (*A* through *D*) Perfusion Golgi-Kopsch procedure. (*E*) and (*F*) Comparison between relation of spiny dendritic branches and synaptic axons in the case of Purkinje cells in cerebellar cortex and in dendritic shafts of cerebral cortical pyramidal cells. (*E*) In Purkinje dendrites the parallel fibers cross spiny dendritic branch, D, at a right angle so that each parallel fiber has only one synaptic contact with any Purkinje cell; convergence is about $2 \times 10^5:1$ [6]. (*F*) In dendritic shafts of pyramidal cells of cerebral cortex, arrangement between dendrite, D, and thin axons is parallel; if thin terminal axons are horsetail-shaped branches of the same axon, number of contacts between same presynaptic and postsynaptic neuron might easily come up to order of approximately 10^2 to 10^3 or even above.

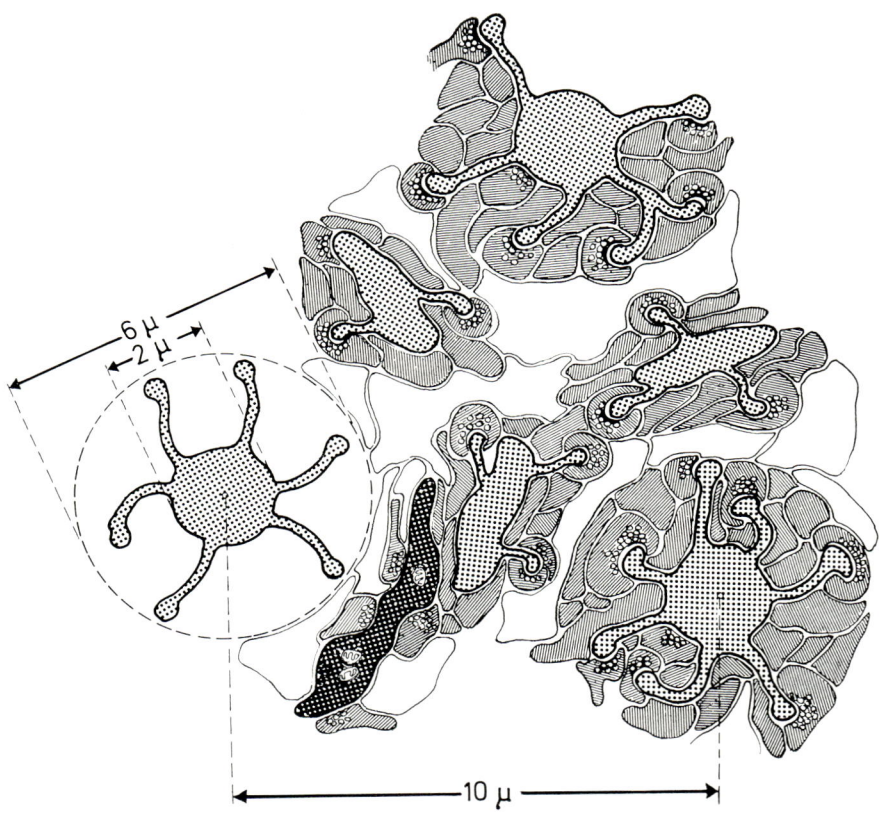

Fig. 2-6. Some aspects of neuropil geometry in lamina 3. Diagram represents 3 apical dendrites of pyramidal cells, arranged in triangular fashion at distances of roughly 10 μ. Each of the dendritic shafts is surrounded by cylindrical neuropil cartridges of 6 μ dia., containing thin axon profiles, dendritic spines, and synapses. Space between cartridges is occupied by other pyramidal cell dendrites (basal and branches of apical dendrites) with their surrounding, more irregular envelopes of synaptic neuropil. Pyramidal cell dendrites and their spines are indicated by stippling, axons by hatching, and a stellate dendrite profile devoid of spines by crosshatching. Empty astrocytic profiles are predominantly arranged in interspaces between neuropil cartridges or envelopes of pyramidal cells, and more closely attached to stellate dendrites. Diagram should be visualized as sectioning plane perpendicular to that shown in Fig. 2-4.

proach to neuropil geometry must be considered preliminary and oversimplified, requiring correction as new information develops.

BASIC NEURON CIRCUIT

Numerous attempts have been made to explain cerebral cortex structure in terms of operating neuron circuits [3, 19, 25, 31]. The diagram shown in Fig. 2-7 lacks certain known details, incorporation of which would make it unintelligible, even for those familiar with involved neuron-circuit diagrams, without discussing details of possible structural bases of the columnar organization [15, 16, 17, 21] of the cerebral cortex done recently [3, 31]; the diagram takes this major principle of organization into consideration.

In spite of no direct proof for spatial arrangement of collateral inhibition, indirect evidence of interneurons giving basket-type pericellular synapses with ovoid vesicles to pyramidal or star-pyramidal cells, and the analogy to similar inhibitory mechanisms in the hippocampus [1] and the cerebellar cortex [2], permit postulation of such mechanisms. Two such basket interneurons are shown in full black in Fig. 2-7. The different tangential spread in different layers of such connections, recognized by Ramón y Cajal [25], might be of considerable interest. In lamina 2, these neurons have an axonal spread of only a few cells in width, whereas this span is much wider (up to 500 μ) in the third and fourth laminae and might well reach still larger distances in the deeper layers. Collateral inhibition

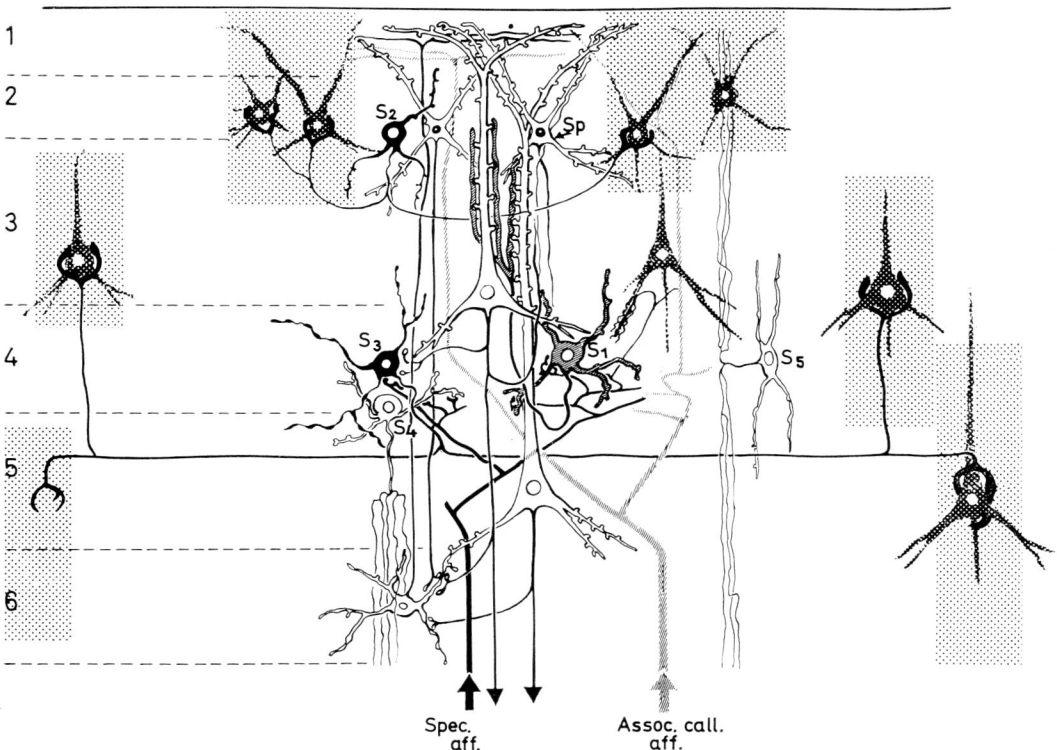

FIG. 2-7. Semidiagrammatic drawing of most important cell types of neocortex in general and interconnections discussed. Pyramidal cells, one in lamina 3 and one in lamina 5, are placed in center of drawing. They can be reached fairly directly and probably with relatively powerful synaptic connections from specific afferents over the S_1 type of stellate interneuron and cartridge synapses established around apical dendrites (hatched). Associative and callosal fibers, as well as stellate or inverse pyramidal neurons having ascending axons, feed into tangentially oriented first lamina, where relatively loose synaptic neuropil is established with final branches of pyramid dendritic shafts and ascending dendrites of star-pyramidal cells of the second lamina. Basket-type stellate interneurons (S_2) establish short-range pericellular connections in this layer. If basket synapses are assumed to be inhibitory, this would secure a mechanism of short-range collateral inhibition within stratum indicated by the stippled territories. Larger basket interneurons of deeper layers (S_3) may secure longer range (500 μ and above) collateral inhibition (stippled areas) in laminae 3 and 4 and perhaps even longer in deeper layers of cortex. An interneuron is shown at S_4 (similar to one shown in Fig. 2-5B) with receiving (dendritic) surface restricted to small space and descending axon breaking up into horsetail-shaped terminal arborization for deep strata. At S_5 is the stellate cell described by Ramón y Cajal as "cellule à double bouquet dendritique," which might secure spread of excitation (or, less likely, inhibition) over the whole depth of the cortex.

might therefore be operating at much smaller distances in the superficial layers and at increasingly larger ones in the deep layers. This is shown by shadowed areas on both sides, although we know almost nothing about tangential connections in the deeper strata. From the operational point of view, this might indicate that the upper laminae act as the "fine grain resolution mechanism," whereas the lower strata would operate on a "coarse grain basis."

Otherwise, in Fig. 2-7, emphasis is on an entirely different feature of neuron connectivity: the possibility of having rather specific through-connections from any given afferent (or group of afferents) to one or more neighboring pyramidal cells by means of the hatched stellate interneuron (S_1), or perhaps even monosynaptically by afferent horsetail synapses on pyramidal-cell basal dendrites (shown right from center in third lamina). The synaptic cartridges of the pyramidal neuron dendritic shafts might be considered as the structural basis of such selective through-conduction. This also indicates that the stellate cells cannot be simply generalized as inhibitory elements. Also incorporated are some other known stellate cell types (S_4, S_5), which might secure the predominantly vertical spread of excitation (or, less likely, inhibition) as required by the columnar concept [3], although not much can be said of their specific position in the circuit.

The ambiguously stellate (or sometimes inverse pyramid) cells of the sixth layer (also of the fifth) undoubtedly have a major role in projecting back into the first layer [3, 28, 31]. These elements have the best opportunity to receive the collaterals of outgoing axons.

ECHELON PROCESSING

Whatever the neuronal machine of the cortex may be, or its general or specific local circuitry or modes of information processings within any finite fraction of its tissue, it is to be hoped that understanding the neuronal machine will lead to understanding of the functions of the cortex as a whole. The most essential feature of its structural design rests not in the local neuron-network of the cortex itself but in the number of its mosaiclike high-order units (the columns) and particularly in wealth and specificity [14] of their interconnections. Compare this latter feature with the diametrically opposite architecture of the cerebellar cortex. The relations between two distant parts of the tissues are restricted to rather sparse connections established by recurrent Purkinje collaterals, which might suggest slightly an association between some folia within a narrow strip in the sagittal plane [6]. In any case, predominance of inhibitory connections would suppress the persistence of earlier excitatory states.

Information processing in the cerebellum is, as expressed by Sir John Eccles [5], provisional and piecemeal. The cerebellar cortex, in other words, processes all incoming information according to the momentary situation. Whatever the output, it comes into relation with the cerebellar cortex again only as part of the information of the next time-fraction of the *evolving movement* [5]. The mode of operation is exactly the reverse in the cerebral cortex. Output from any part of the cerebral-cortical tissue in overwhelming part goes to other regions of the cortex, both neighboring and distant. Only a very negligible fraction of the output is directed toward subcortical structures; even a large part of this serves again only to control the gates of the input channel (as in the descending pathways to thalamus and geniculate bodies) or purposes of more complex association between cortical areas conveyed by specific association nuclei of the thalamus. Information is needed on these nuclei: nucleus lateralis posterior and pulvinar, which show spectacular increase in tissue mass, parallel with development of the neocortex. These appear to have little input except from cortical areas, nor do they lead to structures other than cortex. Fibers from widely different cortical areas converge here not only upon the same cells but upon the same synaptic sites of a single cell [20], and the outcome of this integration is then fed back into the cortex.

The most essential principle of information processing in the cerebral cortex is that it occurs stepwise, in successively arranged layers (but not the cortical layers) or echelons, each of which appears to be specifically constructed to extract some meaningful element of information from the general input. This is particularly well exemplified by the columns of Hubel and Wiesel [17] of the visual cortex having simple, complex, or hypercomplex receptive fields. Incoming channels of the simple columns appear to be arranged in a highly specific way, a specificity well established at birth [16].

The complexity of wiring probably increases with each step further toward the higher echelons. Associative connections are more abundant to the surface strata (Fig. 2-1C), and perhaps to other layers that directly feed into them, where neuronal mechanisms seem to be available for some "finer grain processing" than is the case in layers receiving direct subcortical input.

Performance of the brain, of memory and learning, and the ultimate riddle of the inner self depend less on integrated circuits of the cortex than on the manner in which they are interconnected.

REFERENCES

1. Andersen, P., Eccles, J. C., and Løyning, Y. Recurrent inhibition in the hippocampus with identification of the inhibitory cells and its synapses. *Nature* (London) 198:541, 1963.
2. Andersen, P., Eccles, J. C., and Voorhoeve, P. E. Postsynaptic inhibition of cerebellar Purkinje cells. *J. Neurophysiol.* 27:1138, 1964.
3. Colonnier, M. L. The Structural Design of the Neocortex. In Eccles, J. C. (Ed.), *Brain and Conscious Experience.* New York: Springer, 1966.
4. Colonnier, M. L. Synaptic patterns on different cell types in the different laminae of the cat visual cortex. *Brain Res.* 9:268, 1968.
5. Eccles, J. C. Circuits in the cerebellar control of movement. *Proc. Nat. Acad. Sci. U.S.A.* 58:336, 1967.
6. Eccles, J. C., Ito, M., and Szentágothai, J. *The Cerebellum as a Neuronal Machine.* New York: Springer, 1967.
7. Eccles, J. C., Llinás, R., and Sasaki, K. Excitation of cerebellar Purkinje cells by the climbing fibers. *Nature* (London) 203:245, 1964.
8. Fink, R. P., and Heimer, L. Two methods for selective silver impregnation of degenerating axons and their synaptic endings in the central nervous system. *Brain Res.* 4:369, 1967.
9. Fox, C. A., Hillman, D. E., Siegesmund, K. A., and Dutta, C. R. The Primate Cerebellar Cortex: A Golgi and Electron Microscope Study. In Fox, C. A., and Snider, R. S. (Eds.), *The Cerebellum. Progress in Brain Research,* vol. 25. New York: American Elsevier, 1967, pp. 174–225.
10. Globus, A., and Scheibel, A. B. Synaptic loci on visual cortical neurons of the rabbit: The specific afferent radiation. *Exp. Neurol.* 18:116, 1967.
11. Hámori, J. Electron microscopy of axosomatic and axo-dendritic synapses of the pyramidal cells. In preparation.
12. Hámori, J., and Szentágothai, J. The "crossing-over" synapse: An electron microscope study of the molecular layer in the cerebellar cortex. *Acta Biol. Acad. Sci. Hung.* 15:95, 1964.
13. Hámori, J., and Szentágothai, J. Participation of Golgi neuron processes in the cerebellar glomeruli: An electron microscope study. *Exp. Brain Res.* 2:35, 1966.
14. Heimer, L., Ebner, F. F., and Nauta, W. J. H. A note on the termination of commissural fibers in the neocortex. *Brain Res.* 5:171, 1967.
15. Hubel, D. H., and Wiesel, T. N. Receptive fields, binocular interaction and functional architecture in the cat's visual cortex. *J. Physiol.* (London) 160:106, 1962.
16. Hubel, D. H., and Wiesel, T. N. Receptive fields of cells in striate cortex of very young, visually unexperienced cats. *J. Neurophysiol.* 26:994, 1963.
17. Hubel, D. H., and Wiesel, T. N. Receptive fields and functional architecture in two nonstriate visual areas (18 and 19) of the cat. *J. Neurophysiol.* 28:220, 1965.
18. Lorente de Nó, R. La corteza cerebral del ratón. *Trab. Lab. Invest. Biol. Univ. Madrid* 20:41, 1922.
19. Lorente de Nó, R. The Cerebral Cortex;

Architecture, Intracortical Connections and Motor Projections. In Fulton, J. F., *Physiology of the Nervous System.* London, New York, Toronto: Oxford 1938, pp. 291–321.

20. Majorossy, K., Réthelyi, M., and Szentágothai, J. The large glomerular synapse of the pulvinar. *J. Hirnforsch.* 7:415, 1965.

21. Mountcastle, V. B. Modalities and topographic properties of single neurons of cat's sensory cortex. *J. Neurophysiol.* 20: 408, 1957.

22. Nauta, J. H. Terminal distribution of some afferent fiber systems in the cerebral cortex. *Anat. Record,* 118:333, 1954.

23. Palkovits, M., and Magyar, P. In preparation.

24. Poljakov, G. I. On the fine structure of the human cerebral cortex and functional relations between its neurons (Russian). *Arkh. Anat.* 30:48, 1953.

25. Ramón y Cajal, S. *Histologie du système nerveux de l'homme et des vertèbres,* vol. 2. Paris: Maloine, 1911.

26. Sholl, D. A. Dendritic organization in the neurons of the visual and motor cortices of the cat. *J. Anat.* 87:387, 1953.

27. Sholl, D. A. *The Organization of the Cerebral Cortex.* London: Methuen, 1956.

28. Szentágothai, J. On the synaptology of the cerebral cortex (Russian). In Sarkissov, S. A. (Ed.) *Structure and Function of the Nervous System.* Moscow: Medgiz, 1962, pp. 6–14.

29. Szentágothai, J. The Use of Degeneration Methods in the Investigation of Short Neuronal Connections. In Singer, M., and Schadé, J. P. (Eds.), *Degeneration Patterns in the Nervous System,* Progress in Brain Research, vol. 14. New York: American Elsevier, 1965, pp. 1–32.

30. Szentágothai, J. The synapse of short local neurons in the cerebral cortex. In Szentágothai, J. (Ed.), *Modern Trends in Neuromorphology.* Symposia Biologica Hungarica, vol. 5. Budapest: Akadémiai Kiadó, 1965.

31. Szentágothai, J. The anatomy of complex integrative units in the nervous system. In Lissák, K. (Ed.), *Results in Neuroanatomy, Neurochemistry, Neuropharmacology and Neurophysiology,* Recent Development of Neurobiology in Hungary, vol. 1. Budapest: Akadémiai Kiadó, 1967, pp. 9–45.

32. Tömböl, Therese. Short neurons and their synaptic relations in the specific thalamic nuclei. *Brain Res.* 3:307, 1966/67.

33. Uchizono, Koji. Characteristics of excitatory and inhibitory synapses in the central nervous system of the cat. *Nature* (London) 207:642, 1965.

34. Valverde, I. Structural changes in the area striata of the mouse after enucleation. *Exp. Brain Res.* 5:274, 1968.

Discussion

HETEROGENEITY OF THE CEREBRAL CORTEX*

MARC COLONNIER AND SERGE ROSSIGNOL

In his essay entitled "Boarding-House Geometry," the Canadian humorist Stephen Leacock, recalling the miseries of countless sophomores, pessimistically states as his first axiom that "All boarding-houses are the same boarding-house." Anatomists studying the morphology of the cerebellar cortex can similarly assert, but in this case with optimism, that all cerebellar folia are the same cerebellar folium. The situation is not so encouraging when the student of cortical histology addresses himself to the study of the cerebral cortex, for the converse now obtains, and he must rather assume that no two regions of the cerebral covering are identical.

It should not be inferred that "generalized" models of the cerebral cortex are not valid. Indeed they are absolutely essential and, when they are as elegant as the one presented here by Szentágothai [44], they lay the very foundation of subsequent studies elaborating the variations and permutations of the basic plan in the different regions of the cortex.

Nevertheless, it must be emphasized that even this basic plan may be drastically modified in different regions of the cortex. It is important for anatomists to stress these variations on the cortical theme in order that scientists in other disciplines should not be led astray in the interpretation of their data pertaining to the cortex by assuming that the general plan must necessarily and rigorously apply in any cortical region of whatever species they happen to be studying.

The best and most obvious example of this heterogeneity in the cerebral cortex is in the preceding part of this chapter, on the architectural design of the cerebral cortex, restricted to the neocortex. The description obviously does not apply to archicortex. Such a limitation of the subject matter would not have been necessary in a review of the cerebellar cortex. The archicortex and neocortex of the cerebellum are quite similarly organized. The only difference between the two is the site of origin of their afferents. More, the cytoarchitecture of the cerebellum is almost identical throughout the vertebrate series. "L'écorce grise du cervelet présente dans la série animale, une admirable unité de structure, car, malgré les variations de volume et d'aspect macroscopique de cet organe, tous les détails de fine anatomie que l'on y rencontre chez les mammifères se retrouvent exactement chez les vertébrés inférieurs" [27].

In the cerebral cortex not only is there a marked difference of organization between isocortex and allocortex, but the neocortex itself displays a wide variety of organizational patterns from species to species and from area to area in the same species.

In fact, the most invariable feature of cortical histology, the one that can be generalized most easily, is perhaps the classification of neuron types found in the neocortex. A division into pyramidal type and stellate type cells as suggested by Sholl [37, 38, 39] and as presented here [44], or again a similar division in class I and class II cortical neurons as defined by Globus and Scheibel [19], applies quite uniformly throughout the neocortex. Ramon-Moliner [32] was the first to point out that one of the essential criteria distinguishing between these two large groups of cells is the relative absence of spines on the stellate type or class II cells as compared to pyramidal type or class I neurons. It is intriguing that Ramón y Cajal [27] draws more

---

* Supported by a grant from Medical Research Council of Canada.

spines on many of the stellate cell subgroups than one would expect from recent publications [7, 8, 19, 32] as well as from the presentation by Szentágothai [44]. Valverde [46] has also spoken of numerous spines on stellate cell dendrites of the mouse visual cortex and has shown drawings of such dendrites absolutely studded with spines!

Even the multiple subgroups of pyramidal and stellate-type cells seem to be present in all areas. However there are a few "region specific" cortical neurons. Ramón y Cajal [27] does mention *giant stellate cells* of the fourth layer of the visual cortex and so-called *special giant cells* found in all subzonal layers of the auditory cortex as being characteristic of these two regions in gyrencephalic mammals, especially in man. Both possess a long axon reaching into the white matter. On the basis of dendritic tree structure, these cells would most logically belong to the class II or stellate type group of neurons. Yet they do not conform to the generalization that such cells always possess Golgi type II axons, according to Globus and Scheibel [19] in their study of the lissencephalic rabbit cortex. They are an exception to a rule which otherwise seems to apply quite generally to gyrencephalic mammals.

Relative number and size of pyramidal and stellate type cells and their numerous subgroups vary considerably through the depth of the cortex and from area to area. Insofar as they vary with depth they serve as a basis for describing the tangential lamination of the cortex. Their variations from region to region lay the foundation by which so-called cytoarchitectonic areas are defined and which permits designation of histologically different cortical regions.

Brodmann [3] was one of the first to describe cytoarchitecture of the cerebral cortex on a six-layer basis. His main argument for this scheme was that by the sixth month of intrauterine life he could identify six different layers throughout the neocortex without any regional differentiation. Later, some layers regress, others develop and subdivide to give the heterogeneous adult patterns where the six-layer scheme is often far from obvious. Ramón y Cajal [27] originally considered the visual cortex as having nine layers. Later, he reduced the number of laminae to seven in his work on the cat visual cortex [28]. Ramon-Moliner [30, 31] in his two first articles on the histology of the postcruciate gyrus rejects an a priori lamination scheme and relies uniquely on depth from the pial surface in collecting his data. He concludes that the results fit well in a six-layer scheme.

It is important to have a universally accepted scheme if cortical histologists are to communicate significantly but general acceptance of the six-layer pattern is no panacea. Solnitky and Harman [40] reviewed six different interpretations of this scheme by eight different authors for the visual cortex alone. For example, Brodmann's layer IVc corresponds to O'Leary's [25] layer Va and to Sholl's layer IV, while Brodmann's layer IVb is equivalent to O'Leary's layers IVa and IVb and to Sholl's layer III.

O'Leary's scheme will be used here in dealing with area 17 of the cat. Lamina I is the neuron-poor layer immediately underneath the pia. Laminae II and III are the underlying neuron-rich layers, limited inferiorly by a row of rather large pyramidal cells, the so-called *border* cells of O'Leary. They cannot be distinguished one from the other in this area. Lamina IV is characterized by the dominant presence of densely packed stellate type cells. It can be subdivided into a sublayer IVa of large stellate, and a sublayer IVb of smaller stellate cells. Density of neuron packing is considerably reduced in underlying layer V, also formed of two sublayers. Sublayer Va is a narrow zone corresponding to Ramón y Cajal's layer of pyramidal cells with arciform axons. Sublayer Vb consists of a monocellular row of giant pyramidal cells. Layer VI is characterized by the arrangement of neuron somas in vertical palisades.

Detailed description of projection of specific thalamic afferents into these layers can be very different in different species and according to the cytoarchitectonic area under consideration. For example, Ebner [11] has demonstrated that cells of the medial geniculate nucleus project mainly to the first, fifth, and sixth layers of the auditory cortex in the opossum. Benevento [1] has shown a similar pattern of termination of lateral geniculate axons in the visual cortex of the same species.

On the other hand, terminal degeneration is found in all cortical layers of the mouse visual cortex after lesions of the lateral geniculate nucleus [46]. It predominates in the fourth layer but is also quite dense in the third.

The situation is more complex in the cat. Three independent groups of investigators [14, 15, 52] have described many separate cortical areas of projection of the lateral geniculate nucleus, the most important of which are areas 17 and 18.

A study of patterns of degeneration in the cat visual areas after many types of lesions is presently underway, using a variety of modifications of the Nauta technique and electron microscopy as the main tools of observation.

The part of this work dealing with the axonal projections of dorsal lateral geniculate nucleus neurons [34] has shown that the pattern of degenerating fibers in the cortex is not identical in areas 17 and 18 after lesions of the nucleus. In area 17 (Fig. D2-1A), the greatest density of fibers is concentrated in layers IVa and IVb. The main density begins a short distance above the giant pyramidal cells of layer Vb and stops just below the border cells of O'Leary. Some degenerating fibers ramify at the lowermost portion of layer III. Layers II and III are otherwise free of degenerating material except for a few, widely separated, single vertical fibers ascending to layer I where they spread out tangential to the pial surface (Fig. D2-1B).

Degenerating fibers are also seen in layers V and VI. They might conceivably be interpreted only as fibers of passage. However, their appearance is very suggestive of preterminal degeneration. Moreover, their density is somewhat greater in layer VI than in layer V. It must therefore be concluded that some axons or their collaterals terminate at least in this deepest layer. Endings in layer V would probably be fewer in number.

The presence of preterminal degeneration in the subgennarian layers is in perfect accord with Ramón y Cajal [28] and O'Leary [25]. Both have described collaterals of incoming lateral geniculate nucleus axons in layers V and VI.

In area 18, the degenerating debris is more specifically concentrated in layer IV and the lowermost portion of III. It is also more homogeneously coarse than in area 17 where a mixture of fine and coarse silver granules can be seen. This is an interesting parallel to the observations of Garey and Powell [14] that area 17 would receive axons from small and large cells of the lateral geniculate nucleus while area 18 receives only large cell axons. Fibers ascending vertically through layers II and III to reach layer I are extremely rare. Density of degeneration is minimal in layers V and VI and is the same for both layers. The degenerating fiber pattern is most reasonably interpreted as representing mainly fibers of passage.

Current electron microscope studies of degenerating terminals in area 17 after similar lesions [9] have confirmed the light microscope description of the terminal distribution of specific afferents. They have also yielded three important complementary observations.

The first is that even in layer IV, where the greatest density of degenerating terminals is found, over 90 percent of the synaptic terminals are normal after the geniculate lesion. This is not as surprising as it might appear. Several authors [5, 25, 27] have mentioned nongeniculate elements in the stria of Gennari. Indeed, Clark [5] has shown that the stria is not only present in undercut monkey visual cortex after long survival periods, but is not even noticeably altered.

The second main observation is that opaque [6] degenerating terminals in layer IV are not restricted to a specific cell type. Some are found establishing axosomatic contacts (Fig. D2-2A) on stellate cells. Others are related to *synapse-studded* dendrites (Fig. D2-2B), interpreted as stellate cell dendrites in a previous study [8]. Most degenerating terminals are best interpreted as ending on spines, (Fig. D2-2C, D, E, G).

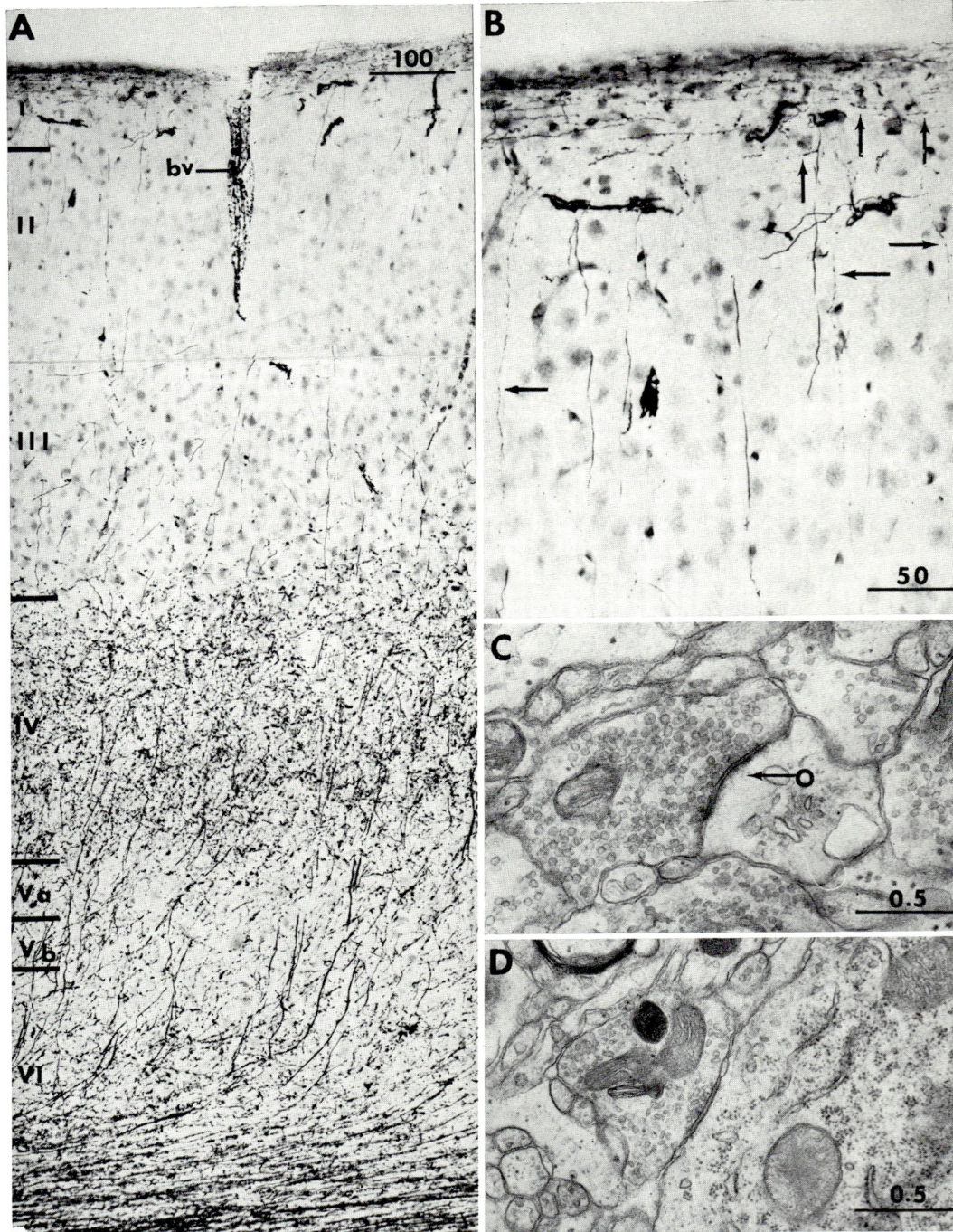

Fig. D2-1. (A) Degenerating fibers in area 17 of the cat cerebral cortex after lesion of the dorsal lateral geniculate nucleus. Upper lip of splenial sulcus; bv, blood vessel. (B) Degenerating fibers (see arrows) in cortical area 17 of the cat after lesion of the dorsal lateral geniculate nucleus, layers I and II. (C) Asymmetrical synapse with spheroidal vesicles from the normal cat area 17; O, postsynaptic opacity. (D) Symmetrical synapse with flattened vesicles from the normal cat area 17. (Digits appearing above calibration lines should all be read in microns.)

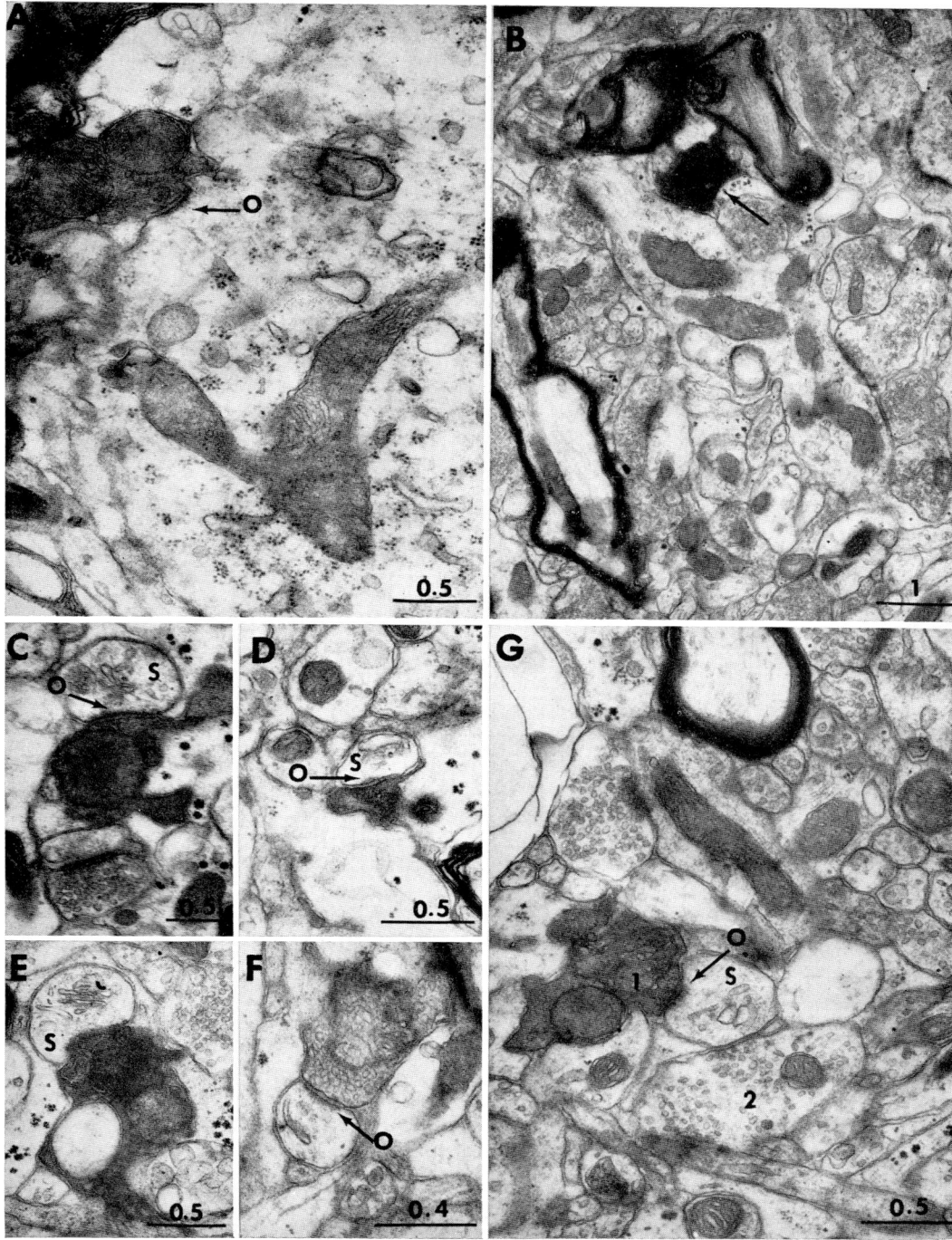

Fig. D2-2. Degenerating synapses in layer IV of cat area 17 after lesion of the lateral geniculate nucleus. (A) Degenerating axosomatic contact; O, postsynaptic opacity. (B) Degenerating axodendritic contact (see arrow). (C), (D), (E) Degenerating synapses contacting dendritic spines; S, spine; O, postsynaptic opacity. (F) Degenerating synapse with distorted vesicles; O, postsynaptic opacity. (G) At 1 is shown degenerating synapse on spine, S, associated with a postsynaptic opacity, O. At 2 is shown normal symmetrical contact with flattened vesicles on the same spine. (Digits appearing above calibration lines should all be read in microns.)

Still others are found on small neural profiles difficult to identify.

Electron microscopy thus confirms the dual termination of specific afferents presented by Szentágothai [44]. The presence of degenerating terminals on spines is in agreement with observations of Globus and Scheibel [18] and Valverde [46] on the disappearance of spines from portions of apical dendrites passing through the fourth layer after lesions of the lateral geniculate nucleus in the rabbit, and after enucleation in the mouse. Thus, corticopetal axons from the lateral geniculate nucleus have direct access to class I or pyramidal type cells whose axons characteristically leave the cortex to enter the white matter.

The finding of degenerating terminals on stellate cell bodies and dendrites supports the classic concept that specific thalamic afferents end on these cells which predominate in the fourth layer, cells which, as a class, possess Golgi type II axons. (In the cat visual cortex, as stated above, there are giant stellate cells in layer IVa whose axons would also proceed toward and into the white matter.)

The third point is related to the types of synapses which degenerate after the lesion. Two main types of synapses have been described in the normal visual cortex of the cat in material that has been formalin fixed and stained with lead citrate [8, 49]. The first is the so-called asymmetrical type with spheroidal vesicles characterized by presence of the spheroidal type of vesicle population [2, 45, 47] in the presynaptic profile, associated with a dense, compact opacity in the cytoplasm immediately underlying the postsynaptic membrane (Fig. D2-1C). The presynaptic profile of the second type contains the flattened type of vesicle population [2, 45, 47] and is not associated with a specialized postsynaptic opacity (Fig. D2-1D). It has been referred to as a symmetrical synapse with flattened vesicles.

The asymmetrical synapse with spheroidal vesicles has been found mainly on pyramidal cell spines. Each spine seems to receive only one such contact. This contact has also been seen on the dendritic trunks bearing the spines and on stellate cell bodies and dendrites. As emphasized by Szentágothai [44], these contacts have never been seen on pyramidal cell bodies. The symmetrical synapse with flattened vesicles is present on pyramidal and stellate cell bodies and dendritic trunks. They are extremely rare on dendritic spines and in these cases are typically coupled to a synapse of the other type.

All the evidence so far suggests that the degenerating terminals in layer IV after lesions of the lateral geniculate nucleus are mainly of the asymmetrical type with spheroidal vesicles. However, this is very difficult to assess. The criteria for identifying degenerating terminals include changes in the morphology of vesicles [6]. Synaptic membrane differentiation, that is, the presence or absence of a postsynaptic opacity must then serve as the main criterion for differentiating between the two main types of synapses described in the normal cerebral cortex. This criterion is useful except that there is no proof that postsynaptic differentiation is not altered during degeneration. Moreover, it might be difficult to distinguish a symmetrical contact from simple contiguity in degenerating material. Nevertheless, the site of termination of the degenerating terminals under discussion correlates well with that of asymmetrical contacts with spheroidal vesicles as described in normal material. A definite postsynaptic opacity is commonly seen (Fig. D2-2A, C, D, F, G). Some terminals whose cytoplasm is probably dense enough to be considered in the initial stages of degeneration have been seen possessing somewhat distorted vesicles most readily interpreted as of the spheroidal type (Fig. D2-2F).

The conclusion that many specific afferents form asymmetrical contacts (analogous to Gray's type I [20]) is an interesting parallel to Szentágothai's observation [43] that Gray's type II axosomatic contacts are the least affected by undercutting the cortex.

At this point it may be interesting to recall the hypothesis that asymmetrical contacts with spheroidal vesicles would be excitatory and symmetrical synapses with flattened vesicles, inhibitory in nature [45]. The electron microscope observations interpreted in the light of this hypothesis are in agreement with physiological observations that monosynaptic geniculate nucleus input to the cortex would be mainly excitatory [48]. They do not exclude the possibility of direct inhibitory projections in the form of symmetrical contacts with flattened vesicles, especially in laminae other than IV, which have not been extensively studied.

It has been suggested that the coupling of synapses of opposite types on spines represents an elegant substratum for remote inhibition [36]. After lesions of the lateral geniculate nucleus, a few degenerating endings, related to a dense postsynaptic opacity, have been seen on spines also related to a still-normal symmetrical synapse with flattened vesicles (Fig. D2-2G). This would suggest the possibility of remote inhibition in the immediate vicinity of specific afferent fiber-terminals.

It must be stressed that these electron microscope observations apply only to layer IV in area 17. Too few terminals have so far been seen in other layers to conclude anything more than their presence. Area 18 has not yet been studied under the electron microscope. Light microscopy suggests that differences are probable, since the morphology of degenerating debris is somewhat different from that seen in the same layer of area 17.

It is important to note that not all of the degenerating terminals necessarily belong to axons of cells in the lateral geniculate nucleus. Some could be the termination of fibers of passage through the nucleus. Moreover, since the lesions were rather large and sometimes encroached upon surrounding white matter, some degenerating terminals may be those of fibers passing in the white matter immediately around the nucleus.

The central theme of this presentation on heterogeneity in the cerebral cortex is perhaps best illustrated by the sites of termination of callosal fibers. Their distribution varies considerably in different cytoarchitectonic areas. The work of Ebner and Myers [12] has demonstrated, for example, that very few callosal fibers project to area 17 and to the somatic sensory arm and distal hindlimb areas. Area 18 and the proximal leg and face areas, on the other hand, receive massive contributions. Rossignol [33] has been able to confirm that, in the cat, area 17 receives virtually no fibers from the contralateral occipital region while area 18 receives callosal fibers throughout its extent, but unevenly distributed in different cortical layers depending on the region of 18 considered. After removal of the contralateral areas 17, 18, and 19, two massive vertical bands of degenerating fibers can be seen at the junction of areas 17 and 18 and at the junction of areas 18 and 19. The preterminal degeneration at these sites extends from layer VI through to layer I. In the central portion of area 18, degeneration is mainly concentrated in the inferior layers. These observations were made on preparations stained by the classic Nauta-Gygax [24] technique only. However, even in an undercut gyrus lateralis, stained by the Fink and Heimer [13] technique, area 18 shows a remarkable sparsity of degenerating material in layers II and III of the central portion of area 18 [33].

This distribution corresponds extremely well with the myeloarchitecture of these areas as recently described by Sanidez and Hoffman [35]. Their PaV area (18) is limited on each side by two dense vertical bands of myelinated fibers extending through all layers. Inferior layers of the center portion are also more densely myelinated than those of his Kv (17) area.

According to Sanidez and Hoffman [35], the inner stria of Baillarger is much denser in area 18 than in area 17. This increase in density begins a bit medial to the limits of area 18, a few millimeters within area 17. A fortunate perpendicular slit lesion through the layers of area 17, approximately two millimeters from the 17–18 border, has made it possible to demonstrate one of the components of this stria. On the medial side of the slit, away from area 18, there was remarkable absence of degenerating debris as described by Szentágothai [41, 42] with this type of lesion. On the lateral side, however, a definite streaming of degenerating axons, tangential to the pial surface, could be seen in the fifth layer. They extended for at least two millimeters to reach area 18. It was impossible to visualize the further course of these tangential axons for, at this point, they were joined by U fibers (from the lesioned area) ascending from the white matter into area 18. Another tangential stream could be seen at the bottom of layer III, but the fibers were fewer and the bundle less convincing. A few axons in layer I extended much further lateral to the lesion to reach the bottom of the posterolateral sulcus.

Differences in the manner of termination of callosal fibers has recently been emphasized in the rat by Heimer, Ebner, and Nauta [21] using the new modification of the Nauta technique [13]. Again in this species and with this technique, they found that area 17 receives very few callosal fibers. Degenerating material can be found mainly in layers I, II, and III in some regions. They are more evenly distributed throughout the layers in others. From their observations, the authors conclude that "callosal fibers distribute in regionally variable laminar patterns."

The finding of specific thalamic and callosal fibers up to layer I in no way contradicts Szentágothai's [41, 42] demonstration that most fibers in layer I are of intracortical origin in the areas studied. Undercutting of areas 17 and 18 reveals only widely scattered tangential fibers in layer I [33] thereby confirming that the great majority of layer I fibers are of intracortical origin. Indeed the density of degeneration through all the layers after undercutting of the gyrus is never much greater than in layer IV after a geniculate lesion, suggesting that most terminals in all layers of the cortex are of intracortical origin!

The organization of neural processes in the form of synaptic cartridges surrounding the apical dendrites of pyramidal cells is one which has completely escaped us in our own electron microscope observations of the cerebral cortex. However, quantitative data have been obtained [10] on synaptic patterns of pyramidal cells of the second and third layers of the cat visual cortex area 17 which are a useful complement to the concepts presented by Szentágothai.

These quantitative data were compiled from large montages of sections through thirty pyramidal cell somas including the initial portion of their apical dendrites. Measurements were also made on eighty spine-bearing dendrites found in layers I, II, and III.

The study confirms that all axosomatic contacts on pyramidal cells of these layers are of the symmetrical type with flattened vesicles [8]. They occupy only 10 percent of the membrane surface. From the data, it was possible to estimate that the number of axosomatic contacts on an "average" pyramidal cell is of the order of fifty to one hundred.

All the contacts found on the initial spine-free portion of the apical dendrites as well as on the parent stem of the basal dendrites were of the same variety. They occupy only 5 percent of the dendritic surface.

Some of the contacts on the dendritic trunks of the eighty spine-bearing dendrites were also of the symmetrical type with flattened vesicles. Others were of the asymmetrical type with spheroidal vesicles. This has already been noted in a previous study [8]. The quantitative data show that the symmetrical synapses with flattened vesicles outnumber the others by a ratio of approximately four to one. The two types together occupy only 2 percent of the dendritic trunk surface.

Contacts on the spines were nearly all (92 percent) of the asymmetrical type with spheroidal vesicles. Only 3 percent were of the symmetrical type with flattened vesicles; and 5 percent could not be characterized.

An important corollary to the described synaptic distribution on pyramidal cells of the second and third layers of the cat area 17 is the theoretical importance one should ascribe to spines. It has been suggested that the function of spines is to increase the surface area available for synaptic contacts [26]. That this is not the case is suggested by the fact that only 2 percent of the spine-bearing dendritic trunk membrane is occupied by contacts. It rather implies that the spines (and perhaps the spine apparatus) have some very special function. Chang [4] has suggested that the fine stem of the spine may be a site of "high ohmic resistance."

Consider momentarily the hypothesis that asymmetrical contacts with spheroidal vesicles are excitatory and that symmetrical contacts with flattened vesicles are inhibitory in nature. The number of spines found on pyramidal cells are of the order of several hundred to a few thousand per dendritic tree. Most of these receive only one contact, usually of the *excitatory* type. Some have two contacts, and they are then of opposite types. The pyramidal cell bodies receive only 50 to 100 contacts. They are of the *inhibitory* type.

Excitatory impulses thus arrive mainly on the dendritic spines of pyramidal cells. If Chang's hypothesis is correct, each excitatory synapse is relatively inefficient, and the neuron then responds only to multiple sets of impulses probably arriving in various specific patterns.

The inhibitory synapses are more strategically placed around the cell body, to prevent cell firing. Other inhibitory synapses on the origin of dendritic trunks could selectively "shut off" separate dendrites. A few on dendritic spines could inhibit individual excitatory impulses. They are the best candidates for "remote inhibition." One of the excitatory axonal components so linked to inhibitory synapses on spines are some of the geniculate projections to layer IV of area 17.

The class II or stellate type cells receive a quite different synaptic array [8]. In the context of the same functional hypothesis, they receive excitatory and inhibitory synapses on both cell body and dendritic trunk. They possess virtually no spines. Some of these cell bodies and dendrites are more densely covered with contacts than are those of pyramidal cells. They might be considered as "lock-on" cells responding readily to a more limited number of afferents.

Thus, even if more specific afferent fibers contact dendritic spines of pyramidal cells than stellate cell bodies and dendritic trunks, the latter might still be more readily fired by the afferents. Because of the spines, pyramidal cells would not respond to the same volley unless other afferents were having some subliminal, concomitant action on other synaptic sites.

Whatever is thought of these specious speculations, it remains clear that spines must exist for a specific reason other than for the purpose of increasing membrane surface area.

Westrum, White, and Ward [50] have shown that there is disappearance of spines from pyramidal cells in epileptic foci adjacent to injections of alumina cream. Significance of this loss with respect to the epileptic phenomenon is difficult to estimate since the injection per se would certainly result in Wallerian degeneration in surrounding cortical tissue. The literature now abounds with evidence [16, 17, 18, 22, 23, 46, 51] that spines disappear after section and degeneration of their afferents. This phenomenon may not be universal, however, since Westrum has electron microscopic evidence that spines remain intact in the pyriform cortex after removal of the olfactory bulb [36].

The Scheibels [36], however, have recently reported that spines are diminished on pyramidal cells in cases of human epilepsy. This is a strong argument in favor of Westrum's [50] concept linking the spine loss to epileptic foci. But here again it may only reflect a partial deafferentation or the lack of certain specific circuits normally ending on these spines, the spine loss being a secondary, telltale, accessory phenomenon.

Relative absence of spines in human or experimental epilepsy would be much more significant if it could be shown that spines were primarily affected by the pathology without direct and previous involvement of their synaptic terminals. Spines could conceivably not grow or be resorbed in human epilepsy or after experimental manipulation, pulling their intact synaptic knobs closer to the dendritic trunk. In the context of the Chang hypothesis on spine function, this transformation of axospine into axotrunk contacts would increase the efficiency of synaptic volleys to fire pyramidal cells and might lead to anarchic patterns of firing. This morphological hypothesis can be verified by determining in electron microscopy if the spine loss in epileptic foci is accompanied by an increase of direct axotrunk contacts.

The complete story of epileptic morphology is surely extremely complex, but probably no more so than the complete elucidation of the normal cytoarchitecture of the cerebral cortex. In his last major publication, Ramón y Cajal [29] warns the neurologist that "clarification of the manner of connection between the innumerable centrifugal and centripetal, terminal and collateral branches emanating from the thalamic, callosal, and association fibers constitutes at present an overwhelming problem. In it many generations of future neurologists will put their sagacity and their patience to the test." Considering all the evidence pointing to the heterogeneity of the cerebral cortex, the problem is compounded in that the "clarification of the manner of connection" will to a great extent require separate studies for each cortical region of a great many species.

ACKNOWLEDGMENTS

We wish to thank Professor J.-P. Cordeau and Professor H. Jasper for their constant encouragement and advice, Mr. K. C. Watkins for his excellent technical assistance, and Mr. M. Smith for his valuable photographic help.

REFERENCES

1. Benevento, L. A. Organization of visual cortex in the opossum. *Anat. Rec.* 160: 313, 1968.
2. Bodian, D. Electron-microscopy: Two major synaptic types on spinal motor-neurons. *Science* 151:1093, 1966.
3. Brodmann, K. *Vergleichende Lokalisationslehre des Grosshirnrinde in ihren Prinzipien dargestellt auf Grund des Zellenbaues.* Leipzig: J. A. Barth, 1909.
4. Chang, H. T. Cortical neurons with particular references to the apical dendrites. *Sympos. Quant. Biol.* 17:189, 1952.
5. Clark, W. E. LeGros, and Sunderland, S. Structural changes in isolated visual cortex. *J. Anat.* 73:563, 1939.
6. Colonnier, M. Experimental degeneration in the cerebral cortex. *J. Anat.* 98:47, 1964.
7. Colonnier, M. The tangential organization of the visual cortex. *J. Anat.* 98:327, 1964.
8. Colonnier, M. Synaptic patterns on different cell types in the different laminae of the cat visual cortex. An electron microscope study. *Brain Res.* 9:268, 1968.
9. Colonnier, M., and Rossignol, S. An electron microscope study of degenerating terminals in the cat cortex after lesions of the lateral geniculate nucleus. In progress.
10. Colonnier, M., and Watkins, K. A quantitative study on the synaptology of cortical pyramidal cells of the second and third layers of cat area 17. In preparation.
11. Ebner, F. F. Medial geniculate nucleus projections to telencephalon in the opossum. *Anat. Rec.* 157:238, 1967.
12. Ebner, F. F., and Myers, R. E. Distribution of corpus callosum and anterior commissure in cat and raccoon. *J. Comp. Neurol.* 124:353, 1965.
13. Fink, R. P., and Heimer, L. Two methods for selective silver impregnation of degenerating axons and their synaptic endings in the central nervous system. *Brain Res.* 4:369, 1967.
14. Garey, L. J., and Powell, T. P. S. The projection of the lateral geniculate nucleus upon the cortex in the cat. *Proc. Roy. Soc.* [Biol.] 169:107, 1967.
15. Glickstein, M., King, R. A., Miller, J., and Berkley, M. Cortical projections from the dorsal lateral geniculate nucleus of cats. *J. Comp. Neurol.* 130:55, 1967.
16. Globus, A., and Scheibel, A. B. Loss of dendritic spines as an index of presynaptic terminal patterns. *Nature* (London) 212:463, 1966.
17. Globus, A., and Scheibel, A. B. Sites of specific sensory and commissural synaptic arrays on cortical pyramids. *Physiologist* 9:3, 1966.
18. Globus, A., and Scheibel, A. B. Synaptic loci on visual cortical neurons of the rabbit: The specific afferent radiation. *Exp. Neurol.* 18:116, 1967.
19. Globus, A., and Scheibel, A. B. Pattern and field in cortical structure: The rabbit. *J. Comp. Neurol.* 131:155, 1967.
20. Gray, E. G. Axo-somatic and axo-dendritic synapses in the cerebral cortex: An electron microscope study. *J. Anat.* 93: 420, 1959.
21. Heimer, L., Ebner, F. F., and Nauta, W. J. H. A note on the termination of

commissural fibers in the neocortex. *Brain Res.* 5:171, 1967.
22. Jones, H., and Thomas, D. B. Changes in the dendritic organization of neurons in the cerebral cortex following deafferentation. *J. Anat.* 96:375, 1962.
23. Mathieu, A. M., and Colonnier, M. Electron microscopic observations in the molecular layer of the cat cerebellar cortex after section of the parallel fibers. *Anat. Rec.* 160:391, 1968.
24. Nauta, W. J. H., and Gypax, P. A. Silver impregnation of degenerating axons in the central nervous system: A modified technique. *Stain Technol.* 29:91, 1954.
25. O'Leary, J. L. Structure of the area striata of the cat. *J. Comp. Neurol.* 75:131, 1941.
26. Ramón y Cajal, S. Le bleu de méthylène dans les centres nerveux. *Rev. Trimest. Microgr.* 1:21, 1896.
27. Ramón y Cajal, S. *Histologie du système nerveux de l'homme et des vertèbres,* vol. 2. Madrid: Consejo Superior de Investigaciones Científicas, Instituto Ramón y Cajal, 1952.
28. Ramón y Cajal, S. Textura de la corteza visual de gato. *Trab. Lab. Invest. Biol. Univ. Madrid.* 19:113, 1923.
29. Ramón y Cajal, S. *Neuron Theory or Reticular Theory.* Madrid: Consejo Superior de Investigaciones Científicas, Instituto Ramón y Cajal, 1954.
30. Ramon-Moliner, E. The histology of the postcruciate gyrus in the cat, I. *J. Comp. Neurol.* 117:43, 1961.
31. Ramon-Moliner, E. The histology of the postcruciate gyrus in the cat, II: A statistical analysis of the dendritic distribution. *J. Comp. Neurol.* 117:63, 1961.
32. Ramon-Moliner, E. The histology of the postcruciate gyrus in the cat, III: Further observations. *J. Comp. Neurol.* 117:229, 1961.
33. Rossignol, S. Unpublished data, 1968.
34. Rossignol, S., and Colonnier, M. A light microscope study of degenerating patterns in the cat cortex after lesions of the lateral geniculate nucleus. In preparation.
35. Sanidez, F., and Hoffman, J. Cyto- and myeloarchitecture of the visual cortex of the cat and of the surrounding integration cortices. *J. Hirnforsch.* In press.
36. Scheibel, M. E., and Scheibel, A. B. On the nature of dendritic spines—Report on a workshop. *Communications in Behavioral Biology,* Part A, 1:231, 1968.
37. Sholl, D. A. Dendritic organization in the neurons of the visual and motor cortices of the cat. *J. Anat.* 87:387, 1953.
38. Sholl, D. A. The organization of the visual cortex in the cat. *J. Anat.* 89:33, 1955.
39. Sholl, D. A. *The Organization of the Cerebral Cortex.* London: Methuen, 1956.
40. Solnitky, O., and Harman, P. J. The regio occipitalis of the lorisiform lemuroid *Galago dimidovii. J. Comp. Neurol.* 84:339, 1946.
41. Szentágothai, J. On the synaptology of the cerebral cortex. In Sarkissov, S. A. (Ed.), *Structure and Function of the Nervous System.* Moscow: State Publishing House for Medical Literature, 1962.
42. Szentágothai, J. Short connexions of the cerebral cortex. In Szentágothai, J. (Ed.), *Symposia Hungarica.* Budapest: Akadémiai Kiado, 1965.
43. Szentágothai, J. The synapses of short local-neurons in the cerebral cortex. *Sympos. Biol. Hung.* 5:251, 1965.
44. Szentágothai, J. Architecture of the Cerebral Cortex. In Jasper, H. H., Ward, A. A., Jr., and Pope, A. (Eds.), *Basic Mechanisms of the Epilepsies.* Boston: Little, Brown, 1969.
45. Uchizono, K. Characteristics of excitatory and inhibitory synapses in the central nervous system of the cat. *Nature* (London) 207:642, 1965.
46. Valverde, F. Structural changes in the area striata of the mouse after enucleation. *Exp. Brain Res.* 5:274, 1968.
47. Walberg, F. Elongated vesicles in terminal boutons of the central nervous system, a result of aldehyde fixation. *Acta Anat.* (Basel) 65:224, 1967.
48. Watanabe, S., Konishi, M., and Creutzfeldt, O. D. Postsynaptic potentials in the cat's visual cortex following electrical stimulation of afferent pathways. *Exp. Brain Res.* 1:272, 1966.
49. Westrum, L. E. On the origin of synaptic vesicles in cerebral cortex. *J. Physiol.* (London) 174:4P, 1965.
50. Westrum, L. E., White, L. E., Jr., and Ward, A. A., Jr. Morphology of the experimental epileptic focus. *J. Neurosurg.* 21:1033, 1964.

51. White, L. E., Jr., and Westrum, L. E. Dendritic spine changes in prepyriform cortex following olfactory bulb lesions in the rat. *Anat. Rec.* 148:410, 1964.

52. Wilson, M. E., and Cragg, B. G. Projections from the lateral geniculate nucleus in the cat and monkey. *J. Anat.* 101:677, 1967.

3
Biophysics of Nerve Membrane[*]

J. WALTER WOODBURY

ROLE OF EXCITABLE MEMBRANES IN EPILEPSY

Nerve-impulse generation and conduction and synaptic transmission processes are the mode of operation of the nervous system at the information-handling level. Hence, alteration in the properties of excitable or synaptic membranes or both are the most probable causes of the epileptic discharge. At this level, the epileptic discharge can result from either or both of two mechanisms. (a) Damaged neurons are changed into pacemakers (inherently rhythmic), generating impulses at abnormally high frequencies or in abnormal places or both. Normal variations in internal environment might then produce conditions conducive to spread of this abnormal activity. (b) Damage to, or alterations in, nerve cells and their processes, particularly synaptic terminals, might lead to the formation of abnormal circuits with maintained circulation of impulses. In either case, the excitable membrane has a central role in epilepsy, and any study of the basic mechanisms must take account of the properties of excitable membranes. Obviously, there are manifold supportive mechanisms (for example, active ion transport) which maintain the conditions requisite for excitable behavior.

This chapter is aimed at describing those properties of excitable cells and their membranes having relevance to the initiation, generation, and aftereffects of the epileptic process. There are three broad categories: (a) the prerequisites for excitability: adequate Na^+ and K^+ concentration gradients across the membrane and a sufficiently high resting potential; (b) the membrane properties responsible for excitable behavior; and (c) variations in the membrane and the solutions bathing it which may lead to spontaneous firing.

The first two major sections of this chapter, *Prerequisites for Excitability,* and *Excitability,* are based on and adapted from two of my chapters, "The Cell Membrane: Ionic and Potential Gradients and Active Transport," and "Action Potential: Properties of Excitable Membranes," in *Physiology and Biophysics,* T. C. Ruch and H. D. Patton, editors [64]. Additionally, short sections from a chapter "Bioelectrochemistry" by Woodbury and co-workers [65] are quoted with minor alterations.

THE NERVE IMPULSE: PHENOMENA OF EXCITATION AND CONDUCTION

Information in the nervous system is transmitted from one place to another by means of nerve impulses. The information content depends directly on the number of impulses per second on any fiber and on the number of active fibers concerned. The strength of a sensory stimulus (light, sound, touch) is signaled to the brain by the combined number of impulses per second on all of the nerve fibers made active by the stimulus.

A nerve impulse is a stereotyped, phasic wave of changes in transmembrane potential and associated ion fluxes, heat production, and other quantities. The use of the word "wave" is exact for an impulse propagates at constant speed

---

[*] In large part based on and adapted from Woodbury [64] and Woodbury et al. [65].

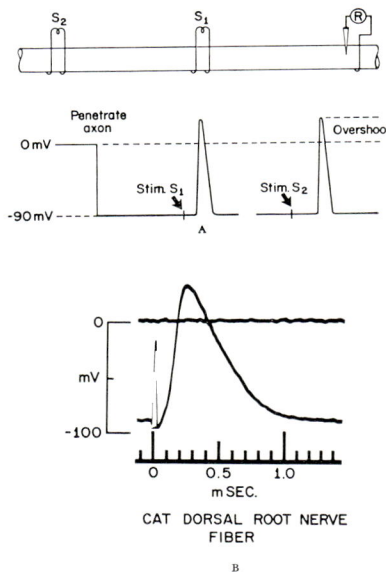

Fig. 3-1. (A) Upper: Method for studying electrical activity of nerve fibers. Nerve trunk containing hundreds of individual nerve fibers is dissected from frog or cat; such trunk is 10–20 cm long. Two pairs of chlorided Ag-stimulating electrodes, S_1 and S_2, are applied to nerve trunk at different distances from recording microelectrode (far right); microelectrode is inserted into one fiber in trunk. Lower: sketch of sequence of potential changes recorded by microelectrode when inserted into a single fiber and when nerve trunk is stimulated by sufficiently strong, short (100 μsec) shocks applied first at S_1 and then at S_2. ABSCISSA: time (a few milliseconds); ORDINATE, transmembrane potential (about 100 millivolts). When microelectrode is inserted into nerve fiber (penetrating axon), potential, recorded as a function of time, changes abruptly from 0 to about −70 to −90 mV. Following stimulation at S_1 (indicated in recording by stimulus "escape" or "artifact"), an action potential, AP, is recorded after short but definite time delay. AP rises rapidly to a peak (depolarization) and then recovers somewhat more slowly to the initial, steady value (repolarization). At peak of AP, transmembrane potential has reversed in sign. After a pause of about a second, indicated by break in line, nerve is stimulated at S_2. An identical AP is recorded but time delay following stimulus is longer. (B) Tracing of action potential recorded from cat dorsal-root fiber. Conduction distance about 1 cm. Photograph is double exposure, consisting of one sweep when microelectrode was in fiber and one sweep immediately after

and shape along the fiber. Since transmembrane potential changes are the most easily measured, the nature of the impulse has been elucidated primarily from electrical measurements; ion tracer and other measurements have also contributed.

The sequence of transmembrane potential changes accompanying a nerve impulse is called an *action potential,* AP. Figure 3-1A is a diagrammatic representation of how an AP can be initiated and recorded; Fig. 3-1B shows the action potential of a mammalian myelinated nerve fiber. Several unique properties of the action potential are shown in Fig. 3-1: (a) The duration of the AP is about 0.7 milliseconds (values range from 0.5 to a few milliseconds and are highly temperature dependent). (b) The total potential change is about 120 millivolts, 30 mV greater than the steady or *resting* potential of −70 to −90 mV. (c) When the stimulus is applied at S_2 rather than S_1, the sequence of events is exactly the same, except that the *latency,* the time between the delivery of the stimulus and the beginning of the AP, is longer. Further investigation shows that the latency is directly proportional to the conduction distance. Hence the action potential is a brief (0.5–1.0 msec) phasic change in membrane potential of fixed shape and amplitude traveling along the nerve fiber at constant speed, i.e., a wave. The conduction speed of large (20 μ diameter) mammalian myelinated nerve fibers is 120 meters per second and that of a squid giant axon (500 μ diameter) is 20 m/sec. The faster speed of the mammalian nerve fiber is due to the myelin sheath and to higher temperature.

Another property of the AP not shown in Fig. 3-1 is *threshold*. If a stimulus is *suprathreshold*, a full size action potential is initiated at the stimulating site (negative terminal of stimulating electrode pair) and propagates along the fiber in both directions. If the stimulus is *subthreshold*, an AP is not initiated and the voltage changes occurring at the stimulus site die out in a few millimeters. This is called *threshold-all-or-nothing* behavior; a sufficient stimulus elicits a full response, an insufficient one, no regenerative response. Threshold and all-or-nothing behavior are two aspects of the same underlying process. A simple example of such a process is a brick standing on end; following a small displacement of the top of the brick, in a horizontal direction, the brick will return to its

electrode was withdrawn from fiber and stimulus turned off, taken as zero potential. (From Ruch, T. C., and Patton, H. D. (Eds.), [64].)

original position. A suprathreshold stimulus tips the brick over.

RÉSUMÉ OF ACTION POTENTIAL GENERATION AND PROPAGATION. The action potential is an explosive or regenerative process. When the membrane is depolarized to threshold, an inward (depolarizing) current through the membrane increases regeneratively, and the depolarization proceeds to a limiting value. An analogous situation is the burning of a line of gunpowder. A match brought near the line at one point sets it on fire at that point (heat liberated is greater than heat losses to surroundings); in turn, the liberated heat sets adjacent regions on fire, and so the flame travels rapidly in both directions.

Upstroke of the AP (Depolarization). In nerve, a reduction in the size of the resting potential (inside made less negative) causes an increase in the membrane's permeability to Na+ ions, which in turn results in an increased inflow of Na+ ions down their electrochemical gradient (from outside to inside). This permeability increase is an intrinsic property of the membrane, which confers excitability. In turn the increased entry of Na+ neutralizes some of the negative charges on the inside of the membrane and thus further reduces the size of the potential. If the Na+ entry is large enough, the process is regenerative and continues until a maximum Na+ permeability is reached and the transmembrane potential, ε_m, approaches the Na+ equilibrium potential, ε_{Na}. This process, termed the Hodgkin cycle, can be diagrammed as shown in Fig. 3-2 [24]. This process accounts

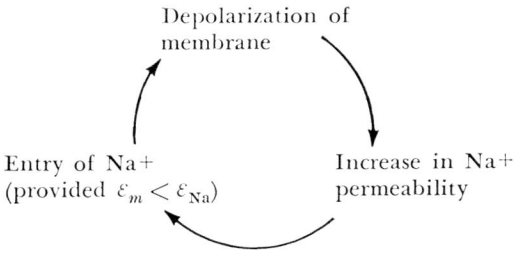

FIG. 3-2. THE HODGKIN CYCLE

for the reversal of membrane polarity during the action potential; ε_m approaches ε_{Na} as P_{Na} becomes much larger than P_K.

Transmembrane potential, ε_m, is defined as the potential of the inside solution, ε_i, minus the potential of the outside solution, ε_o:

$$\varepsilon_m = \varepsilon_i - \varepsilon_o$$

Depolarization is a reduction of the amount of charge separated by the membrane (the inside becoming less negative), and *hyperpolarization* is an increase in internal negativity. A depolarization large enough to reverse membrane charge polarity is still called depolarization.

Repolarization. If the Hodgkin cycle mechanism were a maintained process, ε_m would remain near ε_{Na} until the entering Na+ came into a new steady state with the active Na+ extrusion process. However, the increased P_{Na} induced by depolarization is transient; even if depolarization is maintained by external current flow, the inward Na+ current decays to near zero in a few milliseconds, and the membrane polarizes concomitantly. If this were the only mechanism operating to produce repolarization, it would occur at a rate determined approximately by the time constant (resistance times capacity) of the resting membrane; this would take several milliseconds in nerve (and as much as 200 msec in skeletal muscle). However, repolarization is speeded by a depolarization-induced, but delayed, increase in P_K. Thus the depolarization caused by the Hodgkin cycle mechanism automatically initiates the development of an increasing outward K+ current which restores ε_m to its resting value. Following rapid repolarization and because of the persistence of the increased P_K, the membrane hyperpolarizes for a few milliseconds, and then, as P_K decays, ε_m approaches the resting potential, ε_r. The ability of the membrane to increase its P_{Na} in response to depolarization (via the Hodgkin cycle) recovers after a few milliseconds in the repolarized state and another action potential can then be initiated.

Propagation. The AP propagates along a fiber at constant speed because a current flows through the cell plasm from an active (high P_{Na}), depolarized region (positive inside) to an adjacent, inactive (low P_{Na}), polarized region (negative inside), out through the membrane and back through the interstitial fluid (cf. Fig. 3-3E). The outward current through resting membrane depolarizes it, and, when threshold is reached, the previously inactive membrane becomes active. This process is repeated successively and continuously at each point in unmyelinated nerve fibers and at nodes of Ranvier in myelinated fibers. Hence, the action potential is propagated by means of this *local circuit* current. The local circuits in nerve serve the same function as heat conduction and radiation do in a gunpowder train; both set the adjacent regions on "fire." However, nerve recovers back to the original state so that another impulse can be generated shortly after the end of the previous one [65].

These mechanisms will be reconsidered in greater detail subsequently, after a description of the prerequisites for excitability.

Most of the concepts presented were developed during the past 20 years, largely through the efforts of A. L. Hodgkin, A. F. Huxley, and their co-workers [3, 4, 24, 25, 26, 28, 29, 30, 31, 32, 33, 34, 35, 36] and K. S. Cole and collaborators (cf. [14]). There are numerous other books and reviews [13, 40, 55, 59, 62, 64, 65] and symposia [1, 2, 10] on various aspects of this subject.

PREREQUISITES FOR EXCITABILITY

The maintenance of an adequate resting potential is essential to excitable behavior. Depolarization leads to a transient increase in Na permeability; hence a sufficient, maintained decrease in the size of the resting potential inactivates the Hodgkin cycle. The inward flow of Na^+ during the upstroke of the AP and the outflow of K^+ during repolarization require that the concentration ratios $[Na^+]_o/[Na^+]_i$ and $[K^+]_i/[K^+]_o$ be much greater than one. The subscripts i and o refer to internal and external solutions respectively. The most immediate prerequisites for excitability are thus a sufficiently large resting potential difference and Na^+ and K^+ concentration differences across the excitable membrane. In turn the maintenance of these conditions requires (a) an active transport process that extrudes Na^+ and takes up K^+, and (b) a membrane with a much greater permeability to K^+ than to Na^+ in the resting state. The rest of this section is devoted to an exposition of these requirements.

ELECTRIC POTENTIALS AND ION CONCENTRATION IN CELLS. Any animal tissue such as muscle or brain is composed of closely packed cells and the solution surrounding and bathing them. The cell plasm or intracellular fluid and the interstitial fluid are similar; both consist largely of water and both fluids have about equal numbers of particles per unit volume dissolved in them. The functional boundary between the intracellular and interstitial is the membrane, a thin (75 Å), highly organized, lipoprotein layer which severely restricts the interchange of materials. The differences between the intracellular and interstitial fluids are more striking than their similarities. Two of these are: (a) The concentrations of ions are markedly different, $[Na^+]$ and $[Cl^-]$ are much higher in the interstitial fluid than in the intracellular fluid; the reverse holds for $[K^+]$ (Table 3-1). (b) There is an electric potential difference between the intracellular and interstitial fluids. In nerve cells, the intracellular fluid is about 70 mV negative to the interstitial fluid. Although the cell interior is highly organized, containing the nucleus, nucleolus, mitochondria, endoplasmic reticulum, and other organelles, it is convenient and usually meaningful to regard the cell fluid as a single, aqueous phase when discussing ion exchange across cell membranes.

Two properties of the cell membrane are largely responsible for the observed concentration and potential differences: (a) Ions tend to diffuse from regions of high to regions of low concentration, but their rate of diffusion through the membrane is a minute fraction of their rate through water. This barrier to diffusion is a result of the nonpolar, hydrophobic nature of the lipid portion of the membrane. In most cell membranes, the rate of diffusion of Na^+ is much slower than is the diffusion rate of K^+ and Cl^-. (b) Energy derived from metabolism is used by cells to transport Na^+ out of the cell and K^+ into the cell. These ionic movements just balance, on the average, the passive diffusion of Na^+ into and K^+ out of the cell. This *active transport* of Na^+ and K^+ maintains the intracellular Na^+ concentration at low values and the intracellular K^+ at high values. The voltage arises because potassium permeates the membrane much more readily than does sodium.

DETERMINANTS OF ION MOVEMENTS THROUGH MEMBRANES—Passive Forces. If

TABLE 3-1. Typical Concentrations of Major Ions in Mammalian Interstitial Fluid and Muscle* Intracellular Fluid, T = 37°C. After Woodbury [64].

Ion	$[S]_o$ Concentration interstitial fluid, o (μmoles/cm³)	$[S]_i$ Concentration intracellular fluid, i (μmoles/cm³ cell water)	$\dfrac{[S]_o}{[S]_i}$	$\varepsilon_S = \dfrac{61}{z} \log \dfrac{[S]_o}{[S]_i}$ mV
Na+	145	12	12.1	66
K+	4	150	1/36.6	−96
Cl−	116	3.9**	30	−90
HCO−$_3$	29	12	2.4	−23
A−***		146/1.25		
Resting potential, ε_r	0	−90 mV		

* Values for nerve cells are much the same.
** Calculated as $[Cl^-]_i = (116)(10^{-90/61})$. Direct measurements are inaccurate.
*** A− is used to denote the organic anions which balance excess of inorganic cations in intracellular fluid. A− are organic phosphates, amino acids, and derivatives. Average valence of about −1.25 is necessary to give osmotic equality with interstitial fluid and electroneutrality of intracellular fluid.

the concentration of a substance, S, in a solution is higher in one region than in an adjacent one, there will be a net diffusion of the substance from the region of higher to the region of lower concentration. Thus, from Table 3-1 and Fig. 3-3A, it can be seen that Na+ and Cl− tend to diffuse into cells, and K+ tends to diffuse out of cells. The rates of diffusion of these substances through the membrane depend not only on the concentration difference but also on the ease with which they penetrate the membrane. The cell membrane so severely limits the rate at which substances diffuse through it that the rate of movement is determined solely by the membrane. That is, diffusion of ions through water is so much faster than through the membrane that the ion concentrations near the membrane differ by negligible amounts from those in the surrounding bulk medium.

If the substance is ionized, the transmembrane potential also affects the rate of diffusion of the substance through the membrane. This effect is exerted because a transmembrane potential difference means that electric charges are separated by the cell membrane. This follows from the definition of electric potential difference between two points as the work done against electrical forces in carrying a unit positive charge from one point to the other. No electrical work is done in carrying a charge through the membrane unless charges are separated by the membrane. These separated charges (inside negative) exert a force on any ions in the membrane as diagrammed in Fig. 3-3B. This force tends to drive cations into the cell and anions out of the cell; any cations which enter the membrane are attracted by the negative charges on the inside and are repelled by the plus charges on the outside of the membrane.

K+ tends to diffuse out of the cell because of its high internal concentration, but it tends to diffuse into the cell because of the electric charges separated by the membrane. These two tendencies nearly, but not quite, cancel each other, so that there is a slight tendency for K+ to diffuse out of the cell. A similar argument holds for Cl−, but in this instance the tendency for Cl− to diffuse into the cell because of its high external concentration is exactly balanced by the tendency of the electric forces to keep the negatively charged Cl− from entering the cell. Since there is no net tendency for Cl− to diffuse through the membrane, the inside and outside concentrations of Cl− are in *electrochemical* equilibrium.

Active Transport. The situation is different for Na+: both the concentration and potential differences act to drive Na+ into

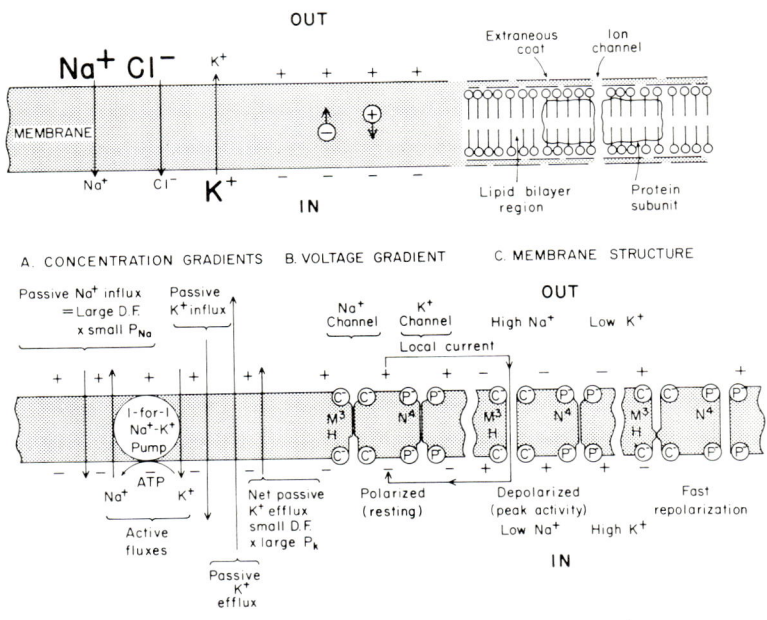

Fig. 3-3. Factors determining ion fluxes through membranes. (A) and (B) passive forces; (C) membrane structure (D) active ion transport; (E) voltage control of cation permeability.

(A) Concentration gradients. Size of ion symbol indicates magnitude of that ion's concentration in fluids bathing membrane. Concentration differences (gradients) generate inward forces on Na^+ and Cl^- and outward on K^+. Organic internal anions are not represented.

(B) Voltage gradient. Voltage difference across membrane is indicated by $+$ and $-$ symbols, signifying electric charge separation; a cation in the membrane has an inward force exerted on it due to repulsion of $+$ charges on outside and attraction of negative charges on inside of membrane. Transmembrane voltage is electrical work to carry unit plus charge across membrane.

(C) Sketch of possible membrane structure. Membrane is represented as consisting mostly of lipid bilayer regions, left and right, interrupted at rare intervals by lipoprotein complexes (protein subunits) embedded in the basic bilayer structure. Mucoprotein extraneous coat is indicated. Ion penetration probably occurs almost entirely at the specialized, hydrophilic regions here shown as interstice between four protein subunits arranged in a square (two shown).

(D) Steady state Na^+ and K^+ ion fluxes and transmembrane potential. Lengths of arrows indicate magnitude of various influxes and effluxes. A one-for-one Na^+-for-K^+ pump actively extrudes Na^+ and takes up K^+. The active Na^+ efflux is balanced by an equal, passive influx of Na^+: Transmembrane voltage builds up until passive forces (concentration and voltage gradients) are sufficient to drive Na^+ inward at this rate despite low P_{Na}: passive Na^+ influx = large driving force (DF) times small permeability, P_{Na}. Similarly, net passive efflux of K^+ is equal to active influx of K^+ because of low driving force on K^+ (difference between outward concentration gradient force and inward voltage gradient force) and high P_K. Passive efflux of Na^+ is negligible. Net passive K^+ efflux consists of difference between a large influx and an even larger efflux. *Phrase attached to right arrow should read: Net passive K^+ efflux = small DF × large P_K.*

(E) Factors controlling ion-permeability of excitable membranes. Two types of ion channels are shown: Na^+ (early, transient current) channels and K^+ (late, maintained current) channels. Ion-selectivity mechanism of these channels is represented by different types of fixed negative charges guarding entrances to channel. C^- represents carboxyl groups, which may give selectivity characteristics of Na^+ channels; P^- represents unknown groups, which may give selectivity characteristics of K^+ channels. Left-hand diagram (separated by wavy gap from middle diagram) shows that Na^+ and K^+ channels are closed in the polarized, resting membrane. Note that lower portion (H factor) of Na^+ channel is open (activated). Middle diagram shows Na^+ channels open (M process) and K^+ channels still closed at peak of action potential when membrane polarity is

the cell. There is also a strong tendency for A^- (see Table 3-1) to diffuse out of the cell. However, the membrane is believed to be impermeable to A^-. Although the membrane is much less permeable to Na^+ than to K^+, there is still an appreciable steady leakage of Na^+ into cells. Despite this leakage, the concentration of Na^+ remains at low values in living cells. Therefore, some mechanism present in the cell must carry Na^+ out of the cell as fast as it enters, on the average. Since work must be done to carry Na^+ from a region of lower to a region of higher concentration and from a lower to a higher electric potential, it must be concluded that energy derived from cellular metabolism is used to expel Na^+ from the cell interior. This extrusion of a Na^+ is usually accompanied one-for-one by the uptake of a K^+ (cf. Fig. 3-3D), and is usually referred to as active Na^+ transport, as the Na^+-K^+ pump or, more simply, as the Na^+ pump. The word *pump* denotes that metabolic energy is required by the process. The linkage of K^+ uptake to Na^+ extrusion accounts for the slight imbalance in the distribution of K^+; the net outward diffusion of K^+ is balanced by the inward pumping of K^+.

Diffusion. The random motion of a solute molecule is such that the rate at which molecules diffuse out of a small volume is proportional to the concentration (moles per liter or better moles per cm³) of the substance in the small volume. In a solution where the concentration of a substance varies from one region to another, there will be a net movement of solute particles from regions of higher to regions of lower concentration. This net diffusion is expressed quantitatively in terms of the *flux*, M, defined as the number of moles per second passing through an area of 1 cm² oriented perpendicularly to the direction of flow. The flux is directly proportional to the change of concentration with distance, the *concentration gradient*.

In a one-dimensional case such as diffusion through a membrane, the concentration gradient is $d[S]/dx$ and the flux of S, M_S, is thus proportional to $-d[S]/dx$, where x is distance measured perpendicular to the membrane. The minus sign is used because diffusion is from high to low concentrations. For a given concentration gradient, M_S depends on the ease with which the molecules of S move through the solvent; the greater the ease of movement (the less the frictional resistance to flow), the greater the flux. The measure of the ease of motion is called the *diffusion constant*, D. Therefore, $M_S = (-D_S)d[S]/dx$ for nonionized substances or for ions in regions with no electric field.

The rate of diffusion of most substances through the membrane is so slow that a negligibly small concentration gradient in the aqueous media suffices to bring the substance up to the membrane as rapidly as it diffuses through the membrane. Thus, appreciable changes in concentration occur only in and near the membrane. Therefore, the rate of penetration of a substance depends on the properties of the membrane and on the concentration gradient of the substance in the membrane. Since the membrane is a thin, fixed structure and the concentration gradient in the solution is negligible, the average concentration gradient through the membrane is obtained by dividing the difference in concentration between the interstitial and intracellular fluids by the thickness of the membrane, δ. Thus, in the membrane, $d[S]/dx = ([S]_o - [S]_i)/\delta$. (Distance increases in the direction from inside to outside.)

Permeability. The net efflux, M_S, of a nonionized substance through the membrane is thus

---

reversed (compare with Fig. 3-6B). Right-hand diagram shows condition when membrane is about two-thirds repolarized: most Na^+ channels have closed at lower end because of inactivation process (H going to H'), while upper ends are still open. K^+ channels are now open (N process). A short time later when repolarization is completed (not shown), Na^+ channels are closed throughout entire pore. This is followed by reactivation, the opening up of lower, H, portions of Na^+ channels, which restores original conditions as shown in left-hand diagram. K^+ channels also close following repolarization, but this is delayed. Local-circuit current is shown by arrows connecting polarized region (left) with active region (center); Na^+ current (center) in active region removes charges in inactive region, thus makes it active via the Hodgkin cycle.

$$M_S = -(D_S/\delta)([S]_o - [S]_i) = P_S([S]_i - [S]_o) \tag{3-1}$$

The ratio D_S/δ is called the *permeability*, P_S, of the membrane to the substance S. P_S depends only on the properties of the membrane and of the substance S. Permeability is a measure of the ease with which a substance can penetrate the membrane. In nerve cells, the permeability of the membrane to K^+, P_K, is about 10^{-6} cm per sec, whereas P_{Na} is about 10^{-8} cm per sec. The permeability to K^+ of a layer of water of the same thickness as the membrane (75 Å) is about 10 cm per sec, or ten million times greater than the P_K of the cell membrane. This ratio indicates the extreme effectiveness of the cell membrane in limiting the flow of ions.

MEMBRANE STRUCTURE AND ION PERMEATION. As sketched in Fig. 3-3C, the cell membrane probably consists of outer and inner monomolecular layers of mucoprotein separated by a bimolecular lipid layer. In the lipid layer, the long, thin lipid molecules are closely packed with their long axes parallel and oriented perpendicular to the membrane. The nonpolar ends of the lipid molecules are opposed. The mucoprotein layers are bonded to the lipids at their polar ends. Since lipids are hydrophobic, the penetration of ions through lipid regions is probably negligible. This is supported by the finding that artificial bi-lipid layer membranes have resistances up to 10^5 times larger than those of cell membranes. This result fits in well with other evidence indicating that cell membranes have protein subunits dissolved in the bi-lipid layer, as shown in Fig. 3-3C. If the junctions between four or more of these subunits are hydrophilic or if there are hydrophilic regions in the central portion of a subunit, then conditions would be appropriate for ion penetration, and this would account for the lower resistances of cell membranes.

It is useful to suppose that ions penetrate protein regions of the membrane through small-diameter (about 7 Å), water-filled pores. Most ions have diameters less than this and hence could diffuse through these pores rapidly (hydrated Na^+, about 5 Å; K^+, about 4 Å). The small size of ionic fluxes is attributed mainly to the comparatively small number of pores per unit area of membrane and secondarily to the restrictive effects of small-size pores on ion passage. The temperature coefficients (Q_{10} of 1–1.5) of passive ion fluxes show that ions are only weakly bound to the membrane when they are in it; once an ion enters a pore, it traverses it rapidly, and there is generally no more than one ion in a pore at a time. (K^+ fluxes through squid axon membranes act as though there are three to four ions in each channel, *in-file* behavior [35]). On a kinetic basis, the low fluxes of ions through membranes are due to the improbability of an ion striking the membrane at one of the few regions where there are channels or pores.

ELECTRICAL PROPERTIES OF MEMBRANES. The existence of an electric potential difference across the cell membrane means that the electric charges are separated by the membrane and hence that the movements of ions through the membrane are affected. A cation traversing a pore or channel will be repelled by the positive charges on the outside surface of the membrane and attracted by the negative charges on its inside surface and vice versa for an anion as shown in Fig. 3-3B.

Certain concepts of electricity which are assumed to be part of the biomedical researcher's armamentarium are: charge; electrical potential (voltage); voltage gradient; and Ohm's law. An elementary textbook of physics or *Physiology and Biophysics* [64] should be consulted for detailed exposition. Concepts of electricity which have significant and direct implication in the neurosciences are reviewed briefly below.

Capacitors. A conductor is a substance in which charges are free to move. Electrolyte solutions are good conductors because their solute particles are charged (ionized) and can move freely in the solvent. Because charges are able to move freely in a conductor, no electric field can exist inside an insulated conductor; if the conductor contained a field, it would exert forces on the free charges, and some of them would move into positions on the surface of the conductor to such an extent that the field would be reduced to zero. Since the field must be zero in a conductor, all points in and on it must be at the same potential, for no electric work is required to move a charge through a region where the electric field is zero.

An insulator is any material in which there are no free charges, such as a vacuum. In an insulating material called a *dielectric*, all electrons are bound to their nuclei and cannot migrate under the influence of an external electric field. The charges in a dielectric are not rigidly fixed, however, so they separate slightly in an external electric field.

In a static situation, the existence of a potential difference, ε_{AB}, between two points, A and B, means that $+$ and $-$ charges have been separated. The greater the amount of charge separated, the greater the electric field and the greater is ε_{AB}. In particular, if $+$ charges are put on an insulated fixed conductor, A, and an equal number of $-$ charges are put on a second fixed conductor, B, the potential difference between the two conductors is directly proportional to the amount of charge on the conductors. Any arrangement of two conductors, A and B, separated by an insulator is called a *capacitor*. The proportionality constant relating charge to voltage is called the capacitance, C, of a capacitor and is given by the equation $C = q/\varepsilon_{AB}$, where q is the total amount of charge on a conductor.

The capacitance of a capacitor depends on the geometry of the conductors (that is, on their spatial extent and separation) and on the dielectric constant of the insulating material (a measure of the extent that the molecules are distorted by an applied electric field). The less the work per unit charge required to place a fixed amount of charge on a capacitor, the higher its capacitance. Hence, the closer two conductors are together, the higher the capacitance between them, for less work is required to move a unit charge through the shorter distance. In addition, the higher the dielectric constant of the insulating material, the larger the capacitance. It follows that the capacitance is high between two closely spaced, parallel conducting sheets or plates separated by an insulator. The opposite charges on the plates of a capacitor attract each other, so they must be on the facing surfaces of the conductors. The charges are prevented from recombining by the insulator separating the conductors. However, if the insulation is not perfect—if some charge can move through the insulator—charges placed on one conductor will leak through the insulator at a rate proportional to the amount of charge still on the conductors.

The unit of capacitance is the farad, F. A capacitor has a capacitance of 1 F if 1 coulomb of charge taken from one plate and placed on the other produces a potential difference of 1 volt, V, between the plates. In terms of physical size, a 1-F capacitor is large; the capacitors commonly encountered have capacitances of about 1 microfarad (1 μF = 10^{-6} F).

Cell Membrane Capacitance and Charge. A nerve cell and its surrounding fluids form a capacitor: two conductors, the interstitial and intracellular fluids, are separated by an insulator, the cell membrane. Since ions can penetrate the membrane to a limited extent, the cell is not a perfect capacitor. Membrane capacitance is high because the membrane is extremely thin. It is convenient to express membrane capacitances in terms of capacitance per unit area (C_m, μF per cm^2), because the capacitance of a capacitor is proportional to its surface area and cells vary considerably in surface area. Nearly all cell membranes studied have capacitances of about 1 μF per cm^2 (cf. [14]).

The amount of charge, q, *separated* by 1 cm^2 area of nerve cell membrane, is the product of the steady potential difference, ε_r, across the cell membrane and the capacity (C_m) $q = C_m\varepsilon_r$. For a nerve cell, $\varepsilon_r = -70$ mV, so $q = 7 \times 10^{-7}$ coulombs per cm^2. This can be converted to moles of monovalent ion (equivalents) per cm^2 by dividing q by the farad, 96,500 coulombs per equivalent. The result is that there are only 7.5×10^{-12} M of ions separated by 1 cm^2 of cell membrane. By comparison, 1 cm^3 of interstitial or intracellular fluid contains 155×10^{-6} M of cations. This shows that the separation of chemically small amounts of charge generate rather substantial voltage differences even when the distance of charge separation is small. Despite the extremely small changes in ion concentration required to charge the membrane capacity, it is worth emphasizing that the law of macroscopic electroneutrality does not apply to macroscopic parts of the intracellular fluid–membrane–interstitial fluid system. The whole system is electrically neutral, but the intracellular fluid contains a slight excess of anions and the interstitial fluid an equal excess of cations. These excess charges are, of course, attracted to each other and thus are near the membrane. Since like charges repel each other, the charges on each surface are uniformly distributed.

Electric Current. As mentioned above, when charges are brought near a conductor (that is, an electric field is applied), charges flow in a manner which neutralizes the applied field. Unless energy is supplied to keep $+$ and $-$ charges separated, the field in the conductor rapidly decreases to zero. In order to keep charges separated, positive charges must be taken continuously from the negative region and supplied to the positive region by an appropriate energy source, such as a battery or generator. Work must be done on + charges to move them from the negatively to the positively charged region. If this is done, charges move continuously: a current flows in a conductor under the influence of a maintained electric field.

The size of a current is defined as the amount of charge (coulombs) passing per unit time (1 sec) through a cross section of the conductor perpendicular to the direction of flow of charge or, more simply, as the time-rate of flow of charge, $I = dq/dt$. Direction of flow is defined as that of positive charges. The unit of current is the ampere (1 coulomb per second). The net passage of 6.25×10^{18} unitary charges (electrons, sodium ions) per second is an ampere. For convenience, charge flow through membranes is expressed as current per unit area (current density, amperes per cm^2), rather than as current. Current density is directly proportional to ionic flux, M; flux is moles per cm^2-sec; current density is coulombs per cm^2-sec. The relationship is thus $I = FzM$, where F is the farad, I is membrane current density, and z is the ion's valence.

ELECTRODIFFUSION. Ionic Equilibrium. Both concentration and voltage gradients exert forces on ions in solution; hence it is expected that ion concentration gradients can generate voltage gradients and vice versa. The simplest physical example of such action is two solutions of differing ionic concentrations separated by a membrane permeable to only one ion. Suppose that the two solutions are interstitial and intracellular fluids and that these are separated by a membrane permeable only to K+. The situation can be visualized with the aid of Fig. 3-3A and B, where the concentration of each ionic species in the interstitial and intracellular fluid is shown qualitatively by the size of its symbol.

Even if it is supposed that there is no potential difference (no charges separated) across the membrane at some instant, a voltage will be generated immediately thereafter by the diffusion of K+ outward down their concentration gradient. As each K+ diffuses out of the cell, it cannot be accompanied by a corresponding movement of A− (not shown in Fig. 3-3A), nor can an equal number of Na+ move inward in exchange for outflowing K+ because the membrane is permeable only to K+. Thus K+ ions reach the outside of the membrane alone, and the outside acquires a net positive charge and the inside a net negative charge. Note that, despite the electrical attraction between the K+ and A−, movement of the K+ back into the cell is counteracted by the concentration gradient of K+, which exerts an outward force on them. The voltage retards outward diffusion of K+ and speeds inward diffusion because any positively charged ion in the membrane is acted upon by the membrane charges (Fig. 3-3B). This process is self-limiting, and eventually a state will be reached (equilibrium) in which the efflux (one-way outward flux) equals influx and net flux is zero. At equilibrium, the tendency for K+ to diffuse out, resulting from the high value of $[K^+]_i$, is exactly balanced by the tendency for them to diffuse inward due to the electric field in the membrane and the low $[K^+]_o$.

The equilibrium condition for the distribution of uncharged molecules across a membrane is simply that the internal and external concentrations be equal (Eq. 3-1). The equilibrium condition for ions is more complicated: both the concentrations and the voltage applied to the membrane must be known in order to calculate the potential energy difference between the inside and outside and thus the equilibrium condition. Any inside concentration of an ionic species may be brought into equilibrium with any outside concentration by applying the appropriate transmembrane voltage. *The transmembrane potential which equalizes fluxes for a particular ion is called the equilibrium potential for that ion.* Its value depends on the ratio of the internal and external concentration of the ion.

Electrochemical Potential. Relationship between the external and internal concentrations of an ion and the transmembrane potential at equilibrium is obtained by setting to zero the expression for the total transmembrane potential energy difference for that ion. This total potential energy difference per mole of ion is called the *electrochemical potential difference*, $\Delta\mu$, and is the sum of the electrical and concentration energy differences across the membrane for that ion.

The *electric potential energy difference* of 1 mole of K+ is the work that must be done solely against electric forces to carry 1 mole of K+ across the membrane, from outside to inside, with the transmembrane potential held at its original value. This work (W_e) is simply the product of ε_m, the transmembrane voltage (joules per coulomb), F, the farad (number of coulombs of charge per mole and z_K, the valence of the K+ ion: $W_e = z_K F \varepsilon_m$. The *concentration potential energy difference*, W_C, is the work required to carry 1 mole of K+ from outside to inside solely against the concentration gradient, with the external and internal K+ concentrations held at their original values. W_C is not as easily calculable, but it can be shown that W_C is proportional to the difference between the logarithms of the internal and external concentrations rather than directly proportional to their difference:

$$W_C = RT(\log_e [K+]_i - \log_e [K+]_o)$$

where R is the universal gas constant and T is the absolute temperature. (Strictly speaking, activities rather than concentrations should be used. However, the activities appear only as ratios, and these ratios are close to the equivalent concentration ratios in value. Thus, the error is not large and does not affect the conclusions reached here.) Thus the electrochemical potential difference for K+ is

$$\Delta \mu_K = W_e + W_C = z_K F \varepsilon_m + RT \log_e \frac{[K+]_i}{[K+]_o}$$

(3-2)

If ε_m, $[K+]_o$, and $[K+]_i$ are such that $\Delta\mu_K = 0$, then K+ are equilibrated across the membrane. If $\Delta\mu_K$ is not zero, it is a measure of the net tendency of K+ to diffuse through the membrane. The larger $\Delta\mu_K$, the greater the net efflux of K+.

Nernst Equation. The condition for K+ equilibrium is obtained by setting $\Delta\mu_K = 0$ (Eq. 3-2). Replacing ε_m by ε_K and solving for ε_K gives the Nernst equation for K+:

$$\varepsilon_K = (RT/Fz_K) \log_e [K+]_o/[K+]_i$$

(3-3a)

The term ε_K indicates that this equation determines the value that ε_m must have if K+ are to be in equilibrium, and ε_K is called the *potassium equilibrium potential*. By substituting the values $R = 8.31$ joules per mole-degree abs, $T = 310$ degrees abs (37°C), $F = 96,500$ coulombs per mole, and $z_K = +1$. Converting to logarithms to the base 10 and expressing ε_K in millivolts (mV) a useful form of the Nernst equation is obtained:

$$\varepsilon_K = 61 \log_{10} [K+]_o/[K+]_i \quad (mV)$$

(3-3b)

Note that if $\varepsilon_K = 0$, the equilibrium condition for ions reduces to that for neutral substances, that is, $[K+]_o = [K+]_i$. The Nernst equation can be written for every ion present in the system.

An ion whose equilibrium potential is equal to the resting membrane potential (equilibrated) is said to be distributed *passively*. This means that there is no net active transport of the ion. The Nernst equation makes it possible to determine which ions in a cell's environment are distributed passively. The requisite numbers for mammalian skeletal muscle are given in Table 3-1.

Potassium Ions. From Table 3-1, $[K+]_o = 4$ and $[K+]_i = 150$ μmoles per cm³; Therefore

$$\varepsilon_K = 61 \log_{10} (4/150) = -96 \text{ mV}$$

This value is close to but significantly different from the measured resting potential of -90 mV.

Chloride Ions. The extracellular concentration of chloride is high, and its intracellular concentration is low. Because of the negative valence of Cl−, the electric and concentration forces affecting Cl− act in opposite directions. It is difficult to estimate $[Cl-]_i$ from analyses of the chloride content of tissues, but indirect evidence is good that chloride is equilibrated in frog skeletal muscle [27]. Although Keynes [41] has shown that the giant axon of the squid actively accumulates Cl−, distribution of Cl− is probably passive in vertebrate neurons. The value of $[Cl^-]_i = 3.9$ μmoles per cm³ in Table 3-1 was calculated on this assumption, that is,

$$\varepsilon_{Cl} = \varepsilon_r = -90 \text{ mV}$$

Sodium Ions. Sodium is distributed far out of equilibrium; both the concentration and voltage gradients act to drive Na+ into the cell. Since $\varepsilon_{Na} = +66$ mV, it would be necessary for ε_m to be +66 mV (inside positive) in order to counteract the inward concentration force on Na+, whereas ε_r is actually −90 mV.

Membrane Ionic Flux, Current, and Conductance. If Eq. 3-3a for ε_K is substituted in Eq. 3-2 for electrochemical potential difference, the result is

$$\Delta\mu_K = z_K F\left(\varepsilon_m - \frac{RT}{z_K F}\log_e \frac{[K^+]_o}{[K^+]_i}\right) = z_K F(\varepsilon_m - \varepsilon_K) \quad (3\text{-}4)$$

where ε_K is the K+ equilibrium potential. Thus in a cell where the equilibrium potential of K+ is not zero, the voltage used in Ohm's law should be $(\varepsilon_m - \varepsilon_K)$, rather than ε_m, and similarly for other ions. A convenient form of Ohm's law in dealing with fluxes is thus

$$I_K = M_K z_K F = g_K(\varepsilon_m - \varepsilon_K) \quad (3\text{-}5)$$

where I_K is the current density of K+ (amps per cm²) and the proportionality factor, g_K, is called the specific membrane conductance to potassium or simply potassium conductance (units: mhos per cm²).

Equation 3-5 expresses the rate of movement of an ion species through the membrane in terms of its ease of penetration and the difference between the actual membrane potential and the equilibrium potential for that ion. Ion current is zero when $\varepsilon_m = \varepsilon_K$, which is, of course, the equilibrium condition. Similarly, the greater the difference between the two potentials, the greater the ion movement through the membrane.

Membrane Ionic Conductance. Membrane ionic conductance is a measure of the ease with which an ion penetrates the membrane, that is, the measurement is made when the ions are driven by an electrical force. On the other hand, permeability is a measure of the ease with which a substance penetrates the membrane when driven by a concentration force; ion conductance and ion permeability are closely related quantities. However, the relationship between them is not simple, depending, among other things, on the transmembrane voltage itself. Equation 3-5 is most frequently used for describing ion fluxes through membranes because conductances are usually easier to measure experimentally than permeabilities, and the relationship is easy to visualize.

ACTIVE SODIUM TRANSPORT. Na+ is distributed so far from equilibrium that it poses forcefully the question of how this disequilibrium is maintained in living cells. There are at least two possibilities: If Na+ ions are unable to penetrate the membrane, the disequilibrium would persist indefinitely. If Na+ can penetrate the membrane, other than passive factor terms must be included in calculation of the expected Na+ distribution. The first possibility is simple, therefore attractive. However, it must be rejected, since studies with radioactive Na+ have shown that these ions penetrate the membrane, although not so readily as do K+ and Cl−. Hence the second possibility must be explored.

There are three apparently contradictory facts about the behavior of Na+ in tissues which must be considered. (a) The distribution of Na+ in tissues is far from equilibrium. (b) Na+ can penetrate the cell membrane. (c) This disequilibrium is maintained by living cells; $[Na^+]_i$ remains low despite an appreciable influx of Na+. Thus for some reason, Na+ efflux must equal Na+ influx, in other words, it is necessary to postulate that some force other than voltage and concentration gradients is expelling Na+ from the cell at an average rate equal to the rate of passive entry.

Since Na+ enters spontaneously, work must be done to carry Na+ out of cells. Further, Na+ is entering constantly, so work must be continuously expended to eject the entering Na+ and maintain a low

$[Na^+]_i$. The power (time-rate of supplying energy or of doing work) to eject Na^+ continually must come ultimately from the oxidation of glucose or other metabolites by the cell. The process whereby the cell continuously uses metabolic energy to maintain an efflux of Na^+ is called *active Na^+ transport* or, colloquially, *the Na^+ pump*.

The term *active transport* implies that the transport process requires a continuous supply of energy; the diffusion of a substance down its electrochemical gradient (*passive transport*) occurs spontaneously and dissipates energy. Although the detailed mechanisms of active Na^+ transport are not known, there is considerable direct experimental evidence that such a mechanism exists in many types of cells, particularly excitable cells [10, 34, 55, 59].

Energy Requirements for Active Sodium Transport. The postulate that disequilibrium of Na^+ between cells and bathing medium is maintained through the expenditure of metabolic energy is subject to a stringent yet simple experimental test. Minimum power required to transport Na^+ out of a cell at the observed rate must be less than the rate of energy production of the cell. The rate of energy production can be calculated from the oxygen consumption of the cell. The minimum transport power is the product of the transport work per mole of Na^+, and the number of moles of Na^+ transported per second. Keynes and Maisel [43] have made the necessary measurements on frog skeletal muscle. Assuming 100 percent efficiency, they found that about 10 percent of the oxygen consumption of a noncontracting muscle must be used to pump Na^+. Pumping efficiency is likely to be about 50 percent, but only about half of the Na^+ efflux is active, the remainder being exchange diffusion [44, 59] so that about 10 percent of resting oxygen consumption goes for Na^+ transport. Hence the energy demands of the Na^+ pump are not excessive.

Active Sodium-Potassium Exchange. Although the detailed mechanism of the Na^+ pump is not yet known, the process has been studied in many tissues, and some of the broad characteristics of Na^+ pumping have been defined. These characteristics seem to be much the same in all the tissues studied. Hodgkin and Keynes [34] carefully investigated Na^+ and K^+ movements in giant axons (150 to 300 μ in diameter) of *Sepia* (cuttlefish) and *Loligo* (squid).

These findings form a compact summary of the general characteristics of the Na^+ pump. (a) Na^+ efflux is a direct function of $[Na^+]_i$. (b) Na^+ efflux is decreased to values near zero by the addition, at appropriate concentrations, of metabolic inhibitors to the bathing medium. (c) K^+ influx is greatly reduced by metabolic inhibitors. These inhibitors produce about equal decreases in K^+ influx and Na^+ efflux. (d) Na^+ influx and K^+ efflux are not greatly affected by metabolic inhibitors. (e) Na^+ efflux is greatly reduced, but not abolished, by removal of K^+ from the external bathing medium and increases when $[K^+]_o$ is increased. (f) Na^+ efflux and K^+ influx are highly temperature dependent; a reduction in temperature markedly decreases the fluxes (Q_{10} of 3 to 4). On the other hand, Na^+ influx and K^+ efflux are relatively insensitive to temperature changes (Q_{10} from 1.1 to 1.4).

These findings are strong evidence for existence of an active Na^+ transport process in cells. Further, the findings suggest that there is also active uptake of K^+ and that this uptake is coupled with Na^+ extrusion. A reduction in the amount of available energy, either by metabolic inhibitors or by temperature reduction, reduces Na^+ efflux and K^+ influx equally. A coupled Na^+-K^+ exchange mechanism is also suggested by the reduction in Na^+ efflux when all the K^+ is removed from the bathing medium and the increase in Na^+ exit when $[K^+]_o$ is increased. However, linkage between Na^+ and K^+ is not rigid.

Dependence of Na^+ extrusion on $[K^+]_o$ has been observed in a number of tissues, and the existence of such relationship is presumptive evidence of a one-for-one Na^+-K^+ exchange. It will be assumed hereafter that Na^+ pumping is coupled with an equal uptake of K^+. This assumption, although not strictly true, simplifies, without invalidating, deductions on the consequences of active Na^+-for-K^+ exchange.

Since the existence of active Na^+-K^+ transport is well established, it is reasonable to ask how the cell does use metabolic energy to extrude Na^+ and take up K^+. Caldwell [10] has carefully reviewed the applicability of a carrier hypothesis to active Na^+-K^+ transport. This model explains most experimental findings with reasonable accuracy. Mechanisms regulating the Na+ pumping rate and their role in epilepsy will be discussed below.

MAINTENANCE OF STEADY STATE CONCENTRATION AND POTENTIALS. If all the important factors affecting the movements of ions have been analyzed in the previous sections, then it should be possible to explain the observed transmembrane ion concentration and voltage differences of cells solely in terms of these factors: A one-for-one Na+-K+ exchange pump *is* sufficient to maintain voltages and concentrations at their observed steady-state values.

Maintenance of Ionic Concentrations. The term *steady state* means that ion concentrations and voltages are unvarying in time—net fluxes are zero—but that the system is not in equilibrium. Energy must be continuously expended to maintain the steady state; the influx equals the efflux, but one of the one-way fluxes consists of both active and passive components.

As shown in Fig. 3-3D, the one-way flux of an ion equals the sum of the passive and active fluxes. The influx of K+ consists of a passive component, K+ driven inward by the voltage gradient, and an active component, the inward leg of the Na+-K+ exchange pump. K+ efflux is passive and balances the sum of the passive and active influxes. If the steady-state membrane potential, ε_r, were just equal to the K+ equilibrium potential, ε_K, the passive fluxes would be equal; the active influx would thus be unbalanced, and $[K^+]_i$ would be increasing at a rate determined by the pumping rate and cell volume. Therefore, in the steady state, ε_r cannot be as large a number as ε_K. In other words, $[K^+]_i$ must be larger than predicted from the Nernst equation in order to make the passive efflux equal to the summed passive and active influxes. Table 3-1 shows that ε_K is 6 mV more negative than ε_r. The difference (driving force) need be no greater than this in the steady state because of the relatively high permeability of the membrane to K+. A small increase in $[K^+]_i$ suffices to increase K+ efflux enough to match the active influx.

Qualitatively, Na+ distribution across the membrane is a mirror image of K+ distribution (Fig. 3-3A, D). Thus, arguments concerning K+ fluxes apply equally well to Na+ fluxes simply by interchanging the words *influx* and *efflux*. However, the membrane is about 100 times more permeable to K+ than to Na+ [27, 33], and so $[K^+]_i$ needs to be only slightly higher than at equilibrium for net passive efflux to balance the active influx but, $[Na^+]_i$ must fall to levels much lower than its equilibrium value before the net inward driving force is large enough to make the passive influx equal active efflux (passive efflux is negligible). This shows that the steady-state transmembrane potential must be near ε_K because P_K is much greater than P_{Na} but does not reveal what causes charge separation across the membrane.

Steady-State Transmembrane Potential. Since the membrane is permeable to the major ionic constituents of the body fluids, the existence of a steady-state transmembrane potential must ultimately be due to active ion-transport processes; without these, internal and external concentrations would equalize, and the cell would swell and burst as $[Cl^-]_i$ increased with decreased ε_m. The pump maintains $[Na^+]_i$ and $[K^+]_i$ relatively constant so that size of the steady-state potential is determined mainly by the ratio P_{Na}/P_K. In the steady state, the net flux of each ion must be zero. For M_{Na} and M_K, active fluxes must be included. There is insufficient knowledge to specify active Na+, M^*_{Na} and K+, M^*_K fluxes as functions of ε_m and ion concentrations (cf. [8, 10, 37, 38, 42, 44]).

However, the experimentally well-founded assumption that $M^*_{Na} = -M^*_K$, that is, active efflux of Na+ is accompanied one-for-one by active uptake of K+, simplifies matters: It is easy to show [65] that ε_r is given by an equation similar to the Nernst equation:

$$\varepsilon_r = \frac{RT}{F} \log_e \frac{p[Na^+]_o + [K^+]_o}{p[Na^+]_i + [K^+]_i}$$

(3-6)

where $p = P_{Na}/P_K$. Since Cl− is not actively transported, $[Cl^-]_i/[Cl^-]_o = \exp(F\varepsilon_r/RT)$. Thus ε_r is determined by P_{Na}/P_K and by external and internal [K+] and [Na+]. The latter, in turn, are determined by the kinetics of the active transport process. Experimentally it is found that $[Na+]_i$ and $[K+]_i$ are much the same in all animal tissues regardless of ε_r and p. Hence p is the main determinant of ε_r (cf. [63]). An explicit expression can be obtained for ε_r by assuming that $M^*_{Na} = -M^*_K = \text{const } [Na+]_i^n$ [63].

The reason that ε_r depends on p can be seen qualitatively from considering the charge separation process that builds up ε_r when it is momentarily reduced to zero. In the first jiffy thereafter, about 100 times more K+ will exit from the cell than Na+ will enter because the driving forces are roughly the same size, opposite in direction, and $P_{Na} \simeq 0.01\ P_K$. The result is a net exit of positive charges which develops an ε_m closer to ε_K and further from ε_{Na}. This process continues until current is zero at ε_r. (Quoted from [65].)

EXCITABILITY

The preceding sections explained how a cell develops and maintains a steady transmembrane potential. In addition, the membranes of some cells, notably nerves, possess the highly distinctive property of being *excitable*. In excitable cells, an environmental change (a *stimulus*) brings about transient depolarization usually by increasing the permeability of the membrane to Na+ or to Na+ and K+. Influx of Na+ depolarizes the membrane, thereby in turn increasing Na+ permeability, which leads to further depolarization, and so on in a regenerative manner as already described (Hodgkin cycle). Depolarization is followed shortly by a spontaneous recovery or repolarization process which restores the original state. This sequence of changes is termed an *impulse*, and the accompanying voltage change is termed an *action potential*. The definitive property of an excitable membrane is regenerative interaction between depolarization and permeability to Na+.

Most excitable cells are long and thin, such as the axons and dendrites. In elongated cells, an impulse once initiated by a stimulus is propagated rapidly from the stimulus site to adjacent regions of the membrane and thus spreads or propagates as a wave over the membrane of the entire cell. The properties of excitability and propagation adapt nerve cells for their function, transmitting information from one part of the body to another.

The description of the unique properties of excitable cells falls into three categories: (a) response of long, thin cells to applied currents (cable properties, electrotonus); (b) intrinsic properties of excitable membranes and how these are measured; and (c) possible molecular mechanisms of excitability. The possible relationships between excitable properties and the epileptic discharge is another category for discussion.

CABLE PROPERTIES OF ELONGATED CELLS. A weak current flowing through a nerve fiber may or may not initiate an action potential; nevertheless, there are always local changes in transmembrane potential. The effects of electric currents are particularly prominent in nerve and muscle fibers because these fibers are approximately cylindrical and have lengths many thousands of times their diameters. With this geometry, the cell plasm is highly resistant to current flow, and different potentials exist at different distances from a point current source. The combination of cell-plasm resistance and membrane resistance and capacitance found in nerve fibers acts in a typical manner to attenuate in distance and slow in time the effects of a locally applied current on membrane potential. This behavior of a nerve cell is denoted by the term *cable properties*. This term is used because an undersea telephone cable may have very similar electrical characteristics. The term *electrotonus* is also used to describe this behavior.

Measurement of Cable Properties. Figure 3-4A and B shows an experimental arrangement for measuring the effects of current flow on the transmembrane potentials of a giant axon or a skeletal muscle fiber. Two microelectrodes are inserted into a cell (Fig. 3-4B); an abruptly applied current (Fig. 3-4A) is passed out through one electrode, and the other is used to record the resulting changes in the transmembrane potential ($\Delta\varepsilon_m = \varepsilon_m - \varepsilon_r$). Current flows out of the electrode into the axoplasm and then out through the membrane by the lowest resis-

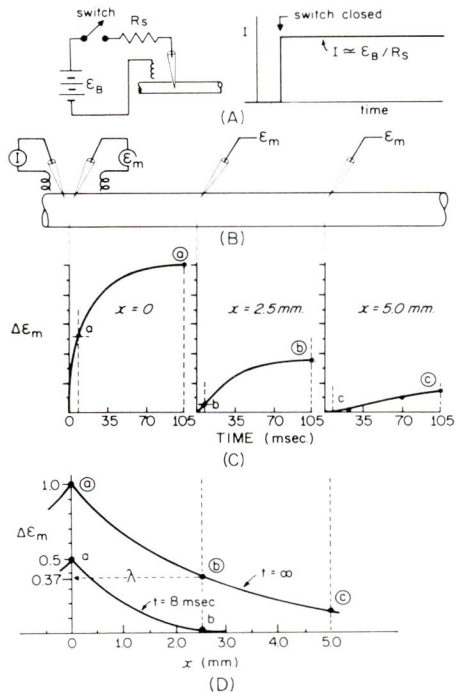

FIG. 3-4. Experimental measurement of cable properties in a skeletal muscle fiber.

(A) Left: Generation of a constant current and its application to a fiber via an intracellular electrode. A battery whose voltage, ε_B, is hundreds of times larger than transmembrane potential is connected to fiber through a resistor, R_S, whose resistance is much greater than that of the microelectrode. Current flows when switch is closed and is $I \simeq \varepsilon_B/R_S$. Right: Applied current as a function of time, zero with switch open and constant with switch closed.

(B) Constant current is suddenly applied to fiber at extreme left ($x = 0$) via intracellular electrode labeled with circled I. Changes in transmembrane potential, $\Delta\varepsilon_m$, at several points along fiber are measured with another intracellular electrode system, ε_m.

(C) Transmembrane potential changes as a function of time after switch closures are recorded at distances indicated by dashed upward extensions of ordinate lines. Note that, as distance increases, potential rises progressively more slowly and reaches lower final value. Rate of rise of $\Delta\varepsilon_m$ at any distance is determined by the membrane time constant, τ, and $\tau \equiv R_m C_m$, the product of membrane resistance and capacitance. In this case, $\tau = 35$ msec, typical for muscle. In nerve, $\tau \simeq 1$ msec; the shape of the curve is the same, the time scale is faster.

tance path available. As a function of time, $\Delta\varepsilon_m$ is recorded at one position of the recording electrode. This electrode is then removed from the cell and reinserted at another distance from the current-applying electrode (Fig. 3-4B). In this way, different measurements for $\Delta\varepsilon_m$ are recorded at several distances. The results of such an experiment, conducted on fibers of a frog sartorius muscle, are shown in Fig. 3-4C. These results are typical of those obtained for all long, thin cells—myelinated and unmyelinated nerve and skeletal, cardiac, and smooth muscle cells. However, the time scale for nerve cells is faster; 35 msec in muscle is equivalent to 1 msec in nerve. In response to an abruptly applied constant current (internal electrode positive), $\Delta\varepsilon_m$ measured at $x = 0$ increases rapidly at first and then gradually levels off to a fixed value (Fig. 3-4C). $\Delta\varepsilon_m$ rises progressively more slowly and reaches a smaller final value as the recording electrode is moved farther from the current electrode in either direction (Fig. 3-4C, $x = 2.5$, $x = 5.0$ mm).

Figure 3-4D ($t = \infty$) shows the way the final, maximum voltage change varies with distance from the current-applying electrode. The curve for $t = 8$ msec shows that the voltage changes are much more closely confined to the region of the current electrode shortly after the current is turned on than at longer times.

Cable Properties. Cable properties are inherent in the structure of long thin cells.

(a) Although the cell plasm is a relatively good conductor, the cell is so long with respect to its diameter that plasm resistance plays an

(D) Replot of data shown in (C). Voltage change is plotted as function of distance along fiber on same scale as in (B) and for two different times, $t = 8$ msec (lower curve) and t greater than 150 msec (labeled $t = \infty$, upper curve). Lettered points in (D) correspond to the same lettered points in (C). Spatial spread at early times is much less than at later times. Space constant, λ, is defined as the distance where the final value of $\Delta\varepsilon_m$ has fallen to $1/\varepsilon = 0.37$ of its initial value. The value shown, $\lambda = 2.5$ mm, is typical of nerve and muscle fibers. (From Ruch, T. C., and Patton, H. D., (Eds.), [64].)

important role in determining the pattern of current flow. (b) The cell plasm is separated from the interstitial fluid by the thin, insulating membrane, forming the membrane capacitor. (c) Ions can penetrate the membrane; hence it is an imperfect insulator and has a high electrical resistance.

The slowing of the time rate of change in transmembrane potential at a distance from the current electrode (Fig. 3-4C) is a consequence of membrane capacitance; it takes time for an applied current to change the amount of charge on the membrane. The diminution of the final $\Delta \varepsilon_m$ with distance (Fig. 3-4D) is a consequence of both protoplasmic and membrane resistance.

Precise understanding of cable properties requires an analysis of the complicated network of resistors and capacitors which is electrically equivalent to a fiber. The properties of a cable are described mathematically by the cable differential equation which specifies the variation of transmembrane voltage with distance and time [36, 58]. The cable equation is a mathematical statement of the seemingly trivial physical law that the current entering the membrane from whatever sources is equal to the current flowing through the membrane.

There are two sources that can supply current to a given patch of membrane (a patch is a length of axon much shorter than the space constant) in a nerve fiber.

(a) Current (i_a) from external sources, that is, via an intracellular electrode; (b) local current (i_L) from adjacent regions of membrane (cf. Fig. 3-3E); if two adjacent regions of membrane have different values for ε_m, then current will flow from one region to the other via the interstitial and intracellular fluids. The sum, $i_a + i_L$, is the total current entering a given patch of membrane from sources outside the patch.

Current can traverse the membrane in two ways: (a) ionic current, i_i, carried by the actual traversal of the membrane by ions; (b) membrane capacitative current, i_C. This is current that changes the amount of charge on the membrane. Charges do not traverse the membrane; for example, + charges moving to the inside of the membrane due to current from an intracellular electrode neutralize some of the − charges on the inside of the membrane. In turn, + charges on the outside of the membrane are released and carry the current in the extracellular fluid. This capacitative current is the time rate of change of membrane charge. Since $q = C_m \varepsilon_m$ and $i_C = C_m (d\varepsilon_m/dt)$, the total current through the membrane is the sum of ionic and capacitative currents: $i_i + i_C = i_i + C_m(d\varepsilon_m/dt)$.

The current flowing up to a patch of membrane is equal to the current through the patch, $i_a + i_L = i_i + i_C$. Since it is customary to express current, i, through membranes as a current density, I, in amperes per cm², dividing the currents through a patch by the area of the patch gives the result:

$$I_a + I_L = I_i + I_C = I_i + C_m(d\varepsilon_m/dt) \tag{3-7}$$

where C_m is the capacitance of 1 cm² of membrane.

Cable properties can be understood from Eq. 3-7. If a constant current is suddenly applied to an axon at $x = 0$ (Fig. 3-4), at first all the current flow is capacitative and directly through the membrane near $x = 0$. Until the charge on the membrane at that point is changed, ε_m cannot change; no current will flow laterally through the plasm or directly through the membrane until ε_m is altered. As time passes $\Delta \varepsilon_m$ changes and some of the applied current is diverted to adjacent regions of membrane, and some of the membrane current near $x = 0$ is carried by ions. As the charge and ε_m rise in immediately adjacent regions (the current spreads to still greater distances), this current is capacitative at first and later carried by ions. Finally, after a long time, the membrane reaches its final charge at each point and all the applied current is carried through the membrane by ions. There are bigger voltage changes near the current electrode because the plasm-resistance limits axial current flow and thus forces current out through the membrane. This outflow decreases exponentially with distance. The cable responses of different fibers differ only in scale. The distance scale is given by λ, the space constant defined in Fig. 3-4D, and the time scale by the time constant $\tau = R_m C_m$, where R_m (ohms per cm²) is the resistance of 1 cm² of membrane. The time constant is independent of fiber diameter but the space constant is proportional to the square root of both diameter and R_m.

INTRINSIC PROPERTIES OF EXCITABLE MEMBRANES. The cable properties of a fiber are such that a signal in the form of membrane hyperpolarization or depolarization at one point is undetectable more than a few space constants (a few millimeters) away (Fig. 3-4D). Since signals are transmitted along nerve fibers for distances of up to two meters in man, some method of boosting the signal at least every few millimeters is needed. The energy for boosting the signal comes from the sodium concentration difference across the membrane. The signal is kept to a fixed height by means of the threshold, all-or-nothing regenerative mechanism already described. The boost occurs at all points in unmyelinated nerve fibers and in muscles and at nodes of Ranvier in myelinated nerve fibers.

Propagation occurs because an "all" depolarization in one region causes current flow to adjacent resting regions, which depolarizes them, eventually to the threshold where the increasing inward Na+ current exceeds the outward K+ current. The previously resting region is now "active," and the procedure is repeated at each region of the membrane successively (cf. Fig. 3-3E).

Voltage Clamping. It is difficult to learn the detailed kinetics of an explosive process such as the action potential by studying explosions. A better way is to control a critical variable so that threshold all-or-nothing characteristics are eliminated. For example, the threshold all-or-nothing behavior of a brick can be eliminated by applying sufficient external force to the brick (by holding it) so that its position at any time is determined by the experimenter rather than by the force of gravity. The kinetics of the process which gives rise to threshold behavior can then be obtained in detail by measuring the force required to hold the brick in a particular position as a function of that position. Initially, a push is required to displace the brick from its upright position. The push required to hold the brick decreases steadily as the brick is tipped and reaches zero at the threshold, an unstable equilibrium point. Thereafter a pull rather than a push is required. This pull increases steadily and then drops to zero when the brick is flat. The threshold behavior of the unimpeded brick is reflected in the shape of the force versus brick-rotation curve, which increases from zero, reaches a maximum, decreases through zero to a negative minimum then increases abruptly to zero. This N-shaped characteristic is typical of regenerative processes.

In nerve, the equivalent of brick position is transmembrane voltage; the equivalent of applied force is applied current. Thus, it has been found that threshold behavior can be eliminated by holding or *clamping* the voltage at a fixed value. The relation between membrane voltage and membrane ionic current is measured by supplying to the nerve, from an external source, whatever current is required to maintain the membrane voltage constant—that is, connecting it to a battery—and then repeating this procedure for different values of the battery voltage. For small depolarizations, an outward current must be supplied to carry K+ outward. The required external current is zero when voltage is maintained at the threshold value and is directed inward to carry sodium ions at larger depolarizations where increased sodium permeability makes inward sodium current exceed outward potassium current. In other words, the dependence of Na+ current, and hence sodium permeability, on ε_m and on time can be measured directly using the voltage-clamp technique; obviously, holding ε_m constant prevents regenerative interactions between ε_m and P_{Na}.

The sources and paths of membrane current given in Eq. 3-7 show what experimental procedures must be used to voltage clamp.

The objectives of voltage clamping are to (a) eliminate regenerative behavior by controlling ε_m and (b) make direct measurements of membrane ionic current. Holding ε_m constant makes capacitance current, $I_C = 0$ because $d\varepsilon_m/dt = 0$; hence Eq. 3-7 becomes $I_a + I_L = I_i$. If the voltage is held constant at only one point of a fiber, there will be substantial current flow from adjacent regions when the clamped region is held at a different voltage. Hence it is necessary to measure or control I_L, preferably by making $I_L = 0$. This can be done in squid giant axons by inserting a wire along the axis of the fiber. The low resistance wire connects all portions of the fiber together so that ε_m must be everywhere the same (Fig. 3-5A). If ε_m is uniform spatially, I_L is zero because a potential difference is necessary to cause a current flow from one region of the fiber to another. Thus a squid axon equipped with an axial wire and an appropriate external electrode can be voltage clamped, in principle, by connecting internal and external leads to a battery. In this case Eq. 3-7 reduces to $I_a = I_i$ because I_L and I_C are zero.

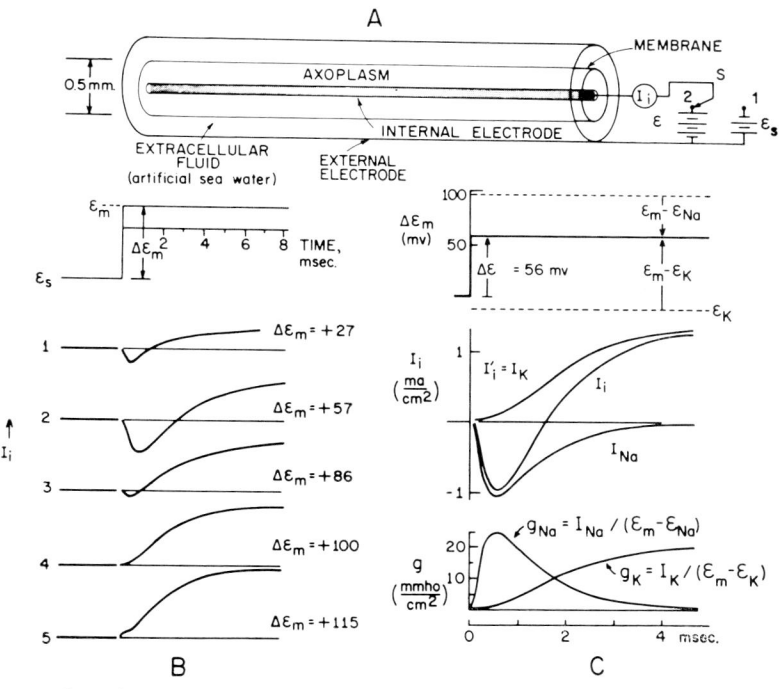

FIG. 3-5. Voltage clamping in the squid giant axon.

(A) Transmembrane voltage, ε_m, is held constant over length of the axon by connecting internal and external media to battery through long electrodes. It is possible to change ε_m suddenly from ε_s (where $\varepsilon_s = \varepsilon_r$ and where ionic current, $I_i = 0$) to any other value by flipping switch, S, from position 1 to position 2. Total current, I_i, through membrane is measured as function of time by an ammeter (cathode ray oscilloscope).

(B) Transmembrane current flow as function of time after sudden change in ε_m. Uppermost curve is ε_m as function of time. Curves 1 to 5 show membrane current which flows after membrane is depolarized, by amounts (in millivolts) shown at right ($\Delta\varepsilon_m = \varepsilon_m - \varepsilon_s$). In curve 4, depolarization was to ε_{Na} and, in curve 5, ε_m was greater than ε_{Na}. Thus, for all but largest depolarizations, early component of current flows in direction opposite to that expected from change in ε_m and late current flows in the same direction. Time scale at top applies to all records in (B).

(C) Components of total membrane current and conductance. Top curve: ε_m as function of time; ε_{Na} and ε_K are indicated by dashed lines. Middle curve: total membrane ionic current, I_i, for $\Delta\varepsilon_m = 56$ mV broken up into its two components, I_{Na} and I_K. (Other ion currents are small and neglected here.) Separation was made (in principle) by reducing $[Na^+]_o$ to a value at which a depolarization of 56 mV equaled ε_{Na}. Since $I_{Na} = 0$ under these conditions, total ion current, I'_i is equal to I_K as labeled. Bottom curve: g_{Na} and g_K as functions of time for step change in ε_m shown in top curve. Conductances are same shape as current curves because they are calculated, as shown, by dividing ion current by effective driving voltage on ion (indicated in top curves). Time scale at bottom applies to all records in (C). Part (B) after Hodgkin and Huxley [31]; part (C) after Hodgkin [25]. (From Ruch, T. C., and Patton, H. D. (Eds.), [64].)

This method has proved a powerful means of studying the properties of membranes. Voltage clamping was developed by Cole [14] and initially exploited by Hodgkin and Huxley [28, 29, 30, 31, 32], who measured and analyzed the ionic currents under voltage clamp and successfully predicted all the excitable properties of the unclamped axon. Other techniques for voltage clamping fibers of smaller diameter have been developed [14].

The principle of the voltage clamp is illustrated in Fig. 3-5A. Spatial variations in voltage are eliminated by the long internal electrode; connecting the internal and external electrodes to a battery holds the voltage constant in time. The experimental maneuver is to hold ε_m constant at some value (usually the resting potential) and then to switch to another value. Throwing the switch from 1 to 2 in Fig. 3-5A causes a large short surge of capacitative current followed by the membrane ionic current (Fig. 3-5B).

When the potential of the battery is set equal to ε_r, no current will flow through the membrane (switch in position 1 of Fig. 3-5A; ε_r is labeled ε_s) because ε_r is the voltage at which the net flow of charge is zero. When the switch is flipped to position 2, current will flow from the battery and bring ε_m to the new voltage, ε. This is true only if the resistance between the long internal and external electrodes is mostly in the membrane, that is, if resistance of axoplasm and external bathing fluid and resistance between electrodes and solution are negligible compared to the membrane resistance. In practice, resistance between the internal electrode and axoplasm is large, and rather elaborate measures are necessary to circumvent this and other difficulties [14, 32].

When the switch is thrown to position 2, the membrane potential is abruptly changed to a new value. In order to change ε_m, it is necessary to change the charge on the membrane capacity. This process, however, is brief because the low radial resistance of the axoplasm allows a high current flow from the battery to the membrane capacitance. Membrane conductance does not change immediately after a sudden change in ε_m; therefore, there is an immediate membrane current proportional to $\Delta\varepsilon_m$; that is, K+ flows outward and Cl− inward. This change is reflected in a sudden small initial jump in outward current (visible in I'_i curve middle record, Fig. 3-5C). Shortly after sudden depolarization and consequent outward current, the total membrane ionic current, I_i, begins to decrease, passes through zero, reaches a negative peak in about 1 msec, then slowly changes back to a large, maintained, positive value (Fig. 3-5B, curves 1, 2, 3). Contributions of Na+ and K+ to the total current at various times can be deduced by varying the amount of depolarization and the external Na+ concentration.

Sodium Ion Current. The curves of membrane current versus time for different depolarizations differ in detail, but the sequence of events in each curve is nearly the same until $\Delta\varepsilon_m$ exceeds about 100 mV (curves 4 and 5, Fig. 3-5B). The early inward current disappears at a particular $\Delta\varepsilon_m$ (about 95 mV), and an early outward current hump appears at larger depolarizations (curve 5). From measurements of [Na+]$_i$ and [Na+]$_o$, the value for ε_{Na} can be calculated. Such analysis demonstrates that the early current hump changes sign when

$$\varepsilon_m = \varepsilon_{Na} \quad \text{or} \quad \Delta\varepsilon_m = \varepsilon_{Na} - \varepsilon_r$$

This finding, together with the finding that changes in the early current-reversal voltage vary exactly with changes in ε_{Na} (varied by replacing some of the Na+ in the artificial seawater bathing solution by choline+ ions), leads to the conclusion that early membrane current is carried by Na+. *The crucial evidence is that this current reverses sign at exactly the ε_m at which the driving force on* Na+ *changes sign* [28].

Potassium Ion Current. The late, maintained outward current is carried largely by K+ [28]. Direct evidence for this conclusion has been obtained only recently because [K+]$_i$ could not be changed conveniently and rapidly until the recent development of a technique for internal perfusion of squid axons. The plasm of squid giant axons can be either squeezed or washed out and replaced by artificial solutions [3, 52]. Resting and action potentials are close to normal when the inside of the axon is perfused with high [K+] solutions and the outside bathed in seawater [56]. Hence, the repolarizing current is due mainly to an outward movement of cations or an inward movement of anions. The latter can be ruled out since the size and shape of the AP is not greatly affected by the complete replacement of external chloride by other anions. Perfused axons can also be voltage clamped [11, 12, 46, 49].

Hodgkin and Huxley [28, 29, 31] devised methods for separating the total ionic current into Na+, K+, and leak, l, (mostly Cl−) components. Hence

$$I_i = I_{Na} + I_K + I_l \quad (3\text{-}8)$$

Sodium and Potassium Ion Conductances. The total ionic current can be separated into Na+ and K+ currents by analyzing the manner in which changes in [Na+]$_o$ affect the shapes of curves relating current to time. Hodgkin and Huxley [28] found that changes in [Na+]$_o$ change I_{Na} but not I_K. Thus, the change in I_i due to a change in [Na+]$_o$ is carried by Na+. Figure 3-5C shows the partition of I_i into Na+ and K+ currents for a depolarization of 56 mV. The value of I_{Na} rises rapidly along an S-curve, reaches a peak in about 0.5 msec, then declines to near zero in another 2 msec. The value of I_K also rises along an S-curve, but much more slowly, and then levels off at a high-maintained value in about 4 msec. If Na+ and K+ components are correctly identified, the membrane conductance, g_{Na}, of Na+, and the membrane conductance, g_K, of K+ as functions of time can be determined by dividing the ionic current by the driving force on that ion. Solving Eq. 3-5 for g_K gives

$$g_K = I_K/(\varepsilon_m - \varepsilon_K)$$

similarly,

$$g_{Na} = I_{Na}/(\varepsilon_m - \varepsilon_{Na})$$

In voltage clamp, ε_m is held constant, so g_{Na} and g_K have the same shape as I_{Na} and I_K, respectively (Fig. 3-5C). The total ionic current (Eq. 3-8) can thus be written as

$$I_i = g_{Na}(\varepsilon_m - \varepsilon_{Na}) + g_K(\varepsilon_m - \varepsilon_K) + g_l(\varepsilon_m - \varepsilon_l) \quad (3\text{-}9)$$

where g_l is the conductance of the leakage channel and ε_l its equilibrium voltage. The leak conductance is a constant, but g_{Na} and g_K are functions of both voltage and time.

Voltage Dependence of g_{Na} and g_K. The dependence of g_{Na} (equivalent to P_{Na}) on voltage can be measured quantitatively from voltage-clamp experiments by making a series of measurements of g_{Na} as a function of time for different clamping voltages and plotting the peak g_{Na} against the voltage [29, 30, 31]. The curve is S-shaped. Small depolarizations (0–10 mV from ε_r) have little effect on g_{Na}, moderate depolarizations (10–70 mV) cause large increases in g_{Na}, and larger depolarizations have little further effect. The final value of g_K depends on ε_m in much the manner that peak g_{Na} does.

Activation and Inactivation of g_{Na}. A suddenly applied, fixed depolarization produces a large increase in Na+ conductance. However, despite continuance of the depolarization, conductance falls rapidly (Fig. 3-5C). This drop is called *inactivation* of Na+ conductance. The properties of this inactivation process can be determined by experiments using two-step changes in voltage or two short, depolarizing pulses spaced at different intervals [30]. Such experiments show that inactivation begins as soon as the membrane is depolarized; the greater the depolarization, the faster the rate of inactivation.

Fast depolarization of the membrane has two effects which relate to Na+ conductance: g_{Na} increases rapidly, and the *rate* at which inactivation of g_{Na} proceeds increases immediately. Repolarization of the membrane has the reverse effects; any g_{Na} not already inactivated will be turned off rapidly. Simultaneously the rate of inactivation decreases and the rate in reverse increases. There is an important difference between the decrease in Na+ conductance due to inactivation and that due to polarization of the membrane. Time is required to reactivate inactivated g_{Na}, whereas a decrease in g_{Na} brought about by polarization is immediately available; that is, a depolarization shortly following a repolarization will cause an increase in g_{Na}. Inactivation is the main cause of the refractory period (see below).

Model of Na+ Conductance Inactivation. The activation-inactivation process is the most difficult, also the most crucial, concept in understanding action potential generation and the refractory period. This process is also one of the major factors which can cause rhythmic discharge of impulses under appropriate circumstances. Hodgkin and Huxley [31] developed a hypothetical model accurately describing variations of g_{Na} with time and voltage in terms of two separate but interacting rate processes. They supposed that a membrane channel or pathway through which Na+ can pass relatively easily is formed when three M molecules and one H molecule are situated at specific sites in the membrane. Sodium conductance is assumed to be proportional to the number of these channels per cm^2 of membrane. The steady-state probability that an M or H molecule is at the proper site for channel formation depends *only* on the transmembrane voltage. Such variation in probability can be explained by supposing that M and H molecules are charged or dipolar, so that the molecules' position or orientation is affected by membrane voltage.

At the resting potential, the kinetics of the M substances are such that most of these molecules are not at the proper site for channel formation (that is, block the channel). If M designates molecules at effective sites and M' those at blocking sites, then the reaction $M = M'$, is equilibrated far to the right at $\mathcal{E}_r$. This situation is represented in Fig. 3-3E, left; the upper (M^3) portion of the channel is closed showing that the 3 M molecules are in the M' (blocking) position. A large depolarization greatly increases the rate of movement of M' molecules to the M position and greatly decreases the opposite reaction, the equilibrium of the $M = M'$ is thus now far to the left. The time required for equilibration is well under 1 msec but depends on the final voltage. Three M molecules must be in place to form a channel; only one needs to be put out of place to block the channel. Thus on sudden depolarization, the number of channels having three M molecules in place increases slowly at first and then more rapidly (third order kinetics); the rise in g_{Na} is S-shaped (Fig. 3-5C, rising phase of g_{Na} curve). Repolarization closes the channels rapidly because only one M need move out of place. Figure 3-3E middle and right shows the M^3 portions of the membrane open in the depolarized state.

The kinetics of the H molecules are the same as those of the M molecules except that the variation of the forward and backward rate constants with voltage is reversed; the reaction $H = H'$ is equilibrated far to the left at the resting potential; most of the H are in position (H portion of the Na+ channel, Fig. 3-3E, left). The equilibration rate of the H reaction is about 10 times slower than for M, several milliseconds being required (Fig. 3-5C, falling phase of g_{Na} curve). The fraction of H molecules at effective sites might be termed *activation* of g_{Na} but, more commonly, the fraction of H in blocking sites, H', is termed *inactivation* [30, 31]. Under circumstances of the Hodgkin-Huxley voltage-clamp experiments, the resting potential was somewhat depressed and the resting inactivation was about 0.4. Maintained hyperpolarization decreases inactivation to zero (all H form), and it is increased to 1.0 (all H' form) by maintained depolarization (Fig. 3-3E, right).

A sudden depolarization thus has two effects on sodium conductance: M molecules move rapidly into effective sites and establish Na+ channels at sites where H molecules are in position; hence g_{Na} rises rapidly (Fig. 3-3E, center). Even as M molecules are moving into position, H molecules are moving out, but at a much slower rate. Thus g_{Na} rises to a peak as M molecules move into place in channels unblocked by H' and then falls over a period of several milliseconds as the H' molecules block them (Fig. 3-5C, g_{Na} curve; Fig. 3-3E, Na+ channels). When the membrane is repolarized after inactivation is completed, there is little change in the already low g_{Na}, but M molecules move out of place rapidly and H molecules move into place slowly. Thereafter, another depolarization would produce an increase in g_{Na} proportional to the fraction of H molecules that had moved back into place during the period of polarization. The possible molecular basis of such changes will be considered below.

Kinetics of Potassium Conductance

Changes. The kinetics of g_K are much the same as those for M, only about 10 times slower. A potassium channel is formed when four N molecules are at four effective (nonblocking) sites simultaneously. At rest the reaction $N = N'$ is equilibrated far right (Fig. 3-3E, left, K+ channels); depolarization shifts the equilibrium to the left. Thus depolarization produces an S-shaped increase in g_K, fourth order kinetics (Fig. 3-5C), but much slower than that of g_{Na} (Fig. 3-3E, middle and right). Repolarization produces an uninflected, rapid fall to low levels. Hodgkin and Huxley [31] expressed these ideas in mathematical form as follows:

$$g_{Na} = \bar{g}_{Na} m^3 h \quad \text{and} \quad g_K = \bar{g}_K n^4 \quad (3\text{-}10a)$$

where $\bar{g}_{Na}$ and $\bar{g}_K$ are maximum values of g_{Na} and g_K and m, h, and n are the probabilities that M, H, and N molecules are in position. Also

$$dp/dt = \alpha_p(1 - p) - \beta_p p \quad (3\text{-}10b)$$

where p stands for m, h, or n and α_p and β_p are rate constants whose values depend only on ε_m.

PREDICTION OF ACTION POTENTIAL FROM VOLTAGE-CLAMP DATA. Hodgkin and Huxley [31] expressed their voltage-clamp data from squid giant axons in mathematical form. The model described above was used in formulating the differential equations describing the variations of g_{Na} and g_K with voltage and time. These equations (3-10a and b) together with Eq. 3-7 and 3-9 form a complete set which can be solved for the appropriate boundary conditions. The solutions of these equations were found to predict accurately the size and shape of the action potential (Fig. 3-6A), the refractory period, the existence and size of threshold, conduction speed, and other properties of the nerve impulse. The analysis permitted calculation of the time-course of the changes in g_{Na} and g_K during the action potential (Fig. 3-6B) and the degree of inactivation of g_{Na}, quantities which are not directly measurable but are the *essence* of the impulse. These calculations are also the basis of the statements made above concerning the sequence of events during the action potential. Frankenhaeuser and Huxley [19] have shown that the same type of analysis accurately predicts the excitable properties of frog myelinated nerve fibers.

Depolarization. Calculated conductance and voltage changes during the propagated action potential are shown in Fig. 3-6. The experimentally measured action potential (Fig. 3-6A, bottom) is noticeably but not significantly different from the calculated one (top). The differences are mainly in the falling phase. The regenerative sequence of changes in g_{Na} and membrane voltage (Hodgkin cycle) which generate the rising phase was described at the beginning of this chapter and is depicted in Fig. 3-6B. Note that g_{Na} does not start to rise rapidly until the membrane has been considerably depolarized. This is because of current flow from the recording region into the depolarized region (high g_{Na}) of the approaching impulse; the recording region must be depolarized to threshold before g_{Na} rises rapidly. Figures 3-6B shows that g_{Na} reaches its peak slightly before the voltage does. Also note that g_{Na} has fallen to about one-sixth of its peak value at a time when repolarization is only half completed. This indicates, and direct calculation confirms, that the major factor acting to decrease Na+ conductance at this time is inactivation (H'), not repolarization (M').

The calculated conduction speed of the top action potential in Fig. 3-6A is 18.8 meters per second; the measured value is 21.2 meters per second. This is remarkably good agreement considering the uncertainties in the measurements and calculations.

Repolarization. The regenerative nature of the depolarization process ensures that it proceeds at the fastest possible rate. Repolarization, on the other hand, is a *degenerative* process; the greater the degree of repolarization, the more slowly it proceeds. The delayed increase in g_K (Fig. 3-6B) is the membrane change responsible for rapid repolarization. If g_K did not increase during activity, nearly complete repolarization would still occur because of the inactivation of g_{Na} but the rate of repolarization would be several times slower.

The sequence of events in repolarization is as follows. At the peak of depolarization g_{Na} is falling because of inactivation, and g_K is beginning to increase (Fig. 3-6B). The resulting increase in K+ efflux and decrease in Na+ influx bring about a rapid repolarization. This voltage change in turn hastens the decrease in g_{Na} and, after a delay, in g_K. As a consequence, g_K is still above normal when repolarization is complete, and thus the membrane hyperpolarizes, that is, the potential goes nearer to ε_K than is the resting potential. Thereafter, g_K and ε_m fall slowly back to their resting values.

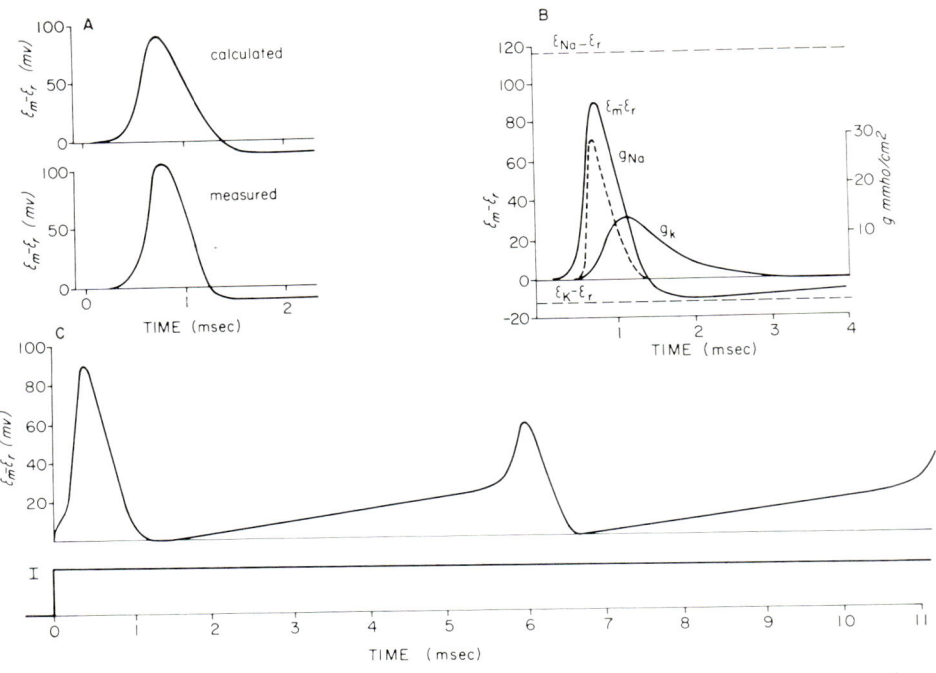

FIG. 3-6. (A) Top: Propagated action potential calculated from Hodgkin-Huxley equations. Calculated conduction speed, 18.8 m/sec; temperature = 18.5°C. Bottom: Propagated action potential in an axon. Measured conduction speed 21.2 m/sec. Calculated and measured action potentials differ somewhat, but resemblance is striking. (After Hodgkin and Huxley [31].)

(B) Calculated time courses of membrane voltage change ($\varepsilon_m - \varepsilon_r$), sodium conductance, g_{Na}, and potassium conductance, g_K, in squid giant axon. Note that there is substantial depolarization before g_{Na} increases appreciably and causes rapid depolarization. Early depolarization is due to local circuit current. Delayed rise in g_K and simultaneous fall in g_{Na} cause rapid repolarization. Delay in fall of g_K causes afterhyperpolarization. (After Hodgkin [25]. (A) and (B) from Ruch, T. C., and Patton, H. D. (Eds.), [64].)

(C) Generation of repetitive discharge in a squid giant axon by a maintained depolarizing current. Upper: Approximate time course, calculated from Hodgkin-Huxley equations, of transmembrane voltage changes at site of current application. Lower: Time course of current applied via an intracellular electrode. Current is turned on at $t = 0$; current turn-on depolarizes membrane to threshold and a propagated action potential is generated. Repolarization process is opposed by maintained current so that voltage returns only momentarily to resting level (no afterhyperpolarization), and then a long, sustained, nearly linear depolarization ensues. This is due to slow decay in g_K and slow turn-on of g_{Na}. Threshold is much higher in second (and succeeding) APs because inactivation occurs during slow depolarization. This also accounts for small size of AP. Despite small size, second and succeeding APs propagate along fiber and are full size 1 cm away from stimulus site. APs are generated as long as current is applied. (After Cooley, J. W., and Dodge, F. A., Jr. [16], and Stein, R. B. [54].)

The conductance changes which occur during propagation can be compactly summarized on the basis of the hypothetical scheme described above and depicted in Fig. 3-3E. This scheme also aids in understanding the refractory period.

Threshold. Threshold is one of three values of ε_m at which the inward Na+ current just equals the outward K+ current (neglecting Cl− and other leak currents). The other two values are the resting potential and the peak of the action potential. When a membrane is depolarized by current outflow, g_{Na} increases and the inflow of Na+ increases. The net efflux of K+ also increases because reduction in ε_m has increased the electrochemical gradient on K+ ($\varepsilon_m - \varepsilon_K$ increases). If the net movement of ionic charges through the membrane is zero (if net Na+ influx equals net K+ efflux), the membrane voltage does not change. However, at threshold, the potential would stay constant only until inactivation of g_{Na} reduced Na+ influx. The potential would then fall to ε_r. On the other hand, if the applied depolarizing current were made slightly larger, the net Na+ influx through the membrane would slightly exceed the net K+ efflux, and the action potential upstroke would ensue via the Hodgkin cycle.

Refractory Period. Since inactivation of g_{Na} is almost complete at the end of the action potential, a depolarizing current applied at this time will not cause much increase in g_{Na}. Therefore, the fiber is refractory (inexcitable); a stimulating current, no matter how strong, cannot initiate a regenerative response. A little later, after some reactivation has occurred, a depolarizing current will cause a larger increase in g_{Na}; then an action potential smaller than normal may be generated. The required depolarizing current is greater than normal because the available g_{Na} is low (threshold voltage elevated) and because g_K is still above normal and more current is required to produce a given depolarization. These effects die out in a few milliseconds, and the threshold returns to normal.

Propagation of the Impulse: Local Circuits. Once an action potential has been initiated at a point, the g_{Na} is high in that region and the membrane potential is near the Na+ equilibrium potential. The potential of adjacent inactive membrane is near the K+ equilibrium potential. There is a potential difference between these regions; consequently, current flows from the active region through the intracellular fluid to the inactive region (arrow directed to left in Fig. 3-3E, left and center), discharges the membrane capacitor, and returns through the interstitial fluid to the active region (arrows directed to right in Fig. 3-3E) and through the membrane as inward Na+ current driven by ε_{Na}. This *local circuit* current reduces membrane charge and voltage in the inactive region. When threshold is reached there, g_{Na} increases rapidly, and the inactive region becomes active. Thus, by *local circuit current flow* an active region stimulates the adjacent inactive regions, and an impulse is conducted away from the stimulus site in both directions at a constant speed.

Accommodation and Block. A brief subthreshold stimulus (depolarizing current) applied to a point on a nerve fiber increases excitability (lowers threshold) in the region of application, because the fiber remains depolarized in that region for a few milliseconds and a second stimulus need not be of normal strength to reach threshold voltage. A maintained, subthreshold depolarizing current first increases excitability, but this is followed by a fall of excitability toward normal as inactivation of g_{Na} occurs.

The steady-state relation between the fraction of available g_{Na} and ε_m is a steep, S-shaped curve. The maximum slope is near threshold so a moderate maintained depolarization can greatly reduce the available g_{Na}. In the squid giant axon, normally available g_{Na} is only about 60 percent. Hence a maintained depolarization reduces available g_{Na} and thus increases the threshold voltage (toward zero). This rise in threshold is called *accommodation*. The delayed increase in g_K also contributes to the fall in excitability since a given current produces less depolarization.

Since a maintained depolarization of 20 mV will decrease available g_{Na} to near zero, it follows that conduction can be blocked at a point on a nerve fiber by a sufficiently strong depolarizing current. If the current is suddenly applied, impulses may be initiated before the block occurs. The blockage of impulse conduction by depolarizing current occurs only in a small region on either side of point of current application; impulses will propagate on either side of the blocked region, but not through it. This method of blocking impulse conduction is called *cathodal block, depolarization block,* or *inactivation block.*

Depolarization block can be produced in many ways other than by applying current. Since a sufficient increase in $[K^+]_o$, ischemia, anoxia, and injury all depolarize the membrane, they all block impulse conduction. An expected characteristic of depolarization blocking agents is that these increase excitability when they do not depolarize sufficiently to block. Local anesthetics block conduction in nerve by increasing g_{Na} inactivation without altering membrane voltage [57]. Depolarization block, no matter how induced, is relieved by a hyperpolarizing current because it increases the absolute value of ε_m and reactivates g_{Na}.

A sufficient hyperpolarization of the membrane can also block conduction in a nerve. Block occurs if ε_m is made so large that local circuit flow from the hyperpolarized region into an approaching active region is insufficient to depolarize the hyperpolarized region to threshold. This phenomenon is called *anodal* or *hyperpolarization block.*

Ion Exchange during Activity. It has been stressed repeatedly that the rising phase of the action potential is brought about by a sudden, large influx of Na^+ ions and repolarization by an efflux of K^+ ions. It might be supposed that these "large" fluxes greatly change the internal concentrations of Na^+ and K^+. Actually, the concentration changes are very small, the reason being that, although the fluxes are high, they flow only for a short time, and, chemically speaking, the amount of ions necessary to charge the membrane is small. The minimum net influx of Na^+ required during activity is simply the amount of charge necessary to change the voltage across the membrane capacitor from ε_K to ε_{Na}. An equal net efflux of K^+ suffices to recharge the membrane. For squid giant axon, the minimum Na^+ entry (or K^+ exit) during one impulse is 1.6 picamoles per cm² (1.6 × 10^{-12} moles per cm²) of membrane. A crucial test of the Na^+-K^+ theory of the action potential is that measured net fluxes of Na^+ and K^+ during the AP must be greater than the minimum required because, as can be seen from Fig. 3-6B, there is considerable simultaneous inflow of Na^+ and outflow of K^+ during the action potential. The measured net Na^+ influx in the squid giant axon is about 4.0, and the net K^+ efflux about 3.0 pmoles per cm²-impulse. These values are greater than the minimum and about that which is predicted by the Hodgkin-Huxley [31] equations.

The change in internal concentrations during an impulse depends not only on the net entry or loss of the ion, but also on the volume of axoplasm in which the extra ions distribute themselves. The bigger the fiber, the smaller the concentration change per impulse. For example, in a squid axon 500 μ in diameter, the net Na^+ entry of 3 pmoles per cm²-impulse raises the internal concentration by only 1.2 × 10^{-10} moles per cm³. The internal concentration of Na^+ in the squid is about 50 μmoles per cm³, some 300,000 times greater. The fractional increase per impulse in $[Na^+]_i$ in a 20-μ myelinated fiber is only one part in a million because of the low capacity of the internodal region. Thus, even with the Na^+ pump turned off, one million impulses would be required to double $[Na^+]_i$. The $[Na^+]_i$ change per impulse in axon terminals 0.1 μ in diameter is much larger; one impulse will increase internal Na^+ concentration by about 10 percent. Hence, in these fibers, the Na^+ pumping rate must be quickly responsive to activity.

MOLECULAR MECHANISMS OF EXCITABILITY

Since a nerve fiber does not fire unless adequately stimulated and since the epileptic discharge involves abnormal, spontaneous discharge of neurons, it is worth considering those changes in intrinsic membrane properties or in the cell's environment which may give rise to spontaneous discharge in nerve cells. The squid membrane's characteristics must be used in this consideration since these are the only ones which have been quantitatively described. (The frog node of Ranvier membrane has nearly identical properties [19].) Unfortunately, little is known of the molecular mechanisms of excitability, so that it is not possible to specify what molecular changes in membranes (if any) give rise to epileptic discharge. Nevertheless, vague outlines of the molecular basis of excitability are beginning to emerge and this forms a framework for considering epileptic mechanisms.

SEPARABILITY OF Na^+ AND K^+ CHANNELS. The low ion permeability of cell membranes and other data strongly indicate that ions penetrate membranes through rare, specialized, hydrophilic regions. These specialized regions are probably protein or lipoprotein molecules embedded in the membrane at wide intervals compared with membrane thickness (Fig. 3-3C). The special nature of these regions is partially indicated by the voltage clamp results described above. A depolarization causes independent and widely differing changes in the membrane's permeability to Na^+ and K^+. The implication is that some regions of the membrane are specialized for Na^+ and others for K^+ penetration. This implication is rather firmly established by the recent findings (cf. [50, 51]) that extremely low concentrations (10^{-8} M) of the puffer fish poison, tetrodotoxin, selectively block the depolarization-induced increase in g_{Na} without altering the increase in g_K.

Tetrodotoxin has no effect when it is added to the solution bathing the inside of the membrane. Moore et al. [50] found that no more than about 15 molecules of tetrodotoxin per μ^2 of membrane are required to block the early current. Thus, it appears that (a) Na^+ and K^+ channels are separate entities, (b) the inside and outside entrances to the Na^+ channel are chemically different, and (c) the fraction of surface area occupied by Na^+ channels is very small. (Quoted from [65].)

Further, the M and H portions of Na^+ channels can be separately altered by drugs.

Koppenhöfer and Schmidt [45] found that scorpion venom acts mainly to reduce the rate and amount of sodium inactivation (H system) with little effect on the M system.

The most likely structural candidates for Na^+ and K^+ channels are the protein subunits of the membrane (Fig. 3-3C). In this view, ions penetrate such a *pore protein* moiety through hydrophilic (charged) regions either at the junction of four or more units or through a charged region near the center of a single unit. This picture, though reasonable, is highly speculative, but will be used henceforth as a basis for discussion. Although Na^+ pore protein and K^+ pore protein have some common characteristics, they also must be distinctly different as preceding and following considerations show.

DISTINCTIVE CHARACTERISTICS OF Na^+ AND K^+ CHANNELS—*Variation of Permeability with Voltage.* As mentioned, the peak value of g_{Na} and the final value of g_K depend dramatically on the size of the step depolarization under voltage clamp conditions. The plot of conductance as a function of voltage is S-shaped, with the inflection point at a depolarization of about 30 mV from the resting potential for both g_{Na} and g_K. For lesser depolarizations, the relationship is approximately exponential; g_{Na} varies as exp ($\varepsilon_m/4$) and g_K as exp ($\varepsilon_m/5$), indicating that the channels are distinct.

The significance of this finding can be seen from the following argument of Hodgkin and Huxley [31]: A depolarization could cause Na^+ and K^+ channels to open because some negatively charged molecules previously at the outside of the membrane move to the inside. (There must be relatively few such channels with many ions moving through each channel because the inward migration of the negatively charged molecules immediately following a step depolarization constitutes an outward current flow at early times. This is not observed experimentally even at depolarizations to V_{Na} where such a current would be particularly obvious.) Suppose that there are N molecules of valence z per unit area in the membrane and that specific ion permeability is proportional to the number, N_i, on the inside surface of the membrane, the remainder, $N_o = N - N_i$, being on the outside surface. If N_i is 0.5 when $\varepsilon_m = 0$, then $N_i/N_o =$ exp ($-Fz\varepsilon_m/RT$) and hence

$$N_i = 1/[\exp(-Fz\varepsilon_m/RT) + 1] \quad (3\text{-}11)$$

For large negative values of $Fz\varepsilon_m/RT$, this expression reduces to $\exp(Fz\varepsilon_m/RT)$. Experimentally g_{Na} varies as $\exp(\varepsilon_m/4)$; hence $z = 25/4 = 6$. Thus six charges (or a triply charged dipole) must move through the full transmembrane potential to account for the observed variation of sodium conductance with voltage. For potassium the magnitude of the valence is 4 to 5. However, the situation is not this simple; the observed dependences of g_{Na} and g_K on ε_m are not accurately described by Eq. 3-11; the more complicated relationship of the Hodgkin-Huxley equations is required. (Quoted from [65].)

Special Characteristics of the K+ Channel. The time delay before I_K starts increasing rapidly following a step depolarization is long; the maximum rate of rise is large (Fig. 3-5C) compared with other mechanisms (such as diffusion) showing delay behavior. Hodgkin and Huxley [31] used fourth order kinetics, n^4, to describe this delay. Cole and Moore [15] found that approximately thirtieth order kinetics, n^{30}, were required to give the requisite time delay if the membrane was first hyperpolarized and then depolarized. They also concluded that the shape of the I_K-vs.-t curve depends only on the final ε_m, that is, ε_m is a state variable. Another important property of the K+ channel is that K+ influxes and effluxes interact in the manner expected if K+ have to traverse the membrane through a long, narrow channel containing about 3 K+ ions [35]. This is termed *in-file* behavior. Na+ channels appear to contain no more than one Na+ at a time; they obey the independence principle [28, 29].

Temperature Dependence of g_{Na} and g_K. The rate of rise of g_{Na} and g_K are relatively slow processes, and the rates depend sensitively on temperature (Q_{10} about 3). This means that changes in membrane structure leading to changes in values for g have high activation energies. The values of Q_{10} for the final values of g_{Na} and g_K are much lower, about 1.3, so that ion transit through an open channel is not greatly impeded.

Effects of Calcium Concentration on g_{Na} and g_K. The electrical properties of excitable cells depend sensitively on $[Ca^{++}]_o$ [7, 18, 22, 39]. Changing $[Ca^{++}]_o$ shifts the curves relating g_{Na} and g_K to voltage along the voltage axis by amounts proportional to $\log[Ca^{++}]_o$. The shift is such that increasing $[Ca^{++}]_o$ increases the threshold. However, the coefficient of $\log[Ca^{++}]_o$ is only about half of RT/zF. One possible interpretation is that Ca^{++} binds to the membrane and alters the electric field near Na+ and K+ penetration sites. Na+ channels are more affected by changes in $[Ca^{++}]$ than are K+ channels.

Selectivity of Na+ and K+ Channels. Most cell membranes are much more permeable to cations than to anions (erythrocytes are an exception) and are much more permeable to K+ than to Na+. This is also true of excitable membranes in the resting state, but not in the excited state, where g_{Na} is much greater than g_K. However, it would be surprising if "Na+ channels" completely excluded all other ions, for example, K+ should be able to traverse a Na+ channel although not as easily as Na+, and vice versa for K+ channels. Internal-perfusion techniques have permitted determination of the cation selectivity sequences of the Na+ channel:

$$P_{Li}:P_{Na}:P_K:P_{Rb}:P_{Cs} = 1.1:1.0:0.083:0.025:0.016$$
(cf. [47]); hence $P_{Na} = 12\, P_K$.

It is generally agreed that the selectivity mechanism is based on the differential binding properties of a specific charge group for the various ions. These charge groups are presumably side groups of the pore proteins with the charge near the entrance to the Na+ and K+ channels. It is not known how the selection process occurs [17], but it is probably significant that the binding sequences of carboxyl groups for cations is exactly the reverse of the selectivity sequence of the Na+ channel [65]. Although the ion-binding ratios are lower than the ion-selectivity ratios, coincidence of the sequences is good presumptive evidence that Na+ channels are "guarded" by carboxyl and K+ channels by phosphate groups, somewhat as depicted in Fig. 3-3E.

A MODEL OF THE Na+ CHANNEL. The previous sections show that there are at least two distinct functional components of Na+ and K+ channels: (a) a selectivity mechanism and (b) a voltage-sensitive gating or valving mechanism. The former selects the appropriate ion, and the latter opens or shuts the channel depending on the voltage and immediate past history in the manner described by the Hodgkin-Huxley equations. There are two possible classes of gating mechanisms: (a) a channel is either open or shut, the fraction of open channels being dependent on the voltage and time; (b) the permeability of one channel varies continuously with voltage. The open-shut type of behavior was assumed by Hodgkin and Huxley: three M molecules and one H molecule need to be in place for a Na+ channel to be open and four N molecules for a K+ channel. The open-shut model is adequate for Na+ channels, but the large time-delay characteristics of the K+ channel require such high order kinetics that the possibility of a continuously variable valve cannot be excluded. The original formal model of Hodgkin and Huxley for Na+ conductance can be given a simple molecular basis:

A Na+ channel may consist of a hole or pore passing through the lipid-protein matrix of the membrane as described above (Fig. 3-3C, E). This pore or channel is about 6 Å in radius and is likely guarded at one or both ends by carboxyl groups. Since tetrodotoxin blocks Na+ channels only when applied on the outside, the outer and inner entrances are different [51].

When a Na+ enters a channel, the ion presumably interacts with one or more carboxyl groups in a way to produce the observed selectivity. However, this interaction is not a simple binding of the ion to a carboxyl group at the channel entrance [65].

As the Na+ moves through the channel it progresses over a series of potential energy barriers until it exits; that is, the ion may loosely bind to fixed negative charges occurring at 10 to 15 Å intervals. These charge groups are probably positioned by loops of protein encasing the channel. The lumen of the channel is hydrophilic, presumably filled with water.

Voltage-Induced Conformation Change in the Na+ Channel. Since the essence of the excitable process in nerve is that depolarization causes a large, rapid, and transient increase in Na+ conductance and since ions probably penetrate through protein regions, it is reasonable to suppose that permeability or conductance changes are due to voltage-induced changes in the shape or conformation of the protein. Changes in the concentrations of certain constituents can cause protein conformation changes, so that it is not unreasonable to suppose that voltage can have the same effect. The most accurately known example is the conformation change of hemoglobin; oxygenation decreases the distance between marked regions of the hemoglobin beta-chains from 40 to 33 Å. Thus, it is attractive to suppose that the opening of a Na+ channel (or a K+ channel) is the result of a conformation change in the pore protein induced by depolarization of the membrane. An increase in chain spacings of 7 Å could easily change a channel from closed to open. A change, $\Delta \varepsilon$, in the voltage across the membrane is equivalent to a change in concentration of an ion from C to $C \cdot \exp(\alpha \Delta \varepsilon F z / RT)$ where α is the fraction of the voltage change acting on charges of valence z in the protein [20].

Since the nature of protein conformation changes is not well understood, this molecular model cannot be put on a quantitative basis. If the pore protein changes conformation in the same way as does hemoglobin, a satisfying but not unique picture of the permeability changes of the Na+ channel results:

Suppose that the pore proteins consist of four more or less parallel chains that extend through the membrane. Each chain has two equilibrium positions, C (closed) and O (open). A Na+ channel is open if and only if all four chains are in the O-position but closed when one or more chains are in the C-position. There are three M-chains and one H-chain. When the membrane is polarized, the M-chains in each channel are mostly in the C-position and the H-chains mostly in the O. An abrupt depolarization has two effects: the M-chains quickly move in a cooperative manner to the O-position, and the H-chains start moving slowly into the C-position; most Na+ channels are thus transiently open, and it is clear the model has the kinetics of the Na+ channel. However, this molecular model suffers from the same defect as the original model of Hodgkin and Huxley [31]: the experimentally determined voltage dependences of the rate constants (α_m, β_m) describing the M-part of the Na+ channels are not described by the simple charge or dipole hypothesis outlined above (Eq. 3-11). However, the H portion (activation-inactivation) is described by Eq. 3-11. K+ channels cannot be described by this model since they open with thirtieth or higher order kinetics.

The effects of changes in $[Ca^{++}]_o$ in shifting the g_{Na}-vs.-$\mathcal{E}_m$ curve are explained by supposing that Ca^{++} combines with some site on the Na+ pore protein and shifts the equilibrium of the O–C reaction for a given voltage.

SPONTANEOUS FIRING OF NEURONS

Obviously, a listing of the types of changes in membrane properties and in the extracellular and intracellular environments of cell which can give rise to spontaneous firing in nerve cells is also a listing of many of the changes which might initiate an epileptic discharge. In general, spontaneous discharge may be initiated by any change that makes the resting potential equal to or more positive than the threshold potential; many types of changes can do this.

MECHANISM OF SPONTANEOUS FIRING. Experimentally, the simplest way to induce rhythmic firing in some types of excitable cells (cf. [23]) is to apply a fixed depolarizing current of appropriate size. If a constant current is applied suddenly to a nerve fiber at one point, the membrane potential follows a time course like that shown in Fig. 3-6C. When the current is turned on at time zero, the membrane depolarizes initially in a manner dictated by cable properties. As threshold is approached, the Hodgkin cycle, supplying an inward Na+ current, causes the voltage-time curve to turn upward, and the stereotyped action potential sequence ensues (Fig. 3-6A, B). Repolarization is brought about by the delayed increase in g_K but the applied current opposes this process with the result that $\mathcal{E}_m$ returns only to about $\mathcal{E}_r$ instead of hyperpolarizing. As the increased g_K dies out, the membrane is again depolarized by the applied current. The depolarization is slow and nearly linear because of the decreasing g_K and increasing g_{Na}. However, since inactivation of g_{Na} is also occurring concomitantly, threshold is moving upward also. There is a range of current strengths where threshold is reached and another, much smaller, AP is generated. Despite its smaller size, this AP is propagated and has reached normal amplitude one centimeter away from the site of current application [16, 54].

The slow depolarization (pacemaker potential), the "cause" of the spontaneous firing, is compounded of a decaying g_K and an increasing g_{Na}. If the applied current is too small, the pacemaker potential will not reach threshold after the first AP; if the current is too large, inactivation of g_{Na} will proceed too far and produce depolarization block. Between these lower and upper limits, the rate of firing depends directly but not sensitively on the strength of the current. Stein [54] studied the behavior of the Hodgkin-Huxley equations under these circumstances and found that the discharge frequency changed only from 200 to 275 per second with a current change from 1.75 to 4 μamp. No continued firing occurs above or below these currents. This behavior is a poor model of spontaneous discharge rates in some axons, which can fire at rates as low as a few per second in response to weak currents [23].

Stein investigated possible changes in the parameters of the Hodgkin-Huxley equation which might improve these equations as a model of spontaneous discharge. The resting potential was increased, and the g_{Na} activation-versus-voltage curve was shifted to increase the activation at the resting potential. These changes gave a repetitive firing range of 30 to 140 per second, which was still inadequate. On the basis of these and other calculations, Stein concluded that the Hodgkin-Huxley equations are not adequate to describe spontaneous discharge in many types of axons in response to applied currents. This is not surprising since the Hodgkin-Huxley equations are a description of data at short times, and any long time effects which might give rise to low firing rates are not necessarily included. Nevertheless, the Hodgkin-Huxley equations do give considerable insight into the types of processes which can give rise to spontaneous firing.

CONSEQUENCES OF REPETITIVE FIRING. Repetitive action potential generation, no matter how caused, results in considerable ion-concentration changes in the fluids bathing the membrane. If it is supposed that in the resting neuron the internal [Na+] and [K+] are initially at steady-state values, with active fluxes balancing passive fluxes, the sudden initiation of repetitive firing will cause increased passive influx of Na+ and efflux of K+ and hence $[K^+]_i$ will decrease and $[Na^+]_i$ increase. As pointed out above, the concentration changes per impulse are small. However, if the nerve cell is to remain excitable, the rate of active Na+-for-K+ transport must eventually increase until a new steady state is reached with zero net K+ and Na+ fluxes. Thus the energy consumption of the cell must also increase and may be quite large; roughly speaking, resting Na+ and K+ fluxes (moles per cm² sec) are the same as the Na+ and K+ fluxes of one impulse (moles per cm² impulse) so that a transition from rest to 50 impulses per second necessitates a fiftyfold increase in pumping rate.

Since active transport requires about 10 percent of resting metabolism in muscle [43], a fiftyfold increase in pump rate requires at least a fivefold increase in total metabolism. There is no need for an immediate increase in pumping rate since the Na+ and K+ concentration cells store enough energy to generate up to 10^6 impulses, depending on fiber diameter.

REGULATION OF Na+-K+ PUMPING RATE. Clearly some aspect of impulse conduction must stimulate the Na+-K+ pump. The most obvious possibility is that the pump rate is a direct function of internal Na+ concentration; as $[Na^+]_i$ increases with impulse firing, the pump rate increases, that is, a feedback system to regulate $[Na^+]_i$ at near normal levels. Another possibility is membrane depolarization [37, 38].

Role of Internal [Na+]. There is much evidence that pumping rate depends on $[Na^+]_i$ [8, 9, 34, 42]. The functional relationship between pump rate and $[Na^+]_i$ is probably S-shaped. At low $[Na^+]_i$ values, M^*_{Na} varies as $[Na^+]_i^N$ where M^*_{Na} is active Na+ efflux and N is a low integer. At higher values, the curve straightens out and finally must saturate at some maximum M^*_{Na} determined by the maximum metabolic rate of the cell. Woodbury [63] has calculated the steady-state transmembrane potential and internal [Na+] and [K+] of frog skeletal muscle as a function of impulse frequency for various values of N. These calculations show that even moderate firing rates cause inordinately large increases in $[Na^+]_i$ and decreases in $[K^+]_i$ for $N = 1$, large changes for $N = 2$, and moderate changes for $N = 3$. Keynes [42] found that $N = 3$ in frog skeletal muscle for normal or low $[Na^+]_i$. The method of regulation of the pump is not completely determined, but it must keep $[Na^+]_i$ at fairly low values. This follows from the foregoing arguments but much more directly from the experimental findings that $[Na^+]_i$ is low in central nervous tissue despite continual impulse generation and conduction.

Role of [K+]$_o$. Experimentally, it is found that M^*_{Na} is directly dependent on $[K^+]_o$, a result indicating the coupling of K+ uptake with Na+ extrusion. Caldwell [10] has reviewed the evidence relevant to a carrier model of the Na+-K+ pump with loose coupling. In terms of maintaining excitability in the face of rapid repetitive firing, a dependence of M^*_{Na} on $[K^+]_o$ is desirable. Loss of K+ into the confined interstitial space of brain probably causes comparatively large increases in $[K^+]_o$. If this is not to depolarize the membrane and thus block impulse generation by inactivating g_{Na}, then mechanisms must be available for maintaining $[K^+]_o$ at nonblocking levels. During normal, near steady-state activity the K+ lost is reabsorbed by the nerve cells but it seems quite probable that, during periods of intense activity, some of the excess interstitial K+ is taken up by glia and gradually released when activity falls. K+ accumulation in interstitial fluid is possibly an important factor in terminating an epileptic discharge and partially responsible for postictal depression.

Pump Inhibition. Since cardiac glycosides inhibit the pump, it is not surprising that these produce convulsions when introduced into the cerebrospinal fluid; inhibition of the pump causes K+ loss, depolarization, and, initially, spontaneous discharge. This discharge and lack of pumping increases $[K^+]_o$ and causes depolarization block. In general, as $[K^+]_o$ increases, there is at first an increase in excitability, which is followed by spontaneous discharge and finally by block at higher concentrations.

MEMBRANE EPILEPTIC AND ANTIEPILEPTIC MECHANISMS

Although spontaneous firing of a nerve cell may be induced by a sufficient depolarizing current, pertinency of this phenomenon to epilepsy depends on the existence of natural means of depolarizing membranes to the spontaneous firing-range since these may initiate the epileptic discharge. The mechanism of spread is almost certainly synaptic.

INCREASED MEMBRANE IONIC PERMEABILITY. The transduction process at sense organs probably results in an increase in P_{Na} or in P_{Na} and P_K of a portion of the terminal membrane. This increase causes an increased net influx of Na+ and consequent depolarization and spontaneous firing. Much the same process occurs at excitatory synapses. If the transmitter action persists or there is continued presynaptic firing, the postsynaptic cell fires at a rate dependent on the amount of depolarization. It is possible that the microscopic and ultramicroscopic changes in brain structure at the focus of an epileptic lesion include changes which increase P_{Na}, for example, denervation hypersensitivity and consequent firing in response to low ambient transmitter concentrations.

DECREASED THRESHOLD. Spontaneous firing can also be caused by any membrane change that lowers the threshold potential to the resting potential. The most direct means of lowering threshold,

$$\Delta \varepsilon_{th} \equiv \varepsilon_{th} - \varepsilon_r,$$

is to reduce $[Ca^{++}]_o$. In many excitable tissues this causes spontaneous firing because reducing $[Ca^{++}]_o$ slides the curves relating g_{Na} and g_K to ε_m along the ε_m axis without affecting $\bar{g}_{Na}$ or $\bar{g}_K$. If this shift is large enough, then the Hodgkin cycle is regenerative at ε_m, and spontaneous firing will occur providing there is not too much inactivation. Frog myelinated nerve fibers do not fire spontaneously in low $[Ca^{++}]_o$ solutions but do so if tetraethylammonium (TEA) ion is added to a low $[Ca^{++}]_o$ solution [5]. Since TEA selectively blocks K+ channels in frog nodes [21], repetitive firing is due primarily to the kinetics of the Na+ channels, rather than a combination of Na+ and K+ channels as in the squid axon.

The processes represented by M, H, and N are distinct and independently modified by drugs [45, 51] so it is possible that pathological processes might alter neuron-membrane properties so that spontaneous firing occurs with normal internal and external environments. In terms of the model of Na+ channel given above, spontaneous activity would become more probable if (a) the number of Na+ pore proteins per unit area increased (increase in $\bar{g}_{Na}$); (b) changes in protein kinetics that duplicated the changes caused by reduction in $[Ca^{++}]_o$.

ANTICONVULSANT ACTION OF DIPHENYLHYDANTOIN. The long-term consequence of a decreased Na+ pumping rate in neurons is a decrease in the size of the resting potential (depolarization) even if P_{Na} and P_K are unchanged. As mentioned above, K+ will accumulate in the interstitial fluid if the pump is slowed or stopped, and thus depolarizes the membrane. A maintained, small depolarization causes an increase in excitability and could thus be epileptogenic.

Conversely, a maintained increase in pumping rate causes some hyperpolarization and a decrease in excitability (cf. [53]). There is evidence [61] that diphenylhydantoin stimulates active Na+ transport in brain. If there is sufficient stimulation to appreciably increase the size of the resting potential, the decreased excitability could account for the anticonvulsant activity of diphenylhydantoin. There are two ways in which an increased pumping rate could cause hyperpolarization of neural membranes: (a) The increased K+ concentration gradients in the cell increases the size of ε_K and hence of ε_r. (b) An increased pumping rate in the choroid plexus might reduce the interstitial [K+] and thus hyperpolarize all membranes bathed by the cerebrospinal fluid.

The effects of membrane hyperpolarization on brain excitability are not clear-cut. Hyperpolarization of nerve terminals may cause a considerable increase in transmitter release and more than compensate for the increased threshold. Hence, it could also be argued that diphenylhydantoin should cause more transmitter release and hence (if the excess transmitter is excitatory), increased brain excitability. One possibility is that the hyperpolarization is large enough to cause conduction-block at terminal branches [60] and thus a reduction in transmitter release. Perhaps diphenylhydantoin has all three actions, but the excitability decreasing actions certainly outweigh the excitability increasing ones.

ANTICONVULSANT ACTION OF BROMIDE. Chloride is believed to be passively distributed across the nerve cell membrane and so makes no permanent contribution to resting potential, nor does the value of ε_{Cl} alter ε_{th}, the threshold voltage. However, if P_{Cl} is appreciable, chloride current tends to hold ε_m at ε_{Cl} during synaptic or action potentials or both. The value of ε_{Cl} is determined by a weighted average of ε_m when APs are being generated and is thus likely to be more positive than ε_m. The amount of current necessary to depolarize to threshold is decreased if ε_{Cl} is more positive than ε_{th} and increased if ε_{Cl} is more negative than ε_{th}. The resting potential of a neuron cell-body is about -70 mV, and ε_{th} is about -55 mV. If the neuron fires 50 times per second, ε_{Cl} is about -64 mV. Hence, in most instances, chloride current tends to stabilize cells by increasing the threshold current.

The magnitude of the stabilization depends directly on P_{Cl}. A large P_{Cl} ($P_{Cl} \simeq P_K$) can have an appreciable effect; average firing rate would be decreased by an increase in P_{Cl}. It follows, then, that replacement of a substantial fraction of the chloride in cerebrospinal fluid (CSF) by bromide would have a stabilizing, anticonvulsant effect if $P_{Br} > P_{Cl} \simeq P_K$. Consider the sequence of events as [Br−] builds up in the CSF: as I_{Br} becomes appreciable with respect to I_K, during the AP, the firing rate is decreased in the epileptic locus (and elsewhere) and thus could reduce the probability that a convulsion will occur. This simple hypothesis is easily testable; it is, comparatively speaking, easy to measure P_{Br}/P_{Cl} for neurons. I do not know whether or not such measurements have been made; if not, they should be.

REFERENCES

1. Adelman, W. J., Jr., (Ed). Physical and mathematical approaches to the study of the electrical behavior of excitable membranes. *J. Cell. Physiol.* 66(Supp. 2):1, 1965.
2. Anon. Cell membrane biophysics. *J. Gen. Physiol.* 51:1s, 1968.
3. Baker, P. F., Hodgkin, A. L., and Shaw, T. I. Replacement of the protoplasm of a giant nerve fibre with artificial solutions. *Nature* (London) 190:885, 1961.
4. Baker, P. F., Hodgkin, A. L., and Shaw, T. I. The effects of changes in internal ionic concentrations on the electrical properties of perfused giant axons. *J. Physiol.* (London) 164:355, 1962.
5. Bergmann, C., Nonner, W., and Stämpfli, R. Sustained spontaneous activity of Ranvier nodes induced by the combined actions of TEA and lack of calcium. *Pflueger. Arch. Ges. Physiol.* 302:24, 1968.
6. Binstock, L., and Lecar, H. Ammonium ion substitutions in the voltage clamped squid axon. *Biophys. Soc. Abs.* 11th Annual Meeting, Abs. WC 4, 1967.
7. Blaustein, M. P., and Goldman, D. E. Competitive action of calcium and procaine on lobster axon. *J. Gen. Physiol.* 49:1043, 1966.

8. Brinley, F. J., Jr. Sodium and potassium fluxes in isolated barnacle muscle fibers. *J. Gen. Physiol.* 51:445, 1968.
9. Brinley, F. J., Jr. Sodium, potassium, and chloride concentrations and fluxes in the isolated giant axon of *Homarus*. *J. Neurophysiol.* 28:742, 1965.
10. Caldwell, P. C. Factors governing movement and distribution of inorganic ions in nerve and muscle. *Physiol. Rev.* 48:1, 1968.
11. Chandler, W. K., Hodgkin, A. L., and Meves, H. The effect of changing the internal solution on sodium inactivation and related phenomena in giant axons. *J. Physiol.* (London) 180:821, 1965.
12. Chandler, W. K., and Meves, H. Voltage clamp experiments on internally perfused giant axons. *J. Physiol.* (London) 180:788, 1965.
13. Cole, K. S. Electrodiffusion models for the membrane of squid giant axon. *Physiol. Rev.* 45:340, 1965.
14. Cole, K. S. *Membranes, Ions and Impulses*. Berkeley, Calif.: U. Calif. Press, 1968.
15. Cole, K. S., and Moore, J. W. Potassium ion current in the squid giant axon: Dynamic characteristic. *Biophys. J.* 1:1, 1960.
16. Cooley, J. W., and Dodge, F. A., Jr. Digital computer solutions for excitation and propagation of the nerve impulse. *Biophys. J.* 6:583, 1966.
17. Eisenmann, G., Bates, R., Mattock, G., and Friedman, S. M. *The Glass Electrode*. New York: Wiley, 1968.
18. Frankenhaeuser, B., and Hodgkin, A. L. The action of calcium on the electrical properties of squid axons. *J. Physiol.* (London) 137:218, 1957.
19. Frankenhaeuser, B., and Huxley, A. F. The action potential in the myelinated nerve fibre of *Xenopus laevis* as computed on the basis of voltage clamp data. *J. Physiol.* (London) 171:302, 1964.
20. Hill, T. L. Electric fields and the co-operativity of biological membranes. *Proc. Nat. Acad. Sci. U.S.A.* 58:111, 1967.
21. Hille, B. The selective inhibition of delayed potassium currents in nerve by tetraethylammonium ion. *J. Gen. Physiol.* 50:1287, 1967.
22. Hille, B. Charges and potentials at the nerve surface. *J. Gen. Physiol.* 51:221, 1968.
23. Hodgkin, A. L. The local electric changes associated with repetitive action in a non medullated axon. *J. Physiol.* (London) 107:165, 1948.
24. Hodgkin, A. L. The ionic basis of electrical activity in nerve and muscle. *Biol. Rev.* 26:339, 1951.
25. Hodgkin, A. L. The Croonian Lecture: Ionic movements and electrical activity in giant nerve fibres. *Proc. Roy. Soc.* [Biol.] 148:1, 1958.
26. Hodgkin, A. L. *The Conduction of the Nervous Impulse*. Springfield, Ill.: Thomas, 1964.
27. Hodgkin, A. L., and Horowicz, P. The influence of potassium and chloride ions on the membrane potential of single muscle fibres. *J. Physiol.* (London) 148:127, 1959.
28. Hodgkin, A. L., and Huxley, A. F. Currents carried by sodium and potassium ions through the membrane of the giant axon of *Loligo*. *J. Physiol.* (London) 116:449, 1952.
29. Hodgkin, A. L., and Huxley, A. F. The components of membrane conductance in the giant axon of *Loligo*. *J. Physiol.* (London) 116:473, 1952.
30. Hodgkin, A. L., and Huxley, A. F. The dual effect of membrane potential on sodium conductance in the giant axon of *Loligo*. *J. Physiol.* (London) 116:497, 1952.
31. Hodgkin, A. L., and Huxley, A. F. A quantitative description of membrane current and its application to conduction and excitation in nerve. *J. Physiol.* (London) 117:500, 1952.
32. Hodgkin, A. L., Huxley, A. F., and Katz, B. Measurements of current-voltage relations in the membrane of the giant axon of *Loligo*. *J. Physiol.* (London) 166:424, 1952.
33. Hodgkin, A. L., and Katz, B. The effect of sodium ions on the electrical activity of the giant axon of the squid. *J. Physiol.* (London) 108:37, 1949.
34. Hodgkin, A. L., and Keynes, R. D. Active transport of cations in giant axons from *Sepia* and *Loligo*. *J. Physiol.* (London) 128:28, 1955.
35. Hodgkin, A. L., and Keynes, R. D. The potassium permeability of a giant nerve fibre. *J. Physiol.* (London) 128:61, 1955.
36. Hodgkin, A. L., and Rushton, W. A. H. The electrical constants of a crustacean nerve fiber. *Proc. Roy. Soc.* [Biol.] 133:444, 1946.

37. Horowicz, P., and Gerber, C. J. Effects of external potassium and strophanthidin on sodium fluxes in frog striated muscle. *J. Gen. Physiol.* 48:489, 1965.

38. Horowicz, P., and Gerber, C. J. Effects of sodium azide on sodium fluxes in frog striated muscle. *J. Gen. Physiol.* 48:515, 1965.

39. Huxley, A. F. Ion movements during nerve activity. *Ann. N.Y. Acad. Sci.* 81:221, 1959.

40. Katz, B. *Nerve, Muscle and Synapse.* New York: McGraw-Hill, 1966.

41. Keynes, R. D. Chloride in the squid giant axon. *J. Physiol.* (London) 169:690, 1963.

42. Keynes, R. D. Some further observations on the sodium efflux in frog muscle. *J. Physiol.* (London) 178:305, 1965.

43. Keynes, R. D., and Maisel, G. W. The energy requirements for sodium extrusion from a frog muscle. *Proc. Roy. Soc.* [Biol.] 142:383, 1954.

44. Keynes, R. D., and Swan, R. C. The effect of external sodium concentration on the sodium fluxes in frog skeletal muscle. *J. Physiol.* (London) 147:591, 1959.

45. Koppenhöfer, E., and Schmidt, H. Incomplete inactivation in nodes of Ranvier treated with scorpion venom. *Experientia* 24:41, 1968.

46. Lecar, H., Ehrenstein, G., Binstock, L., and Taylor, R. E. Removal of potassium negative resistance in perfused squid giant axons. *J. Gen. Physiol.* 50:1499, 1967.

47. Meves, H. Experiments on internally perfused squid giant axons. *Ann. N.Y. Acad. Sci.* 137:807, 1966.

48. Meves, H., and Chandler, W. K. Ionic selectivity in perfused giant axons. *J. Gen. Physiol.* 48:31, 1965.

49. Moore, J. W. Voltage clamp studies on internally perfused axons. *J. Gen. Physiol.* 48:11, 1965.

50. Moore, J. W., Narahashi, T., and Shaw, T. I. An upper limit to the number of sodium channels in nerve and membrane? *J. Physiol.* (London) 188:99, 1967.

51. Narahashi, T., and Moore, J. W. Neuroactive agents and nerve membrane conductances. *J. Gen. Physiol.* 51:93S, 1968.

52. Oikawa, T., Spyropoulos, C. S., Tasaki, I., and Teorell, T. Methods for perfusing the giant axon of *Loligo pealii*. *Acta Physiol. Scand.* 52:195, 1961.

53. Ritchie, J. M., and Straub, R. W. The hyperpolarization which follows activity in mammalian non-medullated fibres. *J. Physiol.* (London) 136:80, 1957.

54. Stein, R. B. The frequency of nerve action potentials generated by applied currents. *Proc. Roy. Soc.* [Biol.] 167:64, 1967.

55. Stein, W. D. *The Movements of Molecules across Cell Membranes.* New York: Academic, 1967.

56. Tasaki, I., Singer, I., and Takenaka, T. Effects of internal and external ionic environment on excitability of squid giant axon. *J. Gen. Physiol.* 48:1095, 1965.

57. Taylor, R. E. Effect of procaine on electrical properties of squid axon membrane. *Amer. J. Physiol.* 196:1071, 1959.

58. Taylor, R. E. Cable Theory. In Nastuk, W. L. (Ed.), *Physical Techniques in Biological Research,* vol. IV, part B. New York: Academic, 1963.

59. Ussing, H. H., Kruhøffer, P., Hess Thasen, J., and Thorn, N. A. *The Alkali Metal Ions in Biology.* Berlin: Springer-Verlag, 1960.

60. Wall, P. D., and Johnson, A. R. Changes associated with post-tetanic potentiation of a monosynaptic reflex. *J. Neurophysiol.* 21:148, 1958.

61. Woodbury, D. M. Effect of diphenylhydantoin on electrolytes and radiosodium turnover in brain and other tissues of normal, hyponatremic and postictal rats. *J. Pharmacol. Exp. Ther.* 115:74, 1955.

62. Woodbury, J. W. Cellular Electrophysiology of the Heart. In Hamilton, W. F. (Ed.), *Handbook of Physiology, Section 2, Circulation, Volume I.* Washington, D. C.: American Physiological Society, 1962.

63. Woodbury, J. W. Interrelationships between ion transport mechanisms and excitatory events. *Fed. Proc.* 22:31, 1963.

64. Woodbury, J. W. The Cell Membrane: Ionic and Potential Gradients and Active Transport, and Action Potential: Properties of Excitable Membranes. In Ruch, T. C., and Patton, H. D. (Eds.), *Physiology and Biophysics* (19th ed.). Philadelphia: Saunders, 1965, chaps. 1 and 2.

65. Woodbury, J. W., White, S. H., Mackey, M. C., Hardy, W. L., and Chang, D. B. Bioelectrochemistry. In Eyring, H., Henderson, D., and Jost, W. (Eds.), *Electrochemistry.* New York: Academic, 1969.

Discussion

VOLTAGE CLAMP ANALYSIS OF A REPETITIVELY FIRING NEURON*

CHARLES F. STEVENS

Because the field of membrane biophysics is large and complex, I shall focus on one aspect of the problem of neuronal excitability rather than attempt to comment on the whole of J. W. Woodbury's excellent and comprehensive treatise [18]. Mechanisms of repetitive discharge appear to be of particular interest in the present context; therefore this discussion will concentrate on some recent results bearing on neuronal mechanisms which permit depolarized nerve cells to discharge long trains of action potentials.

Should epileptic discharge arise from some defect in the membrane-excitability mechanisms of nerve cells, then an understanding of epileptic pathophysiology will turn on knowledge of the excitation process in central nervous system neurons. Although there has been a great increase in information about mechanisms of excitable membranes outside the central nervous system [see 18], technical difficulties so far have precluded adequate analysis of those processes—such as repetitive firing—which characterize the behavior of many mammalian central neurons. This chapter contains a preliminary analysis of data obtained in collaboration with Dr. John Connor on a molluscan model of the mammalian central neuron.

As Woodbury has indicated [18], the Hodgkin-Huxley equations, or simple modifications, do not provide adequate explanation for the type of repetitive firing generally observed in the central nervous system; nor do most of the preparations to which a voltage-clamp analysis may be readily applied exhibit the appropriate behavior. On the other hand, voltage-clamp records from mammalian central neuron somas are difficult to interpret because of loss of current through axons or dendrites whose voltage is not under control. Giant neurons found in many gastropod molluscs would seem to be a favorable preparation in which to study the mechanisms underlying repetitive firing. The reasons are: (1) they exhibit behavior typical of that observed in the mammalian nervous system, (2) they are large and hardy cells which can be penetrated by two or more microelectrodes under visual control, and (3) they have favorable geometry in that the soma is approximately spherical, synapse free, and generally gives rise to only a single, small neurite.

Like other neurons, molluscan neuron somas respond to a large step depolarization with a brief inward current followed by a prolonged outward current. In the voltage region between the resting potential and the firing level, however, the region of the "pacemaker potentials," the molluscan neuron's behavior is dominated by a potassium activation and inactivation to be described in the remainder of this discussion. The mechanism of the action potential is much like that of the squid or frog node, then, but potentials in the interspike interval appear to be controlled by an additional set of processes.

Molluscan Cells

Cells from *Aplysia, Helix,* and a variety of nudibranch molluscs have been examined, but most of the data reported here were obtained from large (4–8 inch) specimens of

---

* This work supported by PHS Research Grant NB05934 from National Institute of Neurological Diseases and Stroke and PHS Research Resources Grant FR00374 from Division of Research Facilities and Resources.

Archidoris collected near Friday Harbor, Washington. The cluster of ganglia forming the brain is removed from the animal and pinned in a chamber filled with sea water maintained at about 9°C. A tough connective tissue sheath encases the ganglia, and this sheath is generally softened with pronase for about 5 minutes before it is dissected free, although in some experiments the nerve cells have been exposed by sharp dissection alone. The preparation is not a difficult one, and isolated brains have been maintained in apparently good condition for up to 3 days.

The typical molluscan neuron (Fig. D3-1A) has a nearly spherical soma and a single neurite which branches in the underlying neuropil. Neurons with a soma diameter of approximately 300 μ are generally selected for the studies described here; smaller cells do not withstand the required procedures well, and the larger cells demand excessively large currents to control their voltage. Because a loss of current down this neurite would make the voltage-clamp record difficult to interpret, it is necessary to isolate the soma from its axo-dendritic tree. This is generally done by tying a fine, silk ligature around the neurite approximately 300–600 μ from the soma [15]. When the soma is thus isolated, 2 KCl-filled glass microelectrodes (resistance 5–10 megohms) are inserted through the soma membrane. The general arrangement is illustrated schematically in Fig. D3-1B.

Voltage-Clamping Techniques. Voltages are led from the recording microelectrode through a field-effect transistor, negative-capacity amplifier into the oscilloscope and into the voltage-clamping amplifiers (Fig. D3-1B). The negative-capacity amplifier is constructed with the input transistor mounted next to the microelectrode in order to reduce the input capacitance, and the capacity negation permits a rise time to injected current steps of less than 10 μsec for a 10-megohm electrode. The voltage-clamping amplifiers themselves are constructed from high frequency response, operational amplifiers, and a final amplifier stage with a 0 to ±50 V operating range is used to drive the required currents through the microelectrode. Proper operation of this arrangement requires careful shielding between the voltage recording and the current-passing electrodes. Current is measured with a field-effect transistor, operational amplifier whose feedback maintains the bath at essentially ground potential. Under ideal conditions, a rapid change in voltage from one level to another is accomplished in 200–500 μsec, but the usual settling times are generally 1–2 msec; under extremely bad conditions, the desired voltage is not established accurately in less than 10 or 20 msec. Experiments using two recording electrodes have shown that the soma is isopotential to within about 5 percent.

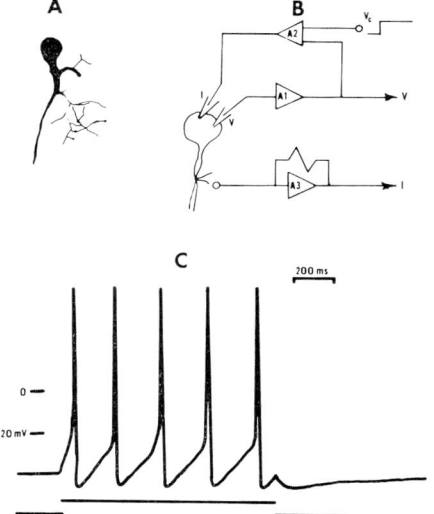

FIG. D3-1. (A) Projection drawing of neuron from *Anisodoris* prepared by rapid Golgi technique. Soma of neuron about 30 μ in diameter; thus neurite is much larger in comparison to soma diameter than is case for neurons employed in this study. (B) Schematic representation of experimental arrangement. A neuron whose ligated axon is penetrated by 2 microelectrodes; electrode designated V records voltage and that designated I is used to pass current. A1 represents negative capacity preamplifier and A2 the voltage-clamping amplifier which amplifies difference between membrane potential and desired voltage V_c. Current is measured with amplifier A3. (C) Typical response of a molluscan neuron to constant current stimulation. Upper trace gives membrane potential as function of time; lower trace indicates current applied through a second electrode.

Apparently normal cells in the gastropod molluscs have a resting potential (under the conditions of these experiments) in the range of −35 to −60 mV, with the most commonly observed values between −40 and −45 mV. At the peak of an action potential, the membrane voltage attains a value between +40 and +60 mV, so that typical action potentials are approximately 90 mV in amplitude. The firing level of these cells is generally between −20 and −30 mV, with −25 mV being a typical value. Those neurons with a resting potential more positive than −50 to −60 mV always exhibit an afterhyperpolarization which lasts approximately 1 sec. This afterhyperpolarization generally reaches −55 to −60 mV and has a decay course which appears to be exponential. The cells we study generally have resistances in the range of 0.5–2 megohms, and cell time constants from about 40–70 msec. In preparations maintained at 9°C, spike durations of approximately 30–35 msec are typical.

Discharge Frequencies. Most healthy molluscan neurons will exhibit a maintained repetitive discharge when subjected to a constant suprathreshold current (Fig. D3-1C). In some instances, nerve-impulse frequency (reciprocal interspike interval) is constant from the first interval onward while, in other instances, the initial interval is shortest and frequency decreases—approximately exponentially—to its steady value. Plots of steady-state frequency as a function of current intensity are invariably linear over a considerable range, although sufficiently large depolarizations damage the cell and cause a deviation from this linear relationship. At 9°C, steady frequencies as slow as 0.1 per second are observed, and the linear relation holds from these low frequencies up to 5 or 10 per second or more. If time is scaled to make spike durations comparable to those observed in the mammalian nervous system, this would correspond to a frequency range of about 1 per second to 50 to 100 per second.

If the membrane potential is changed stepwise from approximately −40 mV to −20 mV or above, an inward-outward current sequence is observed which appears to be qualitatively like that seen in other neurons (Fig. D3-2A). The rate of rise and peak amplitude of the inward current increase rapidly with increasing depolarizations; total duration of the inward current is on the order of 20 msec. The outward current similarly increases with depolarizations, and reaches its final value with a time constant

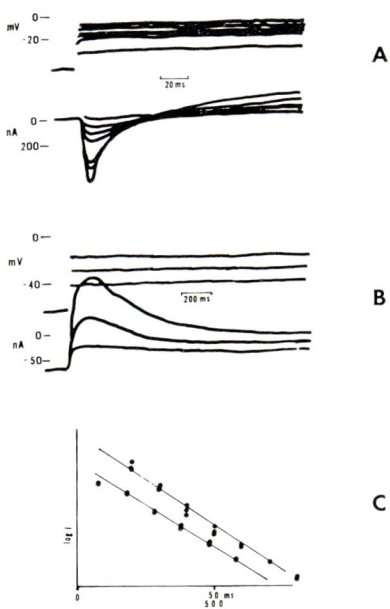

FIG. D3-2. (A) Response of the membrane to voltage steps from −40 mV to −25 mV and above. Upper traces show membrane voltage, and lower traces give membrane current. Downward deflection indicates inward current. (B) Response of membrane to voltage steps from −60 to the voltage region between resting potential and firing level. Rectangular upper traces give membrane potential, and lower traces give membrane current; upward deflection indicates outward current. (C) Semilogarithmic plot of deviation of membrane current from its final value as a function of time. Abscissa of this graph is arbitrary to within an additive constant. Lower curve gives "scaled" currents from declining phase of responses similar to those shown in (B) above. Points from currents caused by 8 different voltage levels are superimposed, but scaled values are so close to the same that it is impossible to distinguish points from separate records. Time scale for this graph is 0–500 msec. Upper graph gives fourth root of currents during rising phase of records similar to those shown in (B) above. Records from 4 different voltage levels were used and scaled to cover same range. Time scale for upper curve is 0–50 msec.

in the range of 80–300 msec. In some preparations, this outward current decreases slowly with time in a manner reminiscent of the potassium inactivation behavior of squid [5], frog nodes [6], puffer supermedullary neurons [11], and frog skeletal muscle [1]. The apparent equilibrium potential of this outward current is in the vicinity of −55 mV, and the ion carrying this current is, as in other membranes, probably predominately potassium. In summary, the voltage-clamp behavior of these gastropod neurons is, in the range of membrane potentials between −40 and 0 mV, qualitatively similar to the original Hodgkin-Huxley analysis of a cephalopod axon.

The results of step-voltage changes in the range from −60 to −20 mV (the potassium equilibrium potential to the firing level) yield quite different results (Fig. D3-2B). A relatively rapid outward current decreases almost to zero or in some cases actually becomes inward (Fig. D3-2B). This inward current develops with a time constant of approximately 30 msec (at 9°C) and decays with a time constant about one order of magnitude higher—approximately 300 msec. Because the equilibrium potential of this conductance change is normally around 60 mV and depends on the outside potassium concentration (but not on sodium or chloride), it would seem that a potassium activation-inactivation sequence constitutes the active membrane response in the subthreshold voltage range.

Unlike the traditional delayed rectification potassium conductance, the time constants of this subthreshold potassium activation-inactivation sequence are not membrane-potential dependent over the voltage range from −60 to −20 mV. It is apparent from Fig. D3-2C that no detectable change in the activation or inactivation time constant is apparent over the range of voltages from −60 to −20 mV. Furthermore, inactivation appears to develop with a single time constant, whereas activation is best fitted by an exponential raised to the third or fourth power; for many purposes, however, this activation process may be adequately approximated by the simple exponential. Amplitude of the activation process seems to increase with the square of the voltage and shows no saturation over the range of voltages extending to −20 mV. On the other hand, the steady-state value of the inactivation is close to 1 at membrane potentials of −60 mV, and approaches zero for membrane potentials in the vicinity of −30 mV. In most cells, then, this second potassium system is largely inactivated at the resting potential. For this reason, step changes from −40 up to −20 mV or above show predominately the typical, delayed rectification currents (Fig. D3-2) and do not reveal the rapid component of potassium activation directly.

Activation and Inactivation Processes. The voltage-clamp data may be described by a quantitative model similar to the first proposed by Hodgkin and Huxley for the squid axon [18]. If attention is restricted to the subthreshold voltage range, only the potassium activation-inactivation process need be described. Differential equations which specify the course of activation and inactivation are found without difficulty (see Appendix) and the solution of these equations is in agreement with the observed behavior of the cell. The solid lines in Fig. D3-3 represent the membrane potential recorded from a neuron which was first hyperpolarized and then depolarized by constant current stimulation through an intracellular electrode. The open circles give the response predicted from equations (and

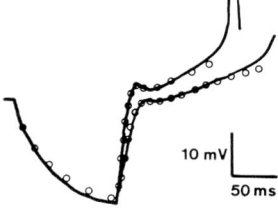

FIG. D3-3. Two superimposed membrane-potential traces as a function of time. Cell was first hyperpolarized (downward deflection in curves above) and then depolarized by a varying amount. Open circles are predictions of membrane potential derived from a voltage-clamp analysis of this same cell. Notice that observed and predicted traces deviate for larger depolarizations because calculations did not include effect of inward-current mechanism. Form of equations giving these predicted responses is in the Appendix to this discussion.

constants) determined by the voltage-clamp behavior of the same cell. The agreement between the predicted and the observed responses is evidence that the subthreshold behavior of the cell is adequately explained by the potassium activation-inactivation mechanisms described above.

If a spike is elicited and if voltage control is then instituted at the termination of the spike, it is possible to study conductance changes which normally follow in the wake of the action potential. Such studies reveal a high conductance immediately after the spike which (after a faster initial change) returns to normal with a time constant of approximately 200–300 msec. This conductance is associated with an equilibrium potential of approximately −60 mV, which (together with results from studies on the effect of various potassium concentrations in the bathing medium) indicates that most of the current is carried by the potassium ion. Currents associated with afterhyperpolarization are thus produced by variations in the potassium conductance and presumably reflect the return to normal of the delayed rectification potassium conductance which has increased during the spike, together with a recovery from inactivation (depending on the membrane potential) of the rapid potassium-activation channels. It is interesting to note that the time constant for delayed rectification potassium activation and the time constant of inactivation for the rapid potassium conductance channels are, at the resting potential, approximately the same.

Although analysis is not yet sufficiently complete to yield equations describing the entire range of behavior exhibited by these molluscan neurons, a clear qualitative picture does emerge of the mechanisms underlying repetitive discharge. Immediately after one spike, the membrane is driven to the vicinity of the potassium equilibrium potential by the large, delayed rectification potassium conductance. As this conductance decays toward resting values, the membrane potential moves toward the firing level, and, as the firing level is approached, potassium inactivation increases the cell's resistance; this resistance increase causes applied currents—synaptic or through a microelectrode —to produce increased depolarizations. The total effect of all of these changes is a membrane potential of nearly linear rise to the firing level. A qualitative description of these processes based on voltage-clamp data will presumably permit accurate prediction of the entire course of membrane potential between one spike and the next.

Possible Role in Mammalian Nervous System

It may, indeed, be wondered to what extent the processes described here also play a role in the mammalian nervous system. Just as analysis of the action potential in squid has carried over to the vertebrate nervous system, so is there some evidence that processes such as those described earlier also occur in the mammalian central nervous system. One consequence of the potassium inactivation near the firing level is a phenomenon known as *anomalous rectification*. Because the potassium channels inactivate, cell resistance is larger for depolarizing pulses than for hyperpolarizing pulses, and a given magnitude of current thus causes a larger membrane-potential deviation in the depolarizing direction than in the hyperpolarizing direction. This phenomenon of anomalous rectification, first described in nerve cells by Kandel and Tauc [8], has now been observed in cat spinal motoneurons [7, 13], cat cortical pyramidal cells [17], hippocampal pyramidal cells [16], and inferior olive neurons [4]. Although it has not yet been demonstrated that anomalous rectification in these neurons is the result of potassium inactivation, this is certainly the most parsimonious explanation. Cat spinal motoneurons [7] and cortical pyramidal cells [9, 10] have both been shown to respond to subthreshold currents in ways not expected from their passive electrical properties. A qualitatively similar deviation occurs, as a result of potassium activation-inactivation in the neurons described in this discussion (Fig. D3-3). Altogether then, it would appear that the processes we have described in the molluscan neurons are probably also present in the vertebrate central nervous system, although direct proof of this supposition will, of course, be required.

Potassium Inactivation. Potassium inactivation occurs in a number of systems. The inactivation described in the squid axon [5], the frog node [6], frog muscle membrane [1], and puffer supermedullary neurons [11] is much slower than that found in the present work and generally seems to be associated with the delayed rectification mechanism. Electroplaques [2, 12] and heart Purkinje fibers [14] also show a potassium "inactivation," but in both instances this process occurs—within the limits of experimental error—instantaneously. If pentyltriethylammonium iodide ions are injected into the squid axon, a more rapid potassium inactivation occurs, which is in some respects similar to that described here [13]. The relationship between all of these forms of potassium inactivation must, however, await further investigation.

In summary, the subthreshold behavior of a repetitively firing gastropod model of central neurons is dominated by voltage sensitive variations in potassium conductance. In addition to the delayed-rectification type of potassium conductance which produces the afterhyperpolarization seen in many neurons, a second potassium activation-inactivation mechanism is present which can play an important role in subthreshold behavior. At the membrane level, then, defects in any of the three mechanisms—sodium activation-inactivation, delayed rectification potassium activation, and the potassium activation-inactivation sequence described here—could conceivably be altered to produce unstable behavior of the neuron and initiate mass epileptic discharge. For example, if the potassium inactivation approached zero for potentials more negative than the normal cell resting potential, a neuron could become so sensitive to slight depolarizing synaptic currents that spike discharge would be elicited with almost any excitatory input. Alternatively, if the time constants for the delayed rectification potassium activation and the potassium inactivation described here were decreased, neurons would tend to discharge more rapidly for the same synaptic input; such an increased discharge also could, in the context of complex neuronal circuits, conceivably give rise to the type of instabilities seen in epilepsy.

The fact that pharmacological agents can cause quite dramatic changes in various of the parameters which describe neuronal behavior implies that disease states could *in principle* produce the instabilities of neuronal behavior seen in epilepsy. If we are to understand the pathophysiology of disorders at the level of the excitable membrane, whether these disorders be disease or drug induced, then a knowledge of the normal mechanisms of the types described here is prerequisite.

Appendix

The equations described here serve as a quantitative specification of the neuronal properties discussed in the body of the discussion. Only the subthreshold behavior is considered; thus membrane voltage must be more negative than -20 to -30 mV for these equations to apply.

A Hodgkin-Huxley equivalent circuit for the soma membrane gives the basic voltage-current relation:

$$C \frac{dV}{dt} + g_K(V(t) - V_K) + g_o(V(t) - V_o) = i_A(t) \quad \text{(D3-1)}$$

Here C is the membrane capacitance; $V(t)$ the deviation of the membrane potential from the resting potential at time t; g_K the potassium conductance; V_K the potassium equilibrium potential; g_o the lumped conductance of all other ions; V_o the lumped equilibrium potential of all other ions; and $i_A(t)$ the current applied at time t. The potassium conductance g_K depends on voltage and time through two terms, $A(V,t)$ (activation) and $B(V,t)$ (inactivation), according to the relation

$$g_K = A(V,t)[1 - B(V,t)]\bar{g}_K \quad \text{(D3-2)}$$

A and B vary between 0 and 1, and $\bar{g}_K$ is a constant which specifies the maximum possible potassium conductance. The dependence of A and B on voltage and time is given by

$$\tau_A \frac{dA(V,t)}{dt} = \overline{A}(V) - A(V,t) \quad \text{(D3-3)}$$

$$\tau_B \frac{dB(V,t)}{dt} = \overline{B}(V) - B(V,t) \quad \text{(D3-4)}$$

The time constants τ_A and τ_B (in contrast to analogous parameters in the Hodgkin-Huxley equations) do not depend on voltage. The parameter $\overline{A}(V)$ depends on voltage but not on time, and the precise dependence is determined empirically; this factor increases approximately as the square of the voltages. In a more accurate description, it would be necessary for $A(V)$ to enter as the third or fourth power in Eq. D3-2. Like $\overline{A}(V)$, the term $\overline{B}(V)$ depends on voltage but not on time, in a manner determined from experiment. Generally, $\overline{B}(V)$ increases in a sigmoid fashion from nearly zero from voltages 30 mV more negative than the resting potential to nearly one at depolarization (relative to the resting potential) of 10 mV. Solution of these equations by machine computation produced the predicted responses in Fig. D3-3.

REFERENCES

1. Adrian, R. H., Chandler, W. K., and Hodgkin, A. L. Voltage clamp experiments in striated muscle fibers. *J. Gen. Physiol.* 51:188, 1968.
2. Bennet, M. V. L., and Grundfest, H. Analysis of depolarizing and hyperpolarizing inactivation responses in gymnotid electroplaques. *J. Gen. Physiol.* 50:141, 1966.
3. Chandler, C. M. Induced inactivation of the potassium permeability of squid axon membrane. *Nature* (London) 219:1262, 1968.
4. Crill, W. E. Unitary multiple spiked responses in the cat inferior olive nucleus. *J. Neurophysiol*, in press.
5. Ehrenstein, G., and Gilbert, C. L. Slow changes of potassium permeability in the squid giant axon. *Biophys. J.* 6:555, 1966.
6. Frankenhaeuser, B., and Waltman, B. Membrane resistance and conduction velocity of large myelinated nerve fibers from *Xenopus laevis*. *J. Physiol.* (London) 148:677, 1959.
7. Ito, M., and Oshima, T. Electrical behavior of the motoneurone membrane during intracellularly applied current steps. *J. Physiol.* (London) 180:607, 1965.
8. Kandel, E. R., and Tauc, L. Anomalous rectification in the metacerebral giant cells and its consequences for synaptic transmission. *J. Physiol.* (London) 183:287, 1966.
9. Koike, H., Okada, Y., Oshima, T., and Takahashi, K. Accommodative behavior of cat pyramidal tract cells investigated with intracellular injection of currents. *Exp. Brain Res.* 5:173, 1968.
10. Koike, H., Okada, Y., and Oshima, T. Accommodative properties of fast and slow pyramidal tract cells and their modification by different levels of their membrane potential. *Exp. Brain Res.* 5:189, 1968.
11. Nakajima, S. Analysis of K inactivation and TEA action in the supramedullary cells of Puffer. *J. Gen. Physiol.* 49:629, 1966.
12. Nakamura, Y., Nakajima, S., and Grundfest, H. Analysis of spike electrogenesis and depolarizing K inactivation in electroplaques of *Electrophorus electricus*, L. *J. Gen. Physiol.* 49:321, 1965.
13. Nelson, P. G., and Frank, K. Anomalous rectification in cat spinal motoneurons and effect of polarizing currents on excitatory postsynaptic potentials. *J. Neurophysiol.* 30:1097, 1967.
14. Noble, D., and Tsien, R. W. The kinetics and rectifier properties of the slow potassium current in cardiac Purkinje fibres. *J. Physiol.* (London) 195:185, 1968.
15. Oomura, Y., and Maeno, T. Does the neurone soma actually generate action potentials? *Nature* (London) 197:358, 1963.
16. Purpura, D. P., Prelevic, S., and Santini, M. Hyperpolarizing increase in membrane conductance in hippocampal neurons. *Brain Res.* 7:310, 1968.
17. Takahashi, K. Slow and fast groups of pyramidal tract cells and their respective membrane properties. *J. Neurophysiol.* 28:908, 1965.
18. Woodbury, J. W. Biophysics of Nerve Membrane. In Jasper, H. H., Ward, A. A., Jr., and Pope, A. (Eds.), *Basic Mechanisms of the Epilepsies*. Boston: Little, Brown, 1969.

4
Cerebral Energy Metabolism and Membrane Phenomena*

HENRY McILWAIN

THIS CONTRIBUTION concerns major aspects of the flux of chemical substances during cerebral activities. Energy-yielding and energy-utilizing processes are especially involved and the passage of ions between intracellular and extracellular compartments of the brain. Table 4-1 lists several of the processes involved, in the order in which they will be discussed.

The human brain takes considerable part in the energy turnover of the body as a whole [54], and concepts of energy and material flux were much involved in Hughlings Jackson's [34] characterization of the epilepsies about a century ago. The "excessive, rapid and local discharge," by which he described the conditions, he saw as an expenditure of energy, drawing appropriate analogies in chemical terms to muscular activities. The "instabilities of cerebral grey matter" in epileptic conditions were chemical instability and successive exhaustion of the parts first and most convulsed, and contributed to his explanation of the "Jacksonian march." Indeed Jackson and some of his contemporaries had a qualitative understanding of energy relationships in the brain, which can be seen today as quite appropriate and enlightened [25, 34, 50, 55].

ENERGY-YIELDING PROCESSES

Detailed metabolic studies of the mammalian brain in vivo and of preparations from it in vitro have repeatedly emphasized its specialization to glucose as main energy source and have afforded consistent data regarding the many enzymic stages involved in glucose utilization by respiration and glycolysis [3, 44, 45, 54]. This utilization is expressed in Table 4-1 as the equivalents of energy-rich phosphate links formed; the sites and mechanisms of their formation will not be discussed in the present account but emphasis given to alterations induced by excitation.

Cerebral Respiration

Respiration of the brain in situ has been studied more extensively in man than in experimental animals. The value (Table 4-1) of 3.3 ml O_2 absorbed per 100 grams of brain per hour refers to man and specifically to normal young adult subjects [40, 54, 78]; it is derived by analysis of arterial and cerebral venous blood. Cerebral respiratory rate so measured can be independent of cerebral blood flow over a considerable range of values, but may undergo a three-fold variation according to the level of activity in the brain. In particular, cerebral respiration can be halved during surgical anesthesia and increased by extreme apprehensiveness or by perfusion of adrenaline.

During convulsive episodes, also, cerebral respiration is greatly increased. With convulsions induced experimentally in monkeys [75], oxygen uptake cerebrally was observed to double in rate with increased output of carbon dioxide, but in

* Supported by the research fund of Bethlem Royal Hospital and Maudsley Hospital.

TABLE 4-1. Major Processes of Cerebral Energy Metabolism

I Energy-yielding		II Intermediates		III Energy-consuming	
(i)	Respiration: Normally, 3.3 ml O_2/ 100 g/hr: 530 $\sim$P	(i)	Adenosinetriphosphate, phosphocreatine: Utilization, 1250 $\sim$P	(i)	Active cation movements Na, K–ATPase 1060 $\sim$P
(ii)	Glycolysis: Normal, 30 $\sim$P Maximal, 2000 $\sim$P	(ii)	Na, K: Downhill movements maximal, 1500	(ii)	Synthetic processes

(a) Quantitative data are approximate and given in µEq per gram of cerebral tissue per hour unless otherwise specified.

(b) $\sim$P represents bond energy available on hydrolysis of the terminal phosphate of adenosinetriphosphate. Formation of 1 mole of lactate from glucose is regarded as yielding 1 $\sim$P, and uptake of 1 mole O_2 as yielding 6 $\sim$P.

the postconvulsive state, to fall below normal. Increase in cerebral respiration and in CO_2 output has also been shown during generalized grand mal seizures [63, 64]. These were induced in epileptic subjects by hyperventilation or by 3-ethyl-3-methylglutarimide, were accompanied by generalized, high-voltage multiple spikes seen electroencephalographically and by a large increase in blood flow. Increased cerebral CO_2 output was also observed to accompany *electrodecremental seizures* which occurred spontaneously in a subject suffering post-traumatic epilepsy. This involved movements occurring in a Jacksonian series, but without loss of consciousness and with no postictal confusion [63]. Before initiation of overt seizures, some degree of electroencephalographic activation may occur and also be associated with increased cerebral oxygen uptake [63].

Human cerebral tissues taken from the temporal cortex of six cases of psychomotor epilepsy, but not including visible lesions, were examined metabolically in vitro [46]. With glucose as substrate, tissues respired at rates not significantly different from those of human neocortical samples, also apparently normal, obtained during operation for other illnesses [29, 46]. A few of the temporal specimens were examined with other substrates but without finding characteristics peculiar to the illness of the patients from whom they were obtained. Many of these tissue samples, as well as other cerebral tissues from man and from experimental animals, increased in respiratory rate on electrical excitation in vitro [46, 48, 49, 60]. Sustained increase in respiratory rate to 180–200 percent of the unstimulated value was found and was maintained for at least 30–60 minutes. Extent of the increase depended on frequency, duration, and potential of the applied pulses [47], and stimulated tissues were significantly different from unstimulated in their susceptibility to a number of drugs [49, 60]. Among anticonvulsants, diphenylhydantoin, methylethylphenylhydantoin, and trimethyloxazolidinedione were without action on neocortical samples respiring with a number of substrates, but they wholly or partly prevented increase in respiration caused by electrical stimulation [26]. Relatively low concentrations acted, but were without effect on tissue respiration comparably increased by potassium chloride, guanidine, or 2:4-dinitrophenol. Some specificity was shown in relation to stimulating pulses of different electrical characteristics, and the data gave assurance that anticonvulsants had direct cerebral actions.

Glycolysis

This second major process of deriving energy-rich phosphates from glucose, in converting it to lactate by the glycolytic sequence, can during brief periods yield the phosphates at rates greater than that of their normal formation by respiration (Table 4-1). In 1887, indication of increased lactate formation on excitation of spinal cord or brain by strychnine or electrical

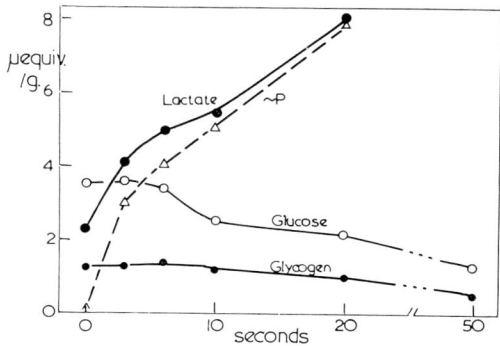

FIG. 4-1. Effects of one second electrical stimulation on components of outer portions of the cerebral hemispheres of mice [42]. Animals were transferred to freezing liquids at times specified. Calculated change in energy utilization from this and other data is given as P equiv. (See Table 4-1.)

stimulation was given [85]. The most accurate information on change in level of glycolysis with cerebral excitation is derived from experimental animals and by techniques of rapid in situ fixation (Fig. 4-1). Indeed these techniques were developed in order to obtain dependable values for the glucose, glycogen, and lactic acid of the brain [39]. Determination of these substances by many investigations in five animal species [54] has shown very large increase in glycolysis to accompany excitation of the brain by convulsive drugs and by direct electrical stimulation.

In mice, the lactate formed during a few seconds' electrical stimulation is greater than could be produced from the glucose, glycogen, and intermediates already present in the brain plus the glucose normally arriving from the bloodstream [42]; it appears, therefore, that entry of glucose to the brain is accelerated during convulsions. Convulsive activity can indeed be prolonged in experimental animals by raised blood-glucose concentrations. Most of the glucose of the brain is extracellular [3], and its entry to the cellular compartments, even in isolated tissues, is subject to inhibition in a fashion suggesting carrier mediation [24]. With normal levels of blood glucose in mice, cerebral lactate increased during the first few seconds of electrical stimulation at rates corresponding to formation of 3000–4000 μmoles per gram of cortex per hour. These extremely high rates can result in doubling cerebral lactate content in 3–6 sec [42], but are not sustained nor reflected in correspondingly large and rapid increase of lactate in cerebral venous blood. Administration of general depressants prior to excision of cerebral tissues from experimental animals preserved much glycogen, which otherwise would have been converted to lactate [61]; on electrical stimulation, phenobarbital but not secobarbital retarded conversion [42].

During convulsive activity in some epileptic subjects, analysis of arterial and cerebral venous blood has suggested an increased acidity to which cerebral lactate formation may contribute [63]. Human cerebral tissues in isolation, in common with those from other species examined, form lactate from glucose [46, 54, 61] at rates similar to those obtaining in the brain in vivo. Moreover, the formation can be increased by electrical excitation [60, 61]. Again, the greatest rates are obtained in the first few seconds of stimulation [61], but, in addition, a sustained increase in tissue glycolysis accompanied the sustained increase in respiration, which was noted above to result from electrical excitation during periods of an hour or more. Increased lactate formation was found in cerebral samples from temporal lobes of subjects suffering psychomotor epilepsy [46].

INTERMEDIATES AND ENERGY-STORES

In his descriptions of epileptic conditions, Hughlings Jackson repeatedly wrote of the abilities of nerve tissue or of the brain to store up and expend energy, which was described as the potential energy from the blood or from nutrient fluids of the brain and as a reservoir of molecular motion [34]. Some sixty years elapsed before the molecules concerned were chemically identified. Then, following characterization of adenosinetriphosphate and phospho-

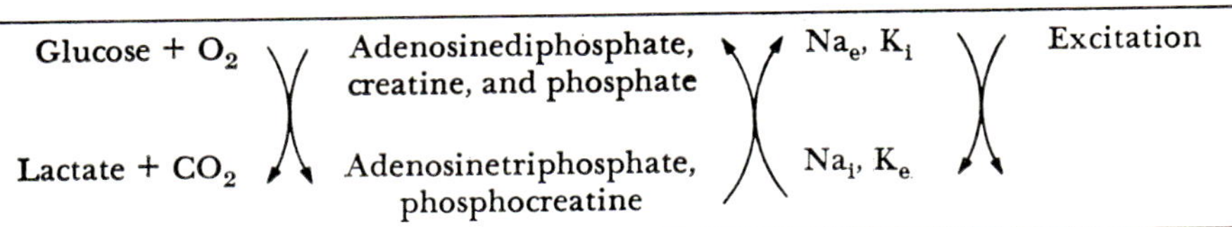

```
Glucose + O₂        Adenosinediphosphate,      Naₑ, Kᵢ         Excitation
                    creatine, and phosphate
Lactate + CO₂       Adenosinetriphosphate,     Naᵢ, Kₑ
                    phosphocreatine
```

FIG. 4-2. Linkage between processes of Table 4-1. Subscript e, extracellular; i, intracellular. Processes are linked in the sense that increased Na_i and K_e resulting from excitation stimulate breakdown of adenosinetriphosphate, which restores the cations and yields adenosinediphosphate and phosphate, which accelerate glucose utilization, which resynthesizes adenosinetriphosphate.

creatine as representing the rapidly available energy sources in muscle, these same compounds and also glycogen were identified in the brain. As befits their role in supporting cerebral activities, changes in these compounds on central excitation can be extremely rapid, and their determination has depended on methods of rapid fixation. A major fashion in which the energy-rich compounds support cerebral activities is adumbrated in Fig. 4-2; from this figure and Table 4-1, it can be seen that the reservoir of molecular motion would now be expressed largely in terms of ion gradients and phosphate-bond energy.

Adenosinetriphosphate and Phosphocreatine

These substances form a minority, about 10 percent, of phosphate derivatives of the brain [54] but are those which undergo the greatest changes in cerebral excitation (Fig. 4-3). Detailed information of their alteration with changed level of cerebral activity has come largely from experimental animals either fixed for analysis in vivo or used as a source of tissues for examination in vitro; the latter techniques are applicable also to human cerebral tissues. The two substances are linked by the enzyme creatine phosphokinase:

$$\text{P-creatine} + \text{ADP} \rightleftharpoons \text{ATP} + \text{creatine}$$

The phosphokinase is highly active in mammalian cerebral tissues and from this source has received extensive purification and characterization [87]. Equilibrium at the kinase is such that adenosinediphosphate formed from the triphosphate is largely rephosphorylated while phosphocreatine is available. Consequently, excitation frequently causes greater changes in the cerebral level of phosphocreatine than of adenosinetriphosphate, although the triphosphate is the compound first utilized. Fig. 4-3 gives an example.

In Vivo. Determination of adenosinetriphosphate and phosphocreatine in the brain of five animal species by many investigators [54] has shown depletion of the compounds to follow disturbance of normal energy-yielding processes of the brain: in hypoxia and hypoglycemia and on administering sodium cyanide, when the development of electroencephalographically observed abnormalities was correlated with loss of phosphocreatine and accumulation of cerebral lactate [68]. Depletion of phosphocreatine and adenosinetriphosphate follows also when convulsions are induced by a number of agents; this is shown in more detail in the case of electrical stimulation, in Fig. 4-3 [65]. This and subsequent data [42, 45] have shown that brief electrical excitation can initiate loss of energy-rich phosphate derivatives ($\sim$P), which continues during and immediately after stimuli at rates up to 2000–3000 µEq P per gram of tissue per hour. Again, the limited cerebral reserves of phosphocreatine and adenosinetriphosphate allow these high rates to operate for only a few seconds. Some 30 sec after the precipitous fall in $\sim$P caused by electroshock of mice, recovery occurred, and the animals showed increasing alertness while their cerebral phosphocreatine and adenosinetriphosphate were half to two-thirds of their normal concentrations [42].

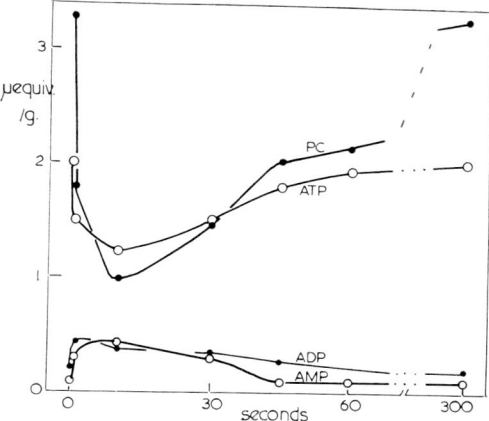

Fig. 4-3. Adenosinephosphates (ATP, ADP, and AMP) and phosphocreatine (PC) in the brain of rats after application of electroshock for one second [65].

It should be emphasized that the large initial changes of Figs. 4-1 and 4-3 do not represent disorganization of cerebral metabolism as a result of convulsive activity. Rather, they indicate adjustments which take place when utilization of adenosinetriphosphate is excessive in a system which normally remains fully capable of recovery. The changes of Figs. 4-1 and 4-3 are part of a complex series of alterations which occur in many metabolites, which have been examined as a means of adjusting energy metabolism to functional need; they may merit more detailed study in tissue from epileptogenic foci. One aspect only is noted in Fig. 4-2: adenosinediphosphate and inorganic phosphate produced in the course of utilizing energy-rich phosphate of adenosinetriphosphate accelerate the respiration and glycolysis which re-form adenosinetriphosphate.

Cerebral stimulation by a characteristically different type of excitant, methamphetamine, also depleted cerebral energy-rich phosphates, and glycogen [20], although at a rate much slower than that following electroshock. Anticonvulsants opposed the actions of electrical excitation on tissue phosphates: in mice, phenobarbital diminished both the overt effects of electroshock, and the diminution of phosphocreatine and adenosinetriphosphate [42].

In Vitro. Many of the preceding observations have been reproduced with isolated tissues from the brain [26, 51, 54], and this contributes greatly to demonstrating the autonomy of such tissues. Although in the course of preparing tissues, their $\sim P$ content falls rapidly, incubation in oxygenated glucose salines largely restores the adenosinetriphosphate and phosphocreatine; restoration is aided by also providing creatine and adenosine in incubating salines, and is diminished by various metabolic inhibitors. The resynthesized phosphocreatine and adenosinetriphosphate are susceptible to extremely rapid loss on electrical stimulation of the tissue, the initial fall occurring at some 1500 μEq of $\sim P$ per gram per hour. Cessation of stimulation was followed by prompter recovery of $\sim P$ than occurred in vivo, presumably because the isolated tissue shows only limited ongoing electrical activity. Recovery proceeded at some 150 μEq of $\sim P$ per gram per hour, which was appreciably less than the $\sim P$ equivalent to the additional energy-yielding processes available. But, as is indicated below, $\sim P$ is being utilized also in other recovery processes, of which a major part concerns the cations now to be discussed.

Sodium and Potassium

Extracellular, interstitial fluids comprise some 20–25 percent of the volume of the mammalian brain [51, 54, 56, 83] and are of composition similar to cerebrospinal fluid. Thus, they differ markedly from the intracellular fluids of cerebral cells, especially in their content of the simple ions Na^+, K^+, and Cl^-. It is to these differences and to permeability characteristics of external nerve-cell membranes that cerebral cells owe their membrane potentials and the many properties which depend on such potentials.

The microscopically visible, external nerve-cell membranes of the brain comprise some 820,000 mm^2 per gram [54, 57], and electron microscopy suggests the true area to be some 5–10 times this value; it also indicates the fundamental barrier between intracellular and extracellular phases to be a bimolecular lipid layer with associated protein layers. Across this great area of minutely thin membrane is deployed a forty-fivefold difference in K^+ concentration and sevenfold difference in Na^+. Here indeed is Hughlings Jackson's or Gowers' potential energy of the nerve centers, poised for discharge in a fashion which was appropriately likened to the discharge of electric fishes or electric batteries.

In Vivo Measurements. Cerebral excitation does indeed involve large transmembrane movements of Na and K, as amply shown by techniques which study fluids in immediate contact with parts of the brain. Only with difficulty, however, is change determined in Na and K by analysis of blood entering and leaving the brain. This is so partly because of the considerable Na and K content of blood and its change in response to activities of other organs of the body. However, it is also because specific mechanisms exist, as part of blood-brain barrier systems, which control and often minimize electrolyte movements to and from the brain [5, 36, 57, 82, 83].

A recent study [63] involving continuous recording of electrolytes of arterial and cerebral venous blood with electrodes that are sensitive to Na^+ and K^+, made it probable that during one type of epileptic seizure, Na entered the brain and K was lost, although rates of movement were not available. Rates can be given from experiments in which the substances were determined in the brain of rats, some of which received electrical stimulation [51, 88]. Here cerebral Na increased at about 1–2 μEq per gram per minute during excitation and convulsive activity, with subsequent return to normal values. Outflow of ^{42}K from the neocortex of the rabbit into a small cup of fluid held in contact with the cortical surface has been detected as occurring during spreading depression [7], which features an initial phase of excitation.

In Vitro Measurements. The data just recounted necessarily contrast with the precise and detailed information obtained for Na and K movements in squid and crustacean nerve fibers examined in vitro.

The contrast does not reflect fundamentally different ion mechanisms, but experimental choice. By also examining mammalian neural systems under satisfactory metabolic conditions in vitro, correspondingly high rates of cation movement were found (Table 4-1). Such experiments were indeed first carried out with samples of mammalian neocortical tissues [59]; subsequently similar rates were observed in a peripheral nonmyelinated fiber tract [41].

Isolated tissues from several parts of the brain maintain, during in vitro incubation, Na and K contents approaching their values in vivo. By applying electrical stimuli to such tissues and determining Na and K contents after chosen periods, minimum values are obtained for movements which are induced by stimulation in the two ions (Fig. 4-4). The values are described as minimal because, as can be judged by preceding data, recovery processes are already in progress. Recovery processes are readily displayed by interrupting stimulation when tissue composition returns toward its previous values. During initial excitation, both rate and extent of cation change were found to depend on electrical characteristics of stimuli applied. Optimal parameters for in vitro change were close to those required

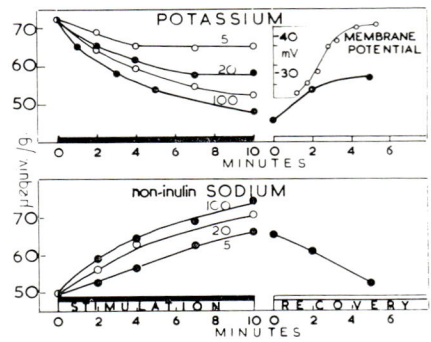

FIG. 4-4. Movements of Na and K of isolated cerebral tissues on electrical stimulation and during subsequent recovery period without stimuli [30, 53, 59]. Stimulating pulses gave a potential gradient of about 1 V/mm, were of duration 0.4 msec and of frequency/sec given by numbers adjacent to curves. Membrane potentials during recovery are also quoted [30].

for inducing motor movements or seizures in vivo. By choosing pulses of duration and potential in slight excess of minimal values needed for maximal response, dependence on pulse-frequency was found to be of the type shown in Fig. 4-4. For frequencies up to about 15 pulses per second, the cation movements were proportional to frequency and corresponded to gain of Na and loss of K, each at 5–6 mµEq per gram of tissue for each stimulating pulse [59].

Even in the absence of stimulation, use of isotopically labeled Na and K showed the two ions in cerebral tissues to be undergoing rapid exchange with the tissue's environment [37, 38]. With suitable experimental arrangements, entry of ^{24}Na to cellular regions of the tissue was separable from its movements in extracellular spaces, and found to occur at some 250 µEq per gram of tissue per hour. This rate increased fourfold to sixfold on electrical stimulation of tissue, when entry occurred at some 1100 µEq per gram per hour. Thus, one-third of the tissue's intracellular Na exchanged each minute. It was significant in judging mechanisms concerned that stimulation increased Na efflux as well as Na influx: tissue permeability was increased by stimulation, rather than unidirectional transfer.

Movements of potassium ions observed isotopically in isolated cerebral preparations are also considerable in absence of applied stimuli, giving values of 330–400 µEq of K per gram per hour [15]. Again, electrical stimulation greatly increased the movements, efflux now exceeding influx and reaching rates of 750 µEq per gram per hour. Thus the effect of stimulation was to increase permeability of the tissue to K ions. Further, such permeability change appeared to be close to a primary action of the stimulating pulses rather than depending on some of the metabolic consequences already described as resulting from stimulation: K was lost from the stimulated tissue under a variety of circumstances, including incubating conditions which provided no glucose.

Modification by Added Agents. The Na and K movements described are essential features of mammalian neural systems and comment is thus merited on agents which affect and contribute to chemical specification of the mechanisms involved. Glutamic acid, the first of these substances, is a normal cerebral constituent and is excitatory when applied to the surface of the brain [16] at concentrations of 0.1 mM or greater. Its intracellular level is some 5 mM, and it has been thought that the substance could play a role in relation to certain forms of excitation in vivo. An in vitro counterpart to the excitatory action of the acid was found by measuring cerebral membrane potentials: at about 0.2 mM, glutamic acid causes rapid depolarization [6, 23]. This was found to be due to entry of Na$^+$ [6, 27] at a sufficiently rapid rate to explain the depolarization and excitatory action.

Tetrodotoxin, a naturally occurring cyclic guanidine, which is highly potent in blocking a number of neural systems [35, 66], inhibits responses to excitation of cerebral preparations at about 20 mµM. This was found to be due to inhibition of the Na entry which occurred on electrical excitation; 1 molecule of tetrodotoxin probably blocked the entry of 5 or more Na ions per stimulating impulse. Tetrodotoxin has now been found to antagonize also the entry of Na$^+$ which is induced by glutamate [62]. In explanation, both the toxin and glutamic acid have been considered to act by combination with a membrane component concerned with Na entry; structures are such that this may be a phosphatidylserine-protein complex [62, 84]. Among cerebral constituents, however, ganglioside components had previously proved most effective in antagonizing an inhibition of cation movement caused by a different blocking agent [51]; conceivably this affected a different site of ion movement. Lipid bimolecular layers between liquid phases give promising model systems for appraising such interactions.

Of therapeutic agents examined for action on cation movements of neocortical tissues in the present systems [30, 52, 60], phenobarbital partly inhibited at 0.3 mM, and the electrically stimulated tissue was more susceptible to chlorpromazine and haloperidol. Actions of phenobarbital and chlorpromazine on potassium movements were correlated with their effects on membrane potential. A normal mechanism controlling cerebral excitability may also operate at this level, for γ-aminobutyrate is inhibitory and its accumulation [86] in hypoxia has been judged protective.

Cellular Membrane Potentials

The rapid adjustments of cellular permeability just described are comparable to those invoked in interpretation of the nerve action potential in neural systems generally [32, 54]. They imply that the tissue preparations contain cellular components which, in their unstimulated state, are more permeable to K^+ than to Na^+ and that this order of permeability changes on stimulation.

Evidence that the ion gradients of cerebral tissues in vitro are manifested as membrane potentials was obtained by micropipette electrodes [23, 31, 43]. In neocortical tissues, values of -60 mV were observed, comparable to those found in vivo. These values are less negative than the -83 mV which is the equilibrium potential corresponding to the measured gradient in K, assuming cellular uniformity. Contributing to this difference is the Na gradient, which would afford an opposing potential. The potentials observed in vitro diminished rapidly on electrical stimulation [30] and on increasing the extracellular concentration of K^+ [23], indicating their dependence on a transmembrane gradient in K^+.

Spike potentials were also observed in the in vitro preparations, occurring spontaneously on mechanical stimulation and in response to electrical excitation [30, 43, 70, 91]. In most cases the discharges included positive overshoots, and at these points it may be judged that the effect of the Na gradient preponderates. It has been deduced, making certain assumptions, that the relative permeability of Na to K ions in the resting cells is about 0.06, this ratio becoming much larger on stimulation [23].

Excitability and characteristics of responses given by the isolated tissues are greatly altered by modifying the composition of incubating media. Exploration of cerebral characteristics by employing these systems [56] is as yet in its infancy, although their potential value is great. Among simple components already examined, it may be noted that diminution in chloride content has resulted in multiple spike-discharges. These were observed first in sections from the hippocampus of the guinea pig [89, 90], in the neocortex [70], and in the piriform cortex [71], stimulating and recording in each case with surface electrodes. In normal media, the hippocampal preparation afforded a discrete negative response to stimulation, but when Cl^- of the medium was replaced by propionate, a long train of spike discharges resulted with a latency of about 40 msec. Subsequent return to normal media restored the simple response. It was concluded that in absence of Cl^-, certain inhibitory processes of the normal tissue no longer operated; this is consistent with some previous suggestions [19], which ascribed to chloride ions a role in inhibitory postsynaptic responses.

In the olfactory cortex maintained in vitro and stimulated from the lateral olfactory tract, diminished Ca^{2+} in incubating media increased the complexity of response, an effect also lost on transfer to normal media; changes in Mg^{2+} and Ca^{2+} had interacting effects on the discharges resulting from stimulation [71]. This preparation allows ready differentiation of presynaptic from a number of postsynaptic responses, and several depressant drugs including phenobarbital inhibited postsynaptic responses at concentrations which were without action presynaptically [9, 91].

ENERGY-CONSUMING REACTIONS

The two categories which receive comment are active transport and synthetic processes.

Active Cation Transport

The major identified energy-consuming process of the brain again concerns the common ions Na^+ and K^+ (Fig. 4-5). Its enzymic aspects can be observed as an adenosinetriphosphatase activated by sodium and potassium ions: an Na,K-ATPase. Work with neural preparations

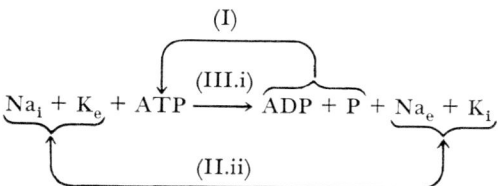

FIG. 4-5. Cation transport by Na,K-ATPase (III.i). The numbers have the same significance as in Table 4-1. Subscript e, extracellular; i, intracellular.

[77] pioneered investigation of this system, which has since been investigated in many organs of the body; in such organs, activity of the Na,K-ATPase has been correlated with performance of active Na transport over a wide range of values [4]. In 1961, the Na,K-ATPase was characterized in preparations from the mammalian brain [18]. Here, as elsewhere, the system has been found to be firmly associated with microsomal membrane-structures and to exhibit properties which indicate the components of the reaction to operate at different sites, which are differentiated in terms of the inside and outside of cells from which the microsomes are derived.

Relevant properties exhibited by cerebral microsomal preparations are shown in Fig. 4-6. Sensitivity to Na and K is prominent and is clearly so to different concentration-ranges of the two ions. The low [K+] required corresponds to the concentration range of K extracellularly rather than intracellularly (which is >100 mM). The [Na+] required, however, is below that of extracellular fluids (about 160 mM) and corresponds, rather, to intracellular [Na+]. The microsomal system is thus sensitive to ion concentrations in regions in which Na and K are at lowest concentration and from which they are being removed: this is understandable for an active transport system. Susceptibility of the Na,K-ATPase to the glycoside ouabain (Fig. 4-6B) has proved useful in characterizing the system [33]; inhibition is competitive with K+ and occurs extracellularly. Mechanisms of action have been suggested for the Na,K-ATPase [1, 51]; the findings of Fig. 4-6C are part of such investigations and suggest that components of the microsomal membrane system become transiently phosphorylated during their action as an ATPase. Purification has afforded great enrichment of the ATPase system while retaining or enhancing its sodium and potassium requirement [13, 21, 67].

The cerebral content of Na and K is normally maintained with little variation despite the rapid cation movements described under *Intermediates and Energy-Stores*. To this aspect of homeostasis the Na and K sensitivity of the ATPase clearly contribute [51], but are not fully adequate without further specification. This can be appreciated when the speed of breakdown

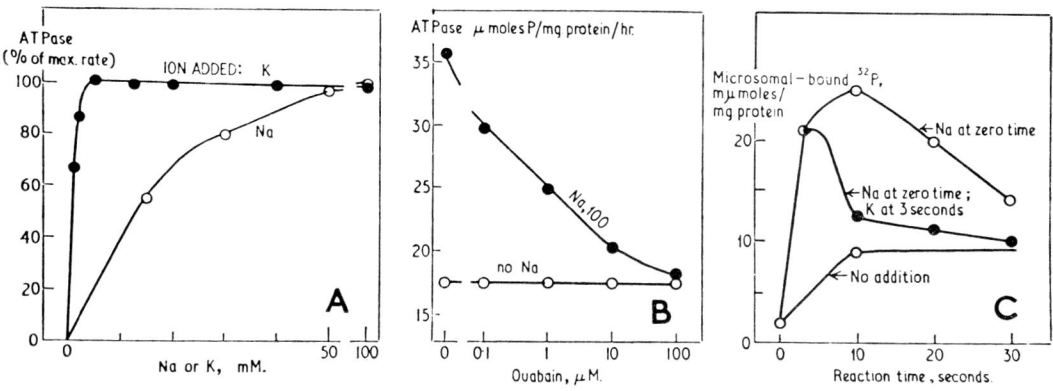

FIG. 4-6. Properties of the Na,K-ATPase of cerebral microsomal membrane-structures [76, 79, 80]. (*A*) Requirement for Na and K. (*B*) Inhibition by ouabain. (*C*) Formation of a ^{32}P-microsome derivative transitorily during the course of reaction [28, 72].

of adenosinetriphosphate and phosphocreatine is recalled (Fig. 4-3). The breakdown is quite large within 1–2 sec of initial stimulation and in this time only 0.2–0.5 µEq of Na will have entered per gram of tissue, with a similar loss of K. These very small changes are inadequate for significant acceleration of the Na,K-ATPase if the ions concerned are distributed over the tissues' intracellular and extracellular phases respectively. Thus for the entering Na to be an effective stimulant, it must be supposed to be present in not more than 1/50 of the tissue volume; there it could afford an increase of 10 or 25 mM. Supposing the tissue's extracellular space to be 20 percent of its volume and the cellular portion to consist of equal volumes of neurons and glia, the neuronal volume then forms 40 percent; of this, half may be perikarya and larger axons, thus the finer processes which receive most Na comprise 20 percent of the total tissue volume. A further tenfold enrichment, on a basis at present unspecified, would be required to give the suggested increase in local concentration. Other possibilities are listed in Table 4-2; the ATPase and its substrates and activators are ionized, thus membrane depolarization (iii, Table 4-2) may allow interactions previously inhibited.

TABLE 4-2. Initiation of ∼P-Utilization on Cerebral Stimulation

A stage of the following sequence may initiate:
  (i)   The membrane change which allows Na entry
  (ii) Na which has entered
  (iii) The resultant depolarization
  (iv) The membrane change which allows K loss
  (v)   The lost K, extracellularly.

Considering process (ii):
  (a) Resting ∼P turnover, about 500 µEq/g/hr; this increases twofold to threefold within 2 sec of commencing stimulation.
  (b) Na entering at about 1000 µEq/g/hr has increased by about 0.5 µEq/g in 2 sec; initial value, 25–30 µEq/g.
  (c) This 1–2 percent increase in intracellular Na is inadequate to account for the ∼P utilization, *unless* the Na is highly localized.

Other Energy-consuming Processes

In a broad sense, these processes include synthesis or assimilation of almost every cerebral constituent; in the present account they can be exemplified only. Several categories, especially those involving neuroendocrine and transmitting agents, are the concern of other contributors.

Comment may be made on the synthesis of glycogen, which in excitation is so rapidly depleted. Enzymic mechanisms of its resynthesis are largely understood, together with aspects of their control [54]. It is noteworthy, however, that resynthesis is often quite slow, occupying some hours, and may be correlated with other slow adjustments after cerebral excitation [53]. One instance concerned conditioned reflexes established in rats in runways, where they received electric shocks or food [8]. During slow recovery of their glycogen content, the energy-reserves of cells concerned are in this respect subnormal.

Much in cerebral functioning involves lipid and protein constituents, and components of both these categories undergo turnover at appreciable rates. Among lipids, the phosphatidyl inositols include the compounds of most rapid turnover, requiring adenosinetriphosphate for their resynthesis. Protein synthesis is demonstrated as an adenosinetriphosphate-requiring process in the brain as elsewhere [54]. In isolated neocortical tissues the synthesis is diminished on electrical stimulation [69]. Supposing that these relationships hold locally when specific nerve cells or nerve terminals are stimulated, basis is provided for persistent changes in the brain which reflect recent activities of its components; proposals regarding lasting effects of some centrally acting drugs have been based on this reasoning [58]. At least part of cerebral protein-synthesis is mitochondrial, and the distribution of mitochondria, which includes their presence in nerve terminals [2], can thus have added significance.

Instances of cerebral adaptive processes which are disturbed when protein synthesis is inhibited are summarized in Table 4-3.

TABLE 4-3. Inhibitors of Protein Synthesis on Cerebral Adaptive Processes

Process	Inhibited by	Notes
Tolerance to morphine [12, 14]	Actinomycin-D mice, 0.1–1 µg/kg, i.p. rats, 10 µg/kg/hr, i.v. 1 µg/kg/hr, i.c.	Acts at RNA polymerase Metabolic consequences [81]
	Puromycin	At amino acid/t-RNA
	Cycloheximide	At ribosome/m-RNA
Sustained increase in cortical firing by surface-positive polarization [22]	Cycloheximide 1–10 µg/liter superfused Neomycin, 1 mM	Not inhibited by puromycin At t-RNA
Retention of induced behavioral change [11, 17]	Puromycin, 170 µg, i.c. Acetoxycycloheximide, 20 µg, i.c.	Not inhibited by cytosine arabinoside, acting at DNA [10]

As several of these become established within a few hours, attention is directed to the cerebral proteins of more rapid turnover. It is unlikely that synthesis of such proteins consumes more than one percent or so of energy turnover of the brain, but the portion so involved is of great importance in conditioning cerebral performance. The energy-utilizing processes of the brain which a therapeutically oriented investigator would most desire to control are indeed the syntheses which at specific regions condition nerve-terminal functioning. Some successful anticonvulsants probably act at synaptic regions but require continued administration for a continuing disorder. For "renewed growth aright" in this situation, last century's suggested molecular basis still lacks the necessary chemical specification.

REFERENCES

1. Albers, R. W. Biochemical aspects of active transport. *Ann. Rev. Biochem.* 36: 727, 1967.
2. Bachelard, H. S. Amino acid incorporation into the protein of mitochondrial preparations from cerebral cortex and spinal cord. *Biochem. J.* 100:131, 1966.
3. Bachelard, H. S., and McIlwain, H. Carbohydrate and Oxidative Metabolism in Neural Systems. In Florkin, M., and Stotz, E. H. (Eds.), *Comprehensive Biochemistry*, 17. Amsterdam: Elsevier, 1969.
4. Bonting, S. L. Na,K-Activated ATPase and Active Cation Transport. In de Graeff, J., and Leijnse, B. (Eds.), *Water and Electrolyte Metabolism*. Amsterdam: Elsevier, 1964.
5. Bradbury, M. W. B., and Davson, H. The transport of potassium between blood, cerebrospinal fluid and brain. *J. Physiol.* (London) 181:151, 1965.
6. Bradford, H. F., and McIlwain, H. Ionic basis for the depolarization of cerebral tissues by excitatory acidic amino acids. *J. Neurochem.* 13:1163, 1966.
7. Brinley, F. J., Kandel, E. R., and Marshall, W. H. Potassium outflux from rabbit cortex during spreading depression. *J. Neurophysiol.* 23:246, 1960.
8. Bureš, V. J. Discussion. In Steinberg, H., de Reuck, A. V. S., and Knight, J. (Eds.), *Animal Behavior and Drug Action*. London: Churchill, 1964, p. 330.
9. Campbell, J., McIlwain, H., Richards, C. D., and Somerville, A. Responses in vitro from the piriform cortex of the rat, and their susceptibility to centrally acting drugs. *J. Neurochem.* 14:939, 1967.
10. Casola, L., Lim, R., Davis, R. E., and Agranoff, B. W. Behavioural and biochemical effects of intracranial injection of cytosine arabinoside. *Proc. Nat. Acad. Sci. U.S.A.* 60:1389, 1968.
11. Cohen, H. D., and Barondes, S. H. De-

layed and sustained effect of acetoxycycloheximide on memory in mice. *Proc. Nat. Acad. Sci. U.S.A.* 58:157, 1967.

12. Cohen, M., Keats, A. S., Krivoy, W., and Ungar, G. Effect of actinomycin-D on morphine tolerance. *Proc. Soc. Exp. Biol. Med.* 119:381, 1965.

13. Cooper, J. R., and McIlwain, H. The sodium-plus-potassium ion-activated adenosine triphosphatase of cerebral microsomal fractions: treatment with disrupting agents. *Biochem. J.* 102:675, 1967.

14. Cox, B. M., and Ginsburg, M. Is There a Relationship between Protein Synthesis and Tolerance to Analgesic Drugs? In Steinberg, H. (Ed.), *Scientific Basis of Drug Dependence*. London: Churchill, 1969.

15. Cummins, J. T., and McIlwain, H. Electrical pulses and the potassium and other ions of isolated cerebral tissues. *Biochem. J.* 79:330, 1961.

16. Curtis, D. R. The Actions of Amino Acids upon Mammalian Neurons. In Curtis, D. R., and McIntyre, A. K., *Studies in Physiology*. Berlin: Springer, 1965, p. 34.

17. Davis, R. E., and Agranoff, B. W. Stages of memory formation: evidence for an environmental trigger. *Proc. Nat. Acad. Sci. U.S.A.* 55:555, 1966.

18. Deul, D. H., and McIlwain, H. Activation and inhibition of adenosine triphosphatases of subcellular particles from the brain. *J. Neurochem.* 8:246, 1961.

19. Eccles, J. C. *The Physiology of Synapses.* Berlin: Springer, 1964.

20. Estler, C.-J., and Ammon, H. P. T. The influence of propanolol on the methamphetamine-induced changes of cerebral function and metabolism. *J. Neurochem.* 14:799, 1967.

21. Fijuta, M., Nagano, K., Mizuno, N., Tashima, Y., Nakao, T., and Nakao, M. Ouabain-sensitive Mg^{++}-ATPase, K^+-ATPase and Na^+-ATPase activities accompanying a highly specific Na^+-K^+-ATPase preparation. *J. Biochem.* (Tokyo) 61:473, 1967.

22. Gartside, I. B. Mechanisms of sustained increases of firing rate of neurons in the rat cerebral cortex after polarization: role of protein synthesis. *Nature* (London) 220:383, 1968.

23. Gibson, I. M., and McIlwain, H. Continuous recording of changes in membrane potential in mammalian cerebral tissues in vitro: recovery after depolarization by added substances. *J. Physiol.* (London) 176:261, 1965.

24. Gilbert, J. C. Mechanism of sugar transport in brain slices. *Nature* (London) 205:87, 1965.

25. Gowers, W. R. *Epilepsy and Other Chronic Convulsive Diseases: Their Causes, Symptoms and Treatment.* London: Churchill, 1881.

26. Greengard, O., and McIlwain, H. Anticonvulsants and the metabolism of separated mammalian cerebral tissues. *Biochem. J.* 61:61, 1955.

27. Harvey, J. A., and McIlwain, H. Excitatory acidic amino acids and the cation content and sodium ion flux of isolated tissues from the brain. *Biochem. J.* 108:269, 1968.

28. Heald, P. J. Studies on the phosphoproteins of brain: 2. Partial purification of a phosphoprotein attached to subcellular particles. *Biochem. J.* 78:340, 1961.

29. Heller, I. H., and Elliott, K. A. C. The metabolism of normal brain and human gliomas in relation to cell type and density. *Canad. J. Biochem. Physiol.* 33:395, 1955.

30. Hillman, H. H., Campbell, W. J., and McIlwain, H. Membrane potentials in isolated and electrically stimulated mammalian cerebral cortex. Effects of chlorpromazine, cocaine, phenobarbitone and protamine on the tissue's electrical and chemical responses to stimulation. *J. Neurochem.* 10:325, 1963.

31. Hillman, H. H., and McIlwain, H. Membrane potentials in mammalian cerebral tissues in vitro: dependence on ionic environment. *J. Physiol.* (London) 157:263, 1961.

32. Hodgkin, A. L. *The Conduction of the Nervous Impulse.* Liverpool: University Press, 1965.

33. Hokin, L. E., Prokotoff, M., and Kupcham, S. M. Alkylation of a brain transport adenosinetriphosphatase at the cardiotonic steroid site by strophanthidin-3-haloacetates. *Proc. Nat. Acad. Sci. U.S.A.* 55:797, 1966.

34. Jackson, John Hughlings. *Selected Writings on Epilepsy and Epileptiform Convulsions*, edited by J. Taylor. London: Hodder & Stoughton, 1931.

35. Kao, C. Y. Tetrodotoxin, saxitoxin and their significance in the study of excitation phenomena. *Pharmacol. Rev.* 18:997, 1966.

36. Katzman, R., Graziani, L., and Ginsburg, S. Cation exchange in blood, brain and CSF. *Progr. Brain Res.* 29:283, 1968.

37. Keesey, J. C., and Wallgren, H. Movements of radioactive sodium in cerebral cortex slices in response to electrical stimulation. *Biochem. J.* 95:301, 1965.

38. Keesey, J. C., Wallgren, H., and McIlwain, H. The sodium potassium and chloride of cerebral tissues: maintenance, change on stimulation and subsequent recovery. *Biochem. J.* 95:289, 1965.

39. Kerr, S. E. The carbohydrate metabolism of brain: 1. The determination of glycogen in nerve tissue. *J. Biol. Chem.* 116:1, 1936.

40. Kety, S. S., Woodford, R. B., Harnel, M. H., Freyan, F. A., Appel, K. E., and Schmidt, C. F. Cerebral blood flow and metabolism in schizophrenia: the effects of barbiturate and semi-narcosis, insulin coma and electroshock. *Amer. J. Psychiat.* 104:765, 1948.

41. Keynes, R. D., and Ritchie, J. M. The movement of labelled ions in mammalian nonmyelinated nerve fibres. *J. Physiol.* (London) 179:333, 1965.

42. King, L. J., Lowry, O. H., Passonneau, J. V., and Venson, V. Effect of convulsants on energy reserves in the cerebral cortex. *J. Neurochem.* 14:599, 1967.

43. Li, C.-L., and McIlwain, H. Maintenance of resting membrane potentials in slices of mammalian cerebral cortex and other tissues in vitro. *J. Physiol.* (London) 139:178, 1957.

44. Lowry, O., and Passonneau, J. V. Relationships between substrates and enzymes of glycolysis in brain. *J. Biol. Chem.* 239:31, 1964.

45. Lowry, O., Passonneau, J. V., Hasselberger, F. X., and Schulz, D. W. Effect of ischemia on known substrates and cofactors of the glycolytic pathway in brain. *J. Biol. Chem.* 239:18, 1964.

46. McIlwain, H. Substrates which support respiration and metabolic response to electrical impulses in human cerebral tissues. *J. Neurol. Neurosurg. Psychiat.* 16:257, 1953.

47. McIlwain, H. Characteristics required in electrical pulses for stimulation of the respiration of separated mammalian cerebral tissues. *J. Physiol.* (London) 124:117, 1954.

48. McIlwain, H. Study of human cerebral biopsy specimens in an electrically excited condition. *Arch. Neurol. Psychiat.* 71:488, 1954.

49. McIlwain, H. Electrically excited metabolism of separated mammalian cerebral tissues. *Electroenceph. Clin. Neurophysiol.* 6:93, 1954.

50. McIlwain, H. *Maudsley, Mott and Mann on the Chemical Physiology and Pathology of the Mind.* London: Lewis, 1955.

51. McIlwain, H. *Chemical Exploration of the Brain. A Study of Cerebral Excitability and Ion Movement.* Amsterdam: Elsevier, 1963.

52. McIlwain, H. Actions of haloperidol, meperidine, and related compounds on the excitability and ion content of isolated cerebral tissue. *Biochem. Pharmacol.* 13:523, 1964.

53. McIlwain, H. Intermediation between administered drugs and behavioural effects. In Steinberg, H., de Reuck, A. V. S., and Knight, J. (Eds.), *Animal Behavior and Drug Action.* London: Churchill, 1964, p. 314.

54. McIlwain, H. *Biochemistry and the Central Nervous System* (3d ed.). London: Churchill, 1966.

55. McIlwain, H. Henry Maudsley, molecular biologist. *Bethlem-Maudsley Hospital Gazette* 9:10, 1967.

56. McIlwain, H. Membrane functioning in preparations from the mammalian brain. *Brit. Med. Bull.* 24:174, 1968.

57. McIlwain, H. Ion movements in isolated preparations from the mammalian brain. *Progr. Brain Res.* 29:273, 1968.

58. McIlwain, H. Metabolic approach to interpreting animal exploratory activity. *Nature* (London) 220:889, 1968.

59. McIlwain, H., and Joanny, P. Characteristics required in electrical pulses of rectangular time-voltage relationships for metabolic change and ion movements in mammalian cerebral tissues. *J. Neurochem.* 10:313, 1963.

60. McIlwain, H., and Rodnight, R. *Practical Neurochemistry.* London: Churchill, 1962.

61. McIlwain, H., and Tresize, M. A. The glucose, glycogen and aerobic glycolysis of isolated cerebral tissues. *Biochem. J.* 63:250, 1956.

62. McIlwain, H., Harvey, J. A., and Rod-

riguez, G. Tetrodotoxin on the sodium and other constituents of cerebral tissues excited electrically and with glutamate. *J. Neurochem.* 16:363, 1969.

63. Meyer, J. S., Gotoh, F., and Favale, E. Cerebral metabolism during epileptic seizures in man. *Electroenceph. Clin. Neurophysiol.* 21:10, 1966.

64. Meyer, J. S., Gotoh, F., and Tazaki, Y. Inhibitory action of carbon dioxide and acetazoleamide in seizure activity. *Electroenceph. Clin. Neurophysiol.* 13:762, 1961.

65. Minard, F. N., and Davis, R. V. The effects of electroshock on the acid-soluble phosphates of rat brain. *J. Biol. Chem.* 237:1283, 1962.

66. Moore, J. W., and Narahashi, T. Tetrodotoxin's highly selective blockage of an ionic channel. *Fed. Proc.* 26:1655, 1967.

67. Nagano, K., Mizuno, N., Fujita, M., Tashima, Y., Nakao, T., and Nakao, M. On the possible role of the phosphorylated intermediate in the reaction mechanism of (Na^+-K^+)-ATPase. *Biochim. Biophys. Acta* 143:239, 1967.

68. Olsen, N. S., and Klein, J. R. Effect of cyanide on the concentration of lactate and phosphates in brain. *J. Biol. Chem.* 167:739, 1947.

69. Orrego, F., and Lipmann, F. Protein synthesis in brain slices. *J. Biol. Chem.* 242:665, 1967.

70. Richards, C. D., and McIlwain, H. Electrical responses in brain samples. *Nature* (London). 215:704, 1967.

71. Richards, C. D., and Sercombe, R. Electrical activity observed in guinea pig olfactory cortex maintained in vitro. *J. Physiol.* (London) 197:667, 1968.

72. Rodnight, R. Phosphoprotein metabolism in the brain. In *The Scientific Basis of Medicine, Annual Reviews.* London: Athlone Press, 1967, p. 304.

73. Sacktor, B., Wilson, J. E., and Tiekert, C. G. Regulation of glycolysis in brain in situ during convulsions. *J. Biol. Chem.* 241:5071, 1966.

74. Samson, F. E., Balfour, W. M., and Dahl, N. A. Rate of cerebral ATP utilization in rats. *Amer. J. Physiol.* 198:213, 1962.

75. Schmidt, C. F., Kety, S. S., and Pennes, H. H. The gaseous metabolism of the brain of the monkey. *Amer. J. Physiol.* 143:33, 1945.

76. Schwartz, A., Bachelard, H. S., and McIlwain, H. The sodium-stimulated adenosinetriphosphatase activity and other properties of cerebral microsomal fractions and subfractions. *Biochem. J.* 84:626, 1962.

77. Skou, J. C. The relationship of a (Mg^{2+} + Na^+)-activated, K^+-stimulated enzyme or enzyme system to the active, linked transport of Na^+ and K^+ across the cell membrane. In *Symposium on Membrane Transport and Metabolism.* Prague: Czechoslovak Academy of Sciences, 1961, p. 228.

78. Sokoloff, L. Metabolism of the central nervous system in vivo. In Field, J., Magoun, H. W., and Hall, V. E. (Eds.), *Neurophysiology,* 1843. Washington, D.C.: American Physiological Society, 1960.

79. Swanson, P. D., Bradford, H. F., and McIlwain, H. Stimulation and solubilization of the sodium ion–activated adenosine triphosphatase of cerebral microsomes by surface-active agents, especially polyoxyethylene ethers: actions of phospholipases and neuraminidase. *Biochem. J.* 92:235, 1964.

80. Swanson, P. D., and McIlwain, H. Inhibition of the sodium-ion-stimulated adenosine triphosphatase after treatment of isolated guinea pig cerebral cortex with ouabain and other agents. *J. Neurochem.* 12:877, 1965.

81. Takemori, A. E. Studies on cellular adaptation to morphine and its reversal by nalorphine in cerebral cortical slices of rats. *J. Pharmacol.* 135:89, 1962.

82. Tower, D. B. *Neurochemistry of Epilepsy.* Springfield, Ill.: Thomas, 1960.

83. Van Harreveld, A. *Brain Tissue Electrolytes.* London: Butterworth, 1966.

84. Watkins, J. C. Pharmacological receptors and general permeability phenomena of cell membranes. *J. Theor. Biol.* 9:37, 1965.

85. Winterstein, H. Der Stoffwechsel des Zentralnervensystems. In Bethe, A. (Ed.), *Handbuch der Normalen und Pathologischen Physiologie.* Berlin: Springer, 1927, p. 566.

86. Wood, J. D., Watson, W. J., and Ducker, A. J. The effect of hypoxia on brain γ-aminobutyric acid levels. *J. Neurochem.* 15:603, 1968.

87. Wood, T. Adenosine triphosphate-creatine phosphotransferase from ox brain: purification and isolation. *Biochem. J.* 87:453, 1963.

88. Woodbury, D. M. Effect of diphenylhydantoin on electrolytes and radiosodium turnover in brain and other tissues of normal, hyponatremic and postictal rats. *J. Pharmacol.* 115:74, 1955.
89. Yamamoto, C., and Kawai, N. Presynaptic action of acetylcholine on thin sections from the guinea pig dentate gyrus in vitro. *Exp. Neurol.* 19:176, 1967.
90. Yamamoto, C., and Kawai, N. Seizure discharge evoked in vitro in thin sections from guinea pig hippocampus. *Science* 155:341, 1967.
91. Yamamoto, C., and McIlwain, H. Electrical activities in thin sections from the mammalian brain maintained in chemically defined media in vitro. *J. Neurochem.* 13:1333, 1966.

Discussion

ENERGY METABOLITES IN EXPERIMENTAL SEIZURES*

JANET V. PASSONNEAU

A convulsive seizure, to the extent that it is associated with increased neuronal activity, must result in increased energy expenditure by the brain.

The relationships between clinical manifestations, neuronal activity, and energy metabolism are difficult to study in epilepsy but this is possible in experimental convulsive states. Electroshock, for example, has been shown to increase neuronal discharge, metabolic rate, and the use of energy reserves. The relationships between neuronal activity and energy expenditure are well documented. Increased oxygen consumption, as a result of electric stimulation, has been observed in frog sciatic nerve [1, 4] and sympathetic ganglia [9]. In the case of ganglia, glucose consumption was also shown to be increased. Increased oxygen uptake and decreases in ATP, P-creatine, and glucose have been observed following electric stimulation of guinea pig brain slices [6, 11, 12]. Convulsive agents and electroshock effect decreases in ATP, glucose, and glycogen in cat brain [8]. P-creatine and ATP also decrease in rat brain following electroshock [13]. Not only is energy expended more rapidly during seizures but, conversely, an adequate energy supply appears to be needed to maintain a seizure. Thus, convulsive activity in dogs following pentylenetetrazol administration was prolonged when O_2 was substituted for air [15]. Paradoxically, however, anoxia or hypoxia can also produce convulsions.

The following discussion will focus on the effects of various convulsants on energy expenditure in brain and on the status of energy reserves. Considering the high metabolic rate of brain, the energy reserves are remarkably low. They consist primarily of ATP, P-creatine, glucose, and glycogen.

ELECTRICAL STIMULATION

Electrical stimulation of mouse brain was shown to cause a large increase in metabolic rate [7]. Changes in ATP, P-creatine, glucose, glycogen, and lactate following a 1 sec stimulus indicated at least a threefold increase in metabolic rate during the first 3 sec. Lactate increase exceeded the disappearance of glucose and glycogen to an extent that indicated a fivefold to tenfold acceleration of glucose entry into the brain. Changes in ATP and P-creatine following electroshock were much greater than those shown by an equal period of complete anoxia. Prevention of clinical signs of seizure with secobarbital (50 mg/kg) had only a minor influence on chemical changes in the brain. Changes in P-creatine with and without secobarbital are shown in Fig. D4-1. Sedation with chlorpromazine (50 mg/kg) also had little effect, while a subanesthetic dose of phenobarbital (100 mg/kg) modified the seizure and diminished some of the chemical changes. The effect on electroshock on the use of $\sim P$ and the modification of this by drugs are shown in Fig. D4-2. It is surprising that anesthesia, which prevents most of the symptoms of electroshock, does not necessarily prevent the metabolic evidence of massive neuronal discharge. Assuming that the anesthetic acts primarily at synapses, there are two possible explanations. First, electrical stimulus may have directly stimulated most of the neurons, making synaptic transmission irrelevant. Second, the bulk of cortical synapses may be relatively insensitive to the anesthetic agent employed (secobarbital), even though it is sufficiently inhibitory at lower levels to prevent somatic expression by a massive discharge.

* Supported in part by Grant P–78 from American Cancer Society.

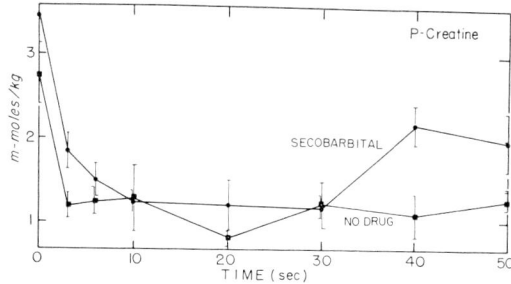

FIG. D4-1. Effect of electrical stimulation on P-creatine in control and anesthetized mice. Secobarbital was given at a level of 50 mg/kg 10 min before stimulation, at which time the mice were asleep with absent righting reflex. Stimulus was applied for 1 sec to all but zero-time animals. Mice were rapidly frozen at times shown. Value for each time interval represents average for 5 animals. Vertical lines represent ± 1 SEM. (From King et al. [7].)

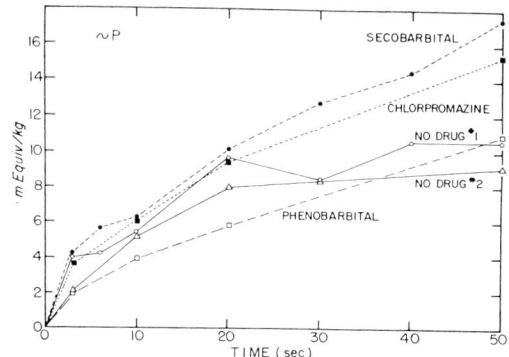

FIG. D4-2. Calculated minimum changes in energy expenditure following electrical stimulation. Calculations are based on changes in ATP, P-creatine, and lactate levels. Extra energy expenditure is calculated as molar equivalent of $\sim$P, i.e., one equivalent of $\sim$P for each mole of lactate that accumulated, one equivalent of each mole of P-creatine that disappeared, and two equivalents for each mole of ATP that disappeared. This calculation does not include any changes that may have occurred in energy production as the result of possible changes in oxygen consumption. (From King et al. [7].)

Convulsants

Stone [15] observed that seizures induced by pentylenetetrazol were prolonged if O_2 rather than air was respired. A similar experiment was conducted using mice; measurements were made of energy reserves. Mice injected with 80 mg/kg of pentylenetetrazol developed irregular clonus [7], especially in the forelimbs and head, beginning 1 min after injection and lasting 7 or 8 min after injection. If the mice are placed in pure O_2 after injection, they continue to exhibit irregular clonus for 15 min. The increased period of convulsion is in agreement with Stone. ATP and P-creatine levels were somewhat reduced 15 min after administration of the drug (Table D4-1). Lactate had greatly increased and glycogen had fallen to one-third of the initial level, while glucose showed some increase. Substitution of O_2 for air resulted in significant increase in ATP, but P-creatine was significantly lower than in the control group.

The fact that ATP increased but P-creatine decreased suggests that the role of O_2 in maintaining seizures may not be limited to maintenance of energy reserves. Lactate levels were somewhat higher, but the difference is not statistically significant. The difference in glucose levels between the groups in O_2 and air is probably due to differences in plasma glucose levels (Table D4-1). Seizures occurred in animals kept in O_2 even though no detectable change was seen in ATP. This is in contrast to the

TABLE D4-1. Effect of Pentylenetetrazol on Brain Metabolites

Subject	ATP	P-Creatine	Lactate	Glucose	Glycogen
Control	2.13	3.63	3.85	1.57	1.73
15 min room air	1.55	2.61	9.32	3.26	0.61
15 min 100% O_2	2.20	1.95	12.90	0.86	0.46

Mice (four in each group) were given 80 mg/kg of pentylenetetrazol intraperitoneally and rapidly frozen 15 min later. Mean values are shown (mmoles/kg). Serum glucose was measured in blood collected from three other groups of mice (four in each group) given similar drug treatment. The respective values (mmoles/liter) were 8.1, 10.3, and 3.0. (From King et al. [7].)

finding with electrically induced seizures in which ATP fell to 50 percent of normal. These observations tend to dissociate ATP levels and seizure generation.

Chemical changes in brain following audiogenic seizures have been contrasted with changes produced by electroshock [2]. When seizures were induced by a 2 sec audiogenic stimulus, the change in rate of $\sim$P use was much less than that produced by electrically induced seizures (Fig. D4-3). ATP did not change significantly from the control values at any time. P-creatine showed significant decrease at 15 sec after the stimulus when tonic extension was observed in the mice, thereafter returned to the original level. The small increase seen in $\sim$P use is due largely to increase in lactate production (1 mM/kg increase in 20 sec). Thus, whatever increase in energy requirements may have occurred was presumably small enough to be met by increased O_2 consumption and therefore did not diminish the energy stores. As in the case of pentylenetetrazol seizures, $\sim$P stores and seizures do not seem to be related.

Hypoglycemic seizures would be expected to result from pure shortage in energy supply. However, mice given a large dose of insulin (125 unit/kg) suffered from no loss of ATP or P-creatine [5, 7] in spite of the fact that they went through all the stages of hypoglycemia. Glucose and all the intermediates of the citric-acid cycle except oxaloacetate were significantly lowered [5].

Similarly, ATP and P-creatine levels were not depressed by fluoroacetate administration (100 mg/kg of sodium monofluoroacetate) even during the convulsive period, 40 min after injection [5]. (In the case of fluoroacetate, citrate levels rose to 3.5 times the normal level of 327 µM.) Whatever the cause of seizure may be, generalized lack of $\sim$P does not seem to be a factor.

Methionine sulfoximine (MSO) was administered intraperitoneally to mice in a dose of 300 mg/kg [3]. When methionine was used to prevent seizures, it was given with the MSO in a molar ratio of 3:1. Levels of ATP, P-creatine, glucose, glycogen, lactate, glutamate, and ammonia in the brain were measured at intervals after administration of the convulsive agent. The first signs of toxicity appeared at about 3 hours, and seizures started between 3 and 5 hours. Animals for analysis were frozen during the second seizure. ATP and P-creatine levels were unchanged throughout, even during the most severe convulsions (Table D4-2). Lactate rose moderately during seizures (65 percent). Glucose and glycogen rose progressively to levels more than

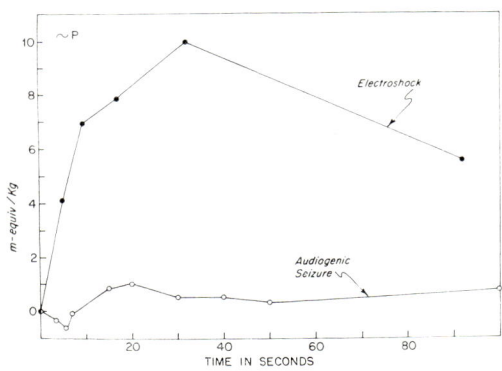

FIG. D4-3. Calculated minimum changes in energy expenditure following electrical stimulation or audiogenic stimulation. Audiogenic stimulus was a 2-sec ringing of a 4-inch doorbell. Clonic convulsions at 5 sec after stimulation are followed by tonic flexion and extension lasting for 10–15 sec. At 30 sec after stimulation, the mice recover; each point represents 4 or 5 mice. Energy expenditure is calculated as in Fig. D4-2. (From J. A. Ferrendelli and D. B. McDougal, unpublished data.)

TABLE D4-2. The Effect of MSO on Metabolites in the Cerebral Cortex of Mice

Metabolite	Controls	MSO (seizures) 3.7–5.2 hr	MSO plus methionine (no seizures) 3.7–5.2 hr
ATP	3.02	2.90	3.04
P-creatine	4.42	4.61	4.66
Glucose	1.12	2.59	2.06
Glycogen	2.10	4.78	4.94
Lactate	0.80	1.32	0.81

Results are expressed as mmoles/kg wet weight. Mice were frozen at indicated intervals after MSO administration. Methionine (last column) was injected at the same time as MSO. (From Folbergrova et al. [3].)

100 percent of control values. When seizures were prevented, lactate accumulation was prevented; however, the glucose and glycogen were increased to the same degree as when MSO was given alone. Measurement of related metabolites (glucose-6-P, UDP-glucose, and glucose-1,6-P_2) showed no effect of MSO. The ratio of brain to serum glucose increased, indicating substantial increase of intracellular glucose.

An estimation of the metabolic rate in the brain was made by measuring rate of change of energy reserves when the animals were decapitated as previously described. The $\sim$P use based on ATP, P-creatine, and lactate changes in the first 20 sec of ischemia was found to be 14 mmoles/kg^{-1}/min^{-1} in controls and 17 mmoles/kg^{-1}/min^{-1} during seizure. It seems unlikely therefore that a decrease in metabolism during seizures could account for the elevated glucose and glycogen levels in the brain.

Somewhat parallel with increases in glucose and glycogen, there occurred a three to fourfold increase in ammonia (Table D4-3, Fig. D4-4). The increase was apparent in 1 hour, and by 2 hours, long before onset of convulsions, maximal levels had been reached. Increases in ammonia were associated with small, but statistically significant, decreases in cerebral and cerebellar glutamate levels (Table D4-3).

In the case of MSO, not only are ATP and P-creatine maintained at normal levels but carbohydrate levels are increased. There appears to be no correlation between the energy supply available and seizure generation.

TABLE D4-3. Effect of MSO on Glutamate and Ammonia Levels in Mouse Brain

	Controls	MSO	Δ	P
Cerebrum				
glutamate	1.8	9.7	−2.1	<0.01
ammonia	0.24	1.18	+0.94	<0.001
Cerebellum				
glutamate	8.7	7.9	−0.8	<0.02
ammonia	0.28	1.02	+0.74	<0.001

Mice were given MSO and killed 3.4 to 5 hours later during convulsions. Results are expressed as mmoles/kg. (From Folbergrova et al. [3].)

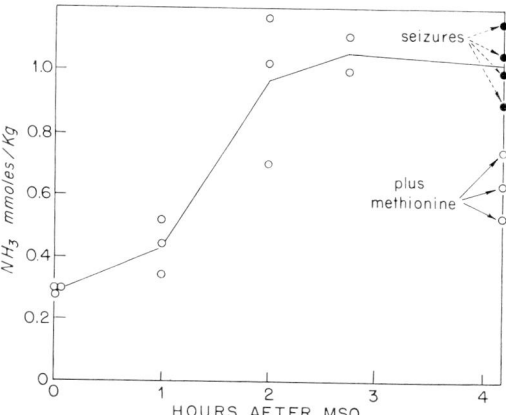

FIG. D4-4. Effect of MSO on ammonia in mouse cerebellum. Mice were frozen at indicated intervals after MSO injection (300 mg/kg). All mice were free of seizures except the 4 mice indicated at the last time interval. Mice receiving methionine as well as MSO are indicated by "plus methionine." These mice remained free of seizures and were killed at time shown. (From Folbergrova et al. [3].)

Hypoxia and Anoxia

Convulsions are induced when an animal is deprived of O_2. Experiments were carried out to determine the effect of decreased O_2 tensions on major energy reserves in the brain [14]. Animals were placed in atmospheres of 7, 5, and 4 percent O_2 and 100 percent N_2. Increased respiratory activity was seen for about 5 min in the animals in 7, 5, and 4 percent O_2. One out of five animals in 4 percent O_2 convulsed and was not used for analysis. In 100 percent N_2 the mice go through an excitement stage, followed by clonic contractions and gasping progressing to apnea at 40 sec. A second group of animals was anesthetized with phenobarbital (150 mg/kg) for one hour before being placed in low oxygen atmospheres.

In spite of prolonged exposure to low O_2 tension, ATP levels were well maintained in the nonanesthetized mice (Table D4-4). P-creatine showed small but progressively greater decreases as O_2 tension was lowered. In 100 percent N_2, ATP was slightly lower and P-creatine fell to half the control values. Glucose levels were higher in mice exposed to low O_2 tension,

TABLE D4-4. The Effect of Anoxia on Major Energy Reserves in Mouse Brain

Treatment	ATP	P-creatine	Glucose	Glycogen	Lactate
Nonanesthetized					
Control, room air	2.95	3.44	1.63	2.40	1.05
7% O_2, 30 min	2.91	2.94	1.67	1.51	4.77
5% O_2, 15 min	2.88	2.54	2.00	1.31	10.49
4% O_2, 15 min	2.87	2.51	2.18	1.50	13.78
100% N_2, 0.7 min	2.66	1.59	0.50	2.66	5.80
Anesthetized					
Control, room air	2.79	3.48	2.21	2.50	0.64
7% O_2, 30 min	2.93	3.14	4.20	2.55	6.10
5% O_2, 15 min	2.83	2.15	2.40	1.87	11.33
4% O_2, 15 min	2.81	2.48	2.04	2.62	7.89
100% N_2, 0.7 min	2.85	1.92	1.29	2.13	3.70

Animals were subjected to different oxygen tensions for time intervals noted and frozen whole in dichlorodifluoromethane chilled to $-150°$. Values are for 5 animals in each group. Anesthetized animals were given 150 mg/kg phenobarbital one hour before freezing. (From Nelson et al. [14].)

but only 30 percent of the normal value in 100 percent N_2. Glycogen was significantly lower than control values in all the experimental groups. Increasing levels of lactate were observed with decreasing O_2 tension. The elevated lactate in the 100 percent N_2 atmosphere represents a sixfold increase in glycolysis.

ATP and P-creatine levels in the anesthetized mice were very similar to the nonanesthetized animals. Glucose levels were elevated by anesthesia as observed by Mayman et al. [10] in air or 7 percent O_2. In the other gas mixtures, glucose levels were the same as those of the nonanesthetized animals. Glycogen was increased in all the anesthetized animals as compared with control groups and did not decrease as much in 100 percent N_2. Lactate in the anesthetized animals increased in similar fashion to the nonanesthetized group. Increase in glycolysis in the anesthetized animals in 100 percent N_2 was fivefold greater than for animals in room air.

The animals with seizures (100 percent N_2) showed far greater changes in energy reserves than hypoxic animals without seizures. However, as in the case of seizures induced by convulsant agents, no clear correlation between energy supply and convulsions can be seen. ATP levels were normal in both nonanesthetized and anesthetized animals. The P-creatine, glucose, and lactate levels were alike in animals with seizures and those where seizures were prevented with phenobarbital.

SUMMARY AND DISCUSSION. Changes in energy metabolites have been observed in experimental convulsive states induced by various agents. Differentiation should be made between biochemical events which elicit seizures and those which occur as a result of convulsive activity. In the case of convulsions induced by electroshock, there is rapid depletion of P-creatine and ATP and marked increase in lactate. These chemical changes were not affected by secobarbital but were diminished by phenobarbital.

When convulsive states were induced by pentylenetetrazol, insulin, fluoroacetate, methionine sulfoximine, or audiogenic stimulation, P-creatine and ATP were maintained at normal levels. Convulsive states induced by anoxia showed decreased levels of P-creatine and carbohydrate stores, but ATP levels were not affected. When seizures were prevented by phenobarbital, P-creatine and glucose showed similar decreases to the nonanesthetized groups, but changes in glycogen were diminished. Hypoxic states (7 to 4 percent O_2) resulted in progressively decreasing levels of P-creatine, glucose, and glycogen and increasing levels of lactate.

The results tend to dissociate ATP levels with seizure generation or termination.

When insulin is given, a marked fall in glucose, glycogen, and lactate was observed; increases in these metabolites occurred following fluoroacetate and MSO administration. No chemical changes were observed which are common to all convulsive states.

REFERENCES

1. Cheng, S.-C. J. Metabolism of frog nerve during activity and recovery. *J. Neurochem.* 7:278, 1961.
2. Ferrendelli, J. A., and McDougal, D. B. Unpublished data.
3. Folbergrova, J., Passonneau, J. V., Lowry, O. H., and Schulz, D. W. Glycogen, ammonia and related metabolites in the brain during seizures evoked by methionine sulfoximine. *J. Neurochem.* 16:191, 1969.
4. Gerard, R. W. Studies on nerve metabolism: II. Respiration in oxygen and nitrogen. *Amer. J. Physiol.* 82:381, 1927.
5. Goldberg, N. D., Passonneau, J. V., and Lowry, O. H. Effects of changes in brain metabolism on the levels of citric acid cycle intermediates, *J. Biol. Chem.* 241:3997, 1967.
6. Heald, P. J. Rapid changes in creatine phosphate level in cerebral cortex slices. *Biochem. J.* 57:673, 1954.
7. King, L. J., Lowry, O. H., Passonneau, J. V., and Venson, V. Effects of convulsants on energy reserves in the cerebral cortex. *J. Neurochem.* 14:599, 1967.
8. Klein, R. J., and Olsen, N. S. Effect of convulsive activity on the concentration of brain glucose, glycogen, lactate, and phosphate. *J. Biol. Chem.* 167:747, 1947.
9. Larrabee, M. G. Oxygen consumption of excised sympathetic ganglia at rest and in activity. *J. Neurochem.* 2:81, 1958.
10. Mayman, C. I., Gatfield, P. D., and Breckenridge, B. McL. The glucose content of brain in anesthesia. *J. Neurochem.* 11:483, 1964.
11. McIlwain, H. Anaerobic glycolysis of cerebral tissues and a second, electrically-induced metabolic defect. *Biochem. J.* 63:257, 1956.
12. McIlwain, H., and Joanny, P. Characteristics required in electrical pulses of rectangular time-voltage relationships for metabolic change and ion movements in mammalian cerebral tissues. *J. Neurochem.* 10:313, 1963.
13. Minard, F. N., and Davis, R. V. The effects of electroshock on the acid-soluble phosphate of rat brain. *J. Biol. Chem.* 237:283, 1962.
14. Nelson, S. R., Passonneau, J. V., and Lowry, O. H. Unpublished data, 1966.
15. Stone, W. E., Webster, J. E., and Gurdjian, E. S. Chemical changes in the cerebral cortex associated with convulsive activity. *J. Neurophysiol.* 8:233, 1945.

5
Central Synaptic Transmitters

DAVID R. CURTIS

A REVIEW of the substances operating as transmitters at synapses in the mammalian central nervous system is relevant to consideration of basic mechanisms of the epilepsies. Abnormalities of transmitter function, at presynaptic or postsynaptic sites, leading to excessive excitation or inadequate inhibition, may be responsible for initiation of disordered and excessive neuronal activity within an epileptogenic *focus*. Subsequent development and spread of paroxysmal activity almost certainly involves synaptic processes; associations have been established between seizure states and alterations of cerebral levels of substances suspected of having a transmitter function [223, 240]. Some anticonvulsants may possibly act in a specific fashion at certain synapses.

Current evidence for the function of acetylcholine, catecholamines, 5-hydroxytryptamine, and amino acids as transmitters, particularly in the cerebral cortex will be summarized here. The general problems associated with transmitter identification have been discussed in relation to amino acids [54]. Factors for consideration are: presence of the substance in the appropriate nerve endings together in that portion of the nervous system with enzymes for synthesis, and enzymic or other mechanisms for inactivation of the transmitter; postsynaptic action identical to that of the synaptically released transmitter, including antagonism by compounds acting in a specific fashion at postsynaptic receptors; and evidence for release of the substance by impulses in appropriate nerve fibers.

None of these factors can independently establish transmitter function [see also 232] and reliance on each is determined to some extent by the investigator. Without detracting from the importance of neurochemical, histochemical, or other types of neuropharmacological evidence, experimental observations of the excitation or depression of single neurons by compounds suspected of being transmitters will be stressed here, as well as antagonism of these effects by substances which also block the appropriate synaptic process in a specific fashion. Information has been derived mainly from investigations in which substances were administered microelectrophoretically close to physiologically and anatomically identified neurons; the uses and disadvantages of this technique have been published recently [50].

ACETYLCHOLINE

The extensive literature concerned with distribution of acetylcholine (ACh), choline acetyltransferase (ChAc), and acetylcholinesterase (AChE) in the mammalian central nervous system [see 104, 128, 236] makes it readily apparent that only a fraction of the total neurons in the brain and spinal cord can be cholinergic or ACh-releasing [see 86]. Nor has the presence been established of any other choline ester or of any other cholinomimetic compound [107, 124, 154]. A reasonable correlation usually exists between levels of ACh, ChAc, and AChE within a given region; areas of particular interest include the cerebral cortex, hippocampus, caudate nucleus, thalamus, spinal cord, and cerebellum. Comparatively high levels of AChE in relation to low levels of both ACh and the transferase characterize the cerebellum. ACh, ChAc, and AChE are associated with a proportion of the nerve endings isolated from brain tissue [67, 69, 166, 237]: ACh as a component of synaptic vesicles, ChAc as a cytoplasmic constituent, and AChE attached to membranes. However, the proportion of cortical synaptic terminals which contain ACh remains unknown; subcellular fractionation techniques have yet to provide evidence for the presence of ACh in terminals of a particular pathway.

In the absence of specific histochemical methods for demonstrating either ACh (but see [2]) or ChAc, considerable use has been made of the distribution of AChE as an indicator of cholinergic function [81, 119, 209]. Some brain-stem reticular and tegmental nuclei give rise to AChE-containing fibers which project extensively to cortical and subcortical structures [204, 206]. More precise localization of the enzyme in the vicinity of synapses will be provided by electron microscopic studies [147, 203, 205, 209], of importance considering differences in opinion on the significance of intracellular AChE [see 209]. Certainly in the hippocampus the fimbria contain both ChAc and AChE [149], and undercutting of suprasylvian or pericruciate areas of the cerebral cortex reduces the levels of both enzymes [105]. In the rat hippocampus, sites of dense AChE staining correspond to aggregations of AChE-containing fibers rather than to concentrations of synaptic endings [205]; there has been caution regarding interpretation of the possible function of intracellularly located AChE [209]. AChE located extracellularly in the immediate vicinity of synapses may be more significant as an indicator of a synaptic function for ACh.

Microelectrophoretic studies have shown that some central neurons are excited and others depressed by ACh [50]. As in the periphery, both nicotinic and muscarinic receptors have been detected on central neurons, but whether the presence of acetylcholine receptors necessarily indicates a direct relationship with synaptic mechanisms is questionable. Specific antagonists of the central actions of ACh have been found, and in a few instances the appropriate antagonist also blocks synaptic action exerted by impulses in particular afferent pathways.

Such observations help to establish the cholinergic nature of the transmission process, although difficulties may exist in demonstrating specific antagonism of synaptic transmission by drugs. Substances administered electrophoretically probably influence only a small proportion of the surface membrane of any one cell and concentrations will usually be much higher in the vicinity of the soma, presumably the commonest site of recording, than at more distant receptors. In order to achieve concentrations of an antagonist at these distant sites adequate to block action of a synaptically released transmitter, concentrations closer to the soma may be more than sufficient to produce membrane effects unrelated to specific antagonism of the same transmitter. On the other hand, if antagonists are administered systemically to achieve a more uniform concentration, there may be problems related to penetration of the blood-brain barrier and to effects at other synapses along the particular afferent pathways being tested.

With regard to the collection of acetylcholine released from central synapses, it is at least possible to administer anticholinesterases as a means of reducing inactivation by AChE. Of necessity, ACh can be collected only at some distance from the site of release, from the surface of tissue, from appropriate veins, or from an artificially created tissue space [170, 220]. It may be hard to determine if the ACh actually originated from nerve terminals [see 32].

CEREBRAL CORTEX, RHINENCEPHALON

Current evidence for the operation of ACh as a cortical transmitter relates to the distribution of ACh, ChAc, and AChE in cortical tissue, the effect of ACh on cortical neurons, the action of ACh antagonists on the synaptic excitation or inhibition of these cells, and the release of ACh from the cortical surface.

A high proportion of the ACh and ChAc of neocortical tissue can be isolated in as sociation with nerve-ending particles [67, 237]; the pyriform cortex, the amygdala, and the hippocampus also contain ChAc [108]. Within the sensory-motor cortex (cats, monkeys) some AChE-containing fibers are located superficially in layer I, but the majority occur deeply in relation to the pyramidal cells of layer V and the polymorph cells of layer VI [139]. Some of these fibers originate from adjacent or more distant areas of the cortex; others, of subcortical origin, originate from the septal region, the striatum, and the midbrain reticular formation [139, 140, 206].

AChE-containing fibers are more uniformly distributed in the pyriform cortex, those of the amygdala occur particularly in the central and basal nuclei [139]. Hippocampal AChE-containing fibers are concentrated in a superficial and deep layer, the pyramidal cells of Ammon's horn and the granule cells of the dentate gyrus containing very little of the enzyme. As with the neocortex, these fibers are derived largely from other cortical areas, subcortical nuclei, and the brain stem; the hippocampal formation receives fibers from the medial septum and diagonal band [139, 148].

ACh Effects. Acetylcholine, administered electrophoretically, excites a proportion of neurons in the feline neocortex; the most consistently sensitive cells are deep pyramidal cells including those of primary sensory areas and the cells of origin of the corticospinal tract, which exhibit irregular spontaneous activity of the *projection* type [41, 131, 210, 211].

The excitatory effect of ACh is slow in onset and maximum firing rates are attained in 10–40 sec after a latent period, during which spontaneous activity is often temporarily depressed; firing persists for 15–60 sec after termination of the ACh ejection. Receptors are of muscarinic type: carbamylcholine, acetyl-β-methylcholine, and muscarine are powerful excitants; the action of ACh can be blocked by atropine administered intravenously or electrophoretically [41, 132]. In addition to enhancing the effect of ACh, anticholinesterases such as edrophonium and neostigmine excite cortical neurons. Similar muscarinic receptors associated with excitation by ACh have also been detected on some neurons throughout the pyriform cortex [143], in the amygdala [216], and on a proportion of hippocampal pyramidal cells [20, 111, 212].

Cortical and subcortical ACh receptors are also evidenced by experiments where cholinomimetics and other substances, acting upon ACh receptors, are administered into the cortical subarachnoid space, intraventricularly [84, 85], or by direct injection into brain tissue [11, 158].

In addition to excitation, acetylcholine depresses some cortical neurons, particularly those located in layers II, III, and IV of the sensorimotor region [179, 188]. This depression is blocked by atropine [179, 188] and strychnine [180], and the receptors involved may also have nicotinic properties [182], although the significance of nicotinic receptors in cortical inhibition is questionable [7].

Acetylcholine may be a transmitter at both excitatory and inhibitory synapses within the cortex, although distribution of AChE-containing fibers does not always correlate well with that of acetylcholine-sensitive cells [209]. Relating these effects of ACh to the operation of particular afferent pathways to the neocortex has been attempted. Transcallosal fibers and short latency pathways from midline and specific thalamic nuclei are probably not cholinergic since many cells fired by impulses in these fibers are not sensitive to ACh [131]; in addition, systemically administered atropine does not block short latency discharges resulting from stimulation of specific thalamic nuclei [132, see also 218]. On the other hand, many neurons fired by ACh exhibit prolonged, repetitive *afterdischarge* following stimulation of peripheral sensory nerves or specific thalamic nuclei [131]; atropine administered systemically tends to block this repetitive firing [132].

Atropine Effects. Effects of atropine may not provide reliable evidence for a transmitter function for ACh at terminals upon deep pyramidal cells; the sensitivity to ACh of subcortical neurons (including those of the striate complex and thalamus, which may be involved in repetitive firing pathways) is also reduced by atropine. The late repetitive firing and the spontaneous projection activity of deep pyramidal cells are not affected by atropine administered electrophoretically near single neurons [18, 41]; the synapses involved in these types of firing may however be located distally from the somatic site of recording and atropine ejection, and remain largely unaffected by the antagonist. Cortical neurons fired by ACh can also be activated from the mesencephalic reticular formation [130], an area from which cortical *arousal* can be evoked with desynchronized activation of the electroencephalogram; arousal response can be suppressed by intravenously administered atropine [30, 125].

The firing of cortical neurons of layers II, III, and IV depressed by ACh has been related to the presence of cholinergic inhibitory interneurons in the cortex. The long-lasting inhibitory effects of repetitive stimulation of the pyramidal tract, mesencephalic reticular formation, lateral hypothalamus, or the cortical surface are reduced by electrophoretically administered atropine or strychnine [179–181]. The inhibitory effect of cortical surface stimulation on ACh-sensitive neurons is also reduced by dihydro-β-erythroidine or D-tubocurarine [182]; it is difficult to specify the type of receptor involved in the inhibitory process.

In the presence of an anticholinesterase, ACh is released continuously from the exposed cerebral cortex in both anesthetized [77, 155, 169] and unanesthetized [30, 36, 208] mammals. ACh can also be detected by means of a push-pull cannula inserted superficially into the cortex, release being negligible at depths greater than 3 mm and from white matter following cortical removal [170].

Convulsant and Anesthetic Agents. The spontaneous release rate of ACh, which is higher from the sensorimotor cortex than from parietal, auditory, and visual cortexes, is enhanced by convulsants [15, 30] and reduced by anesthetic agents; halothane and diethyl ether are less effective in this respect than are barbiturates, which do not lower the levels as much as does chloralose [176]. Significantly, the cortical content of ACh is higher in anesthetized than in unanesthetized (particularly convulsing) animals. For any one cortical area, the release rate is roughly proportional to the *integrated electrical activity* of that region, and is higher in the presence of electroencephalographic arousal than with more synchronized patterns of the EEG [30, 208].

Highest release rates are observed in unanesthetized intact animals, with progressive reductions following sequential high cervical (encéphale isolé) or midpontine pretrigeminal section, midcollicular section (cerveau isolé), and undercutting of the cortex leaving the blood supply intact; under the latter circumstance, release is virtually abolished [14, 30, 155, 208, but see 219].

Unilateral midbrain transection in midpontine pretrigeminal preparations causes synchronization of the EEG on that side and a marked ipsilateral increase in the cortical content of ACh [175]; a similar lesion in an encéphale isolé preparation results in an ipsilateral reduction in ACh release from the cortex [208]. Furthermore, the cortical release rate of ACh is enhanced by direct cortical stimulation, by afferent volleys in transcallosal or primary afferent pathways [35, 109, 169, 176], and by stimulation of subcortical structures, particularly when this results in electroencephalographic evidence of arousal [30, 125, 219].

Stimulation of a specific afferent pathway increases the rate of ACh release from both the appropriate primary receiving area and other areas of the cortex: following retinal or lateral geniculate stimulation the release from the visual cortex is two to three times that from other parts of the cortex [33]. Such great differences have not been reported for cutaneous, auditory, or visual stimulation [176].

The experimental findings [see also 125] have led to the proposal that a reticulocortical pathway, projecting widely to the cortex and associated with cortical arousal, and a more specific thalamocortical pathway, responsible for augmenting and repetitive afterdischarge responses and probably distinct from the direct short-latency thalamocortical fibers, are both cholinergic [27, 35, 36]. This proposal does not completely exclude intracortical cholinergic neurons from contributing to cortical ACh release: the spontaneous release from undercut cortical slabs, although very low, can be raised to approximately one-fourth that of the intact cortex when the slab and the intact tissue are stimulated directly [35]. This figure is in reasonable agreement with the finding that the undercut cortex retains approximately 17 percent of its normal level of ChAc [105].

When atropine or hyoscine is administered systemically, the cortical content of ACh falls [98] and stimulation of the mesencephalic reticular formation fails to desynchronize the EEG. At the same time, the rate of ACh release from the cortex is enhanced [14, 30, 169, see also 183]; similar results have been observed after topical administration of atropine [14, 76, 217]. No completely satisfactory explanation has been provided for the enhanced release of ACh by atropine in association with a presumably postsynaptic block of the cholinergic activating system.

Cortically Released ACh. That the cortically released ACh originates from synaptic terminals has been evidenced by several types of experiment. Reduction of calcium content in the fluid bathing the cortex reduces the release rate [109, 187], a condition which also reduces the release of ACh at peripheral cholinergic synapses. Addition of hemicholinium-3 to the bathing fluid decreases both the release of ACh [218] and the cortical ACh content [153, see also 71]; and reticular formation stimulation, which enhances cortical ACh release, does not enhance the release of urea previously applied to the exposed cortex [37].

On the basis of these results, strong claims can be made for a predominantly rostrally projecting cholinergic system, originating from reticular and tegmental nuclei and other forebrain structures, distributed to practically all cortical and subcortical structures, and which is possibly identical to the ascending reticular activating system [139, 148, 206, see also 24, 130, 150, 241]. There is also evidence for a cholinergic thalamocortical pathway, associated with augmenting and the late repetitive responses evoked by afferent impulses, and for some cholinergic intracortical neurons associated with prolonged inhibition, but the actual pathways involved have not been described.

The possible sites of origin of all these postulated cholinergic systems are not readily amenable to investigation by electrical stimulation; all the pathways appear to be characterized by prolonged conduction times, due to many synapses or to very small fibers, or both. A remarkable feature of the cholinergic system, presumably vital in the control of cortical function, is that the release of ACh tends to exceed the rate of synthesis, a phenomenon not apparent in peripheral cholinergic systems. However this conclusion [see 153], drawn from the relation between the cortical content of ACh and the release of ACh under experimental conditions, may not be completely justified because of the nonphysiological nature of the stimuli used.

Despite the lack of a full understanding of the role of ACh in the cortex, a synaptic function at both excitatory and inhibitory synapses is not unlikely. It may be significant that atropine reportedly has both anticonvulsant [96, 207] and convulsant [17, 168] properties.

BASAL GANGLIA

The caudate nucleus contains particularly high levels of ACh, ChAc, and AChE [104, 119, 128, 200, 203]. A high rate of ACh turnover is indicated by rapid reduction in ACh levels following intracaudate injection of hemicholinium [106]. AChE levels are high in most striatal regions except the claustrum [139], some AChE-containing fibers originating in the ventral-tegmental portion of the mesencephalic reticular formation and the substantia nigra [206].

A proportion of caudate neurons is excited by electrophoretically administered cholinomimetics, particularly cells located toward the ventricular and ventrolateral surfaces [22, 164]. Other cells are depressed, and similar excitant and depressant effects have been observed in the putamen and the globus pallidus [243]. Receptors are of muscarinic type, the ACh action being readily blocked by atropine: results are consistent with effects which follow direct injection of muscarinic agents into the caudate [see 118]. In the cat, effects of ACh on single caudate neurons are paralleled by electrical stimulation of the thalamic nucleus ventralis anterior; synaptic excitation and inhibition are likewise blocked by electrophoretically or systemically administered atropine [164].

Significantly, spontaneous release of ACh from the caudate nucleus [171] can be enhanced by stimulating this thalamic nucleus [161], as well as a portion of the anterior sigmoid cortex or the caudate nucleus itself [171]. ACh, probably of caudate origin, can also be detected in ventricular fluid [183, 184]; the rate of release is increased by afferent cutaneous and auditory volleys and by electrical stimulation of the substantia nigra.

Evidence exists for cholinergic synapses in the feline striatal complex, possibly concerned with both excitation and inhibition. Although the presence of cholinergic synapses in the human striatum provides an explanation for beneficial effects of atropine in Parkinson's disease, the sites of origin of the cholinergic fibers have not been ascertained in primates. A major portion of this system may originate in the mesencephalic reticular formation.

Thalamus

The mammalian thalamus, including geniculate bodies, contains moderate amounts of ACh, ChAc, and AChE [28, 86, 108]. Histochemically, few of the cells contain AChE, which is present mainly in nerve fibers originating from the mesencephalic reticular formation via the dorsal tegmental pathway [rat, 204, 206]. The brachium conjunctivum, projecting to the ventrolateral nucleus, also contains ChAc and AChE and may contain some cholinergic fibers [8, 86, 108].

Neurons fired by acetylcholine administered electrophoretically are found throughout the various thalamic nuclei, and the receptors contain mixed nicotinic-muscarinic properties; depression by ACh also has been reported [50]. Based on the absence of effects of acetylcholine antagonists, spinothalamic, optic, or corticothalamic pathways would not be cholinergic. In contrast, a cholinergic process is evidenced by the firing of neurons in the ventrobasal complex, in the ventrolateral nucleus, and in the lateral geniculate nucleus by stimulating the mesencephalic reticular formation [160, 177; see also 63]. Acetylcholine is released spontaneously in dorsal and ventrobasal thalamic nuclei, and the rate of release is enhanced by stimulating visual and cutaneous afferents as well as by stimulation of the mesencephalic reticular formation [178]. The finding that the excitation of some ventrolateral thalamic neurons by impulses in the brachium conjunctivum is depressed by atropine [88, 160] supports proposals that some of the brachium fibers may be cholinergic.

Spinal Cord

ACh and ChAc levels are higher in ventral than in dorsal roots [104], but differences in levels of AChE are less marked. The few available figures indicate a higher level of ACh in dorsal than ventral gray matter, the levels in gray being higher than those of white matter [153]. AChE activity is weak in all fiber tracts of the cord, and within the gray matter the enzyme is concentrated in the ventral horn, the intermediomedial and intermediolateral columns, and the substantia gelatinosa [97, 119]. AChE has been localized at the surface of physiologically identified Renshaw cells, and is presumably that associated with the synapses of motor-axon collateral fibers [83].

Renshaw cells are readily excited by acetylcholine; the predominant receptor type is nicotinic, and clear evidence shows that ACh is the excitatory transmitter released by collateral branches of spinal-motor axons [57–59, 73, 74, 186]. Firing produced by ACh reaches a peak frequency within 1–3 sec of the beginning of the electrophoretic current and ceases within 1 sec of its termination. Excitation is suppressed by dihydro-β-erythroidine, which also blocks the synaptic excitation of Renshaw cells by axon-collateral volleys, and is enhanced and prolonged by anticholinesterases, which have a similar potentiating effect on synaptic excitation. Hemicholinium-3, after prolonged repetitive stimulation of axon-collateral fibers, progressively reduces and finally abolishes synaptic excitation by such volleys, presumably by reducing the amount of ACh released without altering either the sensitivity of Renshaw cells to ACh or the firing produced by afferent fibers other than axon collaterals. Antidromic stimulation of alpha motor fibers increases the amount of ACh in the effluent of the perfused spinal cord of the cat, and the rate of release is not modified by dihydro-β-erythroidine [141].

Cholinomimetics also excite Renshaw cells by interaction with muscarinic receptors; excitation is blocked by atropine, but an association of these sites with synaptic excitation has not been established. Acetylcholine has relatively weak excitatory and depressant effects upon some spinal interneurons [60, 80, 229], but, again, cholinergic pathways have not been identified to account for the presence of synaptically significant ACh receptors. It is relevant that afferent impulses cause enhanced release of ACh from the feline spinal cord, which is unlikely to result from excitation of motoneurons [see 141]. In addition to motor-axon collaterals, there may be other cholinergic fibers in the spinal cord, perhaps of both local and descending origin [100, 227].

Cerebellum

The possibility that ACh operates as a transmitter in the cerebellar cortex is controversial [see 209]; the cerebellum contains little ACh and ChAc but comparatively high levels of AChE. There are marked species differences in occurrence and distribution of AChE, as well as differences between various cerebellar regions within the one species. Histochemical analyses of AChE distribution do not always correspond with biochemical evidence for presence of the enzyme. In the cat, Purkinje cells [40], granule cells [159], and cells of the intracerebellar nuclei [31] have been excited by electrophoretically administered ACh; sensitivity of the granule cells may be associated with cholinergic mossy fibers originating in the brain-stem reticular formation. Firing of Purkinje cells may be unrelated to the function of ACh as a transmitter, but further investigation is obviously required, particularly in other animals where distribution of AChE differs from that of the cat. Results of these experiments will be of considerable relevance to the proposition that AChE-containing fibers are necessarily of cholinergic function.

CATECHOLAMINES, 5-HYDROXYTRYPTAMINE

Transmitter functions for norepinephrine (NE), dopamine (DA), and 5-hydroxytryptamine (5-HT) are suggested by regional differences in the intracerebral distribution of these substances and associated enzymes [29, 82, 117], the isolation of catecholamine-containing and 5-HT-containing nerve terminals from brain tissue [68, 167, 174, 238], and particularly by fluorescent histochemical demonstrations of NE, DA, and 5-HT within nerve fibers and terminals [94, 113, 114]. There is neuropharmacological evidence for excitation and depression of neurons by these substances [23, 50, 157, 194, 197, 213, 230]. Recent investigations have been concerned with correlating the sensitivity of single neurons to NE, DA, and 5-HT with the presence in their vicinity of very fine unmyelinated fibers containing relatively high concentrations of the monoamines within varicosities. The major proportion of the monoamine content of the brain is stored within these varicosities, presumably presynaptic structures specialized for synthesis, storage, and release of amines; the cell bodies and nonterminal axons contain only very low concentrations. Characteristic differences have been described between catecholamine-containing (NE, DA) and 5-HT-containing neurons, including the nature of the fluorescence observed, the location of the parent cell bodies, the distribution and features of axons and varicosities, and the effects of drugs which enhance or reduce the store of a particular amine [92, 94, 113, 114]. Few of these investigations have been carried out on primates.

Neurons giving rise to catecholamine-containing fibers are localized almost exclusively in the lower brain stem. Most of the NE cell bodies are in the pons and medulla, particularly within the locus caeruleus and the ventrolateral portion of the medullary reticular formation. These cells give rise to two bulbospinal systems and to ascending fibers which distribute widely via the medial forebrain bundle to the hypothalamus, the preoptic area, the septal area, the gyrus cinguli, the neocortex, the amygdaloid cortex, the hippocampus, and the thalamus. Fibers containing DA arise mainly from two groups of neurons in the ventral cranial portion of the mesencephalon: the pars compacta of the substantia nigra projecting to the caudate nucleus and the putamen, and a group of cells dorsal to the interpeduncular nucleus, some of which send axons to the hypothalamus. On the other hand, 5-HT neurons lie mainly in the lower brain stem, almost exclusively in the midline raphe complex, sending axons to forebrain structures via the medial forebrain bundle and to the spinal cord.

Widely distributed systems of fibers containing NE, DA, and 5-HT originate mainly from brain-stem nuclei. With the possible exception of the substantia nigra, these nuclei are not readily accessible to investigation by electrical stimulation. Analysis of synaptic events so evoked is complicated by slow conduction velocity of axons and temporal dispersion of volleys.

Cerebral Cortex, Rhinencephalon

Nerve terminals and varicosities containing NE or 5-HT are present in practically all cortical areas including the hippocampus and cerebellum [90, 93], the majority of terminals in the neocortex making axo-dendritic contacts in the more superficial layers. Cortical content of DA is very low. Although both excitation and depression have been observed when NE, DA, or 5-HT are administered electrophoretically near neurons in the cerebral cortex [133, 193], pyriform cortex, amygdala [143, 215, 216], septum [110], and the hippocampus [20, 111, 212], depressant effects usually predominate, except for 5-HT, which has marked excitatory effects on some cortical neurons [193]. Apart from antagonism of 5-HT-excitation of cortical neurons by lysergic acid diethylamide [193], no specific antagonists of central depressant effects of NE, DA, or 5-HT have been found.

Depressant effects of NE and 5-HT on neurons in the olfactory bulb; antagonism between dibenamine, phentolamine, lysergic acid diethylamide, 2-bromo-(+)-lysergic acid diethylamide, and NE; reduction by these antagonists of inhibition of mitral cells by lateral-olfactory tract stimulation; and the presence of fibers containing NE and 5-HT in the bulb have suggested that these amines are transmitters in this region [197].

Subcortical Structures

Microelectrophoretically administered amines have both excitant and depressant effects on neurons in the mammalian brain stem, hypothalamus, thalamus, and striate complex [25, 50, 197, 230]; experiments have yet to be carried out on primates.

Considerable interest has centered on involvement of nigro-neostriatal, DA-containing pathways in the pathogenesis of Parkinson's disease [29, 91, 117]. The DA content of the caudate nucleus is high; approximately 25 percent can be recovered in isolated nerve endings [238]. The action of electrophoretically administered DA on caudate and globus pallidus-putamen neurons is predominantly depression, although excitation of a low proportion of cells has also been reported [22, 112, 165, 242, 243]. Depression of some caudate neurons by DA is blocked by phenoxybenzamine, which also frequently suppresses the inhibition of these cells evoked by stimulating the thalamic nucleus centromedianus [165, 242]; stimulation of this nucleus increases release of DA from the caudate nucleus [161]. On the other hand, electrical stimulation of the substantia nigra results in excitation [3, 38, 89, 165, 242] of some caudate neurons and inhibition [3, 38] of others. It may be doubtful that the large cells of pars compacta, which give rise to DA-containing terminals, are associated with the shortest latency nigro-caudate projection [89].

Although stimulation of the substantia nigra does not enhance release of DA within the caudate nucleus of the cat [161], there is an increased release of homovanillic acid, the major metabolite of DA, into the lateral ventricle [185]. Stimulation of the substantia nigra, but not of the thalamic nucleus centromedianus, increases release of DA from the feline putamen [162].

SPINAL CORD

All terminals containing NE or 5-HT in the spinal cord are derived from descending pathways [113]; their importance in controlling operation of spinal neurons has been suggested by profound alterations in spinal reflexes which follow systemic administration of dihydroxyphenylalanine, 5-hydroxytryptophan, inhibitors of aromatic amino acid decarboxylase, antagonists of 5-HT and NE receptors, or reserpine [13, 76, 78, 79, 151, 152]. Although NE shows a predominantly depressant action on spinal motoneurons, interneurons, Renshaw cells, and autonomic preganglionic neurons when administered electrophoretically [65, 66, 80, 229], failure to find a specific antagonist of this depression [19, 80], together with associated difficulties in stimulating the cells of origin of the descending *noradrenergic* pathway so far have prevented full investigation of NE action in the spinal cord [49]. Similar difficulties exist with 5-HT, which has both depressant and excitant actions on spinal neurons [80, 229]; 5-HT excites sympathetic [65] but not parasympathetic [66] preganglionic neurons.

AMINO ACIDS

Disturbances of cerebral amino acid levels, particularly of glutamine, glutamic acid, aspartic acid, and gamma-aminobutyric acid (GABA), have long been associated with convulsive disorders [102, 223, 228]. In view of the involvement of such compounds in cerebral oxidative metabolism, it has not been established clearly whether the altered levels are responsible for, or result from, the abnormal neuronal activity.

When administered extracellularly in amounts to produce concentrations of the order of one percent of the normal overall brain levels, acidic amino acids excite and neutral amino acids related to GABA depress neurons [62]. Extracellular concentrations of these pharmacologically active amino acids presumably are maintained at very low levels; alterations sufficient to excite or depress groups of neurons may not be detectable by analysis of the whole tissue. Such neurochemical investigations of cerebral amino acid levels under a variety of conditions have provided valuable information on the function of these compounds. While a discussion of amino acid metabolism is outside the scope of this review, recent evidence [54] for participation of some of these substances as transmitters is highly relevant to the problem of epilepsy.

Whether or not transmitter functions can be established conclusively, alterations of distribution of amino acids between intracellular and extracellular phases in a localized region of the CNS may be adequate to affect excitability of a group of neurons, regardless of their involvement in functionally different neuronal networks. Such a condition, resulting from inhibition or malfunction of enzymes, or disturbances of membrane-uptake mechanisms, may well be the basis of a *biochemical* lesion resulting in epilepsy. The excitant amino acids, glutamic and aspartic acids, and the depressant neutral amino acids, GABA and glycine will be considered in more detail; other excitant and depressant amino acids may also be of importance in connection with convulsive or other states associated with inborn errors of amino acid metabolism.

The vertebrate nervous system contains appreciable amounts of free amino acids, a high proportion presumably being concerned with metabolism and maintenance of cellular water and ion levels. Differences in concentrations between gray and white matter, differences in regional distribution, or association with particular types of neurons may provide significant indications of transmitter function. Few investigations of this type have been made, although histochemical techniques have been used to demonstrate enzymes associated with the metabolism of some amino acids.

Subcellular distribution studies have not indicated specific localization of excitant or depressant amino acids in synaptic terminals isolated from cortical tissue [156, 195, 231], even though synaptic vesicles contain appreciable amounts of these substances [239]. Such results would be expected of a transmitter which either has other intracellular functions and is evenly distributed throughout the cytoplasm, or can be synthesized very rapidly within presynaptic terminals. The relatively crude techniques used during isolation of nerve endings may fail to separate sufficient intact endings containing amino acid from cell bodies to provide significant evidence of a presynaptic amino acid store.

Considerable information is available regarding uptake of amino acids by brain slices or homogenates, and apparently there are structurally specific systems for a wide range of these compounds [21, 146]. Uptake mechanisms differ from membrane processes associated with depressant or depolarizing actions of these compounds [188, 189]. Although in vivo cellular uptake of amino acids provides a ready explanation for maintenance of low extracellular levels and also, perhaps, for rapid removal after synaptic release, the relevance of in vitro studies to processes taking place in vivo in a tissue with complex metabolic and ionic requirements remains to be determined.

Amino Acid Distributions

L-*Glutamic*. The amino acid most abundant in the brain is L-glutamic acid [222]; levels are highest in the cerebral hemispheres and fall progressively toward the spinal cord [202], where higher concentrations occur dorsally than ventrally, suggesting that L-glutamic acid may be the excitatory transmitter of primary afferent fibers [99]. On the other hand, L-aspartic acid, more uniformly distributed in the CNS, is concentrated slightly more in the ventral gray quadrant of the spinal cord than dorsally [99]. Following temporary aortic occlusion in the cat and anoxic destruction of spinal interneurons, correlation is significant between the decrease in concentration of aspartic acid in spinal gray matter and the loss of interneurons; aspartic acid has been proposed as an excitatory transmitter released from spinal interneurons [64]. Widespread distribution of L-glutamic and L-aspartic acids may well indicate that both are involved as excitatory transmitters throughout the mammalian central nervous system.

GABA. Numerous investigations have been concerned with GABA, an amino acid which occurs uniquely in the CNS, particularly in gray matter, where regional differences in concentration correspond roughly to density of neurons [87, 189, 190]. The related substance, β-hydroxy-GABA, might also be considered a possible inhibitory transmitter [103]. GABA is derived principally from L-glutamic acid, and the enzyme L-glutamic acid decarboxylase (GAD) is found only in the CNS, again largely in gray matter and more highly concentrated in nerve endings [12, 196, 231]. On the other hand, GABA-α-ketoglutarate transaminase (GABA-T), which catalyzes the reversible transamination of GABA with α-ketoglutarate, is also found chiefly in gray matter but largely as a cytoplasmic constituent [190]. The GABA-transaminase-succinic semialdehyde dehydrogenase system (GABA-T-S) can be visualized histochemically [224].

In the cerebral cortex, GABA levels are highest in the outer layer [115], but in the cerebellum both the GABA and GAD content of the Purkinje cell layer are higher than those of the molecular or granule-cell layers [190]. GABA content of isolated Purkinje cell bodies, on a weight-per-volume basis, exceeds that of excitatory neurons such as spinal motoneurons and ganglion cells [172], a particularly significant finding in view of the inhibitory nature of Purkinje cells [75]. Other cerebellar neurons, including basket and Golgi cells, are also inhibitory neurons, and an unknown proportion of the Purkinje cell GABA may be present in the terminals of neurons synapsing upon the Purkinje cells.

Cerebellar GABA-T-S is found within neurons which receive inhibitory synapses —Purkinje cells, Golgi cells, and mossy fiber terminals [190, 224]. High levels of GABA-T-S are also found in brain-stem and spinal motoneurons and in synaptic endings of possible inhibitory function surrounding hippocampal-pyramidal cells [225]. In the spinal cord, GABA levels are higher dorsally than ventrally [87], higher in dorsal gray than ventral gray, lower but approximately equal in dorsal and ventral white segments, and very low in dorsal and ventral roots [99]. Higher concentrations of GABA in the dorsal horn correspond to the high levels of GAD [4] and the low levels of glutamic-γ-aminobutyric transaminase [199]. The intraspinal distribution of GABA is not altered significantly after anoxic destruction of predominantly centrally located spinal interneurons [64], supporting, perhaps, an association between GABA and inhibitory terminals located upon dorsal horn interneurons.

Glycine. Of considerable interest as a possible spinal inhibitory transmitter [6], glycine concentrations in the medullary, cervical, and lumbar spinal enlargements of cats and rats are considerably higher than those in the cerebral hemispheres and the diencephalon; cerebellar levels are particularly low [5]. Within the cat's lumbar spinal cord, glycine is more concentrated in the ventral gray matter than in other regions [99, 123]. This distribution would correspond to that of an inhibitory transmitter released from interneurons having synaptic terminals predominantly on spinal motoneurons; glycine content of white matter may be associated with propriospinal fibers [99]. Evidence for an association between glycine and spinal interneurons is supported by correlation between a reduced number of small neurons which follows temporary aortic occlusion and the fall in spinal glycine levels [64].

Other amino acids as possible central transmitters include L-α-alanine, serine, taurine, and cystathionine. Levels of α-alanine and serine are somewhat higher in the gray matter than elsewhere in the spinal cord [123, 233], but cystathionine appears to be evenly distributed [123] and may be of significance in supraspinal regions [see 234]. Alterations in brain cystathionine levels, perhaps in association with production of homocysteic acid, may be important in homocystinuria. Spinal taurine levels are low in comparison with those found in the cerebral hemispheres and cerebellum [123, 202].

Many of the enzymes concerned with amino acid metabolism are pyridoxal dependent, are inhibited by hydrazines, hydrazides, other carbonyl trapping agents, and pyridoxal antagonists. Both GAD and GABA-T are particularly susceptible to these substances [192], and brain GABA levels can be altered by administration of various inhibitors, including thiosemicarbazide, hydroxylamine, and amino-oxyacetic acid.

Thiosemicarbazide depresses cerebral GABA levels while hydroxylamine and amino-oxyacetic acid usually raise GABA levels. When GABA levels are reduced by thiosemicarbazide, presumably a consequence of GAD inhibition, animals are more susceptible to seizures; alterations in cortical seizure threshold do not always correspond to the content of GABA, particularly when levels are increased by hydroxylamine or amino-oxyacetic acid [142, 190, 192, 221]. This is not unexpected in view of the probable greater significance of extracellular amino acid concentrations (rather than the overall level) in controlling nerve cell excitability. Seizures may result from alteration in activity of very few neurons; causative disturbances of amino acid levels in a restricted area of the CNS may not be detectable biochemically. Similar considerations may be applied to production of convulsions by methionine sulphoximine, an inhibitor of glutamine synthetase [see 70].

Amino Acid Actions

L-Glutamic and L-Aspartic Acids. When administered microelectrophoretically to the external surface of neurons, L-glutamic acid reversibly depolarizes both spinal motoneurons [55] and cortical neurons [129, 136]. Such an alteration in membrane potential explains the enhanced excitability or actual firing of all other types of central neurons by this and related amino acids [50, 62]. Intracellular ejection of L-glutamic acid has little or no effect on neurons [39], hence the depolarization results from a change in membrane properties which follows interaction of the amino acid with external membrane receptors.

Depolarization is accompanied by increased membrane conductance, indicative of movement of ions through the membrane. Since the membrane effect of excitatory synaptic transmitters is also one of depolarization, identification of amino acids as transmitters requires the demonstration that the two types of depolarization be generated by the same membrane processes. There are considerable difficulties in determining the ionic events generating excitatory postsynaptic potentials, and in comparing them with ionic changes produced by electrophoretically administered substances; nevertheless, the reversal potentials for both types of depolarization are at a more depolarized level than the resting potential [40, 48]. Intracellular injections of potassium or chloride ions into motoneurons, which produce profound changes in inhibitory postsynaptic potentials, cause no appreciable changes in excitatory synaptic or amino acid depolarizations. The ionic mechanism of depolarization by amino acids may be similar to that of synaptic excitation, probably involving an increase in membrane permeability to sodium and potassium ions [72].

No substances have yet been found which, when administered electrophoretically, either antagonize in a specific fashion or prolong the excitatory effect of amino acids. Failure to prolong amino acid excitation by a variety of enzyme inhibitors, and the similar time courses of action of D- and L-enantiomorphs, may indicate that intracellular uptake is important in removing these substances from the extraneuronal space. Finding specific antagonists is an essential urgent requirement for establishing the role of glutamic and aspartic acids in synaptic excitation [see 54].

In general, relative potencies of excitant amino acids such as N-methyl-D-aspartic acid, DL-homocysteic acid, and L-glutamic acid retain a constant relationship when assessed on different types of neurons, within the limitations of microelectrophoretic technique [see 61]. It was reported recently [163] that neurons in the thalamic nucleus ventralis lateralis are more sensitive to L-glutamic acid, relative to sensitivity to DL-homocysteic and N-methyl-DL-aspartic acids, than are more superficially located neurons. Such investigations should be extended to include other neurons and amino acids, particularly aspartic acid.

GABA and Glycine. Earlier experiments failed to detect alterations of membrane potential of spinal and cortical neurons by GABA, but it has now been established that, when administered extracellularly, GABA hyperpolarizes and increases the membrane conductance of cortical neurons [137], Deiters' neurons [173], and spinal motoneurons [53]. Glycine hyperpolarizes cortical neurons [53] and spinal motoneurons [53, 235]; the ionic mechanism of the effect on motoneurons is indistinguishable from that of GABA. Neuroglial cells [136] and spinal axons are not hyperpolarized by amino acids, and probably the action of these substances is confined to synapses. Similar hyperpolarizing action presumably accounts for depression of the excitability of all types of neurons throughout the CNS by these and related neutral amino acids.

The hyperpolarizing action of GABA and glycine on spinal motoneurons can be reversed to depolarization by increasing the membrane potentials of these cells; the reversal potential is similar to that of inhibitory postsynaptic potentials [53, 233, 235]. Amino acid and synaptic hyperpolarizations, and their reversal potentials, are altered in the same fashion by manipulation of the intracellular content of potassium, or of anions of small hydrated diameter. The ionic mechanism of spinal synaptic inhibition has been analyzed in considerable detail by injecting ions of differing hydrated diameter into motoneurons [72]. The alteration of receptor membrane permeability by the inhibitory transmitter has been described as a sievelike mechanism, where pores can be measured by determining if ions of different hydrated size pass through the membrane. The critical pore diameter of the membrane when activated by synaptically released transmitter is slightly less than that of the hydrated sodium ion, and is apparently similar if not identical to that when the membrane is activated by electrophoretically administered GABA or glycine [53].

The reversal potential for GABA hyperpolarization of cortical neurons is also close to that of inhibitory potentials evoked by direct cortical stimulation [137]; elevation of the intracellular chloride ion concentration has the same effect on both types of hyperpolarization. It has been generally assumed that the ionic mechanism of synaptic inhibition is the same throughout the mammalian CNS, namely an increase in membrane permeability to potassium and chloride ions [72]. But recent analysis suggests that, in contrast to spinal motoneurons, relatively large anions, some of which have a greater hydrated ion diameter than sodium ions, contribute to the membrane current of cortical neurons during synaptic inhibition [127]. If these results can be substantiated, the effect of GABA on cortical neurons apparently differs from that on spinal neurons.

At present, within limitations of available techniques, GABA and glycine appear to have the same postsynaptic action on central neurons as do synaptically released inhibitory transmitters. Differences in relative sensitivity of different neurons to these two amino acids suggest that they may be involved as transmitters in two different inhibitory systems. In general, glycine is a more potent depressant of spinal motoneurons and interneurons than is GABA. The reverse is true for cortical neurons, whereas glycine and GABA are approximately equipotent as depressants of Renshaw cells and cuneate neurons [54]. These results indicate that glycine may be more important as an inhibitory transmitter in the spinal cord, and GABA in the cerebral cortex and cerebellum, a separation of amino acid function which gathers support from a study of the effects of strychnine.

Strychnine. Strychnine in low concentrations reversibly blocks the postsynaptic inhibition of motoneurons and other spinal neurons by impulses in a number of spinal and descending pathways [46, 49]. It has been observed that this alkaloid and other substances of related and diverse structure, all of which diminish spinal inhibition, also reversibly suppress hyperpolarization and depression of spinal neurons by glycine without affecting that produced by GABA. This is of considerable significance in establishing glycine as a major spinal inhibitory transmitter [52, 53].

On the basis of strychnine antagonism and presence in spinal tissue, glycine, as well as L-α-alanine, cystathionine, serine, and taurine, all require consideration as possible spinal inhibitory transmitters. The importance of glycine is perhaps indicated by its abundance and distribution in the spinal cord. Apart from strychnine and related substances which also block the effect of glycine on cortical neurons, no other glycine antagonist was found in a study of compounds which included picrotoxin, pentamethylenetetrazol, and a series of glycine analogues. Tetanus toxin, which blocks spinal inhibitions of the strychnine-sensitive type [26], does not influence the inhibitory action of glycine (or GABA) upon spinal Renshaw cells; presumably it diminishes the amount of transmitter released from spinal inhibitory terminals [51].

Strychnine does not influence the depressant effect of GABA upon cortical and spinal neurons, or the synaptic inhibition of cortical cells, or Deiters' neurons [52, 53, 135, 173]. Exhaustive search has not revealed any antagonist of either GABA or these supraspinal synaptic inhibitions [52, 135, 138], but it might be unwise to accept these negative results as evidence that GABA is the actual transmitter.

AMINO ACID INACTIVATION

Further support for the transmitter function of an amino acid would be provided by the action of a substance that prolonged both the effect of the artificially administered amino acid and the synaptic process with which its effect is being equated. Depressant actions of glycine and GABA on spinal neurons are rapidly reversible after electrophoretic administration, but they are not prolonged by a series of amino acid analogues or enzyme inhibitors, which might be expected to block enzymic or uptake mechanisms involved in the maintenance of low extracellular levels of these amino acids [52, 138, 173].

Significant potentiation of the depressant action of glycine on spinal neurons was obtained with *p*-hydroxymercuribenzoic acid [52], and more recently with *p*-chloromercuriphenylsulphonic acid. These substances in higher concentration also increase the effectiveness of GABA, L- and D-α-alanine, and β-alanine as depressants. It appears unlikely that mercury derivatives inhibit specific enzymes which inactivate glycine in spinal tissue, but further investigation of these compounds is warranted. Considerable technical difficulties associated with these experiments have so far prevented any adequate assessment of the effect of *p*-chloromercuriphenylsulphonic acid on synaptic inhibition.

Release of Amino Acids

Demonstrating the release of an amino acid from nervous tissue, related to the activity of excitatory or inhibitory neurons, would provide supporting evidence for a transmitter function. However, it might be expected that inactivating mechanisms, including cellular uptake, would remove amino acids rapidly from the site of release; this would limit the amount available for detection either on the surface of the tissue, within an artificially created tissue space, or in the bloodstream. Considering the metabolic importance of amino acids and difficulties associated with stimulating systems of excitatory or inhibitory neurons in isolation, it might not be possible to show that the released amino acid is related to the firing of particular excitatory or inhibitory neurons, or is of synaptic origin.

The importance of GABA and L-glutamic acid as cortical transmitters may be indicated by studies of release of these substances from the cortical surface [121, but see 120]. When the pia-arachnoid is perforated, an EEG pattern indicative of arousal is accompanied by a high rate of release of glutamic acid and a low release rate of GABA. In contrast, electroencephalographic evidence of sleep is associated with a reduced rate of glutamic acid release and an increase in GABA release. There is no similar correlation between EEG patterns and the release of glutamine and aspartic acid. Stimulation of the mesencephalic reticular formation in a cerveau isolé preparation enhances cortical release of both ACh and L-glutamate; stimulation of thalamic nuclei produces significantly increased release of ACh only [122]. GABA can be detected when the fourth ventricle is perfused; increased amounts found when the cerebellar cortex is stimulated may originate from Purkinje cell terminals in Deiters' and cerebellar nuclei lying close to the ventricle [172].

Transmitter Function of Amino Acids

Glutamic and aspartic acids, glycine, and GABA are present in the mammalian CNS. Although distribution of glycine in the spinal cord is that expected of an inhibitory transmitter and distribution of glutamic acid that of an excitatory transmitter released by primary afferent fibers, the relationship of the other amino acids to excitatory or inhibitory interneurons may be obscured by their association with cellular metabolic processes. It might be claimed that these and related amino acids are present in nervous tissue *primarily* as transmitter substances, that metabolic processes in which they participate are concerned predominantly with transmitter synthesis, storage, and inactivation.

Glutamic and aspartic acids depolarize nerve cells, and the ionic mechanism of this depolarization appears similar to that of synaptic excitation. Similarly, hyperpolarization of neurons by GABA and glycine probably involves the same alteration in membrane permeability as that which occurs during synaptic inhibition. The lack of effect of amino acids on neuroglial cells and axons indicates an action confined to synapses, but it is yet to be established that excitant and depressant amino acids act only at excitatory and inhibitory synapses respectively.

Specific antagonists have not been found for glutamic acid, aspartic acid, or GABA. Strychnine and strychnine-like substances which block spinal postsynaptic inhibition reversibly block the hyperpolarizing action of glycine. It has not been possible to prolong action of an amino acid, or the synaptic process with which it may be associated, either by inhibiting enzymes or interfering with amino acid uptake mechanisms.

Results suggest that glycine could be the transmitter of strychnine-sensitive inhibitory synapses, particularly in the spinal cord and medulla. On the other hand, GABA may be the major inhibitory transmitter in supraspinal regions, including the cerebral cortex, the cerebellum, and sites of synaptic termination by Purkinje cells. Glutamic and aspartic acids may be excitatory transmitters released at central terminations of the major afferent and efferent pathways, the former particularly in the cerebral cortex and by primary afferent fibers, the latter in the spinal cord.

OTHER SUBSTANCES PROPOSED AS
CENTRAL TRANSMITTERS

Other substances have been proposed as central transmitters, but in most instances definitive evidence of transmitter function has yet to be established.

Adenosinetriphosphate (ATP). Suggested as an excitatory transmitter released from primary afferent terminals [116], but, apart from effects ascribed to the chelation of calcium ions (cuneate neurons [95]), ATP does not excite neurons [56].

Ergothioneine. Present particularly in the cerebellum [45] and identified as the *cerebellar excitatory factor* [43, 44], ergothioneine increases the electrical activity of the rabbit cerebellum when injected into the carotid bloodstream. Neither cerebral cortical [134] nor cerebellar [42, 134] neurons are influenced by electrophoretically administered ergothioneine, although a proportion of brain-stem neurons are excited by this compound, particularly when administered by a microtap [9].

Histamine. Present in the mammalian brain, particularly in the hypophysis in association with mast cells, high levels of histamine also occur in the mammillary bodies and ventral hypothalamus [1]. Subcellular-distribution studies of the nonmast-cell histamine indicate localization in nerve endings [126]. Electrophoretically administered histamine does not affect spinal interneurons [56] and is a weak depressant of cortical [133] and cuneate [95] neurons.

Substance P. A complex of polypeptides extracted from brain and other tissues [34, 145, 214, 244], substance P has a subcellular distribution in cortical tissue similar to that of ACh [237]. A substance like substance P is released from the somatosensory cortex of anesthetized cats, and the rate of release is enhanced by analeptic drugs, particularly during the period of cortical vasodilatation [201]. An enzyme found in bovine brain inactivates substance P [33]. Inconsistent effects upon central neurons have been reported after intraventricular or intracerebral injection of partially purified samples of substance P [10, 101, 226]; electrophoretically administered substance P does not influence the firing of dorsal horn interneurons [47] or cuneate neurons [95]. It appears unlikely that substance P is the excitatory transmitter released by primary afferent fibers [144].

Prostaglandins. Present in mammalian brain tissue, prostaglandins are released from the cortical surface and influence the firing of neurons when injected into lateral ventricles or microelectrophoretically into the brain stem [see 16]. A transmitter function at particular synapses has yet to be established.

SUMMARY

The evidence has been reviewed for the involvement of acetylcholine, norepinephrine, dopamine, 5-hydroxytryptamine, glutamic and aspartic acids, glycine, and GABA and some other substances present in nervous tissue as synaptic transmitters in the mammalian central nervous system. Specific antagonists have not been found for excitatory transmitters released at terminals of major central afferent and efferent pathways; the excitant amino acids, L-glutamic and L-aspartic, may well be transmitters at these synapses. Glycine is probably the transmitter at strychnine-sensitive inhibitory synapses; GABA may be involved at strychnine-insensitive inhibitory synapses, particularly in the cerebral cortex, although a specific antagonist is required in order to establish clearly a transmitter function for this amino acid.

Acetylcholine is the excitatory transmitter released at nicotinic synapses upon spinal Renshaw cells by motor-axon collateral terminals; it may also be the excitatory transmitter of the ascending reticular activating system which projects to cortical and subcortical structures and terminates at synapses of a predominantly muscarinic nature. Widely distributed systems of fibers containing norepinephrine, dopamine, and 5-hydroxytryptamine arise from brain-stem nuclei. These amines have central excitant and depressant effects, but absence of specific antagonists has prevented pharmacological identification of the majority of proposed aminergic pathways.

REFERENCES

1. Adam, H. M., and Hye, H. K. A. Concentration of histamine in different parts of brain and hypophysis of cat and its modification by drugs. *Brit. J. Pharmacol.* 28:137, 1966.
2. Akert, K., and Sandri, C. An electron-microscopic study of zinc iodide-osmium impregnation of neurons. I. Staining of synaptic vesicles at cholinergic junctions. *Brain Res.* 7:286, 1968.
3. Albe-Fessard, D., Raieva, S., and Santiago, W. Sur les relations entre substance noire et noyau caude. *J. Physiol.* (Paris) 59:324, 1967.
4. Albers, R. W., and Brady, R. O. Distribution of glutamic decarboxylase in the nervous system of the Rhesus monkey. *J. Biol. Chem.* 234:926, 1959.
5. Aprison, M. H., Shank, R. P., Davidoff, R. A., and Werman, R. The distribution of glycine, a neurotransmitter suspect in the central nervous system of several vertebrate species. *Life Sci.* 7:583, 1968.
6. Aprison, M. H., and Werman, R. The distribution of glycine in cat spinal cord and roots. *Life Sci.* 4:2075, 1965.
7. Armitage, A. K., and Hall, G. H. Nicotine, smoking and cortical activation. *Nature* (London) 219:1179, 1968.
8. Austin, L., and Phillis, J. W. The distribution of cerebellar cholinesterases in several species. *J. Neurochem.* 12:709, 1965.
9. Avanzino, G. L., Bradley, P. B., Comis, S. D., and Wolstencroft, J. H. A comparison of the actions of ergothioneine and chlorpromazine applied to single neurones by two different methods. *Int. J. Neuropharmacol.* 5:331, 1966.
10. Baile, C. A., and Meinardi, H. Action of substance P on the central nervous system of a goat. *Brit. J. Pharmacol.* 30:302, 1967.
11. Baker, W. W., and Benedict, F. Analysis of local discharges induced by intrahippocampal microinjection of carbachol or diisopropylfluorophosphate (DFP). *Int. J. Neuropharmacol.* 7:135, 1968.
12. Balazs, R., Dahl, D., and Harwood, J. R. Subcellular distribution of enzymes of glutamate metabolism in rat brain. *J. Neurochem.* 13:897, 1966.
13. Banna, N. R., and Anderson, E. G. The effects of 5-hydroxytryptamine antagonists on spinal neuronal activity. *J. Pharmacol. Exp. Ther.* 162:319, 1968.
14. Bartolini, A., and Pepeu, G. Investigations into the acetylcholine output from the cerebral cortex of the cat in the presence of hyoscine. *Brit. J. Pharmacol.* 31:66, 1967.
15. Beleslin, D., Polak, R. L., and Sproull, D. H. The effect of leptazol and strychnine on the acetylcholine release from the cat brain. *J. Physiol.* (London) 181:308, 1965.
16. Bergström, S., and Samuelsson, B. *Prostaglandins*. Stockholm: Almqvist and Wiksell, 1967.
17. Bernard, P. J., Piette, Y., Delaunois, A. L., and de Schaepdryver, A. F. Action of atropine and atropine methylnitrate on cortical epilepsy in the rabbit. *Arch. Int. Pharmacodyn.* 172:224, 1968.
18. Biscoe, T. J., and Curtis, D. R. Unpublished data, 1966.
19. Biscoe, T. J., Curtis, D. R., and Ryall, R. W. An investigation of catecholamine receptors of spinal interneurones. *Int. J. Neuropharmacol.* 5:429, 1966.
20. Biscoe, T. J., and Straughan, D. W. Micro-electrophoretic studies of neurones in the cat hippocampus. *J. Physiol.* (London) 183:341, 1966.
21. Blasberg, R., and Lajtha, A. Hetero-

geneity of the mediated transport systems of amino acid uptake in brain. *Brain Res.* 1:86, 1966.

22. Bloom, F. E., Costa, E., and Salmoiraghi, G. C. Anesthesia and the responsiveness of individual neurons of the caudate nucleus of the cat to acetylcholine, norepinephrine and dopamine administered by microelectrophoresis. *J. Pharmacol. Exp. Ther.* 150:244, 1965.

23. Bloom, F. E., and Giarman, N. J. Physiologic and pharmacologic considerations of biogenic amines in the nervous system. *Ann. Rev. Pharmacol.* 8:229, 1968.

24. Bradley, P. B., and Fink, M. Anticholinergic drugs and brain functions in animals and man. *Progress in Brain Research,* vol. 28. London: Elsevier, 1968.

25. Bradley, P. B., and Wolstencroft, J. H. Actions of drugs on single neurones in the brain stem. *Brit. Med. Bull.* 21:15, 1965.

26. Brooks, V. B., Curtis, D. R., and Eccles. J. C. The action of tetanus toxin on the inhibition of motoneurones. *J. Physiol.* (London) 135:655, 1957.

27. Brownlee, W. C., and Mitchell, J. F. The pharmacology of cortical repetitive afterdischarges. *Brit. J. Pharmacol.* 33:217P, 1968.

28. Burgen, A. S. V., and Chipman, L. M. Cholinesterase and succinic dehydrogenase in the central nervous system of the dog. *J. Physiol.* (London) 114:296, 1951.

29. Carlsson, A. Morphologic and Dynamic Aspects of Dopamine in the Central Nervous System. In Costa, E., Côté, L. J., and Yahr, M. D. (Eds.), *Biochemistry and Pharmacology of the Basal Ganglia.* New York: Hewlett, Raven Press, 1966, pp. 107–113.

30. Celesia, G., and Jasper, H. H. Acetylcholine released from cerebral cortex in relation to state of activation. *Neurology* (Minneap.) 16:1053, 1966.

31. Chapman, J. B., and McCance, I. Acetylcholine sensitive cells in the intracerebellar nuclei of the cat. *Brain Res.* 5:535, 1967.

32. Chase, T. N., and Kopin, I. J. Stimulus-induced release of substances from olfactory bulb using the push-pull cannula. *Nature* (London) 217:466, 1968.

33. Claybrook, D. L., and Pfiffner, J. J. Purification and properties of a substance P–inactivating enzyme from bovine brain. *Biochem. Pharmacol.* 17:281, 1968.

34. Cleugh, J., Gaddum, J. H., Mitchell, A. A., Smith, M. W., and Whittaker, V. P. Substance P in brain extracts. *J. Physiol.* (London) 170:69, 1964.

35. Collier, B., and Mitchell, J. F. The central release of acetylcholine during stimulation of the visual pathway. *J. Physiol.* (London) 184:239, 1966.

36. Collier, B., and Mitchell, J. F. The central release of acetylcholine during consciousness and after brain lesions. *J. Physiol.* (London) 188:83, 1967.

37. Collier, B., and Murray-Brown, N. Validity of a method measuring transmitter release from the central nervous system. *Nature* (London) 218:484, 1968.

38. Connor, J. D. Caudate unit responses to nigral stimuli: Evidence for a possible nigro-neostriatal pathway. *Science* 160:899, 1968.

39. Coombs, J. S., Eccles, J. C., and Fatt, P. The specific ionic conductances and the ionic movements across the motoneuronal membrane that produce the inhibitory post-synaptic potential. *J. Physiol.* (London) 130:326, 1955.

40. Coombs, J. S., Eccles, J. C., and Fatt, P. Excitatory synaptic action in motoneurones. *J. Physiol.* (London) 130:374, 1955.

41. Crawford, J. M., and Curtis, D. R. Pharmacological studies on feline Betz cells. *J. Physiol.* (London) 186:121, 1966.

42. Crawford, J. M., Curtis, D. R., Voorhoeve, P. E., and Wilson, V. J. Acetylcholine sensitivity of cerebellar neurones in the cat. *J. Physiol.* (London) 186:139, 1966.

43. Crossland, J., Garven, J. D., and Mitchell, J. F. Characterization and distribution in the central nervous system of the cerebellar excitatory factor. *J. Physiol.* (London) 148:20P, 1959.

44. Crossland, J., and Mitchell, J. F. The effect on the electrical activity of the cerebellum of a substance present in cerebellar extracts. *J. Physiol.* (London) 132:391, 1956.

45. Crossland, J., Mitchell, J. F., and Woodruff, G. N. The presence of ergothioneine in the central nervous system and its probable identity with cerebellar factor. *J. Physiol.* (London) 182:427, 1966.

46. Curtis, D. R. The pharmacology of central and peripheral inhibition. *Pharmacol. Rev.* 15:333, 1963.

47. Curtis, D. R. The Actions of Amino Acids upon Mammalian Neurones. In Curtis,

D. R., and McIntyre, A. K. (Eds.), *Studies in Physiology, Presented to J. C. Eccles.* Heidelberg: Springer, 1965, p. 34.
48. Curtis, D. R. Unpublished data, 1965.
49. Curtis, D. R. Pharmacology and Neurochemistry of Mammalian Central Inhibitory Processes. In von Euler, C., Skoglund, S., and Söderberg, U. (Eds.), *Structure and Function of Inhibitory Mechanisms.* Oxford: Pergamon, 1968, p. 429.
50. Curtis, D. R., and Crawford, J. M. Central synaptic transmission—microelectrophoretic studies. *Ann. Rev. Pharmacol.* vol. 9, 1969, in press.
51. Curtis, D. R., and de Groat, W. C. Tetanus toxin and spinal inhibition. *Brain Res.* 10:208, 1968.
52. Curtis, D. R., Hösli, L., and Johnston, G. A. R. A pharmacological study of the depression of spinal neurones by glycine and related amino acids. *Exp. Brain Res.* 6:1, 1968.
53. Curtis, D. R., Hösli, L., Johnston, G. A. R., and Johnston, I. H. The hyperpolarization of spinal motoneurones by glycine and related amino acids. *Exp. Brain Res.* 5:238, 1968.
54. Curtis, D. R., and Johnston, G. A. R. Amino Acid Transmitters. In Lajtha, A. (Ed.), *Handbook of Neurochemistry*, vol. 2. New York: Plenum Press, 1968.
55. Curtis, D. R., Phillis, J. W., and Watkins, J. C. The chemical excitation of spinal neurones by certain acidic amino acids. *J. Physiol.* (London) 150:656, 1960.
56. Curtis, D. R., Phillis, J. W., and Watkins, J. C. Cholinergic and non-cholinergic transmission in the mammalian spinal cord. *J. Physiol.* (London) 158:296, 1961.
57. Curtis, D. R., and Ryall, R. W. The excitation of Renshaw cells by cholinomimetics. *Exp. Brain Res.* 2:49, 1966.
58. Curtis, D. R., and Ryall, R. W. The acetylcholine receptors of Renshaw cells. *Exp. Brain Res.* 2:66, 1966.
59. Curtis, D. R., and Ryall, R. W. The synaptic excitation of Renshaw cells. *Exp. Brain Res.* 2:81, 1966.
60. Curtis, D. R., Ryall, R. W., and Watkins, J. C. The action of cholinomimetics on spinal interneurones. *Exp. Brain Res.* 2:97, 1966.
61. Curtis, D. R., and Watkins, J. C. Acidic amino acids with strong excitatory actions on mammalian neurones. *J. Physiol.* (London) 166:1, 1963.
62. Curtis, D. R., and Watkins, J. C. The pharmacology of amino acids related to gamma-aminobutyric acid. *Pharmacol. Rev.* 17:347, 1965.
63. David, J. P., Murayama, S., Machne, X., and Unna, K. R. Evidence supporting cholinergic transmission at the lateral geniculate body of the cat. *Int. J. Neuropharmacol.* 2:113, 1963.
64. Davidoff, R. A., Graham, L. T., Jr., Shank, R. P., Werman, R., and Aprison, M. H. Changes in amino acid concentrations associated with loss of spinal interneurons. *J. Neurochem.* 14:1025, 1967.
65. De Groat, W. C., and Ryall, R. W. An excitatory action of 5-hydroxytryptamine on sympathetic preganglionic neurones. *Exp. Brain Res.* 3:299, 1967.
66. De Groat, W. C., and Ryall, R. W. The identification and characteristics of sacral parasympathetic preganglionic neurones. *J. Physiol.* (London) 196:563, 1968.
67. De Robertis, E. *Histophysiology of Synapses and Neurosecretion.* Oxford: Pergamon, 1964.
68. De Robertis, E. Adrenergic endings and vesicles isolated from brain. *Pharmacol. Rev.* 18:413, 1966.
69. De Robertis, E. Ultrastructure and cytochemistry of the synaptic region. *Science* 156:907, 1967.
70. De Robertis, E., Sellinger, O. Z., Rodriguez de Lores Arnaiz, G., Alberici, M., and Zieher, L. M. Nerve endings in methionine sulphoximine convulsant rats, a neurochemical and ultrastructural study. *J. Neurochem.* 14:81, 1967.
71. Dren, A. T., and Domino, E. F. Effects of hemicholinium (HC-3) on EEG activation and brain acetylcholine in the dog. *J. Pharmacol. Exp. Ther.* 161:141, 1968.
72. Eccles, J. C. *Physiology of Synapses.* Berlin-Heidelberg: Springer, 1964.
73. Eccles, J. C., Eccles, R. M., and Fatt, P. Pharmacological investigations on a central synapse operated by acetylcholine. *J. Physiol.* (London) 131:154, 1956.
74. Eccles, J. C., Fatt, P., and Koketsu, K. Cholinergic and inhibitory synapses in a pathway from motor-axon collaterals to motoneurones. *J. Physiol.* (London) 126:524, 1954.
75. Eccles, J. C., Ito, M., and Szentágothai, J.

The Cerebellum as a Neuronal Machine. New York: Springer, 1967.

76. Ellaway, P. H., and Pascoe, J. E. Noradrenaline as a transmitter in the spinal cord. *J. Physiol.* (London) 197:8P, 1968.

77. Elliott, K. A. C., Swank, R. L., and Henderson, N. Effect of anesthetics and convulsants on acetylcholine content of brain. *Amer. J. Physiol.* 162:469, 1950.

78. Engberg, I., Lundberg, A., and Ryall, R. W. The effect of reserpine on transmission in the spinal cord. *Acta Physiol. Scand.* 72:115, 1968.

79. Engberg, I., Lundberg, A., and Ryall, R. W. Is the tonic decerebrate inhibition of reflex paths mediated by monoaminergic pathways? *Acta Physiol. Scand.* 72:123, 1968.

80. Engberg, I., and Ryall, R. W. The inhibitory action of noradrenaline and other monoamines on spinal neurones. *J. Physiol.* (London) 185:298, 1966.

81. Eränkö, O. Histochemistry of nervous tissues: catecholamines and cholinesterases. *Ann. Rev. Pharmacol.* 7:203, 1967.

82. Erspamer, V. Occurrence of Indolealkylamines in Nature. In Eichler, O., and Farah, A. (Eds.), *Handbook of Experimental Pharmacology*, vol. 19. Berlin: Springer, 1966, p. 132.

83. Erulkar, S. D., Nichols, C. W., Popp, M. B., and Koelle, G. B. Renshaw elements: Localization and acetylcholinesterase content. *J. Histochem. Cytochem.* 16:128, 1968.

84. Feldberg, W. *A Pharmacological Approach to the Brain from its Inner and Outer Surface.* London: Edward Arnold, 1963.

85. Feldberg, W., and Fleischhauer, K. A new experimental approach to the physiology and pharmacology of the brain. *Brit. Med. Bull.* 21:36, 1965.

86. Feldberg, W., and Vogt, M. Acetylcholine synthesis in different regions of the central nervous system. *J. Physiol.* (London) 107:372, 1948.

87. Florey, E., and Florey, E. Studies on the distribution of Factor I in mammalian brain. *J. Physiol.* (London) 144:220, 1958.

88. Frigyesi, T. L., and Purpura, D. P. Acetylcholine sensitivity of thalamic synaptic organizations activated by brachium conjunctivum stimulation. *Arch. Int. Pharmacodyn.* 163:110, 1966.

89. Frigyesi, T. L., and Purpura, D. P. Electrophysiological analysis of reciprocal caudato-nigral relations. *Brain Res.* 6:440, 1967.

90. Fuxe, K. Evidence for the existence of monoamine neurons in the central nervous system. III. The monoamine nerve terminal. *Z. Zellforsch.* 65:573, 1965.

91. Fuxe, K., and Anden, N.-E. Studies on Central Monoamine Neurons with Special Reference to the Nigro-Neostriatal Dopamine Neuron System. In Costa, E., Côté, L. J., and Yahr, M. D. (Eds.), *Biochemistry and Pharmacology of the Basal Ganglia.* New York: Raven Press, 1966, p. 107.

92. Fuxe, K., Dahlström, A., and Hillarp, N.-Å. Central monoamine neurons and monoamine neuro-transmission. *XXIII Int. Physiol. Cong.* 4:419, 1965.

93. Fuxe, K., Hamberger, B., and Hökfelt, T. Distribution of noradrenaline nerve terminals in cortical areas of the rat. *Brain Res.* 8:125, 1968.

94. Fuxe, K., Hökfelt, T., and Ungerstedt, U. Localization of Indolealkylamines in CNS. In Garattini, S., and Shore, P. A. (Eds.), *Advances in Pharmacology*, vol. 6. New York: Academic, 1968, p. 235.

95. Galindo, A., Krnjević, K., and Schwartz, S. Micro-iontophoretic studies on neurones in the cuneate nucleus. *J. Physiol.* (London) 192:359, 1967.

96. Gastaut, H. *The Epilepsies.* Springfield, Ill.: Thomas, 1954.

97. Gerebtzoff, M. A. *Cholinesterases.* Oxford: Pergamon, 1959.

98. Giarman, N. J., and Pepeu, G. The influence of centrally acting cholinolytic drugs on brain acetylcholine levels. *Brit. J. Pharmacol.* 23:123, 1964.

99. Graham, L. T., Jr., Shank, R. P., Werman, R., and Aprison, M. H. Distribution of some synaptic transmitter suspects in cat spinal cord: Glutamic acid, aspartic acid, γ-aminobutyric acid, glycine and glutamine. *J. Neurochem.* 14:465, 1967.

100. Gwyn, D. G., and Wolstencroft, J. H. Ascending and descending cholinergic fibers in cat spinal cord: Histochemical evidence. *Science* 153:1543, 1966.

101. Haefely, W., and Hürlimann, A. Substance P, a highly active naturally occurring polypeptide. *Experientia* 18:297, 1962.

102. Hayashi, T. *Neurophysiology and Neuro-*

chemistry of Convulsion. Tokyo: Dainihon-Tosho, 1959.

103. Hayashi, T. Gamma-Aminobutyric Acid and Its Derivatives in Mental Health. In Martin, G. J., and Kisch, B. (Eds.), *Enzymes in Mental Health.* Philadelphia: Lippincott, 1966, p. 160.

104. Hebb, C. O. Formation, Storage and Liberation of Acetylcholine. In Koelle, G. B. (Ed.), *Handbuch der Experimentellen Pharmakologie,* vol. 15: *Cholinesterases and Anticholinesterase Agents.* Berlin: Springer, 1963, p. 56.

105. Hebb, C. O., Krnjević, K., and Silver, A. Effect of undercutting on the acetylcholinesterase and choline acetyltransferase activity in cat's cerebral cortex. *Nature* (London) 198:692, 1963.

106. Hebb, C. O., Ling, G. M., McGeer, E. G., McGeer, P. L., and Perkins, D. Effect of locally applied hemicholinium on the acetylcholine content of the caudate nucleus. *Nature* (London) 204:1309, 1964.

107. Hebb, C. O., and Morris, D. Parallel bioassay as a method of identifying acetylcholine. *Nature* (London) 214:284, 1967.

108. Hebb, C. O., and Silver, A. Choline acetylase in the central nervous system of man and some other mammals. *J. Physiol.* (London) 134:718, 1956.

109. Hemsworth, B. A., and Mitchell, J. F. The characteristics of acetylcholine release mechanisms in the auditory cortex. *Arch. Pharmak. Exp. Pathol.* 259:209, 1968.

110. Herz, A., and Gogolak, G. Mikroelektrophoretische Untersuchungen am Septum des Kaninchens. *Pflueger Arch. Ges. Physiol.* 285:317, 1965.

111. Herz, A., and Nacimiento, A. C. Über die Wirkung von Pharmaka auf Neurone des Hippocampus nach mikroelektrophoretischer Verabfolgung. *Arch. Exp. Path. Pharmak.* 251:295, 1965.

112. Herz, A., and Zieglgänsberger, W. The influence of microelectrophoretically applied biogenic amines, cholinomimetics and procaine on synaptic excitation in the corpus striatum. *Int. J. Neuropharmacol.* 7:221, 1968.

113. Hillarp, N.-Å., Fuxe, K., and Dahlström, A. Demonstration and mapping of central neurons containing dopamine, noradrenaline, and 5-hydroxytryptamine and their reactions to psychopharmaca. *Pharmacol. Rev.* 18:727, 1966.

114. Hillarp, N.-Å., Fuxe, K., and Dahlström, A. Central Monoamine Neurons. In von Euler, U. S., Rosell, S., and Uvnäs, B. (Eds.), *Mechanisms of Release of Biogenic Amines.* Oxford: Pergamon, 1966, p. 31.

115. Hirsch, H. E., and Robins, E. Distribution of γ-aminobutyric acid in the layers of the cerebral and cerebellar cortex. Implications for its physiological role. *J. Neurochem.* 9:63, 1962.

116. Holton, P. The liberation of adenosine triphosphate on antidromic stimulation of sensory nerves. *J. Physiol.* (London) 145:494, 1959.

117. Hornykievicz, O. Dopamine (3-hydroxytyramine) and brain function. *Pharmacol. Rev.* 18:925, 1966.

118. Hull, C. D., Buchwald, N. A., and Ling, G. Effects of direct cholinergic stimulation of forebrain structures. *Brain Res.* 6:22, 1967.

119. Ishii, T., and Friede, R. L. A comparative histochemical mapping of the distribution of acetylcholinesterase and nicotinamide adenine dinucleotide-diaphorase activities in the human brain. *Int. Rev. Neurobiol.* 10:231, 1967.

120. Iversen, L. L., and Neal, M. J. Uptake of ^{3}H-gamma-aminobutyric acid (GABA) by rat cerebral cortex. *Brit. J. Pharmacol.* 33:216, 1968.

121. Jasper, H. H., Khan, R. T., and Elliott, K. A. C. Amino acids released from the cerebral cortex in relation to its state of activation. *Science* 147:1448, 1965.

122. Jasper, H. H., and Koyama, I. Amino acids released from the cortical surface in cats following stimulation of the mesial thalamus and mid-brain reticular formation. *Electroenceph. Clin. Neurophysiol.* 24:292, 1968.

123. Johnston, G. A. R. The intraspinal distribution of some depressant amino acids. *J. Neurochem.* 15:1013, 1968.

124. Johnston, G. A. R., Lloyd, H. J., and Stone, N. Liquid cation exchange extraction of cholinomimetic activity from brain. *J. Neurochem.* 15:361, 1968.

125. Kanai, T., and Szerb, J. C. Mesencephalic reticular activating system and cortical acetylcholine output. *Nature* (London) 205:80, 1965.

126. Kataoka, K., and De Robertis, E. Histamine in isolated small nerve endings and synaptic vesicles of rat brain cortex. *J. Pharmacol. Exp. Ther.* 156:114, 1967.

127. Kelly, J. S., Krnjević, K., Morris, M. E., and Yim, G. K. Anionic permeability of cortical neurones during inhibition. *J. Physiol.* (London) 196:120P, 1968.

128. Koelle, G. B. Cytological Distributions and Physiological Functions of Cholinesterases. In Koelle, G. B. (Ed.), *Handbuch der Experimentellen Pharmakologie,* vol. 15: *Cholinesterases and Anticholinesterase Agents.* Berlin: Springer, 1963, p. 187.

129. Krnjević, K. Micro-iontophoretic studies on cortical neurones. *Int. Rev. Neurobiol.* 7:41, 1964.

130. Krnjević, K. Chemical transmission and cortical arousal. *Anesthesiology,* 28:100, 1967.

131. Krnjević, K., and Phillis, J. W. Acetylcholine sensitive cells in the cerebral cortex. *J. Physiol.* (London) 166:296, 1963.

132. Krnjević, K., and Phillis, J. W. Pharmacological properties of acetylcholine-sensitive cells in the cerebral cortex. *J. Physiol.* (London) 166:328, 1963.

133. Krnjević, K., and Phillis, J. W. Actions of certain amines on cerebral cortical neurones. *Brit. J. Pharmacol.* 20:471, 1963.

134. Krnjević, K., Randić, M., and Straughan, D. W. Ergothioneine and central neurones. *Nature* (London) 205:603, 1965.

135. Krnjević, K., Randić, M., and Straughan, D. W. Pharmacology of cortical inhibition. *J. Physiol.* (London) 184:78, 1966.

136. Krnjević, K., and Schwartz, S. Some properties of unresponsive cells in the cerebral cortex. *Exp. Brain Res.* 3:306, 1967.

137. Krnjević, K., and Schwartz, S. The action of γ-aminobutyric acid on cortical neurones. *Exp. Brain Res.* 3:320, 1967.

138. Krnjević, K., and Schwartz, S. The Inhibitory Transmitter in the Cerebral Cortex. In von Euler, C., Skoglund, S., and Söderberg, U. (Eds.), *Structure and Function of Inhibitory Neuronal Mechanisms.* Oxford: Pergamon, 1968, p. 419.

139. Krnjević, K., and Silver, A. A histochemical study of cholinergic fibres in the cerebral cortex. *J. Anat.* 99:711, 1965.

140. Krnjević, K., and Silver, A. Acetylcholinesterase in the developing forebrain. *J. Anat.* 100:63, 1966.

141. Kuno, M., and Rudomin, P. The release of acetylcholine from the spinal cord of the cat by antidromic stimulation of motor nerve. *J. Physiol.* (London) 187:177, 1966.

142. Kuriyama, K., Roberts, E., and Rubinstein, M. K. Elevation of γ-aminobutyric acid in brain with amino-oxyacetic acid and susceptibility to convulsive seizures in mice: A quantitative re-evaluation. *Biochem. Pharmacol.* 15:221, 1966.

143. Legge, K. F., Randić, M., and Straughan, D. W. The pharmacology of neurones in the pyriform cortex. *Brit. J. Pharmacol.* 26:87, 1966.

144. Lembeck, F. Zur Frage der zentralen Übertragung afferenter Impulse. III. Das Vorkommen und die Bedeutung der Substanz P in den dorsalen Wurzeln des Rückenmarks. *Arch. Exp. Path. Pharmak.* 219:197, 1953.

145. Lembeck, F., and Zetler, G. Substance P, a polypeptide of possible physiological significance, especially within the nervous system. *Int. Rev. Neurobiol.* 4:159, 1962.

146. Levi, G., Kandera, J., and Lajtha, A. Control of cerebral metabolite levels. I. Amino acid uptake and levels in various species. *Arch. Biochem.* 119:303, 1967.

147. Lewis, P. R., and Shute, C. C. D. The distribution of cholinesterase in cholinergic neurons demonstrated with the electron microscope. *J. Cell Sci.* 1:381, 1966.

148. Lewis, P. R., and Shute, C. C. D. The cholinergic limbic system: Projections to hippocampal formation, medial cortex, nuclei of the ascending cholinergic reticular system, and the subfornical organ and supra-optic crest. *Brain* 90:521, 1967.

149. Lewis, P. R., Shute, C. C. D., and Silver, A. Confirmation from choline acetylase analyses of a massive cholinergic innervation to the rat hippocampus. *J. Physiol.* (London) 191:215, 1967.

150. Longo, V. G. Behavioural and electroencephalographic effects of atropine and related compounds. *Pharmacol. Rev.* 18:965, 1966.

151. Lundberg, A. Monoamines and Spinal Reflexes. In Curtis, D. R., and McIntyre, A. K. (Eds.), *Studies in Physiology, Presented to J. C. Eccles.* Berlin: Springer, 1965, p. 186.

152. Lundberg, A. Integration in the Reflex Pathway. In Granit, R. (Ed.), *Muscular Afferents and Motor Control.* Stockholm: Almqvist and Wiksell, 1966, p. 275.

153. MacIntosh, F. C. The distribution of acetylcholine in the peripheral and the central nervous system. *J. Physiol.* (London) 99:436, 1941.

154. MacIntosh, F. C. Synthesis and storage of acetylcholine in nervous tissue. *Canad. J. Biochem.* 41:2555, 1963.
155. MacIntosh, F. C., and Oborin, P. E. Release of Acetylcholine from Intact Cerebral Cortex. In XIX Int. Physiol. Congr., *Abstracts of Communications*. 1953, p. 580.
156. Mangan, J. L., and Whittaker, V. P. The distribution of free amino acids in subcellular fractions of guinea-pig brain. *Biochem. J.* 98:128, 1966.
157. Mantegazzini, P. Pharmacological Actions of Indolealkylamines and Precursor Aminoacids on the Central Nervous System. In Eichler, O., and Farah, A. (Eds.), *Handbook of Experimental Pharmacology*, vol. 19. Berlin: Springer, 1966, p. 424.
158. Marczynski, T. J. Topical application of drugs to subcortical brain structures and selected aspects of electrical stimulation. *Ergebn. Physiol.* 59:86, 1967.
159. McCance, I., and Phillis, J. W. Discharge patterns of elements in cat cerebellar cortex, and their responses to iontophoretically applied drugs. *Nature* (London) 204:844, 1964.
160. McCance, I., Phillis, J. W., and Westerman, R. A. Acetylcholine-sensitivity of thalamic neurones: Its relationship to synaptic transmission. *Brit. J. Pharmacol.* 32:635, 1968.
161. McLennan, H. The release of acetylcholine and of 3-hydroxytyramine from the caudate nucleus. *J. Physiol.* (London) 174:152, 1964.
162. McLennan, H. The release of dopamine from the putamen. *Experientia* 21:725, 1965.
163. McLennan, H., Huffman, R. D., and Marshall, K. C. Patterns of excitation of thalamic neurones by amino-acids and by acetylcholine. *Nature* (London) 219:387, 1968.
164. McLennan, H., and York, D. H. Cholinergic mechanisms in the caudate nucleus. *J. Physiol.* (London) 187:163, 1966.
165. McLennan, H., and York, D. H. The action of dopamine on neurones of the caudate nucleus. *J. Physiol.* (London) 189:393, 1967.
166. Michaelson, I. A. The subcellular distribution of acetylcholine, choline acetyltransferase and acetyl cholinesterase in nerve tissue. *Ann. N.Y. Acad. Sci.* 144:387, 1967.
167. Michaelson, I. A. Discussion of the Neuronal Compartmentation of 5-Hydroxytryptamine Stores. In Garattini, S., and Shore, P. A. (Eds.), *Advances in Pharmacology*, vol. 6. New York: Academic, 1968, p. 271.
168. Minvielle, J., Cadilhac, J., and Passouant, P. Action of atropine on epileptics. *Electroenceph. Clin. Neurophysiol.* 6:162, 1954.
169. Mitchell, J. F. The spontaneous and evoked release of acetylcholine from the cerebral cortex. *J. Physiol.* (London) 165:98, 1963.
170. Mitchell, J. F. Acetylcholine Release from the Brain. In von Euler, U. S., Rosell, S., and Uvnäs, B. (Eds.), *Mechanisms of Release of Biogenic Amines*, vol. 5. Oxford: Pergamon, 1966, p. 425.
171. Mitchell, J. F., and Szerb, J. C. The Spontaneous and Evoked Release of Acetylcholine from the Caudate Nucleus. In XXII Int. Congr. Physiol. Sci., *Proceedings*, vol. 2. New York: Excerpta Medica, (1962-64), Abst. No. 819.
172. Obata, K. Unpublished data, 1966.
173. Obata, K., Ito, M., Ochi, R., and Sato, N. Pharmacological properties of the postsynaptic inhibition of Purkinje cell axons and the action of γ-aminobutyric acid on Deiters neurones. *Exp. Brain Res.* 4:43, 1967.
174. Pellegrino de Iraldi, A., Zieher, L. M., and Etcheverry, G. J. Neuronal Compartmentation of 5-Hydroxytryptamine Stores. In Garattini, S., and Shore, P. A. (Eds.), *Advances in Pharmacology*. New York: Academic, 1968, p. 257.
175. Pepeu, G., and Mantegazzini, P. Midbrain hemisection: Effect on cortical acetylcholine in the cat. *Science* 145:1069, 1964.
176. Phillis, J. W. Acetylcholine release from the cerebral cortex: Its role in cortical arousal. *Brain Res.* 7:378, 1968.
177. Phillis, J. W., Tebècis, A. K., and York, D. H. A study of cholinoceptive cells in the lateral geniculate nucleus. *J. Physiol.* (London) 192:695, 1967.
178. Phillis, J. W., Tebècis, A. K., and York, D. H. Acetylcholine release from the feline thalamus. *J. Pharm. Pharmacol.* 20:476, 1968.
179. Phillis, J. W., and York, D. H. Cholinergic inhibition in the cerebral cortex. *Brain Res.* 5:517, 1967.
180. Phillis, J. W., and York, D. H. Strychnine block of neural and drug-induced

inhibition in the cerebral cortex. *Nature* (London) 216:922, 1967.

181. Phillis, J. W., and York, D. H. An intracortical cholinergic inhibitory synapse. *Life Sci.* 7:65, 1968.

182. Phillis, J. W., and York, D. H. Nicotine, smoking and cortical inhibition. *Nature* (London) 219:89, 1968.

183. Polak, R. L. Effect of hyoscine on the output of acetylcholine into perfused cerebral ventricles of cats. *J. Physiol.* (London) 181:317, 1965.

184. Portig, P. J., and Vogt, M. Search for substances released on stimulation of the caudate nucleus in the cat. *J. Physiol.* (London) 186:131P, 1966.

185. Portig, P. J., and Vogt, M. Activation of a dopaminergic nigrostriatal pathway. *J. Physiol.* 197:20P, 1968.

186. Quastel, D. M. J., and Curtis, D. R. A central action of hemicholinium. *Nature* (London) 208:192, 1965.

187. Randić, M., and Padjen, A. Effect of calcium ions on the release of acetylcholine from the cerebral cortex. *Nature* (London) 215:990, 1967.

188. Randić, M., Siminoff, R., and Straughan, D. W. Acetylcholine depression of cortical neurones. *Exp. Neurol.* 9:236, 1964.

189. Roberts, E. *Inhibition in the Nervous System and Gamma-Aminobutyric Acid.* New York: Pergamon, 1960.

190. Roberts, E., and Kuriyama, K. Biochemical-physiological correlations in studies of the γ-aminobutyric acid system. *Brain Res.* 8:1, 1968.

191. Roberts, E., and Sano, K. The Specific Occurrence of the γ-Aminobutyric Acid System in Nervous Tissue of Animals. In Mayia, D., and Tyler, A. (Eds.), *General Physiology of Cell Specialization.* New York: McGraw-Hill, 1963, p. 323.

192. Roberts, E., Wein, J., and Simonsen, D. G. γ-Aminobutyric acid (γABA), vitamin B_6, and neuronal function—a speculative synthesis. *Vitamins Hormones* 22:503, 1964.

193. Roberts, M. H. T., and Straughan, D. W. Excitation and depression of cortical neurones by 5-hydroxytryptamine. *J. Physiol.* (London) 193:269, 1967.

194. Rothballer, A. B. The effects of catecholamines on the central nervous system. *Pharmacol. Rev.* 11:494, 1959.

195. Ryall, R. W. The subcellular distributions of acetylcholine, substance P, 5-hydroxytryptamine, γ-aminobutyric acid and glutamic acid in brain homogenates. *J. Neurochem.* 11:131, 1964.

196. Salganicoff, L., and De Robertis, E. Subcellular distribution of the enzymes of the glutamic acid, glutamine and γ-aminobutyric acid cycles in rat brain. *J. Neurochem.* 12:287, 1965.

197. Salmoiraghi, G. C. Central adrenergic synapses. *Pharmacol. Rev.* 18:717, 1966.

198. Salmoiraghi, G. C., and Nicoll, R. A. Effects of Drugs on Responses in the Olfactory Bulb. In Herxheimer, A. (Ed.), *Drugs and Sensory Functions.* London: Churchill, 1968, p. 73.

199. Salvador, R. A., and Albers, R. W. The distribution of glutamic-γ-aminobutyric transaminase in the nervous system of the Rhesus monkey. *J. Biol. Chem.* 234:922, 1959.

200. Sattin, A. The synthesis and storage of acetylcholine in the striatum. *J. Neurochem.* 13:515, 1966.

201. Shaw, J. E., and Ramwell, P. W. Release of a substance P polypeptide from the cerebral cortex. *Amer. J. Physiol.* 215:262, 1968.

202. Shaw, R. K., and Heine, J. D. Ninhydrin positive substances present in different areas of normal rat brain. *J. Neurochem.* 12:151, 1965.

203. Shimizu, N., and Ishii, S. Electron microscopic histochemistry of acetylcholinesterase of rat brain by Karnovsky's method. *Histochemie* 6:24, 1966.

204. Shute, C. C. D., and Lewis, P. R. Cholinesterase-containing system of the brain of the rat. *Nature* (London) 199:1160, 1963.

205. Shute, C. C. D., and Lewis, P. R. Electron microscopy of cholinergic terminals and acetylcholinesterase-containing neurones in the hippocampal formation of the rat. *Z. Zellforsch.* 69:334, 1966.

206. Shute, C. C. D., and Lewis, P. R. The ascending cholinergic reticular system: Neocortical, olfactory and subcortical projections. *Brain* 90:497, 1967.

207. Sie, G. Extractum belladonnae as an adjuvant to luminal in the therapy of epilepsy with a possible explanation in neurophysiological and neurochemical terms. *Proc. Aust. Ass. Neurol.* 5:113, 1968.

208. Sie, G., Jasper, H., and Wolfe, L. Rate of ACh release from cortical surface in

encéphale and *cerveau isolé* cat preparations in relation to arousal and epileptic activation of the ECoG. *Electroenceph. Clin. Neurophysiol.* 18:206, 1965.

209. Silver, A. Cholinesterases of the central nervous system with special reference to the cerebellum. *Int. Rev. Neurobiol.* 10:58, 1967.

210. Spehlmann, R. Acetylcholine and prostigmine electrophoresis at visual cortex neurons. *J. Neurophysiol.* 26:127, 1963.

211. Stefanis, C. Electrophysiological properties of cortical motoneurones during iontophoretic application of chemical substances. *Physiologist* 7:263, 1964.

212. Stefanis, C. Hippocampal neurons: Their responsiveness to microelectrophoretically administered endogenous amines. *Pharmacologist*, 6:171, 1964.

213. Stefanis, C. Discussion of Serotonin Effects on Central Neurons. In Garattini, S., and Shore, P. A. (Eds.), *Advances in Pharmacology*, vol. 6. New York: Academic, 1968, p. 414.

214. Stern, P. Substance P as a sensory transmitter and its other central effects. *Ann. N.Y. Acad. Sci.* 104:403, 1963.

215. Straughan, D. W. The Actions of Various Biological Amines on Single Neurones in the Limbic System. In Himwich, H. E., Kety, S. S., and Smythies, J. R. (Eds.), *Amines and Schizophrenia*. Oxford: Pergamon, 1967, p. 219.

216. Straughan, D. W., and Legge, K. F. The pharmacology of amygdaloid neurones. *J. Pharm. Pharmacol.* 17:675, 1965.

217. Szerb, J. C. The effect of tertiary and quaternary atropine on cortical acetylcholine output and on the electroencephalogram in cats. *Canad. J. Physiol. Pharmacol.* 42:303, 1964.

218. Szerb, J. C. Averaged evoked potentials and cholinergic synapses in the somatosensory cortex of the cat. *Electroenceph. Clin. Neurophysiol.* 18:140, 1965.

219. Szerb, J. C. Cortical acetylcholine release and electroencephalographic arousal. *J. Physiol.* (London) 192:329, 1967.

220. Szerb, J. C. Model experiments with Gaddum's push-pull cannulas. *Canad. J. Physiol. Pharmacol.* 45:613, 1967.

221. Tapia, R., and Awapara, J. Formation of γ-aminobutyric acid (GABA) in brain of mice treated with L-glutamic acid-γ-hydrazide and pyridoxal phosphate-γ-glutamyl hydrazone. *Proc. Soc. Exp. Biol. Med.* 126:218, 1967.

222. Tallan, H. H. A Survey of Amino Acids and Related Compounds in Nervous Tissue. In Holden, J. T. (Ed.), *Amino Acid Pools*. Amsterdam: Elsevier, 1962, p. 471.

223. Tower, D. B. *Neurochemistry of Epilepsy*. Springfield, Ill.: Thomas, 1960.

224. van Gelder, N. M. The histochemical demonstration of γ-aminobutyric acid metabolism by reduction of a tetrazolium salt. *J. Neurochem.* 12:231, 1965.

225. van Gelder, N. M. A comparison of γ-aminobutyric acid metabolism in rabbit and mouse nervous tissue. *J. Neurochem.* 12:239, 1965.

226. Vogler, K., Haefely, W., Hürlimann, A., Studer, R. O., Lergier, W., Strässle R., and Bernus, K. H. A new purification procedure and biological properties of substance P. *Ann. N.Y. Acad. Sci.* 104:378, 1963.

227. Waldron, H. A. Cholinergic fibres in the spinal cord of the rat. *Brain Res.* 4:113, 1967.

228. Watkins, J. C. Metabolic derangements and other causative factors in toxic convulsions. *Biochem. J.* 106:4P, 1968.

229. Weight, F. F., and Salmoiraghi, G. C. Responses of spinal cord interneurons to acetylcholine, norepinephrine and serotonin administered by microelectrophoresis. *J. Pharmacol. Exp. Ther.* 153:420, 1966.

230. Weight, F. F., and Salmoiraghi, G. C. Serotonin Effects on Central Neurones. In Garattini, S., and Shore, P. A. (Eds.), *Advances in Pharmacology*, vol. 6. New York: Academic, 1968, p. 395.

231. Weinstein, H., Roberts, E., and Kakefuda, T. Studies of subcellular distribution of γ-aminobutyric acid and glutamic decarboxylase in mouse brain. *Biochem. Pharmacol.* 12:503, 1963.

232. Werman, R. Criteria for identification of a central nervous system transmitter. *Comp. Biochem. Physiol.* 18:745, 1966.

233. Werman, R., and Aprison, M. H. Glycine: The Search for a Spinal Cord Inhibitory Transmitter. In von Euler, C., Skoglund, S., Söderberg, U. (Eds.), *Structure and Function of Inhibitory Neuronal Mechanisms*. Oxford: Pergamon, 1968, p. 473.

234. Werman, R., Davidoff, R. A., and Aprison, M. H. The inhibitory action of cystathionine. *Life Sci.* 5:1431, 1966.
235. Werman, R., Davidoff, R. A., and Aprison, M. H. Inhibitory action of glycine on spinal neurons in the cat. *J. Neurophysiol.* 31:81, 1968.
236. Whittaker, V. P. Identification of Acetylcholine and Related Esters of Biological Origin. In Koelle, G. B. (Ed.), *Handbuch der Experimentellen Pharmakologie*, vol. 15: *Cholinesterases and Anticholinesterase Agents*. Berlin: Springer, 1963, p. 1.
237. Whittaker, V. P. The application of subcellular fractionation techniques to the study of brain function. *Progr. Biophys.* 15:39, 1965.
238. Whittaker, V. P. Catecholamine storage particles in the central nervous system. *Pharmacol. Rev.* 18:401, 1966.
239. Whittaker, V. P. The Subcellular Distribution of Amino Acids in Brain and Its Relation to a Possible Transmitter Function for These Compounds. In von Euler, C., Skoglund, S., and Söderberg, U. (Eds.), *Structure and Function of Inhibitory Neuronal Mechanisms*, vol. 10. Oxford: Pergamon, 1968, p. 487.
240. Wolfe, L. S., and Elliott, K. A. C. Chemical Studies in Relation to Convulsive Disorders. In Elliott, K. A. C., Page, I. H., and Quastel, J. H. (Eds.), *Neurochemistry*. Springfield, Ill.: Thomas, 1962.
241. Yamamoto, K., and Domino, E. F. Cholinergic agonist-antagonist interactions on neocortical and limbic EEG activation. *Int. J. Neuropharmacol.* 6:357, 1967.
242. York, D. H. The inhibitory action of dopamine on neurones of the caudate nucleus. *Brain Res.* 5:263, 1967.
243. York, D. H. A microiontophoretic study of neurones in the globus pallidus-putamen complex. *Aust. J. Exp. Biol. Med. Sci.* 46:3, 1968.
244. Zetler, G., and Baldauf, J. Chromatographische Analyse eines Substanz-P-Präparates aus Gehirn. *Arch. Pharmak. Exp. Path.* 256:86, 1967.

Discussion

TRANSMITTER ACTION AND MULTIPLE DISCHARGE*

MOTOY KUNO

Professor Curtis [2] has presented an extensive survey on central synaptic transmitters from chemical and pharmacological aspects. In relation to the basic problems of epilepsies, this discussion is devoted principally to the transmitter action causing multiple discharge in central neurons.

There is general agreement that synaptic transmission in mammalian central neurons is mediated by chemical transmitters. The transmitter released by presynaptic impulses acts on central neurons and produces an increase in conductance of the postsynaptic membrane as long as the transmitter action lasts. Therefore, synaptic depolarization in central neurons may be determined by the time course as well as by the magnitude of transmitter action.

It is common experience that a single afferent volley often evokes multiple discharges in central neurons. This implies that the transmitter action is continuously maintained during the repetitive firing so that the duration of multiple discharge may be considered as a manifestation of the duration of the transmitter action. It has been postulated that multiple discharge in central neurons is due to the prolonged transmitter action exerted by individual presynaptic impulses [4]. The purpose of this study is to test whether the prolonged transmitter action is the only condition necessary for multiple discharge in central neurons.

STUDY MATERIALS—PROCEDURES AND RESULTS

Dorsal spinocerebellar tract (DSCT) neurons of the cat anesthetized with sodium pentobarbital were selected for this study. Intracellular recording from DSCT neurons was identified by action potentials (Fig. D5-1Ba) produced by antidromic stimulation of the ipsilateral dorsolateral funiculus (S_1 of Fig. D5-1A). These neurons receive monosynaptic connections from primary afferent fibers [13], as do spinal motoneurons. Consequently, stimulation of an appropriate dorsal root (S_2 of Fig. D5-1A) or muscle nerve (S_4) evoked monosynaptic discharges in DSCT neurons (Fig. D5-1Bb) as well as in spinal motoneurons (Fig. D5-1Cb). The response in DSCT neurons was often characterized by a double or triple spike to a single afferent volley. This contrasts with the behavior of motoneurons which usually discharge only once in response to the same afferent volley. Since the afferent input is common to these two types of neurons, the difference in their response patterns provides a favorable condition to analyze the factors responsible for multiple discharge in central neurons.

Time Course of Synaptic Potential

The underlying synaptic depolarization which causes multiple discharges in DSCT neurons may be disclosed by hyperpolarization of the cell membrane to prevent initiation of the spike discharge (Fig. D5-1Bc). The excitatory postsynaptic potential (EPSP) so observed showed a rapidly developing depolarization followed by a slow phase of decay, and the time course was virtually independent of the amplitude when the intensity of afferent stimulation was gradually reduced. The general features of the EPSPs in DSCT neurons were thus qualitatively comparable to those of monosynaptic EPSPs observed in spinal moto-

---

* This work supported in part by PHS Research Grants NB05667, NB06891, NB07938, NB07391, NB05244, NB04553 from National Institute of Neurological Diseases and Stroke, and Grant R17764 from United Cerebral Palsy Foundation.

Time Course of Synaptic Current

It is generally assumed that the time-to-peak of the EPSP gives an approximate measure of the duration of transmitter action whereas decay of the EPSP is largely determined by the electrical properties of the postsynaptic membrane. A comparison of monosynaptic EPSPs shown in Fig. D5-1Bc and D5-1Cc suggests that duration of transmitter action in DSCT neurons does not differ significantly from that in spinal motoneurons. This suggestion can be tested further by measurement of the time course of synaptic current, which should be approximately identical with the time course of transmitter action.

If the synaptic current producing the monosynaptic EPSP is uniformly distributed over the entire soma and dendrites, the time course of synaptic current may be calculated, based on the time constant of the postsynaptic membrane [3]. Dotted curves in Fig. D5-2 show the time course of synaptic current so calculated for monosynaptic EPSPs (solid curves) in a DSCT neuron (A) and a motoneuron (B). It is clear that the transmitter action virtually ceases within 2 msec after its onset in both DSCT neurons and spinal motoneurons. This value agrees with the time course of synaptic current previously estimated on spinal motoneurons [1, 3].

The active phase of synaptic action on DSCT neurons was also measured by extracellular recording techniques in which the microelectrode was placed very close to the neuron so that the flow of *synaptic depolarizing current* could be observed [12]. The results again, were comparable to that shown in Fig. D5-2A.

It may be argued that the time course of excitatory synaptic current might have been underestimated by the presence of inhibitory impulses admixed in the afferent volley. This possibility was unlikely, since the synaptic current produced by stimulation of a single afferent fiber was similar in time course to that elicited by a synchronous afferent volley [12]. Therefore, it can be concluded that the transmitter action on DSCT neurons is approximately identical

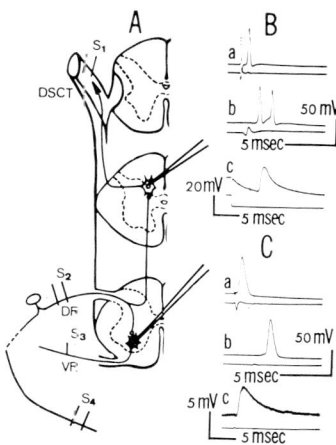

FIG. D5-1. (A) Schematic representation of experimental arrangement. Intracellular recording from DSCT neurons (upper microelectrode) made at third lumbar segment and identified by antidromic stimulation of the ipsilateral dorsolateral funiculus (S_1). Activity of spinal motoneurons recorded at the seventh lumbar segment (lower microelectrode). S_2, for stimulation of dorsal root; S_3, for stimulation of ventral root; S_4, for stimulation of appropriate muscle nerves. (B) Intracellular potentials from a DSCT neuron. (a) antidromic response; (b) response to stimulation of the seventh lumbar dorsal root; (c) same as (b) but with postsynaptic hyperpolarization to isolate the EPSP. (C) Intracellular potentials from a spinal motoneuron. (a) antidromic response; (b) response to stimulation of the biceps-semitendinosus muscle nerve; (c) same as (b) but with reduced stimulus intensity. (Unpublished results by M. Kuno and J. T. Miyahara.)

neurons (Fig. D5-1Cc). Evidently, the multiple discharge in DSCT neurons (Fig. D5-1Bb) is due to a synchronous monosynaptic volley rather than to delayed synaptic bombardment through polysynaptic pathways. It should be noted that DSCT neurons also show repetitive discharges as a consequence of temporal dispersion of presynaptic volleys through polysynaptic pathways [12]. However, the multiple discharges due to the delayed arrival of presynaptic impulses were longer in duration and discharge interval than those initiated by synchronous monosynaptic volleys.

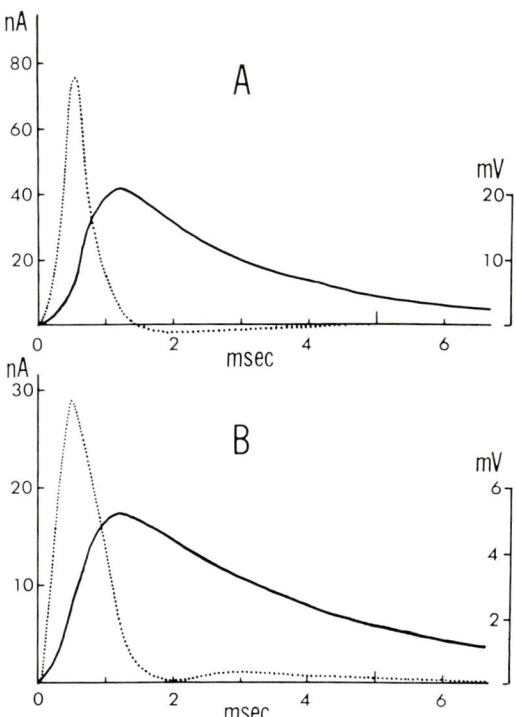

FIG. D5-2. Relation between the EPSP (solid curves) and synaptic current (dotted curves) calculated from the time constant of the postsynaptic membrane. (A) for a DSCT neuron; (B) for a spinal motoneuron. (Unpublished results by M. Kuno and J. T. Miyahara.)

in duration with that on spinal motoneurons.

Factors Responsible for Multiple Discharge

From the foregoing analysis, it appears clear that single and multiple discharges in different central neurons can be produced by transmitter actions having identical time courses. But it should be pointed out that monosynaptic EPSPs in DSCT neurons are much greater in amplitude than the EPSPs observed in spinal motoneurons (Figs. D5-1 and D5-2). Monosynaptic EPSPs evoked in DSCT neurons by maximum stimulation of a dorsal root ranged up to 65 mV [12], while the largest monsynaptic EPSP never exceeded 12 mV in motoneurons [5]. When the intensity of afferent stimulation was decreased so that the EPSP amplitude was reduced to less than 15 mV, no multiple discharge was observed in DSCT neurons. A question then arises if the occurrence of multiple discharge in central neurons is entirely dependent on the magnitude of transmitter action.

To test this question, depolarizing pulses were applied across the postsynaptic membrane in DSCT neurons (Fig. D5-3A) and in motoneurons (Fig. D5-3B). An increase in current intensity caused repetitive discharges both in DSCT neurons and motoneurons. Maximum discharge frequency observed in DSCT neurons with current pulses of more than $30–50 \times 10^{-9}$ A was 800–1000/sec (Fig. D5-3Ab). In contrast, the maximum discharge evoked in motoneurons by similar depolarizing pulses was

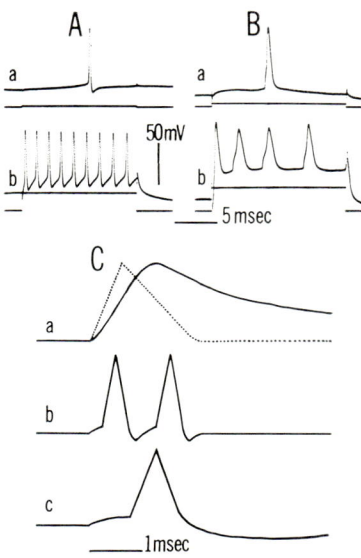

FIG. D5-3. Responses of a DSCT neuron (A) and a spinal motoneuron (B) to depolarizing pulses applied through intracellular electrodes. (a) Responses to rheobasic currents; (b) responses to strong depolarizing currents. 50 mV calibration also indicates 62.5×10^{-9} A for current (lower beams). (C) Schematic drawing of synaptic current (a, dotted curve) and monosynaptic EPSP (a, solid curve). Transmitter actions with identical time courses may cause multiple discharge in DSCT neurons (b) and single discharge in motoneurons (c). (Unpublished results by M. Kuno and J. T. Miyahara.)

300–500/sec (Fig. D5-3Bb; also see [11]). In Fig. D5-3 (also see Fig. D5-1), it is clear that the duration of spike potentials and hence of the refractory period is significantly shorter in DSCT neurons (about 0.5 msec) than in motoneurons (about 1 msec). Nor was there any evidence to indicate that DSCT neurons are subject to recurrent inhibitory action [6, 12]. Furthermore, DSCT neurons showed a smaller after-hyperpolarization following each spike and a less prominent adaptative process than spinal motoneurons. Obviously, these factors provide favorable conditions for the high frequency discharge in DSCT neurons.

Figure D5-3C is a diagrammatic representation of synaptic responses evoked in DSCT neurons (b) and motoneurons (c) by single afferent volleys. The monosynaptic EPSPs (Fig. D5-3Ca, solid curve) may be generated by the transmitter action (dotted curve), which lasts for about 2 msec. The first spike of a DSCT neuron would be initiated nearly at onset of the EPSP because of the intense synaptic action. Since the spike duration is short, synaptic depolarization may be rebuilt sufficiently to reach the threshold level to initiate the second spike before the transmitter action is terminated. Since DSCT neurons are able to discharge at frequencies up to 1000/sec, the short-lasting transmitter action can thus produce two or three repetitive spikes. On the other hand, the discharge of spinal motoneurons (Fig. D5-3Cc) may be initiated nearly at the peak of the EPSP because of relatively weak synaptic action. As the spike potential is approximately 1 msec in duration, transmitter action would be practically dissipated when the discharge subsides. It should be noted that even when spinal motoneurons are subjected to intense synaptic action, there would be no multiple discharge because of the limited frequency at which motoneurons can discharge. Thus, presence of large EPSPs alone is not sufficient for generation of multiple discharges in central neurons.

Structural Characteristics

It has recently been shown that the amplitude of monosynaptic EPSPs produced by impulses in a single afferent fiber is considerably larger in DSCT neurons than in spinal motoneurons [9, 12]. The high synaptic efficacy in DSCT neurons was obviously due to the large amount of transmitter released by one impulse [12]. Since the amount of transmitter released by presynaptic impulses should depend entirely on the properties of presynaptic elements, it is conceivable that presynaptic terminals on DSCT neurons may be different in structure from those on spinal motoneurons.

Figure D5-4 shows an electron micrograph of presynaptic terminals (T) located on dendrites (D) of a DSCT neuron. In agreement with previous observations by light microscope [14], a substantial number of presynaptic terminals on DSCT neurons were 5–15 μ in diameter. This contrasts with spinal motoneurons in which the diameter of presynaptic terminals usually ranges from 0.5 to 3 μ [10]. A likely possibility is that the difference in size of presynaptic terminals may account for the difference in synaptic efficacy between DSCT neurons and spinal motoneurons. In this regard, Eccles and Jaeger [7] have suggested that diffusion of transmitters out of the synaptic cleft may account sufficiently for rate of decay of the central transmitter action. This implies that clearance of the transmitter from the synaptic cleft is retarded at *giant* synaptic contacts on DSCT neurons [8]. However, present observations clearly show that there is no significant difference in the time course of transmitter action between DSCT neurons and spinal motoneurons (Fig. D5-2). Therefore, it is suggested that termination of the transmitter action on central neurons must be due to some mechanism(s) other than elimination of the transmitter by diffusion.

CONCLUSION

In contrasting the synaptic transmission in DSCT neurons and in spinal motoneurons, the observations provide certain conclusions.

● There is no need to postulate a prolonged transmitter action to account for multiple discharge of central neurons to single afferent volleys.

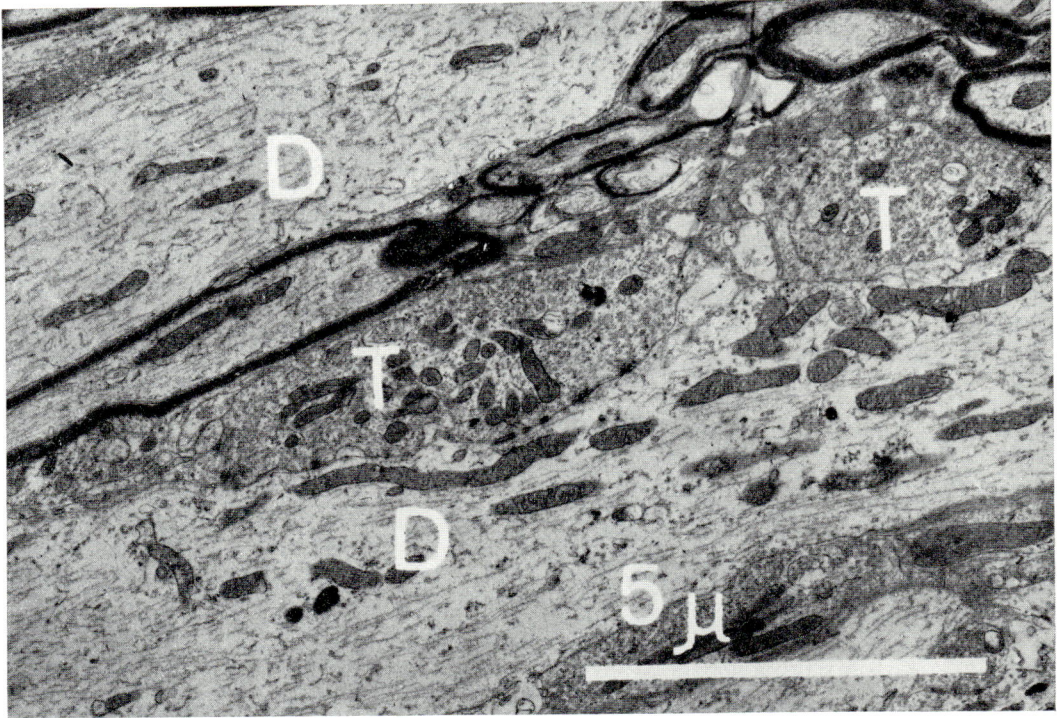

Fig. D5-4. Electron micrograph taken from the region of Clarke's column of the cat, third lumbar segment; (*D*) dendrites; (*T*) presynaptic terminals. Tissues were fixed by perfusion with glutaraldehyde followed by postosmication and stained with lead. (Unpublished results by M. Kuno and J. T. Miyahara.)

- Presence of an intense synaptic action is a necessary but not a sufficient condition for generation of multiple discharge in central neurons.
- Occurrence of multiple discharge is also dependent on the maximum frequency at which the central neurons can discharge.
- Termination of transmitter action in central neurons is due to some mechanism other than diffusion of the transmitter out of the synaptic cleft.

Acknowledgments

I wish to thank Dr. J. T. Miyahara for his collaboration throughout the present study and for granting me the use of our unpublished results. I am also indebted to Mrs. L. L. L. DeKorver for her technical assistance in electron microscopic studies.

REFERENCES

1. Araki, T., and Terzuolo, C. A. Membrane currents in spinal motoneurons associated with the action potential and synaptic activity. *J. Neurophysiol.* 25:772, 1962.
2. Curtis, D. R. Central Synaptic Transmitters. In Jasper, H. H., Ward, A. A., Jr., and Pope, A. (Eds.), *Basic Mechanisms of the Epilepsies*. Boston: Little, Brown, 1969.
3. Curtis, D. R., and Eccles, J. C. The time courses of excitatory and inhibitory synaptic actions. *J. Physiol.* (London) 145:529, 1959.
4. Eccles, J. C. *Physiology of Synapses*. Berlin-Heidelberg: Springer, 1964.

5. Eccles, J. C., Eccles, R. M., and Lundberg, A. The convergence of monosynaptic excitatory afferents onto many different species of alpha motoneurones. *J. Physiol.* (London) 137:22, 1957.
6. Eccles, J. C., Hubbard, J. I., and Oscarsson, O. Intracellular recording from cells of the ventral spino-cerebellar tract. *J. Physiol.* (London) 158:486, 1961.
7. Eccles, J. C., and Jaeger, J. C. The relationship between the mode of operation and the dimensions of the junctional regions at synapses and motor end-organs. *Proc. Roy. Soc.* [Biol.] 148:38, 1958.
8. Eccles, J. C., Oscarsson, O., and Willis, W. D. Synaptic action of Group I and II afferent fibres of muscle on the cells of the dorsal spino-cerebellar tract. *J. Physiol.* (London) 158:517, 1961.
9. Eide, E., Fedina, L., Jansen, J., Lundberg, A., and Vyklický, L. Unitary excitatory postsynaptic potentials in Clarke's column neurones. *Nature* (London) 215:1176, 1967.
10. Haggar, R. A., and Barr, M. L. Quantitative data on the size of synaptic end-bulbs in the cat's spinal cord. *J. Comp. Neurol.* 93:17, 1950.
11. Kernell, D. High-frequency repetitive firing of cat lumbosacral motoneurones stimulated by long-lasting injected currents. *Acta Physiol. Scand.* 65:74, 1966.
12. Kuno, M., and Miyahara, J. T. Factors responsible for multiple discharge of neurons in Clarke's column. *J. Neurophysiol.* 31:624, 1968.
13. Lundberg, A. Ascending Spinal Hindlimb Pathways in the Cat. In Eccles, J. C., and Schadé, J. P. (Eds.), *Progress in Brain Research*, vol. 12. Amsterdam: Elsevier, 1964.
14. Szentágothai, J., and Albert, A. The synaptology of Clarke's column. *Acta Morph. Acad. Sci. Hung.* 5:43, 1955.

6
Ultrastructural Neurochemistry*

EDUARDO DE ROBERTIS, GEORGINA RODRIGUEZ DE LORES ARNAIZ, AND MARTHA ALBERICI

THE PAROXYSMAL FIRING of neurons which characterizes epileptic activity may result from an intrinsic enhancement of the normal excitability, due to multiple factors, or from exogenous stimuli, which either increase synaptic excitatory bombardment or decrease the effect of inhibitory synapses [60]. Since convulsant drugs may produce simulation of some of the pathological states in the human, their experimental use may be of considerable interest in learning about the basic mechanisms of epilepsies. In the past few years our laboratory has been engaged in studying the action of certain drugs which may induce seizure activity. For this purpose, in a combined approach we used: (a) the electron microscope, to demonstrate the ultrastructural changes occurring in situ, or in the subcellular particles isolated after cell fractionation, and (b) biochemical methods to study the changes in transmitter content or in key enzymes involved in the mechanism of synaptic excitation or inhibition.

We shall summarize, first, some of the findings obtained in the study of the normal brain regarding the ultrastructure and cytochemistry of the synaptic region, which may be pertinent to the problem of epilepsies; and second, mention some of the results obtained with the convulsant drugs methionine sulfoximine (MSO), allylglycine, and pentylenetetrazol.

MORPHOLOGICAL AND NEUROCHEMICAL STUDIES IN SYNAPTIC REGION OF NORMAL BRAIN

Current theories of chemical transmission are based on the assumption that specific transmitters are synthesized and stored in nerve endings and that these are released upon the arrival of the nerve impulse. It is also postulated that the transmitter reacts with chemical receptors situated in the second neuron or postsynaptic element and that from this reaction a change in ionic permeability and a new bioelectric phenomenon originates. Such mechanisms are found both in excitatory and inhibitory synapses and the end result—excitation or inhibition—depends upon the chemical nature of the transmitter, the molecular structure of the receptor, and the ionic species that migrate through the postsynaptic membrane [26].

AMINERGIC AND NONAMINERGIC NERVE ENDINGS

With the introduction of the cell fractionation methods to the study of brain, a more direct approach to the fine localization of transmitters and other active substances, as well as of the enzymes involved in their synthesis or inactivation and of the chemical receptors, was made available. Gray and Whittaker [29] and De Robertis

---

* Original research supported by grant from Consejo Nacional de Investigaciones Científicas y Técnicas, and PHS Research Grant NB06953–03 from National Institute of Neurological Diseases and Stroke.

et al. [20] were able to demonstrate independently that the mitochondrial fraction of brain contained isolated nerve endings. Use of a sucrose density gradient on this fraction permitted the separation of three layers of nerve endings from brain in addition to myelin and mitochondria (Fig. 6-1). In these various submitochondrial fractions of brain, study of distribution of biogenic amines, acetylcholine (ACh), 5-hydroxytryptamine, norepinephrine, dopamine, and histamine, together with those of some enzymes related to their metabolism such as cholineacetylase (ChAc), acetylcholinesterase (AChE), and 5-hydroxytryptophane and dopa-decarboxylase (5-HTP-D), demonstrated that nerve endings could be separated into two main subfractions. One of these groups contained the aminergic nerve endings, rich in biogenic amines, while the other large subfraction of nerve endings was essentially nonaminergic and lacked these active biogenic amines (Table 6-1). Monoaminoxidase (MAO), an enzyme involved in the catabolism of active monoamines, was found tightly bound to mitochondria [49]. Using a gradient of Ficoll it was found that catechol-O-methyltransferase (COMT) paralleled distribution of ChAc, indicating that this enzyme, of the catecholamine system, is also contained in isolated nerve endings [2].

NONAMINERGIC NERVE ENDINGS AND INHIBITORY SYNAPSES

In 1963 Salganicoff and De Robertis [51] demonstrated that the two main enzymes of the γ-aminobutyric acid (GABA) system, i.e., glutamic acid decarboxylase (GAD) and GABA-aminotransferase (GABA-AT), had very different localizations in the submitochondrial fractions (Table 6-1). GAD, the enzyme that catalyzes the formation of GABA from L-glutamic acid, was found to be concentrated in the nonaminergic fraction of nerve endings; on the other hand, GABA-AT, the enzyme that reversibly transaminates GABA with α-ketoglutarate to succinic semialdehyde, is preferentially localized in neuronal mitochondria. Because of the strict parallelism existing between GAD and GABA [55] and the irreversibility of the reaction catalyzed by GAD, it was postulated that this amino acid should be localized in nonaminergic nerve endings and should play an inhibitory presynaptic role [51]. See Fig. 6-2.

These findings are related to the current

TABLE 6-1. Distribution of the Biogenic Amines and Some Enzymes

	Myelin A	Aminergic Nerve Endings		Nonaminergic Nerve Endings D	Mitochondria E
		B	C		
Amines					
Acetylcholine [20]	0.24	2.02	4.11	0.67	0.27
5-Hydroxytryptamine [67]	0.61	0.78	2.17	0.76	0.48
Norepinephrine [68]	0.32	2.05	1.66	0.77	0.72
Dopamine [68]	0.79	1.85	1.13	0.91	0.71
Histamine [33]	0.72	2.70	1.56	0.44	0.70
Enzymes related to amines					
ChAc [24]	0.10	1.88	0.98	1.00	0.59
AChE [20]	0.15	2.24	2.99	0.94	0.58
5-HTP-D [50]	0.05	1.05	2.05	1.22	0.26
MAO [2]	—	—	0.17	1.16	2.28
Enzymes related to GABA					
GAD [51]	0.02	0.49	1.22	2.00	0.40
GABA-AT [51]	0.15	0.11	0.29	1.10	8.00

(A-E) submitochondrial fractions isolated by gradient centrifugation as in Fig. 6-1. Results are expressed as the relative specific concentration of amine or of enzymatic activity recovered divided by the percentage of protein recovered. (Numbers in brackets refer to references.)

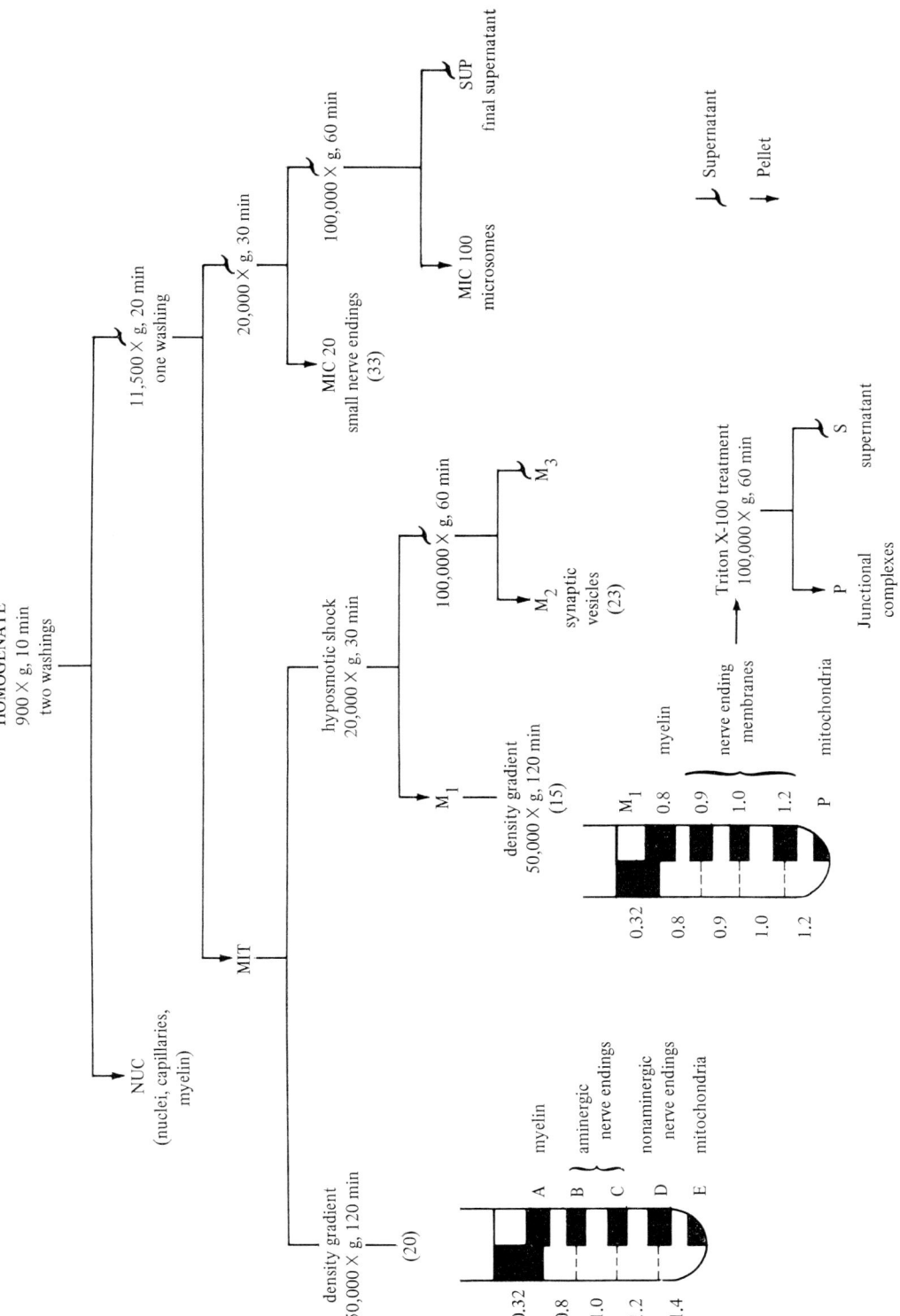

FIG. 6.1. Cell fractionation techniques used for separation of nerve endings, nerve-ending membranes, synaptic vesicles, junctional complexes, and other subcellular components of the central nervous system. (Numbers in parentheses refer to references.)

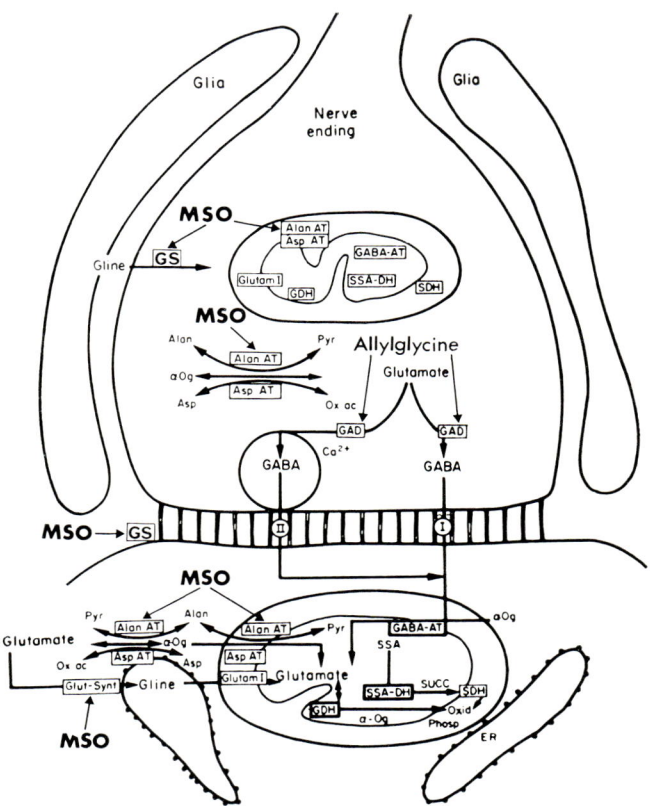

FIG. 6-2. Possible role of GABA as an inhibitory transmitter. Structural and biochemical organization of an inhibitory synaptic ending indicating possible sites of action of convulsant drugs methionine sulfoximine (MSO) and allylglycine. Localization of enzymes of glutamate, glutamine (Gline), and GABA cycles in different compartments and subcompartments of nerve ending and neuron are indicated. (For a more detailed description, see [52].) MSO inhibits preferentially glutamine synthetase (GS) and alanine-aminotransferase (Alan-AT); allylglycine acts exclusively on glutamic acid decarboxylase (GAD).

concept that amino acids may have an important function in synaptic transmission of central synapses. In 1965 Krnjević [34] summarized existing evidence which indicated that in the cerebral cortex, glutamate, GABA, and other amino acids could have an important role in transmission. According to this viewpoint the cholinergic system, coming from subcortical projections, has a rather restricted distribution in cortical synapses. More recently the role of GABA as a cortical transmitter was strongly supported [8, 35] and glycine was shown to be an inhibitory transmitter in the spinal cord [64].

SYNAPTIC VESICLES AND QUANTAL RELEASE OF TRANSMITTER

Discovery of the synaptic vesicles as constant components of chemical synapses led to the concept that they could be the storage sites of the transmitter substances [17, 18] and could represent the units for quantal release in synaptic transmission [9]. Population of vesicles within the nerve ending was thought to be the result of a steady state between their production and disintegration after release, and this is an important point in the interpretation of ultrastructural changes in seizure activity. Experiments with electrical stimulation in peripheral synapses demonstrated that reduction in number was obtained only after sustained stimuli of high frequency [10]. The rapid rate at which vesicles could be released led to the interpretation that they could be used more than once in successive firings. This concept received recent support from turnover studies with ^{3}H-leucine in which a mean life of 21 days for synaptic vesicles of the central nervous system was calculated [63]. Also, the fact that the protein [6] and lipid composition [39] of synaptic vesicles differs from that of membranes of the nerve ending rules out the possibility that the vesicles could be fusing with the membrane or that they were being re-formed from it. Recently, Pellegrino de Iraldi and De Robertis [43], in working with compressed nerve endings, brought out new morphological evidence that vesicles could be rapidly formed from neurotubules.

We shall not discuss here the variety of morphologically different synaptic vesicles which have been described in different parts of the peripheral and central nervous system [10, 12]. However, special mention should be made of the so-called *elliptical* or *flattened* vesicles, first found by Pellegrino de Iraldi et al. [44] in the hypothalamus of rats fixed with aldehydes, which have been interpreted by Uchizono [61, 62] as corresponding to inhibitory synapses. De Robertis [14] has reported that nerve endings containing elliptical-shaped vesicles were more abundant in the nonaminergic fraction of the cat cortex which, as mentioned, corresponds to the GAD-rich fraction and probably represents a population of inhibitory nerve endings.

ISOLATION OF SYNAPTIC VESICLES AND
CONTENT OF BIOGENIC AMINES

In 1962 it was found in our laboratory [23] that nerve endings underwent considerable swelling and disruption in hypotonic solutions; this permitted separation of the synaptic vesicles, the nerve-ending membranes, and other components of the synaptic ending in different fractions (Fig. 6-1). As shown in Table 6-2, the various biogenic amines were found to be concentrated in fraction M_2, which contains

TABLE 6-2. Content in Biogenic Amines of Synaptic Vesicles

Amine		M_1	M_2	M_3
Acetylcholine	(23–24)	0.55	2.85	1.20
5-Hydroxy-tryptamine[a]		0.47	1.84	2.31
Norepinephrine	(68)	0.40	2.56	1.93
Dopamine	(68)	0.46	2.46	1.72
Histamine	(33)	0.39	2.24	2.27

Content of biogenic amines in the bulk fraction (M_1), in synaptic vesicles (M_2), and in the soluble fraction (M_3). The crude mitochondrial fraction of the brain was shocked osmotically and then centrifuged as indicated in Fig. 6-1. The results are expressed in relative specific concentrations.

[a] Recalculated from data of Maynert et al. [40].

the synaptic vesicles. This confirmed the early postulate that the synaptic vesicles were the storage site of transmitters [17].

In relation to the GAD-containing nerve endings, it is of interest that this enzyme, although being rather free in the cytoplasm, could be bound to the vesicles by a small concentration of Ca^{2+} [51]. This suggests that, in the living condition, the enzyme might be fixed to the outer surface of the synaptic vesicles in a way similar to that of ChAc in cholinergic synapses [24, 41]. As in the occurrence with ACh, the GABA formed could be collected into the vesicles to play a synaptic role as a true transmitter.

ISOLATION OF CHOLINERGIC AND
NONCHOLINERGIC NERVE-ENDING
MEMBRANES

The study of nerve-ending membranes with attached junctional complex is of particular interest in understanding the primary function of neurons and how these may be altered in convulsant states. The limiting membrane of the ending, a continuation of the axolemma, regulates the passage of ions, metabolites, and other small molecules, maintaining a special milieu for the metabolic activities of this part of the neuronal compartment. Across this membrane, ionic fluxes take place from which the resting and action potentials originate. Since the junctional complex includes the subsynaptic membrane, belonging to the second neuron, its isolation may presumably lead to a better knowledge of the chemical receptor involved in nerve transmission.

The osmotic shock of the nerve endings, used to separate the synaptic vesicles, may also be employed to isolate the nerve-ending membranes. In the method used in this laboratory, the nerve-ending membranes are separated in fractions M_1 0.9; M_1 1.0; and M_1 1.2 (Fig. 6-1). Under the electron microscope, nerve-ending membranes are characterized by size, which corresponds to that of the nerve terminals, and the observation, in many profiles, of the attached junctional complexes. The various membrane populations in the gradient of M_1 are separated on the basis of their specific gravity, which depends on the lipid-protein ratio. These membranes are also characterized by other differences in chemical composition, particularly in the content of gangliosides, by a group of membrane-bound enzymes, and by their different binding capacity for radioactive biogenic amines and blocking agents [15, 48].

Membrane-Bound Enzymes

The determination of AChE in the various membranous fractions indicates that it is concentrated in the membranes of M_1 0.9 and M_1 1.0, while those of M_1 1.2 have small quantities of this enzyme and probably belong to the noncholinergic nerve endings (Table 6-3). The localization of Na^+-K^+ activated adenosinetriphosphatase (ATPase) in these M_1 subfractions is of particular interest, considering the activity of this enzyme in transphosphorylations and cation transport. Several investigations suggest that the final step in the action of ATPase could involve a K^+ activated phosphatase.

Albers et al. [4] found that both enzymes are closely associated with the membranous components of the nerve endings, and Hosie [31] made similar observations for ATPase. Table 6-3 shows that, while Na^+-K^+ activated ATPase is more closely associated with the membranes rich in AChE, the K^+ activated p-nitrophenylphosphatase is also in the M_1 1.2 fraction, which has little AChE. Glutamine synthetase (GS) is mainly concentrated in microsomal membranes [52]; however, there is a definite portion of this enzyme associated with nerve-ending membranes, especially of the noncholinergic type [48]. By synthesizing glutamine, an amino acid that easily crosses the nerve-ending membrane, GS may regulate the concentration of glutamate (and GABA) within nerve endings, and may play a role in some convulsant states, which will be indicated later.

Adenyl cyclase is an enzyme which reaches its highest concentration in the cerebral cortex and by catalyzing the production of cyclic adenosine monophosphate (3'5'AMP), is involved in the regulation of various cell activities. Another enzyme, cyclic phosphodiesterase, may function as a modulator of adenyl cyclase, acting on the intracellular concentration of 3'5'AMP [58]. Adenyl cyclase is bound to microsomal membranes but is more concentrated in the isolated nerve-ending membranes [22] (Table 6-3). Cyclic phosphodiesterase, while partly free, is also bound to the same nerve-ending membranes (Table 6-3). The localization of these two enzymes favors the view that 3'5'AMP may be important in the metabolic regulation of synaptic endings, but the exact nature of this participation is still unknown.

Receptor Properties of Nerve-Ending Membranes

A basic assumption of the chemical theory of synaptic transmission is that the subsynaptic membrane should contain the chemical receptors for the various transmitters. Since this membrane remains attached to the nerve-ending membrane, the expectation was that it should also have the receptor properties. Investigations were performed mainly with radioactive drugs that act as blocking agents for the transmitters, and some labeled biogenic amines were also used.

Using a technique in vitro in which the subcellular fractions of the rat cerebral cortex were exposed to minimal concentrations (10^{-7} to $10^{-6}M$) of dimethyl-^{14}C-D-tubocurarine (^{14}C-DMTC), this drug became preferentially bound to the AChE-rich nerve-ending membranes of fractions

TABLE 6-3. Distribution of Various Enzymes and Binding Capacity for Dimethyl-^{14}C-D-tubocurarine (^{14}C-DMTC). (See Fig. 6-1.) The results are expressed as in Table 6-1. Data from [15, 22, 48].

Subfraction	Structure	AChE	Na+-K+-ATPase	K+p-Nitro-phenylphos-phatase	Glutamine Synthetase	Adenyl Cyclase	Phospho-diesterase	MAO	^{14}C-DMTC
M_1 0.8	myelin	1.68	1.37	0.56	0.66	1.06	1.32	0.44	2.14
M_1 0.9	nerve-ending membranes	3.22	2.28	2.41	0.96	2.04	1.77	0.33	4.16
M_1 1.0	nerve-ending membranes	2.13	3.16	1.39	2.04	2.46	2.68	0.23	6.88
M_1 1.2	nerve-ending membranes	0.98	1.40	2.53	1.74	1.95	1.03	0.65	3.00
M_1 P	mitochondria	0.15	0.17	0.30	0.73	0.31	0.43	1.56	1.60

M_1 0.9 and M_1 1.0 [15] (Table 6-3). The AChE-poor membranes of fraction M_1 1.2 showed much less binding capacity. Results indicated that AChE and the cholinergic receptor were associated in the same type of nerve-ending membranes. More recently, the nerve-ending membranes of the basal ganglia and brain stem were found to bind preferentially the α-adrenergic blocking agent ^{14}C-Sy28 (N-α-naphthylmethyl-N-ethyl-β-bromoethylamine) and ^{14}C-dibenamine [28], the β-blocking drug ^{14}C-propranolol, and also ^{3}H-chlorpromazine, ^{14}C-LSD, and ^{14}C-serotonin.

Isolation of the Chemical Receptor

The uptake in vitro of radioactive blocking agents by the nerve-ending membranes provided a good starting point to attempt isolation of the molecular species involved in the binding. De Robertis et al. [19] found that after an extraction with chloroform, methanol (2:1), which produced complete inhibition of AChE, the ^{14}C-DMTC was recovered in the organic phase. With the use of thin-layer chromatography it could be demonstrated that radioactivity remained at the point of origin, together with the proteolipids, while very little was recovered in the various lipids. Furthermore, by means of column chromatography with Sephadex-L_{20} the ^{14}C-DMTC was eluted, together with a protein peak. All these findings suggested that the receptor for this cholinergic blocking agent is a proteolipid which, in itself, is only a small proportion of the total protein present in the nerve-ending membrane.

Essentially similar findings have been obtained so far with ^{14}C-serotonin and with the adrenergic α-blocking agent ^{14}C-Sy28, in the nerve-ending membranes isolated from basal ganglia and brain stem of the rat and cat [28]. In experiments with nerve-ending membranes treated with alkyl aryl polyether alcohol (Triton X-100) it was shown that the receptor properties for ^{14}C-DMTC remained with the junctional complexes represented principally by the subsynaptic membranes, while most of the limiting membranes of the endings, together with the bound enzymes, were solubilized [16]. These findings indicate that the proteolipid receptors are probably localized at the subsynaptic membrane. At present it is not possible to establish that these findings may have some bearing on the epilepsies, but it is evident that changes in the receptor proteins may influence neuronal excitability and could play a role in abnormal synaptic transmission. For example, changes in the receptor proteins may explain the hypersensitivity of a denervated epileptic neuron. A more detailed description of the cytochemistry of the normal synaptic region has been published [13, 21].

ULTRASTRUCTURAL AND NEUROCHEMICAL STUDIES IN CERTAIN EXPERIMENTAL CONVULSIVE STATES

The ultrastructural and neurochemical methods already described have been applied to the study of the cerebral cortex of rats undergoing seizures resulting from injections of the convulsant drugs methionine sulphoximine, allylglycine, and pentylenetetrazol. The two first drugs produce convulsions after a rather prolonged, latent period (1.5–4 hours) while pentylenetetrazol acts immediately, producing a convulsive shock similar to that induced by insulin or electric currents. A brief summary of findings is presented; more detailed information has been published [3, 25].

Methionine Sulfoximine (MSO)

Because of the similarity between convulsions induced by MSO and those of human epilepsy, this drug has been the object of numerous physiological and neurochemical studies [65]. The studies pointed toward a possible causal relationship between MSO and a disequilibrium in the glutamine–glutamic acid–GABA metabolism. Peters and Tower [45] found a marked inhibition of glutamine synthesis in brain slices of MSO-treated cats. In vitro a competitive inhibition of the enzyme GS [54] was reported, and Lamar and Sellinger [37] found that this drug inhibits GS irreversibly in vivo.

One of our first experiments was aimed

at learning the localization of the drug within the subcellular compartments of the cerebral cortex. Subarachnoidally, ^{14}C-MSO was administered to rats and 1–1.5 hours later (at the start of convulsions) the cerebral cortex was fractionated as indicated in Fig. 6-1. It was found that 61.2 percent of the bound ^{14}C-MSO went to the crude mitochondrial fraction and that 81.7 percent of this was recovered in the three nerve-ending fractions (B + C + D) pooled together.

Action of MSO on Enzymes and Biogenic Amines. After intraperitoneal administration of MSO (400–800 mg per kg), the rats were killed 4 hours later and studied for enzyme activity and content of biogenic amines. Practically no effect was observed on ChAc, AChE, and MAO, but there was some increase in COMT (Table 6-4). Of the enzymes related to the metabolism of glutamine-glutamate and GABA, no effect was found on glutamate dehydrogenase, aspartate-aminotransferase, and GABA-AT. GAD showed some inhibition while alanine-aminotransferase and GS were very significantly inhibited (Table 6-4).

In regard to the biogenic amines, the ACh content of whole brain remained unchanged while the free and bound amine showed a small decrease. Norepinephrine and 5-hydroxytryptamine showed a certain decrease. Dopamine remained unchanged in whole brain, but there was an increase in the bound portion of this amine. While the results on catechol and indolamines warrant further studies, negative findings in the various components of the cholinergic system tend to disprove involvement of this type of transmission in MSO convulsions [25].

Electron Microscope Observations on the Effect of MSO in Brain. Harris [30] observed glial swelling in MSO-treated cats and rabbits under the electron microscope. In our material the slices of brain cortex, fixed at the beginning of convulsions, showed a variety of changes, especially in synaptic areas. However, at certain points, a definite swelling of the glial processes was observed. Comparison with similar parts of the cortex from normal control rats showed that in the neuropil region and near the nerve cell perikarya there were numerous synaptic endings which had lost most of their synaptic vesicles; only a few of the synapses showed an approximately normal content. Synapses devoid of or containing few synaptic vesicles could be recognized by the presence of special differentiations of the synaptic membrane and associated structures which constitute the junctional complex [13]. Such ultrastructural changes of synapses are more clearly observed after fractionation of the cortex in convulsant rats.

Contrasted with that found in the normal control where all nerve endings are filled with vesicles, in the crude mitochondrial fraction of the MSO-treated rats, a higher proportion of nerve endings lost, to a greater or lesser extent, the synaptic vesicles. In the nerve-ending fraction C, and particularly in D, the effect of MSO on some synaptic complexes is very notable, and the various changes described in the intact cortex and in the crude mitochondrial fraction may be observed. For example, in fraction D, corresponding to the noncholinergic nerve endings, only few nerve endings contained vesicles, while the

TABLE 6-4. Percentage Change in Activity of Enzymes Related to Biogenic Amines or Glutamate and Glutamine after Injection of MSO.

Enzyme	Percentage of Change[a]
Related to biogenic amines	
ChAc	− 3 (6)
AChE	− 8 (2)
COMT	+37 (3)
MAO	+ 6 (5)
Related to glutamate and glutamine	
GDH	+ 2 (2)
Asp-AT[b]	− 9 (3)
Alan-AT[c]	−60 (2)
GABA-AT	+ 8 (3)
GS	−66 (3)

[a] Numbers of experiments in parentheses.
[b] Aspartate-aminotransferase.
[c] Alanine-aminotransferase.
The enzymes were studied in rats injected intraperitoneally with 400 mg per kg of MSO and decapitated 4 hours later.

others were swollen and mostly deprived of synaptic vesicles. More detailed information on the effect of MSO has been published. See Figs. 6-1 to 6-5 in [25].

Possible Mechanism of Action of MSO. It is difficult at present to establish the initial cause of convulsions in the MSO-treated rat and the exact chain of events by which this drug causes disequilibrium in amino acid metabolism. However, several significant points may be inferred from the findings. The subcellular distribution of bound ^{14}C-MSO indicates that the drug is preferentially localized in nerve endings. The strong inhibition of GS and alanine-aminotransferase and, to a lesser extent, of GAD may produce considerable changes in the many interconnected reactions of the glutamate-glutamine and GABA metabolism (Fig. 6-2). Salganicoff and De Robertis [52] found that nerve endings maintained in isotonic conditions are permeable to glutamine but not to glutamate or aspartate. By diminishing the accessibility of glutamine to the nerve ending and intrasynaptic mitochondria, the MSO could reduce the formation of glutamate and GABA thus impairing inhibitory synapses. Since alanine passes freely into the nerve ending, an inhibition of alanine-aminotransferase may alter the metabolism in the same direction, producing a reduction in glutamate and indirectly in GABA. The presence of GS in the nerve-ending membrane may also be of interest since, in an excitatory synapse using glutamate, the enzyme could play a postsynaptic role, and its inhibition could cause an increase in the depolarizing effect of glutamate (Fig. 6-2).

The observation that most nonaminergic nerve endings of subfraction D are profoundly changed in the convulsant animal is in line with previous findings that such endings contain the GABA system and are probably involved in inhibitory functions in brain. This conclusion is also supported by the fact that the cholinergic system is not altered by MSO and that the subfractions containing aminergic nerve endings are less affected by the convulsant drug. It is of interest that in convulsions induced by thiosemicarbazide, involving a decrease in GABA content, the ACh content of the brain also remains unchanged [46].

ALLYLGLYCINE

The convulsant properties of the 2-amino 4-pentenoic acid

$$[CH_2=CH—CH_2—CH(NH_2)COOH]$$

allylglycine were described by Schneider et al. [53], and a study of the dose-response relationship of this drug and protection by barbiturates was made by McFarland and Wainer [42]. Recently we studied the cerebral cortex of rats, convulsing after administration of allylglycine, for the activity of the main enzymes associated with the metabolism of glutamine, glutamate, and GABA [3]; the study was complemented with optical and electron microscope observations on the cerebral and cerebellar cortex of rats undergoing convulsions.

Action of Allylglycine on Enzymes and Free Amino Acids. When adult rats were injected intraperitoneally with DL-C-allylglycine at a dose of 150 mg per kg, after a period of latency of 2 to 2.5 hours, there

TABLE 6-5. In Vivo and In Vitro Action of Allylglycine on Enzymes Related to GABA

Enzyme	Control	Allylglycine	% Inhibition
In vivo			
GAD	68.0 ± 4.2 (3)	50.3 ± 2.3 (8)	25
GABA-AT	122.4 ± 4.7 (2)	113.6 ± 8.8 (9)	8
In vitro			
GAD	25.8 ± 2.8 (6)	10.9 ± 1.9 (6)	58
GABA-AT	108.0 ± 10.1 (5)	108.0 ± 10.0 (5)	0

The enzymes were determined in individual homogenates from the cerebral cortex of untreated controls and in convulsant rats, 2 hours after the administration of 150 mg per kg allylglycine. In the in vitro experiment, the enzymes were determined in individual homogenates of the cerebral cortex with allylglycine; it was added in equimolecular concentration with respect to that of the substrate (10 mM for GAD and 31 mM for GABA-AT).

Results are expressed as units per gram and percent inhibition with respect to the control. The number of experiments is in parentheses.

was considerable excitation, with running and jumping, followed by convulsions and rigidity of the animals. At this time they were decapitated and the brain studied. Table 6-5 shows that in vivo there was a definite inhibition of GAD which became more evident (58 percent) when the drug was added in vitro to the homogenate. No appreciable changes were observed in GABA-AT and in the other enzymes studied, such as GS and aspartate-aminotransferase; only alanine-aminotransferase showed a certain inhibition in vitro.

Table 6-6 shows preincubation of the homogenate with allylglycine, which resulted in an 80 percent inhibition of GAD. This inhibition being less marked when the homogenate is preincubated with the buffer substrate suggests that the drug and the substrate compete for the active sites of GAD. It is interesting that the effect of other convulsants acting on the GABA system (i.e., thiosemicarbazide) is at variance with allylglycine, which does not act by way of the cofactor pyridoxal phosphate. This finding agrees with the fact that pyridoxine given in vivo before or simultaneously with allyglycine has no protective effect on the convulsions [42].

The assay of free amino acids in the convulsant rat showed that there were practically no changes in aspartate, glutamate, glycine, glutamine, and alanine while the content of GABA was reduced by 40 percent.

Ultrastructural Changes in Nerve Endings Induced by Allylglycine. Electron microscope observations on neuropil regions of the cerebral cortex of convulsant rats showed that most nerve endings had normal aspects. A few showed striking alterations characterized by swelling of the axoplasm, reduction in number of vesicles, some swelling of the intraterminal mitochondria, and sometimes extensive vacuolization of the nerve ending. Similar to the MSO-treated rats, in the crude mitochondrial fraction, altered nerve endings among normal ones could be observed. Furthermore, the fraction of nonaminergic endings showed mostly altered nerve endings. The effect of allylglycine has been illustrated by Alberici et al. [3]. See Figs. 6-1 through 6-3.

Structural Changes by Allylglycine in the Cerebellar Cortex. The neurochemical findings which pointed toward a direct effect of allylglycine on the GABA system prompted investigation of the structural changes occurring in cells, known to be inhibitory by way of GABA. The extensive neurophysiological investigations on the cerebellum [5, 27, 32] led to the conclusion that the efferent fibers from the Purkinje cells are entirely inhibitory and mediated by GABA. It has been estimated that isolated Purkinje cells contain a high content of GABA, several times larger than that in motoneurons or spinal ganglion cells [8]. Roberts [47] found that the GAD activity and GABA content in the Purkinje layer is higher than in other layers of the cerebellar cortex. The results obtained so far are consistent with the view that GABA in the cerebellum may be presynaptically liberated from cells and axon terminals

TABLE 6-6. GAD Inhibition by Allylglycine in Various Conditions of Preincubation

Preincubation	Addition after Preincubation	Units per gram	% Inhibition
H	BS	28.8	—
H + A-gly	BS	5.7	80
H + BS	—	26.6	—
H + BS + A-gly	—	13.3	50
H + BS	A-gly	21.8	18
H + PP	B + Glut	43.8	—
H + PP + A-gly	B + Glut	17.5	60
H + PP	B + Glut + A-gly	15.1	65

Fresh homogenates from rat cerebral cortex were preincubated for 30 min at 37°C in the conditions indicated. The final concentrations for glutamate and allylglycine were 10 mM. Results are expressed in absolute values and as percentage inhibition with respect to the corresponding control. H, homogenate; BS, buffer substrate mixture; PP, pyridoxal phosphate; B, buffer phosphate; A-gly, allylglycine; Glut, glutamate.

having an inhibitory function, i.e., Purkinje cells, stellate cells, and Golgi type II cells [47].

In the cerebellar cortex of rats undergoing allylglycine-induced convulsions, dramatic changes are observed in the Purkinje cells which are already evident at the level of the optical microscope and may be differentiated from the controls (Fig 6-3). Figures 6-4 and 6-5 show that among Purkinje cells having a rather normal aspect, others show different degrees of retraction and condensation. Such irregularly shaped cells are surrounded by clear spaces, the main dendrites are also very much condensed, and the astrocytes found in the same layer show a certain degree of swelling. These alterations contrast with the rather normal aspect of the granular layer.

At the electron microscope level, the alterations of the Purkinje cells are striking (Figs. 6-6 and 6-7). Condensation of the nucleus and the cytoplasmic matrix is very dense, as if it had undergone considerable loss of fluid. The mitochondria appear in the negative as clear regions within the matrix. The ribosomes are packed together and are rather uniformly distributed (not in polysome arrangements as in the control, Fig. 6-6). The cisternae of the Golgi complex and endoplasmic reticulum show some degree of dilatation. The main dendrites of the Purkinje cells show similar changes, predominantly the extreme condensation of the matrix. The base of the Purkinje cells appears surrounded by (a) distorted axons and terminals, which in most cases have lost the synaptic vesicles or show vacuolization, and (b) clear spaces due to the swollen glial processes (Fig. 6-7). In contrast, the glomerular regions of the granular layer of the convulsant rats show practically no alterations with the exception of a few processes situated at the periphery of the glomeruli, which may correspond to Golgi II axons (Fig. 6-8).

Possible Mechanism of Convulsions by Allylglycine. To interpret the mechanism of action of allylglycine, an important consideration is the great reduction in GABA observed at the time of convulsions, which contrasts with the normal levels of the other free amino acids. GABA concentration is mainly determined by the activities of GAD and GABA-AT, the latter enzyme being localized in mitochondria [51]. In our experiments the convulsant rats had practically no inhibition of GABA-AT and no changes were found in vitro. That GAD is inhibited by allylglycine, both in vitro and in vivo, suggests that reduction in GABA is directly determined by the effect of the convulsant on the synthesizing enzyme. This should be correlated with the ultrastructural changes observed in a certain number of nerve endings of the cerebral cortex which consist of swelling, reduction in number of synaptic vesicles, and vacuolization, which were corroborated by similar observations of isolated nerve endings [3]. More altered nerve endings were found in the nonaminergic fraction, which also supports the idea that the mechanism of allylglycine is accompanied by its action on GAD, which is contained in the nerve endings of the cortex.

Remarkable structural changes observed in the Purkinje cells and basket synapses of the cerebellum also agree with the foregoing interpretation; evidence favors the view that these neurons are of inhibitory nature and mediated by GABA. The final stage of allylglycine convulsions is followed by considerable rigidity, which is reminiscent of the hypertonicity after total cerebellar ablation in rats. The ultrastructural changes point toward a considerable loss of water and of electrolytes from these neurons with a shift toward the glial cells. Astroglial swelling appears to be a phenomenon accompanying convulsions and, as will be shown later, reaches maximal expression in

---

FIGS. 6-3, 6-4, 6-5. Light micrographs of the cerebellar cortex of rats. Sections of tissues 1 μ in diameter were embedded in Epon 812 stained as described by Lane and Europa [38]. Figure 6-3 is from a control rat ($\times$ 3600). Figures 6-4 and 6-5 from an allylglycine convulsant rat ($\times$ 4200). Symbols: aP, altered Purkinje cell; aPd, altered Purkinje cell dendrite; dg, dilated astroglia; g, astroglia; gl, glomerulus; gr, granular cell; P, Purkinje cell; Pd, Purkinje dendrite.

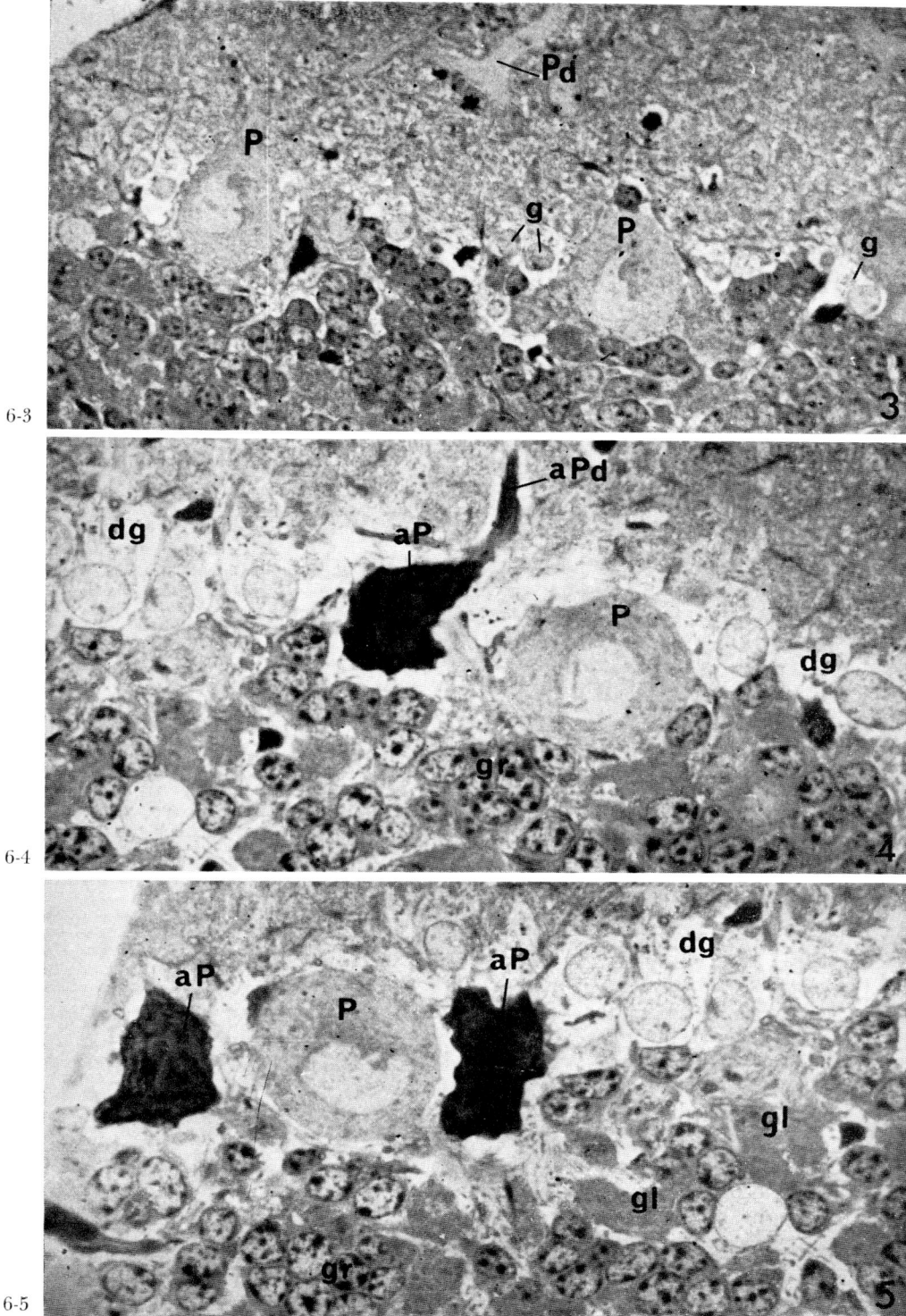

150 ULTRASTRUCTURAL NEUROCHEMISTRY

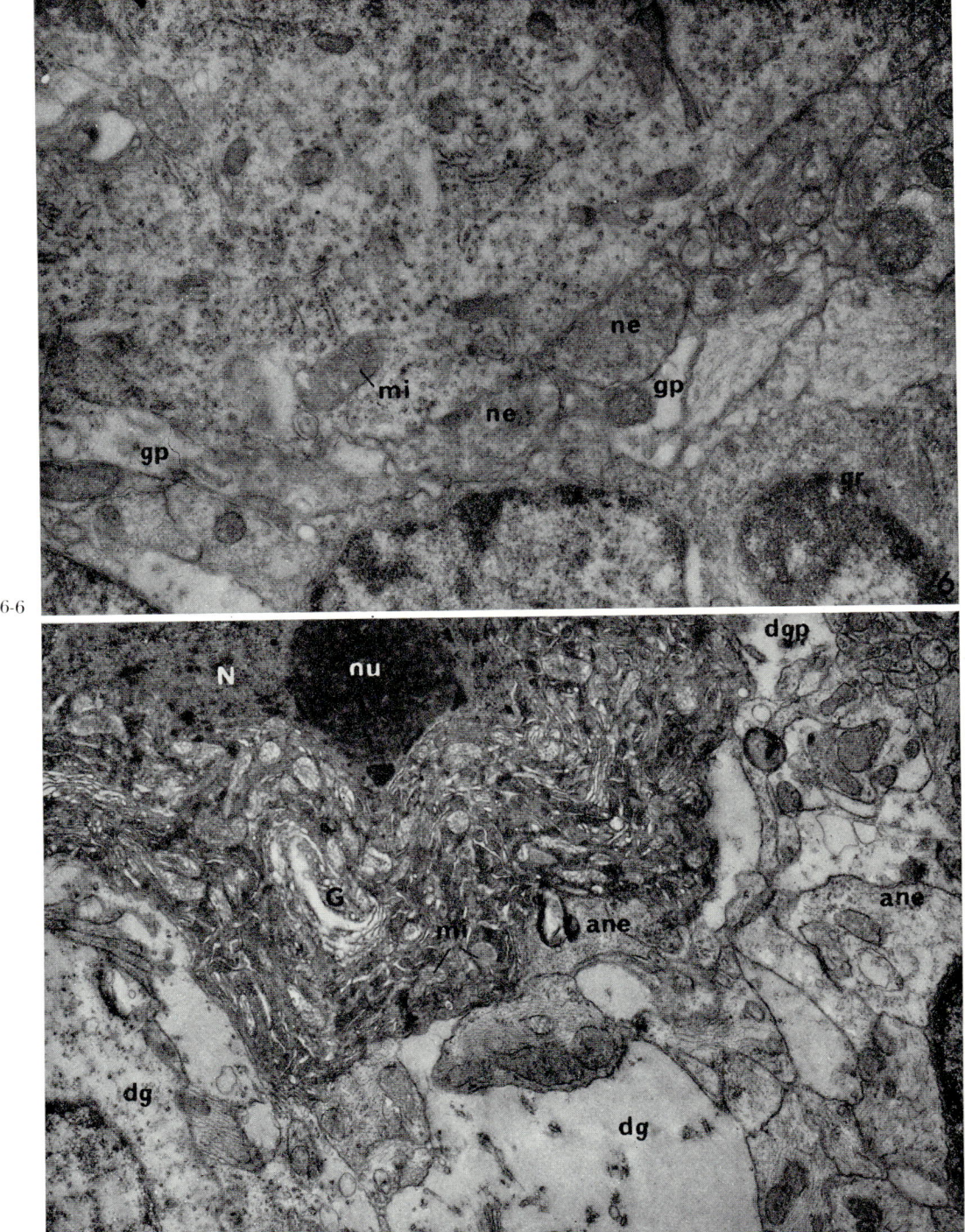

6-6

6-7

acute convulsive states such as those induced by pentylenetetrazol.

Pentylenetetrazol

Pentylenetetrazol has been extensively used as a convulsant agent. After injection intraperitoneally in the rat, seizures appear very rapidly and coincide with a decrease in content of ACh [7]. Stone [57] proposed that pentylenetetrazol induces excitation by way of certain noncholinergic neurons which in turn activate the cholinergic pathways, reducing the content of ACh.

Our studies were concentrated mainly on the acute effects of a convulsant lethal dose of pentylenetetrazol (150 mg per kg) on rats. At the onset of seizures—between 3 and 5 minutes—the rats were decapitated and the brains studied by means of electron microscopy and cell fractionation as indicated above. The most striking observation was an acute astroglial swelling in the cerebral cortex, which led to a study of the action of pentylenetetrazol on the phosphohydrolases.

Astroglial Swelling after Pentylenetetrazol. In the cerebral cortex of these acutely convulsant rats, the electron microscope revealed great enlargement of the astrocyte perikarya and processes accompanied by considerable reduction in electron density. This was at variance with the relative increase in electron density of neuronal somata, dendrites, axons, and nerve endings; the changes were most striking in the pericapillary regions where the vascular feet of the astrocytes are attached (Figs. 6-9 and 6-10). Here the bulging of the swollen processes compressed the lumen of the capillary, reducing the blood flow, and the endothelium and basement membranes became folded. It should be noted that while there was such an abrupt increase in volume in the astrocytes, the neuronal compartment appeared denser, as if the water content was reduced. On the other hand, the intercellular spaces remained practically unaltered (Fig. 6-10).

These morphological findings led to the investigation of possible changes in water and cations, particularly Na^+ and K^+. Since the results obtained on the total cerebral cortex were negative, it was concluded that the localized swelling of astroglia probably resulted from water and ion transfer from the neuronal compartment.

Action of Pentylenetetrazol on Phosphohydrolases. These findings suggested the study of the action of pentylenetetrazol on the various phosphohydrolases related to cation transport in nerve tissue [56]. As summarized in Table 6-7, the main results were an activation of the Na^+-K^+-stimulated ATPase, while the Mg^{2+}-dependent

TABLE 6-7. In Vivo and In Vitro Action of Pentylenetetrazol on Cation-Stimulated ATPases

Enzyme	Control	Pentylenetetrazol	% Variation
In vivo			
Na^+-K^+-ATPase	65 ± 5 (5)	106 ± 13 (4)	+63
Mg^{2+}-ATPase	291 ± 9 (5)	276 ± 16 (4)	− 5
In vitro			
Na^+-K^+-ATPase	73	89	+22
Mg^{2+}-ATPase	193	72	−63

The enzymes were determined according to Albers et al. [4] in individual homogenates from the cerebral cortex of controls and convulsant rats, 3–5 min after the injection of 150 mg per kg pentylenetetrazol. In the in vitro experiments the homogenates were preincubated with pentylenetetrazol, 30 min at 37°C during the assay; the final concentration of pentylenetetrazol was 40 mM.

Results are expressed in μmoles ATP hydrolyzed per hour per gram fresh tissue and percent variation with respect to the corresponding control.

Figs. 6-6 and 6-7. Electron micrographs, basal region of Purkinje cells of rat cerebellum. Figure 6-6 is from a control rat (× 18,500), and Fig. 6-7 from an allylgylcine-convulsant rat (× 12,500). Symbols: ane, altered nerve ending; dg, dilated astroglia; dgp, dilated astroglial process; G, Golgi complex; gp, astroglial process; gr, granular cell; mi, mitochondria; N, nucleus; ne, nerve ending; nu, nucleolus.

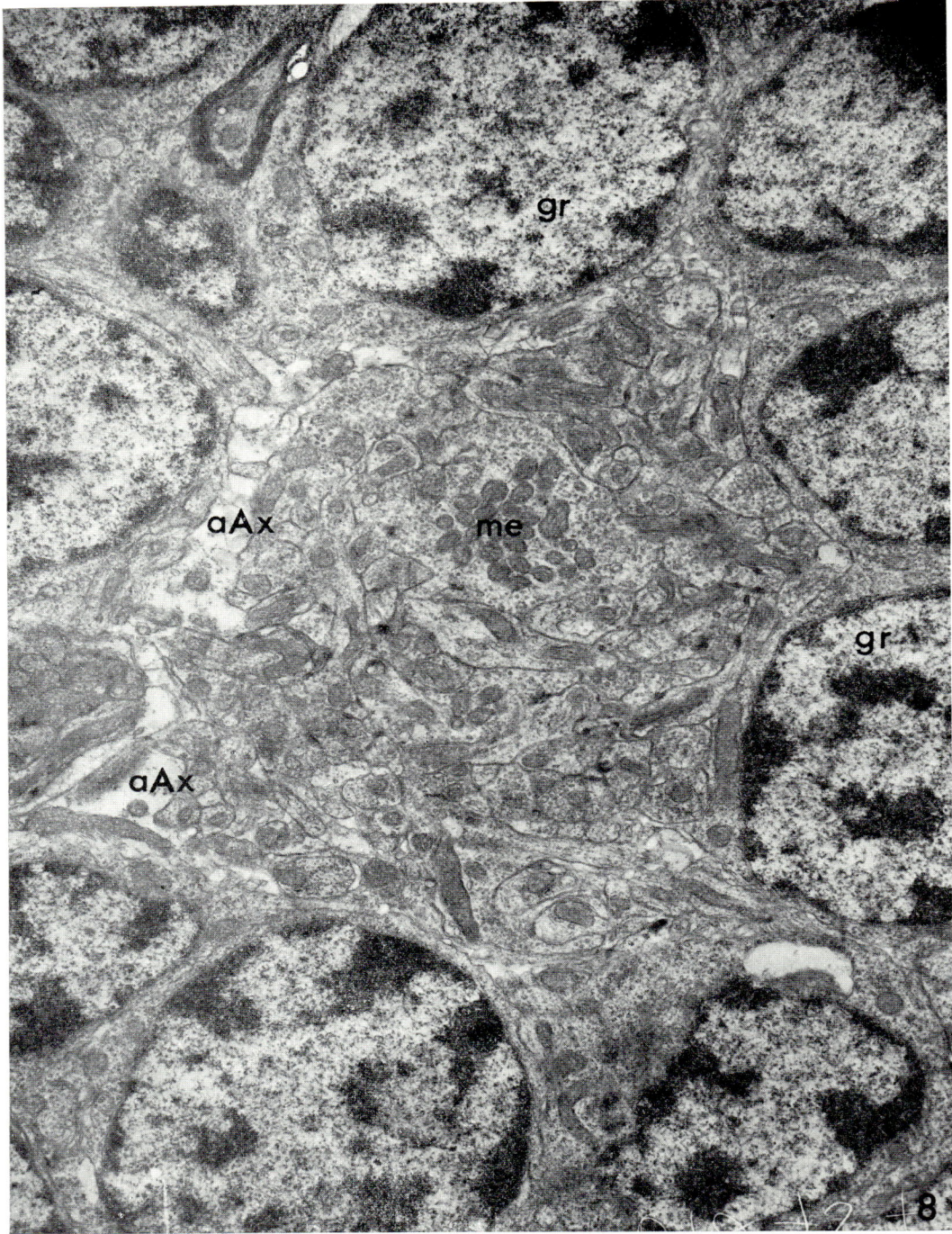

Fig. 6-8. Electron micrograph, glomerular synapse of cerebellum and surrounding granular cells (gr) of an allylglycine-convulsant rat. Endings of mossy fibers are normal (me). The only altered axons are indicated (aAx). × 12,500.

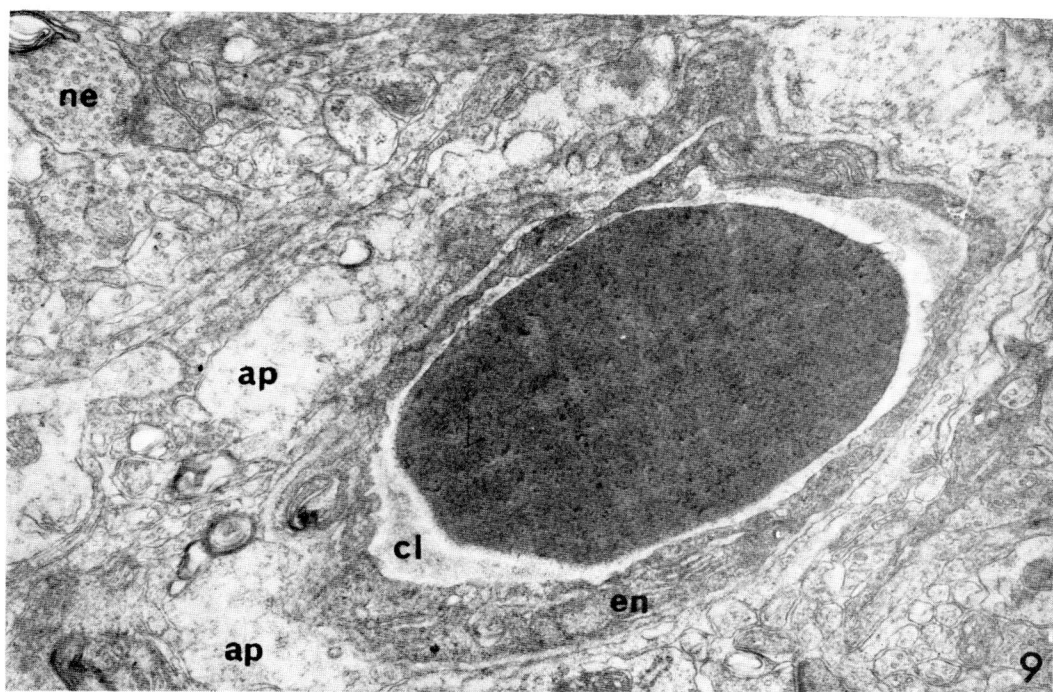

Fig. 6-9. Electron micrograph, blood capillary and surrounding neuropil region in cerebral cortex of a control rat. The lumen is widely open, contains a red blood cell. × 22,000.

ATPase did not change in vivo but was greatly inhibited after preincubation with pentylenetetrazol. Another positive result was the activation *in vitro* of the K^+-stimulated *p*-nitrophenylphosphatase.

Although these findings suggest involvement of the phosphohydrolases in the altered water and cation distribution in convulsant animals, at present they are certainly not conclusive. One of the difficulties stems from limited knowledge of the distribution of phosphohydrolases in neurons and glial cells of the central nervous system. Using cell fractionation methods, it was shown previously in this laboratory that the Na^+-K^+-stimulated ATPase is present mainly in nerve endings and nerve-ending membranes [4]. Differences in the fine subcellular localization between Na^+-K^+-ATPase and K^+-*p*-nitrophenylphosphatase were also observed [48] (Table 6-3). There is evidence in the literature that some cation-stimulated phosphohydrolases may be present in glial cells [1]. Torack [59] has reported that the histochemical reaction for Mg^{2+}-ATPase present in astroglial membranes is inhibited by triethyl-tin, a drug that produces considerable swelling of the astrocytes.

Interpretation of the Astroglial Swelling by Pentylenetetrazol. In his monograph, Tower [60] mentions some data of the literature in which seizures induced by electrical stimulation or pentylenetetrazol resulted in decrease of K^+ and increase of Na^+. It is possible that our negative results on the content of these ions may be due to the acute character of our experiments.

The finding of astroglial swelling in convulsions by pentylenetetrazol is also in line with previous observations [11] where it was demonstrated that glial cells behave as a specially active osmotic compartment which can retain appreciable quantities of water and ions. This was particularly evident in experiments done in vitro on isolated frog brains where the increase in water and electrolytes was accompanied by glial swelling, while there was no change in the inulin space [66].

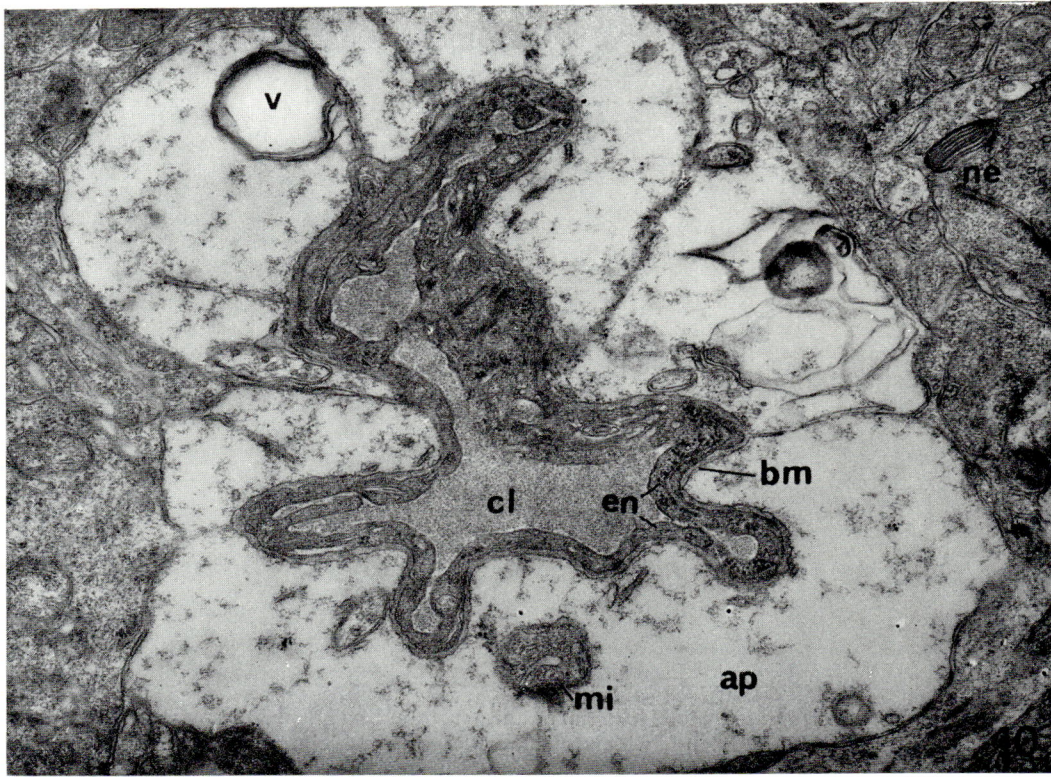

FIG. 6-10. Similar to Fig. 6-9, but from a pentylenetetrazol-convulsant rat, showing reduction and star shape of lumen. Neuropil appears more condensed than in the control ($\times$ 16,000). Symbols: ap, astroglial process; bm, basement membrane; cl, capillary lumen; en, endothelium; mi, mitochondria; ne, nerve ending; v, vacuole.

The Na^+-K^+-ATPase which appeared significatively activated in vivo may suggest an increase in the extrusion of Na^+ and water from the neuronal compartment which may be taken up by the astroglial cells. Kuffler and co-workers [36] have suggested that glial cells may act as *spatial buffers* for K^+, by the uptake of this cation from the intercellular clefts when it is in excess and by releasing it back when there is a lower K^+ concentration. According to this interpretation of glial function, it could be postulated that the extensive depolarization of neurons during convulsions could be accompanied by considerable release of K^+ and its retention by the astroglial cells. In these water and ion interchanges, the cation-stimulated hydrolases could also play an important role. The swelling of astrocytes in pentylenetetrazol convulsions may thus be a consequence of the extensive depolarization caused by the neuronal activation. This acute and localized edema may have a deleterious effect causing anoxia of the cerebral cortex, by impairment of cerebral blood flow, and death.

CONCLUDING REMARKS

The first part of this presentation reviews the main results obtained on the ultrastructural and biochemical organization of the synaptic region by the use of cell-fractionation methods. Findings that may have a bearing on the problem of the epilepsies are emphasized.

The complex population of nerve endings in the central nervous system is demonstrated by their separation into aminergic, i.e., rich in biogenic amines (ACh, norepinephrine, dopamine, 5-hydroxytryptamine, histamine), and nonaminergic nerve endings which contain the system synthesizing γ-aminobutyric acid (GABA) and probably represent inhibitory synapses. Separation of the synaptic vesicles has also been achieved, and their content in transmitter substances demonstrated.

Dissection of the synaptic region has led to the separation of different types of nerve-ending membranes and of the junctional complexes integrated by the synaptic membranes. In these membranes a series of important bound enzymes was demonstrated, as well as their receptor properties, by the binding of radioactive biogenic amines and blocking agents. A special proteolipid receptor has been isolated from the nerve-ending membranes.

The methods and concepts used for the normal brain were applied to three experimentally induced convulsant states:

(a) In the convulsions induced by methionine sulfoximine (MSO), the drug binds preferentially to nerve endings, the enzymes glutamine synthetase and alanine-aminotransferase are strongly inhibited, while the ACh system is unaffected. Considerable ultrastructural changes were observed in synapses particularly in those of the nonaminergic group. The possible mechanism of action of this drug is discussed in relation to the several interconnected reactions of the glutamate-glutamine and GABA metabolism in brain.

(b) It is demonstrated that the convulsant drug allylglycine acts by inhibiting glutamic acid decarboxylase (GAD) and reducing the levels of GABA. This inhibition is caused by competition with the substrate and not by way of pyridoxal phosphate. Only some of the nerve endings of the cerebral cortex were found altered, and these were separated mainly in the nonaminergic fraction. Purkinje cells of the cerebellum, which are inhibitory and mediated by GABA, are considerably altered by allylglycine. In the light of these findings, the possible mechanism of these convulsions is discussed.

(c) The rapid convulsions which are induced by pentylenetetrazol cause an acute swelling of the astrocytes, which compress the capillary and may impair cerebral blood flow. These changes are probably due to water and ion shifts from the neuronal compartment. In addition to its known effect on the cholinergic system, pentylenetetrazol may stimulate Na^+-K^+-ATPase and inhibit Mg^{2+}-ATPase. The effect on these and other phosphohydrolases is discussed in relation to the possible mechanism of astroglial swelling due to pentylenetetrazol. Brain edema is probably a condition frequently associated with the different types of epilepsies.

REFERENCES

1. Adams, C. W. M. Histochemistry of the Cells in the Nervous System. In Adams, C. W. M. (Ed.), *Neurohistochemistry*. Amsterdam: Elsevier, 1965.

2. Alberici, M., Rodríguez de Lores Arnaiz, G., and De Robertis, E. Catechol-O-methyltransferase in nerve endings of rat brain. *Life Sci.* 4:1951, 1965.

3. Alberici, M., Rodríguez de Lores Arnaiz, G., and De Robertis, E. Glutamic acid decarboxylase inhibition and ultrastructural changes by the convulsant drug allylglycine. *Biochem. Pharmacol.* 18:137, 1969.

4. Albers, R. W., Rodríguez de Lores Arnaiz, G., and De Robertis, E. Sodium-potassium-activated ATPase and potassium-activated p-nitrophenylphosphatase: a comparison of their subcellular localizations in rat brain. *Proc. Nat. Acad. Sci. U.S.A.* 53:557, 1965.

5. Andersen, P., Eccles, J., and Voorhoeve, P. E. Inhibitory synapses on somas of Purkinje cells in the cerebellum. *Nature* (London) 199:655, 1963.

6. Cotman, C. W., and Mahler, H. R. Resolution of insoluble proteins in rat brain subcellular fraction. *Arch. Biochem.* 120:384, 1967.

7. Crossland, J. The significance of brain acetylcholine. *J. Ment. Sci.* 99:247, 1953.

8. Curtis, D. R. Pharmacology and Neuro-

chemistry of Mammalian Central Inhibitory Processes. In von Euler, C., Skoglund, S., and Söderberg, U. (Eds.), *Structure and Function of Inhibitory Neuronal Mechanisms*. Oxford: Pergamon, 1968.

9. Del Castillo, J., and Katz, B. Biophysical aspects of neuromuscular transmission. *Progr. Biophys.* 6:121, 1956.

10. De Robertis, E. *Histophysiology of Synapses and Neurosecretion*. Oxford: Pergamon, 1964.

11. De Robertis, E. Some New Electron Microscopical Contributions to the Biology of Neuroglia. In De Robertis, E., and Carrea, R. (Eds.), *Biology of Neuroglia*. Amsterdam: Elsevier, 1965.

12. De Robertis, E. Adrenergic endings and vesicles isolated from brain. *Pharmacol. Rev.* 18:413, 1966.

13. De Robertis, E. Ultrastructure and cytochemistry of the synaptic region. *Science* 156:907, 1967.

14. De Robertis, E. Isolation of Inhibitory Nerve Ending from Brain. In von Euler, C., Skoglund, S., and Söderberg, U. (Eds.), *Structure and Function of Inhibitory Neuronal Mechanisms*. Oxford: Pergamon, 1968.

15. De Robertis, E., Alberici, M., Rodríguez de Lores Arnaiz, G., and Azcurra, J. M. Isolation of different types of synaptic membranes from the brain cortex. *Life Sci.* 5:577, 1966.

16. De Robertis, E., Azcurra, J. M., and Fiszer, S. Ultrastructure and cholinergic binding capacity of junctional complexes isolated from rat brain. *Brain Res.* 5:45, 1967.

17. De Robertis, E., and Bennett, H. S. Submicroscopic vesicular component in the synapse. *Fed. Proc.* 13:35, 1954.

18. De Robertis, E., and Bennett, H. S. Some features of the submicroscopic morphology of synapses in frog and earthworm. *J. Biophys. Biochem. Cytol.* 1:47, 1955.

19. De Robertis, E., Fiszer, S., and Soto, E. Cholinergic binding capacity of proteolipids from isolated nerve-ending membranes. *Science* 158:928, 1967.

20. De Robertis, E., Pellegrino de Iraldi, A., Rodríguez de Lores Arnaiz, G., and Salganicoff, L. Cholinergic and non-cholinergic nerve endings in rat brain. I. Isolation and subcellular distribution of acetylcholine and acetylcholinesterase. *J. Neurochem.* 9:23, 1962.

21. De Robertis, E., and Rodríguez de Lores Arnaiz, G. Structural Components of the Synaptic Region. In Lajtha, A. (Ed.), *Handbook of Neurochemistry*. I. New York: Plenum, in press.

22. De Robertis, E., Rodríguez de Lores Arnaiz, G., Alberici, M., Butcher, R. W., and Sutherland, E. W. Subcellular distribution of adenyl cyclase and cyclic phosphodiesterase in rat brain cortex. *J. Biol. Chem.* 242:3487, 1967.

23. De Robertis, E., Rodríguez de Lores Arnaiz, G., and Pellegrino de Iraldi, A. Isolation of synaptic vesicles from nerve endings of the rat brain. *Nature* (London) 194:794, 1962.

24. De Robertis, E., Rodríguez de Lores Arnaiz, G., Salganicoff, L., Pellegrino de Iraldi, A., and Zieher, L. M. Isolation of synaptic vesicles and structural organization of the acetylcholine system within brain nerve endings. *J. Neurochem.* 10:225, 1963.

25. De Robertis, E., Sellinger, O. Z., Rodríguez de Lores Arnaiz, G., Alberici, M., and Zieher, L. M. Nerve ending in methionine sulphoximine convulsant rats, a neurochemical and ultrastructural study. *J. Neurochem.* 14:81, 1967.

26. Eccles, J. C. *The Physiology of Synapses*. Berlin: Springer, 1964.

27. Eccles, J. C. Postsynaptic Inhibition in the Central Nervous System. In von Euler, C., Skoglund, S., and Söderberg, U. (Eds.), *Structure and Function of Inhibitory Neuronal Mechanisms*. Oxford: Pergamon, 1968.

28. Fiszer, S., and De Robertis, E. Subcellular distribution and nature of the α-adrenergic receptor in the CNS. *Life Sci.* 7:1093, 1968.

29. Gray, E. G., and Whittaker, V. P. The isolation of nerve ending from brain: an electron-microscopic study of cell fragments derived by homogenization and centrifugation. *J. Anat.* 96:79, 1962.

30. Harris, B. Cortical alterations due to methionine sulfoximine. *Arch. Neurol.* (Chicago), 11:388, 1964.

31. Hosie, R. J. A. The localization of adenosine triphosphatase in morphologically characterized fractions of guinea-pig brain. *Biochem. J.* 96:404, 1965.

32. Ito, M., and Yoshida, M. The cerebellar-evoked monosynaptic inhibition of Deiters' neurons. *Experientia* 20:515, 1964.

33. Kataoka, K., and De Robertis, E. Hista-

mine in isolated small nerve endings and synaptic vesicles of rat brain cortex. *J. Pharmacol. Exp. Ther.* 156:114, 1967.
34. Krnjević, K. Transmitters in the Cerebral Cortex. In *XXIII International Congress of Physiological Sciences*, Tokyo, Sept. 1965, p. 435.
35. Krnjević, K., and Schwartz, S. The Inhibitory Transmitter in the Cerebral Cortex. In von Euler, C., Skoglund, S., and Söderberg, U. (Eds.), *Structure and Function of Inhibitory Neuronal Mechanisms*. Oxford: Pergamon, 1968.
36. Kuffler, S. W., Nicholls, J. G., and Orkand, R. K. Physiological properties of glial cells in the central nervous system of amphibia. *J. Neurophysiol.* 29:768, 1966.
37. Lamar, C., and Sellinger, O. Z. The inhibition in vivo of cerebral glutamine synthetase and glutamine transferase by convulsant methionine sulfoximine. *Biochem. Pharmacol.* 14:489, 1965.
38. Lane, B., and Europa, D. L. Differential staining of ultrathin sections of epon-embedded tissues for light microscopy. *J. Histochem. Cytochem.* 13:579, 1965.
39. Lapetina, E., Soto, E., and De Robertis, E. Lipids and proteolipids in isolated subcellular membranes of rat brain cortex. *J. Neurochem.* 15:437, 1968.
40. Maynert, E. W., Levi, R., and De Lorenzo, A. J. The presence of norepinephrine and 5-hydroxytryptamine in vesicles from disrupted nerve-ending particles. *J. Pharmacol. Exp. Ther.* 144:385, 1964.
41. McCaman, R., Rodríguez de Lores Arnaiz, G., and De Robertis, E. Species differences in subcellular distribution of choline acetylase in the CNS. A study of choline acetylase, acetylcholinesterase, 5-hydroxytryptophane decarboxylase and monoamine oxidase in four species. *J. Neurochem.* 12:927, 1965.
42. McFarland, D., and Wainer, A. Convulsant properties of allylglycine. *Life Sci.* 4:1587, 1965.
43. Pellegrino de Iraldi, A., and De Robertis, E. The neurotubular system of the axon and the origin of granulated and nongranulated vesicles in regenerating nerves. *Z. Zellforsch.* 87:330, 1968.
44. Pellegrino de Iraldi, A., Farini-Duggan, H., and De Robertis, E. Adrenergic synaptic vesicles in the anterior hypothalamus of the rat. *Anat. Rec.* 145:521, 1963.
45. Peters, E. L., and Tower, D. B. Glutamic acid and glutamine metabolism in cerebral cortex after seizures induced by methionine sulfoximine. *J. Neurochem.* 5:80, 1959.
46. Roa, D., Tews, J. K., and Stone, W. E. A neurochemical study of thiosemicarbazide seizures. *Biochem. Pharmacol.* 13:477, 1964.
47. Roberts, E. Some Biochemical-Physiological Correlations in Studies of γ-Aminobutyric acid. In von Euler, C., Skoglund, S., and Söderberg, U. (Eds.), *Structure and Function of Inhibitory Neuronal Mechanisms*. Oxford: Pergamon, 1968.
48. Rodríguez de Lores Arnaiz, G., Alberici, M., and De Robertis, E. Ultrastructural and enzymic studies of cholinergic and non-cholinergic synaptic membranes isolated from brain cortex. *J. Neurochem.* 14:215, 1967.
49. Rodríguez de Lores Arnaiz, G., and De Robertis, E. Cholinergic and non-cholinergic nerve endings in the rat brain. II. Subcellular localization of monoaminoxidase and succinate dehydrogenase. *J. Neurochem.* 9:503, 1962.
50. Rodríguez de Lores Arnaiz, G., and De Robertis, E. 5-Hydroxytryptophan decarboxylase activity in nerve endings of the rat brain. *J. Neurochem.* 11:213, 1964.
51. Salganicoff, L., and De Robertis, E. Subcellular distribution of glutamic decarboxylase and gamma-aminobutyric alpha-ketoglutaric transaminase. *Life Sci.* 2:85, 1963.
52. Salganicoff, L., and De Robertis, E. Subcellular distribution of the enzymes of the glutamic acid, glutamine and γ-aminobutyric acid cycles in rat brain. *J. Neurochem.* 12:287, 1965.
53. Schneider, J. H., Cassir, R., and Chordikian, F. Inhibition of incorporation of thymidine into deoxyribonucleic acid by amino acid antagonists in vivo. *J. Biol. Chem.* 235:1437, 1960.
54. Sellinger, O. Z., and Weiler, P., Jr. The nature of the inhibition in vitro of cerebral glutamine synthetase by the convulsant methionine sulfoximine. *Biochem. Pharmacol.* 12:989, 1963.
55. Sisken, B., Roberts, E., and Baxter, C. F. γ-Aminobutyric and Glutamic Decarboxylase Activity in the Brain of the Chick. In Roberts, E. (Ed.), *Inhibition in the Nervous System and GABA*. Oxford: Pergamon, 1960.

56. Skou, J. C. Enzymatic basis for active transport of Na+ and K+ across cell membrane. *Physiol. Rev.* 45:596, 1965.
57. Stone, W. E. The role of acetylcholine in brain metabolism and function. *Amer. J. Phys. Med.* 36:222, 1957.
58. Sutherland, E. W., Øye, I., and Butcher, R. W. The action of epinephrine and the role of the adenyl cyclase system in hormone action. *Recent Progr. Hormone Res.* 21:623, 1965.
59. Torack, R. M. Electron Histochemistry of the Nervous System. In Adams, C. W. M. (Ed.), *Neurohistochemistry*. Amsterdam: Elsevier, 1965.
60. Tower, D. B. *Neurochemistry of Epilepsy*. Springfield, Ill.: Thomas, 1960.
61. Uchizono, K. Characteristics of excitatory and inhibitory synapses in the central nervous system of the cat. *Nature* (London) 207:642, 1965.
62. Uchizono, K. Inhibitory and Excitatory Synapses in Vertebrate and Invertebrate Animals. In von Euler, C., Skoglund, S., and Söderberg, U. (Eds.), *Structure and Function of Inhibitory Neuronal Mechanisms*. Oxford: Pergamon, 1968.
63. von Hungen, K., Mahler, H. R., and Moore, W. J. Turnover of protein and ribonucleic acid in synaptic subcellular fractions from rat brain. *J. Biol. Chem.* 243:1415, 1968.
64. Werman, R., and Aprison, M. H. Glycine: The Search for a Spinal Cord Inhibitory Transmitter. In von Euler, C., Skoglund, S., and Söderberg, U. (Eds.), *Structure and Function of Inhibitory Neuronal Mechanisms*. Oxford: Pergamon, 1968.
65. Wolfe, L. S., and Elliott, K. A. C. Chemical Studies in Relation to Convulsive Conditions. In Elliott, K. A. C., Page, I. H., and Quastel, J. H. (Eds.), *Neurochemistry* (2d ed.). Springfield, Ill.: Thomas, 1962.
66. Zadunaisky, J. A., Wald, F., and De Robertis, E. Osmotic Behaviour and Glial Changes in Isolated Frog Brains. In De Robertis, E., and Carrea, R. (Eds.), *Biology of Neuroglia*. Amsterdam: Elsevier, 1965.
67. Zieher, L. M., and De Robertis, E. Subcellular localization of 5-hydroxytryptamine in rat brain. *Biochem. Pharmacol.* 12:596, 1963.
68. Zieher, L. M., and De Robertis, E. Distribución subcelular de noradrenalina y dopamina en cerebro de rata. In *VI Congreso de la Asociación Latinoamericana de Ciencias Fisiológicas,* Viña del Mar, Chile, Nov. 1964, p. 150.

Discussion

NEUROTRANSMITTERS IN NORMAL AND ISOLATED CORTEX*

K. KRNJEVIĆ

NEUROCHEMISTRY OF NORMAL BRAIN

The valuable studies of De Robertis and colleagues reviewed here [8], together with extensive investigations by Whittaker and collaborators [46], have thrown a great deal of light on the subcellular distribution of many neurochemical agents; they are of interest in regard to normal cerebral function as well as in the present context of abnormal seizure activity.

The greatest single achievement in this series of studies is probably the effective separation of nerve endings [10, 15, 16] as morphological and even functional entities, *synaptosomes* [46], whose behavior and properties can now be examined in isolation.

Although this work has been quite successful, certain interpretations arising from it lead to some difficulties. For example, it has often been taken for granted that cholinergic transmission must play a major role in the brain; much emphasis has been placed on the presence of bound ACh in synaptosomes. Evidence for cholinergic transmission in the brain, while suggestive, is still far from conclusive [22]. It is quite possible that the role of ACh in cerebral function is of relatively secondary importance, that the main excitatory transmitter is a dicarboxylic amino acid, closely related to L-glutamate [21].

The role played by catecholamines and 5-HT in the brain is by no means yet clear. Only in the striatum is there reasonably good evidence for a possible aminergic mechanism: nigro-striatal ascending projections apparently moderate the activity of caudate neurons through the release of dopamine [5, 35, 36, 39].

Considerable evidence has been accumulated showing that GABA or some close derivative, but not glycine [18], could be an inhibitory transmitter in the cerebral cortex [19, 23, 28], also in other parts of the brain [38]. Although it is well known that GABA occurs in the brain in relatively large amounts [2, 41], it has not yet been possible to demonstrate conclusively its release from nerve endings during inhibitory activity.

The technique described by Whittaker and by De Robertis has revealed the presence in synaptosomes of functionally significant amounts of GABA and some other amino acids [34]. Minute quantities of extracts of synaptosomes produce definite inhibitory effects when tested on cortical neurons [32].

Quite marked excitatory effects are also obtained with similar extracts of nerve endings, which can be accounted for by their dicarboxylic amino acid content [32]. Thus, although only a rather small fraction of the total excitatory and inhibitory amino acid content of the brain is present in synaptosomes, and most of it is not bound as is ACh, the nerve endings undoubtedly contain a sufficient supply for significant synaptic action. Since nerve endings are also provided with the enzymes needed for synthesis of the active amino acids [8], this lends further support to the conclusion.

The greatest drawback at present to this experimental approach is the lack of any definite means of separating excitatory from inhibitory endings. Although De Robertis' more recent work has progressed toward overcoming this handicap, it is clear that no satisfactory solution is yet at hand. The possibility of distinguishing inhibitory end-

---

* Supported by Canadian Medical Research Council and United Cerebral Palsy Research and Educational Foundation.

ings by the shape of their vesicles may become a useful tool [8, 45].

Synaptic Vesicles

De Robertis' and Bennett's [9] discovery of synaptic vesicles led to the widely accepted hypothesis that the vesicles are the morphological correlate of quantal transmission [cf. 7]. Although suspensions of vesicles can be shown to contain ACh [8, 46], their content in amino acids is relatively low [34]. Most of the excitatory and inhibitory effects evident when extracts of synaptosomes are applied to single neurons from micropipettes can be ascribed to the cytoplasmic subfraction [32]. It remains to be proved that vesicles can be equated with quanta of transmitter.

Convulsive States

In his review, De Robertis [8] suggests two possible causative mechanisms operating in convulsive disorders: first, a loss of normal inhibitory mechanisms and, second, an increased excitability of neuronal elements, caused by chemical supersensitivity (which would result from the presence of an excess of membrane "receptors"). These hypotheses can be put to experimental test. Most of the remainder of this discussion gives a preliminary description of some relevant observations on cortical tissue with convulsive properties [26, 27].

Experiments on Long-Isolated Cortical Slabs

Long-isolated slabs are of much interest because they readily give very prolonged, apparently self-sustained seizure discharges [12]. In the normal or just-isolated suprasylvian cortex, a convulsive afterdischarge can be elicited only by repetitive stimulation at a relatively high frequency, >10 Hz, and the effects last only a few seconds; in the long-isolated slab, stimulation at frequencies as low as 3–4 Hz may trigger a convulsive discharge lasting many minutes [14, 42]. The properties of cells and neuronal mechanisms in such slabs may throw much light on the generation of convulsive activity, and this is clearly an excellent means for testing the two hypotheses mentioned above.

Extracellular Studies

The present study was performed on cats. In most preliminary operations, relatively shallow slabs of cortical tissue were isolated within the suprasylvian gyrus by the method of Burns [3]. In some cases larger portions of the suprasylvian or pericruciate cortex were isolated by deeper and wider cuts, overlapping adjacent gyri. The properties of the cells in the isolated cortex were analyzed mostly 3–8 weeks later, either under anesthesia or in the unanesthetized cerveau isolé.

The experiments, performed with multibarreled micropipettes as described by Krnjević and Phillis [23], involved a search for neurons which were firing spontaneously or could be excited with L-glutamate or ACh released from the microelectrode by iontophoresis. When such neurons were found, we noted the minimal amount of glutamate required to produce a discharge and tested their sensitivity to GABA released from another barrel. In several experiments where the cortical surface was stimulated with single shocks, we looked for the normal marked and prolonged inhibitory effect which is easily detected as a silent period against a background of firing evoked with glutamate [25]. In all cases, as a partial control, parallel observations were made in the corresponding area of the contralateral cortex.

Preliminary analysis leads to various conclusions about the properties of long-isolated cortical tissue.

Presence of Neurons. Very few active neurons are encountered, particularly in the small slabs, and there is a total absence of discharges which definitely cannot be attributed to mechanical stimulation by the microelectrode.

Excitation by L-Glutamate. Discharges are readily evoked with a local iontophoretic release of L-glutamate. Although they usually have the normal rapid onset and termination (Fig. D6-1), the spikes are often relatively small, and the discharge is sometimes poorly maintained. The mean threshold dose of glutamate is either unchanged or somewhat higher than normal.

Excitation by ACh. In small slabs, unusually few cells show clear excitation by

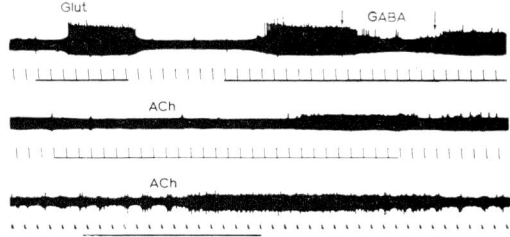

Fig. D6-1. Microelectrode recording. Upper trace: neuron in isolated suprasylvian slab (at 7 weeks) excited by applications of glutamate during times indicated by black lines—iontophoretic doses 14 and 28 nanoamperes (nA); second discharge was blocked by release of GABA between arrows (14 nA). Middle trace: excitation of neuron in same long-isolated slab by ACh (140 nA). Lower trace: neuron in slab of contralateral suprasylvian cortex, only few hours after isolation; dose of ACh was 28 nA. Time marks indicate seconds.

ACh (only 4 percent vs 20 percent on control side), and the responses tend to be poorly developed (Fig. D6-1). In some cases ACh may initiate a very prolonged discharge, not unlike normal spontaneous activity. With most other cells, ACh gives only a mild depression of discharges evoked by glutamate (eserine is a much more potent depressant). In larger slabs there is no obvious deficiency of ACh-excited cells, and there is some evidence of an increased sensitivity to ACh.

Effects of GABA. Brisk firing generated by a release of glutamate is in all cases readily blocked by GABA, in doses comparable with or somewhat lower than those required on the normal side (Fig. D6-1).

Inhibition Evoked by Surface Shocks. A strong inhibitory effect is readily obtained by surface shocks (Fig. D6-2). It appears to last even longer than normal, possibly because of the absence of spontaneous or extraneous activity. The threshold for inhibition is more often somewhat greater than on the control side; there is some evidence of an enhanced early phase of excitation immediately after the surface shock.

Convulsive Discharges. Convulsive firing can be elicited by repetitive surface stimulation. Once started, the discharge of

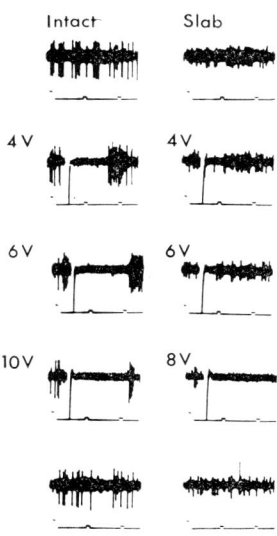

Fig. D6-2. Microelectrode recording. Inhibition of glutamate-evoked discharge, in intact cortex (left-hand column) and isolated suprasylvian slab (right-hand column). Intensity of surface shocks is indicated. Upper and lower traces are controls in absence of surface stimulation. Time marks 100 msec. Several sweeps are superimposed in each trace.

bursts may go on at a relatively regular rate (1–3 Hz) for many minutes; between bursts the neurons are refractory to glutamate. Microiontophoretic applications of GABA reduce unit firing during bursts without affecting the sequence of bursts. However, the seizure can be stopped by an intravenous infusion of GABA.

Intracellular Observations. These experiments were performed on small suprasylvian slabs, with conventional, fine micropipettes filled with either 1 M potassium citrate or potassium acetate. The usual precautions were taken to reduce movements and the cats were paralyzed by intravenous succinylcholine.

Neurons. Very few neurons can be found; the resting potentials are low, and they decay rapidly.

Inhibition. Inhibitory postsynaptic potentials (IPSPs) can be elicited by surface shocks (Fig. D6-3). In most respects, such as duration, polarity, and conductance

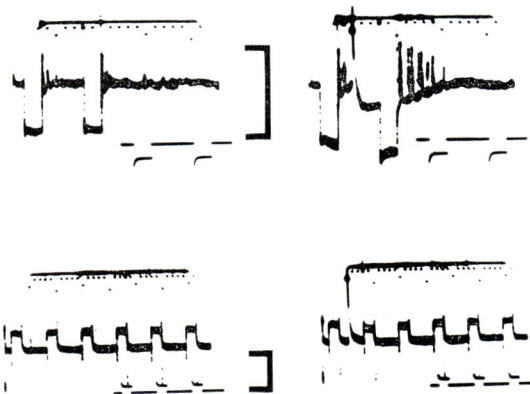

FIG. D6-3. Microelectrode recording. IPSPs and inhibitory conductance changes recorded intracellularly in suprasylvian slab (cerveau isolé). Left-hand records show pulses measuring membrane resistance in absence of surface shock as well as testing current pulses (displaced to right). Right-hand records show effect of a 12 V surface shock. Upward deflections are positive. Time marks 10 + 100 msec. Calibrations indicate 50 mV and 2 nA.

change, they do not differ obviously from those seen in normal cortex.

Unresponsive Cells. Exceptionally large numbers of cells are encountered which have particularly high and stable resting potentials but cannot be excited and have no IPSPs. Strong tetanic stimulation of the cortical surface has a slowly reversible depolarizing effect on some, but not on all the cells tested.

HISTOLOGICAL AND HISTOCHEMICAL
OBSERVATIONS

Many neurons show chromatolytic changes. Neuroglia are particularly abundant throughout the slab.

There is an almost total loss of the normal acetylcholinesterase (AChE) content of the small slabs, with no staining of any recognizable neuronal elements (fibers or cells). The larger isolated portions of cortex preserved much of the normal acetylcholinesterase distribution.

DISCUSSION

Denervation Supersensitivity. The present observations lend no support to the idea that partially denervated neurons necessarily become supersensitive to chemical stimulation [4, 11, 12, 43], and it is unlikely that the convulsive tendency can be due to this phenomenon. There is either no change or a reduction in the sensitivity to glutamate. In the small slabs, there is a marked reduction in the number of cells excited by ACh which is particularly significant, since the histochemical evidence confirms previous observations of disappearance of AChE-containing fibers [11, 13, 17, 30]. The small isolated slab is therefore comparable to the cortex of the newborn kitten. At this stage of development, the cortex has not yet been fully invaded by AChE-containing elements [31], and neuronal responses to ACh are either absent or poorly developed [24]; this is clearly quite different from the situation in fetal and denervated skeletal muscle [37].

Inhibitory Mechanisms. The convulsive tendency of the long-isolated cortex cannot be attributed to disappearance of inhibitory mechanisms in general or a loss of the cells' sensitivity to GABA in particular. On the other hand the inhibitory mechanism, although clearly operative, is somewhat more difficult to elicit than usual, possibly because of the lower density of neurons.

These observations do not exclude the possibility of a reduced efficiency of the inhibitory system. This could lead to exhaustion of the inhibitory control during repetitive activity. Low efficiency might result from inadequate synthesis of inhibitory transmitter due to a loss of the required enzymes (cf. synaptosomes in convulsive states [8]).

The tendency toward unusually pronounced, early excitation after a surface shock may thus be due to less effective inhibition. On the other hand, it could be caused either by an increased efficiency of excitatory synapses or by a greater excitability of the neurons.

Condition of Neurons. The low levels and high lability of resting potentials suggest that restorative processes in the isolated neurons have a reduced efficiency. This factor may enhance excitability and favor any tendency toward inactivation by depolarization; it could also partly reduce the efficiency of the inhibitory mechanisms by allowing a rise in internal Cl content.

Density of Glia. The abundance of glia suggests a disruption of the normal organization of the cortex, which could be of significance. The large number of unresponsive cells found during intracellular recording confirms previous evidence that these cells are mostly neuroglia [20, 29]. Their high resting potentials and absence of any periodic fluctuations in potential during seizures is evidence against substantial accumulation of extracellular K [29, 33], except possibly in some cases immediately after a particularly strong tetanus.

Blood-Brain Barrier. The fact that systemic doses of GABA can block a seizure in isolated cortex may be of some importance; on the one hand, it supports the hypothesis of an inadequate supply of inhibitory transmitter; on the other, it is in keeping with comparable observations on epileptiform discharges in cortex damaged by freezing [40, 44] and thus points to a possibly significant link between changes in the permeability of the blood-brain barrier and the development of a convulsive tendency. This also brings to mind earlier suggestions of the importance of a disordered blood-brain barrier in the etiology of epileptic phenomena [1]. It cannot be decided at present without further studies whether the greater permeability of the blood-brain barrier causes abnormal behavior by permitting an unfavorable change in the precisely controlled environment of the neurons [6] or whether it is the result of a general running-down of active mechanisms essential for the maintenance of normal cellular function, caused by reduced vascular supply or by prolonged neuronal inactivity.

REFERENCES

1. Aird, R. B., and Strait, L. Protective barriers of the central nervous system: an experimental study with Trypan red. *Arch. Neurol. Psychiat.* 51:54, 1944.
2. Awapara, J., Landua, A. J., Fuerst, R., and Seale, B. Free γ-aminobutyric acid in brain. *J. Biol. Chem.* 187:35, 1950.
3. Burns, B. D. Some properties of isolated cerebral cortex in the unanaesthetized cat. *J. Physiol.* (London) 112:156, 1951.
4. Cannon, W., and Rosenblueth, A. *The Supersensitivity of Denervated Structures.* New York: Macmillan, 1949.
5. Connor, J. D. Caudate unit responses to nigral stimuli: evidence for a possible nigro-neostriatal pathway. *Science* 160:899, 1968.
6. Davson, H. The cerebrospinal fluid. *Ergebn. Physiol.* 52:20, 1963.
7. Del Castillo, J., and Katz, B. Biophysical aspects of neuromuscular transmission. *Progr. Biophys. Biophys. Chem.* 6:121, 1956.
8. De Robertis, E. Ultrastructural Neurochemistry. In Jasper, H. H., Ward, A. A., Jr., and Pope, A. (Eds.), *Basic Mechanisms of the Epilepsies.* Boston: Little, Brown, 1969.
9. De Robertis, E., and Bennett, H. S. Submicroscopic vesicular component in the synapse. *Fed. Proc.* 13:35, 1954.
10. De Robertis, E., Pellegrino de Iraldi, A., Rodríguez de Lores Arnaiz, G., and Salganicoff, L. Cholinergic and noncholinergic nerve endings in rat brain. I. Isolation and subcellular distribution of acetylcholine and acetylcholinesterase. *J. Neurochem.* 9:23, 1962.
11. Duncan, J. A., Rutledge, L. T., and Domino, E. F. Acetylcholinesterase activity in partially isolated cerebral cortex after prolonged intermittent stimulation. *Exp. Neurol.* 20:268, 1968.
12. Echlin, F. A. The supersensitivity of chronically "isolated" cerebral cortex as a mechanism in focal epilepsy. *Electroenceph. Clin. Neurophysiol.* 11:697, 1959.
13. Echlin, F. A., and Battista, A. Baisse de la cholinestérase dans les zones du cortex cérébral "isolés" de manière chronique et hypersensibles à l'épilepsie. *C.R. Soc. Biol.* (Paris) 156:450, 1962.
14. Grafstein, B., and Sastry, P. B. Some preliminary electrophysiological studies on chronic neuronally isolated cerebral cortex. *Electroenceph. Clin. Neurophysiol.* 9:723, 1957.

15. Gray, E. G., and Whittaker, V. P. The isolation of synaptic vesicles from the central nervous system. *J. Physiol.* (London) 153:35P, 1960.
16. Gray, E. G., and Whittaker, V. P. The isolation of nerve endings from brain: an electronmicroscopic study of cell fragments derived by homogenization and centrifugation. *J. Anat.* 96:59, 1962.
17. Hebb, C. O., Krnjević, K., and Silver, A. Effect of undercutting on the acetylcholinesterase and choline acetyltransferase activity in the cat's cerebral cortex. *Nature* (London) 198:692, 1963.
18. Kelly, J. S., and Krnjević, K. Effects of γ-aminobutyric acid and glycine on cortical neurones. *Nature* (London) 219:1380, 1968.
19. Kelly, J. S., Krnjević, K., and Dreifuss, J. J. Cortical inhibition and γ-aminobutyric acid. *Exp. Brain Res.* In press, 1969.
20. Kelly, J. S., Krnjević, K., and Yim, G. K. W. Unresponsive cells in cerebral cortex. *Brain Res.* 6:767, 1967.
21. Krnjević, K. Microiontophoretic studies on cortical neurons. *Int. Rev. Neurobiol.* 7:41, 1964.
22. Krnjević, K. Central cholinergic pathways. *Fed. Proc.* 28:113, 1969.
23. Krnjević, K., and Phillis, J. W. Iontophoretic studies of neurones in the mammalian cerebral cortex. *J. Physiol.* (London) 165:274, 1963.
24. Krnjević, K., Randić, M., and Straughan, D. W. Unit responses and inhibition in the developing cortex. *J. Physiol.* (London) 175:21P, 1964.
25. Krnjević, K., Randić, M., and Straughan, D. W. An inhibitory process in the cerebral cortex. *J. Physiol.* (London) 184:16, 1966.
26. Krnjević, K., Reiffenstein, R., and Silver, A. Inhibition in long-isolated cortical slabs. *Fed. Proc.* 28:521, 1969.
27. Krnjević, K., Reiffenstein, R., and Silver, A. Properties of neurons in long-isolated cortical slabs. *J. Physiol.* (London), in press, 1969.
28. Krnjević, K., and Schwartz, S. The action of γ-aminobutyric acid on cortical neurones. *Exp. Brain Res.* 3:320, 1967.
29. Krnjević, K., and Schwartz, S. Some properties of unresponsive cells in the cerebral cortex. *Exp. Brain Res.* 3:306, 1967.
30. Krnjević, K., and Silver, A. A histochemical study of cholinergic fibres in the cerebral cortex. *J. Anat.* 99:711, 1965.
31. Krnjević, K., and Silver, A. Acetylcholinesterase in the developing forebrain. *J. Anat.* 100:63, 1966.
32. Krnjević, K., and Whittaker, V. P. Excitation and depression of cortical neurones by brain fractions released from micropipettes. *J. Physiol.* (London) 179:298, 1965.
33. Kuffler, S. W., and Nicholls, J. G. The physiology of neuroglial cells. *Ergebn. Physiol.* 57:1, 1966.
34. Mangan, J. L., and Whittaker, V. P. The distribution of free amino acids in subcellular fractions of guinea pig brain. *Biochem. J.* 98:128, 1966.
35. McLennan, H. The release of acetylcholine and of 3-hydroxytyramine from the caudate nucleus. *J. Physiol.* (London) 174:152, 1964.
36. McLennan, H., and York, D. H. The action of dopamine on neurones of the caudate nucleus. *J. Physiol.* (London) 189:393, 1967.
37. Miledi, R. Induction of Receptors. In Mongar, J. L., and Reuch, A. V. S. (Eds.), *Ciba Foundation Symposium on Enzymes and Drug Action.* Boston: Little, Brown, 1962, pp. 220-238.
38. Obata, K., Ito, M., Ochi, R., and Sato, N. Pharmacological properties of the postsynaptic inhibition by Purkinje cell axons and the action of γ-aminobutyric acid on Deiters neurones. *Exp. Brain. Res.* 4:43, 1967.
39. Poirier, L. J., and Sourkes, T. L. Influence of the substantia nigra on the catecholamine content of the striatum. *Brain* 88:181, 1965.
40. Purpura, D. P., Girado, M., Smith, T. G., and Gomez, J. A. Effects of systemically administered ω-amino and guanidino acids on spontaneous and evoked cortical activity in regions of blood-brain barrier destruction. *Electroenceph. Clin. Neurophysiol.* 10:677, 1958.
41. Roberts, E., and Frankel, S. γ-Aminobutyric acid in brain: its formation from glutamic acid. *J. Biol. Chem.* 187:55, 1950.
42. Sharpless, S. K., and Halpern, L. M. The electrical excitability of chronically iso-

lated cortex studied by means of permanently implanted electrodes. *Electroenceph. Clin. Neurophysiol.* 14:244, 1962.
43. Stavraky, G. W. *Supersensitivity Following Lesions of the Nervous System.* Toronto: Univ. of Toronto Press, 1961.
44. Strasberg, P., Krnjević, K., Schwartz, S., and Elliott, K. A. C. Penetration of blood-brain barrier by γ-aminobutyric acid at sites of freezing. *J. Neurochem.* 14:755, 1967.
45. Uchizono, K. Synaptic organization of the Purkinje cells in the cerebellum of the cat. *Exp. Brain Res.* 4:97, 1967.
46. Whittaker, V. P. The application of subcellular fractionation techniques to the study of brain function. *Prog. Biophys. Biophys. Chem.* 15:39, 1965.

7
Mechanisms of Action of Convulsants*

DON W. ESPLIN AND BARBARA ZABLOCKA-ESPLIN

A GREAT MANY SUBSTANCES of natural or synthetic origin are capable of producing convulsions in man and laboratory animals. This list of drugs is considerably extended if agents are included such as morphine, the general anesthetics, and many autonomic drugs, which often produce marked excitation of the central nervous system as one facet of their action in certain dosages and in some species. Stimulant drugs will not be cataloged here or their effects described; a survey of the extensive literature on this subject indicates that the mechanisms of action of most convulsants are completely obscure. Ways by which stimulation of the central nervous system may be accomplished and a review within this framework of information concerning a few prototype convulsants will be considered.

GENERAL MECHANISMS OF CONVULSANT DRUG ACTION

Normal neural functions are accomplished within balance between excitatory and inhibitory processes. Excessive neural activity leading to convulsions results either from increase in the efficiency of transmission in excitatory pathways or from decrease in effectiveness of inhibitory action. This serves only to provide a logical framework within which to list the potential mechanisms by which inhibitory or excitatory processes may be modified.

Block of Inhibition

Three distinct inhibitory processes have been demonstrated in animals: presynaptic inhibition, postsynaptic inhibition, and electrogenic pump inhibition. Inhibition accomplished by electrical coupling, occasionally found in some lower animals, is not known to occur in mammals.

The three types of inhibition are all accomplished by specific chemical transmitters. On the basis of knowledge of drug action on neurotransmitter mechanisms in the peripheral nervous systems, several ways by which each type of inhibition may be blocked are possible. Table 7-1 lists the more probable of such mechanisms; it is conceivable that a drug could cause selective blockade of conduction in the inhibitory path. Such an action presupposes some site in the conductile elements of the inhibitory pathway, such as a region of low safety factor, at which conduction in the inhibitory pathway is selectively blocked by an agent affecting conductile tissue in general. The list could be further expanded by inclusion of other possible but unlikely drug actions, such as enhancement in the rate of dissipation of the inhibitory transmitter.

Enhancement of Excitation

Synaptic excitation may be accomplished by one or several transmitters in the central nervous system. Excitatory processes in both the peripheral and central nervous systems have certain basic common fea-

---

* Unpublished work referred to was performed in Department of Pharmacology, University of Utah College of Medicine, and supported by PHS Grants NB00872 and 5–PO1–NB04553 from National Institute of Neurological Diseases and Stroke and 2–TO1–GM00153 from National Institute of General Medical Sciences.

TABLE 7-1. Potential Mechanisms of Convulsant Drug Action

Block of Inhibition	Enhancement of Excitation
1. Decrease in the amount of inhibitory transmitter available	1. Increase in the amount of excitatory transmitter available
2. Block of release of the inhibitory transmitter	2. Increase in the amount of transmitter released by each nerve impulse
3. Postsynaptic block of the inhibitory transmitter	3. Prolongation of the action of the transmitter, as by blocking its destructive enzyme
4. Change in properties of postsynaptic membrane to reduce effectiveness of the inhibitory transmitter	4. Increasing the sensitivity of the postsynaptic membrane to the transmitter—labilization
	5. Increase in resistance of the postsynaptic membrane
	6. Decrease in the firing level
	7. Decrease in membrane potential of the postsynaptic cell
	8. Decrease in synaptic recovery time

tures. From greater understanding of junctional transmission and of drug action in the periphery, listing may be made again of the principal potential mechanisms by which synaptic excitation in the central nervous system may be enhanced. The first five mechanisms listed in Table 7-1 can be better understood by a brief consideration of the biophysics of excitatory synaptic transmission.

The nerve impulse reaching the presynaptic terminal causes the release of a certain number, m, of quanta of excitatory transmitter. The number of quanta released is a function of the number of quanta or packets available, n, in the nerve terminal and of the probability, p, of release of each packet, such that

$$m = np$$

The depolarization produced by one quantum, v_1, is given by

$$v_1 = i_1 Rm$$

which is the product of the unitary synaptic current and the membrane resistance of the postsynaptic cell. The depolarization (excitatory postsynaptic potential, EPSP) produced by many quanta is, in its simplest expression, therefore

$$\text{EPSP} = m i_1 Rm \quad \text{or} \quad \text{EPSP} = n p i_1 Rm$$

The final expression gives terms for each process that can be manipulated through mechanisms 1 to 5. The terms n, p, and Rm are related to mechanisms 1, 2, and 5, respectively. Drugs that prolong transmitter action (mechanism 3) or that alter the sensitivity of the postsynaptic membrane to the transmitter (by *labilization*, mechanism 4) would produce changes in the unitary current, i_1, or in its effectiveness.

Whether the transmitter released by a synchronous volley invading the presynaptic terminals produces a depolarization sufficient to initiate postsynaptic discharge depends upon the voltage required to reach threshold. Two principal factors (cf. mechanisms 6 and 7) contribute to threshold: the absolute voltage required to initiate discharge (the firing level) and the existing membrane potential. Thus, a decrease in the firing level without a change in membrane potential or a decrease in membrane potential for a given firing level would lead both to a reduction in threshold and an enhanced probability of synaptic discharge for a given amount of excitatory transmitter.

Following synaptic discharge there is a period of depression (ranging from milliseconds to seconds depending upon the synapse) before full synaptic efficacy is restored. This process of *synaptic recovery* is related to mobilization of available transmitter at the presynaptic membrane. Agents that shorten synaptic recovery time would increase the frequency of discharge of repetitively active systems and would thereby increase the level of excitation (mechanism 8). The list in Table 7-1 could be further expanded by inclusion of less probable mechanisms. For example, it is possible that drugs may selectively enhance transmission in excitatory pathways by affecting some critical site of conduction to increase synaptic efficacy.

Drugs That Block Postsynaptic Inhibition

Postsynaptic inhibition was the earliest form of central inhibition described and is the best understood of the several types of inhibition. The ionic mechanisms underlying the inhibitory process are described in the monograph by Eccles [18], and the mechanisms of postsynaptic inhibition are compared with other forms of inhibition in the more recent monograph by Eccles [19]. Postsynaptic inhibition is accomplished by an unknown inhibitory transmitter acting directly upon the postsynaptic membrane to increase the permeability of the membrane to small ions, principally K and Cl. In most cells, membrane potential is slightly less than the equilibrium potential for the inhibitory process; thus, the inhibitory transmitter produces a brief hyperpolarization: the inhibitory postsynaptic potential (IPSP). Postsynaptic inhibition is mediated by so-called "direct" pathways, which presumably contain one interneuron between the motoneuron and the collateral from the group Ia afferent fiber. It is also mediated by a variety of polysynaptic pathways throughout the nervous system as well as by recurrent pathways, such as that containing the Renshaw cell in the spinal cord.

Knowledge of the actions of strychnine on spinal motor reflexes together with information that has accumulated concerning determinants of seizure patterns have given simple and reliable tests that may be used to indicate whether a drug stimulates by blocking postsynaptic inhibition or by some other mechanism. Generalized stimulation of the neuraxis, whether by electrical stimulation or by convulsants such as pentylenetetrazol, produces clonic convulsions when the stimulus is mild or moderate and tonic flexor-extensor convulsions when the stimulus is intense [57]. The flexor-extensor sequence observed with intense, generalized seizure activity in the neuraxis is determined by spinal reflex mechanisms [22, 23, 24, 62]. The explanation for this sequence is, briefly: in most laboratory animals the most powerful limb muscles are the extensors, which serve an antigravity function. Early during the seizure, only flexor motoneurons are activated. Coincident with the onset of extension is the activation of the extensor motoneurons, which is due to a facilitation of extensor motoneurons from peripheral sense organs via afferents that traverse the dorsal roots [23]. Interestingly, this sequence of motor events is exactly reversed in the sloth [24], an animal in which, because of its upside-down existence, the flexors serve an antigravity function.

In contrast to the convulsion patterns produced by generalized stimulation, strychnine and other agents that block postsynaptic inhibition produce a convulsion consisting only of tonic extension and extensor jerks. Seizures may be triggered by any form of sensory stimulation; this pattern is a consequence of blockade of inhibition. Interestingly again, administration of strychnine to the sloth produces immediate tonic flexion of all appendages. All the anti-inhibitory drugs whose convulsion patterns have been described are known to produce extensor convulsions. Conversely, stimulant agents that produce clonic or flexor-extensor convulsions have not been shown to block postsynaptic inhibition.

Strychnine

Strychnine has been the most studied of all of the centrally acting drugs [10]. Sherrington, who postulated central inhibition as an active process, suggested that the excitatory effects of strychnine were due to a decrease in inhibition. After several decades, this suggestion was tested by Eccles and co-workers [8], who showed that strychnine blocked various forms of direct and indirect inhibition in the spinal cord. These workers subsequently showed that it also blocked recurrent inhibition [10]. The drug did not decrease frequency of Renshaw-cell discharges; therefore, the site of action of strychnine was localized to the synapse between the Renshaw cell and the motoneuron.

Strychnine selectively reduces IPSPs and prevents conductance change produced by the inhibitory transmitter. It does this by all routes of administration, including iontophoretic application [9]. These factors localize its site of action to the synaptic region and eliminate the possibility of strychnine action on the postulated interneuron or on conduction elsewhere in the inhibitory pathway.

The precise site of action of strychnine has not been determined. Eccles, in the works referred to above, suggested by analogy with the action of curare in peripheral nervous system, that strychnine acted by postsynaptic blockade of the inhibitory transmitter. Such a mechanism is consistent with available evidence on the action of strychnine, but other conceivable mechanisms are not excluded.

Strychnine is immediate in its effect, which argues against actions of the drug to decrease the availability of the inhibitory transmitter by an effect on synthesis or transmitter mobilization. The possible remaining mechanisms of action are therefore: a presynaptic action of the drug to decrease the amount of transmitter released by the incoming nerve impulse; a postsynaptic blockade of the inhibitory transmitter; or a change in the properties of the postsynaptic membrane to reduce the effectiveness of the inhibitory transmitter. Evidence presently available does not permit a decision with assurance among these three possible mechanisms of action.

Some evidence indicates that strychnine alters properties of the postsynaptic membrane. Araki [2] has suggested that the drug abolished IPSPs by reducing membrane pore size such that even small ions pass with difficulty. Indirect evidence supporting this suggestion comes also from studies of the actions of strychnine on cortical cells [45, 46, 51]. Needed definitive experiments concerning this suggested action have yet to be performed.

Only indirect evidence exists to indicate that strychnine may affect the release of the transmitter in the inhibitory pathways. Until the transmitter substance or substances producing postsynaptic inhibition have been positively identified, definitive experiments concerning the intimate mechanisms of transmitter release may hardly be performed. However, existing evidence is sufficient to make actions on the release mechanism worthy of consideration, for strychnine as well as for other drugs in this category. McKinstry and Koelle [39] have shown that strychnine blocks the release of acetylcholine by nerve impulses in perfused sympathetic ganglia. This observation will be considered in more detail subsequent to presentation of the actions of a variety of cholinergic drugs on postsynaptic inhibitory processes.

Many reports in recent years have described strychnine-resistant postsynaptic inhibition in the central nervous system. Rigid criteria for establishing that the inhibition is truly postsynaptic have rarely been satisfied; it now becomes necessary to show that these strychnine-resistant inhibitions are not due to the recently described electrogenic pump inhibition. Nevertheless, current interpretation is that some forms of postsynaptic inhibition are not blocked by strychnine. This is frequently taken as evidence for more than one postsynaptic inhibitory transmitter [11], but existence of more than one receptor type at the appropriate presynaptic or postsynaptic locus would also satisfy available evidence. The autonomic nervous system provides several examples of different receptors for a single transmitter.

Strychninelike Drugs. Bruceine, an alkaloid of the *Strychnos nux-vomica* plant, is closely related to strychnine structurally and produces similar convulsant effects. The discrete actions of bruceine have been much less studied than those of strychnine. It is not unlikely that a more complete investigation of the action of bruceine and similar alkaloids might yield subtle differences between these agents from which clues concerning mechanism of action may be gained.

Thebaine. One of the most selective stimulants among the opium alkaloids, thebaine has been shown by electrophysiological techniques to block postsynaptic inhibition [44]. Morphine and codeine were without effect on inhibition. Longo and coworkers [37, 38] have studied a number of drugs with strychninelike activity and have shown interesting structural and pharmacological similarities between such agents and analgesic compounds. Two synthetic drugs, diphenyl-diazadamantan (IS-1757), and 4-formyl-4-phenyl-N-methyl piperidine (IS-1762), were shown to block postsynaptic inhibition; other pharmacological properties of these agents will be described.

Cholinergic Agents. The drugs mentioned above have been known for some time to block postsynaptic inhibition. In addition to these agents, a number of drugs having prominent effects upon peripheral cholinergic synapses have recently been shown to affect postsynaptic inhibition. The results obtained in the studies so far completed in our laboratories point to diverse mechanisms by which inhibition may be influenced, and they suggest also that the group Ia inhibitory pathway in the spinal cord possesses certain features in common with peripheral cholinergic junctions.

Coniine. This drug is a poisonous alkaloid of the hemlock *Conium maculatum*. Interest in coniine goes back many centuries. Its depressant or paralyzant effects were described in the accounts of the death of Socrates. Pharmacological studies of the last century established that coniine produced neuromuscular paralysis, and some reports gave indication of both central depressant and central stimulatory effects. De Boer [12] showed that nonlethal amounts of the drug enhanced severity of strychnine convulsions. More recent electrophysiological studies [48] have demonstrated that coniine administered intravenously blocks both autonomic ganglia and the neuromuscular junction but does not affect the response of the nictitating membrane to nerve stimulation or to injected acetylcholine. In doses that block peripheral cholinergic junctions, coniine blocks both group Ia and recurrent postsynaptic inhibition in the spinal cord; blockade of the latter is not associated with reduction in Renshaw-cell discharges. Intracellular recordings have shown that coniine reduces IPSPs selectively over EPSPs [47].

It is significant to contrast the actions of coniine and strychnine. Like strychnine, coniine increases polysynaptic activity, increases spinal reflex excitability, produces spontaneous discharges resembling so-called strychnine waves, and blocks IPSPs. Unlike strychnine, however, the drug causes a delayed decrease in membrane resistance, a slow and reversible decline in membrane potential, and a transitory depression of the monosynaptic reflex response. These results leave little doubt that blockade of inhibition by coniine includes sites in the inhibitory pathway not affected by strychnine. It is important to note that both coniine and strychnine block olivocochlear inhibition; however, actions of the two drugs are quite different [33].

Analysis of coniine actions presents an interesting problem. Because the drug produced neuromuscular paralysis in the same dosage range at which central excitatory effects were seen, tonic extensor convulsions were not seen. Suggestion of an anti-inhibitory action came from the observed summation of the effects of coniine and strychnine [12, 48] and from the slight but equivocal evidences of central stimulation seen in animals prior to or coincident with paralysis. Clear evidence of central stimulation was obtained only through electrophysiological studies.

Pilocarpine. An alkaloid whose well-known action is stimulation of effector organs in the parasympathetic system, pilocarpine has been found to have a variety of effects on the central nervous system [6, 63], including marked decrease in the threshold for strychnine convulsions [64]. In cats pretreated with atropine to protect against the lethal peripheral effects of pilocarpine, the drug produced extensor convulsions, easily triggered by sensory stimuli, that closely resembled those caused by strychnine [65].

In electrophysiological studies in cats [25] it was found that pilocarpine increased monosynaptic and polysynaptic reflex discharges and blocked group Ia and recurrent inhibitions. Recurrent inhibition was blocked by pilocarpine without effect upon Renshaw-cell discharges; effects of pilocarpine were observed immediately after intravenous injection. Unlike coniine, the drug did not decrease the monosynaptic response at any time after administration.

An observation of some interest was that stimulatory effects of pilocarpine, including strychninelike spontaneous activity, occurred as much as 24 hours after administration. It is unlikely that the drug itself was present in a reasonable concentration systemically at such time, as experiments had shown that the parasympathomimetic effects in cats were of much shorter duration. This observation suggested that one of the prolonged effects of the drug might be to cause partial depletion of stores of inhibitory transmitter in the central nervous system. Experiments in mice [58], in which convulsive thresholds for intravenously administered strychnine were determined at various intervals after injection of pilocarpine, showed that pilocarpine did indeed produce a transient reduction in strychnine threshold followed by a period in which the threshold was elevated, and this in turn was followed by a prolonged phase of reduction in strychnine threshold. This triphasic effect is similar to that observed with drugs acting on the adrenergic system to cause release and then depletion of neurotransmitters [41].

Arecoline. A close pharmacological relative of pilocarpine, arecoline was also investigated in intact animals and by electrophysiological techniques [66]. Arecoline did not produce full extensor convulsions in laboratory animals; however, it markedly reduced the threshold dose for strychnine convulsions. Studies of arecoline on postsynaptic inhibition revealed a more complex pattern of effects than that observed with pilocarpine. Intravenous administration of arecoline in cats, with or without the prior administration of protective doses of atropine, caused prompt reduction in the monosynaptic spike that lasted for 10 to 15 minutes. This reduction was not associated with the transient fall in blood pressure observed upon rapid injection of the drug. Following decrease in the monosynaptic spike, response returned to normal, and a block of postsynaptic inhibition ensued. In sharp contrast to effects observed with pilocarpine, the block of inhibition by arecoline was short lasting and appeared to wane before the peripheral cholinergic effects of the drug had disappeared. Polysynaptic activity was increased immediately after administration of arecoline, and this increase lasted for more than an hour. Spontaneous discharges resembling those produced by strychnine were often seen after arecoline, but they could not invariably be produced even with doses of the drug as high as 100 mg per kg. Effects of arecoline on the spinal cord are certainly complicated by actions at a variety of sites [54]. Nevertheless, the unequivocal block of postsynaptic inhibition associated with an increase in polysynaptic discharge and occurring at a time when the monosynaptic response was comparable to that observed during the control period strongly indicates direct actions of arecoline on some step in the postsynaptic inhibitory process. Further investigation of the actions of pilocarpine and arecoline by intracellular recording techniques now under way may reveal clues to their mechanisms and sites of action.

The old observation that strychnine in large doses blocks ganglionic and neuromuscular transmission, as was clearly shown by Lanari and Luco [34], is recalled by the fact that coniine produced ganglionic and neuromuscular blockade in doses affecting postsynaptic inhibition and the observation that pilocarpine produced neuromuscular paralysis [65] in doses similar to those that blocked inhibition. Investigation of this action of strychnine on the frog neuromuscular junction by Alving [1] showed that strychnine acted competitively with acetylcholine in much the same manner as curare. It seemed worthwhile therefore to determine to what extent the other known anti-inhibitory drugs possess the capability of blocking peripheral cholinergic junctions. Accordingly, thebaine, IS-1757, IS-

1762, and arecoline were studied on the superior cervical ganglion and the neuromuscular junction of the cat, and pilocarpine was studied on the ganglion, having been previously shown to block neuromuscular transmission. Evoked postganglionic discharges were recorded electrically in the ganglion experiments. Neuromuscular transmission was studied by recording the tension of the triceps surae muscles during stimulation of the sciatic nerve.

All drugs exhibited the ability to produce complete or partial block at both cholinergic junctions [28]. In all cases, the agents were more potent in blocking neuromuscular transmission than in blocking ganglionic transmission. Arecoline appeared to have the least capacity for blocking these junctions; the dose-effect curve was very flat, and complete block could not be produced by 120 mg per kg, the highest dose used. Convulsive doses and neuromuscular blocking doses of these drugs in the cat are given in Table 7-2.

TABLE 7-2. A Comparison of Convulsive Doses and Neuromuscular Blocking Doses of Anti-Inhibitory Drugs

Drug	A 50% Blocking Dose (mg/kg)	B Convulsive Dose (mg/kg)	A/B
Strychnine[a]	2	0.1	20
IS-1757	0.5	0.4	1.2
Pilocarpine	200	200	1.0
IS-1762	10	10	1.0
Thebaine	3.5	3–4	1.0
Arecoline	~40	~60	~0.7
Coniine	20	50	0.4

[a] Lanari and Luco [34].

It is apparent that very large doses of pilocarpine and arecoline are required to block inhibition and to produce convulsions compared to those that produce parasympathomimetic effects. It might be argued that such large doses of drugs do a variety of things; the important point here is that these large doses do one particular thing in the central nervous system: they block postsynaptic inhibition. This action is accomplished by doses quite similar to those that block peripheral cholinergic junctions, the other feature common to all the anti-inhibitory drugs listed.

The drugs listed in Table 7-2 represent great variation in chemical structure. Nevertheless, three of the agents (IS-1762, arecoline, and coniine) are rather simple piperidine derivatives. In a brief survey of the structural characteristics required for block of postsynaptic inhibition, 13 alkyl derivatives of piperidine were synthesized [61]. Block of inhibition was observed with compounds having alkyl groups in the 4 position. Potency increased with chain length up to the 4-butyl-piperidine and thereafter decreased as more carbons were added. The butyl derivative had a potency comparable to that of thebaine; significantly, this agent also blocked neuromuscular transmission in doses considerably higher than those that produced convulsions.

A correlation of especial interest from this table is the potency ratio for neuromuscular blockade compared to the anti-inhibitory effect. Strychnine shows the greatest selectivity in blocking postsynaptic inhibition, since about 20 times the convulsive dose must be given to produce paralysis. At the other end of the spectrum, it can be seen that coniine and arecoline are more potent as neuromuscular blocking agents than as anti-inhibitory drugs.

Similarities between strychnine and the autonomic agents (coniine, pilocarpine, and arecoline) can be shown in another way [67]. When a small amount of strychnine is injected through an indwelling catheter into the subdural space of the lumbosacral region of the cord, characteristic extensor thrusts are observed in the hindlimbs. These movements may be triggered by stimulation of a restricted area of the body innervated by the segments affected by strychnine. The dose of strychnine required to produce detectable local convulsive activity is 1/30 to 1/50 of the intravenous convulsive dose. Coniine, pilocarpine, and arecoline, in comparable fractions of their estimated intravenous convulsive doses (see Table 7-2), produce similar localized convulsive activity.

Parallelism between actions on postsynaptic inhibition and blockade of cholinergic junctions suggests a cholinergic link at some step in the inhibitory process. Since it appears unlikely that the inhibitory transmitter itself is acetylcholine, it is probable that such a cholinergic link, or a chemical step common to both inhibitory synapses and peripheral cholinergic junctions, is involved in the transmitter release process. The recent observation by McKinstry and Koelle [39] provides additional evidence for this suggestion and indicates the value of further studies of the actions of drugs on the mechanism of release of the inhibitory transmitter.

Drugs Affecting Presynaptic Inhibition

Presynaptic inhibition has been described comparatively recently. In the mammalian central nervous systems, the process is difficult to study directly; consequently, pathways involved in presynaptic inhibition and precise mechanisms by which inhibitory action is exerted become the subject of some controversy. According to the most generally accepted scheme proposed by Eccles [19] on the basis of extensive work, inhibitory pathways, which apparently contain at least two synapses, make axo-axonal connections with terminals of other afferent fibers. The inhibitory transmitter produces depolarization (giving origin to the dorsal root potential) of terminals of the excitatory afferent fibers, with consequent reduction in the amount of excitatory transmitter released by afferent impulses.

In the course of their investigations of presynaptic inhibition, Eccles and co-workers [20] observed that picrotoxin in subconvulsive doses caused marked reduction in presynaptic inhibition of monosynaptic reflex responses. Other convulsants examined, including pentylenetetrazol, strychnine, and bemegride, were without direct actions on presynaptic inhibition. These authors suggested that blockade of presynaptic inhibition was the basis for the convulsant action of picrotoxin, although they expressed reservations that this was solely action of the convulsant because spinal presynaptic inhibition was not abolished by convulsant doses of the drug. This proposed mechanism is appealing because it provides a neurophysiological basis for the distinct differences in effect between strychnine and picrotoxin. However, subsequent studies have cast further doubts upon this as the mechanism of convulsant action of picrotoxin. These studies also raise doubts concerning the importance of presynaptic inhibition in determining general excitability of the central nervous system. It is worthwhile to note briefly the basis for these reservations.

Eccles and colleagues [20] observed that pentobarbital and chloralose markedly intensified presynaptic inhibition. From these observations there appeared to be a reciprocal relation in which the convulsant decreased inhibition and the depressants increased it. Schmidt [49] in a further investigation of several anesthetics on dorsal root potentials proposed that enhancement of presynaptic inhibition was an important mechanism involved in anesthesia. Llinas [36] observed that mephenesin markedly depressed presynaptic inhibition. He suggested that mephenesin decreased inhibition by blocking interneurons in the polysynaptic inhibitory pathway. It is important to note, however, that mephenesin is devoid of excitatory effects that might be expected from blockade of presynaptic inhibition regardless of the mechanism by which the process is depressed.

Systematic study of a variety of depressants has further confounded attempts to correlate increases or decreases in presynaptic inhibition with changes in reflex excitability. Miyahara and colleagues [40] showed that eight general depressants from diverse chemical classes all increased presynaptic inhibition in a manner qualitatively similar to that observed with pentobarbital. Trimethadione, an anticonvulsant with only a weak potentiality for sedation, produced effects similar to the general anesthetics. It is clear therefore that enhancement of presynaptic inhibition may occur in the absence of marked depression of the central nervous system; thus it is unlikely that this is an important basis for anesthesia. Furthermore, carbon dioxide, in concentrations that markedly decreased reflex excitability, had no effect upon presynaptic inhibition.

Inability to correlate changes in presynaptic inhibition with corresponding changes in reflex excitability considerably undermines the attractive hypothesis that picrotoxin causes convulsions by blocking presynaptic inhibition. It would not be profitable to generate the ad hoc assumptions required to make this hypothesis conform with the observations on presynaptic inhibition mentioned above. It would be equally unwise to discard this hypothesis entirely, at the present state of our scanty knowledge of the role of presynaptic inhibition in the function of the central nervous system and of the ways by which this process may be manipulated by drugs.

Drugs Affecting Electrogenic Pumps

Subnormality associated with increased Na-K pump activity following an action potential is well known. However, demonstration that transmitter activation of electrogenic pumps may occur as a direct process and not merely as a consequence of activity is a recent observation [42]. Decreased excitability resulting from such a process falls in the category of true inhibition. Definitive studies on such inhibitory actions have come presently from autonomic ganglia and from synapses in *Aplysia*. Although such actions have not been conclusively demonstrated in the central nervous system, the potential significance of this process is mentioned by Spencer and Kandel (Chap. 21) as well as by others. If this form of inhibition is found to play a prominent role in the function of the central nervous system, then a basis may be provided for understanding the actions of a variety of convulsant drugs.

First to be suggested are the cardiac glycosides; many members of this large group are potent convulsants in species, such as the rat, able to withstand the direct cardiac effects. The cardiac glycosides are cited because of their known action to block Na-K pump activity through inhibition of the ATPase system [50]. In Chap. 22, Tower discusses the convulsant activity of these agents in relation to their inhibition of ionic pumps. In discussing the mechanism of action of diphenylhydantoin Woodbury (Chap. 23) describes antagonism between this anticonvulsant and ouabain; he reviews evidence suggesting actions of diphenylhydantoin to enhance Na-K pumping.

There is little basis at present for mentioning other agents that might operate by affecting this process. Nevertheless, electrogenic pump inhibition provides a link between metabolism, electrical activity, and inhibitory action that fully harmonizes with philosophical themes running through much of the literature [55, 56], attempting to outline the possible mechanisms underlying epilepsy and convulsant and anticonvulsant drug actions.

Drugs That Act by Direct Stimulation

Only few of the known stimulants have been shown to affect central inhibition. By exclusion, therefore, it is presumed that the remaining agents increase excitation by one or more of the mechanisms listed in Table 7-1. Further investigation of electrogenic pumps may reveal that some of the drugs presently presumed to act by direct stimulation produce convulsions by blocking this process. Somewhat surprisingly, very little is known of the mechanism of action of any convulsant drug in this large category, although the literature concerning manifestations of increased excitability is very extensive [26, 29]. Scarcity of this information is partly because it is more difficult to investigate the actions of convulsant drugs on synaptic systems than depressants. Increases in the level of excitability lead to great variation in evoked responses, and frequently spontaneous discharges become troublesome. These especially complicate intracellular investigations. By contrast, depressant drugs reduce background activity, and evoked responses show little variation.

Pentylenetetrazol

Pentylenetetrazol (PTZ) is a valuable diagnostic tool in clinical epilepsy and a useful laboratory tool in studying seizure mechanisms and in drug screening. Knowledge of the mode of action of this agent would provide valuable insights into the mechanisms of seizure discharge and of anticonvulsant drug action. In low doses, the drug produces graded increases in excitability of the central nervous system associated with activation of the electroencephalogram (EEG). Earliest manifestations of convulsive activity in animals are clonic movements of limbs and facial muscles; full convulsions are not triggered by sensory stimulation, as they are in the case of strychnine. At doses above those producing clonic activity, flexor-extensor convulsions are observed.

An antagonism between PTZ and trimethadione is almost unique among convulsant-depressant drug pairs; trimethadione completely reverses the changes in EEG and in spinal reflex excitability produced by PTZ. The antagonism is so complete that several lethal doses of both drugs may be given to an animal with no apparent effect. It is possible that this interaction represents true pharmacological antagonism in which the drugs act at the same receptor sites by opposite mechanisms. Whether this in fact is the case, we can, at our present state of knowledge, make inferences concerning the mechanism of action of PTZ from the actions of trimethadione.

Eyzaguirre and Lilienthal [27] showed that PTZ in large concentrations induced repetitive firing of nerve fibers and shortened the refractory period; the authors proposed a "veratrinic" action for PTZ. A similar action of PTZ was indicated in a study of the interactions of trimethadione and pentylenetetrazol on spinal-cord synaptic systems where trimethadione markedly prolonged the time required for synaptic recovery in the monosynaptic pathway [21]. The drug did not affect posttetanic potentiation. The changes in synaptic recovery and the consequent rapid failure of response during repetitive stimulation were both completely antagonized by PTZ.

In a further investigation, Lewin and Esplin [35] studied effects of PTZ on spinal synaptic systems and the antagonism of these effects by trimethadione. Although it is known that the dose required to produce convulsive activity in the spinal animal is somewhat higher than that producing full seizures in the intact animal, it was found that spinal synaptic systems were affected by convulsive doses of the drug (20–30 mg per kg). It appears reasonable, therefore, to use synaptic systems of the cord as models upon which to investigate actions of PTZ that underlie convulsive activity originating in higher centers. PTZ characteristically increased polysynaptic activity at all doses employed (10–40 mg per kg), and, somewhat paradoxically, the drug consistently decreased the monosynaptic spike elicited by dorsal root stimulation. After PTZ, there was much less response failure during tetanization than in the absence of the drug. Similarly, synaptic recovery time appeared to be shortened by PTZ, although this was difficult to investigate because of the increase in excitability. Trimethadione reversed all the actions of PTZ described.

It is unlikely that decrease in monosynaptic response following PTZ was due to a depressant action; rather, it seemed more reasonable to attribute this to an increase in inhibitory activity on the motoneuron associated with the marked increase in activity of spinal internuncial systems. Such observations suggested an explanation for the selective convulsant action of PTZ on higher centers that did not require the assumption of greater sensitivity of individual cells in the brain. Selectivity could be explained by actions of PTZ on cerebral systems relatively unopposed by inhibition while, in contrast, stimulation of the extensive inhibitory systems of the cord would tend to oppose actions of the drug on excitation.

The studies described gave little indication of the definitive mechanism by which PTZ increases neuronal excitability. Accordingly, microelectrode techniques were employed [4] to attempt to determine which step in the process of excitation is affected by PTZ. In this case also, the motoneuron was used as the principal model. Because of increased response variability in the presence of the convulsant drug, it was neces-

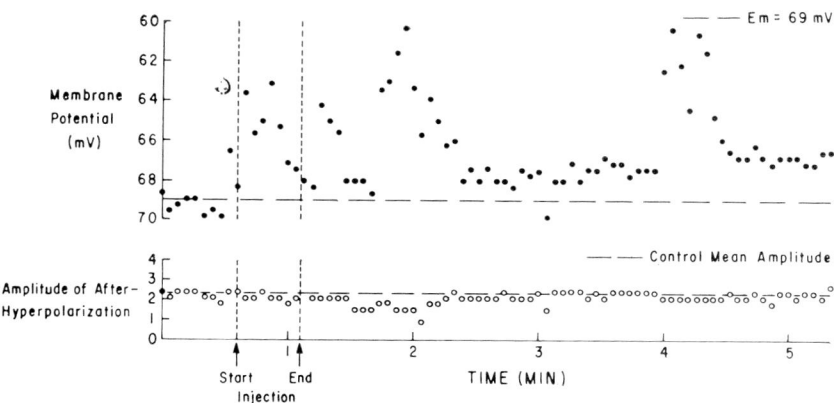

FIG. 7-1. Effects of pentylenetetrazol (40 mg per kg) on motoneuron membrane potential and on afterhyperpolarization following the antidromic spike. Upper graph shows changes in membrane potential with time after injection of pentylenetetrazol. Beginning and end of injection are indicated by arrows on the abcissa common to both graphs. The interrupted line represents the resting membrane potential, E_m, of 69 mV, the average of ten responses prior to drug administration. Lower graph shows changes in peak amplitude of the afterhyperpolarization.

sary to carry out many experiments with individual cells before a clear pattern emerged.

Figure 7-1 shows results of one representative experiment in which membrane potential and afterhyperpolarization of the motoneuron were studied. After intravenous injection of 40 mg per kg of PTZ, the membrane potential showed marked fluctuations; peak depolarizations were as much as 9 mV. Nevertheless, a uniform depolarization was not observed. It is probable that these waves of depolarization underlie periodic bursts of activity recorded in ventral roots following this dose of PTZ [4, 35]. Afterhyperpolarization was also little affected by PTZ. Figure 7-1 shows occasional slight decreases in afterhyperpolarization following the drug, which are associated temporally with waves of depolarization and do not appear to represent direct actions of PTZ on the motoneuron.

Effects of PTZ on EPSP amplitude were studied in many experiments, and Fig. 7-2 illustrates results typically obtained. PTZ characteristically caused a slight reduction in EPSP amplitude and a reduction in the frequency of motoneuron discharge with stimuli near threshold. Figure 7-2 also illustrates another significant feature: the EPSPs in the control series are terminated abruptly by a positive-going wave presumably of inhibitory origin. After PTZ, this positivity is much more pronounced.

Other properties of the motoneuron were also studied. PTZ did not alter resistance of the motoneuron membrane, its firing threshold to depolarizing currents passed through the microelectrode, or the firing level to orthodromic stimulation. Results presented suggest that observed changes in motoneuron response are due primarily to changes in background state of the cell that result from stimulation of both excitatory and inhibitory internuncial systems by PTZ.

Effects of PTZ on background influences on excitability of motoneurons were studied [4] by means of input-output relations in flexor (biceps-semitendinosus) and extensor (triceps surae) motoneuron pools. After PTZ, input-output relations for the flexor pathway were characteristically shifted to the left, reflecting increase in excitability due to increased facilitatory background discharge. On the other hand, PTZ caused a shift to the right in the input-output curves for the extensor pathway, reflecting increase in inhibitory back-

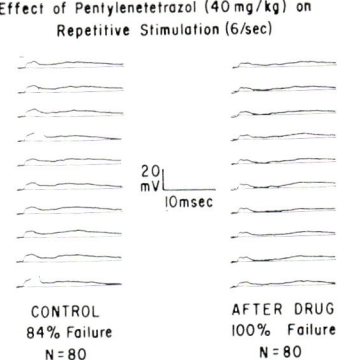

FIG. 7-2. Effects of pentylenetetrazol (40 mg per kg) on motoneuron response during repetitive dorsal root stimulation. Left-hand series of traces shows sampling of 80 responses taken before the drug, and right-hand series shows similar sampling of 80 responses after pentylenetetrazol. Lower trace in each record represents resting membrane potential; upper trace is microelectrode recording from motoneuron innervated monosynaptically by dorsal root, stimulated at 6 per sec. Two motoneuron spikes are illustrated in records on the left. Control failure rate was 84 percent. After the drug, motoneuron firing was not observed.

ground activity. These results, in view of the lack of direct effect upon the monosynaptic pathway, indicate that PTZ primarily excites interneurons in the spinal cord. Extracellular recording with metal electrodes from interneurons at various sites showed that PTZ increased both rate of background discharge and frequency of evoked discharges. However, these experiments do not provide any clues concerning the mechanism of the excitant action on interneurons.

Because of its discrete input, the Renshaw cell appeared to be an appropriate interneuron upon which to examine the excitatory effects of PTZ. Twelve cells were followed before and after PTZ by means of extracellular metal electrodes [5]. In this case also the results were disappointingly and unequivocally negative. PTZ did not alter the spontaneous firing rate of Renshaw cells, and it also failed to increase discharge frequency or the number of discharges in the train evoked by either dorsal root or ventral root stimulation.

Experiments described have failed to point clearly to a mechanism by which PTZ increases neuronal excitability. It is tempting again to reiterate the suggestion supported by many experiments [7, 21, 27, 35] that PTZ may produce convulsive activity by shortening the time required for synaptic recovery. An action on this process would selectively enhance ongoing repetitive activity without appreciably affecting systems that discharge only in response to discrete stimulation. This suggestion is in conformity with the lack of effect of PTZ on the properties of the monosynaptic pathway investigated by intracellular techniques. However, it is not supported by negative results obtained on Renshaw cells. Further experiments to test this proposed mechanism clearly are needed.

Recent experiments by Borys [3] on cells in the *Aplysia* abdominal ganglion give promise of contributing clues to the mechanism of action of PTZ. These experiments employed a concentration of PTZ of 4 mM per liter in the bath, a concentration approximately 10 times that existing in the body water of cats after intravenous administration of 40 mg per kg of the drug. Pacemaker cells were consistently depolarized by PTZ; in some cases, this depolarization was as great as 30 mV. Associated with this depolarization was a marked increase in rate of discharge; in some instances the discharge rate was 2 times that observed prior to the drug. Depolarization of irregularly firing cells was less marked than that of pacemaker cells, but this slight depolarization was again associated with a marked decrease in the interval between discharges. In contrast to the cells mentioned, however, the giant cell was not appreciably depolarized by PTZ; in this respect it resembles the cat spinal motoneuron. Membrane depolarization by PTZ apparently depends upon the presence of certain receptors or upon some special characteristics of the membrane; interestingly, PTZ has been shown to depolarize *Amoeba proteus* [17]. The *Aplysia* ganglion provides a system on which to study the actions of PTZ on membrane and synaptic properties, including the electrogenic pump inhibition referred to above. Results of these experiments may provide further leads in investigating actions of this important drug on the mammalian nervous system.

Convulsant Barbiturates

These compounds have no present clinical application and are little used as laboratory tools. They are of especial interest, however, because their actions are antagonized by the closely related depressant barbiturates. It is particularly opportune to study their actions because, as with the pentylenetetrazol-trimethadione antagonism described above, clues to the mechanisms of actions of the convulsant barbiturates may be obtained from knowledge of the actions of their antagonists, the better-known depressant barbiturates.

Velluz and co-workers [59] in 1951 synthesized and studied an interesting convulsant barbiturate, 5-(2-cyclohexylidene-ethyl)-5-ethyl barbituric acid, hereinafter referred to as CHEB. This agent has recently been the object of a variety of studies in our laboratories. CHEB produces flexor-extensor seizures in mice with a median convulsive dose (CD_{50}) of 3.9 mg per kg, intravenously. Pretreatment with pentobarbital (at a third of its minimal neurotoxic dose) antagonizes the convulsant effect of CHEB. In studies on spinal synaptic systems [16], CHEB (0.5 mg per kg) was found to produce a marked increase in the monosynaptic response. Polysynaptic activity was also increased in a few instances, but this was more variable than the enormous increase in monosynaptic spike amplitude. Again, low doses of pentobarbital (2 mg per kg) prevented the increase in monosynaptic response if given before CHEB and restored the augmented spike to control levels if given during the phase of increased excitability after CHEB. These doses of pentobarbital alone did not depress the monosynaptic spike. The non-barbiturate depressants (diphenylhydantoin, trimethadione, and mephenesin) did not antagonize the effects of CHEB on the monosynaptic response.

Blood pressure was continuously recorded in the spinal cord experiments with CHEB, and it was noted that the drug produced a marked increase in blood pressure of short duration. Phenoxybenzamine pretreatment prevented hypertension following low doses of CHEB but was ineffective against hypertension induced by higher doses of CHEB. These observations suggested direct action of CHEB on smooth muscle. Studies with isolated rabbit aortic strips [30] showed that CHEB did indeed produce a marked and long-lasting contraction of the aortic smooth muscle. Interestingly, this effect was antagonized by equivalent amounts of pentobarbital.

Microelectrode experiments being carried out by Downes [15] give additional insights into the mechanism of action of these convulsant drugs. CHEB acts at a variety of sites in the spinal monosynaptic pathway. Synaptic potentials can be markedly increased after the drug. This is probably due to an increase in the amount of transmitter liberated, but the effects of CHEB on transmitter release are difficult to evaluate because of the changing condition of the postsynaptic membrane. CHEB causes a depolarization of the motoneuron membrane, which in some cells has been as much as 50 mV, after administration of 0.5 mg per kg of the drug. Associated with this depolarization is a marked increase in the electrical excitability of the membrane.

One of the most interesting aspects of the action of CHEB is the production of double motoneuron discharges. In studies of the drug on spinal reflex pathways [16], it was noted that the monosynaptic spike elicited from muscle afferents was often followed at an interval of 3–4 msec by another spike of almost identical configuration. Figure 7-3 shows double discharges of the motoneuron activated antidromically after administration of CHEB; it can be seen in this figure that responses taken early after the drug show lack of complete invasion of the motoneuron. This lack of invasion is associated with a marked depolarization of the motoneuron. By the fourth minute after CHEB, the soma is invaded and double discharges are produced by a single antidromic volley. However, the spikes are smaller than those elicited prior to the drug because of continued slight depolarization.

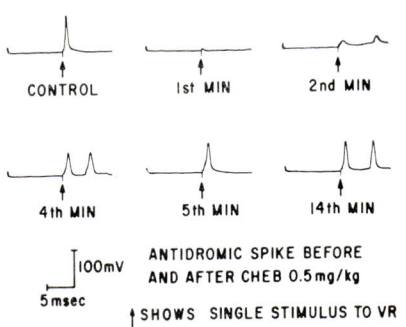

Fig. 7-3. Effect of CHEB on motoneuron response to antidromic stimulation. Successive traces show control response and responses recorded at indicated times after administration of CHEB (0.5 mg per kg). Single stimulus to ventral root is indicated by arrow in each record. Upward deflection at beginning of each trace is an artifact produced by synchronizing signal.

Because convulsant barbiturates are structurally so similar to their depressant relatives and because the depressant barbiturates so antagonize actions of the convulsants, it is tempting to speculate that the two types of drugs act by opposite mechanisms on a common substrate. It is appropriate in this regard to note that in moderate doses the depressant barbiturates are highly selective in depressing transmitter release in the spinal monosynaptic pathway. Weakly [60], who employed the technique developed by Kuno [32], has shown that pentobarbital and thiopental in doses up to 15 mg per kg reduce the number of quanta of transmitter released by impulses in single afferent fibers without affecting the EPSP produced by one quantum of transmitter. In somewhat larger doses, as previous workers have shown, the barbiturates cause a depression of the postsynaptic membrane. The actions of CHEB on transmitter release have not yet been directly investigated. The fact that CHEB acts at a number of sites would appear to argue against a pharmacological antagonism between this drug and the depressant barbiturates. However, this hypothesis may not be discarded until dose-effect relations of CHEB on the spinal monosynaptic pathway have been fully explored, because generalized actions noted with the dose of 0.5 mg per kg may have obscured a more selective action on transmitter release observable with lower doses.

Another convulsant barbiturate of interest is 5-(1,3-dimethylbutyl)-5-ethyl barbituric acid, or DMBB, whose actions were first studied by Swanson [52] and by Swanson and Chen [53]. Effects of this agent on the nervous system have been investigated by various workers [13, 14, 31]. Domino and co-workers [13, 14] noted that while small doses of the agent appeared to be purely excitant, larger doses revealed a depressant facet of the drug. These studies were made with the racemic mixture of the two optical isomers of DMBB. Recently Perry and Downes [43] resolved the two optical isomers of this agent and studied them separately. The + isomer of DMBB is a convulsant agent much like CHEB; it produces tonic flexor-extensor seizures in mice with a CD_{50} of 3.1 mg per kg, intravenously; it also constricts rabbit aortic strips [30]. The − isomer of DMBB, on the other hand, is an anesthetic with a median lethal dose (LD_{50}) of 70 mg per kg in mice and appears to closely resemble pentobarbital. The − isomer does not constrict aortic strips; like pentobarbital, it prevents action of the + isomer on aortic strips and antagonizes the convulsant effects of the + isomer in mice.

These experiments, which have borne fruit in their early stages, point to a common link at the molecular level between drug excitation and drug depression of neuronal activity. Extension of these experiments will doubtless contribute greatly to our understanding of states of excitation in the nervous system and of means by which these can be manipulated pharmacologically.

Summary

The purpose of this brief presentation has been to consider in neurophysiological terms the potential mechanisms by which drugs may produce convulsive activity in the mammalian central nervous system. On this basis, definitive information relating to site and mechanism of action of a few prototype convulsants has been considered. Evaluation of the data concerning mechanisms of action has at the same time indicated some information needed in order to understand actions of the drugs considered. With the exception of agents that act by blocking postsynaptic inhibition, the mechanisms of actions of convulsants are largely unknown. Knowledge of the mode of action of the prototype convulsants of several classes would enormously enhance their usefulness as tools in neuropharmacological investigations.

Much valuable information would also be provided concerning balance between excitatory and inhibitory processes in the central nervous system and basic causes of alterations in this balance in disease states, such as epilepsy. This information would be additionally valuable in the rational search for drugs and procedures to alleviate such states.

REFERENCES

1. Alving, Barbara, O. The action of strychnine at cholinergic junctions. Arch. Int. Pharmacodyn. 131:123, 1961.
2. Araki, T. The Effects of Strychnine on the Postsynaptic Inhibitory Action. Proceedings of the International Union of Physiological Sciences, vol. 4, XXIII International Congress. Amsterdam: Excerpta Medica Foundation, Mouton & Co., 1965.
3. Borys, H. K. Unpublished data, 1969.
4. Borys, H. K., and Esplin, D. W. Unpublished data, 1969.
5. Borys, H. K., and Esplin, D. W. Pentylenetetrazol and Renshaw-cell activity. Int. J. Neuropharmacol. 1969, in press.
6. Boyd, E. M., and Fulford, R. A. Pilocarpine-induced convulsions and delayed psychotic-like reaction. Canad. J. Biochem. 39:1287, 1961.
7. Boyd, E. S., Meritt, D. A., and Gardner, L. C. The effect of convulsant drugs on the transmission through the cuneate nucleus. J. Pharmacol. Exp. Ther. 154:398, 1966.
8. Bradley, K., Easton, D. M., and Eccles, J. C. An investigation of primary or direct inhibition. J. Physiol. (London) 122:474, 1953.
9. Curtis, D. R. The depression of spinal inhibition by electrophoretically administered strychnine. Int. J. Neuropharmacol. 1:239, 1962.
10. Curtis, D. R. The pharmacology of central and peripheral inhibition. Pharmacol. Rev. 15:333, 1963.
11. Curtis, D. R. Synaptic Transmission in the Central Nervous System and its Pharmacology. In Rodahl, K., and Issekutz, B. (Eds.), Nerve as a Tissue. New York: Harper, 1966.
12. De Boer, J. The death of Socrates: A historical and experimental study on the actions of coniine and Conium maculatum. Arch. Int. Pharmacodyn. 83:473, 1950.
13. Domino, E. F. Pharmacological actions of a convulsant barbiturate. II. Effects compared with pentobarbital on cerebral cortex and some brain stem systems of the cat. J. Pharmacol. Exp. Ther. 119:272, 1957.
14. Domino, E. F., Fox, Kaye E., and Brody, T. M. Pharmacological actions of a convulsant barbiturate sodium-5-ethyl-5-(1,3-dimethylbutyl) barbiturate. I. Stimulant and depressant effects. J. Pharmacol. Exp. Ther. 114:173, 1955.
15. Downes, H. Unpublished data, 1969.
16. Downes, H., and Williams, J. K. Effects of a convulsant barbiturate on the spinal monosynaptic pathway. J. Pharmacol. Exp. Ther. 1969, in press.
17. Duff, W. M., and McCashland, B. W. Effect of metrazol upon membrane potential and rate of locomotion in Amoeba proteus. Proc. Soc. Exp. Biol. Med. 115:444, 1964.
18. Eccles, J. C. The Physiology of Nerve Cells. Baltimore: Johns Hopkins Press, 1957.
19. Eccles, J. C. The Physiology of Synapses. New York: Academic, 1964.
20. Eccles, J. C., Schmidt, R., and Willis, W. D. Pharmacological studies on presynaptic inhibition. J. Physiol. (London) 168:500, 1963.
21. Esplin, D. W., and Curto, E. M. Effects

of trimethadione on synaptic transmission in the spinal cord; antagonism of trimethadione and pentylenetetrazol. *J. Pharmacol. Exp. Ther.* 121:267, 1957.

22. Esplin, D. W., and Freston, J. W. Physiological and pharmacological analysis of spinal cord convulsions. *J. Pharmacol. Exp. Ther.* 130:68, 1960.

23. Esplin, D. W., and Laffan, R. J. Determinants of flexor and extensor components of maximal seizures in cats. *Arch. Int. Pharmacodyn.* 113:189, 1957.

24. Esplin, D. W., and Woodbury, D. M. Spinal reflexes and seizure patterns in the two-toed sloth. *Science* 133:1426, 1961.

25. Esplin, D. W., and Zablocka, Barbara. Pilocarpine blockade of spinal inhibition in cats. *J. Pharmacol. Exp. Ther.* 143:174, 1964.

26. Esplin, D. W., and Zablocka, Barbara. Central Nervous System Stimulants. In Goodman, L. S., and Gilman, A. (Eds.), *The Pharmacological Basis of Therapeutics* (3d ed.). New York: MacMillan, 1965.

27. Eyzaguirre, C., and Lilienthal, J. L., Jr. Veratrinic effects of pentamethylenetetrazol (metrazol) and 2,2-bis (*p*-chlorophenyl) 1,1,1 trichloroethane (DDT) on mammalian neuromuscular function. *Proc. Soc. Exp. Biol. Med.* 70:272, 1949.

28. Ferguson, R. K., Zablocka, Barbara, Esplin, D. W., and Williams, J. K. Peripheral cholinergic blockade by drugs that block postsynaptic central inhibition. *Arch. Int. Pharmacodyn.* 1969, in press.

29. Hahn, F. Analeptics. *Pharmacol. Rev.* 12:447, 1960.

30. Hupka, A. L., and Downes, H. Unpublished data, 1969.

31. Knoefel, P. K. Stimulation and depression of the central nervous system by derivatives of barbituric and thiobarbituric acids. *J. Pharmacol. Exp. Ther.* 84:26, 1945.

32. Kuno, M. Quantal components of excitatory synaptic potentials in spinal motoneurones. *J. Physiol.* (London) 175:81, 1964.

33. La Grutta, V., and Desmedt, J. E. Contrastes entre les actions centrales de la coniine et de la strychnine. *Arch. Int. Pharmacodyn.* 151:289, 1964.

34. Lanari, A., and Luco, J. V. Depressant action of strychnine on superior cervical sympathetic ganglion and on muscle. *Amer. J. Physiol.* 126:277, 1939.

35. Lewin, J., and Esplin, D. W. Analysis of the spinal excitatory action of pentylenetetrazol. *J. Pharmacol. Exp. Ther.* 132:245, 1961.

36. Llinas, R. Mechanisms of supraspinal actions upon spinal cord activities. Pharmacological studies on reticular inhibition of alpha extensor motoneurons. *J. Neurophysiol.* 27:1127, 1964.

37. Longo, V. G., and Chiavarelli, S. Neuropharmacological Analysis of Strychnine-like Drugs. In Paton, W. D. M., and Lindgren, P. (Eds.), *First International Pharmacological Meeting.*, vol. 8. New York: MacMillan, 1962.

38. Longo, V. G., and Pinto Corrado, A. A neuropharmacological investigation of the convulsant action of 4-phenyl-4-formyl-N-methyl piperidine. *Proc. Soc. Exp. Biol. Med.* 107:272, 1961.

39. McKinstry, Doris N., and Koelle, G. B. Effects of drugs on acetylcholine release from the cat superior cervical ganglion by carbachol and by preganglionic stimulation. *J. Pharmacol. Exp. Ther.* 157:328, 1967.

40. Miyahara, J. T., Esplin, D. W., and Zablocka, Barbara. Differential effects of depressant drugs on presynaptic inhibition. *J. Pharmacol. Exp. Ther.* 154:119, 1966.

41. Nickerson, M. Drugs Inhibiting Adrenergic Nerves and Structures Innervated by Them. In Goodman, L. S., and Gilman, A. (Eds.), *The Pharmacological Basis of Therapeutics* (3d ed.). New York: Macmillan, 1965.

42. Nishi, S., and Koketsu, K. Analysis of slow inhibitory postsynaptic potential of bullfrog sympathetic ganglion. *J. Neurophysiol.* 31:717, 1968.

43. Perry, R., and Downes, H. Unpublished data, 1969.

44. Pinto Corrada, A., and Longo, V. G. An electrophysiological analysis of the convulsant action of morphine, codeine, and thebaine. *Arch. Int. Pharmacodyn.* 132:255, 1961.

45. Pollen, D. A., and Ajmone-Marsan, C. Cortical inhibitory postsynaptic potentials and strychninization. *J. Neurophysiol.* 28:342, 1965.

46. Pollen, D. A., and Lux, H. D. Conductance changes during inhibitory postsynaptic potentials in normal and strychninized

cortical neurons. *J. Neurophysiol.* 29:369, 1966.

47. Sampson, S. R. Mechanism of coniine-blockade of postsynaptic inhibition in the spinal cord of the cat. *Int. J. Neuropharmacol.* 5:171, 1966.

48. Sampson, S. R., Esplin, D. W., and Zablocka, Barbara. Effects of coniine on peripheral and central synaptic transmission. *J. Pharmacol. Exp. Ther.* 152:313, 1966.

49. Schmidt, R. F. The Pharmacology of Presynaptic Inhibition. In Eccles, J. C., and Schadé, J. P. (Eds.), *Physiology of Spinal Neurons*, Progress in Brain Research, vol. 12. Amsterdam: Elsevier, 1964.

50. Skou, J. C. Enzymatic basis for active transport of Na+ and K+ across cell membrane. *Physiol. Rev.* 45:596, 1965.

51. Stefanis, C., and Jasper, H. Strychnine reversal of inhibitory potentials in pyramidal tract neurones. *Int. J. Neuropharmacol.* 4:125, 1965.

52. Swanson, E. E. Short acting barbituric acid derivatives. *Proc. Soc. Exp. Biol. Med.* 31:963, 1934.

53. Swanson, E. E., and Chen, K. K. The aberrant action of sodium I: 3-dimethylbutylethyl-barbiturate. *Quart. J. Pharm. Pharmacol.* 12:657, 1939.

54. Tang, A. H., and Yim, G. K. W. The effects of arecoline on spinal reflexes of the cat. *Int. J. Neuropharmacol.* 4:309, 1965.

55. Toman, J. E. P. Drugs Effective in Convulsive Disorders. In Goodman, L. S., and Gilman, A. (Eds.), *The Pharmacological Basis of Therapeutics* (3d ed.). New York: MacMillan, 1965.

56. Toman, J. E. P., and Goodman, L. S. Anticonvulsants. *Physiol. Rev.* 28:409, 1948.

57. Toman, J. E. P., Swinyard, E. A., and Goodman, L. S. Properties of maximal seizures, and their alteration by anticonvulsant drugs and other agents. *J. Neurophysiol.* 9:231, 1946.

58. Turkanis, S. A., and Esplin, D. W. Evidence for the release and depletion of the postsynaptic inhibitory transmitter by pilocarpine. *Arch. Int. Pharmacodyn.* 173:195, 1968.

59. Velluz, L., Jequier, R., Teodoru, C., Plotka, C., and Mathieu, J. Analeptiques respiratoires en série barbiturique IV—Activité particulière de l'acide 5-(γ,γ-cyclopentaméthylène-allyl) 5-ethyl barbiturique. *Ann. Pharm. Franc.* 9:292, 1951.

60. Weakly, J. N. Site of action of barbiturates on spinal monosynaptic transmission in the cat. Unpublished data, 1969.

61. Williams, J. K., Zablocka, Barbara, Esplin, D. W., and Turkanis, S. A. Blockade of central inhibition by C-alkylpiperidines. *Pharmacologist* 6:192, 1964.

62. Woodbury, D. M., and Esplin, D. W. Neuropharmacology and neurochemistry of anticonvulsant drugs. *Res. Publ. Ass. Res. Nerv. Ment. Dis.* 37:24, 1959.

63. Zablocka, Barbara. Effects of autonomic agents, alone and in combination with antiepileptic drugs, on electroshock seizures in rats. *Arch. Int. Pharmacodyn.* 142:533, 1963.

64. Zablocka, Barbara, and Esplin, D. W. Central excitatory and depressant effects of pilocarpine in rats and mice. *J. Pharmacol. Exp. Ther.* 140:162, 1963.

65. Zablocka, Barbara, and Esplin, D. W. Central excitatory and neuromuscular paralyzant effects of pilocarpine in cats. *Arch. Int. Pharmacodyn.* 147:490, 1964.

66. Zablocka, Barbara, and Esplin, D. W. Analysis of the effects of arecoline on the central nervous system. *Pharmacologist* 6:192, 1964.

67. Zablocka-Esplin, Barbara, and Esplin, D. W. Unpublished data, 1969.

Discussion

ACTION OF CONVULSANTS: NEUROCHEMICAL ASPECTS*
WILLIAM E. STONE

Convulsants undoubtedly act by mechanisms that bring about changes in characteristics of neuronal membranes with consequent depolarization, Esplin having discussed several of the possible mechanisms. A depolarizing drug might have direct action on membranes of presynaptic elements, it might mimic or potentiate the action of an excitatory transmitter on postsynaptic membranes, or it might act on other parts of the membranes of cell bodies or dendrites. A convulsant of another type might interfere with action of an inhibitory transmitter, either presynaptic or postsynaptic. Some convulsants might act indirectly by altering enzymic activities, thus affecting the rate of removal of a transmitter or metabolic processes concerned with maintenance of membrane polarization or permeability. (These processes include the electrogenic pumps.)

Once a seizure is induced, many chemical changes would be expected to occur in the brain as concomitants of the convulsive discharge. These would be comparable to changes occurring in muscle during contraction, such as hydrolysis of high-energy phosphates releasing energy. Such changes are of interest, but when observed in muscle they reveal nothing about the processes by which the contraction was initiated at the neuromuscular junctions. Thus an observed neurochemical alteration associated with convulsive activity must be interpreted with great caution, particularly if it is not shown to begin before appearance of the electrographic seizure pattern. As a further complication, a convulsant may have metabolic side effects that bear no relation to the excitatory response.

Accordingly, an interpretation of some observations on neurochemical changes induced by convulsant drugs is offered as a supplement to Esplin's presentation; comments on electrophysiological aspects will be limited. As Esplin has suggested, one possible excitatory mechanism is that drugs blocking at known "nicotinic" receptor sites may, by a similar action, block the release of a central inhibitory transmitter. This might explain the fact that such agents, when applied topically to the cerebral cortex, have excitatory actions. The spikes induced by application of strychnine are well known, but some of the common curarizing agents (d-tubocurarine and dihydro-beta-erythroidine, for example) initiate very similar spikes, and gallamine triethiodide induces a fast-frequency spiking activity [1].

Studies in our laboratory over a period of years have been concerned with neurochemical effects of a variety of convulsants. Unfortunately, little can be said about strychnine and other agents thought to block postsynaptic inhibition, since there are so few neurochemical data available relevant to these drugs.

Most of our experiments were done on dogs. The general procedure was to freeze the brain in situ at a time chosen in relation to events recorded electrographically and to analyze specimens from the cerebrum. Morphine was used for analgesia, since it does not antagonize convulsants. Arterial blood pressure was monitored, and adequate oxygenation was ensured by use of a respiration pump when necessary. A few observations on mice will be included; in such experiments motor seizures induced

---

* Supported in part by PHS Research Grants NB00818 and NB3360 from the National Institute of Neurological Diseases and Stroke.

by convulsants were observed, but recordings or artificial respiration were not attempted. The whole animal was frozen in liquid nitrogen, and the specimen for analysis included the cerebrum and the brain stem.

NEUROCHEMICAL CORRELATES OF THE CONVULSIVE DISCHARGE

Energetics. Certain chemical changes related to the energetics of the seizure have been known for many years. These include increases in oxidative metabolism and in brain lactic acid and a hydrolytic cleavage of creatine phosphate. Several different convulsants have been shown to increase the oxygen consumption, and this change is often assumed to occur in every type of seizure [38]. Increase in lactate has been found in seizures induced by many different convulsants; apparently it can be observed whenever the intensity and duration of the seizure are sufficient, except in the case of hypoglycemic convulsions. In hypoglycemia the reduced availability of glucose lowers the lactate level prior to occurrence of seizures, and the level remains below normal when seizure occurs.

Apparently the breakdown of creatine phosphate is observable in all seizures of sufficient intensity and duration. Adenosine triphosphate also shows a tendency toward dephosphorylation, with formation of diphosphate and small amounts of monophosphate, but with older methods these changes were clearly discernible only when the convulsive discharge was massive and creatine phosphate had been considerably depleted. Saktor et al. [26] recently demonstrated these effects in mice convulsed with hexafluorodiethyl ether (Indokolon). They also observed an initial increase in fructose 1,6-diphosphate and a decrease in its precursor, hexose 6-monophosphate, suggesting increased activity of the enzyme phosphofructokinase.

The brain contains relatively little glycogen, but the amount present tends to decrease during seizures. Significant changes have been observed in mice given pentylenetetrazol, picrotoxin, or hexadifluoroethyl ether [4, 26], and in cats given any one of several convulsants [17]. A decrease in brain glucose also has been observed [17, 26], but like the change in glycogen, it is sometimes too small to be apparent. Geiger and his associates [10, 13] held that in pentylenetetrazol seizures the cerebral uptake of glucose from the blood does not increase and that extra oxidative metabolism is supported largely by substrates other than glucose. Presumably these substrates are endogenous.

Ammonia and Amino Acids. Another change occurring in seizures is a small increase in the cerebral ammonia content. This was observed by Richter and Dawson [23] in rats convulsed by picrotoxin or electroshock. In our studies this change was not statistically significant in dogs given picrotoxin [28], but was clearly evident in seizures induced by pentylenetetrazol [29], bemegride [37], thiosemicarbazide [24], and cyclotrimethylenetrinitramine (RDX). This ammonia formation appears to be a consequence of excitation. However, in poisoning by fluoro-fatty acids and other conditions to be discussed later, ammonia production is much greater and precedes the occurrence of seizures; in these conditions ammonia could possibly play a role in the initiation of seizures.

Precursors of the ammonia formed in vivo have not been identified. Glutamic acid is a possible source or intermediate; amide groups of free and protein-bound glutamine also have been suggested. Since normal levels of glutamate and glutamine are high, a decrease equivalent to increase in ammonia would not be statistically significant.

It was found that alanine was increased in seizures induced by pentylenetetrazol, bemegride, thiosemicarbazide, fluoro-fatty acids, and ammonium chloride [24, 29, 32, 37]. This change was too small to be significant with picrotoxin and RDX. In general, alanine tends to vary in the same manner as lactate, increasing in anoxia and decreasing in hypoglycemia. This is not surprising since pyruvate is a precursor of alanine as well as of lactate and occupies a key position in metabolic processes.

The level of aspartic acid tends to decrease during convulsive activity. This change was evident in brief but intensive seizures induced by picrotoxin [29], fluoro-fatty acids [32], ammonium chloride [29], or RDX, and in status epilepticus induced by pentylenetetrazol [37]. The decrease was not statistically significant in shorter periods of status with bemegride as the stimulant, and no change was apparent in pentylenetetrazol [29] or thiosemicarbazide [24] seizures of brief duration. The cerebral glutamic-acid content showed similar but less consistent changes, being decreased in pentylenetetrazol seizures (whether brief or extended) and in fluoro-fatty acid seizures, but not in brief seizures induced by picrotoxin, thiosemicarbazide, ammonium chloride, or RDX. The level increased significantly in extended bemegride seizures.

For each amino acid the observed level may represent an average of two or more pools as well as a complex balance between formation and removal. Tracer studies have shown a rapid metabolic turnover of aspartate, glutamate, and related substances. As precursors of oxaloacetate and α-oxoglutarate, respectively, aspartate and glutamate may feed into the Krebs cycle when the metabolic rate increases during seizures. It is possible that thiosemicarbazide retards these reactions by inactivating pyridoxal phosphate.

Exchanges between amino acid pools and proteins represent another mechanism for alteration of the amino acid levels. Geiger et al. [12] found that the rate of protein turnover is increased by stimulation with pentylenetetrazol, and Chitre et al. [6] observed changes in ribonucleic acid content and turnover.

Also to be considered are possible exchanges between intracellular and extracellular compartments. According to current concepts, aspartate or glutamate might act as an excitatory transmitter, being released and removed in increased quantities during convulsive activity.

Study of pentylenetetrazol-induced status epilepticus [37] revealed changes in other amino acids, observable when intermittent convulsive activity was maintained for 40 minutes. The following essential amino acids were increased: arginine, histidine, leucine, lysine, phenylalanine, and valine. Threonine showed a tendency to increase, but the change was not significant. Four other amino acids increased: γ-aminobutyric (GABA), glycine, serine, and tyrosine. These changes may result from the breakdown phase of the increased protein turnover. In status epilepticus of shorter duration induced by bemegride, only two of these changes were significant: increases in lysine and GABA. Status epilepticus has not been studied with other convulsants.

Lipids. We examined also some cerebral lipid fractions in status epilepticus. With both pentylenetetrazol and with bemegride, decreases were found in the ganglioside fraction and in a fraction consisting of lecithin and sphingomyelin. Gangliosides are thought to play some role in excitatory mechanisms or in maintenance of membrane excitability, and phospholipids may be used in oxidative processes. Torda [34] noted a decrease in brain phospholipid content in mice convulsed with pentylenetetrazol or electroshock.

Acetylcholine. It is well known that the acetylcholine (ACh) content of brain decreases during convulsive activity induced by various means: electroshock, pentylenetetrazol, picrotoxin, fluoro-fatty acids, ammonium carbonate, and perhaps other convulsants. The decrease is attributed to increased release and hydrolysis of ACh at cholinergic synapses during the period of excitation; this view is supported by measurements of ACh diffusing into fluid perfusing the cortical surface [5]. Thus the change in ACh is taken to signify increased transmission, a part of the convulsive response rather than a triggering mechanism. However, there is one important exception to be noted: when an anticholinesterase is injected, provided it can pass the blood-brain barrier, the ACh content increases, and a convulsive response may ensue. This type of seizure is discussed in the next section.

DRUG-INDUCED CONDITIONS
PREDISPOSING TO SEIZURES

When response to a convulsant is preceded by a long enough induction period, it is possible to study neurochemical changes that begin prior to the seizure and may have causal importance. This has been done with certain drugs.

Tetraethyl pyrophosphate (TEPP). A potent anticholinesterase, TEPP was one of the agents chosen [27]. In order to study the central effects of this drug it is necessary to block the peripheral muscarinic effects with a small dose of atropine and to provide artificial respiration. After TEPP is injected, the cerebral ACh increases, presumably because it is being synthesized and released as in normal activity but is not being destroyed. The initial electrographic effect is an intense arousal reaction, a sudden increase in frequency followed by increasing amplitude for a few minutes and then gradually decreasing amplitude. In some dogs the high frequency pattern continues indefinitely, but usually epileptiform convulsive activity supervenes. Both the arousal pattern and the convulsive phenomena can be quickly suppressed by a massive intravenous dose of atropine or hyoscine, the latter being preferred because it has no hypotensive effect.

This suppression serves to distinguish cholinergic seizures from other types, which are not suppressed by these agents. (Convulsants not blocked include pentylenetetrazol, picrotoxin, bemegride, fluoro-fatty acids, thiosemicarbazide, RDX, and hexafluorodiethyl ether.) When TEPP is given and its effects are blocked by hyoscine, subsequent injection of pentylenetetrazol in a dose just above the normal convulsive threshold induces a seizure. Thus the cholinergic pathways appear to be unnecessary for the pentylenetetrazol response.

In this connection it is of interest that the enhancing effect of injected TEPP on auditory evoked potentials (in dogs under pentobarbital) is suppressed by hyoscine, while the enhancing effects of pentylenetetrazol and of hexafluorodiethyl ether are not suppressed [1]. Evoked potentials are not altered by hyoscine in the absence of TEPP.

It seems clear that the TEPP seizure is induced by the action of accumulated ACh on postsynaptic membranes of cholinoreceptive neurons. At present, the cholinergic type of seizure is the only one that can be confidently explained in terms of a neurochemical mechanism.

Convulsant Hydrazides. Another type of seizure is induced by convulsant hydrazides, and these compounds react with and inactivate pyridoxal phosphate, a coenzyme involved in several metabolic reactions. Formation of GABA by decarboxylation of glutamic acid requires pyridoxal phosphate, as does also the further metabolism of GABA by a transamination. GABA, well known as a brain constituent with inhibitory properties, is often regarded as a modulator of excitability since the excitability tends to vary inversely with the GABA level. However, there is recent evidence favoring the earlier view that GABA may act as an inhibitory transmitter [18].

In dietary pyridoxine deficiency, GABA in brain decreases and seizures sometimes occur. Several of the convulsant hydrazides also reduce the level of GABA, presumably by inhibiting its production while not affecting its degradation. Convulsant action of hydrazides was once attributed to decrease in GABA, but it soon developed that seizures can occur in the absence of this change.

Several compounds that react with pyridoxal phosphate tend to block removal of GABA more than its synthesis, thus increasing the GABA level. (The two enzyme systems differ in that the coenzyme is bound tightly to the apoenzyme of the transaminase, but only loosely to that of the decarboxylase [25].) Hydrazine, hydroxylamine, and amino-oxyacetic acid are among agents that raise the GABA level. Effects of these drugs are complex, depending upon dosage and probably other factors; either inhibitory or excitatory actions may predominate.

Experiments with thiosemicarbazide and amino-oxyacetic acid [24] serve to illustrate some of the effects and interactions of such compounds. Thiosemicarbazide at 20 mg per kg intravenously induces seizures in the dog; electroencephalogram (EEG) abnormalities begin to appear about 30 minutes after injection, and epileptiform seizures at about 1 hour. The brain GABA decreases and this change is observable before the seizures begin. Amino-oxyacetic acid at the same dosage has essentially opposite effects; it raises the GABA level, depresses the EEG, and in dogs given no other drugs it induces a state of profound depression and flaccidity, almost a paralysis, lasting several hours. (This condition differs from anesthesia since the animal can be momentarily aroused.) When a 20 mg per kg dose of amino-oxyacetic acid is followed immediately or within 90 minutes by the same dose of thiosemicarbazide, the brain GABA is maintained above the normal level and the convulsant action of thiosemicarbazide is suppressed. However, if the dose of thiosemicarbazide is raised to 60 mg per kg, seizures occur despite a high level of brain GABA.

Thus, decreased GABA is not the only factor concerned in initiating thiosemicarbazide seizures. Amino-oxyacetic acid shows a limited capacity to inhibit the seizures, possibly by raising the GABA level. But a larger dose of amino-oxyacetic acid alone sometimes induces convulsive activity. Seizures were observed in only two such experiments, and in one of them the excitation did not invade the cerebral cortex, but other workers also have noted convulsant effects.

Additional biochemical effects of amino-oxyacetic acid include a rise in blood ammonia with accompanying increases in brain ammonia and glutamine. A decrease in brain aspartate and small increases in lactate and alanine also occur; these may be secondary to the high ammonia. In the dog having a cortical seizure, the ammonia level was elevated to about the same extent as in others showing depression, but increase in GABA was smaller than usual.

It is possible that the convulsive effects of hydrazides and of amino-oxyacetic acid are due to the same unknown stimulating mechanism, with a decrease in GABA potentiating excitation by hydrazides and an increase opposing excitation by amino-oxyacetic acid. Several workers have suggested that the unknown mechanism may be the reduction in the rate of metabolism through the GABA pathway. However, the high level of brain ammonia developing after injection of amino-oxyacetic acid may also play an important role in mediating the actions of this drug. Serious consideration of this possibility is warranted since high brain ammonia occurs in certain other conditions, to be described next, that lead to seizures or depression.

Ammonium Chloride. Several workers have noted that seizures can be induced by injection of ammonium salts. When a dog is given ammonium chloride slowly, by infusion of a buffered solution, the result may be either a seizure or the development of an EEG pattern of depression when a high level of cerebral ammonia is attained [2, 29]. The convulsive response appears to be favored by a rapid rate of infusion; in either seizures or depression, the high ammonia is accompanied by a gradually increasing concentration of glutamine. The glutamic acid tends to decrease only slightly; the GABA level remains unaffected. Presumably γ-oxoglutarate is being diverted from the Krebs cycle to go via glutamate to glutamine. Other changes include increases in alanine, lactate, and histidine, a marked decrease in aspartate, and a slight decrease in valine. McKhann and Tower [20] found that ammonium ions increase anaerobic glycolysis in cat cortex slices in vitro.

Fluoro-Fatty Acids. Fluoroacetic and fluorobutyric acids (and their methyl esters) are potent convulsants. They enter the Krebs cycle and lead to a partial block in the metabolic pathway at the stage of citrate oxidation. Dogs given 1 mg per kg of methylfluoroacetate intravenously develop extremely violent seizures after about an hour [2, 22]. Both citrate and ammonia accumulate in the brain during the preconvulsive period; the increases are nearly equimolar, with the ammonia slightly in the lead. Initial seizure begins when these changes are well advanced, and little further increase occurs thereafter in either constituent; increases in the blood levels are negligible. Changes in brain lactate and creatine phosphate do not precede appearance of the first seizure, which suggests that the excitation is not to be ascribed to failure of oxidative metabolism (although such failure becomes evident in the depressed state that follows an extended series of convulsions).

Goldberg et al. [14] examined the effects of fluoroacetate on Krebs cycle and other intermediates in mouse brain. In an early stage of poisoning, when initial signs of excitation are appearing, the citrate is increased, but subsequent metabolites in the pathway (isocitrate, α-oxoglutarate, succinate, fumarate, malate, and oxaloacetate) are normal or above. Thus, the actual flux in the pathway seems to be maintained at about the normal level. At a later stage (marked by a degree of depression with intermittent seizures) the succinate, fumarate, and malate are below normal, suggesting a decrease in the flux. Glucose 6-phosphate is increased at this time. Pyruvate is decreased even in the earlier stage, indicating a possible inhibitory effect in the pathway to pyruvate.

There is evidence that the fluoro-fatty acids also have an inhibitory action on the synthesis of glutamine from ammonia and glutamate, both in vivo [32] and in vitro [19]. This may account partly for increase in the ammonia level [19], but it seems probable that increased formation also occurs [32].

Although citrate might be expected to induce excitatory effects by sequestering calcium ions, there is considerable evidence that the high citrate is not an important factor in the initiation of seizures. By varying the doses of fluoro compounds, Kandel and Chenoweth [16] found that excitation is not correlated with the citrate level and sometimes occurs when citrate is not measurably increased. Other evidence has been cited by Peters [21].

Whether accumulated ammonia plays a significant role in the development of either excitation or depression in fluoro-fatty acid toxicity remains uncertain. It should be noted that when even higher levels of ammonia are attained by infusion of ammonium chloride, convulsive responses are less frequent and less severe. However, with fluoro-fatty acids the source of the ammonia must be intracellular.

Hypoglycemia. Insulin shock is a condition that in some way predisposes to convulsive phenomena, although full-blown seizures can be elicited less regularly in some species than in others. In dogs prepared under morphine the convulsions are infrequent. The hypoglycemic phase is characterized by gradual EEG depression, the appearance of slow waves and occasional spikes, and finally almost complete cessation of cortical activity. Frequently in the recovery phase (after glucose injection), localized epileptiform or other bizarre patterns appear, usually unaccompanied by visible motor activity. A series described in 1965 [30] witnessed only one generalized convulsion during profound hypoglycemia and none during recovery. More recently seizures have been observed during hypoglycemia in three animals and during the recovery stage in two. These were clonic or tonic-clonic motor seizures with corresponding epileptiform cortical activity. In another hypoglycemic dog, convulsive EEG patterns (perhaps localized) and motor activity were partially dissociated, each being present at times in the absence of the other.

Convulsive activity is believed to originate in limbic structures such as the hippocampus and the amygdala, spreading to other deep structures and sometimes invading the neocortex [3, 33, 35]. Evidently a motor seizure can occur when many parts of the cortex are not involved; conversely, there can be widespread cortical convulsive potentials in the absence of motor activity.

This type of seizure is thought to occur either shortly before the cortex becomes isoelectric or during the recovery stage. This suggests that the precipitating factor may be a decrease in membrane potentials resulting from inadequate but functioning oxidative processes. If it can be assumed that all parts of the brain are subject to changes similar to those in the cortex, analyses of brain frozen in situ might supply additional clues to predisposing factors.

Some chemical changes observed in hypoglycemia [30] appear related rather directly to lack of sufficient glucose as an oxidative substrate. These include decreases in lactate and glycogen and a gradual breakdown of creatine phosphate and nucleotide triphosphate. Decreases in glutamate, glutamine, GABA, alanine, and leucine suggest that these are used as oxidative substrates in this emergency, especially since the ammonia level shows great increase and cerebral arteriovenous differences indicate removal of ammonia by the blood. Whether protein breaks down to provide further substrates is uncertain. Significant increases were found in only two of the free amino acids, aspartic and lysine, but more recent experiments with glucose-^{14}C (unpublished) indicated that during the recovery stage protein synthesis is increased. In the same study the gangliosides and two phospholipid fractions (cephalin and lecithin + sphingomyelin) showed significant decreases in profound hypoglycemia. Geiger [11] has reviewed evidence that the perfused brain of the cat can utilize endogenous substrates for maintenance of function in the absence of glucose.

Within an hour after the hypoglycemia is terminated, some of the altered constituents show partial or complete restitution; these include creatine phosphate, ammonia, and glutamate. Nucleotides are rephosphorylated, but some loss of total nucleotide is evident. Lactate, citrate, GABA, and alanine increase from subnormal to above normal levels, and aspartate drops below normal. Glycine, arginine, and histidine increase during recovery, although they are not altered in hypoglycemia. Glycogen, glutamine, and lysine do not recover rapidly.

Goldberg et al. [14] found that glucose 6-phosphate and pyruvate are decreased in the brain during hypoglycemia. Of seven Krebs cycle intermediates, six are decreased and only oxaloacetate remains at its normal level. The decreased ratio of α-oxoglutarate to oxaloacetate and the concomitantly increased ratio of aspartate to glutamate suggest a shift in equilibrium of transamination involving these metabolites.

The ACh content of the brain tends to decrease during hypoglycemia and to rise above normal during recovery [7, 30]. Since the level of one of its precursors, acetyl coenzyme A, is probably reduced in hypoglycemia, the rate of synthesis of ACh may be reduced. Possibly the decrease in adenosine triphosphate is sufficient to be a contributing factor.

Of the observed changes in levels of cerebral constituents, only two at present can be regarded as excitatory. One of these is the decrease in GABA; however, the decrease is rather small in the hypoglycemic phase, at least in the dog. The level rises quickly during recovery, actually goes above normal before the stage of recovery in which seizures have been recorded. Thus the GABA level does not seem to be a major factor.

The other change to be considered is the increase in ammonia, which is similar in magnitude to that seen in fluoroacetate poisoning. Here also, findings in the recovery stage are instructive, being at variance with the hypothesis that ammonia is a major excitatory factor. Ammonia level decreases to normal within 15 minutes after injection of glucose [30], while seizures seen in the recovery period occurred only after 30 minutes or more. It seems more likely that the ammonia acts as a depressing factor. In the perfused brain deprived of glucose, Geiger and associates found development of EEG depression to be retarded by a very high perfusion rate [11]. They postulated the formation of depressing metabolic products (unidentified) by oxidation of endogenous substrates, products which could accumulate at low perfusion rates but were washed out at higher rates. Ammonia may be such a toxic metabolite.

Methionine Sulfoximine. This agent induces a semichronic state characterized by recurrent epileptiform seizures and other symptoms. Unlike most convulsant drugs, it has a very long latent period of several hours (varying inversely with the dosage). A recent neurophysiological study [15] revealed that gradually increasing excitability in the preconvulsive stage is characterized by alterations in visual-evoked potentials, different from those seen with convulsants such as pentylenetetrazol, picrotoxin, and bemegride.

De Robertis et al. [9] found that methionine sulfoximine induced a loss of synaptic vesicles at endings thought to be noncholinergic (observed in rats killed during convulsions). This and other evidence suggested that the drug acts on synaptic structures.

Methionine sulfoximine has potent inhibitory action on synthesis of glutamine from glutamate and ammonia, reduces formation of glutamate in surviving cortex slices, and is a methionine antagonist [38]. It also inhibits alanine aminotransferase [9].

Available data on in vivo neurochemical effects relate to condition of the brain in the animal subject to intermittent seizures but not actually having a seizure at the moment of sampling. In dogs subject to methionine sulfoximine toxicity, we found numerous alterations in nitrogenous constituents of the brain [31]. Ammonia accumulates, but increases are not as great as those seen in fluoroacetate poisoning and hypoglycemia. Increases occur also in the levels of alanine, lysine, phosphoethanolamine, and serine. Glutamine content is greatly reduced, and there are decreases in aspartate, glutamate, leucine, and the methionine + cystathionine fraction. GABA and valine also show slight decreases, lactate a small increase. It is possible that changes in alanine, aspartate, valine, and lactate are secondary to the high ammonia. Other free amino acids, glucose, glycogen, creatine phosphate, and nucleotides in the brain remain at normal levels, and blood ammonia shows little or no increase.

Thus there is evidence of profound disturbance in the nitrogenous metabolism of the brain, but relationship of metabolic changes to convulsive activity is not clear. Decrease in GABA might be significant as an excitatory factor. Initially we considered the high ammonia level to be of probable importance in the excitation. However, at the same time that our paper appeared, Warren and Schenker [36] also reported this change (in mice treated with methionine sulfoximine), adding the surprising observation that the animals were protected from ammonia toxicity. Injection of ammonium chloride raised the cerebral level, which was already high, by as large an increment as in control animals not given methionine sulfoximine. While the ammonia quickly reached a peak and then declined rapidly in the control mice, it was maintained at a high level in methionine sulfoximine toxicity (due to impairment of the ability to form glutamine). Yet the mice given methionine sulfoximine survived doses of ammonium chloride that were lethal (causing death in coma) in other mice. Possibly the depressing effect of ammonia is opposed by unknown excitatory factors in methionine sulfoximine toxicity. It should be noted that amino-oxyacetic acid, which increases both ammonia and GABA in the brain, protects against methionine sulfoximine [8].

SUMMARY

Neurochemical effects of convulsants are discussed, with emphasis on data obtained by the technique of freezing the brain quickly in situ for analysis.

A number of chemical changes undoubtedly occur as manifestations or results of convulsive activity, appearing during the seizure but not preceding it, bearing no relation to the particular convulsant used, and offering no clues to causal mechanisms. Probably to be included in this group are changes related to the energetics of the seizure: increased oxidative metabolism, increased lactate, partial breakdown of high-energy phosphates, decreased glycogen, changes in hexose phosphates, and increased utilization of noncarbohydrate substrates. Another characteristic change is slight increase in ammonia, possibly related to changes in amino acids. Aspartic and glutamic acid levels tend to decrease in intense or prolonged seizures, suggesting that by transamination and oxidative decarboxylation they may enter the Krebs cycle for oxidation. Proteins and some phospholipids also may be utilized to some extent, and gangliosides show alterations. Decrease in acetylcholine probably is related to increased release and destruction of this transmitter.

Convulsants with long latent periods can be used to investigate conditions predisposing to seizures. A change observed in the preconvulsive stage may be either a manifestation of an excitatory influence or a side effect unrelated to the seizure. Several agents have been used for such studies:

Anticholinesterases have excitatory effects, undoubtedly due to ACh which accumulates in the brain. Seizures so induced are blocked by large doses of atropine or hyoscine, while other types are not. The cholinergic type is the only one that can now be confidently explained in terms of a neurochemical mechanism.

Convulsant hydrazides inactivate the coenzyme pyridoxal phosphate, thereby decreasing the level of GABA. This change tends to be excitatory, but can be prevented without abolishing the convulsive response.

Infusion of *buffered ammonium chloride* may induce either seizures or a state of depression, with a very high level of ammonia in the brain. Likewise in fluoro-fatty acid poisoning, insulin hypoglycemia, and methionine sulfoximine toxicity, cerebral ammonia is greatly increased. Significance of this change is difficult to evaluate; depressing effects may be more important than excitatory actions. Various changes in amino acids and other constituents occur in these conditions, but are not known to be excitatory.

REFERENCES

1. A'Hearn, M. C. Effects of Cortical Stimulants and Cholinolytic Agents on Spontaneous and Evoked Potentials. Ph.D. thesis, University of Wisconsin, 1966.
2. Benitez, D., Pscheidt, G. R., and Stone, W. E. Formation of ammonium ion in the cerebrum in fluoroacetate poisoning. *Amer. J. Physiol.* 176:488, 1954.
3. Berkowitz, E. C., Sundsten, J. W., and Sawyer, C. H. Electrographic and behavioral changes in unrestrained rabbits during insulin hypoglycemia. *Neurology* (Minneap.) 10:355, 1960.
4. Carter, S. H., and Stone, W. E. Effect of convulsants on brain glycogen in the mouse. *J. Neurochem.* 7:16, 1961.
5. Celesia, G. G., and Jasper, H. H. Acetylcholine released from cerebral cortex in relation to state of activation. *Neurology* (Minneap.) 16:1053, 1966.
6. Chitre, V. S., Chopra, S. P., and Talwar, G. P. Changes in the ribonucleic acid content of the brain during experimentally induced convulsions. *J. Neurochem.* 11:439, 1964.
7. Crossland, J., Elliott, K. A. C., and Pappius, H. M. Acetylcholine content of brain during insulin hypoglycemia. *Amer. J. Physiol.* 183:32, 1955.
8. DaVanzo, J. P., Greig, M. E., and Cronin, M. A. Anticonvulsant properties of amino-oxyacetic acid. *Amer. J. Physiol.* 201:833, 1961.
9. De Robertis, E., Sellinger, O. Z., Rodríguez de Lores Arnaiz, G., Alberici, M., and Zieher, L. M. Nerve endings in methionine sulphoximine convulsant rats, a neurochemical and ultrastructural study. *J. Neurochem.* 14:81, 1967.
10. Geiger, A. Chemical Changes Accompanying Activity in the Brain. In Richter, D. (Ed.), *Metabolism of the Nervous System*. London: Pergamon, 1957.
11. Geiger, A. Correlation of brain metabolism and function by the use of a brain perfusion method in situ. *Physiol. Rev.* 38:1, 1958.
12. Geiger, A., Horvath, N., and Kawakita, Y. The incorporation of ^{14}C derived from glucose into the proteins of the brain cortex, at rest and during activity. *J. Neurochem.* 5:311, 1960.
13. Geiger, A., Kawakita, Y., and Barkulis, S. S. Major pathways of glucose utilization in the brain in brain perfusion experiments in vivo and in situ. *J. Neurochem.* 5:323, 1960.
14. Goldberg, N. D., Passonneau, J. V., and Lowry, O. H. Effects of changes in brain metabolism on the levels of citric acid cycle intermediates. *J. Biol. Chem.* 241:3997, 1966.
15. Hřebíček, J., and Koloušek, J. Paroxysmal changes of spontaneous and evoked electrical activity of the cat brain after administration of methionine sulfoximine. *Epilepsia* (Amst.) (Fourth Series) 9:145, 1968.
16. Kandel, A., and Chenoweth, M. B. Metabolic disturbances produced by some fluoro-fatty acids: Relation to the pharmacologic activity of these compounds. *J. Pharmacol. Exp. Ther.* 104:234, 1952.
17. Klein, J. R., and Olsen, N. S. Effect of convulsive activity upon the concentration

of brain glucose, glycogen, lactate and phosphates. *J. Biol. Chem.* 167:747, 1947.

18. Krnjević, K., and Schwartz, S. The action of γ-aminobutyric acid on cortical neurones. *Exp. Brain Res.* 3:320, 1967.

19. Lahiri, S., and Quastel, J. H. Fluoroacetate and the metabolism of ammonia in brain. *Biochem. J.* 89:157, 1963.

20. McKhann, G. M., and Tower, D. B. Ammonia toxicity and cerebral oxidative metabolism. *Amer. J. Physiol.* 200:420, 1961.

21. Peters, R. A. Mechanism of the toxicity of the active constituent of *Dichapetalum cymosum* and related compounds. *Advances Enzym.* 18:113, 1957.

22. Pscheidt, G. R., Benitez, D., Kirschner, L. B., and Stone, W. E. Effects of fluoroacetate poisoning on citrate, lactate and energy-rich phosphates in the cerebrum. *Amer. J. Physiol.* 176:483, 1954.

23. Richter, D., and Dawson, R. M. C. The ammonia and glutamine content of the brain. *J. Biol. Chem.* 176:1199, 1948.

24. Roa, P. D., Tews, J. K., and Stone, W. E. A neurochemical study of thiosemicarbazide seizures and their inhibition by amino-oxyacetic acid. *Biochem. Pharmacol.* 13:477, 1964.

25. Roberts, E., and Eidelberg, E. Metabolic and neurophysiological roles of γ-aminobutyric acid. *Int. Rev. Neurobiol.* 2:279, 1960.

26. Saktor, B., Wilson, J. E., and Tiekert, C. G. Regulation of glycolysis in brain, in situ, during convulsions. *J. Biol. Chem.* 241:5071, 1966.

27. Stone, W. E. The role of acetylcholine in brain metabolism and function. *Amer. J. Phys. Med.* 36:222, 1957.

28. Stone, W. E., Tews, J. K., and Mitchell, E. N. Chemical concomitants of convulsive activity in the cerebrum. *Neurology* (Minneap.) 10:241, 1960.

29. Tews, J. K., Carter, S. H., Roa, P. D., and Stone, W. E. Free amino acids and related compounds in dog brain: Postmortem and anoxic changes, effects of ammonium chloride infusion, and levels during seizures induced by picrotoxin and by pentylenetetrazol. *J. Neurochem.* 10:641, 1963.

30. Tews, J. K., Carter, S. H., and Stone, W. E. Chemical changes in the brain during insulin hypoglycemia and recovery. *J. Neurochem.* 12:679, 1965.

31. Tews, J. K., and Stone, W. E. Effects of methionine sulfoximine on levels of free amino acids and related substances in brain. *Biochem. Pharmacol.* 13:543, 1964.

32. Tews, J. K., and Stone, W. E. Free amino acids and related compounds in brain and other tissues: Effects of convulsant drugs. *Progr. Brain Res.* 16:135, 1965.

33. Tokizane, T., and Sawyer, C. H. Sites of origin of hypoglycemic seizures in the rabbit. *Arch. Neurol. Psychiat.* 77:259, 1957.

34. Torda, C. Effects of corticotropin and various convulsion-inducing agents on the P^{32} content of brain phospholipids, nucleoproteins and total acid-soluble phosphorus compounds. *Amer. J. Physiol.* 177:179, 1954.

35. Van Meter, W. G., Owens, H. F., and Himwich, H. E. Cortical and rhinencephalic electrical potentials during hypoglycemia. *Arch. Neurol. Psychiat.* 80:314, 1958.

36. Warren, K. S., and Schenker, S. Effect of an inhibitor of glutamine synthesis (methionine sulfoximine) on ammonia toxicity and metabolism. *J. Lab. Clin. Med.* 64:442, 1964.

37. Whisler, K. E., Tews, J. K., and Stone, W. E. Cerebral amino acids in drug-induced status epilepticus. *J. Neurochem.* 15:215, 1968.

38. Wolfe, L. S., and Elliott, K. A. C. Chemical Studies in Relation to Convulsive Conditions. In Elliott, K. A. C., Page, I. H., and Quastel, J. H. (Eds.), *Neurochemistry* (2d ed.). Springfield, Ill.: Thomas, 1962.

8
Pharmacology of Synaptic Transmitters*

GEORGE B. KOELLE

MUCH OF WHAT WE KNOW or assume about the pharmacology of central synapses is derived by synthesis of the still relatively limited and indirect observations made at central sites, with a much broader fund of more direct evidence obtained at synapses or neuroeffector junctions of the peripheral nervous system (NS). The theory of neurohumoral transmission, proposed in general terms nearly a century ago by DuBois-Reymond [42], was invoked by Elliot [49] early in the present century to account for activation of autonomic effectors by the sympathetic NS.

The first direct evidence of neurohumoral action was obtained by Löewi [93] for the parasympathetic control of the frog heart. During the early 1930s the concept was extended to the entire mammalian peripheral efferent NS by Dale, Feldberg, Gaddum, Vogt, and others. Apparently, the first suggestion that synaptic transmission in the central nervous system (CNS) might be neurohumoral was made by the late Sir Henry Dale in 1934 [35]. The present status of neurohumoral transmission in the CNS is reviewed in this volume by Curtis [31]. As he has indicated, all present evidence: physiological, pharmacological, histochemical, and electron microscopic, is consistent with occurrence of neurohumoral transmission throughout the mammalian CNS; tight interneuronal junctions, where transmission is undoubtedly electrotonic, have so far been reported only for submammalian species [9, 61, 95]. Yet, as indicated, much of this evidence is based on analogies with the peripheral NS where, because of its relative anatomical simplicity, it has been possible both to satisfy criteria for neurohumoral transmission and to identify the transmitters involved at various sites.

The same contrast between the peripheral NS and the CNS holds for our knowledge of mechanisms of drug action. Actions of most of the important drugs employed either clinically or investigationally for their effects on the peripheral NS and its effector organs can be defined in terms of their modifying some stage of neurohumoral transmission [81]. This is true of a limited number of centrally acting agents, many of which are described in other chapters in this volume [31, 44, 52]. However, it is not possible to relate to known synaptic events the effects of such important and extensive classes of drugs as the general anesthetics, analgesics, and centrally acting skeletal muscle relaxants. The same is largely true of drugs with which we are primarily concerned here, the anticonvulsant agents, which Woodbury [138] and Toman [129] discuss. From our present knowledge, or lack of such, it seems likely that compounds of these varied classes act by modifying the general level of neuronal excitability, rather than the immediate events in synaptic transmission. Actions of a more recently exploited group of drugs, the phrenotropic agents (tranquilizers, antidepressants, and hallucinogens), have been explained at least hypothetically in terms of their effects at central synapses [15].

---

* Original investigations from the author's laboratory mentioned in this review were supported by PHS Research Grant NB00282 from National Institute of Neurological Diseases and Stroke.

The likelihood is not remote of developing more effective anticonvulsants that act by modifying synaptic mechanisms, which seems to be a primary justification for including a general discussion of the pharmacology of central synapses.

NEUROHUMORAL TRANSMITTERS. As Curtis has indicated, there is little doubt that acetylcholine (ACh) and norepinephrine (NE), as well as its immediate precursor, dopamine (DA), are neurohumoral transmitters in the CNS. Neurohumoral functions of several additional centrally occurring compounds seem possible, but are less definitely established; this group includes the excitatory dicarboxylic amino acids (A.A.s), for example, aspartic, glutamic; inhibitory monocarboxylic A.A.s such as glycine and GABA; 5-hydroxytryptamine (5-HT, serotonin); the polypeptide substance P; and a variety of other agents.

Just as in the periphery, the cholinergic and adrenergic systems appear at certain levels of the CNS to maintain a balance by exerting mutually antagonistic effects. This is perhaps best illustrated by nuclei of the corpus striatum and fibers that radiate to them from the substantia nigra. The caudate nucleus and putamen contain the highest concentrations of ACh [94], choline acetylase (ChAc) [58], and acetylcholinesterase (AChE) [17, 75] of any region of the CNS. The same nuclei also contain high concentrations of catecholamine (CA), but mostly in the form of DA rather than its β-OH derivative, NE, which is the predominant CA elsewhere in the peripheral nervous system and CNS [10, 11, 20]. This is of phylogenetic interest, since the corpus striatum represents the highest level of the motor system in submammalian species, and DA is probably the principal adrenergic inhibitory transmitter in the CNS of certain molluscs [63, 73]. Most of the DA of the corpus striatum appears to be present in the terminals of fibers that arise from the substantia nigra [5, 33].

Evidence for the physiological balance maintained by opposing tones of cholinergic and adrenergic (or dopaminergic) systems of the corpus striatum is derived mainly from observations of the symptomatology, pathology, and therapy of Parkinson's disease [25]. This condition is characterized by rigidity, tremor, akinesia, and a variety of other symptoms; regardless of its primary etiology, a consistent pathological finding is evidence of damage to the neurons of the substantia nigra and a marked decrease in their contents of melanin and DA; the concentration of the latter is correspondingly diminished in the nuclei of the corpus striatum [47, 70].

Partial development of this pattern of signs, chiefly akinesia, and loss of DA from the same regions can be produced in monkeys by sectioning the nigrostriatal tracts [123]. An even closer replication of the clinical condition occurs transiently following administration of the centrally acting cholinomimetic agent, oxotremorine, to various laboratory animals [23, 55]. The fact that all the standard drugs used in the symptomatic treatment of Parkinson's disease are anticholinergic agents is consistent with the assumption that the symptoms are based on relative overbalance in cholinergic tone, consequent to diminution of the store of the adrenergic transmitter. Development of a parkinsonian syndrome in patients who have received high doses of potent tranquilizing agents over long periods can be explained in similar terms: through depletion of DA (reserpine) [6] or by α-adrenergic blockade (phenothiazines) [96] or dopaminergic blockade (butyrophenones) [131].

On the basis of the foregoing findings, Birkmayer and Hornykiewicz [12] administered intravenously L-dihydroxyphenylalanine (L-dopa), the immediate precursor of dopamine, to parkinsonian patients and obtained brief but distinct reversal of the major symptoms. This has led more recently to the long-term therapy of Parkinson's disease, currently undergoing trial at several centers, by the oral administration of frequent, high doses of L-dopa [26]. Results to date have been extremely promising and can be expected to lead to development of still more effective antiparkinsonian agents in the form of relatively stable, dopaminomimetic compounds that accumulate more selectively within the CNS or corpus striatum. Beyond illustrating a balance of cholinergic and adrenergic tone at a specific level in the CNS, the foregoing account exemplifies advances in therapy that can result from an understanding of the biochemical or physiological deficits in diseases of the CNS.

EFFECTS OF DRUGS ON THE CNS

Figure 8-1 and its legend have been adapted from a standard textbook [64] to illustrate the dozen or so known mechanisms by which various drugs can act at adrenergic nerve terminals and their effector organs to produce their characteristic effects. While nearly all the proposed mechanisms are based on studies at peripheral sites of adrenergic transmission and the adrenal medulla, it is reasonable to assume that similar actions could occur at adrenergic synapses in the CNS. Indeed, some of the examples mentioned (imipramine, amitriptyline, amphetamine) are drugs that are used exclusively or extensively for their effects on the CNS, where they are assumed to act by the same primary mechanisms as at the periphery.

The greater anatomical complexity of synaptic relationships in the CNS could allow for additional mechanisms of action that have no known peripheral counterparts. Examples of such would include modifications of presynaptic inhibition, relative dominance of effects at sites of axosomatic versus axodendritic transmission, and relatively selective effects on the great numbers of excitatory and inhibitory presynaptic endings that impinge on single central neurons. These aspects are also considered in detail elsewhere in this volume [31, 44, 52, 118].

A few additional points should be emphasized regarding Fig. 8-1. Actions indicated in the diagram for the various drugs are probably their major or primary actions; this by no means excludes the likelihood of their acting also at additional sites in the diagram or elsewhere. In any discussion of this sort, the first adage of pharmacology should be recalled: no drug has a single action. For example, at certain stages of their actions, both guanethidine and bretylium can either promote or prevent release of norepinephrine from adrenergic nerve terminals. At those doses in which they are used clinically to lower blood pressure, guanethidine appears to act predominantly by the former and bretylium by the latter mechanism; hence, they are labeled accordingly in the diagram. Likewise, most of the commonly employed monoamine oxidase (MAO) inhibitors can also block release of norepinephrine by a mechanism unrelated to MAO inhibition; this is probably the basis of their hypotensive effect.

The enzymes involved chiefly in the initial metabolic breakdown of NE, *i.e.*, MAO and catechol-O-methyltransferase (COMT), probably play little or no part in terminating the effects of adrenergic impulses; this appears to be accomplished chiefly by a combination of active uptake of NE by the adrenergic terminals, and simple diffusion. Finally, it is apparent that the majority of mechanisms indicated involve the presynaptic adrenergic terminal, rather than the postjunctional effector site. This is in striking contrast to the situation of a decade or so ago, when the only types of drug actions generally considered at such sites were postjunctional sympathomimetic activation or adrenergic blockade.

Cholinergic and Adrenergic Transmissions. At sites of cholinergic transmission in both the peripheral and central nervous systems, major attention is still focused largely on the postjunctional membrane as the primary locus of drug action. Drugs so encompassed would include the cholinomimetic and cholinergic blocking agents, with their relative specificities for either muscarinic or nicotinic receptors, and the anticholinesterase (anti-ChE) agents. In contradistinction to the adrenergic system, in cholinergic systems the rapid destruction of the transmitter, ACh, by the enzyme acetylcholinesterase, AChE, is of major importance in terminating its action. To what extent equivalent enzymes function in regulating the synaptic actions of the other putative central neurohumoral transmitters is essentially unknown at present.

The first definite indication of presynaptic actions of cholinomimetic, cholinergic blocking, and anti-ChE agents was probably that published by Masland and Wigton [97] in 1940 for the motor end-plate

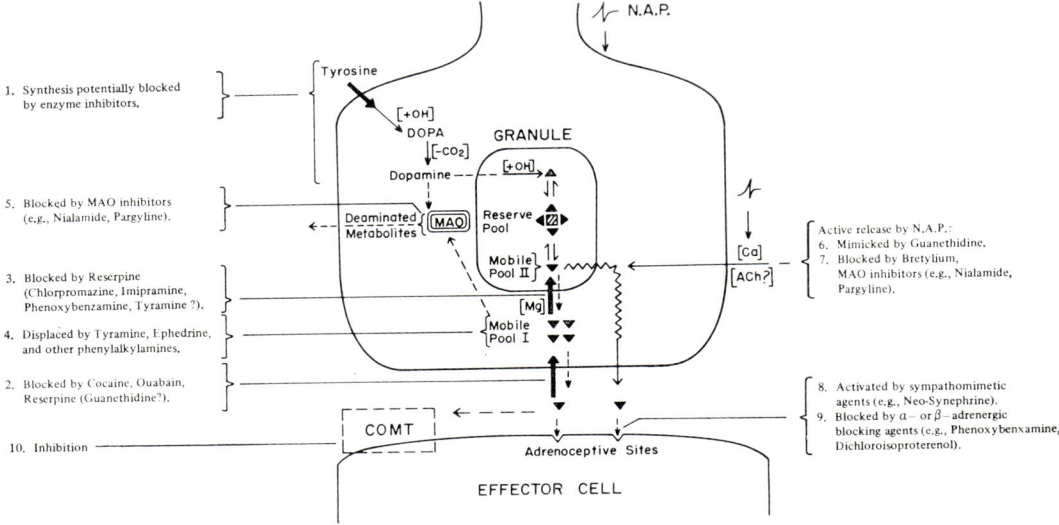

FIG. 8-1. Proposed sites of action of drugs that modify synthesis, uptake, and release of norepinephrine at adrenergic nerve terminals. Norepinephrine (▼) within the nerve terminal is partitioned into a cytoplasmic Mobile Pool I and intragranular pools through equilibria between active transport (heavy arrows), passive diffusion (dash arrows), enzymatic synthesis (light arrows), and destruction (mitochondrial monoamine oxidase, MAO). Intragranular reserve pool consists of catecholamine-ATP (▨) salt (combined in a ratio of 4:1) in equilibrium with an intragranular Mobile Pool II. As shown at right, norepinephrine is discharged rapidly to the exterior by the nerve action potential (NAP) through the mobilization of calcium ion, with possible involvement of acetylcholine—Burn and Rand hypothesis [18]. On the basis of pharmacological data, the norepinephrine released by the NAP is shown to come from Mobile Pool II, but this is by no means proven. Following release of norepinephrine and its action at adrenoceptive sites of effector cells, excess is removed from extracellular region largely by return to axonal terminal through active transport or by enzymatic inactivation by extraneuronal catechol-O-methyltransferase (COMT). Drugs may exert their effects by modifying these processes as follows:

(1) Interference with active uptake of precursor (tyrosine) or synthesis of norepinephrine leading to depletion of reserve pool (e.g., α-methyl-p-tyrosine).

(2) Blockade of active transport from extracellular fluid to cytoplasmic Mobile Pool I, causing augmentation of norepinephrine action at adrenoceptive sites (e.g., cocaine, imipramine).

(3) Blockade of active transport from cytoplasmic I to intragranular II pools, leading to depletion of latter, and enzymatic deamination within cytoplasm by mitochondrial MAO (e.g., reserpine).

(4) Displacement of norepinephrine from cytoplasmic Mobile Pool I, leading to sympathomimetic effects (e.g., tyramine, ephedrine).

(5) Inhibition of MAO, leading to accumulation of norepinephrine at central and possibly other sites (e.g., tranylcypromine). Also see (7).

(6) Active release from intragranular Mobile Pool II, leading to transient sympathomimetic effects followed by depletion of reserve pool (e.g., guanethidine).

(7) Interference with release by NAP, causing block of adrenergic nerve activity (e.g., bretylium, MAO inhibitors).

(8) Activation at adrenoceptive sites of effector cells by sympathomimetic agents (e.g., phenylephrine).

(9) Blockade at adrenoceptive sites by adrenergic blocking agents (e.g., phenoxybenzamine, propranolol).

(10) Inhibition of COMT, leading to enhancement of effects of adrenergic nerve impulses or injected catecholamines. (No important present examples.)

(11) Same site as (1) Synthesis of false neurotransmitters from precursors that undergo same

(MEP) of skeletal muscle. Some of their observations confirmed similar ones made considerably earlier by Langley and Kato [91] and have in turn been amply corroborated and extended since [114, 115, 137].

A series of histochemical observations directed our own interest to the presynaptic terminals of both cholinergic and noncholinergic nerve fibers as potentially important sites of drug action. These findings and the working hypotheses derived from them have been presented in detail elsewhere [78, 79, 80, 82]; accordingly, they will be reviewed only briefly here, with emphasis on some of the more recent work that seems particularly pertinent to the subject of this volume.

One of the strongest lines of evidence for adrenergic transmission in the CNS was the demonstration by Dahlström, Fuxe, and Hillarp [34, 69] of CA-containing central fiber tracts, by means of a highly sensitive formaldehyde vapor, histofluorescence technique [56]. The procedure was based on the earlier one of Eränkö [50], who had employed formaldehyde in solution for localizing the NE-containing cells of the adrenal medulla of various species. This important area will be discussed by A. Dahlström in the presentation that follows.

At the present time, there is no established method for the histochemical demonstration of ACh, or the enzyme involved in the final step of its synthesis, choline acetyltransferase or choline acetylase (ChAc), although investigators are seeking such procedures. Somewhat by default, then, the only available histochemical index of cholinergic function is the localization of acetylcholinesterase (AChE), the enzyme involved specifically in the breakdown of the transmitter. Obviously, this is a less direct criterion than would be the histochemical demonstration of ACh or ChAc. However, with certain exceptions, most areas of the peripheral NS and the CNS of various species show high degrees of correlation between the relative concentrations of ACh, ChAc, and AChE [17, 58, 67, 94]. The outstanding exception is the cerebellum, where concentration of AChE is extremely high relative to those of ACh and ChAc [122]; the reason for this is not clear.

By means of the copper thiocholine technique, known cholinergic neurons of the peripheral NS of the cat were shown to have relatively high concentrations of AChE throughout their somata, dendrites, and axonal terminals, with somewhat lower concentration along the axons themselves; the AChE concentration was found to be considerably lower in the primary afferent neurons of this species and extremely low or absent from most of the adrenergic neurons [76].

AChE—Functional and Reserve. From modifications in AChE staining obtained following treatment in vivo and in vitro with various combinations of anti-ChE agents and related findings, it was postulated that the AChE of cholinergic neurons is composed of a functional fraction, with the active groups oriented externally at the neuronal membrane, and a recently synthesized reserve fraction within the α-cytomembranes of the endoplasmic reticulum [77, 85, 86]. Corroborative pharmacological evidence was obtained for this concept [99].

When the distributions of functional and reserve AChE were compared at various autonomic ganglia of the cat, it was found that in the superior cervical ganglion, essentially all the functional AChE is presynaptic, whereas in the ciliary ganglion it is both presynaptic and postsynaptic [86]. At the other end of the spectrum is the neuromuscular junction or motor end-plate of skeletal muscle, where most of the AChE is postjunctional [27]. Yet even here, recent electron microscopic findings [36] have suggested that the difference is largely due to the considerably greater surface area presented by extensive unfoldings of the post-

---

enzymatic conversions but result in less active end products (e.g., α-methyl-dopa→α-methyldopamine→α-methylnorepinephrine).
(After Euler [54], Trendelenburg [130], Kirshner [74], Axelrod [8], Braunwald et al. [13], Brodie [14], Carlsson et al. [21], and others). (From Goodman, L. S., and Gilman, A. (Eds.), *The Pharmacological Basis of Therapeutics*, p. 424 [64].)

junctional membrane; the intensity of staining for AChE per unit area appears to differ little for the prejunctional and postjunctional membranes of the motor endplate (Fig. 8-2).

In seeking an explanation of the significance of the exclusively presynaptic localization of the AChE in the superior cervical ganglion, with Volle [134] the effects were determined of preganglionic denervation and of inactivation of the ganglionic AChE by diisopropyl phosphorofluoridate (DFP) on the threshold of intra-arterial doses of ACh and its stable analog, carbachol (Car), for producing postganglionic firing. Subsequent investigators have reported evidence both to confirm [66] and to refute [16] our original results; the reasons for the discrepancies are not clear.

Nevertheless, it was concluded that in the normal ganglion the presynaptic terminals have a lower threshold for activation by injected Car or ACh than have the postsynaptic membranes, and that postganglionic firing after threshold intra-arterial doses of either compound is due to release of endogenous ACh from the presynaptic terminals. At the time we were unaware

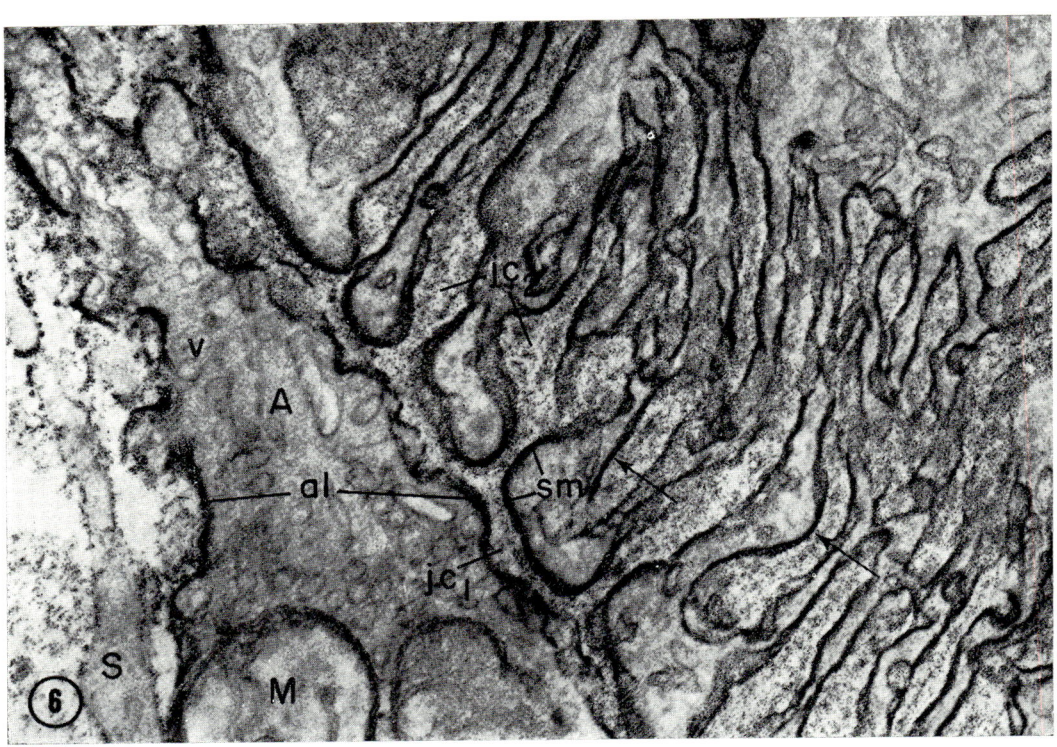

FIG. 8-2. Electron microscopic histochemical localization of acetylcholinesterase at the motor end-plate of mouse intercostal muscle. A high-magnification ($\times 63{,}000$) view of the junctional complex, showing the axonal terminal (A) containing mitochondria (M) and numerous synaptic vesicles (v), the junctional cleft (jc), and junctional folds of the sarcolemma (sm). The electron-dense granules, 40–50 Å in diameter, represent gold sulfide, the reaction product in the gold–thiolacetic acid method for acetylcholinesterase and nonspecific cholinesterase. The axolemma (al) exhibits marked enzymatic activity both on the surface facing the primary junctional cleft (jc_1) and at the surface facing the teloglial Schwann cell sheath (S). The axonal terminal is somewhat separated from the Schwann cell in this micrograph. Where the plane of section is perpendicular to the sarcolemma (arrows), the particles form a dense line about 120–140 Å in thickness. A few particles are also present in the primary (jc_1) and secondary (jc_2) junctional clefts, possibly indicating some diffusion of the reaction product. (From Davis and Koelle [36].)

that Renshaw et al. [113] had suggested several years previously that Car produces its cardiovascular effects by the release of endogenous ACh, a reference that was brought to our attention by Burn. It has been demonstrated more recently that Car, in the same dosage range (0.25–1.0 μg) that produced threshold activation of the normally circulated ganglion, releases ACh from the Ringer-Locke perfused ganglion [101].

PROPOSED DUAL NEUROHUMORAL ROLE OF ACh

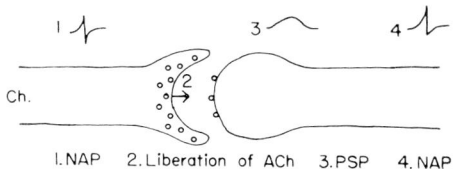

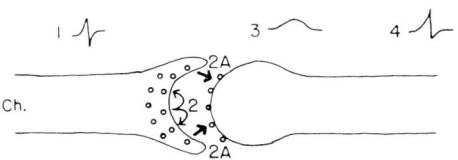

2A. Liberation of additional quanta of ACh from presynaptic site by local action of initially liberated ACh.

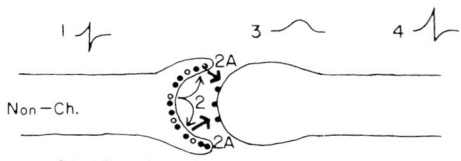

2A. Liberation of another neurohumoral transmitter from presynaptic site by local action of initially liberated ACh.

FIG. 8-3. Proposed presynaptic function of acetylcholine in cholinergic and noncholinergic transmission. Top: Standard concept. Center: Proposed presynaptic function in cholinergic fibers. Acetylcholine considered to act first at terminal from which liberated to activate release of (2A) additional quanta of ACh, which produce the PSP. Bottom: Proposed presynaptic function in noncholinergic fibers. (1) NAP liberates (2) ACh from presynaptic terminals, which acts at same terminals to effect release of (2A) another synaptic transmitter; latter produces (3) PSP, which initiates (4) NAP. (From Koelle [79].)

The foregoing histochemical and pharmacological findings led to the working hypothesis [79] for ganglionic transmission outlined in Fig. 8-3; no attempt has been made to indicate the various intermediary steps, such as the mobilization of Ca^{++} ion or the migration of synaptic vesicles to the axonal terminal membrane.

ACh Release. The quanta of ACh released initially by the nerve action potential (NAP) were proposed to act at the external surface of the same presynaptic membrane, to prolong briefly the depolarized state and thereby amplify the number of quanta released to effect depolarization of the postsynaptic membrane (Fig. 8-3, middle diagram). This is somewhat analogous to the manner in which tetraethylammonium is believed to increase the release of ACh at the motor end-plate [87].

The presynaptic release amplification mechanism is assumed to be terminated by a combination of hydrolysis of the ACh by the functional AChE located at the same site, and possibly by desensitization of the presynaptic cholinoreceptors such as has been shown to occur postjunctionally at the motor end-plate [126]. It has been calculated that termination of the postsynaptic action of the ACh released during transmission in the superior cervical ganglion can be accounted for by diffusion alone [104]. Its ultimate disposal from the ganglionic synaptic clefts probably results chiefly from its hydrolysis by the presynaptically located AChE.

One of the chief objections [43] that has been raised to the foregoing hypothesis is that it has not been possible to record antidromic firing along the preganglionic trunk following intra-arterial injection of cholinomimetic or anti-ChE agents into the ganglion [40] as has been done, although inconsistently, at the somatic motor nerves to motor end-plates under similar conditions [97, 115]. However, this can probably be accounted for by the marked structural differences between the neuromuscular junction and the ganglionic synapses. The former is a well-defined entity in which the diameter of the motor nerve does not change abruptly at its terminal [7]; the localized depolarization of the latter by activation of its cholinoceptive sites can, presumably, generally trigger a propagated antidromic impulse at the adjacent conducting portion of the axon.

In the ganglion, on the other hand, most of the points of synaptic contact occur *en passage* at vesicular swellings of the fine (0.1–0.3 μ in diameter) preganglionic terminals that course along the dendrites of the ganglion cells [48]. The localized depolarization of the vesicular preganglionic swellings by ACh, released from their own stores or administered via the circulation, might be expected to decrease below the activation threshold before reaching the conducting region of the axonal membrane. The only condition under which antidromic preganglionic firing has been recorded has been following infection with pseudo rabies virus [37]. Its suppression, along with the suppression of the synchronous, spontaneous bursts of postganglionic firing, by cholinergic blocking agents, and the amplification of both by physostigmine, suggest that both are initiated by the release of endogenous ACh [38]. A possible explanation for the preganglionic antidromic firing in this condition is that the virus induces a spread of the chemoreceptor area of the preganglionic terminals, just as denervation does at the postjunctional membrane of skeletal muscle [127]. Recently, Koketsu and Nishi [88] have established the presence of cholinoceptive sites at the presynaptic terminals of both amphibian and mammalian sympathetic ganglia; their activation, either by preganglionic impulses or by applied ACh, results in the slow, nonpropagated depolarization of the terminals.

As a corollary to the foregoing hypothesis, it was proposed that in certain AChE-containing noncholinergic fibers, including the neurosecretory cells of the hypothalamico-neurohypophysis [1, 84] and the primary afferent neurons of the vagus [98], the initial release of ACh facilitates the release of another neurohumoral transmitter (Fig. 8-3, lower diagram). This is equivalent to the Burn and Rand [18] hypothesis of a cholinergic link in adrenergic transmission, the arguments for [19] and against

[59] which have been reviewed recently in detail. Interestingly enough, the adrenergic ganglion cells of practically all species examined excepting the cat contain moderate concentrations of AChE [22, 76]. In the rabbit and cat, this distinction appears to extend to the terminals of the adrenergic fibers, where only those of the former were found to contain detectable concentrations of AChE [72]. Hemicholinium ion (HC-3), which interferes with cholinergic transmission by blocking the uptake of choline to replenish the store of ACh, was shown to reduce contraction of the nictitating membrane in response to postganglionic sympathetic stimulation in the rabbit but not in the cat [71]. Thus, the proposal of the participation of ACh in the release of NE by adrenergic fibers could account for the presence of AChE in the adrenergic neurons of most species. If such a mechanism operates in the adrenergic system of the cat, the histochemical findings would suggest that it does so not by individual fibers but through the release of ACh by cholinergic fibers that run parallel with adrenergic fibers, as indicated in the right-hand diagram of Fig. 8-4. A similar arrangement may be the basis for some of the pharma-

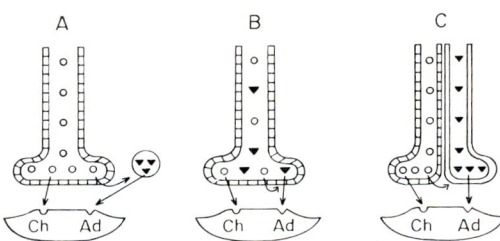

Fig. 8-4. Schematic representation of relationships between distributions of AChE (crosshatching) and NE (filled triangles) in accordance with mechanisms by which ACh (clear circles) might promote release of NE following activation of postganglionic sympathetic fibers. ACh-releasing fibers assumed to contain AChE and effector cells to have both cholinoceptive (Ch) and adrenoceptive (Ad) sites. (*A*) ACh released from fiber activates release of NE from nearby chromaffin or mast cells. (*B*) ACh facilitates release of NE from same fiber. (*C*) ACh facilitates release of NE from adjacent fiber arising from same ganglion. (Adapted from Burn and Rand [18, 19]; Jacobowitz and Koelle [72].)

cological anomolies associated with the sympathetic control of eccrine sweat secretion in several species [92].

Inhibitory Transmission in CNS

Of more direct interest in the context of this volume is the recent extension of the same working hypothesis to certain sites of inhibitory transmission in the CNS. The olivocochlear bundle (OCB) represents part of an efferent inhibitory system whose fibers terminate both at the level of the cochlear nucleus and at the hair cells of the cochlea [111, 112]. Stimulation of the OCB during the course of a series of clicks causes suppression of the passage of afferent impulses from the cochlea [62], apparently by release of a hyperpolarizing transmitter at the terminations of the OCB on the cochlear hair cells [60].

As shown originally by Churchill, Schuknecht, and Doran [24] and confirmed by several other groups [68, 116, 117, 120, 132], the terminals of the OCB are the only structures within the cochlea that stain distinctly for AChE. Yet, from a careful pharmacological analysis employing a variety of muscarinic and nicotinic cholinergic blocking agents, Desmedt and Monaco [39] concluded that ACh is not the transmitter of the OCB. On the other hand, strychnine and some related alkaloids effectively blocked inhibition of afferent auditory impulses produced by OCB stimulation [39, 125].

For many years it has been assumed that strychnine blocks inhibitory transmission from the Renshaw cells to the motor neurons of the lumbar cord by competing with the unidentified hyperpolarizing transmitter at the postsynaptic membrane [29, 46]. This assumption received direct confirmation in the recently reported experiments of Curtis and associates [30], who showed that strychnine blocks also the hyperpolarization of the motor neurons produced by the microiontophoretic application of glycine [32], a present major candidate for the role of the inhibitory transmitter of the Renshaw cells [136]. The same mechanism of strychnine blockade at the OCB was concluded by Desmedt and Monaco [39]. This, of course, omits from consideration any physiological function of the AChE located there. Strychnine has been shown recently to have an additional action, inhibition of the release of ACh from the cat superior cervical ganglion following preganglionic stimulation [100, 102], as well as from the guinea pig ileum during coaxial stimulation [124]. This action may account for the blockade of transmission produced by strychnine at the ganglion [57, 90] as well as at the neuromuscular junction [3]. It could also be the basis, in part or in whole, for strychnine blockade at the OCB, on the assumption that the release of its hyperpolarizing transmitter is mediated by the initial release of ACh and that this step, as at the ganglion, is blocked by strychnine. While this proposal admittedly is inconsistent with the principle of parsimony, or Ockham's razor, it nevertheless takes into account the selective localization of AChE at the terminals of the OCB.

The amacrine cells of the retina apparently perform an inhibitory or integrative function in the visual pathway [108, 109], somewhat analogous to that of the OCB in the auditory system. These cells have been shown by electron microscopy to form a complex series of synaptic contacts with both the bipolar cells and the ganglion cells, with impulses traveling either peripherally or centrally at given points [41]. Like the OCB, the amacrine cells are the only retinal elements that exhibit marked staining for AChE in all species examined; in some species the retinal ganglion cells also show light, inconsistent staining for the enzyme [83, 103]. Although there is pharmacological evidence of cholinergic transmission at some level of the retina [4], the neurohumoral transmitter of the amacrine cells has not been identified.

Likewise unknown is the retinal site or sites of action of strychnine, which was shown many years ago to initiate rhythmic retinal discharges [2] and to block postexcitatory retinal inhibition [65]. In the absence of evidence to the contrary, analogy may be drawn from the preceding analysis to speculate that ACh promotes release of an inhibitory or hyperpolarizing transmitter by the amacrine cells and that strychnine produces blockade at that step.

Renshaw Cells. The Renshaw cell, which represents a negative feedback system between the axon collaterals of the anterior horn cells of the spinal cord and their somata, has been investigated more thoroughly than any other central inhibitory site [29, 43, 46]. The question raised recently, concerning its existence as a separate entity or as the terminal of the axon collateral itself [135], has been discussed extensively [45, 51, 82]. By a modification of the technique employed by Thomas and Wilson [128], Renshaw cells were located in the spinal cord of the cat by intracellular recording and were tagged with fast green FCF; sections of the area were then stained for AChE. Most of the structures so identified were between 5 and 10 μ in diameter and were closely adjacent to anterior horn cells; all showed variable degrees of staining for AChE [51]. Thus, the Renshaw cell represents another central inhibitory neuron, the neurohumoral transmitter of which unquestionably is not ACh [29, 43] but where the presence of AChE suggests a role of ACh in its release.

The extension of the hypothesis of cholinergically mediated transmitter release to the foregoing central inhibitory synapses is depicted in Fig. 8-5.

Cholinergic and Noncholinergic Transmission. In the first general histochemical survey of the distribution of AChE in the CNS of the rat [75], it was found that the neurons of motor nuclei, which are known to give rise to peripheral cholinergic fibers, showed intensive staining for the enzyme, as did certain other sites for which there is indirect evidence of cholinergic transmission, such as the caudate nucleus. In contrast, many groups of neurons appeared to be essentially devoid of AChE, and were presumably noncholinergic. This principle has been utilized to great advantage by Shute and Lewis [121] in their extensive and careful mapping of cholinergic tracts in the CNS. However, a great number of neurons and their processes were found to contain intermediate concentrations of AChE. The distribution of similarly stained tracts is even more extensive in the CNS of the frog [119]. In attempting to interpret mechanisms of drug action in the CNS, it

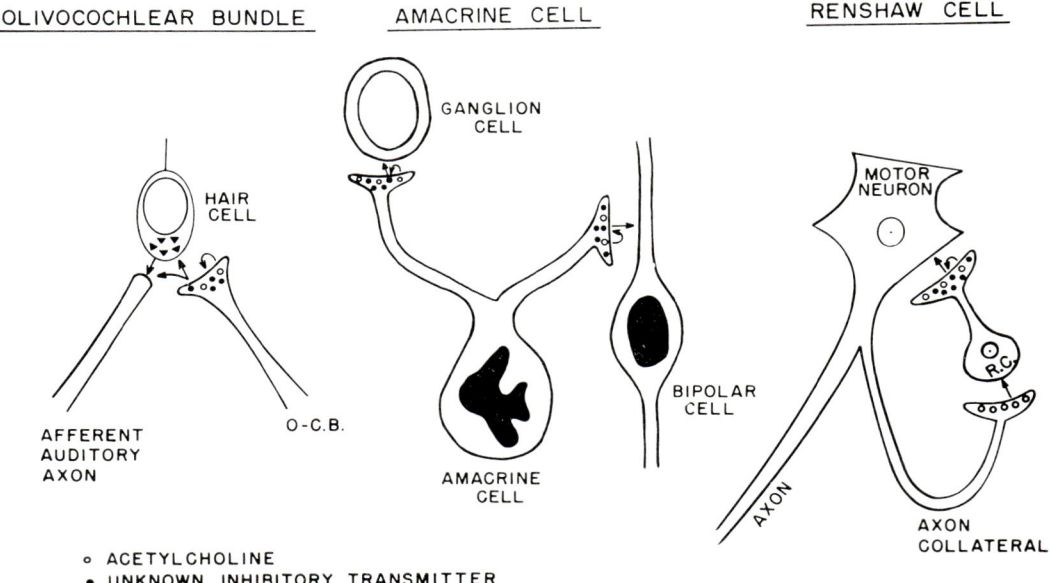

FIG. 8-5. Proposed role of ACh in releasing unidentified inhibitory transmitters from AChE-staining, noncholinergic presynaptic terminals of olivocochlear bundle, amacrine cell, and Renshaw cell. (From Koelle [82].)

seems worth considering the possibility that at many or all such sites, ACh is involved in the release of other agents that serve as the actual excitatory or inhibitory transmitters.

Some additional observations from the literature might be interpreted similarly. As Curtis and Krnjević have pointed out, the excitatory action of ACh when applied iontophoretically at cortical neurons has a characteristically slow onset [28, 89]; this latency might be occasioned by its actually releasing another excitatory transmitter from adjacent presynaptic terminals. The same explanation might be applied to Krnjević's observations that in the isolated cortical slab only one-fifth as many neurons responded to the iontophoretic application of ACh as in the normal cortex [89]. Likewise, blockade of the inhibitory effect of ACh at other cortical neurons by both atropine [106, 110] and strychnine [107] might be due to interference with postsynaptic and presynaptic actions of ACh, respectively, the latter involving a cholinergically activated release mechanism. Finally, in discussing the interrelationships between certain cholinomimetic agents and strychnine, Esplin and Zablocka-Esplin [53] have mentioned the possibility of "a common chemical step in peripheral cholinergic junctions and in the pathways which mediate postsynaptic inhibition."

CONCLUSIONS

It is clear from the foregoing survey that our knowledge of the pharmacology of central synapses is still rudimentary. Attention has been confined here largely to drugs that appear to act primarily by modifying synaptic processes, exclusive of presynaptic inhibition which is covered elsewhere [44, 52]. Similarly omitted have been the anticonvulsant and most convulsant agents, for the same reason, and such engrossing new areas of investigation as the modification by drugs of learning and memory, which seems outside the immediate scope of this volume.

As noted at the beginning of this chapter, we are still forced to draw on analogies with the peripheral NS to a great extent in order to interpret pharmacological findings in the CNS, where anatomical and physiological complexities are vastly greater. This situation is placed in more precise perspective by consideration of how much is still unexplained concerning transmission in the relatively simple superior cervical ganglion [133], an extensively investigated structure that has been called a "microcosmic nervous system" [105].

A great deficit exists not only in knowledge of mechanisms of drug actions in the CNS, but also in regard to specifically acting drugs. In reviewing the evidence that certain amino acids function as central excitatory or inhibitory transmitters, Curtis has indicated that only in the case of glycine and strychnine has a postsynaptic blocking agent been found for a candidate amino acid transmitter. Even here the evidence reviewed above seems convincing that strychnine has an important presynaptic action as well.

In spite of or because of this state of relative ignorance, the outlook for the future treatment of convulsive disorders should be regarded with high optimism. This is because in addition to the types of anticonvulsant therapy now employed, there are so many potential pharmacological resources still untapped. An obvious partial listing, from the data reviewed above, could include drugs with useful degrees of stability and specificity that block excitatory or mimic inhibitory central transmitters; agents that promote or block transmitter release, through a cholinergic mechanism or otherwise; and compounds that inhibit the metabolic destruction of inhibitory transmitters. Every effort should certainly be made to exploit these potentialities. The recent promising advance in the treatment of parkinsonism, mentioned earlier, is a concrete example of what can be accomplished therapeutically by a basic pharmacological approach to diseases of the nervous system.

REFERENCES

1. Abrahams, V. C., Koelle, G. B., and Smart, P. Histochemical demonstration of cholinesterases in the hypothalamus of the dog. *J. Physiol.* (London) 139:137, 1957.
2. Adrian, E. D., and Matthews, R. The action of light on the eye. Part III. The interaction of retinal neurones. *J. Physiol.* (London) 65:273, 1928.
3. Alving, B. O. The action of strychnine at cholinergic junctions. *Arch. Int. Pharmacodyn.* 131:123, 1961.
4. Ames, A., III, and Pollen, D. A. Neurotransmission in central nervous tissue: a study of isolated rabbit retina. *J. Neurophysiol.* 32:424, 1969.
5. Andén, N.-E., Dahlström, A., Fuxe, K., and Larsson, K. Further evidence for the presence of nigro-neostriatal dopamine neurons in the rat. *Amer. J. Anat.* 116:329, 1965.
6. Andén, N.-E., Roos, B.-E., and Werdinius, B. Effects of chlorpromazine, haloperidol and reserpine on the levels of phenolic acids in rabbit corpus striatum. *Life Sci.* 3:149, 1964.
7. Andersson-Cedergren, E. Ultrastructure of motor end plate and sarcoplasmic components of mouse skeletal muscle fiber. *J. Ultrastruct. Res.* Suppl. 1, 1959.
8. Axelrod, J. The Formation, Metabolism, Uptake and Release of Noradrenaline and Adrenaline. In Varley, H., and Gowenlock, A. H. (Eds.), *The Clinical Chemistry of Monoamines*. Amsterdam: Elsevier, 1963.
9. Bennett, M. V. L., Aljure, E., Nakajima, Y., and Pappas, G. D. Electronic junctions between teleost spinal neurons: Electrophysiology and ultrastructure. *Science* 141:262, 1963.
10. Bertler, Å. Occurrence and localization of catechol amines in the human brain. *Acta Physiol. Scand.* 51:97, 1961.
11. Bertler, Å., and Rosengren, E. Occurrence and distribution of dopamine in brain and other tissues. *Experientia* 15:10, 1959.
12. Birkmayer, W., and Hornykiewicz, O. Der L-3,4-Dioxyphenylalanin (=DOPA)-Effekt bei der Parkinson-Akinese. *Wien. Klin. Wschr.* 73:787, 1961.
13. Braunwald, E., Chidsey, C. A., Harrison, D. C., Gaffney, T. E., and Kahler, R. L. Studies on the function of adrenergic nerve endings in the heart. *Circulation* 28:958, 1963.
14. Brodie, B. B. Recent views on mechanisms for lowering sympathetic tone. *Circulation* 28:970, 1963.
15. Brodie, B. B., Spector, S., and Shore, P. A. Interaction of drugs with norepinephrine in the brain. *Pharmacol. Rev.* 11:548, 1959.
16. Brown, D. A. Effects of preganglionic denervation on the sensitivity of sympathetic ganglion cells to stimulant compounds. *J. Physiol.* (London) 196:117P, 1968.
17. Burgen, A. S. V., and Chipman, L. M. Cholinesterase and succinic dehydrogenase in the central nervous system of the dog. *J. Physiol.* (London) 114:296, 1951.
18. Burn, J. H., and Rand, M. J. Sympathetic postganglionic mechanism. *Nature* (London) 184:163, 1959.
19. Burn, J. H., and Rand, M. J. Acetylcholine in adrenergic transmission. *Ann. Rev. Pharmacol.* 5:163, 1965.
20. Carlsson, A. The occurrence, distribution and physiological role of catecholamines in the nervous system. *Pharmacol. Rev.* 11:490, 1959.
21. Carlsson, A., Hillarp, N.-Å., and Waldeck, B. Analysis of the Mg^{++}-ATP dependent storage mechanism in the amine granules of the adrenal medulla. *Acta Physiol. Scand.* Suppl. 215, 59:1, 1963.
22. Cauna, N., Naik, N. T., Leaming, D. B., and Alberti, P. The distribution of cholinesterases in the autonomic ganglia of man and of some mammals. *Bibl. Anat.* 2:90, 1961.
23. Cho, A. K., Haslett, W. L., and Jenden, D. J. The peripheral actions of oxotremorine, a metabolite of tremorine. *J. Pharmacol. Exp. Ther.* 138:249, 1962.
24. Churchill, J. A., Schuknecht, H. F., and Doran, R. Acetylcholinesterase activity in the cochlea. *Laryngoscope* 66:1, 1956.
25. Costa, E., Côté, L. J., and Yahr, M. D. (Eds.), *Biochemistry and Pharmacology of the Basal Ganglia*. Hewlett, N.Y.: Raven Press, 1966.
26. Cotzias, G. C., VanWoert, M. H., and Schiffer, L. M. Aromatic amino acids and modification of parkinsonism. *New Eng. J. Med.* 276:374, 1967.

27. Couteaux, R. Morphological and cytochemical observations on the post-synaptic membrane at motor end-plates and ganglionic synapses. *Exp. Cell Res.* Suppl. 5, 294, 1958.
28. Crawford, J. M., and Curtis, D. R. Pharmacological studies on feline Betz cells. *J. Physiol.* (London) 186:121, 1966.
29. Curtis, D. R. The pharmacology of central and peripheral inhibition. *Pharmacol. Rev.* 15:333, 1963.
30. Curtis, D. R. Acetylcholine, strychnine and spinal inhibition. *Nature* (London) 215:1503, 1967.
31. Curtis, D. R. Central Synaptic Transmitters. In Jasper, H. H., Ward, A. A., Jr., and Pope, A. (Eds.), *Basic Mechanisms of the Epilepsies.* Boston: Little, Brown, 1969.
32. Curtis, D. R., Hosli, L., and Johnston, G. A. R. Inhibition of spinal neurones by glycine. *Nature* (London) 215:1502, 1967.
33. Dahlström, A., and Fuxe, K. Evidence for the existence of monoamine-containing neurons in the central nervous system. I. Demonstration of monoamines in the cell bodies of brain stem neurons. *Acta Physiol. Scand.* Suppl. 232, 62:1, 1964.
34. Dahlström, A., and Fuxe, K. Evidence for the existence of monoamine-containing neurons in the central nervous system. II. Experimentally induced changes in the intraneuronal amine levels of bulbospinal neuron systems. *Acta Physiol. Scand.* Suppl. 247, 64:1, 1965.
35. Dale, H. H. Chemical transmission of the effects of nerve impulses. *Brit. Med. J.* 1:835, 1934.
36. Davis, R., and Koelle, G. B. Electron microscopic localization of acetylcholinesterase and nonspecific cholinesterase at the neuromuscular junction by the gold-thiolcholine and gold-thiolacetic acid methods. *J. Cell. Biol.* 34:157, 1967.
37. Dempsher, J., Larrabee, M. G., Bang, F. B., and Bodian, D. Physiological changes in sympathetic ganglia infected with pseudorabies virus. *Amer. J. Physiol.* 182:203, 1955.
38. Dempsher, J., and Riker, W. K. The role of acetylcholine in virus-infected sympathetic ganglia. *J. Physiol.* (London) 139: 145, 1957.
39. Desmedt, J. E., and Monaco, P. Mode of action of the efferent olivo-cochlear bundle on the inner ear. *Nature* (London) 192:1263, 1961.
40. Douglas, W. W., Lywood, D. W., and Straub, R. W. On the excitant effect of acetylcholine on structures in the preganglionic trunk of the cervical sympathetic: With a note on the anatomical complexities of the region. *J. Physiol.* (London) 153:250, 1960.
41. Dowling, J. E., and Boycott, B. B. Neural connections of the retina: Fine structure of the inner plexiform layer. *Cold Spring Harbor Symp. Quant. Biol.* 30:393, 1965.
42. Du Bois-Reymond, E. Gesammelte Abhandl. d. allgem. *Muskel und Nervenphysik* 2:700, 1877.
43. Eccles, J. C. *The Physiology of Synapses.* Berlin: Springer, 1964.
44. Eccles, J. C. Excitatory and Inhibitory Mechanisms in Brain. In Jasper, H. H., Ward, A. A., Jr., and Pope, A. (Eds.), *Basic Mechanisms of the Epilepsies.* Boston: Little, Brown, 1969.
45. Eccles, J. C. Central cholinergic transmission and its behavioral aspects. Historical introduction. *Fed. Proc.* 28:90, 1969.
46. Eccles, J. C., Fatt, P., and Koketsu, K. Cholinergic and inhibitory synapses in a pathway from motor-axon collaterals to motoneurones. *J. Physiol.* (London) 126: 524, 1954.
47. Ehringer, H., and Hornykiewicz, O. Verteilung von Noradrenalin und Dopamin (3-Hydroxytyramin) im Gehirn des Menschen und ihr Verhalten bei Erkrankungen des Extrapyramidalen Systems. *Klin. Wschr.* 38:1236, 1960.
48. Elfvin, L.-G. The ultrastructure of the superior cervical sympathetic ganglion of the cat. II. The structure of the preganglionic end fibers and the synapses as studied by serial sections. *J. Ultrastruct. Res.* 8:441, 1963.
49. Elliot, T. R. The action of adrenalin. *J. Physiol.* (London) 32:401, 1905.
50. Eränkö, O. The histochemistry of the adrenal medulla of the rat, with special reference to acid phosphatase. *Acta Anat.* (Basel) Suppl. 17, 16:1, 1952.
51. Erulkar, S. D., Nichols, C. W., Popp, M. B., and Koelle, G. B. Renshaw elements: Localization and acetylcholinesterase content. *J. Histochem. Cytochem.* 16:128, 1968.
52. Esplin, D. W., and Zablocka-Esplin, B. Mechanisms of Action of Convulsants. In

Jasper, H. H., Ward, A. A., Jr., and Pope, A. (Eds.), *Basic Mechanisms of the Epilepsies*. Boston: Little, Brown, 1969.

53. Esplin, D. W., and Zablocka, B. Central Nervous System Stimulants. In Goodman, L. S., and Gilman, A. (Eds.), *The Pharmacological Basis of Therapeutics*. New York: Macmillan, 1965, pp. 346–347.

54. Euler, U. S. von. Neurotransmission in the adrenergic nervous system. *Harvey Lect.* 55:43, 1959–1960.

55. Everett, G. M., Blockus, L. E., and Shepperd, I. M. Tremor induced by tremorine and its antagonism by anti-Parkinson drugs. *Science* 124:79, 1956.

56. Falck, B. Observations on the possibilities of the cellular localization of monoamines with a fluorescence method. *Acta Physiol. Scand.* Suppl. 197, 56:1, 1962.

57. Feldberg, W., and Vartiainen, A. Further observations on the physiology and pharmacology of a sympathetic ganglion. *J. Physiol.* (London) 83:103, 1934.

58. Feldberg, W., and Vogt, M. Acetylcholine synthesis in different regions of the central nervous system. *J. Physiol.* (London) 107:372, 1948.

59. Ferry, C. B. Cholinergic link hypothesis in adrenergic neuroeffector transmission. *Physiol. Rev.* 46:420, 1966.

60. Fex, J. Augmentation of cochlear microphonic by stimulation of efferent fibers to cochlea: Preliminary reports. *Acta Otolaryng.* (Stockholm) 50:540, 1959.

61. Furshpan, E. J., and Potter, D. D. Transmission of the giant motor synapses of the crayfish. *J. Physiol.* (London) 145:289, 1959.

62. Galambos, R. Suppression of auditory nerve activity by stimulation of efferent fibers to cochlea. *J. Neurophysiol.* 19:424, 1956.

63. Gerschenfeld, H. M. A non-cholinergic synaptic inhibition in the central nervous system of a mollusc. *Nature* (London) 203:415, 1964.

64. Goodman, L. S., and Gilman, A. (Eds.). *The Pharmacological Basis of Therapeutics* (3d ed.). New York: Macmillan, 1965, p. 424.

65. Granit, R. Some properties of post-excitatory inhibition, studied in the optic nerve with micro-electrodes. *Arkiv. Zool.* 36A:1, 1945.

66. Green, R. D. The sensitivity of the denervated superior cervical ganglion (SCG) to nicotinic and muscarinic stimulants. *Pharmacologist* 10:216, 1968.

67. Hebb, C. O., Krnjević, K., and Silver, A. Effect of undercutting on the acetyltransferase activity in the cat's cerebral cortex. *Nature* (London) 198:692, 1963.

68. Hilding, D., and Wersäll, J. Cholinesterase and its relation to the nerve endings in the inner ear. *Acta Otolaryng.* (Stockholm) 55:205, 1962.

69. Hillarp, N.-Å., Fuxe, K., and Dahlström, A. Demonstration and mapping of central neurons containing dopamine, noradrenaline, and 5-hydroxytryptamine and their reactions to psychopharmaca. *Pharmacol. Rev.* 18:727, 1966.

70. Hornykiewicz, O. Metabolism of Brain Dopamine in Human Parkinsonism: Neurochemical and Clinical Aspects. In Costa, E., Côté, L. J., and Yahr, M. D. (Eds.), *Biochemistry and Pharmacology of the Basal Ganglia*. Hewlett, N.Y.: Raven Press, 1966, p. 171.

71. Jacobowitz, D., Johnson, P., Kitchner, I., and Koelle, G. B. The effect of hemicholinium (HC-3) on sympathetic transmission at the nictitating membrane of the rabbit. *Brit. J. Pharmacol.* 25:527, 1965.

72. Jacobowitz, D., and Koelle, G. B. Histochemical correlations of acetylcholinesterase and catecholamines in postganglionic autonomic nerves of the cat, rabbit, and guinea pig. *J. Pharmacol. Exp. Ther.* 148:225, 1965.

73. Kerkut, G. A., and Walker, R. J. The specific chemical sensitivity of *Helix* nerve cells. *Comp. Biochem. Physiol.* 7:277, 1962.

74. Kirshner, N. Uptake of catecholamines by a particulate fraction of the adrenal medulla. *J. Biol. Chem.* 237:2311, 1962.

75. Koelle, G. B. The histochemical localization of cholinesterases in the central nervous system of the rat. *J. Comp. Neurol.* 100:211, 1954.

76. Koelle, G. B. The histochemical identification of acetylcholinesterase in cholinergic, adrenergic and sensory neurons. *J. Pharmacol. Exp. Ther.* 114:167, 1955.

77. Koelle, G. B. Histochemical demonstration of reversible anticholinesterase action at selective cellular sites *in vivo*. *J. Pharmacol. Exp. Ther.* 120:488, 1957.

78. Koelle, G. B. A proposed dual neurohumoral role of acetylcholine: Its func-

tions at the pre- and post-synaptic sites. *Nature* (London) 190:208, 1961.

79. Koelle, G. B. A new general concept of the neurohumoral functions of acetylcholine and acetylcholinesterase. *J. Pharm. Pharmacol.* 14:65, 1962.

80. Koelle, G. B. Cytological Distributions and Physiological Functions of Cholinesterases. In Koelle, G. B. (Ed.), *Cholinesterases and Anticholinesterase Agents.* Berlin: Springer, 1963, pp. 187–298.

81. Koelle, G. B. Functional anatomy of synaptic transmission. *Anesthesiology* 29:643, 1968.

82. Koelle, G. B. Significance of acetylcholinesterase in central synaptic transmission. *Fed. Proc.* 28:95, 1969.

83. Koelle, G. B., Friedenwald, J. S., Wolfand, L. and Allen, R. A. Localization of specific cholinesterase in ocular tissues of the cat. *Amer. J. Ophthal.* 35:1580, 1952.

84. Koelle, G. B., and Geesey, C. N. Localization of acetylcholinesterase in the neurohypophysis and its functional implications. *Proc. Soc. Exp. Biol. Med.* 106:625, 1961.

85. Koelle, G. B., and Steiner, E. C. The cerebral distributions of a tertiary and a quaternary anticholinesterase agent following intravenous and intraventricular injection. *J. Pharmacol. Exp. Ther.* 118:420, 1956.

86. Koelle, W. A., and Koelle, G. B. The localization of external or functional acetylcholinesterase at the synapses of autonomic ganglia. *J. Pharmacol. Exp. Ther.* 126:1, 1959.

87. Koketsu, K. Action of tetraethylammonium chloride on neuromuscular transmission in frogs. *Amer. J. Physiol.* 193:213, 1958.

88. Koketsu, K., and Nishi, S. Cholinergic receptors at sympathetic preganglionic nerve terminals. *J. Physiol.* (London) 196:293, 1968.

89. Krnjević, K. Neurotransmitters in Normal and Isolated Cortex. In Jasper, H. H., Ward, A. A., Jr., and Pope, A. (Eds.), *Basic Mechanisms of the Epilepsies.* Boston: Little, Brown, 1969.

90. Lanari, A., and Luco, J. V. The depressant action of strychnine on the superior cervical sympathetic ganglion and on skeletal muscle. *Amer. J. Physiol.* 126:277, 1939.

91. Langley, J. N., and Kato, T. The physiological action of physostigmine and its action on denervated skeletal muscle. *J. Physiol.* (London) 49:410, 1915.

92. Lloyd, D. P. C. Cholinergy and Adrenergy in the Neural Control of Sweat Glands. In Curtis, D. R., and McIntyre, A. K. (Eds.), *Studies in Physiology. Presented to John C. Eccles.* New York: Springer, 1965, pp. 169–178.

93. Löewi, O. Über humorale Übertragbarkeit der Herznervenwirkung. *Pflueger Arch. Ges. Physiol.* 189:239, 1921.

94. MacIntosh, F. C. The distribution of acetylcholine in the peripheral and central nervous system. *J. Physiol.* (London) 99:436, 1941.

95. Martin, A. R., and Pilar, G. Transmission through the ciliary ganglion of the chick. *J. Physiol.* (London) 168:464, 1963.

96. Martin, W. R., Riehl, J. L., and Unna, K. R. Chlorpromazine. III. The effects of chlorpromazine and chlorpromazine sulfoxide on vascular responses to L-epinephrine and levarterenol. *J. Pharmacol. Exp. Ther.* 130:37, 1960.

97. Masland, R. L., and Wigton, R. S. Nerve activity accompanying fasciculation produced by prostigmin. *J. Neurophysiol.* 3:269, 1940.

98. Matsumura, M., and Koelle, G. B. The nature of synaptic transmission in the superior cervical ganglion following reinnervation by the afferent vagus. *J. Pharmacol. Exp. Ther.* 134:28, 1961.

99. McIsaac, R. J., and Koelle, G. B. Comparison of the effects of inhibition of external, internal, and total acetylcholinesterase upon ganglionic transmission. *J. Pharmacol. Exp. Ther.* 126:9, 1959.

100. McKinstry, D. N. Effects of drugs on carbachol-induced ganglionic ACh-release. *Fed. Proc.* 24:711, 1965.

101. McKinstry, D. N., and Koelle, G. B. Acetylcholine release from the cat superior cervical ganglion by carbachol. *J. Pharmacol. Exp. Ther.* 157:319, 1967.

102. McKinstry, D. N., and Koelle, G. B. Effects of drugs on acetylcholine release from the cat superior cervical ganglion by carbachol and by preganglionic stimulation. *J. Pharmacol. Exp. Ther.* 157:328, 1967.

103. Nichols, C. W., and Koelle, G. B. Comparison of the localization of acetylcholinesterase and non-specific cholinesterase activities in mammalian and avian retinas. *J. Comp. Neurol.* 133:1, 1968.

104. Ogston, A. G. Removal of acetylcholine from a limited volume by diffusion. *J. Physiol.* (London) 128:222, 1955.

105. Perry, W. L. M. Transmission in autonomic ganglia. *Brit. Med. J.* 13:220, 1957.

106. Phillis, J. W., and York, D. H. Cholinergic inhibition in the cerebral cortex. *Brain Res.* 5:517, 1967.

107. Phillis, J. W., and York, D. H. Strychnine block of neural and drug-induced inhibition in the cerebral cortex. *Nature* (London) 216:922, 1967.

108. Polyak, S. L. *The Retina*. Chicago: University of Chicago Press, 1941.

109. Ramón y Cajal, S. La rétine des vertébrés. *Cellule* 9:121, 1893.

110. Randić, M., Siminoff, R., and Straughan, D. W. Acetylcholine depression of cortical neurones. *Exp. Neurol.* 9:236, 1964.

111. Rasmussen, G. L. The olivary peduncle and other fiber projections of the superior olivary complex. *J. Comp. Neurol.* 84:141, 1946.

112. Rasmussen, G. L. Anatomic Relationships of the Ascending and Descending Auditory Systems. In Fields, W. S., and Alford, B. R. (Eds.), *Neurological Aspects of Auditory and Vestibular Disorders*. Springfield, Ill.: Thomas, 1964, pp. 1–19.

113. Renshaw, R. R., Green, D., and Ziff, M. A basis for the acetylcholine action of choline derivatives. *J. Pharmacol. Exp. Ther.* 62:430, 1938.

114. Riker, W. F., Jr. Actions of acetylcholine on mammalian motor nerve terminal. *J. Pharmacol. Exp. Ther.* 152:397, 1966.

115. Riker, W. F., Jr., Roberts, J., Standaert, F. G., and Fujimori, H. The motor nerve terminal as the primary focus for drug-induced facilitation of neuromuscular transmission. *J. Pharmacol. Exp. Ther.* 121:286, 1957.

116. Rossi, G., and Cottesina, G. The "efferent cochlear and vestibular system" in *Lepus cuniculus, L. Acta Anat.* (Basel) 60:362, 1965.

117. Schuknecht, H. F., Churchill, J. A., and Doran, R. The localization of acetylcholinesterase in the cochlea. *Arch. Otolaryng.* (Chicago) 69:549, 1959.

118. Sharpless, S. K. Isolated and Deafferented Neurons: Disuse Supersensitivity. In Jasper, H. H., Ward, A. A., Jr., and Pope, A. (Eds.), *Basic Mechanisms of the Epilepsies*. Boston: Little, Brown, 1969.

119. Shen, S. C., Greenfield, P., and Boell, E. J. The distribution of cholinesterase in the frog brain. *J. Comp. Neurol.* 102:717, 1955.

120. Shute, C. C. D., and Lewis, P. R. Cholinesterase-containing pathways of the hindbrain afferent cerebellar and centrifugal cochlear fibres. *Nature* (London) 205:242, 1965.

121. Shute, C. C. D., and Lewis, P. R. The ascending cholinergic reticular system: Neocortical, olfactory and subcortical projections. *Brain* 90:497, 1967.

122. Silver, A. Cholinesterases of the central nervous system with special reference to the cerebellum. *Int. Rev. Neurobiol.* 10:57, 1967.

123. Sourkes, T. L., and Poirier, L. J. Neurochemical bases of tremor and other disorders of movement. *Canad. Med. Ass. J.* 94:53, 1966.

124. Takagi, K., and Takayanagi, I. Effects of strychnine, derivatives of phenyl acetate and catecholamines on contraction and acetylcholine output from the cholinergic nerve ending of guinea pig ileum. *Jap. J. Pharmacol.* 16:211, 1966.

125. Tanaka, Y., and Katsuki, Y. Pharmacological investigations of cochlear responses and of olivocochlear inhibition. *J. Neurophysiol.* 29:94, 1966.

126. Thesleff, S. The effects of acetylcholine, decamethonium and succinylcholine on neuromuscular transmission in the rat *Acta Physiol. Scand.* 34:386, 1955.

127. Thesleff, S. Effects of motor innervation on the chemical sensitivity of skeletal muscle. *Physiol. Rev.* 40:734, 1960.

128. Thomas, R. C., and Wilson, V. J. Precise localization of Renshaw cells with a new marking technique. *Nature* (London) 206: 211, 1965.

129. Toman, J. E. P. Further Observations on Diphenylhydantoin. In Jasper, H. H., Ward, A. A., Jr., and Pope, A. (Eds.), *Basic Mechanisms of the Epilepsies*. Boston: Little, Brown, 1969.

130. Trendelenburg, U. Modification of the effect of tyramine by various agents and procedures. *J. Pharmacol. Exp. Ther.* 134:8, 1961.

131. Van Rossum, J. M. The significance of dopamine receptor blockade for the mechanism of action of neuroleptic drugs. *Arch. Int. Pharmacodyn.* 160:492, 1966.

132. Vinnikov, A., and Titova, L. K. Presence and distribution of acetylcholinesterase in the organ of Corti in animals who are in a state of relative rest, and under the conditions of acoustic effect (in Russian). *Dokl. Akad. Nauk. SSSR* 119:164, 1958.

133. Volle, R. L. Muscarinic and Nicotinic Stimulant Actions at Autonomic Ganglia. In Karczmar, A. G. (Ed.), *International Encyclopedia of Pharmacology and Therapeutics.* sec. 12, vol. 1. New York: Pergamon, 1966.

134. Volle, R. L., and Koelle, G. B. The physiological role of acetylcholinesterase (AChE) in sympathetic ganglia. *J. Pharmacol. Exp. Ther.* 133:223, 1961.

135. Weight, F. F. Cholinergic Mechanisms in Recurrent Inhibition of Motoneurons. In Efron, D. H. (Ed.), *Psychopharmacology. A Review of Progress, 1957–1967.* Washington, D. C.: Public Health Service Publication no. 1836, 1968, pp. 69–75.

136. Werman, R., Davidoff, R. A., and Aprison, M. H. Inhibitory action of glycine on spinal neurons in the cat. *J. Neurophysiol.* 31:81, 1968.

137. Werner, G. Generation of antidromic activity in motor nerves. *J. Neurophysiol.* 23:453, 1960.

138. Woodbury, D. M. Mechanisms of Action of Anticonvulsants. In Jasper, H. H., Ward, A. A., Jr., and Pope, A., (Eds.), *Basic Mechanisms of the Epilepsies.* Boston: Little, Brown, 1969.

Discussion

FLUORESCENCE HISTOCHEMISTRY OF MONOAMINES IN THE CNS

A. DAHLSTRÖM

As indicated by Curtis and also mentioned by Koelle, there is little doubt that norepinephrine (NE) and dopamine (DA) are neurohumoral transmitters in the CNS. With the introduction of the histochemical fluorescence method of Hillarp, Falck, and co-workers (see [29]), it was found that NE and DA in the CNS were localized within the perikarya, axons, and nerve terminals of special neurons. It was also found that 5-hydroxytryptamine (5-HT) was localized in the same way within special neurons, and that nerve terminals of these neurons had about the same appearance as those of neurons containing NE or DA. Since it was also found that the 5-HT neurons react pharmacologically much the same way as do the catecholamine (CA) neurons and since it has been possible to release 5-HT from nerve terminals by stimulating the brain areas containing the nerve cell bodies [36], the transmitter action of 5-HT in the CNS appears rather well established.

Morphology of Monoamine (MA) Neurons

Due to the intraneuronal presence and distribution of the respective amines, it has been possible to obtain information on the morphology of these neurons with help of the histochemical formaldehyde fluorescence method for cellular localization of CA and 5-HT [21]. The fluorescent reaction products of NE-formaldehyde and DA-formaldehyde are both green, while the fluorescent product of 5-HT-formaldehyde is greenish yellow to yellow with the filter combinations used [33]. Hence, the CA neurons can be distinguished from the 5-HT neurons, whereas pharmacological methods have so far been necessary in order to distinguish the DA from the NE neurons [33, 34, 52].

In the fluorescence microscope it has been found that these neurons consist of small- to medium-sized cell bodies (20–40 μ in diameter) with several processes (Fig. D8-1). The axons are very thin and unmyelinated (0.2–2 μ in diameter). When axons have reached the areas to be innervated, they branch to form widespread networks of nerve terminals. These nerve terminals are built up of so-called varicosities (0.5–2 μ in diameter) separated by much thinner interparts (Figs. D8-2, D8-3).

Several attempts have been undertaken to identify by electron microscope the neurons containing the CA and 5-HT. In the peripheral sympathetic nervous system a small type of dense-cored vesicle (diam. 400–500 Å) has been found [62, 74, 76]. In order to observe this type of vesicle in the CNS, a special fixation method using potassium permanganate ($KMnO_4$) must be used [75, 91]. Recent studies by Hökfelt [76, 77] have shown good correlation between occurrence of boutons containing these small granular vesicles and distribution of fluorescent MA nerve terminals (Fig. D8-4). This author also demonstrated correlation between presence or absence of the electron dense core and the tissue levels of MA after pharmacological treatment, indicating that the small granular vesicles also in the CNS may represent the main type of storage site of CA and 5-HT. With this fixation technique it has been demonstrated that MA nerve cell bodies contain a low to medium density of small dense-cored vesicles, while the nerve terminals contain high density vesicles [77, 78]. This is in accordance with the intraneuronal MA distribution within these neurons which will be mentioned.

Another type of vesicle, the large dense-cored vesicle (diam. about 1000 Å) has also been observed. By the use of glutaralde-

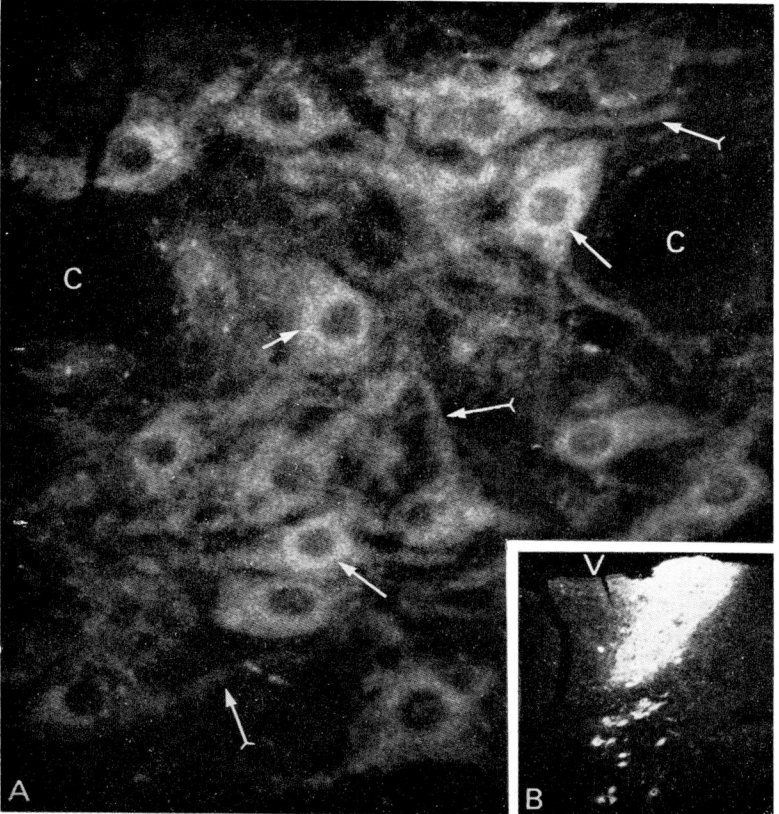

FIG. D8-1. NE-containing nerve cell bodies in locus ceruleus (Group A6 of [33]) of normal rat. (A) Transverse section through the periphery of this nucleus. The cells are often multipolar, and the green fluorescence (reaction product of NE-formaldehyde) in the cytoplasm is accumulated in a zone around the nonfluorescent nucleus (→). The fluorescent processes are indicated (↠). Two small transversely cut vessels are seen (C). ×460 (B) Transverse section, showing the closely packed nerve cells in the floor of the fourth ventricle (V). ×40. (Dahlström and Fuxe, unpublished material.)

hyde-osmium fixation, it was first thought to be the storage site of brain MA. Contradictory results on the effect of MA depleting or increasing treatment on the dense core of those vesicles have been reported [16, 77].

In a recent study by Bloom and Aghajanian [16], the problem was reinvestigated; it was found that large, dense, semidense, and lucent vesicles were more numerous in areas of the brain containing high amounts of NE and 5-HT nerve terminals. However, pharmacological manipulations did not obviously influence the dense core of these vesicles, and it was suggested by these authors that the large vesicles may be a type of organelle, important in MA neurons but not necessarily involved in the storage of amines. However, recent studies by Hökfelt [77] using the $KMnO_4$ fixation technique indicate that the large granular vesicles may also take part in NE and 5-HT storage in the CNS, although the main storage site is presumably represented by the small granular vesicles, as already pointed out.

INTRANEURONAL DISTRIBUTION OF MA

The intraneuronal distribution of the NE and DA, respectively, appears rather similar to that found in the peripheral sympathetic adrenergic neuron [31, 37, 40].

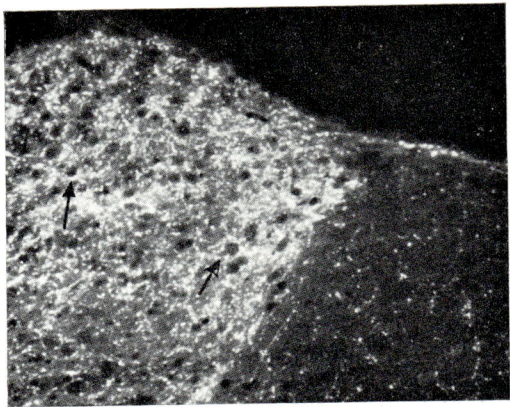

Fig. D8-2. N. motorius dorsalis n. vagi (left) and n. hypoglossus (right) of normal rat. The former nucleus has a dense innervation of strongly green fluorescent nerve terminals, while the n. hypoglossus has a rather low density. Especially in the vagus nucleus it is often seen how nonfluorescent nerve cell bodies are surrounded by green fluorescent nerve terminals (→). ×170 before 18 percent reduction. (Dahlström and Fuxe, unpublished material.)

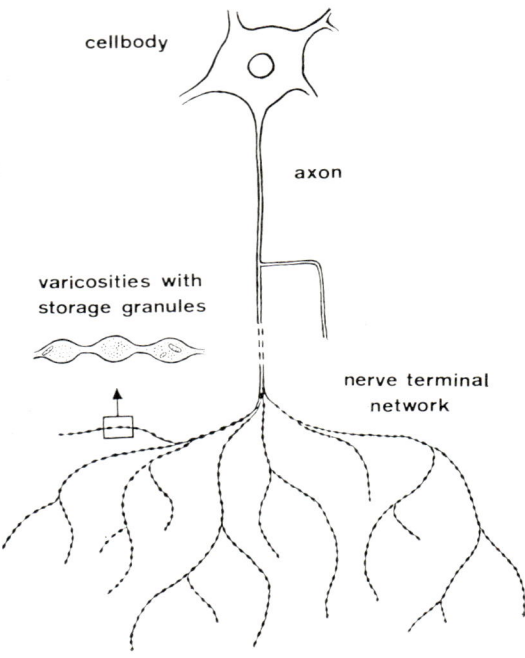

Fig. D8-3. Schematic illustration of the morphology of a MA neuron in the CNS as shown with the fluorescence microscope. The proposed axon collateral has not been directly observed, but some data indicate the existence of such collaterals, (cf. [10]).

Quantitative studies in the CNS have been undertaken so far only on the DA neurons in the nigro-neostriatal DA system [9]. It was calculated that nerve cell bodies contain 0.8–2.5 picograms (pg) (10^{-12} gm) of DA and that the concentration in the cytoplasm was around 60–200 µg per gram wet weight (ww), probably being the same in the axoplasm of the nonterminal axons. Varicosities of the DA nerve terminals in the neostriatum were calculated to contain on the average 2.5×10^{-4} pg of DA, corresponding to a concentration of about 8000 µg per gm ww. The summarized lengths of the terminal arborizations of each neuron in this very densely innervated nucleus was calculated by these authors to be 55–77 cm including on the average 500,000 varicosities per neuron [9].

As for the NE-containing neurons in the CNS, the intraneuronal transmitter distribution seems, as judged from histochemical observations, to be similar to the peripheral NE neuron. Concentration in the cell bodies and axons may be on the order of 10–100 µg per gm ww, and in the nerve terminal varicosities on the order of 1000–3000 µg per gm ww [37, 40]. On the basis of these figures together with quantitative studies on the NE content in the spinal cord [66], it may be suggested that the length of the NE terminals per descending neuron is less than that of the neostriatal DA terminals, approximately 2–10 cm per neuron.

The 5-HT neuron is more difficult to study than the CA neurons, mainly due to high photosensitivity of the 5-HT-paraformaldehyde reaction product. Since varicosities seem to be of very different sizes (mainly large in the spinal cord and mainly rather small in the rest of the CNS), this also adds to difficulties of observing them in certain areas of the brain. It may be mentioned that in normal animals the intraneuronal concentration of 5-HT is probably smaller than the intraneuronal concentration of CA in CA neurons,

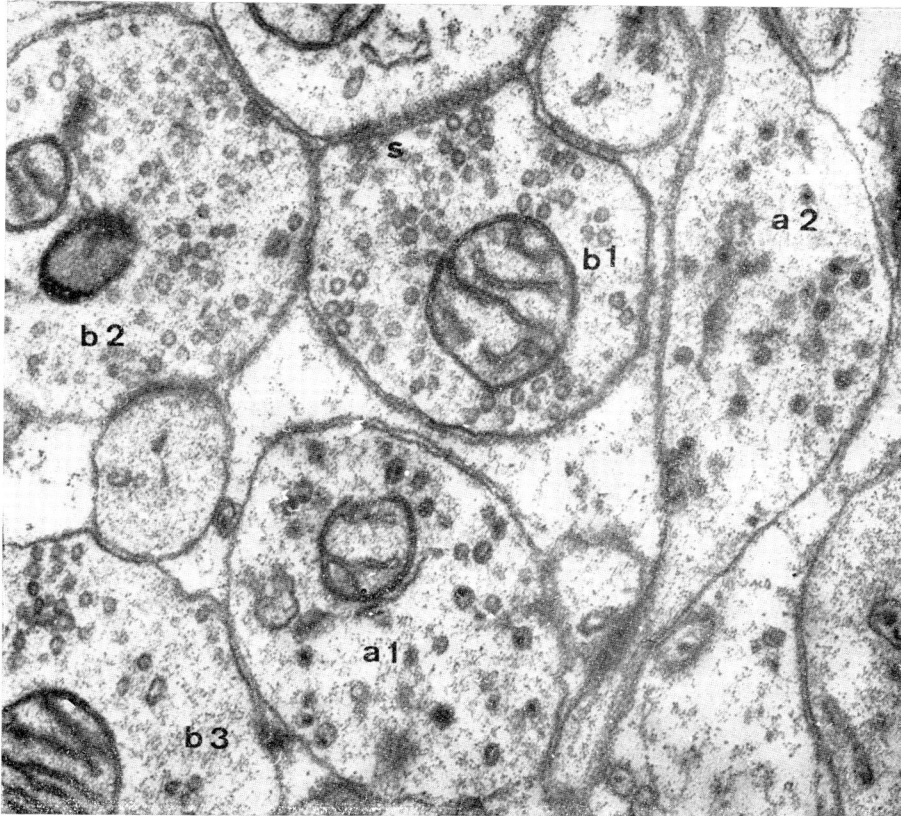

Fig. D8-4. Locus ceruleus of rat. A number of boutons are seen. Small granular vesicles are seen in two boutons (a_1 and a_2), one of which (a_2) probably represents a so-called bouton en passage. The other boutons (b_1, b_2, and b_3) contain agranular vesicles. Bouton b_1 probably makes synaptic contact(s) to a dendrite. × 50,000. (From Hökfelt [75].)

Distribution of MA Neurons

Almost all the MA nerve cell bodies have been found in the lower brain stem [33]. The only known exceptions are the DA neurons in the arcuate nucleus in the ventral hypothalamus [33, 50] and the DA neurons in the retina [67]. It can generally be said that the CA neurons occupy lateral positions, while the 5-HT nerve cell bodies are mainly found within the different raphe nuclei (Figs. D8-5, D8-7) [33]. The NE cell bodies are mainly found in the pons and medulla oblongata, while the DA cells bodies are located in the mesencephalon, especially in the substantia nigra area (Fig. D8-6). The MA cell bodies are usually scattered, seldom forming a well-defined nucleus. However, the NE cell bodies in the locus ceruleus are closely concentrated (Fig. D8-1) and may be suitable for electrophysiological studies. To a certain degree this is also the case for 5-HT cell bodies in some of the raphe nuclei, for example, the nucleus medianus raphe and nucleus dorsalis raphe (Fig. D8-7).

While the cell bodies are found in rather restricted areas, the MA nerve terminals are found in all parts of the brain, from spinal cord [22, 34] to cerebral cortex, in varying concentrations. It is, in fact, easier to enumerate areas devoid of MA innervation than innervated areas. Some areas devoid of both CA and 5-HT nerve terminals are: the olivary complex, the nucleus of the trapezoid body, the nucleus ruber, and the subthalamic nucleus. 5-HT nerve

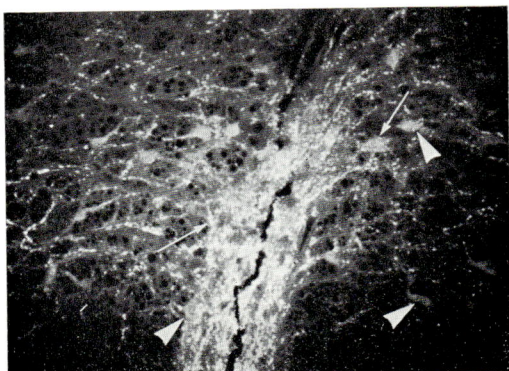

Fig. D8-5. Transverse section through the n. raphe pallidus of rat treated with nialamide (500 mg per kg, 3 hr, intraperitoneally). A large number of rather closely packed, strongly yellow fluorescent 5-HT nerve cells (▶) (Group B1 in [33]) are observed, surrounded by green fluorescent NE nerve terminals (→). The nialamide (MAO inhibitor) treatment was performed in order to increase the intraneuronal 5-HT levels and thereby make the neuron more visible. ×250. (Dahlström and Fuxe, unpublished material.)

terminals appear to be present in most areas receiving CA terminals except for the cerebellum, which contains very little 5-HT. One nucleus receiving 5-HT terminals only has been found in the rat, namely, the suprachiasmatic nucleus in the ventral hypothalamus. Some areas are very densely innervated by MA terminals; some cranial nerve nuclei in the lower brain stem (Fig.

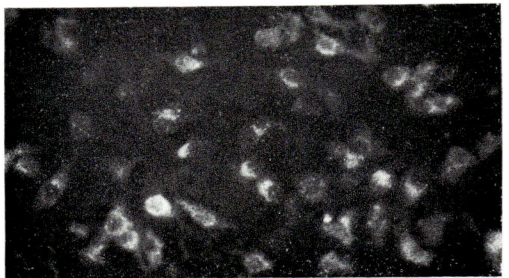

Fig. D8-6. Green fluorescent DA nerve cells in the mesencephalon of normal rat (Group A9 in [33]). Transverse section. Small to medium sized cell bodies, oval or round, can be seen in the substantia nigra. ×180 before 23% reduction. (Dahlström and Fuxe, unpublished material.)

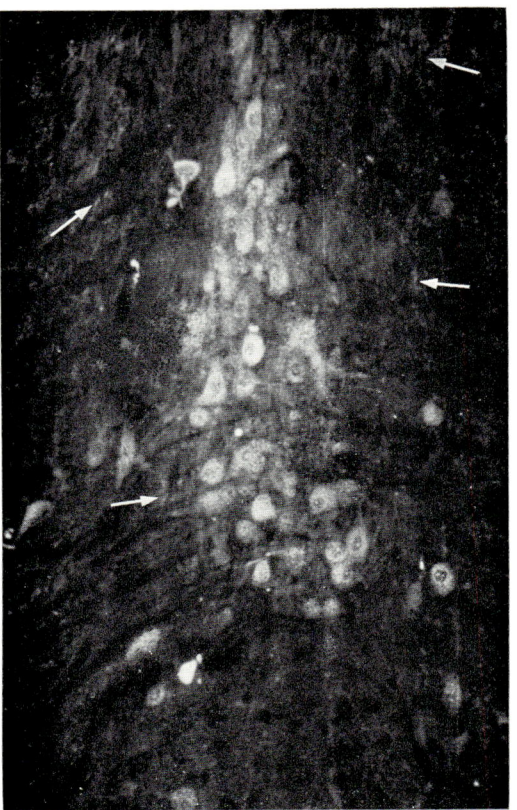

Fig. D8-7. Yellow fluorescent 5-HT nerve cells in the n. raphe medianus (Group B8 in [33]) of nialamide-treated rat pretreated with reserpine. By reserpine treatment all MA are depleted, and the subsequent MAO inhibition causes a strong increase of 5-HT in 5-HT neurons, while the effect on CA neurons is much less. Thus, in this animal only 5-HT neurons are visualized. Transverse section. A large number of small to medium sized round to oval cells of medium to strong yellow fluorescence intensity are found close together. A large number of ascending 5-HT axons, cut transversely and obliquely, can be seen (→). ×170. (Dahlström and Fuxe, unpublished material.)

D8-2) and some areas especially in the ventral hypothalamus. The hippocampal cortex and neocortex receive scattered NE and 5-HT terminals of medium to low density found in all layers (Figs. D8-8, D8-9) [54]. For detailed description of MA nerve terminal distribution see [51, 52].

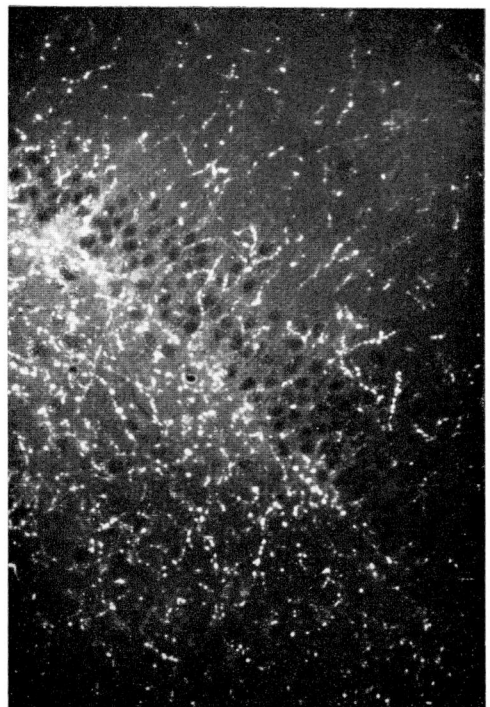 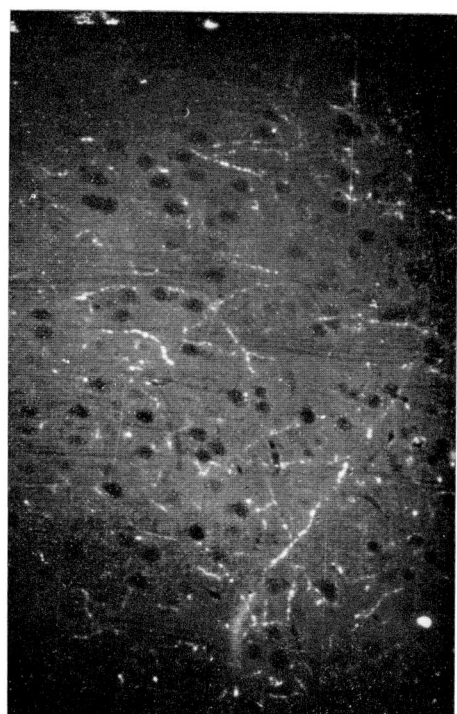

FIG. D8-8. NE nerve terminals in the gyrus dentatus of normal rat. Cross section. A dense plexus of strongly fluorescent NE terminals is seen in the hilus fasciae dentati, while the molecular layer is less dense, and the granular layer contains the lowest density of terminals. ×200. (Blackstad, Fuxe, and Hökfelt, unpublished material.)

FIG. D8-9. NE nerve terminals in the gyrus precentralis of normal rat. Cross section. A scarce network of nerve terminals can be seen all through the cortex. Upper surface at the top of the figure. ×200. (Fuxe, Hamberger, and Hökfelt, unpublished material.)

Mapping Out of Central MA Neuron Systems

The MA-containing nerve cell bodies in the CNS are situated mainly in the lower brain stem and give rise to the NE, DA, and 5-HT terminals in the whole brain and spinal cord. The mapping out of these neuron systems has been done by combining the technique of brain lesions with fluorescent histochemistry and bioassay [6, 7, 8, 10, 72]. Three different types of lesions can be used for the procedure.

(A) The cell bodies can be destroyed. This results in a complete degeneration and disappearance of the nerve terminals belonging to the group of cell bodies destroyed.

(B) The axons can be destroyed. In the CNS three phenomena may be observed after axotomy in MA-containing neurons: (1) accumulations of the transmitter substance in enlarged axons proximal to the lesion [32, 34]; (2) disappearance of nerve terminals distal to the lesion within 7–10 days (see also [71]); (3) retrograde cell body changes, observed as increased fluorescent intensity, a swollen appearance, and often a displaced nucleus [6], occurring after 1–2 days.

(C) Removal of terminal areas by suction or lesion techniques. This results in (1) accumulations of the transmitter substance in the afferent axons and (2) retrograde cell body changes.

By making series of lesions according to this scheme and observing the mentioned phenomena, a gross outline of the MA neuron systems in the CNS has been obtained [7] (Fig. D8-10). Thus, it was found

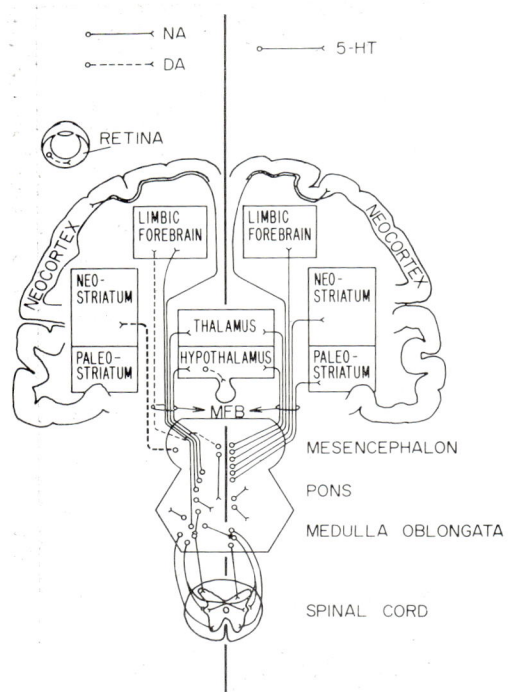

FIG. D8-10. Schematic drawing showing in highly simplified form the main MA neuron systems in the CNS. (From [7].)

that most NE and 5-HT cell bodies in the medulla oblongata send axons down to the spinal cord. Most of the NE and 5-HT cell bodies in the pons and a few in the medulla oblongata send ascending axons, which pass in and close to the median forebrain bundle (MFB) to innervate the hypothalamus, thalamus, limbic forebrain, and neocortex [7, 10, 72]. The 5-HT neurons from these areas also seem to innervate neostriatum and paleostriatum. The fibers to the neocortex ascend from the MFB dorsally into the tractus diagonalis. They then turn caudally to pass in this direction mainly within the outer parts of the white matter and probably also partly within the grey matter, sending up terminals into the cortex.

The DA cell bodies in the mesencephalon send a few fibers down to the pons and the medulla oblongata, but the majority of fibers ascend just lateral to the MFB to innervate the limbic forebrain and the neostriatum. Nerve cell bodies of terminals innervating the neostriatum are found in the substantia nigra in the lateral part of the mesencephalon [6]. This last mentioned pathway has also been verified with silver-stain techniques [46].

PHARMACOLOGY OF CENTRAL MA NEURONS

Koelle has already presented some of the pharmacology of CA neurons, mainly based on results obtained in peripheral sympathetic adrenergic neurons. However, since pharmacological studies have recently been performed in CA and 5-HT containing neurons in the CNS proper, some of these data are presented here. A certain amount of overlapping in information cannot be avoided, since, as Koelle pointed out, many similarities exist between central and peripheral MA neurons. The studies have included the use of brain slices in vitro, intraventricular injections (both techniques in order to get around the blood-brain barrier for NE, DA, and 5-HT), fluorescent histochemistry, bioassay, and to a certain extent also electron microscopy.

In the normal animal (Fig. D8-11), the major part of the amines are stored within the amine storage granules, and thereby also protected from deamination by MAO, probably localized within the mitochondria. The amino acids and the precursors L-DOPA and 5-HTP seem to be taken up through the nerve membrane by an active mechanism, probably different from the uptake mechanism for NE, DA, and 5-HT [17]. Intraneuronally the precursors are decarboxylated to DA and 5-HT, respectively, which are taken up and stored in the granules. In the case of NE neurons, conversion of DA into NE seems to take place in relation to the granules (cf. [68]), which probably contain the enzyme DA-β-hydroxylase [84, 87]. The synthesis of the amines can thus be depressed by special synthesis inhibitors (Table D8-1), or enhanced by the administration of L-DOPA or 5-HTP, since the first step in the transmitter synthesis (tyrosine → DOPA and tryptophane → 5-HTP) seems to be rate limiting [93]. By inhibition of MAO, the extragranular concentrations of amines may be increased,

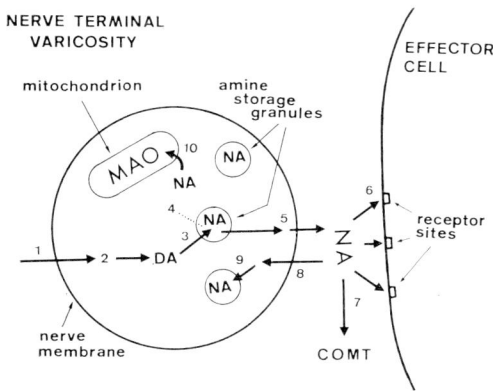

FIG. D8-11. Schematic illustration of the pharmacology of a central MA neuron. The figure indicates a cross-sectioned NE nerve terminal varicosity. (See also [19].)

(1) Uptake into the nerve of tyrosine or L-DOPA or both; in 5-HT neurons, of tryptophane or 5-HTP or both [4, 17, 19].

(2) Synthesis steps:

$$\text{tyrosine} \xrightarrow{\text{tyrosine-hydroxylase}} \text{L-DOPA}$$

$$\xrightarrow{\text{DOPA decarboxylase}} \text{DA}$$

In 5-HT neurons:

$$\text{tryptophane} \xrightarrow{\text{tryptophane-hydroxylase}} \text{5-HTP}$$

$$\xrightarrow{\text{5-HTP-decarboxylase}} \text{5-HT}$$

Cf. [5, 15, 27, 88, 94]. Inhibited by Group B substances (Table D8-1). DOPA-decarboxylase and 5-HTP-decarboxylase probably the same enzyme, e.g. [88].

(3) Uptake of DA into granules. Uptake of 5-HT in 5-HT neurons.

(4) Synthesis of NE from DA by DA-β-hydroxylase, cf. [61, 84], only in NE neurons. Inhibited by a Group B substance (Table D8-1). Storage of NE (DA or 5-HT, respectively) in the storage granules, cf. [19]. Blocked by Group C substances (Table D8-1).

(5) Release of the transmitter at nerve activity, e.g. [4, 18, 47].

(6) Action of the released transmitter on receptor sites at the target cell membrane, cf. [4, 18]. May be blocked by Group G substances (Table D8-1).

(7) Elimination of released transmitter by the enzyme COMT, cf. [4, 18, 47].

The storage function of the granules can be blocked by reserpine (long lasting) or tetrabenazine (short lasting) [19, 35, 39, 65, 90], resulting in leakage of the amines from the granules into the cytoplasm. If the MAO is not blocked, the extragranular amines are deaminated and the neuron becomes depleted of amines (cf. [18, 19]).

The amines released by nerve impulses are thought to influence the postsynaptic membrane at specific receptor sites. Very little is known about how this influence is brought about, but it is not generally thought that the amine binds to the receptor for any long period of time. Many drugs may interfere with this mechanism, either by blockade of the receptor and possibly thereby hindering the access of the amine molecules to it, or by "artificial" stimulation of the receptor. A large part of the released transmitter is probably reaccumulated into the nerve terminal by the very efficient so-called membrane pump, found in nonterminal axons and terminals [4, 58, 59, 69]. This mechanism may be of considerable value for the *economy* of the neurons, since the reaccumulated transmitter is probably reused as has been discussed for the peripheral sympathetic adrenergic neurons (cf. [4, 47]). Thymoleptics of the imipramine type seem to be very efficient in blocking this membrane pump, while the effects of cocaine in the CNS appear to be comparatively weak [69]; its actions seem to be more complex.

Another route for the inactivation of released amines is O-methylation by the enzyme COMT. This enzyme, however, seems to be only of moderate importance quantitatively for amine inactivation [4, 17]. A

---

(8) Elimination of released transmitter via reuptake by the membrane pump in the nerve membrane. Probably the same mechanism for uptake of, e.g., exogenous NE, DA, 5-HT (and adrenaline), administered intraventricularly or in vitro to brain slices, e.g. [24, 25, 59, 69]. May be blocked by Group E substances (Table D8-1).

(9) Reuptake of transmitter into the storage granules.

(10) Deamination of cytoplasmic "free" transmitter by the enzyme MAO, cf. [18]. The MAO may be blocked by Group D substances (Table D8-1).

TABLE D8-1. Main Site of Action of Some Drugs on Neurons Containing CA and 5-HT in the CNS.

Substance	Main Type of Action	Neuron Type Influenced	Effect on MA Transmission
Group A	Transmitter precursors		
L-DOPA (e.g. [15, 27])		DA, NE	+
5-HTP (cf. [86])		5-HT	
Group B	Inhibitors of transmitter synthesis by inhibition of:		−
α-methyl-p-tyrosine NSD-1015	tryosinehydroxylase [15, 93, 94] DOPA-decarboxylase (cf. [95])	DA, NE DA, NE	
sodium diethyldithiocarbamate	DA-β-hydroxylase [26, 61, 84]	NE	
p-chloro-phenylalanine	tryptophane-hydroxylase [81, 86]	5-HT	
Group C	Blockers of granular MA storage function		−
reserpine (e.g. [19, 35, 39])	long-lasting blocker	DA, NE, 5-HT	
tetrabenazine [19, 65, 90]	short-lasting blocker	DA, NE, 5-HT	
Group D	Inhibitors of MAO (cf. [18])	5-HT (DA, NE)	+
nialamide			
iproniazide			
pheniprazine			
tranylcypromine			
Group E	Blockers of the membrane pump		+
imipramine [23, 25, 60] desmethylimipramine [23, 24, 59, 69]		5-HT (NE) NE (5-HT)	
chlorimipramine [20]		5-HT (NE)	
protriptyline [24, 60, 69]		NE (5-HT)	
Group F (For ref. see [4])	Receptor activators		+
NE	natural	NE	
DA	natural	DA	
5-HT	natural	5-HT	
apomorphine	artificial	DA	
LSD	artificial	5-HT	
Group G	Receptor blocking agents (cf. [4])		−
chlorpromazine		DA, NE	
haloperidol		DA, NE	
phenoxybenzamine		NE	
Group H	Releases the natural transmitters by replacement (e.g. [70])		+
amphetamine		DA, NE	

very important inactivation mechanism in the peripheral sympathetic system, the diffusion to the blood, is probably of very little or no importance in the CNS, due to presence of the blood-brain barrier.

For more detailed discussions on monoamine mechanisms and pharmacology, reference is made to a review by Andén, Carlsson, and Häggendal [4].

THE AMINE STORAGE GRANULES. Since storage granules are complex structures, containing a specific storage protein, ATP, Mg^{++}, and also an enzyme (DA-β-hydroxylase in the NE granules), it has been suggested that they are manufactured in the perikaryon with its high amounts of RNA [80] and transported proximodistally to the terminals. Satisfactory evidence for this view has been obtained in the peripheral NS by independent authors [38, 83, 87]. It has been found that large accumulations of presumably storage granules occur proximally to a cut or ligation of adrenergic axons [31, 83, 87] and that the accumulation proceeds linearly with time [38]. The rate of the proximodistal transport was calculated in the rat to be about 5 mm per hour, in the cat about 10 mm per hour. The life span of the granules in the terminals was estimated to be about 4–5 weeks in the rat and 10 weeks in the cat [38]. It was also calculated that turnover of storage granules in the nerve cell body may be rather short, on the order of 1 to 6 hours [31].

Studies on the proximodistal transport and life span of amine storage granules in CNS neurons have been made in the bulbospinal NE neuron system. This system is most suitable for this type of study, since the cell bodies, localized to the medulla oblongata, are well separated from the nerve terminals in the spinal cord. It was found that the proximodistal transport of NE storage granules was slower than in the peripheral NS, the figure of 0.7 mm per hour (in contrast to 5 mm per hour in the peripheral NS) was obtained [66]. The life span of the granules was calculated to be about 30 days, which is very close to the time found in the peripheral NS [38]. Thus, the life span of NE granules seems to be the same in the CNS and peripheral NS. There exists some evidence that 5-HT storage granules and DA storage granules have about the same life span as NE granules in the rat [39].

RELEASE OF MA. The turnover of MA in the CNS nerve terminals is presumably very rapid, on the order of 6 to 12 hours, as indicated by studies using synthesis inhibitors [5, 27]. This is quite a different order of magnitude than the calculated life span of the amine storage granules. It seems very unlikely that whole granules are liberated as transmitter packages on nerve stimulation, as has been suggested for the ACh-containing vesicles in cholinergic neurons [41]. Also, the fact that the amine storage granules contain a specific storage protein and a synthesizing enzyme makes it improbable that such a mechanism would exist, since it would imply a remarkable waste of proteins.

Electron microscopic studies using potassium permanganate fixation on sympathetically stimulated iris in rats pretreated with a synthesis inhibitor of NE (α-methyl-*p*-tyrosine) have shown a disappearance of the dense core in the small granulated vesicles on the stimulated side, while the dense core was unchanged on the unstimulated side [74]. In these animals the NE level was very low at the stimulated side and much higher in the control iris. The total number of 500 Å vesicles was about the same on both sides. The only difference was thus disappearance of the content after stimulation. This indicates that whole granules are not released on nerve activity.

A study by Folkow, Häggendal, and Lisander [47] on the NE release (per nerve stimulus per varicosity) in the peripheral NS, with all inactivation routes so far known blocked or taken into consideration, revealed that at least in the system studied, only 400 molecules of NE, equivalent to about 3 percent of the content of one storage granulum (note granulum, not varicosity), was released per nerve stimulus per average varicosity. This indicates that only a small fraction of the NE content of the granules is mobilized on nerve activity.

ACh Release Compared. This view is not in accordance with the view on release of ACh in the cholinergic neurons, which is considered to imply release of the total ACh content of one vesicle as a transmitter packet ([41], cf. Eccles, Chap. 9). However, even if many similarities may exist between the cholinergic and the monoaminergic neuron, several differences have also been found so far. It would, therefore, not be impossible that the mechanisms for release of the respective transmitters are different, although it would appear reasonable if chemical transmission occurred in about the same way in all neurons working with transmitter substances. For further discussion on CA and 5-HT release on nerve stimulation see Andén [4].

FUNCTION OF THE MA NEURONS

The thin, varicose nerve terminals in the CNS are often seen lying very close to, and in some areas forming basketlike formations surrounding nonfluorescent nerve cell bodies (Figs. D8-2, D8-12b). This is the case especially in some nuclei receiving a rich supply of terminals. In some areas, such as the raphe nuclei of the medulla oblongata and pons, green fluorescent CA terminals can be seen to surround yellow fluorescent 5-HT cell bodies (Figs. D8-5, D8-12a) while, on the other hand, 5-HT terminals close to CA cell bodies have not been observed. The fluorescent microscopic localization of these nerve terminals close to cell bodies is highly suggestive of some synaptic contact between two structures (Fig. D8-12b), but whether this is a direct contact (axosomatic) or indirect contact via an interjacent nerve ending (axoaxonic) cannot be judged in the fluorescent microscope. However, electron microscope studies of areas rich in CA terminals have failed to reveal the presence of axoaxonic contacts [56]. Thus it seems likely that MA nerve terminals in the CNS have direct action on other nerve cells. Also, there is good evidence that nerve terminals containing NE and 5-HT in the spinal cord may function by releasing either of these substances on nerve activity [2, 3, 36], and there are good reasons to believe that the same holds true also for MA nerve terminals in other parts of the CNS.

MA-containing neurons have been found in the CNS of most animals studied so far; in hydrae [96], molluscs [30, 97], worms [85], insects [48, 49], crayfish [42], fish [13], birds [57], and mammals [33, 51, 52, 72, 73], including man (cf. [14] and Fuxe and Roos, unpublished). Thus, they constitute phylogenetically very old systems, which also is indicated by the localization of the cell bodies (in the lower brain stem) in mammalian brain. Therefore, they probably have very important functions in the CNS which are generally expressed as a regulating and modulating action on functions such as spinal reflexes [11, 12, 43], extrapyramidal functions (especially the nigroneostriatal DA pathway) [6–8], sleep and alertness [82], aggressiveness [53], thermoregulation [28, 44, 45], sexual behavior [89], and endocrine functions [55]. Some mental diseases may be more or less connected to the MA neuron systems in the CNS [92].

During hyperbaric oxygen exposure, epilepticlike convulsions occur as a sign of so-called O_2 intoxication. Recent studies by Häggendal [63, 64] on rats exposed to oxy-

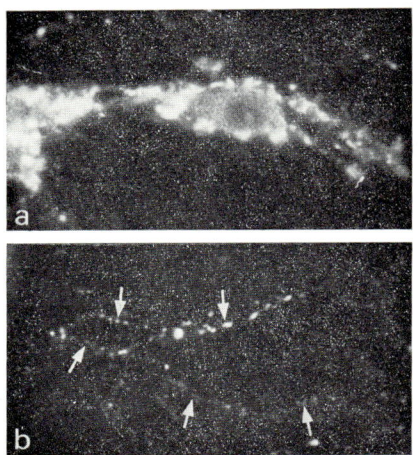

FIG. D8-12. (a) 5-HT nerve cell body from the lateral part of Group B1, in [33], in the medulla oblongata of nialamide-treated rat. The yellow fluorescent cell body is surrounded by strongly green fluorescent NE nerve terminals, forming a basketlike network around the 5-HT cell body. ×520. (b) Nonfluorescent motor neuron from the spinal cord ventral horn of normal rat. Both NE and 5-HT nerve terminals (→) can be observed lying very close to the surface of the motor neuron. ×460. (Dahlström and Fuxe, unpublished material.)

gen at high pressure showed that the onset time of convulsions could be influenced by drugs acting on central MA neurons. Thus, reserpine and tetrabenazine, which deplete the amine stores (Table D8-1), markedly shorten onset time for convulsions, while the administration of an MAO inhibitor (nialamide), which increases the MA levels, significantly prolongs the time before onset of convulsions. It may be of interest to compare this study with the observation made in clinical psychiatry, that drugs interfering with MA transmission in a negative direction (e.g., reserpine, chlorpromazine, see Table D8-1) may induce epileptic seizures in patients with latent epilepsy and aggravate the condition in epileptic patients [1, 79]. This is thus an effect in the same direction as described for the rats exposed to hyperbaric oxygen. It may be speculated that impaired MA transmission may induce a decrease in irritability threshold, normally maintained at a higher level by the CA and 5-HT nerve terminals (cf. [19]).

REFERENCES

1. Aid, F. J. Medical phenothiazide tranquilizers—Eight years of development. Clin. North Amer. 45:1127, 1961.

2. Andén, N.-E., Carlsson, A., Hillarp, N.-Å., and Magnusson, T. 5-Hydroxytryptamine release by nerve stimulation of the spinal cord. Life Sci. 3:473, 1964.

3. Andén, N.-E., Carlsson, A., Hillarp, N.-Å., and Magnusson, T. Noradrenaline release by nerve stimulation of the spinal cord. Life Sci. 4:129, 1965.

4. Andén, N.-E., Carlsson, A., and Häggendal, J. Adrenergic mechanisms. Pharmacol. Rev. 1969, in press.

5. Andén, N.-E., Corrodi, H., Dahlström, A., Fuxe, K., and Hökfelt, T. Effects of tyrosine hydroxylase inhibition on the amine levels of central monoamine neurons. Life Sci. 5:561, 1966.

6. Andén, N.-E., Dahlström, A., Fuxe, K., and Larsson, K. Further evidence for the presence of nigroneostriatal dopamine neurons in the rat. Amer. J. Anat. 116:329, 1965.

7. Andén, N.-E., Dahlström, A., Fuxe, K., Larsson, K., Olsson, L., and Ungerstedt, U. Ascending monoamine neurons to the telencephalon and diencephalon. Acta Physiol. Scand. 67:313, 1966.

8. Andén, N.-E., Dahlström, A., Fuxe, K., and Larsson, K. Functional role of the nigro-neostriatal dopamine neurons. Acta Pharmacol. (Kobenhavn) 23:263, 1966.

9. Andén, N.-E., Fuxe, K., Hamberger, B., and Hökfelt, T. A quantitative study on the nigro-neostriatal dopamine neuron system in the rat. Acta Physiol. Scand. 67:306, 1966.

10. Andén, N.-E., Fuxe, K., and Larsson, K. Effect of large mesencephalic-diencephalic lesions on the noradrenaline, dopamine and 5-hydroxytryptamine neurons of the central nervous system. Experientia 22:842, 1966.

11. Andén, N.-E., Jukes, M. G. M., and Lundberg, A. Spinal reflexes and monoamine liberation. Nature (London) 202:1222, 1964.

12. Andén, N.-E., Lundberg, A., Rosengren, E., and Vyklicky, L. The effect of DOPA on spinal reflexes from the FRA (Flexor Reflex Afferents). Experientia 19:654, 1963.

13. Baumgarten, H. G. Catecholamine in Hypothalamus vom Goldfisch. Z. Zellforsch. 80:246, 1967.

14. Bertler, Å. Occurrence and localization of catecholamines in the human brain. Acta Physiol. Scand. 51:97, 1961.

15. Blaschko, H. The specific action of L-dopa decarboxylase. J. Physiol. (London) 96:50–51P, 1939.

16. Bloom, F. E., and Aghajanian, G. K. An electron microscopic analysis of large granular synaptic vesicles of the brain in relation to monoamine content. J. Pharmacol. Exp. Ther. 159:261, 1968.

17. Bloom, F. E., and Giarman, N. J. Physiologic and pharmacologic considerations of biogenic amines in the nervous system. Ann. Rev. Pharmacol. 8:229, 1968.

18. Carlsson, A. Functional significance of drug-induced changes in brain monoamine levels. Progr. Brain Res. 8:9, 1964.

19. Carlsson, A. Drugs which Block the Storage of 5-Hydroxytryptamine and Related

Amines. In Eichler, O., and Farah, A. (Eds.), *Handbuch der exp. Pharmacol.* Berlin: Springer, 1965, pp. 529–592.

20. Carlsson, A., Corrodi, H., Fuxe, K., and Hökfelt, T. Effect of antidepressant drugs on the depletion of intraneuronal brain 5-hydroxytryptamine stores caused by 4-methyl-α-ethyl-meta-tyramine. *Europ. J. Pharmacol.* 15:357, 1969.

21. Carlsson, A., Falck, B., and Hillarp, N.-Å. Cellular localization of brain monoamines. *Acta Physiol. Scand.* Suppl. 196, 56:1, 1962.

22. Carlsson, A., Falck, B., Fuxe, K., and Hillarp, N.-Å. Cellular localization of monoamines in the spinal cord. *Acta Physiol. Scand.* 60:112, 1964.

23. Carlsson, A., Fuxe, K., Hamberger, B., and Lindqvist, M. Biochemical and histochemical studies on the effect of imipramine-like drugs and (+)-amphetamine on central and peripheral catecholamine neurons. *Acta Physiol. Scand.* 67:481, 1966.

24. Carlsson, A., Fuxe, K., and Hökfelt, T. Effect of desmethylimipramine, protriptyline and (+)-amphetamine on fluorescence of central adrenergic neurons of rats pretreated with α-methyl-DOPA and tetrabenazine or reserpine. *Europ. J. Pharmacol.* 2:196, 1967.

25. Carlsson, A., Fuxe, K., and Ungerstedt, U. The effect of imipramine on central 5-hydroxy-tryptamine neurons. *J. Pharm. Pharmacol.* 20:150, 1968.

26. Carlsson, A., Lindqvist, M., Fuxe, K., and Hökfelt, T. Histochemical and biochemical effects of diethyldithiocarbamate on tissue catecholamines. *J. Pharm. Pharmacol.* 18:60, 1966.

27. Corrodi, H., Fuxe, K., and Hökfelt, T. Refillment of the catecholamine stores with 3,4-dihydroxyphenylalanine after depletion induced by inhibition of tyrosinehydroxylase. *Life Sci.* 5:605, 1966.

28. Corrodi, H., Fuxe, K., and Hökfelt, T. A possible role played by central monoamine neurons in thermo-regulation. *Acta Physiol. Scand.* 71:224, 1967.

29. Corrodi, H., and Jonsson, G. The formaldehyde fluorescence method for the histochemical demonstration of biogenic amines. A review on the methodology. *J. Histochem. Cytochem.* 15:65, 1967.

30. Dahl, E., von Mecklenburg, C., and Myhrberg, H. An adrenergic nervous system in sea-anemones. *Quart. J. Micr. Sci.* 104:531, 1963.

31. Dahlström, A. The Intraneuronal Distribution of Noradrenaline and the Transport and Life-Span of Amine Storage Granules in the Sympathetic Adrenergic Neuron. M.D. thesis, Stockholm, 1966.

32. Dahlström, A., and Fuxe, K. A method for the demonstration of monoamine containing nerve fibres in the central nervous system. *Acta Physiol. Scand.* 60:293, 1964a.

33. Dahlström, A., and Fuxe, K. Evidence for the existence of monoamine containing neurons in the central nervous system. I. Demonstration of monoamines in the cell bodies of brain stem neurons. *Acta Physiol. Scand.* Suppl. 232, 62:1, 1964b.

34. Dahlström, A., and Fuxe, K. Evidence for the existence of monoamine-containing neurons in the central nervous system. II. Experimentally induced changes in the intraneuronal amine levels of bulbo-spinal neuron systems. *Acta Physiol. Scand.* Suppl. 247, 64:1, 1965.

35. Dahlström, A., Fuxe, K., and Hillarp, N.-Å. Site of action of reserpine. *Acta Pharmacol.* (Kobenhavn) 22:277, 1965.

36. Dahlström, A., Fuxe, K., Kernell, D., and Sedvall, G. Reductions of the monoamine stores in the terminals of bulbo-spinal neurons following stimulation in the medulla oblongata. *Life Sci.* 4:1207, 1965.

37. Dahlström, A., and Häggendal, J. Some quantitative studies on the noradrenaline content in the cell bodies and terminals of a sympathetic adrenergic neuron system. *Acta Physiol. Scand.* 67:271, 1966a.

38. Dahlström, A., and Häggendal, J. Studies on the transport and life-span of amine storage granules in a peripheral adrenergic neuron system. *Acta Physiol. Scand.* 67:278, 1966b.

39. Dahlström, A., and Häggendal, J. Recovery of noradrenaline levels after reserpine compared with the life-span of amine storage granules in rat and rabbit. *J. Pharm. Pharmacol.* 18:750, 1966c.

40. Dahlström, A., Häggendal, J., and Hökfelt, T. The noradrenaline content of the varicosities of sympathetic adrenergic nerve terminals in the rat. *Acta Physiol. Scand.* 67:287, 1966.

41. Eccles, J. C. *The Physiology of Synapses.* Berlin: Springer, 1964.

42. Elofsson, R., Nielson, K., and Strömberg, J.-O. Localization of monoaminergic neurons in the central nervous system of

Astacus Astacus Linné (Crustacea). *Z. Zellforsch.* 74:464, 1966.

43. Engberg, I., and Ryall, R. W. The inhibitory action of noradrenaline and other monoamines in spinal neurons. *J. Physiol.* (London) 185:298, 1966.

44. Feldberg, W., Hellon, R. F., and Myers, R. D. Effects on temperature of monoamines injected into the cerebral ventricles of anaesthetized dogs. *J. Physiol.* (London) 186:416, 1966.

45. Feldberg, W., and Myers, R. D. Changes in temperature produced by microinjections of amines into the anterior hypothalamus of cats. *J. Physiol.* (London) 177:239, 1965.

46. Fink, R. P., and Heimer, L. Two methods for selective silver impregnation of degenerating axons and their synaptic endings in the central nervous system. *Brain. Res.* 4:369, 1967.

47. Folkow, N., Häggendal, J., and Lisander, B. Extent of release and elimination of noradrenaline at peripheral adrenergic nerve terminals. *Acta Physiol. Scand.* Suppl. 307, 1967.

48. Frontali, N., and Norberg, K. A. Catecholamine containing neurons in the cockroach brain. *Acta Physiol. Scand.* 66:243, 1966.

49. Frontali, N., and Häggendal, J. Noradrenaline and dopamine content in the brain of the cockroach, *Periplaneta Americana*. To be published 1969.

50. Fuxe, K. Cellular localization of monoamines in the median eminence and infundibular stem of some mammals. *Z. Zellforsch.* 61:710, 1964.

51. Fuxe, K. Evidence for the existence of monoamine containing neurons in the central nervous system. III. The monoamine nerve terminal. *Z. Zellforsch.* 65:573, 1965a.

52. Fuxe, K. Evidence for the existence of monoamine containing neurons in the central nervous system. IV. The distribution of monoamine nerve terminals in the central nervous system. *Acta Physiol. Scand.* Suppl. 247, 64:39, 1965b.

53. Fuxe, K., and Gunne, L.-M. Depletion of the amine stores in brain catecholamine terminals on amygdaloid stimulation. *Acta Physiol. Scand.* 62:493, 1964.

54. Fuxe, K., Hamberger, B., and Hökfelt, T. Distribution of noradrenaline nerve terminals in cortical areas of the rat. *Brain Res.* 8:125, 1968.

55. Fuxe, K., and Hökfelt, T. The Influence of Central Catecholamine Neurons on the Hormone Secretion from the Anterior and Posterior Pituitary. In Stutinsky, F. (Ed.), *Neurosecretion*. Berlin: Springer, 1967, pp. 165–177.

56. Fuxe, K., Hökfelt, T., and Nilsson, O. A fluorescence and electromicroscopic study on certain brain regions rich in monoamine terminals. *Amer. J. Anat.* 117:33, 1965.

57. Fuxe, K., and Ljunggren, L. Cellular localization of monoamines in the upper brain stem of the pigeon. *J. Comp. Neurol.* 125:355, 1965.

58. Fuxe, K., and Ungerstedt, U. Localization of catecholamine uptake in rat brain after intraventricular injection. *Life Sci.* 5:1817, 1966.

59. Fuxe, K., and Ungerstedt, U. Localization of 5-hydroxytryptamine uptake in rat brain after intraventricular injection. *J. Pharm. Pharmacol.* 19:335, 1967.

60. Fuxe, K., and Ungerstedt, U. Histochemical studies on the effect of (+)-amphetamine, drugs of the imipramine group and tryptamine on central catecholamine and 5-hydroxytryptamine neurons after intraventricular injection of catecholamines and 5-hydroxytryptamine. *Europ. J. Pharmacol.* 4:135, 1968.

61. Goldstein, M., Anagnoste, B., Tanber, E., and McKereghan, M. R. Inhibition of dopamine-β-hydroxylase by disulfiram. *Life Sci.* 3:763, 1964.

62. Grillo, M. A. Electron microscopy of sympathetic tissues. *Pharmacol. Rev.* 18:387, 1966.

63. Häggendal, J. Hyperbaric oxygen exposure and monoamine metabolism in central and peripheral tissues of the rat. *Acta Physiol. Scand.* 73:29A, 1968.

64. Häggendal, J. Effect of hyperbaric oxygen on monoamine metabolism in central and peripheral tissues of the rat. *Europ. J. Pharmacol.* 2:323, 1968.

65. Häggendal, J. The depletion and recovery of noradrenaline in the brain and some sympathetically innervated mammalian tissues after tetrabenazine. *J. Pharm. Pharmacol.* 20:364, 1968.

66. Häggendal, J., and Dahlström, A. The transport and life-span of amine storage granules in bulbospinal noradrenaline

67. Häggendal, J., and Malmfors, T. Evidence for dopamine containing neurons in the retina of rabbits. *Acta Physiol. Scand.* 59:295, 1963.

68. Häggendal, J., and Malmfors, T. The effect of nerve stimulation on catecholamines taken up in adrenergic nerves after reserpine pretreatment. *Acta Physiol. Scand.* 75:33, 1969.

69. Hamberger, B. Reserpine-resistant uptake of catecholamines in isolated tissues of the rat. *Acta Physiol. Scand.* Suppl. 295, 1967.

70. Hanson, L. C. F. Evidence that the central action of (+)-amphetamine is mediated via catecholamines. *Psychopharmacologia* (Berlin) 10:289, 1967.

71. Heller, A., and Moore, R. Y. Effect of central nervous system lesions on brain monoamines in the rat. *J. Pharmacol.* 150:1, 1965.

72. Hillarp, N.-Å., Fuxe, K., and Dahlström, A. Demonstration and mapping out of central neurons containing dopamine, noradrenaline and 5-hydroxytryptamine and their reactions to psychopharmaca. *Pharmacol. Rev.* 18:727, 1966a.

73. Hillarp, N.-Å., Fuxe, K., and Dahlström, A. Central Monoamine Neurons. In von Euler, U. S., Rosell, S., and Uvnäs. B. (Eds.), *Mechanisms on Release of Biogenic Amines*. Oxford: Pergamon, 1966a, pp. 31–57.

74. Hökfelt, T. Ultrastructural studies on adrenergic nerve terminals in the albino rat iris after pharmacological and experimental treatment. *Acta Physiol. Scand.* 69:125, 1967a.

75. Hökfelt, T. On the ultrastructural localization of noradrenaline in the central nervous system of the rat. *Z. Zellforsch.* 79:110, 1967b.

76. Hökfelt, T. In vitro studies on central and peripheral monoamine neurons at the ultrastructural level. *Z. Zellforsch.* 91:1, 1968.

77. Hökfelt, T. Electron Microscopic Studies on Peripheral and Central Monoamine Neurons. M.D. thesis, Stockholm, 1968.

78. Hökfelt, T. Distribution of noradrenaline storage particles in peripheral adrenergic neurons as revealed by electron microscopy. *Acta Physiol. Scand.* 1969, in press.

79. Hollister, L. E. Complications from psychotherapeutic drugs. *Clin. Pharmacol. Ther.* 5:322, 1964.

80. Hydén, H. The Neuron. In Brachet, J., and Mirsky, A. (Eds.), *The Cell*, vol. IV. New York: Academic, 1960, pp. 215–323.

81. Jequier, E., Lovenberg, W., Sjoerdsma, A. Tryptophanehydroxylase inhibition, the mechanism by which *p*-chloro-phenylalanine depletes rat brain serotonin. *Molec. Pharmacol.* 3:274, 1967.

82. Jouvet, M., Bobillier, P., Pujol, J.-F., and Renault, J. Suppression du sommeil et diminution de la sérotonine cérébrale par lésion du système du raphae chez le chat. *C. R. Acad. Sci.* [D] (Paris) 264:360, 1967.

83. Kapeller, K., and Mayor, D. The accumulation of noradrenaline in constricted sympathetic nerves as studied by fluorescence and electron microscopy. *Proc. Roy. Soc.* [*Biol.*] 167:282, 1967.

84. Kaufmann, S., and Friedman, S. Dopamine-β-hydroxylase. *Pharmacol. Rev.* 17:71, 1965.

85. Kerkut, G. A., Sedden, C. B., and Walker, R. J. Cellular localization of monoamines by fluorescence microscopy in *Hirudo medicinalis* and *Lumbricus terrestris*. *Comp. Biochem. Physiol.* 21:687, 1967.

86. Koe, B. K., and Weissman, A. *p*-Chlorophenylalanine: A specific depleter of brain serotonin. *J. Pharmacol. Exp. Ther.* 154:499, 1966.

87. Laduron, P., and Belpaire, F. Transport of noradrenaline and dopamine-β-hydroxylase in sympathetic nerves. *Life Sci.* 7:1, 1968.

88. Lovenberg, W., Weissbach, H., and Udenfriend, S. Aromatic L-amino acid decarboxylase. *J. Biol. Chem.* 237:89, 1962.

89. Meyerson, B. J. Central nervous monoamines and hormone induced estrous behaviour in the spayed rat. *Acta Physiol. Scand.* Suppl. 241, vol. 63, 1964.

90. Pletscher, A., Brossi, A., and Gey, K. F. Benzoquinolizine derivatives: A new class of monoamine decreasing drugs with psychotropic action. *Int. Rev. Neurobiol.* 4:275, 1962.

91. Richardson, K. C. Electron microscopic identification of autonomic nerve endings. *Nature* (London) 210:756, 1966.

92. Schildkraut, J. J., and Kety, S. S. Biogenic amines and emotion. *Science* 156:21, 1967.

93. Spector, S., Sjoerdsma, A., and Uden-

friend, S. Blockade of endogenous norepinephrine synthesis by α-methyl-tyrosine, an inhibitor of tyrosinehydroxylase. *J. Pharmacol. Exp. Ther.* 147:86, 1965.

94. Udenfriend, S. Tyrosine hydroxylase. *Pharmacol. Rev.* 18:43, 1966.

95. Udenfriend, S., Zaltzman-Nirenberg, P., Gordon, R., and Spector, S. Evaluation of the biochemical effects produced in vivo by inhibitors of the enzymes involved in norepinephrine biosynthesis. *Molec. Pharmacol.* 2:95, 1966.

96. Welsh, J. H. Distribution of serotonin in the nervous system of various animal species. *Adv. Pharmacol.* 6:171, 1968.

97. Zs.-Nagy, I. Histochemical demonstration of biogenic monoamines in the central nervous system of the lamellibranch mollusc *Anodonta cygnea* L. *Acta Biol. Hung.* 18:1, 1967.

9
Excitatory and Inhibitory Mechanisms in Brain

J. C. ECCLES

EXCITATORY AND INHIBITORY SYNAPSES

It is proposed, first, to give a general account of excitatory and inhibitory mechanisms with special reference to the sites where the pioneering work was done [18, 19]. It will be recognized that the term "excitatory and inhibitory mechanisms" applies to the neuronal pathways as well as to the synapses. Following this initial treatment, there will be an account of excitatory and inhibitory mechanisms in regions more relevant to the problems of epilepsy, namely the hippocampus and the thalamus. Oshima will then give an account of neocortical synaptic mechanisms.

STRUCTURAL FEATURES OF SYNAPSES

The body and dendrites of a nerve cell are specialized for the reception and integration of information which is conveyed as impulses that are fired from other nerve cells along their axons. In the diagrammatic drawing of a nerve cell (Fig. 9-1A) it is seen that impinging on its surface are numerous small knoblike endings of fine fibers which are, in fact, the terminal branches of axons from other nerve cells. Communication between nerve cells occurs at these numerous areas of close contact or *synapses,* the name first applied by Sherrington, who laid the foundations of what is often called *synaptology.* We owe to Dale and Löewi the concept that transmission across synapses is effected by secretion of minute amounts of specific chemical substances that act across the synapse, which has already been described by Curtis and Kuno (Chap. 5). The cablelike transmission of impulses over the surfaces of nerve cells and their axons ceases abruptly at the synaptic contact between cells, but may begin again on the other side of the synapse. It should be mentioned that there are now many examples of synapses in which transmission is effected by the flow of electric currents across the juxtaposed presynaptic and postsynaptic membranes, but none has yet been recognized in the mammalian central nervous system.

The high resolving power of the electron microscope gives essential information on those structural features of synapses that are specially concerned with this chemical phase of transmission. For example, in Fig. 9-1B, C, we can see the membrane, about 70 Å thick, that encloses the expanded axonal terminal or *synaptic knob.* These knobs contain numerous small vesicular structures, the *synaptic vesicles,* that are believed to be packages (quanta) of the chemical substances concerned in synaptic transmission. Some of these vesicles are concentrated in zones on the membrane that fronts the synaptic cleft, which is the remarkably uniform space about 200 Å across, indicated by the arrows in Fig. 9-1B. The chemical transmitter substance is released from the synaptic knob into the cleft and acts on the *subsynaptic membrane.*

Since synaptic transmission must occur across the synaptic cleft that is interposed between the presynaptic and postsynaptic components of the synapse, it might appear that the synaptic cleft is merely a barrier

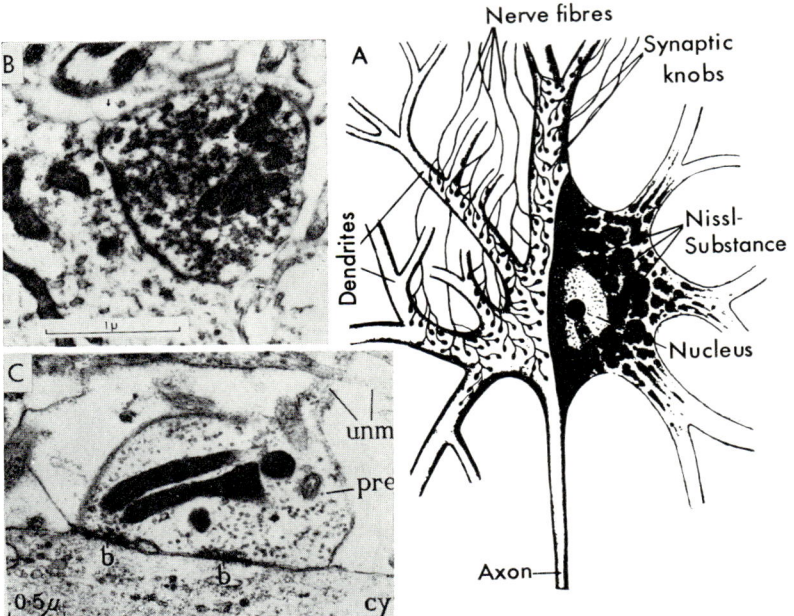

Fig. 9-1. (A) Drawing by Jung [28] of neuron showing dendrites and axon radiating from cell body or soma that contains the nucleus. Several fine nerve fibers branch profusely and end in synaptic knobs on the body and dendrites. (B) Electron micrograph by Palay [42] of synaptic knob separated from subsynaptic membrane of a nerve cell by synaptic cleft (marked by arrows), about 200 Å wide. In some areas, vesicles concentrate close to synaptic surface of knob. There is an associated increase in membrane density on either side of the cleft. (C) Electron micrograph by Hamlyn [26] of an inhibitory synapse formed by synaptic knob (pre) of basket cell on soma (cyt) of a hippocampal pyramidal cell; there are two active sites (b).

to transmission; but it must not be too narrow, or else it will unduly impede the flow of the postsynaptic electric currents (cf. Fig. 9-5A, B) that provide the essential expression of synaptic actions of all kinds. In its dimensional design the synaptic cleft approaches optimal efficiency.

EXCITATORY SYNAPTIC ACTION

A simple example of excitatory synaptic action is illustrated in Fig. 9-2A–C, where a single synchronous synaptic bombardment diminishes the electric charge on the cell membrane. There is a rapid rise to the summit and a slower, approximately exponential decay. This depolarization becomes progressively larger in (A) to (C) as the number of activated synapses increases. There is, in fact, a simple summation of the depolarizations produced by each individual synapse. In the much faster records of (D) to (G), it can be seen that when above a critical size, the synaptic depolarization evokes the discharge of an impulse, similar to that which occurs in peripheral nerve [27, 33], there being the explosive increase in sodium permeability at the double arrows in (E) to (G). The only effect of strengthening the synaptic stimulus in (E) to (G) is the earlier generation of the impulse, which in every case arises when the depolarization reaches 18 mV. The depolarizing potentials that excitatory synapses produce in the postsynaptic membrane are called *excitatory postsynaptic potentials* (EPSPs). Generation of impulses by excitatory synapses is entirely attributable to the depolarization of the EPSPs. An EPSP that failed to generate an impulse can be caused to do so when it is superimposed on an applied depolarizing current so that the threshold level of depolarization is attained.

At this time there has been extensive

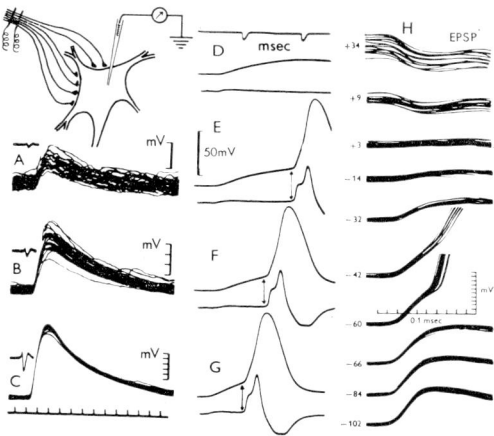

FIG. 9-2. (A) through (C) Excitatory postsynaptic potentials (EPSPs) in a biceps semitendinosus motoneuron with afferent volleys of different size, experimental arrangements shown schematically in inset diagram. Inset records (negativity downward) at left of main records show afferent volley recorded near entry of dorsal nerve roots into spinal cord. Records of EPSPs taken at amplification that decreases in steps from (A) to (C) as response increases. All records formed by superposition of about 40 faint traces. (D) through (G) Intracellularly recorded potentials of gastrocnemius motoneuron (resting membrane potential, −70 mV) evoked by monosynaptic activation that was progressively increased from (D) to (G). Lower traces are electrically differentiated records, double-headed arrows indicating onsets of IS spikes in (E) to (G). (H) Intracellular EPSPs produced by maximum afferent volley as in (C), but at indicated membrane potential which were changed from the resting level of −66 mV by application of steady background currents through one barrel of a double microelectrode, the other used for recording. Spike potentials evoked at membrane potentials of −42 mV and −60 mV. (From Eccles [18].)

investigation of a wide variety of nerve cells in the central nervous system, and in every case synaptic transmission of impulses is due to this same process of production of EPSPs, which in turn generate impulse discharge when attaining a critical level of depolarization. In several species of neurons the EPSP produced by activation of synapses covering the soma and dendrites is effective not by generating an impulse in these regions, but by electrotonic spread of the depolarization to the initial segment, which is the region of the axonal origin. In most species of neurons, the threshold depolarization at the initial segment is much lower than for the somadendritic membrane. Excitatory synapses on the soma and adjacent dendritic regions usually cannot produce a depolarization sufficient for local impulse generation; nevertheless, it may be adequate at the initial segment, the much lower threshold (even less than half) more than compensating for decrement produced by the electrotonic spread.

The synaptic excitation of neurons by a single synchronous volley, as in Fig. 9-2, is a very unphysiological procedure, but is justified because of the light it throws on synaptic mechanisms. Under physiological conditions neurons would be depolarized by prolonged asynchronous synaptic activations produced by impulses discharged from receptor organs or other neurons. To a considerable extent, this depolarization can be modeled by action of a steady depolarizing current applied through an intracellular electrode [17, 37, 38]. Many motoneurons and all cortical pyramidal cells exhibit a slowly adapting response, the frequency declining to a steady, maintained level. With these so-called tonic motoneurons there is an approximately linear relationship between current strength and frequency over a very wide range [37]. The remaining motoneurons are phasic, responding to steady currents with a rapid and large decline in frequency, even to complete cessation of discharge.

The level of the membrane potential of a presynaptic terminal determines the rate of emission of quanta therefrom, the rate rising by as much as a millionfold during invasion by a nerve impulse [32]. Recently tetrodotoxin has been utilized to prevent increase in sodium conductance that normally results from a large depolarization of the nerve fiber and which makes this depolarization self-regenerative. As a consequence, tetrodotoxin completely suppresses production of impulses in presynaptic terminals directly subjected to controlled levels of depolarization [33, 34, 35, 40].

Figure 9-3 shows that with the giant synapse in the squid stellate ganglion, no transmitter is liberated until the directly applied current pulse depolarizes the presynaptic fiber by as much as 40 mV. With larger depolarizations, up to and exceeding 100 mV, there is a large increase in the output of transmitter as measured by the postsynaptic response, a ceiling being reached at about 120 mV. When presynaptic depolarization is measured in close proximity to the synapses, the threshold level for producing a minimal output of transmitter is as low as 25 mV [33, 35].

The other indispensable factor in the release of transmitter is extracellular calcium [34, 36, 41]. Release in response to presynaptic depolarization falls to zero in the absence of calcium and can be restored

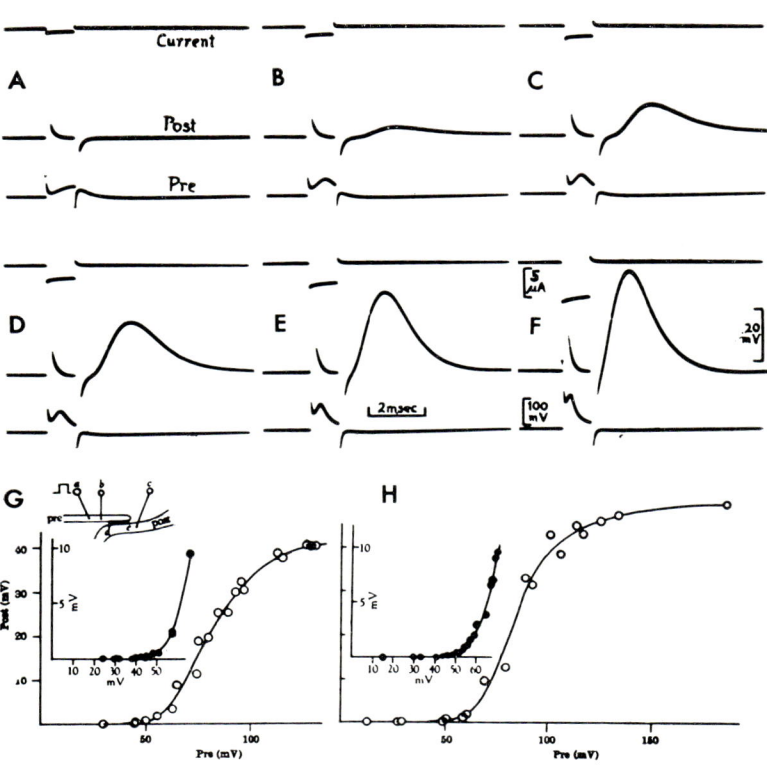

Fig. 9-3. Arrangement of electrodes is shown in upper diagram of (G). Pre: presynaptic terminal. Post: postsynaptic giant axon. Length of synaptic contact d–e, 0.8 mm; a, current-passing electrode; b, "pre"-recording electrode; c, "post"-recording electrode. Distances: a–d, 0.7 mm; b–d, 0.35 mm. (A) through (F) Sample recordings. (G) Input-output relation obtained with 1 msec current pulses. Abscissa, presynaptic depolarization; ordinate, postsynaptic response. Inset, initial part of curve in greater detail. (H) From same synapse after external calcium concentration had been raised from 11 to 58 mM. Temperature in these experiments was about 10°C; concentration of tetrodotoxin 2×10^{-7} gm per ml. (From Katz and Miledi [33].)

in a few milliseconds by electrophoretic injection of calcium just outside the presynaptic terminal. Furthermore, release can be increased several times when extracellular calcium is increased above normal. It has been postulated by Katz and Miledi [34, 36] that release of transmitter must be preceded by the combination of calcium with receptors on the outside of the membrane and by movement of this calcium compound inward across the presynaptic membrane, as is indicated by the arrows in Fig. 9-8. Apparently this activated calcium must act just on the inside of the membrane in close proximity to synaptic vesicles as illustrated in Fig. 9-8. It is an attractive hypothesis that depolarization of the presynaptic terminal is effective in evoking release of transmitter solely because it opens specific gates for calcium ions, which then cross the presynaptic membrane by running down their electrochemical gradient. This postulate is strongly supported by the finding that transmitter release is prevented during a depolarization so large that the electrochemical gradient for calcium is reversed, the release recurring only during recovery from this depolarization [35].

When the postsynaptic membrane potential is displaced in the depolarizing direction by a steady current, the EPSP is reduced in size; eventually when the membrane potential is at about zero potential, the EPSP is also at zero [18]. A still larger background current reverses both the membrane potential and the EPSP (Fig. 9-2H). Hence it has been concluded that the currents producing the EPSP are caused to flow because under the excited synapses there is a virtual short circuit of the membrane potential. The equilibrium potential for excitatory synaptic action may therefore be said to be at about zero membrane potential.

There is relatively little evidence relating to the ionic permeabilities that are responsible for currents generating the EPSPs of nerve cells [21]. By electrophoretic injection through an intracellular electrode, large changes can be made in the ionic composition of motoneurons. These injections of anions or cations may cause considerable decrease in the membrane potential; the EPSP is then diminished correspondingly, but is not otherwise changed. In the light of recent evidence that anions are not appreciably concerned in generation of the end-plate potential (EPP), further investigation is desirable, particularly with isolated preparations, where it will be possible to change extracellular ions in the way done in investigations by Takeuchi and Takeuchi [46, 47] on the EPP. Provisionally it can be assumed that, as with the EPP, the EPSP of neurons is generated by opening the ionic gates for Na^+ and K^+ ions across the subsynaptic membrane. The equilibrium potential for the EPSP at about 0 mV can therefore be attributed to a compromise between the potassium and sodium equilibrium potentials (cf. Fig. 9-5C).

Postsynaptic Inhibitory Action

A second class of synapses that oppose excitation and tend to prevent the generation of impulses by excitatory synapses are called inhibitory synapses. There is general agreement that these two basic modes of synaptic action govern the generation of impulses by nerve cells at the higher levels of the nervous system. As shown in Fig. 9-4A through D, activation of inhibitory synapses causes an increase in the postsynaptic membrane potential. This inhibitory postsynaptic potential or IPSP (Fig. 9-4D) is virtually a mirror image of the EPSP (Fig. 9-4E). The effects of individual inhibitory synapses (Fig. 9-4A–C) on a nerve cell summate in exactly the same way as with the excitatory synapses. As shown in Fig. 9-4J, K, inhibition of neuronal discharge evoked by excitatory synaptic action is accounted for by the opposed action on the potential of the postsynaptic membrane (Fig. 9-4I), hyperpolarization versus depolarization.

Effects produced in the size and direction of the IPSP by varying the initial membrane potential (Fig. 9-4G) correspond precisely to changes that would be expected if the currents generating the IPSP were due to ions moving down their electrochemical gradients, there being a reversal of the current at about −80 mV. These currents would be caused to flow by increases in the ionic permeability of the subsynaptic mem-

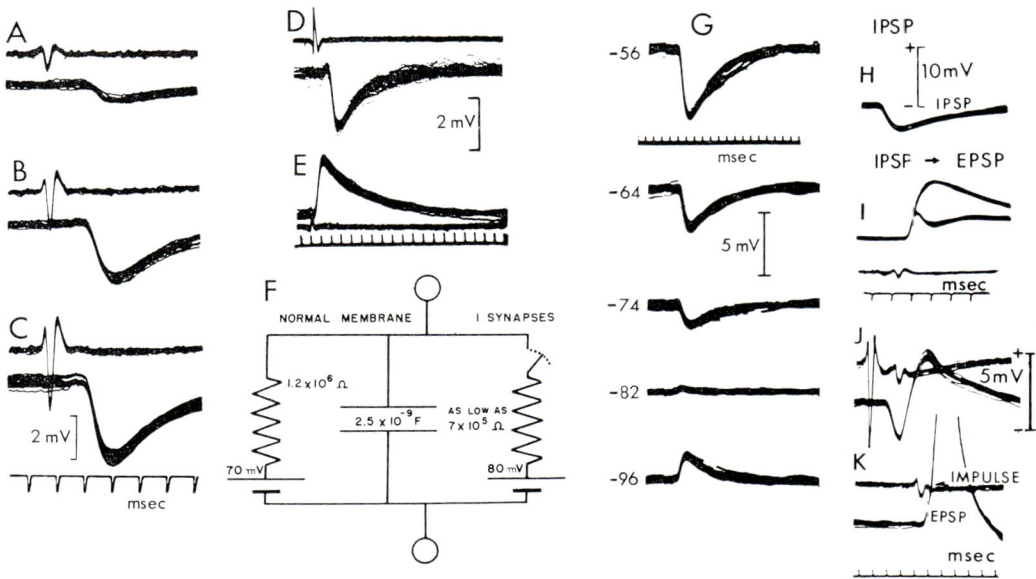

Fig. 9-4. (A) through (C) Lower records give intracellular responses of inhibitory postsynaptic potentials (IPSPs) of motoneuron produced by afferent volley of progressively increasing size, as shown in upper traces which are dorsal-root records, downward deflections signaling negativity. All records formed by superposition of about 40 faint traces. (D) IPSPs similarly recorded at slower sweep speed from another motoneuron, (E) being its monosynaptic EPSPs. (F) Formal electrical diagram of membrane of motoneuron. On left side, normal membrane (as in Fig. 9-2B), on right side, inhibitory subsynaptic areas of membrane that when activated give the IPSP. Maximum activation of these areas would be symbolized by momentary closure of switch. (G) IPSPs recorded intracellularly from motoneuron with double-barreled microelectrode, membrane potential being changed to indicated values by steady background current through one barrel (as in Fig. 9-2H). (H), (I) Interaction of IPSPs and EPSPs. (J), (K) Inhibition of neuronal discharge (K) by a preceding IPSP (J). (From Eccles [18].)

brane that are produced under influence of the inhibitory transmitter substance. Conditions causing generation of an IPSP are depicted in the formal electrical diagram for a motoneuron in Fig. 9-4F, where activation of the synapses closes the switch in the right element of the diagram.

Figure 9-5B shows diagrammatically the flow of current under an activated inhibitory synapse—outward through the subsynaptic membrane along the synaptic cleft and so circling back to hyperpolarize the postsynaptic membrane by inward flow over its whole surface, which is the reverse of that for an excitatory synapse in Fig. 9-5A. The outwardly directed current across the inhibitory subsynaptic membrane could be due to outward movement of a cation such as potassium, or inward movement of an anion such as chloride, or to such a combination of anionic and cationic movements that there is a net outward flow of current driven by a battery of about −80 mV in series with a fairly low resistance.

Figure 9-5C serves to illustrate the simplest findings on the EPSP and the IPSP and their interaction (cf. [19]). Approximate equilibrium potentials for sodium, chloride, and potassium ions are shown by the horizontal lines. The equilibrium potential for chloride ions is assumed to be identical with the resting membrane potential. In the left diagram, the EPSP appears large enough to generate a spike potential, the course of the EPSP in absence of a spike being shown by the broken line. In the right diagram (continuous line), an initial IPSP appears to diminish depo-

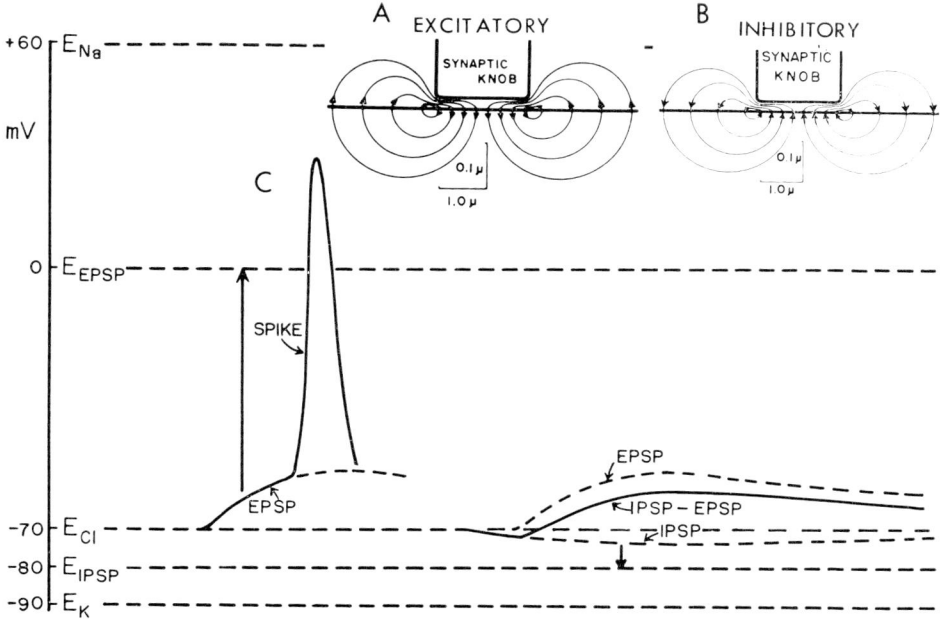

Fig. 9-5. (A) Activated excitatory synaptic knob. Synaptic cleft shown at ten times scale for width as against length. Current passes inward along cleft and across activated subsynaptic membrane. Elsewhere it passes outward across membrane, so generating depolarization of EPSP. (B) Reverse direction of current flow for activated inhibitory synaptic knob. (C) Equilibrium potentials for sodium (E_{Na}), potassium (E_K), and chloride (E_{Cl}) ions together with equilibrium potential for postsynaptic inhibition, (E_{IPSP}) (cf. Fig. 9-4G). Equilibrium potential for EPSP (E_{EPSP}) is shown at zero (cf. Fig. 9-2H). To left, an EPSP is generating a spike potential at depolarization of about 18 mV (see Fig. 9-2E through G). To right of diagram, IPSP and EPSP are shown alone (broken lines), then interacting (continuous line). As a consequence of the depressant influence of the IPSP, the EPSP that alone generated a spike (left diagram) no longer is able to attain the threshold level of depolarization, i.e., the inhibition has been effective.

larization produced by the same synaptic excitation (continuous line) so that it is no longer adequate to generate a spike.

Experimental investigations on ionic mechanisms involve altering the concentration gradient across the postsynaptic membrane for one or another species of ion normally present, and in addition employing a wide variety of other ions in order to test ionic permeability of the subsynaptic membrane. With the inhibitory synapses on invertebrate nerve and muscle cells, investigations are usually performed on isolated preparations. Changes in relative ionic concentration across the postsynaptic membrane are readily effected by altering ionic composition of the external medium. This method is not suitable for neurons in the mammalian central nervous system. Instead, the procedure of electrophoretic injection of ions out of the impaling microelectrode has been used to alter ionic composition of the postsynaptic cell. For example, the species of anions that can pass through the inhibitory membrane have been recognized by injecting one or another species into a nerve cell, to see if the increase in intracellular concentration effects an appropriate change in the inhibitory postsynaptic potential. These injections are accomplished by filling microelectrodes with salts containing anions under investigation. When the microelectrode is inserted into a nerve cell, a given amount of the anion can be injected electrophoretically into the cell by passing an appropriate current through the microelectrode [19, 21].

In Fig. 9-6 the IPSP in (A) was changed

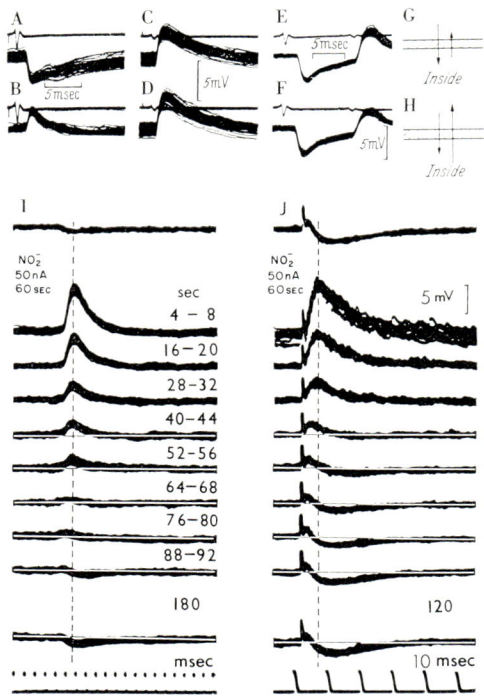

FIG. 9-6. (A) and (B) IPSPs. (C) and (D) EPSPs generated in biceps-semitendinosus motoneuron by afferent volleys (as in Fig. 9-4D and E, respectively). (A) and (C) were first recorded, then hyperpolarizing current of 2×10^{-8} amp was passed through microelectrode which had been filled with 3-M KCl. Note that the injection of chloride ions converted the IPSP from hyperpolarizing (A) to depolarizing response (B), while EPSP was not appreciably changed (C) and (D). Passing much stronger hyperpolarizing current (4×10^{-8} amp for 90 sec) through a microelectrode filled with 0.6-M K_2SO_4 caused no significant change (E) to (F) in either the IPSP or the later EPSP. (G) and (H) represent the assumed fluxes of chloride ions across the membrane before (G) and after (H), the injection of chloride ions, which is shown greatly increasing the efflux of chloride. (I) and (J) Effects of electrophoretic injection of NO_2^- ions into motoneurons. (I) IPSP in motoneuron evoked by quadriceps Ia volley, (J) Renshaw IPSP in motoneuron, innervation of which was not identified, induced by maximal L_7 ventral-root stimulation. Records in top row show control IPSPs at indicated time, identical in (I) and (J), after injection of NO_2^- ions by passage of current 5×10^{-8} amp for 60 sec. Bottom records are IPSPs at end of recovery. Note different time scales of (I) and (J). All records formed by superposition of about 20 faint traces. (From Coombs, Eccles, and Fatt [16].)

to a depolarizing potential (B) by the addition of about 5 picaequivalents of chloride ions to the cell, which would more than triple the intracellular concentration, whereas after more than twice this injection of sulphate ions into another cell the IPSP was unchanged (Fig. 9-6E and F). In both cases the EPSP was virtually unchanged. This simple test establishes that under action of the inhibitory transmitter, the subsynaptic membrane momentarily becomes permeable to chloride ions, but not to sulphate, there being change in chloride movement as illustrated in Fig. 9-6G and H. In Fig. 9-6I and J, it is evident that with two types of inhibitory synaptic action in the mammalian spinal cord, the inhibitory membrane was permeable to nitrite ions, and recovery from the effect of the ionic injection was complete in about 2 minutes.

It is essential to recognize that Fig. 9-6I

and *J* exemplify two quite distinct processes of ionic exchange. First, the ionic permeability of the whole postsynaptic membrane controls intracellular ionic composition and is responsible for recovery after ionic injections that occupies 2 minutes in Fig. 9-6*I* and *J*. Second, the specialized subsynaptic areas under the influence of the inhibitory transmitter develop for a few milliseconds a specific ionic permeability of a much higher order. The second process is responsible for ionic fluxes that give the inhibitory subsynaptic currents which are our present concern.

Potassium ions are normally at a high level in nerve cells. For this reason ion-injection procedures cannot produce large increases or decreases in intracellular potassium concentration, and hence have been indecisive in regard to evidence for or against potassium ion permeability as a contributory factor in production of the IPSP [19, 21]. Nevertheless, there is evidence for a relatively large contribution from potassium ion permeability: the equilibrium potential for potassium is about 20 mV more hyperpolarized than the resting membrane potential (Fig. 9-5*C*), the equilibrium potential for inhibition is similarly in the hyperpolarizing direction, but less so, probably about 6 to 10 mV. The equilibrium potential for chloride is probably slightly in the depolarizing direction because of operation of the postulated inward chloride pump [19]. These considerations suggest that permeability of the activated inhibitory membrane for potassium ions is at least half that for chloride ions; the simplest assumption is equality, the permeability being determined solely by hydrated ion size, but for cations as well as anions, which is of course sufficient to exclude the large hydrated sodium ions [19, 21].

PRESYNAPTIC INHIBITION. The other method of inhibitory control in the central nervous system was recognized by Frank and Fuortes [24], but only very recently have we understood the mechanism of presynaptic inhibition, and appreciated its preeminent role in negative feedback control of the sensory pathways. The mode of operation of presynaptic inhibition is illustrated above the neuron in Fig. 9-7. The presynaptic inhibitory synapse is drawn superimposed on the excitatory synapse and many such synapses have been seen in electron micrographs. By a chemical transmitter action the excitatory synaptic knob is depolarized; consequently, a spike potential in this knob is diminished and the output of excitatory transmitter substance is depressed. It is thus seen that inhibitory action is exerted on excitatory presynaptic terminals and not at all on the postsynaptic membrane, so it is called presynaptic inhibition [19, 20]. Presynaptic inhibition is exerted on all varieties of large afferent fibers that have been examined so far; at the first synaptic relay it is usually of far greater potency than postsynaptic inhibition.

Presynaptic inhibition can be displayed by various experimental procedures. A direct test is to record from the excitatory fiber by an intracellular electrode and observe the depolarization directly, as in the upper right-hand records of Fig. 9-7. Another method is to record intracellularly from the neuron and show that the excitatory postsynaptic potential is reduced because the excitatory transmitter output is depressed, as may be seen in the upper left-hand records of Fig. 9-7. A very convenient way of demonstrating presynaptic inhibition is provided by diminution in the discharge of impulses evoked by a test excitatory input, as is shown to the lower left of Fig. 9-7. All of these tests have been applied systematically. Another way of demonstrating presynaptic inhibition that is particularly valuable is to test the excitability of excitatory fibers, that is, of the primary afferent fibers. When depolarized by the presynaptic inhibitory action, they become more excitable; this effect can be quantitatively estimated by the technique first developed by Wall [49].

Generalizations about Presynaptic Inhibition. First, presynaptic inhibition has no patterned topography. It is widely dispersed over the afferents of a limb with no tendency to focal application. For example, presynaptic inhibitory action by the afferent fibers of a muscle is effective on the

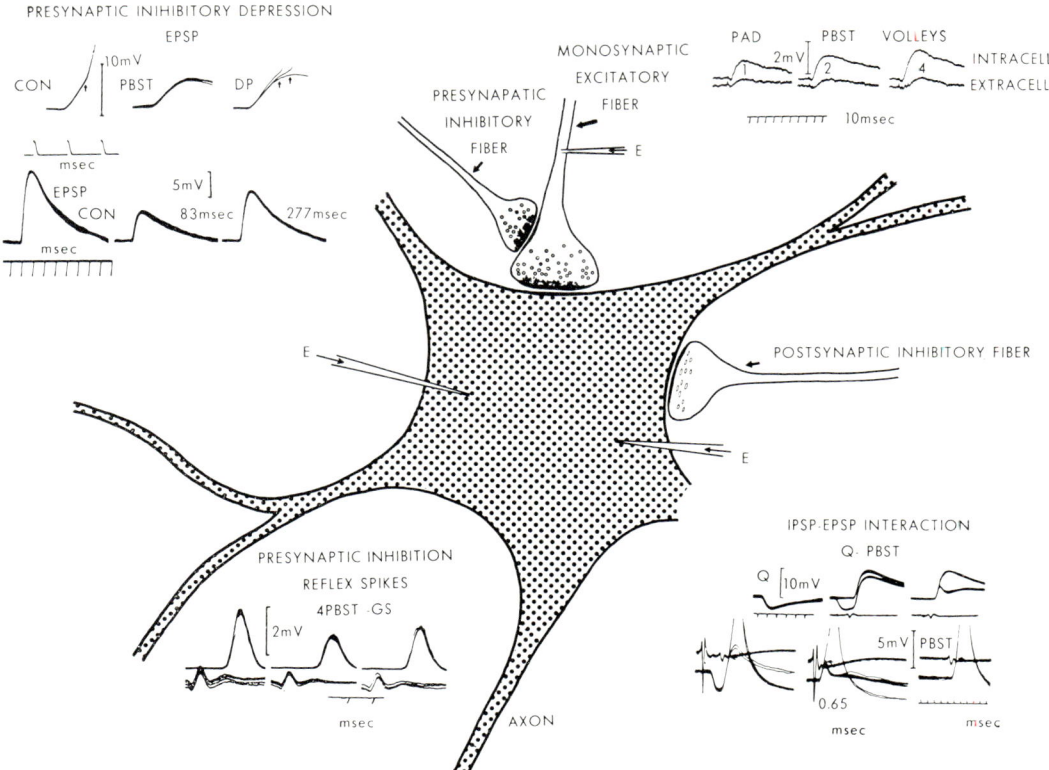

Fig. 9-7. Specimen records of various types of responses associated with synaptic action. On right side, intracellular electrode with specimen records of IPSPs (downward deflections) and EPSPs (upward deflections) and their interactions; two examples of spike inhibition in lower row. Excitatory and inhibitory synapses shown on neuron, also presynaptic inhibitory ending on excitatory fiber, which by intracellular recording (note electrode) is depolarized, shown by difference in intracellular records in upper right traces for 1, 2, and 4 volleys. In upper left quadrant are effects of presynaptic depolarization on its excitatory synaptic action (EPSP), recorded intracellularly. Note large diminution of excitatory potentials in lower row. In upper row presynaptic inhibition depresses excitatory potential so that it often fails to generate spike, as it regularly does in the control (CON record) at the arrow. Lower left quadrant, resultant diminution of reflex spike discharge recorded in ventral roots, the first being the control response.

afferents from all muscles regardless of function. It is not selective on one class of muscle, or on the muscles acting at any one joint of a limb. This widespread, non-specific character is exactly what would be expected for the general suppressor influence of negative feedback. Nevertheless, there is organization or pattern in the distribution of presynaptic inhibition; this pattern depends on the class or modality of the afferent fiber on which the presynaptic inhibition falls (cf. [20]).

Another generalization is that presynaptic inhibition is much more effective at the primary afferent level than at the higher levels of the nervous system. However, it has been shown to exercise an important inhibitory influence on pathways through the thalamus and lateral geniculate body. So far there has been no evidence for presynaptic inhibition at the highest levels of the mammalian brain, the cerebellar and cerebral cortexes, both neocortex and archicortex.

SUMMARY

In conclusion, Fig. 9-8 will serve to summarize diagrammatically the detailed events

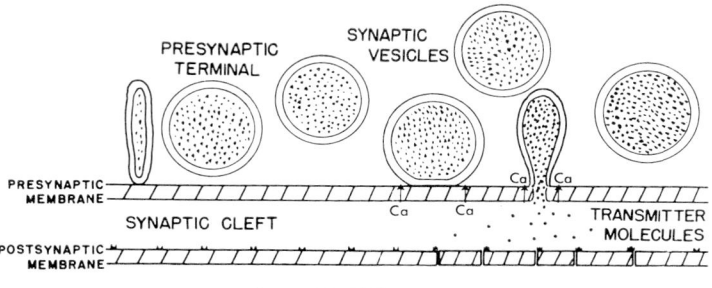

Fig. 9-8. Portion of synaptic cleft with synaptic vesicles in close proximity in presynaptic terminal, one actually discharging transmitter molecules into synaptic cleft. Some molecules shown combined with receptor sites on subsynaptic part of postsynaptic membrane with consequent opening-up of pores through that membrane. Arrows denoted Ca show movement of Ca ions through presynaptic membrane.

which are presumed to occur when an impulse reaches an excitatory or inhibitory presynaptic terminal, which we would expect to see if electron microscopy can be developed with sufficient resolving power. Some of the synaptic vesicles are in close contact with the membrane and one or more are caused by the depolarizing action of the impulse to eject their contained transmitter substance into the synaptic cleft. An essential link in this process of quantal liberation is movement of calcium ions from the synaptic cleft to the inside of the presynaptic membrane, as shown by the arrows. Diffusion of liberated transmitter molecules across and along the cleft, as shown, would occur in a few microseconds for distances of a few hundred angstroms. Some of the transmitter becomes momentarily attached to the specific receptor sites on the postsynaptic membrane, with the consequence of an opening-up of fine channels across this membrane; the subsynaptic membrane momentarily assumes a sievelike character. With excitatory synapses, there is opening of ionic channels specifically permeable to potassium and sodium and closely related ions, the net ionic flux depolarizing the postsynaptic membrane. With inhibitory synapses, the ions, chloride or potassium, or both, move across the membrane thousands of times more readily than normally; this intense ionic flux gives current that produces the IPSP and that counteracts the depolarizing action of excitatory synapses, so effecting inhibition as illustrated in Fig. 9-4H through K.

INHIBITORY AND EXCITATORY PATHWAYS IN CENTRAL NERVOUS SYSTEM

Introduction

An outcome of the recent, intensive investigation of the mammalian central nervous system is the finding that almost all neurons are subjected to antagonistic excitatory and inhibitory synaptic actions. A further, more remarkable outcome is the hypothesis that a neuron itself can exert only one type of synaptic action. If it acts by excitatory synapses at some of its axonal terminals, then it does so at all of its synapses; it can exercise an inhibitory action only through an interpolated interneuron, which itself, likewise, has an inhibitory action at all of the synapses made by its axon. This hypothesis led to the generalization that with the exception of presynaptic inhibitory pathways (see below) there are but two classes of nerve cell in the central nervous system: those purely excitatory and those purely inhibitory. This hypothesis has been developed in relation to the mammalian central nervous system. In fish there is electrical transmission between some motoneurons [10] and in invertebrates the same transmitter, acetylcholine, may have excitatory or inhibitory synapses on different target neurons [14, 15, 29]. However, no evidence for such ambivalency has yet been adduced for the mammalian central nervous system. It can be added in parenthesis that in the mammalian central nervous system there probably is a third class: the presynaptic inhibitory cells responsible for presynaptic inhibition (cf. Fig. 9-7). But the evidence is less convincing because it is still possible, although unlikely, that depolarization of the presynaptic terminals is effected by collaterals of cells belonging to the class of excitatory nerve cells.

THE PATHWAY THROUGH RENSHAW CELLS

Figure 9-9 illustrates a very thoroughly studied example of a simple postsynaptic inhibitory mechanism [23], which can be used as an initial example. Axon collaterals of motoneurons monosynaptically excite fast and prolonged repetitive discharges (Fig. 9-9B) from Renshaw cells by the same excitatory transmitter (acetylcholine) that acts peripherally at the neuromuscular synapses (Fig. 9-9A). These Renshaw cells in turn directly inhibit the motoneuron, producing large and relatively prolonged IPSPs (Fig. 9-9D) that may show the ripple of the Renshaw cell rhythmic discharge of about 1000 per sec (Fig. 9-9C). Latency of the IPSP is determined by comparison of the intracellular and just-extracellular records, the onset at the lower arrow in Fig. 9-9E having a latency of 1.2 msec, which is just sufficient for the pathway of Fig. 9-9A, because the Renshaw cell discharge may commence as soon as 0.65 msec after the entry of an antidromic volley into the spinal cord. Moreover, the repetitive discharge of the Renshaw cell is generated solely by the simple monosynaptic excitatory pathway by motor axon collaterals (Fig. 9-9A). There is no evidence for any polysynaptic excitatory pathway, and continued action of the transmitter liberated by a single synchronous synaptic bombardment is responsible for the repetitive response (Fig. 9-9B).

EXCITATORY AND INHIBITORY PATHWAYS IN HIPPOCAMPUS

One of the most important aspects of hippocampal histology, making this area a preferred target for physiological studies,

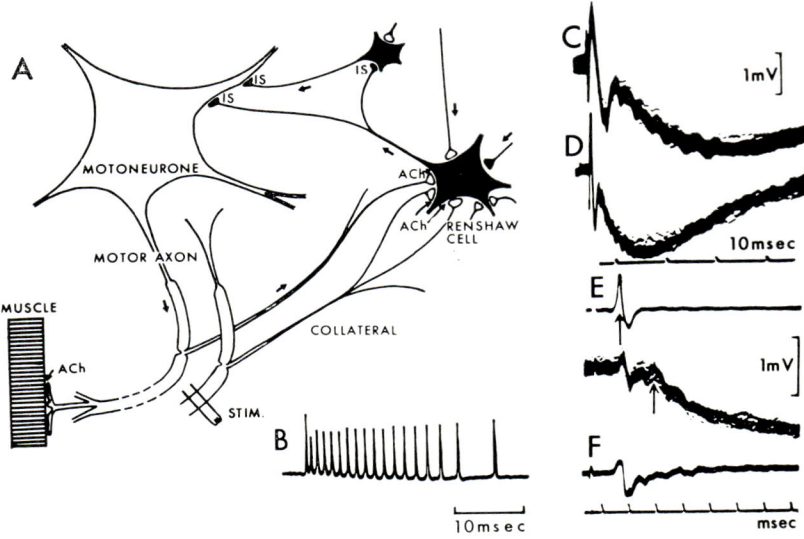

FIG. 9-9. Inhibitory pathways to motoneurons by their axon collaterals and Renshaw cells. (B) Extracellular recording of Renshaw cell being excited by antidromic volley in motor fibers of lateral gastrocnemius muscle. (C), (D) and lower trace of (E) Intracellular responses evoked by antidromic volley in ventral root (fully described in text). The upper trace of (E) gives the potential recorded at site of entry of antidromic volley into spinal cord, which occurs at time of arrow, 1.2 msec before onset of IPSP at arrow in lower trace of (E). (F) Extracellular control for (E). Same time scale for (C), (E), and (F). (From Eccles, Fatt, and Koketsu [23].)

is the zoning of synapses on pyramidal cells. For all practical purposes these cells are arranged in one layer, parallel to each other, and with their long axes perpendicular to the ventricular surface. Since histological investigations have shown that the various afferent systems to the hippocampus form synapses in sharply restricted, band-like structures, parallel to the surface (Fig. 9-10A, B) [11, 12, 26, 39, 44], it may be concluded that a particular afferent route can influence synaptically a restricted part of the pyramids only. For example, the soma itself receives synapses almost exclusively from the basket cells. Since these were the first synapses to be recognized as inhibitory [3, 4, 5], and since the basket cells provide the simplest and clearest examples of inhibitory cells, the hippocampus is worthy of privileged treatment in the story of central inhibitory pathways. The zoning of excitatory pathways on dendrites of pyramidal cells has given Andersen and his colleagues the opportunity for further understanding of regional synaptic action.

Excitatory Mechanisms in Hippocampus

Figure 9-10C shows the principal excitatory pathways that have been investigated by Andersen and his colleagues [1, 7, 8]. A stimulus into the entorhinal area activates the perforant pathway (pp) that excites the dentate cells and their axons, which form the mossy fibers (mf) in Fig. 9-10C that terminate in the basal part of the apical dendrite of CA3 pyramidal cells as in Fig. 9-10A. The axons of the CA3 pyramidal cells give off collaterals, the Schaffer collaterals (Sch), that form synapses on the apical dendrites of the CA1 pyramidal cells. In addition, Fig. 9-10A and B show the ending of many commissural fibers on the basal dendrites and the more proximal zone of the apical dendrite of CA1 pyramidal cells.

Figure 9-11A shows the extracellular records of field potentials generated by CA1 pyramidal cells in response to entorhinal stimulation. At depths of 0.8–0.6 mm there is a large, late negative potential (SN) that has a spike superimposed at 0.6

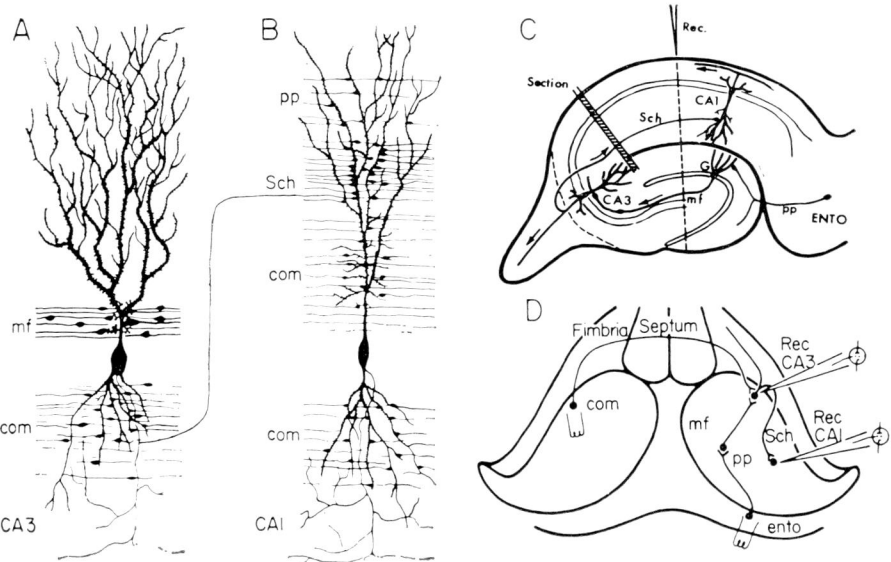

FIG. 9-10. Neuronal system under study. (A) Simplified drawing of pyramidal cell of field CA3 of hippocampus with some of its afferent connections. (B) Similar drawing of CA1 pyramidal cell. (C) Sagittal section through dorsal part of hippocampus indicating relative position of cells and synapses under study. (D) Dorsal view of hippocampal formation with localization of stimulating and recording electrodes. Abbreviations: com, commissural afferent fibers; ento, entorhinal area; mf, mossy fibers (axons of dentate granule cells); pp, perforant path; Sch, Schaffer collaterals of the CA3 pyramids. (From Andersen and Lømo [8].)

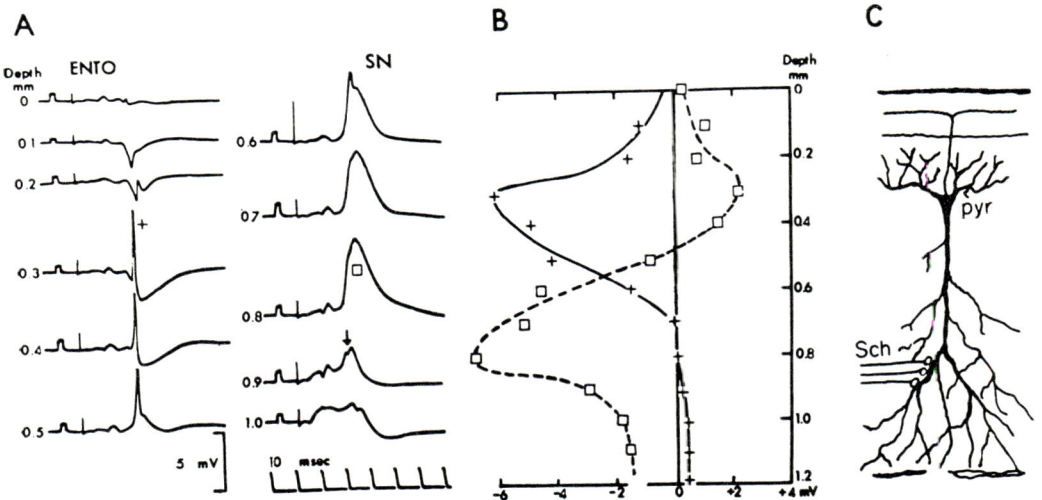

FIG. 9-11. Extracellular potentials recorded from CA1 in response to entorhinal stimulation. (A) Extracellular records obtained at indicated depths below ventricular surface in response to single-shock entorhinal stimulation. Two main components appear: spike (cross) and Schaffer negativity (SN, open square). (B) Amplitudes of these two components plotted against recording depth. (C) Typical CA1 pyramid and its entorhinal input via Sch, drawn to scale to facilitate comparison with records in (A). (From Andersen, Holmqvist, and Voorhoeve [7].)

mm depth. More superficially, at 0.5–0.3 mm there is a large, extracellular spike potential. Measurements of these two potentials, as indicated by the symbols, are plotted in Fig. 9-11B on the same depth profile as the drawing of the CA1 pyramidal cell in Fig. 9-11C. The negative potential at 0.6–0.8 mm clearly can be interpreted as the extracellular counterpart of the synaptic excitatory action of Schaffer collaterals (Sch in Fig. 9-11C). The depth profile corresponds, as may be seen by comparing B and C in Fig. 9-11; and the long latency is, of course, attributable to the two additional synaptic relays plus the long conduction pathway illustrated in Fig. 9-10C. Evidently the spike potential is produced by the Schaffer collateral excitation. At depths of 0.3–0.5 mm, much faster recording than that illustrated in Fig. 9-11A shows that this spike is conducted from the region of the Schaffer collateral synapses towards the soma with a velocity of about 0.4 meter a second. Relationship of the extracellular spike to the slow potential (the sequence from depths of 0.8 to 0.5 mm in Fig. 9-11A) suggests that this spike is generated in the dendrites just on the somatic side of the Schaffer axon synapses.

When recording intracellularly from the somata of the CA1 pyramidal cells, there is usually no trace of an EPSP generated by the Schaffer collateral synapses. For example, in Fig. 9-12B, C, and D there is merely the large IPSP of basket-cell inhibition that is illustrated in Fig. 9-14A through C. However, occasionally as in Fig. 9-12E there is a small initial depolarization that is recorded probably because the electrode was in the large apical dendrite and thus nearer to the excitatory synapses. In Fig. 9-12F, repetitive stimulation potentiated this EPSP and at the same time eliminated the later IPSP.

Synaptic excitation of pyramidal cells by the commissural pathway to the basal dendrites of CA3 pyramidal cells is illustrated in Fig. 9-13. It shows spike potentials in B, C, and D that are not preceded by any appreciable prepotential. In Fig. 9-13A there appears to be only an IPSP as in Fig. 9-12B through D. However, on repetitive stimulation at 10 per sec for several seconds (Fig. 9-13B and C), a synaptically evoked

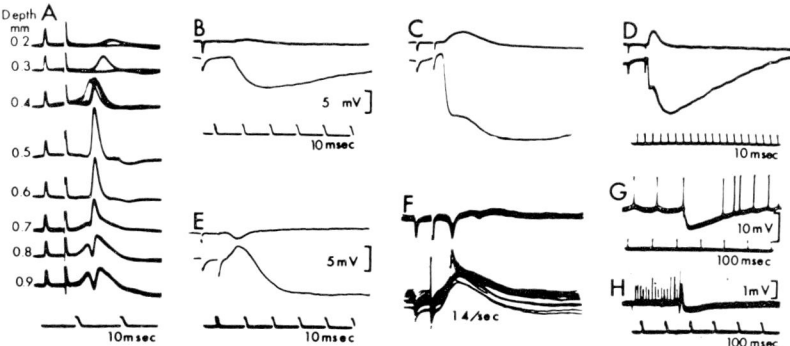

FIG. 9-12. Absence of soma depolarization in response to Schaffer collateral activation. (A) Extracellular records, taken at indicated depth in response to single Schaffer collateral stimulation in cat. (B) and (C) Intracellular records (lower traces) and extracellular records (upper traces) in response to a weak (B) and a stronger (C) activation of Schaffer collaterals. (D) As (C), but slower sweep speed. (E) Record from cell met at depth of 0.6 mm, showing initial depolarization followed by larger hyperpolarization (lower trace). Note that extracellular record (upper trace) shows negativity comparable to intracellular depolarization. (F) Recording from same cell as (E) but at higher stimulus rate (14 sec). (G) and (H) Two examples showing cessation of spontaneous discharges in response to single Schaffer collateral activation. (From Andersen, Holmqvist, and Voorhoeve [7].)

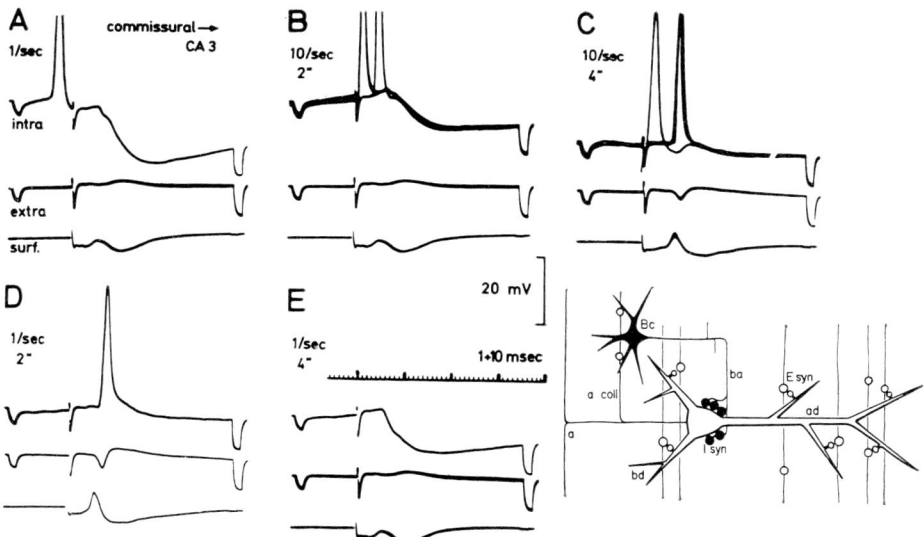

FIG. 9-13. Intracellular records from CA3 pyramidal cell synaptically activated by commissural pathway. (A) Cell firing spontaneously, following commissural volley, IPSP is only response. (B) and (C) Responses following 10-per-sec stimulation for 2 and 4 sec, respectively. Antidromic invasion has short latency; when it fails, synaptic spike occurs, followed by IPSP. Thus, excitatory effect of commissural pathway demonstrated by synaptically driven spikes. Note, no prepotential in front of spike. (D) Excitatory state outlasted tetanic stimulation, taken 2 sec after cessation of tetanus. Again, no prepotential. (E) Normal potential in response to single shock through commissural pathway is IPSP with no preceding sign of excitation. Abbreviations: intra, intracellular records; extra, extracellular records; surf, surface records. Inset, diagram of synaptic connections. (From Andersen, Blackstad, and Lømo [1].)

spike appears without any prepotential and this is observable even for some seconds after reduction of this high rate to the initial 1 per sec frequency (Fig. 9-13D). A small electrotonically transmitted EPSP can be seen in Fig. 9-13C when the antidromic spike prevented the subsequent synaptically evoked spike. The usual failure to record from the soma EPSPs preceding the spike potential (Fig. 9-13B through D) indicates that there is severe electrotonic decrement from the sites of excitatory synaptic action on the dendrites. The evidence is quite conclusive in showing that impulses are generated in the dendrites close to the excitatory synapses and propagate from there down to the soma. In some experiments it was possible to demonstrate local responses that failed to grow to fully propagated spikes [8].

Evidently the excitatory synapses on the hippocampal pyramidal cells are effective in generating impulse discharges in adjacent regions on the dendrites, which is a mechanism very different from generation in the initial segment of motoneurons and many other species of neurons, as shown in Fig. 9-2E through G. Probably neocortical pyramidal cells resemble hippocampal pyramidal cells in this respect, but it has not yet been possible to perform sufficiently discriminative experiments because of the much greater structural diversity in the neocortex.

Inhibitory Mechanisms in Hippocampus

Because of the differences between the upper (extracellular) and lower (intracellular) traces, shown in Fig. 9-14A through C, stimulation of the three separate inputs to the hippocampal cortex (cf. Fig. 9-10D, Com and Septum) regularly produces very large and long IPSPs of the pyramidal cells [4]. Such IPSPs in response

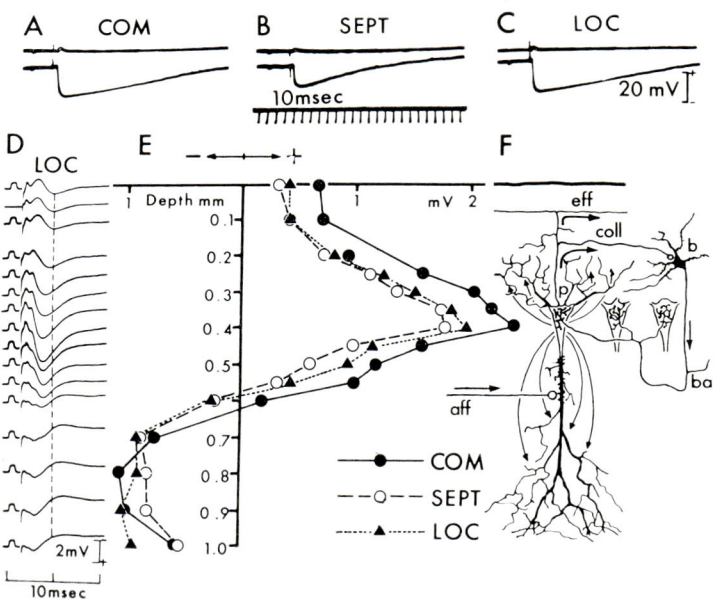

FIG. 9-14. Responses evoked in hippocampus by commissural (COM), septal (SEPT), and local (LOC) stimulation. (A), (B), (C) Lower traces, intracellular records; upper traces, extracellular records taken just outside cell with same gain and polarity as inside recording. (D) Responses recorded by microelectrode penetrating CA3 following local stimulation. (E) Graph in which sizes of positive waves of responses to commissural, septal, and local stimulation are plotted against depth. Positivities are measured at time indicated by stippled line in (D) correspondingly for the other inputs. Same depth scale for (D) and (E). (F) CA3 pyramidal cell, semidiagrammatically drawn to scale to facilitate comparison with (E). Arrows indicate extracellular flow of current generating inhibitory postsynaptic potentials. (From Andersen, Eccles, and Løyning [3].)

to fimbrial stimulation were originally observed by Kandel, Spencer, and Brinley [30], by Kandel and Spencer [31], and by Spencer and Kandel [45]. Figure 9-14D shows an arrangement of the extracellular potentials produced by local stimulation and recorded at various depths along a track that penetrated as deeply as the terminals of apical dendrites of the CA3 pyramidal cells. An initial negativity at superficial levels probably is due to synaptic excitation of basal dendrites of pyramidal cells [8]; but the dominant potential down to 0.5 mm is the large positive wave that attains a maximum at about 5 msec after the stimulus. This wave was measured at the fixed interval (shown in Fig. 9-14D by the broken line), so as to minimize contamination by the initial superficial negativity, and is plotted as filled triangles in Fig. 9-14E. Similarly, measurements for the potentials generated by the other stimulations, commissural and septal, are also plotted in Fig. 9-14E. There is remarkable congruity in these three plots of potential fields, all of which have a sharp maximum at a depth of 0.4 mm.

The interpretation of such potential fields is simplified by recognizing that, because of their length, density, and orientation, pyramidal cells are the only neurons that could generate such large extracellular fields. Furthermore, cell bodies of these neurons are arranged in a sheet at a depth of 0.4–0.5 mm below the surface of the alveus (cf. Fig. 9-10C); the electrode track is perpendicular to this sheet and runs along the length of the cells from their basal to their apical dendrites, which can be understood from Figs. 9-11C and 9-14F. It can thus be concluded that field potentials of Fig. 9-14E must be produced by a powerful source of potential at or near the somata of the pyramidal cells, and that in the extracellular medium, current flows from this source both superficially to the basal dendrites and deeply to the apical dendrites, indicated by the arrows in Fig. 9-14F.

Cells with a very different response pattern were found at depths from the hippocampal surface of 0.2–0.45 mm, from the alveus down into the layer of the pyramidal cell bodies. These were observed more frequently closer to the pyramidal layer than more superficially, and were more difficult to discover with the microelectrode than were the pyramidal cells. In every respect these cells conform with specifications for postulated inhibitory cells. In contrast, an afferent input usually evoked a single-spike response of a pyramidal cell; only rarely was more than one input effective. Impalement by the microelectrode was obtained much more easily with pyramidal cells than with interneurons.

Since these presumed inhibitory cells were never fired by fimbrial stimulation with a latency compatible with antidromic invasion, it can be concluded that their axons do not project to the fimbria and that these cells belong to one or another of the many types of basket cells (Fig. 9-15Ab) [39, 44] which form the large majority of cells in the stratum oriens.

Features of Basket Cells. The variety of the basket cell types stems from the diversity of their dendritic pattern. However, they have one feature in common: the axonal terminals of each (Fig. 9-15Aba) make a dense meshwork of fibers, a basket-like entanglement, around the somata of a large number of pyramidal cells. The synapses formed by these axonal terminals are concentrated on the somatic regions of the pyramidal cells (Fig. 9-15A) in the region that is bare of spines (Fig. 9-10A and B), to the exclusion of virtually all other synapses.

Basket cells fulfill one of the essential, anatomical requirements for an inhibitory interneuron according to physiological findings. There are no precise statements on the degree of distribution of the basket-cell axons. On the assumption that there is uniform distribution of these axons in all directions and a thickness of about 100 μ of the Golgi sections, the drawings of Ramón y Cajal and of Lorente de Nó allow an estimate that one basket cell makes synaptic contact with 200–500 pyramidal cells. This wide axonal distribution fulfills another requirement for the inhibitory interneuron in the hippocampus.

Although there are other types of cells with short axons in the hippocampus, only the basket cell meets the anatomical re-

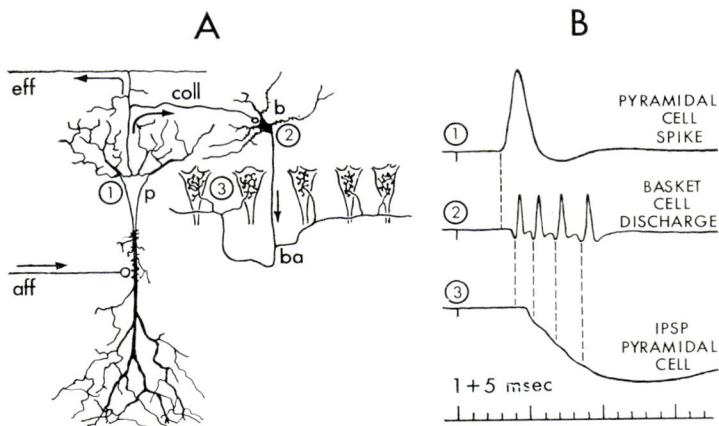

FIG. 9-15. Postulated pathway of postsynaptic inhibition in hippocampus. (A) Cellular elements involved in production of IPSPs in hippocampal pyramidal cells. (B) Responses produced by elements labeled correspondingly in (A). Afferent volley (aff) excites small number of pyramidal cells (p) and brings them to discharge along their axons (eff) (1). Via their axon collaterals (coll) they activate basket cells (b) which respond with short repetitive discharge (2). Terminals of basket-cell axons (ba) produce IPSPs in somata of large number of pyramidal cells (3), which show faint ripple indicative of their production by repetitive synaptic activation. (From Andersen, Eccles, and Løyning [5].)

quirements set by physiological observations. No other cell type has endings on the cell bodies of the pyramidal cells and no other type displays the same wide distribution of axon ramifications. It can be concluded with assurance that basket cells of the hippocampus are the inhibitory cells responsible for producing the IPSPs of the pyramidal cells. Since basket cells are exclusively distributed to the somata of pyramidal cells, it is possible to recognize the morphological characteristics of presumed inhibitory synapses. These synapses have a sparse population of synaptic vesicles and usually conform with the type 2 of Gray [25], having a few small active zones with only moderate increase in opacity of the presynaptic and postsynaptic membrane, although some have an unspecialized appearance [13, 26].

In animals with chronic severence of the fimbria, all orthodromically conducting fibers in this tract to the hippocampus are degenerated. Stimulation restricted to the fimbria will, therefore, activate pyramidal cells only by antidromic invasion from their axons. In such preparations, IPSPs were recorded from pyramidal cells and showed the same latency difference between the antidromic invasion of the pyramidal cells and onset of the IPSP as in animals with intact fimbria. First stated by Spencer and Kandel [45], this indicates that the IPSP is initiated by impulses traveling along axon collaterals of the pyramidal cells, but they made no further statements about the inhibitory pathway.

The latency difference between excitation and inhibition was observed to be about 1.5–2 msec, not only after antidromic stimulation but also after synaptic excitation from the three additional inputs used in the present investigation (Fig. 9-14A, B, and C). The most likely explanation of these observations is that an afferent volley entering the hippocampus initiates the following sequential events (illustrated by the diagrams in Fig. 9-15A and B).

(1) Some pyramidal cells are fired by synaptic excitation described in the preceding section; discharges of these cells are conducted along their axons into the fimbria and also along their axon collaterals within the hippocampal cortex. (2) Synapses of the axon collaterals excite repetitive discharges in a set of inhibitory interneurons, the basket cells, which in turn activate their inhibitory synapses around the cell bodies of a much larger number of pyramidal cells than were excited initially. (3)

The effect of the somatically located basket-cell synapses on the pyramidal cells is to produce the large IPSP recorded by an intracellular electrode. The basket cell (Fig. 9-15Ab) is drawn in black to signify that its action is exclusively inhibitory, in contrast to the excitatory action of pyramidal neurons.

It will be appreciated that the inhibitory pathway of Fig. 9-15A is a simple example of recurrent inhibition to the same class of cell that was originally activated, and that it provides an efficient mechanism for wide distribution of negative feedback. Far more detailed investigation is required before the functional significance of this feedback can be understood.

Andersen, Holmqvist, and Voorhoeve [7] have shown that in the dentate area of hippocampus there is a comparable inhibitory pathway. Numerous axon collaterals of the granule cells ramify in relationship to the dentate basket cells, the axons of these cells ascend to form basketlike terminals around the somata of the dentate granule cells. Identification of the basket cells as inhibitory cells acting on the granule cells depends upon the experimental evidence of Andersen et al. [7], which is comparable with that illustrated above for basket cells and pyramidal cells of hippocampus. Axon collaterals of granule cells are assumed to excite basket cells that in turn give inhibitory synapses to granule cells, to which they are so profusely and widely distributed.

EXCITATORY AND INHIBITORY MECHANISMS IN THALAMUS

The afferent pathway for transmission of somatosensory information to the cerebral cortex passes up the medial lemniscus through the ventrobasal complex of thalamus. Shown diagrammatically in Fig. 9-16K, there is a monosynaptic relay in the thalamus, and the axon collaterals of the thalamocortical relay cells feed back to inhibitory interneurons which exert widespread inhibition of thalamic neurons just as Renshaw cells to motoneurons (Fig. 9-9A) and basket cells to hippocampal pyramidal cells (Fig. 9-15A). The thalamus thus provides a further example of recurrent inhibition [2, 6]; similarly, there is recurrent inhibi-

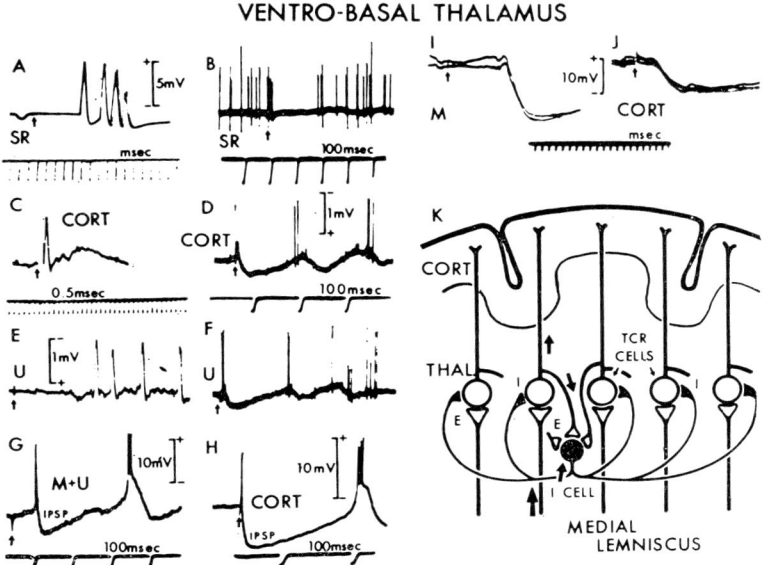

FIG. 9-16. Electrical potentials evoked in ventrobasal thalamus by peripheral nerve and cortical stimulation. SR, U, and M: Responses evoked by single volleys in superficial radial, ulnar, and median nerves respectively. CORT: Responses evoked by stimulation of sensorimotor cortex. Further description in text. (From Andersen, Brooks, Eccles, and Sears [2]; Andersen, Eccles, and Sears [6].)

tion on the pathway from the brachium conjunctivum to the VL thalamus [43]. Experimental evidence for this pathway is illustrated in Fig. 9-16*A* through *J* for the VPL thalamus. Purpura et al. [43] have reported similar evidence for the VL thalamus.

In Fig. 9-16*A* an afferent volley from the superficial radial nerve evokes a brief burst of discharges in thalamocortical relay cells and in Fig. 9-16*B* it can be seen that after this initial burst, the background discharge of all thalamic cells is completely suppressed for a period of almost 200 msec. In another preparation (Fig. 9-16*C*) a single thalamic cell is antidromically invaded at about 0.5 msec after cortical stimulation, which establishes that it is a thalamocortical relay cell. In Fig. 9-16*E* this same cell gives a repetitive burst in response to an afferent volley from the ulnar nerve. In the very slow record of Fig. 9-16*D* the cortical stimulus is followed by a prolonged, extracellular positive wave and there are further spike discharges (some quite small from distant cells) on the declining phase of this wave; again there is a subsequent positive wave and recovery with further spike discharges. In Fig. 9-16*F* a similar sequence of positive waves and spike discharges is seen to be evoked by an afferent volley in the ulnar nerve.

In the diagram of Fig. 9-16*K*, discharges of thalamocortical relay (TCR) cells excite the inhibitory cell (I cell) by axon collaterals; discharges from the I cells in turn give widespread inhibition that causes suppression of all discharges (in Fig. 9-16*B*) and the positive potential waves (in Fig. 9-16*F*). According to this diagram, stimulation of the cortex should likewise activate inhibitory cells by means of antidromic impulses to the same axon collaterals, which explains the first positive wave in Fig. 9-16*D*.

The diagram reveals that each time some thalamic cells discharge impulses, there will be further activation of inhibitory cells with generation of a positive potential (Fig. 9-16*D* and *F*) and suppression of background discharge (Fig. 9-16*B*). Evidence is considerable that the principal feature involved in generation of impulses late on the decline of the positive wave (Fig. 9-16*D* and *F*) is due to postinhibitory rebound. Intracellular recording illustrates that rebound phenomenon very clearly (Fig. 9-16*G*, and *H*), where, after initial activation by an afferent or antidromic volley, there is a prolonged IPSP on which a slowly rising depolarization develops with eventually a burst of spike discharges and subsequently further onset of IPSP. In Fig. 9-16*I* and *J*, the latent periods of IPSPs generated by afferent and cortical stimulation conform to the times expected from circuits illustrated in Fig. 9-16*K*.

The actual diagram of synaptic pathways (Fig. 9-16*K*) is, of course, greatly oversimplified. There are presumably various interneurons responsible for the widespread dispersal of impulses generated by the burst discharges of the postulated pacemaker cells of the rhythmic response. As a consequence of the initial widespread postsynaptic inhibition illustrated in the diagram, both an afferent and an antidromic volley tend to be followed by widespread suppression of thalamocortical cells. Recovery from synchronized IPSPs in this population will occur more or less in phase. The first burst discharge arising during the recovery phase is again widely dispersed to thalamocortical neurons with the consequence that there is a powerful IPSP again cutting off discharges of all these cells, there being a fairly well synchronized cycle of inhibition and recovery to a second burst discharge and so on. In this way it is possible to account for the prolonged succession of positive waves and burst discharges in response to the afferent or antidromic volley [9].

Generation of a phased rhythmic discharge of about 6–10 per second in the thalamus by the mechanism diagrammed (Fig. 9-16*K*) is undoubtedly responsible for a great amount of the rhythmic responses observed in the cortex. Considering the significance of this inhibitory mechanism in regard to the randomized, afferent discharges normally produced by sensory stimulation, it will be appreciated that this negative feedback mechanism functions to depress particularly those synaptic relays in the thalamus that have a weak excitatory action. Hence this inhibitory mechanism serves to sharpen the focus of thalamocortical relay cells in the manner postulated for Renshaw-cell inhibition of motoneuronal pools.

There has been neurohistological evidence for some time for the two main classes of cells in the ventrobasal complex of the thalamus (shown in Fig. 9-16K) [44]. Tömböl [48] has provided more detailed corroboration of the neural connections diagrammed in Fig. 9-16K. She finds that Golgi type II neurons are probably innervated by collaterals of the TCR cells and the Golgi neurons give dense synaptic distribution to TCR cells mostly on the dendrites but to some extent on the soma. These Golgi II neurons have the properties postulated for the inhibitory interneurons. Microelectrode studies by Andersen, Eccles, and Sears [6] have shown that of a total of 167 cells in the ventrobasal complex, 16 had the properties postulated for these postsynaptic inhibitory cells: synaptic activation by cortical stimulation and delayed synaptic stimulation by afferent volleys.

They tended to respond in fast repetitive bursts as do other inhibitory cells (Figs. 9-9B, 9-15B2).

SUMMARY

The illustrative examples of synaptic action in the nervous system point out certain principles of functional design. First, at all transmission sites in the central nervous system there is an inhibitory antagonism to generation of impulse discharge by the excitatory synapses. Almost all species of neurons in the central nervous system that have been adequately investigated exhibit conflict of excitatory and inhibitory synaptic action; never does excitatory synaptic action have the unchallenged power to cause discharge of impulses that in turn have an unchallenged excitatory action upon the next neuronal relay. It can be understood that such unchallenged power would result in an explosive excitation through the neuronal networks of the nervous system which, of course, would appear overtly as a convulsion. This essential inhibitory action is now recognized as due, exclusively, to operation of special-

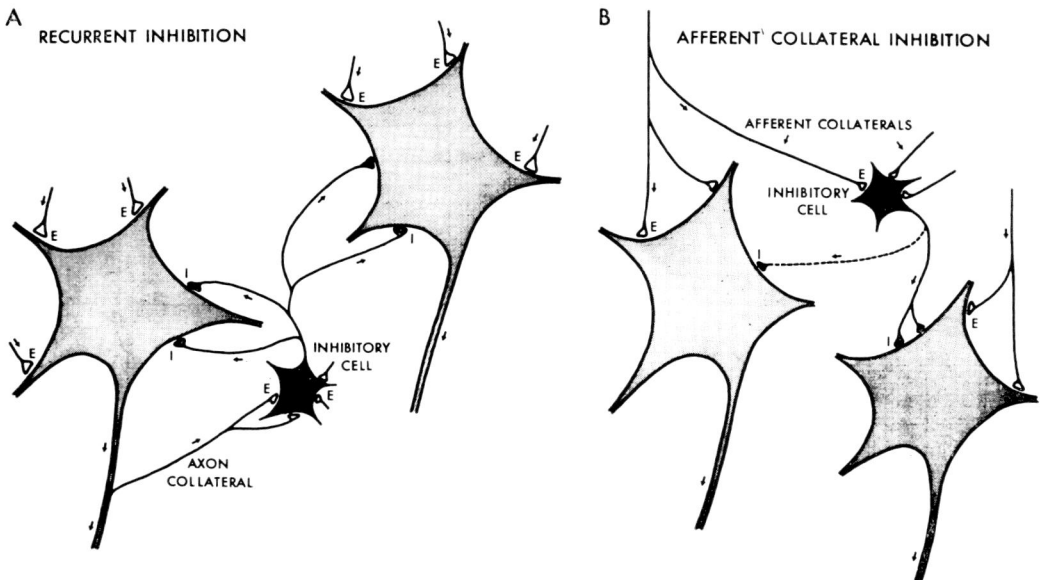

FIG. 9-17. Two types of inhibitory pathways (inhibitory cells shown in black), as described in text.

ized cells which may be called inhibitory neurons, since they have no function other than inhibition. Such generalization is based on detailed study of at least 24 different species of inhibitory interneurons in the mammalian central nervous system [22].

Further, two types of postsynaptic inhibitory pathway can be regarded as elementary constituents of all neuron-inhibitory pathways. In Fig. 9-17A the axon of the nerve cell gives off a recurrent collateral ending in excitatory synapses on a neuron that has widespread inhibitory action. In this way, whenever a nerve cell discharges an impulse, it automatically activates a recurrent inhibitory pathway tending to prevent further discharges from that cell and many other like cells. Examples have been shown diagrammatically in Figs. 9-9A, 9-15A, and 9-16K. In contrast to *recurrent inhibition*, another variety may be termed *afferent collateral inhibition*. In Fig. 9-17B, an afferent nerve fiber, synaptically exciting a nerve cell, gives off a collateral branch which also synaptically excites an inhibitory cell that in turn exerts inhibitory synaptic action on other functionally related neurons. Many examples of this type of inhibition are in the spinal cord, the dorsal-column nuclei, the cerebellum, and probably in the neocortex [22].

REFERENCES

1. Anderson, P., Blackstad, T. W., and Lømo, T. Location and identification of excitatory synapses on hippocampal pyramidal cells. *Exp. Brain Res.* 1:236, 1966.
2. Andersen, P., Brooks, C. McC., Eccles, J. C., and Sears, T. A. The ventro-basal nucleus of the thalamus: potential fields, synaptic transmission and excitability of both presynaptic and post-synaptic components. *J. Physiol.* (London) 174:348, 1964.
3. Andersen, P., Eccles, J. C., and Løyning, Y. Recurrent inhibition in the hippocampus with identification of the inhibitory cell and its synapses. *Nature* (London) 198:540, 1963.
4. Andersen, P., Eccles, J. C., and Løyning, Y. Location of postsynaptic inhibitory synapses on hippocampal pyramids. *J. Neurophysiol.* 27:592, 1964a.
5. Andersen, P., Eccles, J. C., and Løyning, Y. Pathway of postsynaptic inhibition in the hippocampus. *J. Neurophysiol.* 27:608, 1964b.
6. Andersen, P., Eccles, J. C., and Sears, T. A. The ventro-basal complex of the thalamus: types of cells, their responses and their functional organization. *J. Physiol.* (London) 174:370, 1964.
7. Andersen, P., Holmqvist, B., and Voorhoeve, P. E. Excitatory synapses on hippocampal apical dendrites activated by entorhinal stimulation. *Acta Physiol. Scand.* 66:461, 1966.
8. Andersen, P., and Lømo, T. Mode of activation of hippocampal pyramidal cells by excitatory synapses on dendrites. *Exp. Brain Res.* 2:247, 1966.
9. Andersen, P., and Sears, T. A. The role of inhibition in the phasing of spontaneous thalamo-cortical discharge. *J. Physiol.* (London) 173:459, 1964.
10. Bennett, M. V. L. Similarities Between Chemically and Electrically Mediated Transmission. In Carlson, F. D. (Ed.), *Physiological and Biochemical Aspects of Nervous Integration*. Englewood Cliffs, N. J.: Prentice-Hall, 1968.
11. Blackstad, T. W. Commissural connections of the hippocampal region in the rat, with special reference to their mode of termination. *J. Comp. Neurol.* 105:417, 1956.
12. Blackstad, T. W. On the termination of some afferents to the hippocampus and fascia dentata. *Acta Anat.* (Basel) 35:202, 1958.
13. Blackstad, T. W., and Flood, P. R. Ultrastructure of hippocampal axo-somatic synapses. *Nature* (London) 198:542, 1963.
14. Chiarandini, D. J., and Gerschenfeld, H. M. Ionic mechanism of cholinergic inhibition in molluscan neurons. *Science* 156:1595, 1967.
15. Chiarandini, D. J., Stefani, E., and Gerschenfeld, H. M. Ionic mechanisms of cholinergic excitation in molluscan neurons. *Science* 156:1597, 1967.
16. Coombs, J. S., Eccles, J. C., and Fatt, P. The specific ionic conductances and the

ionic movements across the mononeuronal membrane that produce the inhibitory postsynaptic potential. *J. Physiol.* (London) 130:326, 1955.

17. Creutzfeldt, O. D., Lux, H. D., and Nacimiento, A. C. Intracelluläre Reizung corticaler Nervenzellen. *Pflueger Arch. Ges. Physiol.* 281:129, 1964.

18. Eccles, J. C. *The Physiology of Nerve Cells.* Baltimore: Johns Hopkins Press, 1957.

19. Eccles, J. C. *The Physiology of Synapses.* Berlin: Springer, 1964a.

20. Eccles, J. C. Presynaptic Inhibition in the Spinal Cord. In Eccles, J. C., and Schadé, J. P. (Eds.), *Progress in Brain Research.* Amsterdam: Elsevier, 1964b.

21. Eccles, J. C. The ionic mechanisms of excitatory and inhibitory synaptic action. *Ann. N. Y. Acad. Sci.* 137:473, 1966.

22. Eccles, J. C. *The Inhibitory Pathways of the Central Nervous System* (Sherrington lectures). Liverpool: Liverpool Univ. Press, 1969.

23. Eccles, J. C., Fatt, P., and Koketsu, K. Cholinergic and inhibitory synapses in a pathway from motor-axon collaterals to motoneurones. *J. Physiol.* (London) 126:524, 1954.

24. Frank, K., and Fuortes, M. G. F. Presynaptic and postsynaptic inhibition of monosynaptic reflexes. *Fed. Proc.* 16:39, 1957.

25. Gray, E. G. Axo-somatic and axo-dendritic synapses of the cerebral cortex: an electron microscope study. *J. Anat.* 93:420, 1959.

26. Hamlyn, L. H. An electron microscope study of pyramidal neurons in the Ammon's Horn of the rabbit. *J. Anat.* 97:189, 1963.

27. Hodgkin, A. L. *The Conduction of the Nervous Impulse.* Liverpool: Liverpool Univ. Press, 1964.

28. Jung, R. Allgemeine Neurophysiologie. In *Handbuch der Inneren Medizin.* Berlin: Springer, 1953.

29. Kandel, E. R., Frazier, W. T., Waziri, R., and Coggeshall, R. E. Direct and common connections among identified neurons in *Aplysia. J. Neurophysiol.* 30:1352, 1967.

30. Kandel, E. R., Spencer, W. A., and Brinley, F. J. Electrophysiology of hippocampal neurons. I. Sequential invasion and synaptic organization. *J. Neurophysiol.* 24:225, 1961.

31. Kandel, E. R., and Spencer, W. A. Electrophysiology of hippocampal neurons. II. After-potentials and repetitive firing. *J. Neurophysiol.* 24:243, 1961.

32. Katz, B. The transmission of impulses from nerve to muscle, and the subcellular unit of synaptic action. *Proc. Roy. Soc.* [Biol.] 155:455, 1962.

33. Katz, B., and Miledi, R. Input-output relation of a single synapse. *Nature* (London) 212:1242, 1966.

34. Katz, B., and Miledi, R. Release of acetylcholine from nerve endings by graded electric pulses. *Proc. Roy. Soc.* [Biol.] 167:23, 1967a.

35. Katz, B., and Miledi, R. A study of synaptic transmission in the absence of nerve impulses. *J. Physiol.* (London) 192:407, 1967b.

36. Katz, B., and Miledi, R. The role of calcium in neuromuscular facilitation. *J. Physiol.* (London) 195:481, 1968.

37. Kernell, D. Repetitive Discharge of Motoneurones. In Granit, R. (Ed.), *Muscular Afferents and Motor Control.* Stockholm: Almqvist and Wiksell, 1966, pp. 351-362.

38. Koike, H., Mano, N., Okada, Y., and Oshima, T. Repetitive impulses generated in fast and slow pyramidal tract cells by intracellularly applied current steps. 1969, in press.

39. Lorente de Nó, R. Studies on the structure of the cerebral cortex. II. Continuation of the study of the ammonic system. *J. Psychol. Neurol.* 46:113, 1934.

40. Miledi, R. Spontaneous synaptic potentials and quantal release of transmitter in the stellate ganglion of the squid. *J. Physiol.* (London) 192:379, 1967.

41. Miledi, R., and Slater, C. R. The action of calcium on neuronal synapses in the squid. *J. Physiol.* (London) 184:473, 1966.

42. Palay, S. L. The morphology of synapses in the central nervous system. *Exp. Cell Res.*, Suppl. 5, 275, 1958.

43. Purpura, D. P., Frigyesi, T. L., McMurtry, J. C., and Scarff, T. Synaptic Mechanisms in Thalamic Regulation of Cerebello-cortical Projection Activity. In Purpura, D. P., and Yahr, M. D. (Eds.), *The Thalamus.* New York: Columbia Univ. Press, 1966, pp. 153-172.

44. Ramón y Cajal, S. *Histologie du système*

nerveux de l'homme et des vertébrés, vol. II. Paris: Maloine, 1911.

45. Spencer, W. A., and Kandel, E. R. Hippocampal neuron responses to selective activation of recurrent collaterals of hippocampofugal axons. *Exp. Neurol.* 4:149, 1961.

46. Takeuchi, A., and Takeuchi, N. On the permeability of the end-plate membrane during the action of transmitter. *J. Physiol.* (London) 154:52, 1960.

47. Takeuchi, N. Some properties of conductance changes at the end-plate membrane during the action of acetylcholine. *J. Physiol.* (London) 167:128, 1963.

48. Tömböl, T. Short neurons and their synaptic relations in the specific thalamic nuclei. *Brain Res.* 3:307, 1967.

49. Wall, P. D. Excitability changes in afferent fiber terminations and their relation to slow potentials. *J. Physiol.* (London) 142:1, 1958.

Discussion

STUDIES OF PYRAMIDAL TRACT CELLS

TOMOKAZU OSHIMA

The basic concepts of excitatory and inhibitory mechanisms in the brain have been summarized by Eccles. Classifying the excitatory and inhibitory neurons now becomes an essential step for investigation of various structures of the mammalian nervous system. This type of study has been performed effectively with the intracellular recording technique, initiated by Phillips [45, 46], for pyramidal cells projecting into the pyramidal tract; these cells were called pyramidal tract (PT) cells [5]. Until recently such intracellular investigations were restricted to the large PT cells with relatively fast axonal conduction velocities [14], but in 1965 Takahashi was successful in applying the intracellular technique to the small PT cells with slower axonal conduction velocities [52]. Thus, two distinct populations of PT cells have been shown, as suggested by earlier extracellular studies [7, 8, 23, 30, 55]. These two groups of PT cells can be distinguished not only by their axonal conduction velocities, but they also exhibit different biophysical properties and synaptic organizations. Physiologically, they behave as different species of neurons. The first part of this discussion describes the means of differentiating between them with regard to various biophysical properties of their membranes. Second, the excitatory and inhibitory connections of these two categories of PT cells are summarized and the functional significance of spatial patterns of these various neurocircuits are discussed.

CLASSIFICATION AND BIOPHYSICAL PROPERTIES OF PT CELLS

Axonal Conduction Velocity

When PT cells are impaled by a microelectrode, stimulation of the pyramidal tract at various points induces action potentials which are identified as antidromic spike potentials by their sharp onset and fixed latency. For example, Fig. D9-1 shows the spike potentials of two PT cells induced from the cerebral peduncle (A, D, F), the pyramid at the trapezoid level (B, E, G), and the dorsolateral surface of the sixth cervical cord (C, H). As indicated by two time scales, the cell of A through C responds to these stimulations with latencies much briefer than the cell of D through H. A total of 148 PT cells was intracellularly sampled during the peduncle and pyramid stimulations, their axonal conduction velocities were calculated from differences in latencies for antidromic invasion and the distances between the two stimulated sites [25]. A frequency histogram of the conduction velocity (Fig. D9-1I) clearly reveals two populations of PT cells, although the sample may be biased by greater difficulty of penetrating into small PT cells with slower conduction velocities [52]. The critical conduction velocity for separating these two groups is about 20 meters per second.

Resting, and Action Potentials

The resting membrane potentials in relatively uninjured PT cells are between -60 and -80 mV [26, 27]. Within this range of resting potentials, amplitudes of the spike potentials are 62–107 mV in 23 fast PT cells (mean and SD, 79 ± 11.1 mV) and 75–100 mV in 10 slow PT cells (88 ± 8.8 mV). Thus, the overshoot of the spike summit above zero potential level is larger in slow PT cells (19 ± 4.6 mV; range, 8–25 mV) than in fast cells (9 ± 6.6 mV; range, 0–27 mV). All of these spikes exhibit the inflection at the rising phase between the initial segment (IS) and somadendritic (SD) components. By taking the differentiated records of the spikes, the threshold level

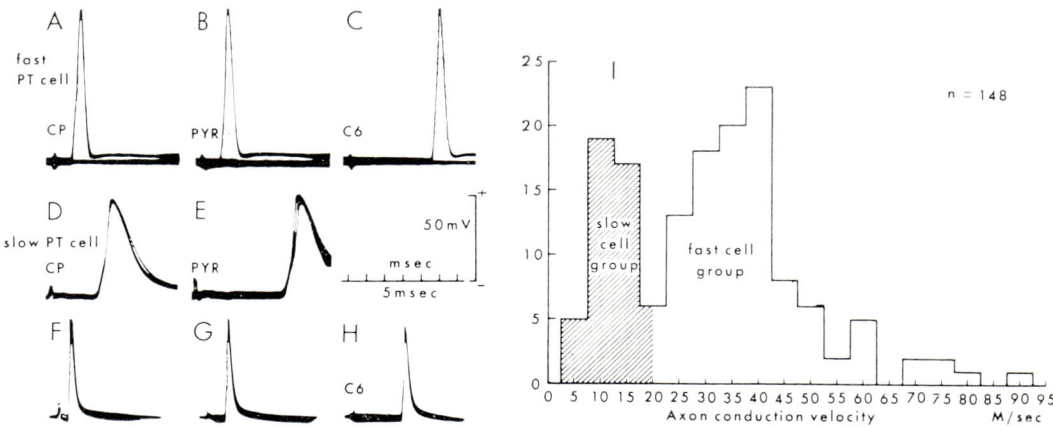

FIG. D9-1. Intracellular antidromic responses evoked by stimulations of cerebral peduncle (CP) and pyramid (PYR) and dorsolateral surface of sixth cervical cord (C6). Former two sites are ipsilateral and latter contralateral to recording site in postcruciate gyrus of cerebral cortex. (A), (B), (C) Spikes from a fast PT cell. (D), (E), (F), (G), (H) Spikes from a slow PT cell in one and the same preparation with a KCl-filled microelectrode. Time scale applies to (A) through (E) as 1 msec, and to (F) through (H) as 5 msec. (I) Frequency histogram of axonal conduction velocity [25].

of depolarization for SD spikes can be measured [12]. These threshold depolarizations are 30–41 mV in 10 PT cells (34 ± 3.6 mV). The thresholds for the initial segment spikes were measured at the foot of sharp-rising spikes which are induced by passing depolarizing pulses without significant artifacts and range from 13 to 20 mV in 7 PT cells (17 ± 1.9 mV) [25, 27]. Significant differences in these threshold values between fast and slow cells are not detectable. Durations of the spike potentials are 0.5–1.2 msec (0.71 ± 0.20 msec) in fast cells and 1.1–2.2 msec (1.52 ± 0.23 msec) in slow cells [52].

As in many other neurons, the spike potential in PT cells is followed by afterdepolarization (ADP) and afterhyperpolarization (AHP). In fast cells, a dip is interposed between the falling phase of the spike and ADP, but not significantly in slow cells [52]. The AHP has larger amplitudes and longer durations in fast cells (amplitude in polarization (ADP) and afterhyperpolariza-13 cells 3.63 ± 2.12 mV; range of peak time, 6–18 msec) than in slow cells (amplitudes in 8 cells, 1.72 ± 0.64 mV; range of peak time, 14–38 msec) [52].

ELECTRICAL PARAMETERS OF THE MEMBRANES

The intracellular application of currents enables further examination of quantitative properties of the PT cell membrane [13, 26, 27, 41, 52]. On application of current steps in both depolarizing and hyperpolarizing directions, the PT cell membrane reveals peculiar potential changes; there is an initial rise and subsequent fall to a certain stabilized level, so that there is in effect an initial overshoot. Reciprocally, break of the current causes an undershoot before the membrane potential recovers to the original resting level. The same observation was made earlier in motoneurons [3, 22] and recently in spinocervical tract cells [20]. These potential changes can be expressed by an electrical model circuit with three time constants [22]. Of these three time constants, the second component is the membrane time constant in the usual sense, is smaller in fast PT cells (range, 7.3–16.3; mean of 6 cells, 12.3 msec) than in slow cells (18.4 and 30.0 msec in 2 cells; mean, 24.2 msec) [26]. Because of the overshoot phenomenon and contribution of dendritic components, the time course of potential changes during current steps is not simply exponential [13, 41, 52]. However, when as a first approximation, the membrane time constant is measured by the time from onset of current to the moment where the polarized potential reaches $1 - (1/e)$ of the summit value, these values are 6.8 ± 1.3 msec in 10 fast cells and 12.3 ± 3.6 msec in 9 slow cells [26].

When a current step is applied across the membrane, the membrane resistance can be measured from the potential changes either at the peak of the overshoot or at the subsequent stabilized level [22, 52]. Both values are lower in fast PT cells than in slow cells. The values calculated for the peak of the overshoot were 5.9 ± 2.8 MΩ in 26 fast cells and 10.1 ± 2.5 MΩ in 10 slow cells [52]. Another measurement for seemingly fast PT cells shows the values of 6.70 ± 1.90 MΩ [41].

When the intensity of depolarizing current steps is sufficiently large, PT cells produce single or repetitive spikes [13, 27]. When PT cells with resting potentials of -60 to -80 mV are sampled, the value of rheobase is larger in fast cells ($1.64 \pm 0.85 \times 10^{-9}$ amp; range, 0.7–3.1×10^{-9} amp in 9 cells) than in slow cells ($0.94 \pm 0.71 \times 10^{-9}$ amp; range, 0.1–2.0×10^{-9} amp in 5 cells) [25, 26]. As already described, the critical depolarization for spike generation is 17 ± 1.9 mV in both groups of PT cells [25, 26, 27]. When the intensity of current steps is larger than rheobase, both fast and slow PT cells reveal the tonic maintenance of repetitive firing [13, 25].

Figure D9-2A and B shows an example of fast PT cells (C). Decrease of discharge frequency (adaptation) occurs during the initial 2 seconds (or up to 5–7 seconds when the frequency is relatively high) [25]. As in motoneurons [18], the stronger the applied current the greater the frequency of discharge [13, 25]. In the two cases of fast and slow cells of Fig. D9-2, the frequencies measured at various periods during current passage are almost linearly related to current intensity over the range tested in Fig. D9-2D and E. The adapted frequency (Fig. D9-2F) is plotted as a function of the current intensity, which is taken as a multiple of the rheobase. Range of frequency change is generally wider in fast cells than slow cells, which implies that fast cells can respond more sensitively to any small changes in stimulus intensity, in other words, in a more phasic manner.

The phasic nature of fast cells is further revealed in the degree of adaptation. When (in Fig. D9-2) the maximum and minimum frequencies respectively in the initial and later (5–6 sec after the make of the current) stages of current passage are measured, it is seen that the frequency decreases to 30.3 ± 2.06 percent of the initial maximum value in 4 trials of the fast cell and to 59.1 ± 9.52 percent in the slow cell. Membranes of fast and slow cells appear to exhibit phasic and tonic properties in their respective patterns of discharge. This is interesting because the separation of fast and slow cell groups was originally based on a time factor, that is, the axonal conduction velocity. Further, on applying linearly rising currents, fast cells revealed more accommodative property than slow cells [26]. When estimated by the ratio between minimum and maximum threshold currents for initiating spikes, the degree of accommodation was 1.33 ± 0.12 for 18 fast cells and 1.14 ± 0.07 for 5 slow cells. These properties may also be favorable for phasic and tonic pattern formation respectively in fast and slow cells.

SUMMARY

The PT cells with an axonal conduction velocity of more than 20 meters per second (fast PT cells) reveal various membrane properties different from those of slower conduction velocity (slow PT cells). It is of particular interest to find differences in their speeds of membrane reaction as revealed by such properties as the rheobase, frequency and pattern of repetitive discharge, and accommodative behavior. Slow PT cells are discharged by weaker stimulating currents than the fast cells, but frequency is maintained in a narrower range in spite of a large increase in current intensity. Further, slow cells adapt less to rectangular currents and display less accommodation during application of linearly

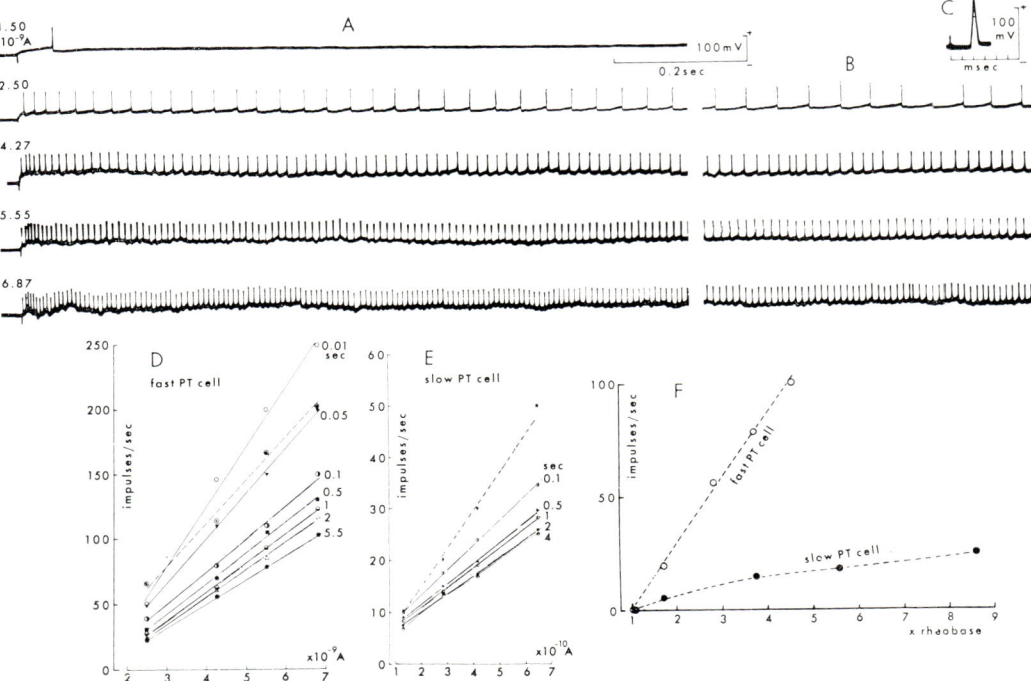

Fig. D9-2. Responses evoked in a PT cell by passage of depolarizing current steps through intracellular microelectrode. Column (A) Responses during the first 1-second of current application. Current intensities given at each trace in 10^{-9} amp. Column (B) Responses during period of 4.5–5.0 sec after current passage, showing adapted frequency of repetitive discharge. (C) Antidromic spike from pyramid. (D) and (E) Relationship of discharge frequency to intensity of applied current in fast and slow PT cells respectively. Broken curves show frequency calculated as a reciprocal of interval between first and second discharges. Other curves plot frequencies similarly calculated from one or several spike-to-spike intervals at indicated times after onset of current. (F) Curves for each of fast and slow PT cells where adapted frequency is plotted as a function of current expressed as multiples of rheobase of each cell [25].

rising currents. These properties suggest that slow cells are related to the threshold or to the perception of impinging stimuli to the cortex, thus maintaining a basic activity level of the neocortex. On the other hand, fast PT cells are phasic in respect to adaptation, both the range of frequency in repetitive firing and the accommodative behavior, suggesting that fast cells are capable of initiating discriminative muscle movements. There has been general suggestion that fine, individual muscle movements in men and primates are related to the increased number of thicker pyramidal tract fibers [36]. These timing properties of the PT cell membrane would be useful in interpreting the spatial synaptic organization which will be described.

SYNAPTIC ORGANIZATION OF PT CELLS

PT Cells as Excitatory Neurons

It is known that in monkeys the activation of PT cells causes monosynaptic excitatory postsynaptic potentials (EPSPs) in spinal motoneurons [31, 47]. Latencies of the EPSPs are so brief that the PT cells with fast axonal conduction velocities must be principally concerned. In the cat there is no evidence for monosynaptic excitation from PT cells to motoneurons. However, polysynaptic excitation of motoneurons is exerted via a chain of spinal interneurons which are at least partly activated directly through the fast-conducting pyramidal tract fibers [19, 24, 35, 37, 38]. All this evidence indicates that fast PT cells uniformly are excitatory neurons.

Slow PT cells are also shown to be excitatory. Thus, during stimulation of the pyramidal tract, monosynaptic EPSPs were recorded in fast PT cells [4, 29, 54] and in red-nucleus neurons [57] through activation of collateral branches of slow PT cell axons. All these EPSPs showed as common characteristics their slow rise time and virtually unchanged size when the membrane potential was greatly altered by intracellular current application. These features suggest that synapses are mainly distributed on dendrites remote from the cell bodies of these neurons. All experimental evidence on the mammalian central nervous system indicates that all axon branches or collaterals of single mammalian neurons exert the same excitatory or inhibitory synaptic actions [15]; hence, from these examples of excitatory collateral actions it can be predicted that slow PT cells are excitatory in nature on all other target neurons.

INTRACORTICAL SYNAPTIC MECHANISMS

Ramón y Cajal [48] has suggested that deeply located pyramidal cells receive convergent excitatory actions via the axon collaterals of pyramidal cells located near the cortical surface. When it is recognized that fast PT cells lie in deeper cell layers than do the slow cells [55, 56], Ramón y Cajal's figure is approximately in agreement with the finding of recurrent monosynaptic excitation from slow PT cells to fast PT cells [54]. Since the population of slow PT cells would be greater than fast cells [58], this excitation probably would converge on single fast PT cells from axons of several slow PT cells. The finely graded manner of recurrent EPSPs to increasing stimulus intensities supports this view of convergent action [54].

There is general agreement that IPSPs are evoked in both fast and slow PT cells during stimulation of the cerebral peduncle or pyramid [4, 28, 46, 49, 50, 51]. These IPSPs are assumed to be due to action of impulses in the axon collaterals of PT fibers. They exhibit a wide range of latencies from the pyramid, 1.8–6 msec, and great sensitivity to additional administration of sodium pentobarbital to the animal. Therefore, it can be presumed that they are produced by polysynaptic pathways. IPSPs with the shortest latency are in accord with a disynaptic path, the inhibitory interneurons being directly excited by the fast PT cell axon collaterals. Corresponding to the recurrent IPSPs intracellularly recorded, a positive potential wave can be recorded extracellularly in various cortical layers; the wave attains a maximum amplitude in the deeper layers of the cortex in which the somata of the most fast PT cells are located [28]. This suggests that inhibitory synapses are located on or close to the somata of PT cells, which thus resemble pyramidal cells of the hippocampus and Purkinje cells of the cerebellum.

Stimulation of sensory pathways gives rise to both excitatory and inhibitory influences on PT cells [33, 34, 39, 40, 43, 59]. Differences in fast and slow PT cells have been found during stimulation of ventralis posteromedialis (VPM) and ventralis lateralis (VL) of the thalamus. Monosynaptic EPSPs with the latency of 1.4–1.7 msec are produced in fast cells [53, 59]. On the other hand, EPSPs recorded from slow PT cells show longer latencies (shortest value, 2.2 msec from VL and 4.5 msec from VPM). The difference in latency of the EPSPs from the thalamus would be relevant to the previous finding that fast cells responded earlier to foot-pad stimulation [55]. These thalamic-induced EPSPs in both fast and slow PT cells are followed by IPSPs with durations of 50–150 msec.

The general statement may be made that in response to an afferent input the inhibitory influences on PT cells have wider distribution than the excitatory influences, with a lateral or "surround" inhibition as a consequence. It has been proposed that the inhibitory neuronal element for this type of inhibition would be the stellate cell with its pericellular nests of axonal terminals on the cortical pyramidal cells in the manner of divergence [11]. The supposed synaptic structures of divergence in inhibition and convergence in recurrent excitation make a clear contrast. Both structures would facilitate sharpening of an activated focus in the cortex, thus supporting partly the columnar organization in the afferent and efferent functioning of the neocortex [6, 9, 10, 32].

CORTICOFUGAL INFLUENCES BY PT CELLS

The early pioneering works of Fritsch and Hitzig [17] and further work showed that a main function of the pyramidal tract would be the control of muscle movements. Contribution of fast PT cells to activation of motoneurons has been shown by the brief latency of action, both in monkeys [31, 47] and in cats [24, 38]. Further, pyramidal tract fibers project onto many nuclei in the brain stem which in turn project down the spinal cord, thus forming the so-called extrapyramidal motor system. For example, monosynaptic EPSPs are evoked in reticulospinal tract cells via the activation of fast PT cell axons [42] and in red-nucleus cells through slow PT cell axons [57]. Disynaptic or polysynaptic inhibitions are also exerted on red-nucleus neurons from fast PT cells [57]. The cerebellar cortex is activated from the pyramidal tract via the precerebellar nuclei such as the pontine and the inferior olive nuclei. Thus, mossy fiber responses of the cerebellum are caused from both fast and slow PT axons, and climbing fiber responses from only slow PT axons [44].

On the other hand, the pyramidal tract controls the activity of many sensory relay nuclei. Differences of effects from fast and slow PT cells were found in the inhibitory influences on transmission in the cuneate nucleus; in this nucleus there are two inhibitory mechanisms: postsynaptic and presynaptic [1, 2]. Recent studies further reveal that postsynaptic inhibition is exerted mainly from fast PT fibers and that presynaptic inhibition is largely from slow PT fibers [21]. Figure D9-3 illustrates one type of these experiments performed in cats where the midbrain is cut bilaterally except for the cerebral peduncle. During stimulation of the cerebral peduncle with various intensities (inset diagram in Fig. D9-3C), the field potentials were recorded both from the cerebral white matter after removing cortical tissues (Fig. D9-3A) and from the dorsal surface of the cuneate nucleus (Fig. D9-3B). The former revealed the fast and slow component waves which were measured separately, thus deriving the numbers, respectively, of fast and slow PT fibers

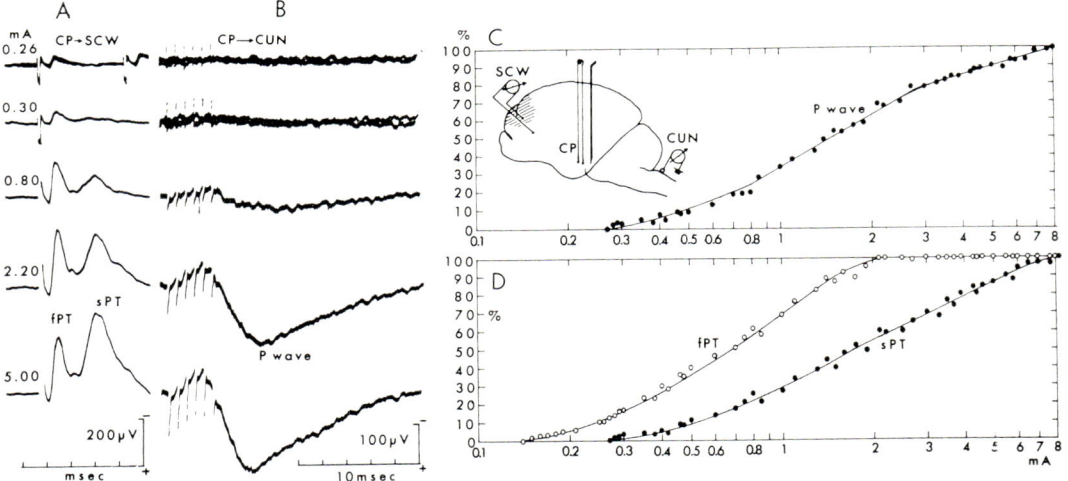

FIG. D9-3. Cuneate surface potentials evoked by stimulation of contralateral cerebral peduncle. (A) Pyramidal tract volleys recorded from subcortical white matter (SCW) after removing overlying cortical tissues. (B) Cuneate N and P waves illustrated in response to increasing stimulus intensities in milliamperes. Duration of pulse stimuli is 0.1 msec. (C) Inset diagram shows experimental design; six stimuli used for evoking maximum P wave response. (C) and (D) Cuneate P wave size and fast (fPT) and slow component sizes (sPT) of pyramidal volleys plotted respectively in (C) and (D) against stimulus intensities [21].

activated. The positive component of the latter (the P wave) was taken as the indicator for presynaptic inhibition [1, 2].

In Fig. D9-3C and D, the P wave shows a threshold and a pattern of increase in amplitude similar to that of the slow PT fibers. Since cuneate nucleus neurons project to PT cells via the ventrobasal complex of the thalamus, inhibitory actions would provide a negative feedback or lateral inhibitory effect in each of the afferent systems to the fast and slow PT cells (cf. [53]). Further, it is interesting to consider the effects on fast PT cell activity exerted from slow PT cells at both the cortical and cuneate levels. Slow PT cells with the lower threshold for firing would give tonic facilitatory influences on fast cells, maintaining the latter at a certain activity level. On the other hand, slow cells may limit afferent inflow from the peripheral receptors to the fast cells. It is thus conceivable that by these dual excitatory and inhibitory mechanisms, slow cells can open the gate to fast cells for excitatory inputs other than the peripheral somatosensory inputs; for example, from the association and visual cortical areas, or the cerebellothalamocortical pathway [16].

Summary

Studies of two types of PT cells have revealed the existence of both inhibitory and excitatory actions in and from the neocortex. Some functional cooperation of these opposite actions is further suggested, if the spatial distribution of these excitatory and inhibitory actions is considered. These hypothetical situations are suggested by two examples. One is a dual sharpening effect on the cortical active site by widespread inhibition and narrowly focused excitation in the pyramidal recurrent system. An elegant example of such a spatial pattern formation of excitation and inhibition has been shown in the cerebellar cortex, where the excitatory connection from granular cells and the inhibitory one via basket cells are combined on Purkinje cells, forming the narrow-strip excitatory zone and its lateral inhibition [16]. The other example is the effect of selective opening for the excitatory gate to fast PT cells by the slow PT cells with their tonic facilitation in the cortical level and their presynaptic inhibitory action on the cuneate transmission of specific somatosensory afferents. The biophysical properties of the PT cell membranes may take part in these operations between fast and slow cells by yielding different timing factors such as axonal conduction velocity, threshold, and pattern of excitation.

In conclusion, the excitatory and inhibitory mechanisms of the brain are now understood not only as an assembly of neural elements with antagonistic actions, but also as an organized cooperation with a certain principle of temporal and spatial patterns of excitation and inhibition. Although data on classification of fast and slow PT cells within the neocortex are still very limited, this concept has already proved useful in interpreting the complicated functional design of the motor cortex.

ACKNOWLEDGMENTS. The author wishes to thank Professor Toshihiko Tokizane and Dr. Hiroshi Shimazu who have organized and encouraged a research group for the studies on fast and slow PT systems.

REFERENCES

1. Andersen, P., Eccles, J. C., Oshima, T., and Schmidt, R. F. Mechanisms of synaptic transmission in the cuneate nucleus. *J. Neurophysiol.* 27:1096, 1964.
2. Andersen, P., Eccles, J. C., Schmidt, R. F., and Yokota, T. Slow potential waves produced in the cuneate nucleus by cutaneous volleys and by cortical stimulation. *J. Neurophysiol.* 27:78, 1964.
3. Araki, T., Ito, M., and Oshima, T. Potential changes produced by application of current steps in motoneurones. *Nature* (London) 191:1104, 1961.
4. Armstrong, D. M. Synaptic excitation and inhibition of Betz cells by antidromic pyramidal volleys. *J. Physiol.* (London) 178:37–38P, 1965.

5. Asanuma, H. Microelectrode studies on the evoked activity of a single pyramidal tract cell in the somatosensory area in cats. *Jap. J. Physiol.* 9:94, 1959.
6. Asanuma, H., and Sakata, H. Functional organization of a cortical efferent system examined with focal depth stimulation in cats. *J. Neurophysiol.* 30:35, 1967.
7. Bishop, P. O., Jeremy, D., and Lance, J. W. Properties of pyramidal tract. *J. Neurophysiol.* 16:537, 1953.
8. Brookhart, J. M., and Morris, R. E. Antidromic potential recordings from the bulbar pyramid of the cat. *J. Neurophysiol.* 11:387, 1948.
9. Brooks, V. B. Some Factors Governing Sensory Convergence in Cat's Motor Cortex. In Curtis, D. R., and McIntyre, A. K. (Eds.), *Studies in Physiology*. Heidelberg: Springer, 1965, pp. 13–17.
10. Brooks, V. B., and Asanuma, H. Recurrent cortical effects following stimulation of medullary pyramid. *Arch. Ital. Biol.* 103:247, 1965.
11. Colonnier, M. L. The Structural Design of the Neocortex. In Eccles, J. C. (Ed.), *Brain and Conscious Experience*. New York: Springer, 1966, pp. 1–23.
12. Coombs, J. S., Curtis, D. R., and Eccles, J. C. The interpretation of spike potentials of motoneurones. *J. Physiol.* (London) 139:198, 1957.
13. Creutzfeldt, O. D., Lux, H. D., and Nacimiento, A. C. Intracelluläre Reizung corticaler Nervenzellen. *Pflueger Arch. Ges. Physiol.* 281:129, 1964.
14. Eccles, J. C. Cerebral Synaptic Mechanisms. In Eccles, J. C. (Ed.), *Brain and Conscious Experience*. New York: Springer, 1966, pp. 24–58.
15. Eccles, J. C. Excitatory and Inhibitory Mechanisms in Brain. In Jasper, H. H., Ward, A. A., Jr., and Pope, A. (Eds.), *Basic Mechanisms of the Epilepsies*. Boston: Little, Brown, 1969.
16. Eccles, J. C., Ito, M., and Szentágothai, J. *The Cerebellum as a Neuronal Machine*. New York: Springer, 1967.
17. Fritsch, G., and Hitzig, E. Über die elektrische Erregbarkeit des Grosshirns. *Arch. Anat. Physiol. Wiss. Med.* 37:300, 1870.
18. Granit, R., Kernell, D., and Shortess, G. K. Quantitative aspects of repetitive firing of mammalian motoneurones caused by injected currents. *J. Physiol.* (London) 168:911, 1963.
19. Hern, J. E. C., Phillips, C. G., and Porter, R. Electrical thresholds of unimpaled corticospinal cells in the cat. *Quart. J. Exp. Physiol.* 47:134, 1962.
20. Hongo, T., and Koike, H. Unpublished data, 1969.
21. Hongo, T., Oshima, T., and Stone, J. Unpublished data, 1969.
22. Ito, M., and Oshima, T. Electrical behavior of the motoneurone membrane during intracellularly applied current steps. *J. Physiol.* (London) 180:507, 1965.
23. Jabbur, S. J., and Towe, A. L. Analysis of the antidromic cortical response following stimulation at the medullary pyramids. *J. Physiol.* (London) 155:148, 1961.
24. Kato, M., Takamura, H., and Fujimori, B. Studies on the effects of pyramidal stimulation upon flexor and extensor motoneurons and gamma motoneurons. *Jap. J. Physiol.* 14:34, 1964.
25. Koike, H., Mano, N., Okada, Y., and Oshima, T. Unpublished data, 1969.
26. Koike, H., Okada, Y., and Oshima, T. Accommodative properties of fast and slow pyramidal tract cells and their modification by different levels of their membrane potential. *Exp. Brain Res.* 5:189, 1968.
27. Koike, H., Okada, Y., Oshima, T., and Takahashi, K. Accommodative behavior of cat pyramidal tract cells investigated with intracellular injection of currents. *Exp. Brain Res.* 5:173, 1968.
28. Kubota, K., Sakata, H., Takahashi, K., and Uno, M. Location of the recurrent inhibitory synapse on cat pyramidal tract cell. *Proc. Jap. Acad.* 41:195, 1965.
29. Kubota, K., and Takahashi, K. Recurrent facilitatory pathway of the pyramidal tract cell. *Proc. Jap. Acad.* 41:191, 1965.
30. Lance, J. W. Pyramidal tract in spinal cord of cat. *J. Neurophysiol.* 17:253, 1954.
31. Landgren, S., Phillips, C. G., and Porter, R. Minimal synaptic actions of pyramidal impulses on some alpha motoneurones of the baboon's hand and forearm. *J. Physiol.* (London) 161:91, 1962.
32. Landgren, S., Phillips, C. G., and Porter, R. Cortical fields of origin of the monosynaptic pyramidal pathways to some alpha motoneurones of the baboon's hand and forearm. *J. Physiol.* (London) 161:112, 1962.

33. Li, C. L. Cortical intracellular synaptic potentials. *J. Cell. Comp. Physiol.* 58:153, 1961.
34. Li, C. L. Cortical intracellular synaptic potentials in response to thalamic stimulation. *J. Cell. Comp. Physiol.* 61:165, 1963.
35. Lloyd, D. P. C. The spinal mechanism of the pyramidal system in cats. *J. Neurophysiol.* 4:525, 1941.
36. Lloyd, D. P. C. Functional Properties of Neurons. In Fulton, J. F. (Ed.), *Howell's Textbook of Physiology* (15th ed.). Philadelphia: Saunders, 1946, pp. 96–120.
37. Lundberg, A., Norrsell, U., and Voorhoeve, P. Pyramidal effects on lumbosacral interneurones activated by somatic afferents. *Acta Physiol. Scand.* 56:220, 1962.
38. Lundberg, A., and Voorhoeve, P. Effects from the pyramidal tract on spinal reflex arcs. *Acta Physiol. Scand.* 56:201, 1962.
39. Lux, H. D., and Klee, M. R. Intracelluläre Untersuchungen über den Einfluss hemmender Potentiale im motorischen Cortex. 1. Die Wirkung elektrischer Reizung unspezifischer Thalamuskerne. *Arch. Psychiat. Nervenkr.* 203:648, 1963.
40. Lux, H. D., Nacimiento, A. C., and Creutzfeldt, O. D. Gegenseitige Beeinflussung von postsynaptischen Potentialen corticaler Nervenzellen nach Reizen in unspezifischen und spezifischen Kernen des Thalamus. *Pflueger Arch. Ges. Physiol.* 281:170, 1964.
41. Lux, H. D., and Pollen, D. A. Electrical constants of neurons in the motor cortex of the cat. *J. Neurophysiol.* 29:207, 1966.
42. Mano, N. Unpublished data, 1969.
43. Nacimiento, A. C., Lux, H. D., and Creutzfeldt, O. D. Postsynaptische Potentiale von Nervenzellen des motorischen Cortex nach elektrischer Reizung spezifischer und unspezifischer Thalamuskerne. *Pflueger Arch. Ges. Physiol.* 281:152, 1964.
44. Oshima, T., Provini, L., Tsukahara, N., and Kitai, S. T. Cerebrocerebellar connections mediated by fast and slow conducting pyramidal tract fibers. *Proc. Int. Union Physiol. Sci.* 7, 1968.
45. Phillips, C. G. Intracellular records from Betz cells in the cat. *Quart. J. Exp. Physiol.* 41:58, 1956.
46. Phillips, C. G. Actions of antidromic pyramidal volleys on single Betz cells in the cat. *Quart. J. Exp. Physiol.* 44:1, 1959.
47. Preston, J. B., and Whitlock, D. G. Intracellular potentials recorded from motoneurons following precentral gyrus stimulation in primate. *J. Neurophysiol.* 24:91, 1961.
48. Ramón y Cajal, S. Nuevo concepto de la histología de los centros nerviosos. *Rev. Cienc. Med. Barcelona,* Tomo 18, Nums. 16, 20, 22 y 23 de 1892.
49. Sawa, M., Maruyama, N., Kaji, S., and Hanai, T. Actions of stimulation to medullary pyramid on single neurons in cat's motor cortex. *Folia Psychiat. Neurol. Jap.* 14:316, 1960.
50. Stefanis, C., and Jasper, H. Intracellular microelectrode studies of antidromic responses in cortical pyramidal tract neurons. *J. Neurophysiol.* 27:828, 1964.
51. Stefanis, C., and Jasper, H. Recurrent collateral inhibition in pyramidal tract neurons. *J. Neurophysiol.* 27:855, 1964.
52. Takahashi, K. Slow and fast groups of pyramidal tract cells and their respective membrane properties. *J. Neurophysiol.* 28:908, 1965.
53. Takahashi, K. Unpublished data, 1969.
54. Takahashi, K., Kubota, K., and Uno, M. Recurrent facilitation in cat pyramidal tract cells. *J. Neurophysiol.* 30:22, 1967.
55. Towe, A. L., Patton, H. D., and Kennedy, T. T. Properties of the pyramidal system in the cat. *Exp. Neurol.* 8:220, 1963.
56. Towe, A. L., Whitehorn, D., and Nyquist, J. K. Differential activity among widefield neurons of the cat postcruciate cerebral cortex. *Exp. Neurol.* 20:497, 1968.
57. Tsukahara, N., Fuller, D. R. G., and Brooks, V. B. Collateral pyramidal influences on the corticorubrospinal system. *J. Neurophysiol.* 31:467, 1968.
58. van Crevel, H., and Verhaart, W. J. C. The 'exact' origin of the pyramidal tract. A quantitative study in the cat. *J. Anat.* 97:495, 1963.
59. Yoshida, M., Yajima, K., and Uno, M. Different activation of two types of pyramidal tract neurons through the cerebello-thalamo-cortical pathway. *Experientia* 22:331, 1966.

10

The Epileptic Neuron: Chronic Foci in Animals and Man*

ARTHUR A. WARD, JR.

THE ELEMENTAL PROBLEM in epilepsy deals with mechanisms underlying the "highly explosive" discharges, as Hughlings Jackson called them, which characterize what he called the "hyper-physiological" state at the epileptogenic focus in the cortex. Although it appears that epilepsy in the human may take many forms, it is reasonable to assume that a thorough understanding of seizures of focal onset in the cortex is necessary before more complex manifestations of human epilepsy can be investigated. In such an endeavor, it is desirable to have an experimental model that may be suitably manipulated and studied.

EXPERIMENTAL MODELS OF EPILEPSY

The relevance of a model is determined by the degree to which it serves as a surrogate for the phenomenon in nature. Since epilepsy in the human is characterized by chronically recurrent, spontaneous clinical seizures, the model in the experimental animal should also exhibit these fundamental properties. Seizures can be induced in a variety of organisms by many techniques [70], but relatively few techniques have been evolved which result in production of clinical seizures which are spontaneously recurrent over extended periods of time.

One of the first experimental models of epilepsy was described by Openchowski [56] in 1883 utilizing local application of cold to the cerebral cortex. These observations were confirmed by Nims et al. [55], and the technique was subsequently modified by Morrell [52], who induced freezing of the cortex by topical application of ethyl chloride spray to visual and motor cortex in rabbits and cats. Morrell noted that spontaneous motor seizures were rare in occipitally placed lesions but were more common if the lesion was made closer to the motor cortex. Seizures were apparently seen for only some hours after production of the lesion although electrographic changes were present for much longer periods of time. Even after the return of EEG normality, the focus could be activated by such agents as pentylenetetrazol for as long as 3 months. This technique has permitted the study of behavior of individual cortical neurons during such acute seizure activity utilizing intracellular recording methods [33]. However, the freezing technique does not induce chronic, recurrent clinical seizures.

It has been more recently reported that intracerebral injection of tetanus toxin may produce convulsive activity and foci of electrical discharge [18]. During the hours preceding onset of large seizures, intracellular recording has demonstrated that recurrent collateral inhibition induced by antidromic pyramidal stimulation is reduced [11]. Following injection of the

---

* This work supported by PHS Research Grant NB04053 from National Institute of Neurological Diseases and Stroke.

toxin, there is a delay of some hours which is dose-related, following which seizures occur which increase in frequency up to 30–60 per minute. Thus the process terminates in an almost continuous convulsive discharge or, with smaller doses, the initial milder changes spontaneously clear without sequelae. Again the technique does not induce chronic, recurrent seizures.

Application of Metals. Various heavy metals have been applied to the cortex, and Dow [24] reported that the application of cobalt powder to rat cortex induced contralateral motor-seizure activity which began about 2 weeks after implantation but lasted only 1 or 2 days. Generalized fits were rare. The EEG focus, however, persisted for 4–6 weeks. Studies of the electrographic changes induced in this fashion have also been reported by Dimov [23], while Fischer et al. [30] induced a more discrete focus utilizing small, cobalt-gelatine sticks introduced into the cortex of rats. Electrographic abnormalities appeared in 6–8 days, but spontaneous seizures were not observed [36].

Kopeloff [40] confirmed that intracerebral injection of cobalt would result in spontaneous clinical seizures of limited duration in the mouse, but Chusid and Kopeloff [19] were unable to induce clinical seizures by this means in the monkey. They also reported that occasional spontaneous clinical seizures, which recurred for 1–6 months, followed intracortical implantation of pellets of the pure metals antimony and nickel. Subclinical EEG foci were induced by implantation of aluminum, antimony, bismuth, cadmium, nickel, tantalum, titanium, tungsten, vanadium, and zirconium. In these instances, seizures could be precipitated by activation with pentylenetetrazol or picrotoxin for periods of 6–18 months after implantation. Neither spontaneous nor induced seizures were induced by beryllium, chromium, cobalt, copper, gold, iron, lead, magnesium, manganese, mercury, molybdenum, silicon, silver, tin, or zinc. In all these studies, Chusid and Kopeloff introduced the pure metal into the motor cortex of the monkey.

The intracortical injection of tungstic acid gel also induces epileptic activity. Blum and Liban [8] reported that injection of this compound into the medial temporal lobe structures results in clinical seizures which usually start 1 day after the injection, and spontaneous attacks usually occurred at least every hour, for "more than 2–3 days" [9]. The physical state of the compound is apparently critical in determining epileptogenic action since only the colloidal form is biologically active. Details of preparation of this form have been reported by Black, Abraham, and Ward [6] who found that its injection into an area of the central nervous system containing neurons is followed, over a period of an hour, by motor and sensory signs of hyperactivity appropriate to the site of injection. Preliminary microelectrode studies indicated that the neurons at the focus exhibited a rapid-burst type of firing activity reminiscent of the epileptic units of Schmidt, Thomas, and Ward [69]. In their experience, clinical seizures continued for up to 12 hours and then cleared, leaving no clinically detectable deficit, in contrast to the somewhat longer duration reported by Blum et al. [9]. Again, chronic, recurrent clinical seizures are not induced by this technique.

In 1942, Kopeloff, Barrera, and Kopeloff [41] reported that application of alumina cream to the motor cortex of monkey brings on development of an epileptogenic focus which results in chronically recurring clinical seizures of focal onset. For the first time, a model was then available that provided an experimental preparation which exhibited spontaneous seizures of focal onset occurring recurrently over a period of months and years. In the initial technique, a specially prepared suspension of aluminum hydroxide was utilized while subsequently alumina cream of commercial origin was found to be equally effective. Initially, the alumina was applied in a disc over the cortex, and the technique subsequently was modified by introducing the compound into the cortical grey matter by injection [42].

Because of the obvious similarities between chronically recurrent seizures in the monkey induced by this technique and the phenomenon of human epilepsy, a major interest in our laboratories has focused on this experimental preparation. We have prepared our primates (primarily *Macaca mulatta*) in the following fashion.

Under aseptic conditions and pentobarbital anesthesia, the sensorimotor cortex is exposed by trephining the bone and incision of the dura. At four points in the sensory and motor hand and face areas, commercial aluminum hydroxide gel is injected into the cortex with a small syringe and 27-gauge hypodermic needle to produce a minimally detectable bolus beneath the pia at each puncture site. Great care is taken to prevent spillage of the alumina onto the pial surface, and a layer of absorbable gelatin film is placed between the cortex and overlying dura as well as between the dura and overlying bone disc to minimize scarring. In such monkeys, spontaneous clinical seizures appear after a variable delay, usually 35–60 days. Electroencephalographic examination reveals abnormalities in the form of spikes or sharp wave activity prior to overt epilepsy. The clinical pattern of seizures is characteristic of location of the scar as in human epilepsy of focal cortical onset. The clinical seizures vary in extent from focal seizures involving portions or all of the contralateral extremities to those seizures which begin focally and rapidly become generalized. Seizures occur spontaneously, and frequency is roughly proportional to the degree of cortical pathology induced. If a large number of focal, punctate injections of alumina are performed, the seizures, once they occur, may increase in frequency to status epilepticus; aggressive treatment with anticonvulsant medication is necessary to maintain a viable preparation. In the majority of animals, once seizures are established, they recur spontaneously almost indefinitely and a relatively constant pattern of seizure frequency has been observed in such monkeys for at least 7 years.

Seizures Recorded. A technique has been developed by Lockard and Barensten [47] utilizing activity chairs which trigger video tape so that all seizures in each monkey under observation can be visually validated. In this fashion each seizure can be recorded as it occurs, twenty-four hours a day continuously for weeks. This provides quantitative information regarding occurrence of seizures in such monkeys which is difficult to obtain even in human epileptic patients. These studies [47] indicate that seizures in some of these monkeys with epilepsy of focal onset have a pronounced diurnal variation and may occur only during certain hours of the night; seizures may cluster in relation to estrus; the frequency may be increased as much as threefold by behavioral stress; and, in some preparations, the monkey appears to be able to abort focal seizures in the hand by voluntary movement of that member [46].

Thus this experimental model exhibits a lag between cortical insult and development of chronic seizures: the seizures are spontaneous, and the frequency is modified in certain specific ways. All these aspects of seizure behavior in the monkey model also characterize human epilepsy of focal cortical origin. Thus an experimental model is available where some of the fundamental mechanisms operating in epilepsy may be profitably investigated.

INTERICTAL ACTIVITY OF EPILEPTIC NEURONS

If seizures arise in a geographically restricted mass of neurons, it must first be determined how the behavior of such neurons at the epileptogenic focus differs from normal neuronal activity. By recording gross electrical activity from either the exposed brain or scalp, it is agreed that the hallmark of the epileptic process is the occurrence of the *epileptic spike*.

In monkeys exhibiting spontaneous clinical seizures some months after the intracortical injection of alumina, the epileptogenic focus is characterized by the occurrence of such epileptic spikes. It is then possible to monitor the spontaneous activity of single units at the focus utilizing extracellular recording with microelectrodes. The random, low-frequency firing patterns of normal cells in unanesthetized monkey cortex are well known. In contrast to this random but well-ordered activity a variety of patterns of neuronal hyperactivity may be observed at the epileptic focus.

Figure 10-1 is an example of the inter-

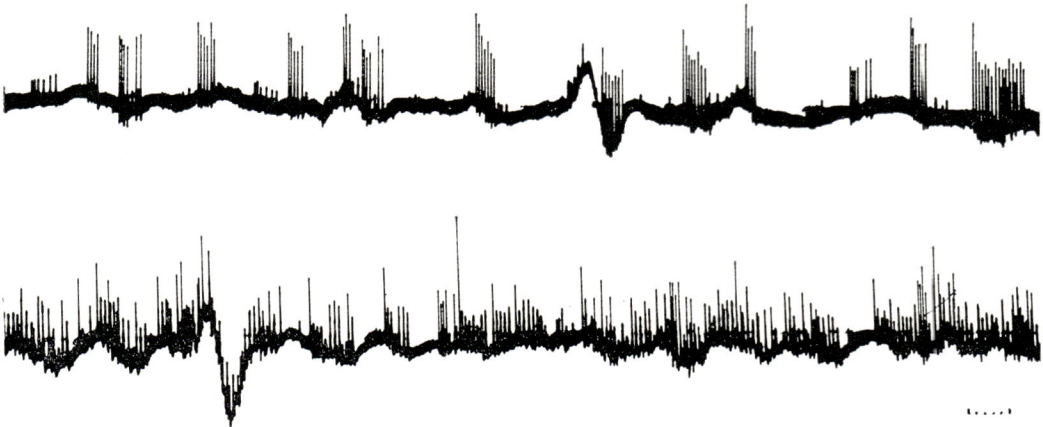

Fig. 10-1. Interictal spontaneous activity of single unit in epileptic cortex of monkey. Time marks, 10 msec.

ictal firing patterns of two epileptic neurons which can be seen as characterized by random, autonomous hyperactivity. The unit in the upper trace exhibits irregular burst firing in which the cell fires 4–21 times in each burst with apparently random intervals between the bursts. The epileptic neuron in the lower trace is an example of tonic discharge, waxing and waning in frequency with occasional silent intervals. In both examples, an epileptic spike occurs; in the upper trace a burst of cell firing appears during the downward deflection of the epileptic spike; in the lower trace, there is no obvious relation of the spike to the unit firing.

Over the past thirteen years, a rather large body of data has been accumulated dealing with patterns of interictal firing of epileptic neurons in such chronic epileptogenic foci [69, 79, 80, 81, 85] and a variety of patterns have been observed. In some instances, there are tonic trains of rapid discharge waxing and waning in frequency while, at random intervals, abrupt cessation of firing may occur for intervals of 100–250 msec. In other cases the unit may fire rather rhythmically or there may be interspersed episodes of tonic firing as well as admixtures of these varieties of hyperactivity. The sustained nature of these high frequency discharges over long periods of time (for hours), as well as patterns of firing and waveform, distinguish such discharges from injury discharges evoked by damage to the cell membrane from the electrode tip. All of these observations were carried out during the course of terminal, acute experiments, with the cortex exposed under local anesthesia in which the monkeys were immobilized with a variety of neuromuscular blocking agents, and ventilation was maintained by means of a respiratory pump.

Since there is evidence that some of the neuromuscular blocking agents can augment cortical excitability [34] and since other factors such as cortical exposure, artificial respiration, and state of arousal may influence the degree of epileptogenicity at the focus, it would be desirable to record the activity of neurons at the focus in intact, awake, undrugged monkeys. This has been accomplished by Sypert and Ward [72] utilizing an implanted chamber to which a microdrive could be attached which permitted chronic recording of neurons at the focus with tungsten microelectrodes introduced transdurally. The most frequently encountered interictal pattern of unit discharge in the epileptogenic focus under these more physiological circumstances is regular, recurrent, high frequency bursts of action potentials. Frequency of burst repetition is remarkably constant for a given unit but may vary from 4 to 8 per sec from cell to cell. Two samples of this type of activity are illustrated in Fig. 10-2 in which grouped firing recurs at intervals of 100 to 130 msec. The number of action potentials in each burst is fairly constant

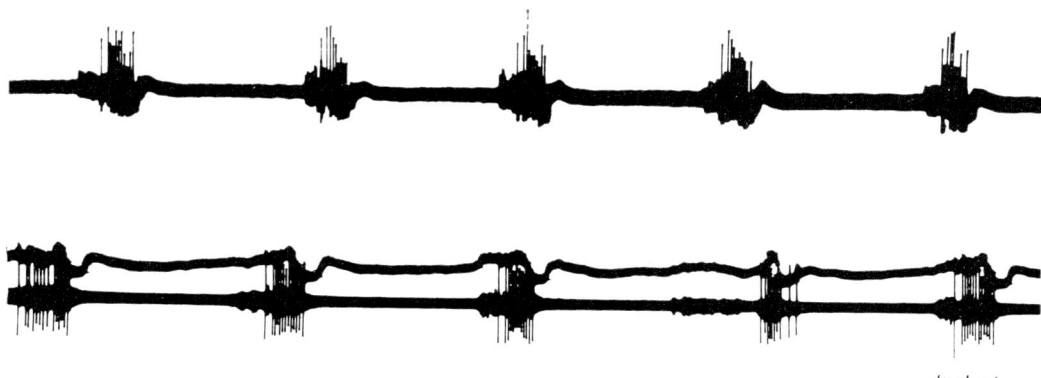

FIG. 10-2. Rhythmic repetitive bursts of unit potentials in epileptic cortex of intact, awake monkeys. Local EEG from overlying cortex on upper beam of lower trace. Time marks, 10 msec.

for a given unit and varies between 9 and 11 for the examples shown. In other instances, between 4 and 15 unit discharges may characterize the burst. Temporal relationship of spikes within the burst remains remarkably constant from one burst to the next. Firing rates in a burst may range from 200 to 900 per sec. Such stereotyped, interictal activity may be observed in the same cell with little change for periods of hours. Although systematic sampling of the population of cells at the focus with multiple microelectrodes has not been undertaken, examples in Fig. 10-2 show, in both instances, that the microelectrode is recording from more than one cell. It was commonly noted that when more than one cell was under observation, the bursting patterns of firing of both units appeared to be temporally related. In Fig. 10-2 the small unit (presumably a cell at some distance from the recording tip) always starts to fire repetitively at variable intervals before the large unit.

In the lower record of Fig. 10-2, the EEG recorded from the immediately adjacent cortex is also displayed on the upper trace. It will be noted that synchronous deflections of the electrocorticogram bear a temporal relationship to unit bursts and that the major electrical events recorded from graded response membrane appear to follow onset of the burst generated in all-or-none membrane. A somewhat similar sequence is also recorded in the upper record of Fig. 10-2, where local extracellular field potentials, as reflected by the baseline of the microelectrode record, exhibit certain positive-negative sequences during and following the burst respectively. However, in other instances, it has proved difficult to correlate local EEG changes with patterns of repetitive patterns of unit firing [78].

Neuronal Firing. The stereotyped bursts of repetitive neuronal firing appear to be typical of the focus in the undrugged, awake animal. Other units were recorded in these preparations in which interictal hyperactivity was manifested by rhythmically recurrent burst activity with less well-defined relationships between spikes within each burst, greater variation in the number of spikes in successive bursts, and lower, intraburst action-potential frequency. These units appeared to surround the area of greatest neuronal and electrographic hyperactivity, representing transition from maximal unit hyperactivity to normal-appearing spontaneous activity seen at approximately 4 mm from the epileptogenic focus in these preparations [72].

Thus these observations in the undrugged, intact, awake monkey indicate that the interictal pattern of firing of neuronal elements in the epileptogenic focus is characterized by regular, repetitive bursts of action potentials which are remarkably constant in number and temporal relationships. This is in contrast to the observations made during acute experiments we previously reported [69] where interictal unit activity was characterized by irregular bursts as well as by long, tonic trains of discharge, waxing and waning in frequency. Presumably the differing patterns are a consequence of different experimental conditions. The acute experiments were carried out as terminal experiments on chronically affected monkeys with wide exposure of the cortex for long periods under local anesthesia and immobilization with neuromuscular blocking agents and artificial ventilation. Whereas observations on undrugged epileptic monkeys were carried out only when they were behaviorally awake, no control of the state of arousal was obviously possible in the acute experiments. One or a combination of these variables could account for the differences observed.

The relevance of such experimental data can be best determined by validation of observations in the human. Patterns of firing of single neuronal elements in the epileptogenic focus have been examined in the human during the course of operations for epilepsy during the past thirteen years [81, 85]. The data are limited since observations have been restricted to those instances where the epileptogenic focus could be clearly delimited to a relatively restricted area, which had to be superficially located in the cortex so that it was accessible to the microelectrode. Most of the operations were carried out under local anesthesia. The epileptogenic focus was delimited by multichannel electrocorticography using silver-ball pial electrodes. The cortical area of maximal epileptic activity was then stabilized with a pressure foot attached to a skull-mounted manipulator and the KCl-filled micropipettes (1–5 µ) were introduced utilizing a hydraulic micromanipulator. Patterns of high frequency firing have been recorded which are indistinguishable from those recorded in the awake, undrugged, epileptic monkeys. Under optimal circumstances, unit activity at the epileptogenic focus in the human is characterized by regular, repetitive bursts of action potentials which may also be remarkably constant [84]. Examples of such repetitive firing in bursts are seen in Fig. 10-3. These records were obtained from a relatively restricted electrographic focus just anterior to a porencephalic cyst in the parietal region in a patient with intractable seizures. The bursts are characterized by 5–26 action potentials in each burst and the frequency of firing within the burst ranges from 280 to 400 per sec. The unit is quiescent between bursts, and the interburst interval varies between 50 and 380 msec. There is no obvious relation between the length of a burst and the interval between bursts. This particular unit was under observation for some 20 min. In contrast to such well-

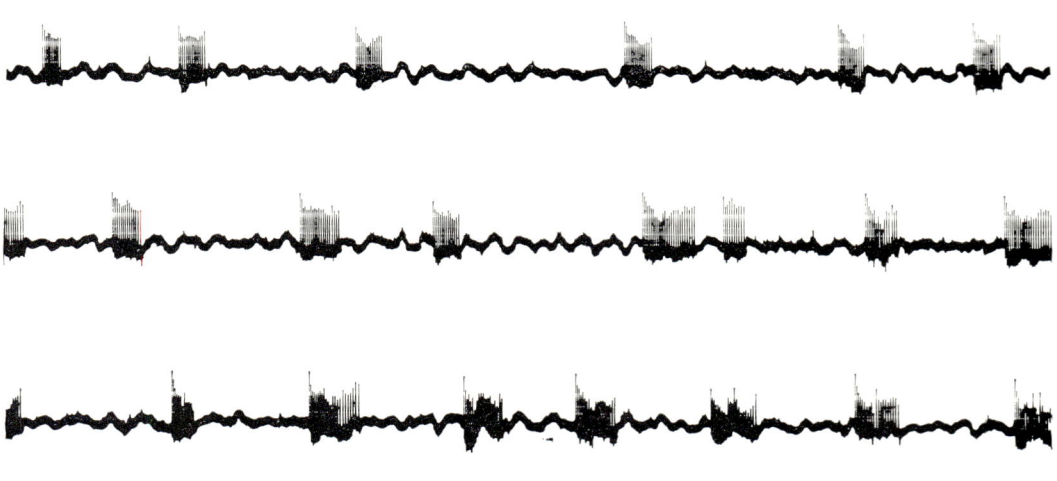

Fig. 10-3. Neuron in epileptogenic focus of human, firing in high frequency, rhythmic bursts.

structured bursts, irregular burst firing has been recorded in other instances [85] with greater variation in the number of spikes per burst and lower frequencies of firing—much like those units in the undrugged, awake epileptic monkey recorded from the transitional zone surrounding the primary area of maximal unit and slow wave hyperactivity.

Systematic observations have not been undertaken dealing with relationship between the high frequency burst firing and slow wave activity in the human. However, the extracellular field potentials recorded with the microelectrode in the human have not revealed any obvious temporal correlations between slow wave activity and unit firing (Fig. 10-3).

Thus it would appear that the interictal patterns of firing of neurons in the epileptogenic focus of the monkey are very similar to those recorded in epileptic man.

Epileptogenic Focus. The data dealing with patterns of firing of epileptic neurons in both the monkey and man are inevitably related to problems of sampling. The behavior of epileptic neurons is said to be peculiar to those neurons in the epileptogenic focus. Delimitation of what we call the focus, on the other hand, is more ambiguous. In the monkey it is not just the area of cortex into which alumina has been injected some months previously; in both monkey and man the focus is defined as the area of maximal epileptic spiking as recorded with gross electrodes. This operational definition of the focus will vary with the technique utilized and the parochial criteria of the observer. There are certain superficial similarities between the epileptic spike and the strychnine spike which can be induced by topical application of strychnine to the cortex. In the case of strychnine, the point of origin of the spike discharge is clearly known. Yet, from examination of the recorded gross electrographic spikes, it may be impossible to distinguish those spikes recorded at the focus from the strychnine spikes recorded from either subcortical conducting pathways or from a recipient area of normal cortex in the same or opposite hemisphere. Similar difficulties arise in terms of distinguishing those epileptic spikes recorded at the focus from those broadcast to distant neuronal aggregates [83].

This problem has been of sufficient concern to lead Meyers [51] to question the validity of the concept of the epileptogenic focus. However, based on the known ability of spikes to propagate over known corticocortical as well as subcortical projections, it is not cause for dismay that spikes may "wander like a will-o'-the wisp" through the brain [51]. In the monkey, spatial distribution of uncertainty can be decreased by producing as small an epileptogenic focus as possible so that the cortical volume to be sampled with a fine microelectrode will be limited. Even so, the sampling problem is sufficiently great so that it is difficult to make negative statements (such as that a certain phenomenon is not seen). This problem assumes rather major proportions when data regarding epileptic neurons are sought in the human. Cortical pathology is always more diffuse and factors of spike propagation and electrotonic conduction make it difficult to obtain unequivocal evidence regarding the geographical location of the epileptogenic focus. The yield of epileptic neurons by microelectrode sampling is therefore low in this circumstance, particularly since the time available is limited during a therapeutic surgical procedure for such observations. This accounts for the rather limited data we have otbained in the human and may account for the failure of others [65, 66] to confirm the presence of "epileptic neurons" in the human focus exhibiting firing patterns such as those in Fig. 10-3.

The sampling problem also has bearing on observations relating the repetitive, burst firing of epileptic neurons to the slow potentials recorded from the pial surface. It is well known that a potent synaptic input to an aggregate of neurons will generate excitatory postsynaptic potentials (EPSPs) in each cell which will evoke all-or-none discharges. Such soma firing will obviously be temporally related to the gross evoked response as recorded either from the pial surface or within the cortex. Neuronal hyperactivity which is fundamental to the process of epilepsy can clearly generate such synaptic inputs on other cells since this is the mechanism of expression of clinical seizures. Such *follower* neurons synaptically related to the focus might well fire in temporal relation to the summed EPSPs recorded in the EEG. We have observed instances of this phenomenon with extracellular recording in the epileptic monkey, which may account for the elegant, intracellular observations recorded from neurons in the alumina focus of monkey by Prince and Futamachi [58]. However, consistent temporal correlation of burst firing characteristic of epileptic neurons with epileptiform surface potentials in either monkey or man has been inconstant in the interictal state [78], though common during spontaneous seizures in our experience [69, 82]. Again, failure to observe a phenomenon in the presence of such ambiguities of sampling makes interpretation difficult.

Finally, we have repeatedly observed that it is most difficult to evoke epileptic units in sensory cortex of the monkey by afferent stimulation [2, 69]. A systematic attempt was made to clarify this point [63], during which observations were carried out on some 50 epileptic units in the sensory cortex of 6 monkeys in which the epileptogenic focus had been induced by intracortical injection of alumina into the arm area of the postcentral gyrus. No unit exhibiting the firing patterns characteristic of epileptic neurons could be evoked by either appropriate cutaneous or peripheral nerve stimulation. Again, the problems of sampling with a microelectrode make interpretation of such negative data tentative.

Deafferentation

The consistent observation that epileptic neurons in sensory cortex are most difficult to evoke by afferent volleys generated by peripheral nerve stimulation is, nevertheless, of interest. This does not appear to be a simple consequence of "busy-line" phenomenon. It appears to be a consequence of reduction of synaptic input on these cells. It is unlikely that all synaptic input is lost since epileptic seizures in the human and monkey can be modified by events that are, presumably, synaptically mediated.

Furthermore, epileptic neurons in the sensory cortex of the monkey can be evoked occasionally by powerful stimulation of the nucleus ventralis posterolateralis of the thalamus [5]. These clues have led to the hypothesis that a fundamental defect in these cells may be related to their partial denervation.

The hypothesis that neurons in the epileptogenic focus are characterized by reduced synaptic input is susceptible to anatomical test. Westrum et al. [89] have investigated this matter utilizing the Golgi-Cox method.

Fresh Golgi preparations of cerebral cortex in the normal monkey yielded a consistent picture of cortical elements which has been abundantly documented in the literature in the past. The normal cortical pyramidal neuron (Fig. 10-4) has a unique dendritic pattern with a prominent apical dendritic shaft which may be devoid of branches for 10–40 μ from the soma and then gives off side branches throughout the rest of its length. At its termination, it divides into a characteristic plume or arborization which may extend parallel to the pial surface for 150–350 μ. Along the surface of the dendritic membrane are numerous outpouchings or spines (Fig. 10-4, #6). They are not seen on the first 20–25 μ of the apical shaft and almost never on the perikaryon. On the apical shaft they increase in density peripherally and may give the appearance of veritable fur (Fig. 10-4, #5). As the branches become particularly fine (1 μ or less), there are fewer spines per unit length. The majority of spines range in size from 1 to 2 μ.

Similar studies were carried out in the epileptogenic focus induced in the monkey cortex by alumina. The primary focus was electrographically localized and excised for study. Histologically, this primary focus was found to be immediately adjacent to the area of alumina injection. At the injection site, there are well-circumscribed deposits of alumina which are bordered by glia and acellular areas. In the adjacent electrographic focus, there is an overall decrease in neuronal elements and an apparent increase in glial forms. In contrast to normal cortex, the superficial layers do

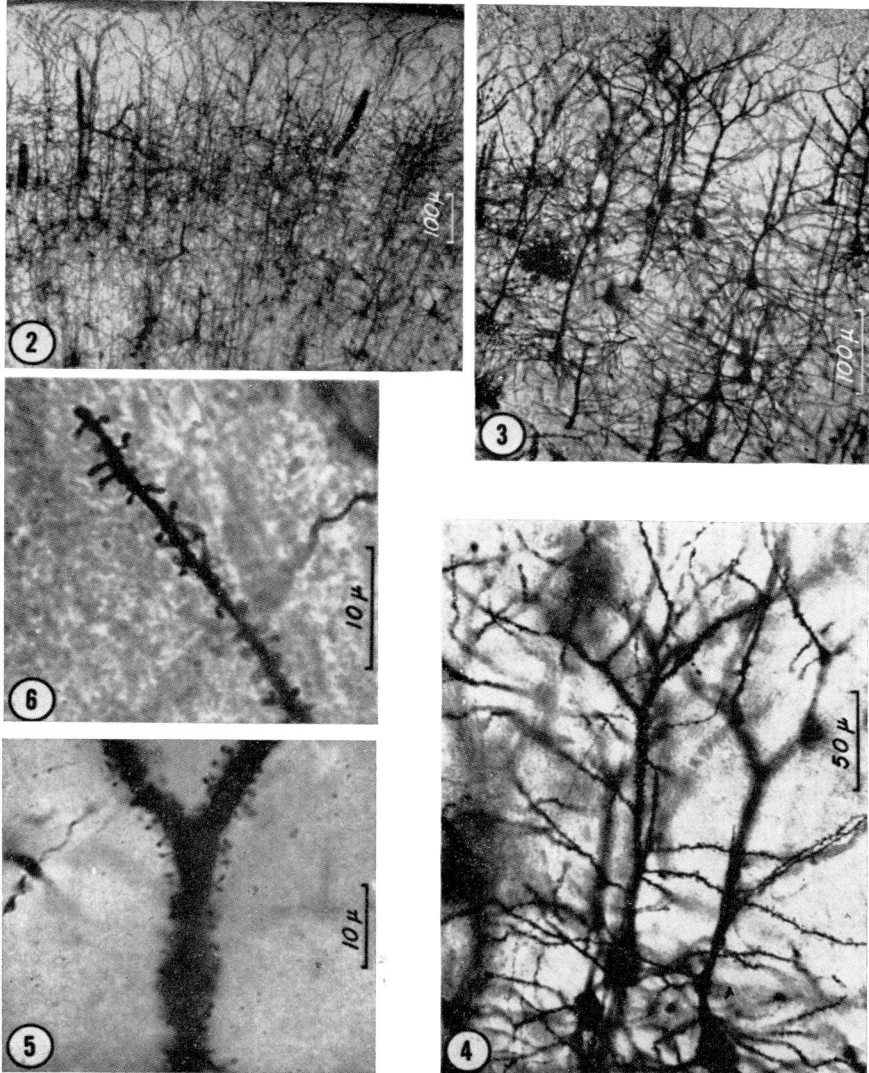

FIG. 10-4. Normal monkey sensorimotor cortex. Golgi-Cox preparations. (2) Low-power scan of superficial layers. Pial surface at top. (3) High-power view of superficial layers to show intricate branching. (4) High-power of individual neuron. (5) Oil-immersion view of apical shaft to illustrate character and extent of spines. (6) Terminal dendritic branch to illustrate finer morphology of spines. (From Westrum, White, and Ward [89].)

not have the intricate pattern of terminal arborizations (Fig. 10-5, #9). The neurons remaining appear to be of intermediate to small size. This may be pertinent in view of observations by Henneman et al. [35] that small cells are easier to discharge. These neurons in the focus have distinct morphological alterations specifically related to the dendrites. There is less dendritic branching, and the course of the apical shaft and its branches is frequently distorted in different planes. Dendrites are marked by irregular varicoselike swelling on both the large shafts and on the finer branches. Closer inspection of the dendritic surfaces reveals that they are relatively

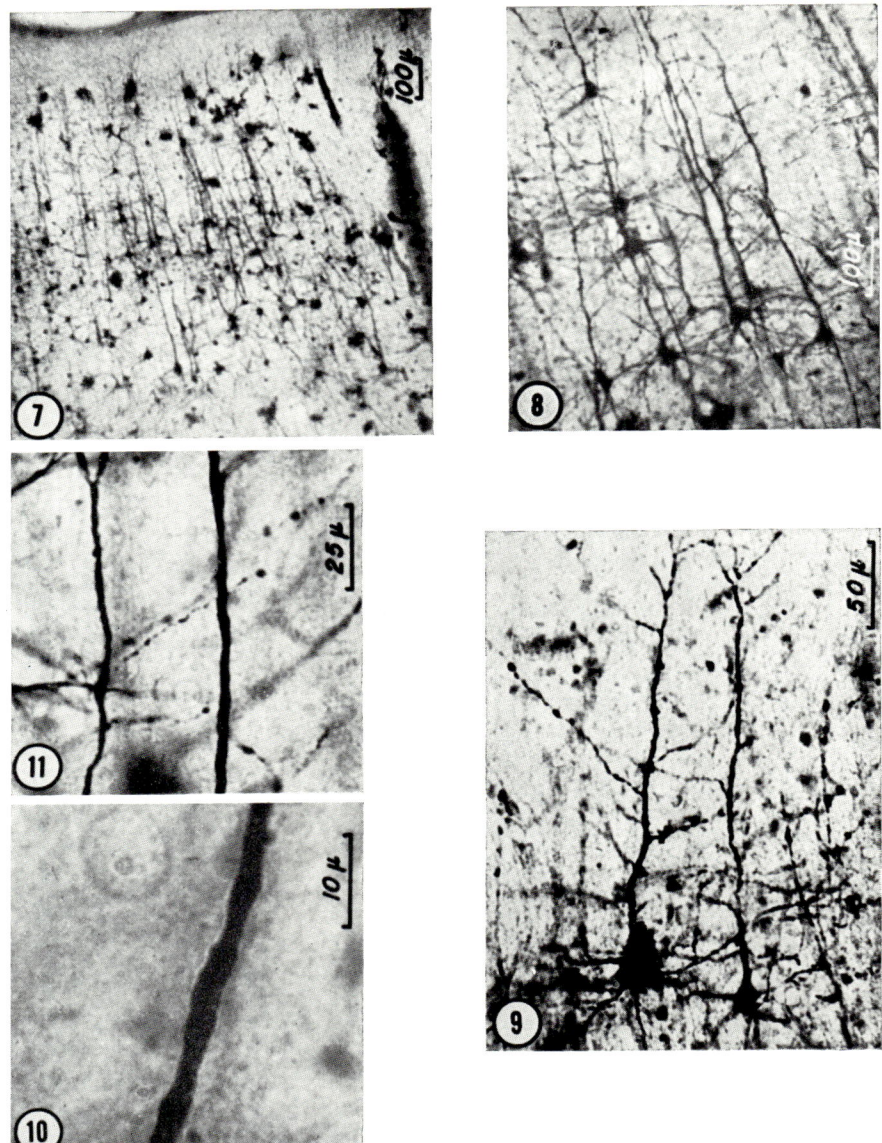

Fig. 10-5. Epileptic cortex. Golgi-Cox preparations. (7) Low-power scan. Small amount of residual alumina to right of field. Note decrease in terminal arborization. (8) High-power view. Note stunted character of individual neurons. (9) Note decreased branching and absence of spines. (10) Oil-immersion view of dendritic branches to show detail of varicose swellings and absence of spines. (From Westrum, White, and Ward [89].)

smooth along most of their course and are almost completely divested of their normal dendritic spines (Fig. 10-5, #10, 11). This finding is most prominent within the area of the electrically active primary focus where many neurons are completely devoid of spines. The apical shafts appear to be most affected and are completely bare. A rare spine is occasionally seen on finer branches.

Dendritic Changes. Radially away from the primary electrographic focus, all of the dendritic changes appear less marked. Dendritic branching becomes denser and increasing numbers of both large and small neurons are seen. At distances of 1 to 4 mm from the primary focus, and particularly in the deeper layers, dendritic shafts and branches again show increasing numbers of spines. These changes appear to continue away from the region of the focus, gradually blending into relatively normal cortex. It is of interest that this geographical distribution of the anatomical changes correlates well with the physiological changes [72] where abnormal patterns of firing show a similar transition to normal unit activity as one moves radially from the focus.

The use of the Golgi stain to study human epileptic cortex was first described by DeMoor in 1898 [22] while morphological changes similar to those described in the monkey have recently been confirmed in man by Scheibel and Scheibel [68]. They observed:

Distortion of dendrites was evident throughout most tissue samples. Apical shafts of pyramids appeared to show the most obvious changes which included nodulation of the processes, and twisted, often corkscrew deformations of the usually vertically organized processes.

Loss of dendritic spines was apparent over most of the dendrite systems and in the majority of dendrites even at some distance from the presumed ictal focus. In some cases, the shaft profiles were entirely smooth except for the nodulation. In many, there were short lengths of dendrite still carrying spiny projections. In these cases, the spines frequently appeared to project from the apices of the dendritic nodules while the inter-nodule portions of the shaft were spine-free.

Although there may be differing interpretations of the fate of postsynaptic membranes in neocortex following degeneration of the presynaptic fiber [68], it would appear that the spine tips remain apparently unaffected [88] when examined with the electron microscope. Thus the exact significance of loss of dendritic spines in the Golgi stain on epileptic cortex remains to be determined. Nevertheless, similarities between changes demonstrated in the epileptic focus in the monkey and in man are striking. Furthermore, in view of evidence indicating that destructive lesions to presynaptic afferents in mature axodendritic synaptic systems are associated with loss of dendritic spines as visualized with the Golgi stain [68], it appears that the morphological information is consistent with the physiological data suggesting that epileptic neurons may be at least partially deafferented.

Deafferentation of Spinal Neurons

The thesis that a reduction in synaptic input can result in autonomous hyperactivity is difficult to test directly in the cerebral cortex where it is not possible to divorce afferent from efferent activity because of the complex geometry of the cortical feltwork. But the anatomy of the spinal cord permits selective deafferentation without manipulation of efferent systems. We have studied this problem in cats [48], where deafferentation was produced by dorsal rhizotomy or hemicordotomy. Spontaneous activity of neurons in the cord was then monitored by extracellular microelectrode recording 14–177 days later. As illustrated in Fig. 10-6, such partial deafferentation resulted in spontaneous hyperactivity and burst firing which was most prominent in smaller neurons of the dorsal horn laminae V, VI, and VII. These second order sensory neurons tended to fire with abnormally prolonged bursts of high frequency. In addition, following L5 through S1 intradural rhizotomy, a prolonged (100 msec) high frequency discharge of presumed spinocerebellar neurons in the dorsal horn could be evoked by a single stimulus to an adjacent intact root. Both dorsal rhizotomy and hemicordotomy lead to partial deafferentation of neurons in the spinal cord.

In 1939, Cannon and Haimovici [17] demonstrated that spinal motoneurons ipsilateral to a cord hemisection are more excitable than are contralateral cells. Teasdall and Stavraky [74] showed that chronic hindlimb deafferentation reduced the threshold and augmented amplitude and duration of the flexor response to pyramidal-tract stimulation while Drake and Stavraky [25] pointed out that dorsal rhizotomy led to hypersensitivity to exogenous acetylcholine or strychnine in the deaf-

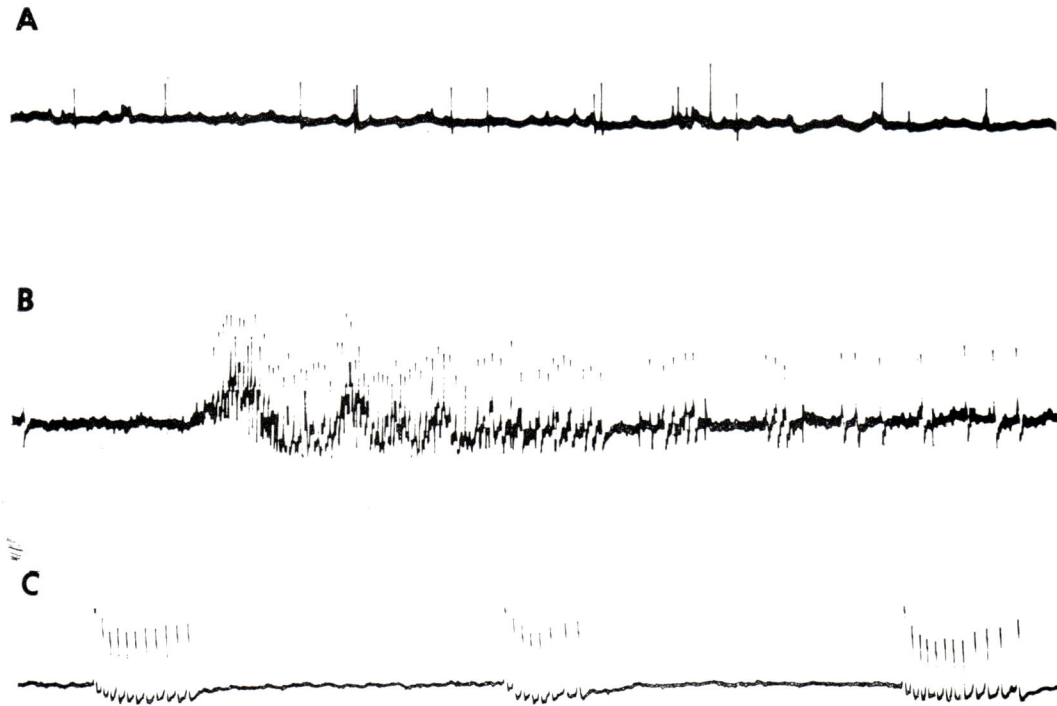

Fig. 10.6. Spontaneous activity in base of dorsal horn of cat spinal cord. Top: normal. Center: after multiple dorsal rhizotomy. Bottom: after hemicordotomy. Time marks, 5 msec. Negativity upward. (From Loeser and Ward [48].)

ferented segments. Thus one of the mechanisms involved might be a hypersensitivity of postsynaptic membrane to transmitter compounds such as acetylcholine.

Teasdall and Stavraky [74] found that polysynaptic reflexes were augmented by cord hemisection and Eccles et al. [28] found that monosynaptic reflexes were augmented by partial deafferentation. There is then ample evidence that reduction of input to spinal cord neurons can lead to augmented output in response to a standard stimulus. Significantly, Kostyuk [43] has shown augmentation of EPSPs evoked by monosynaptic input to partially deafferented motoneurons, and these observations are supported by Bokri et al. [10]. One can infer from the work of Eccles et al. [28] that the motoneuron itself is not altered by partial dorsal rhizotomy. Thus it is most likely that the hyperexcitability which

characterizes deafferented cord segments is not due to changes in motoneuron excitability but is related to events at the interneuronal level. Eccles [28] and Kostyuk [43] have demonstrated no detectable changes in the motoneuron membrane potential, conductance, or resistance after such deafferentation, so it is reasonable to question the role of the motoneuron itself in the production of hyperactivity after deafferentation.

Our results [48] are consistent with the findings of others that the motoneuron itself is not primarily hyperactive. Of course, this might be predicted from the anatomical evidence that less than 2 percent of the synapses upon motoneuron soma are derived from dorsal roots. Under such circumstances, any functional increased output from motoneurons [31, 90] may be a consequence of hyperactivity in interneurons. The majority of hyperactive cells in our studies were found in the base of the dorsal horn and not in those regions of the ventral horn which are richly endowed with motoneurons.

If cells in the cat spinal cord receiving a major synaptic input from dorsal root or suprasegmental projections become hyperactive after lesions of these inputs, it would be useful to determine whether similar changes occur in partially deafferented spinal neurons in more complex nervous systems such as that of man. Limited confirmation of these experimental findings is available [49]. The activity of neurons in the cord was sampled at and just central to a functional cord transection in a patient who had sustained a traumatic paraplegia two years previously. Activity of neurons in the dorsal half of the cord, two segments above the level of transection, exhibited low frequency burst firing; one level above the transection, high frequency burst firing was encountered; while tonic, high frequency firing was recorded from neurons located at the upper border of the segmental level of clinical paraplegia. These patterns of burst firing encountered in grossly normal cord, one segment above the level of transection, were almost indistinguishable from those recorded in the cat after hemisection (Fig. 10-6, lower trace).

Thus partial deafferentation of neurons in the spinal cord of animal and man appears to result in autonomous hyperactivity with patterns of burst firing which are strikingly similar to those recorded from epileptic neurons.

Deafferentation of Trigeminal Spinal Complex

The spinal trigeminal system also lends itself well to the study of neuronal deafferentation since it is supplied by a large nerve containing only sensory fibers. At varying times following retro-Gasserian rhizotomy, microelectrode recordings were made from the trigeminal complex [1]. From 10 to 20 days after rhizotomy, generalized hyperactivity of single cells was found throughout the spinal trigeminal complex (Fig. 10-7). This activity was regular and continued without interruption. At 19 days after rhizotomy, neurons were observed to be firing in brief bursts separated by equally short periods of inactivity. At 31 days after rhizotomy, the hyperactivity became even more pronounced and almost uninterrupted tonic firing was encountered in neurons throughout pars interpolaris and caudalis of the trigeminal spinal complex.

Not only is gross hyperactivity induced in the central trigeminal neurons by the rather massive deafferentation that follows trigeminal rhizotomy, but Black et al. [7] have shown that hyperactivity also is in-

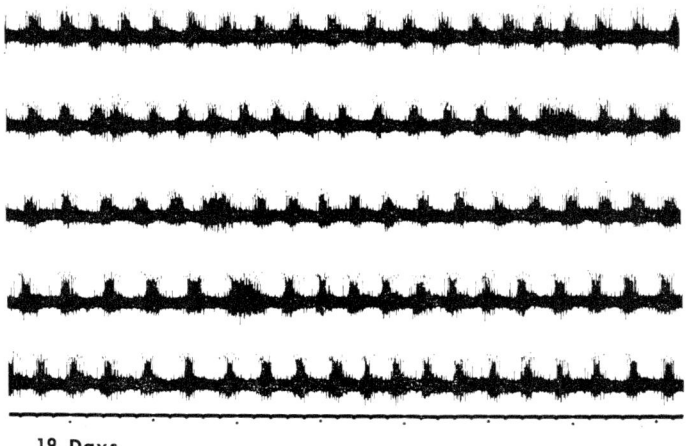

FIG. 10-7. Spontaneous unit activity recorded in nucleus caudalis of the trigeminal spinal complex 19 days after trigeminal rhizotomy.

duced by partial loss of synaptic input that occurs after removal of all the teeth on one side of the animal. Again, some weeks after such partial deafferentation, spontaneous hyperactivity and intermittent high frequency burst firing occurs and afferent volleys induced by stimulation of cutaneous trigeminal afferents evokes prolonged (200 msec) firing of such hyperactive neurons in the nucleus caudalis of the spinal trigeminal complex.

Thus it would appear that the spontaneous activity of single neurons at various levels of the nervous system is appreciably augmented by deafferentation. Patterns of firing of such partially deafferented neurons in spinal cord or brain stem are qualitatively similar to the firing patterns of neurons in the epileptic focus in the cortex where, again, there is both physiological and anatomical evidence to indicate that the synaptic input is altered. From the available evidence it should be noted that, although deafferentation appears to induce hyperactivity in the denervated cell, such cells are not completely devoid of synaptic input. Partial rather than complete deafferentation appears to represent the necessary condition for inducing this phenomenon.

Analysis of Patterns of Burst Firing

Since bursts are such a dominant feature of the spike train in epileptic neurons, there is considerable interest in examining the fine structure of the timing within such burst patterns; this has been undertaken by Calvin et al. [15]. In contrast to the spontaneous firing of normal cortical neurons where there is uncertainty regarding where a normal burst begins or ends, bursts of the epileptic neurons are so stereotyped that there is no problem defining where such a burst starts or stops, even for a computer program. This has enabled bursts to be explicitly analyzed for the first time, utilizing computer techniques developed by Calvin [12].

Since these are extracellular recordings, only the output of the neuron is available, forcing inferences about synaptic input and spike generating mechanisms to be made from the output spike train. Many models have been made in this fashion based on the activity of normal neurons, using interval variability statistics to reason backwards to the kind of input or spike generator, or both, which could have produced such statistics. Such efforts may be hazardous [13, 14]. In epileptic neurons, however, firing patterns are often quite structured rather than random, providing considerable additional information for attempts at modeling, compared to variability information alone.

Utilizing such common methods as the interspike interval histogram and the joint interval density, comparison can be made of the spontaneous firing of normal and epileptic neurons (Fig. 10-8). For the normal, cortical neuron of Fig. 10-8A, these techniques yield displays which give less information about bursts than mere visual inspection of raw data. The interspike-interval histogram of the epileptic neuron (Fig. 10-8E) shows three peaks: 1.6, 4.0, and about 120 msec. The 1.6 msec peak presum-

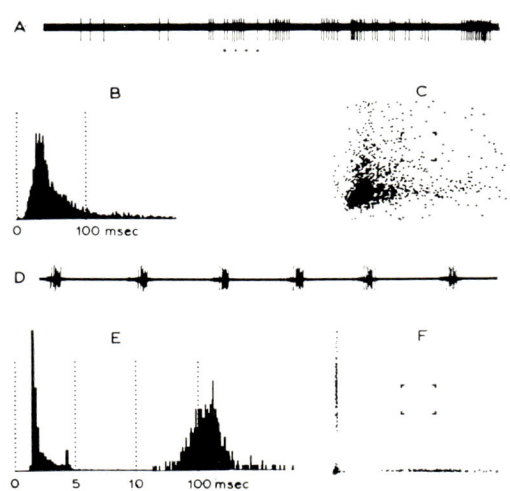

FIG. 10-8. Bursts in normal and epileptic neurons. (A) Normal undrugged cortical neuron in monkey. Time marks, 100 msec. Positive upward. (B) Interspike interval histogram. (C) Joint interval density; brackets at 80 and 120 msec. (D) Epileptic neuron in undrugged monkey. Time scale expanded ×7.5 over (A). (E) Interspike interval histogram. Time scale compressed and probability scale expanded after 10 msec. (F) Joint interval density. (From Calvin, Sypert, and Ward [15].)

ably corresponds to high frequency firing within the burst, and the 120 msec peak to the silent period between bursts. The joint-interval density (Fig. 10-8F) shows a cluster of points near the origin due to short intervals within the burst and the two arms corresponding to the silent period preceded and followed by the burst. There is slight asymmetry to these arms, and it, with the 4 msec peak in the interval histogram, are the only two features of these traditional interspike-interval measures not immediately explicable from visual inspection of the film strips. The variability of the silent period between bursts (Fig. 10-8E) peaking at about 120 msec might be concealing a more fixed process if the number of spikes per burst varied, thus causing the silent period to vary correspondingly. However, a histogram of intervals from the first spike of one burst to the first spike of the next shows no less variability. Thus there is little evidence to suggest that the bursts might be started (or stopped) by some more regular process.

More insight into burst structure can be provided by raster displays and spike densities [12]. By lining up sequential bursts beneath one another, using dots to represent the full height of the spike, it is possible to compact a large amount of raw data so that it can be scanned visually. Aligning all first spikes of the bursts beneath one another, it is apparent both from the raster and the spike density (Fig. 10-9A) that the rest of the burst is not time-locked to the first spike. It is also clear that the interval between the first and second spikes or the "first interval" of the burst is longer and much more variable than are subsequent intervals. If all the second spikes of the bursts are now aligned (Fig. 10-9B), a considerable improvement may then be noted in the way in which subsequent spikes of the burst are synchronized. Peaks of the corresponding spike densities likewise demonstrate that the later spikes of the burst are synchronized with the second spike, not with the first spike of the burst. This would suggest that the first spike and the rest of the burst are somewhat independent of each other; a variable

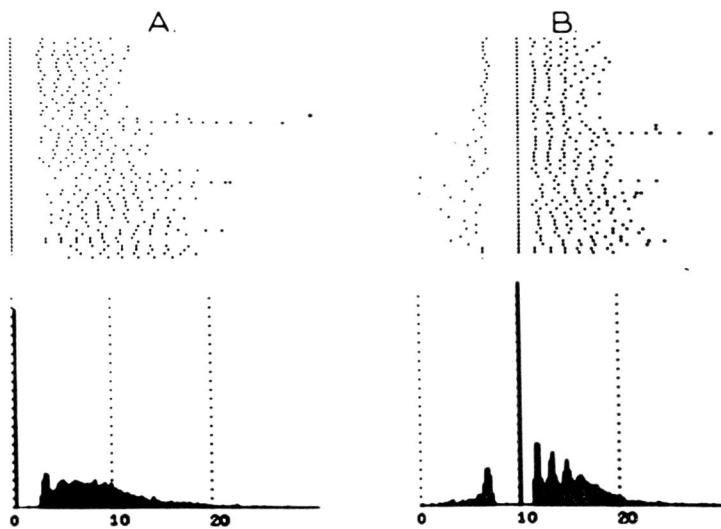

Fig. 10-9. Raster displays and spike densities of epileptic neuron. (A) All first spikes of each burst aligned to a vertical column. Histogram below shows probability of finding a spike relative to first spike of the burst. Height of first spike peak has a probability of one. (B) Second spikes aligned by computer. Note succeeding spikes are more synchronized to second spike than to first. Time scale (in nanoseconds) is same for rasters as in spike densities. (From Calvin, Sypert, and Ward [15].)

time elapses between first and second spikes, but, once the second spike occurs, the burst is stereotyped thereafter.

Thus the general characteristics of epileptic bursts may be summarized as follows: that there is only high frequency firing within the burst, without a marked tapering off in the firing frequency before the end of the burst; that the first interval in a burst is sometimes unusual in its behavior; and that there is a silent period between bursts which is quite variable and which may occasionally be associated with the number of spikes in the next burst.

We may distinguish between bursts which have these long first intervals and bursts without them, that is, where the first interval is typically little different from succeeding intervals. The long first-interval bursts do not occur in the same neuron as the nonspecific bursts. Furthermore, it has been our observation that long first-interval neurons tend to occur only within the area of the major epileptic spike activity as recorded in the surface EEG at the focus. As penetrations are made farther away from this area, only nonspecific bursting neurons are encountered. This marginal region tapers off into regions of cortex where neurons produce firing patterns resembling those of normal control neurons (Fig. 10-8A). This would be consistent with previous physiological [72] and anatomical [89] observations.

We are thus led to focus attention upon the long first-interval bursts, not only because they are more common in the central regions of the epileptogenic focus, but because it appears as if the first spike were in some way a separate process from the rest of the burst. Three types of long first-interval behavior have been observed (Fig. 10-10). Since the first interval is often variable as well as long, the displays align all second spikes of the bursts. Thus, in the spike densities, all points to the left of the second spike peak are necessarily first spikes, providing a reversed histogram of intervals between first and second spikes. In examining these first intervals, it can be seen that the neuron of Fig. 10-10A has a markedly variable time between first and second spikes; the first-interval histogram is unimodal with a smooth decline in probability toward longer first intervals. The neuron of Fig. 10-10B, on the other hand, shows a systematic change in first interval. There seem to be two preferred modes of operation: one with a 4 msec lag and the other with only a 3 msec lag between the

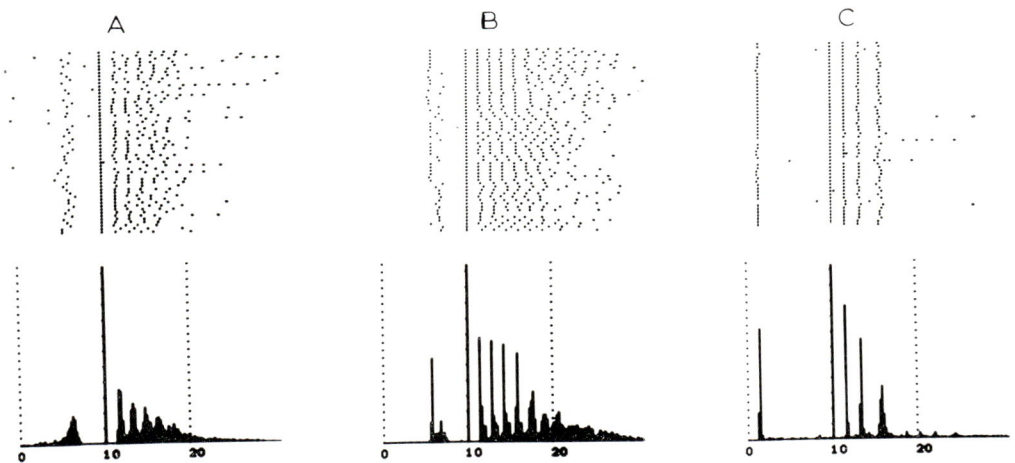

FIG. 10-10. Three different types of long first-interval bursts of epileptic neurons. Raster displays align all second spikes. (A) Interval from first spike to stereotyped rest of burst varies randomly. (B) Long first interval with two preferential modes at 3 msec or 4 msec. (C) This cell shows a very long (8.6 msec) first interval which is remarkably constant. Time in nanoseconds. (From Calvin, Sypert, and Ward [15].)

first spike and the stereotyped part of the burst. This bimodal behavior is reflected in the two peaks of the spike-density histogram of first intervals. Judging from the raster, however, it would seem that the neuron does not randomly jump from one mode to the other, but rather may stay in one mode for a while. It has been our observation that neurons exhibiting bimodality may drift into other modes of behavior indistinguishable from that of Fig. 10-10A.

In the neuron of Fig. 10-10C, the long first interval is quite long (8.6 msec) compared to later intervals in the burst which lie in the 1.6 msec range. Its most puzzling characteristic, however, is lack of variability in the first interval. Nearly all first spikes fall within one 200-μsec bin, and what variability there is could be expected from computer sampling error alone. To have interval variability of less than 2 percent of the mean is an unusual situation for repetitive firing.

Long first-interval neurons, to judge from these examples, therefore seem to have two components to their bursts: a first spike and a group of stereotyped spikes beginning with the second spike. Neither appears alone, always being infallibly associated with each other, but with the long first interval between them exhibiting various forms of behavior. This first interval can be remarkably fixed in duration or it can be quite variable, in some cases with a bimodal behavior. The rest of the burst which follows is merely stereotyped and locked to the second spike, but it begins according to this variable or bimodal behavior of the first interval. While theories of epileptic burst firing must presently be made without benefit of the relevant intracellular potential swings, there are nonetheless a considerable number of constraints placed upon models by this unusual "fine structure" of the spike timing.

MODELS OF THE EPILEPTIC NEURON

Any model of the mechanisms operating at the chronic epileptogenic focus should account for certain observations. It appears that epilepsy of focal onset in the cerebral cortex is induced by damage to neurons in both the human and in the monkey models. Some weeks, months, or years after such an insult, an epileptogenic focus appears and clinical seizures are observed. The epileptogenic focus is characterized morphologically by depopulation of neurons, and the remaining neurons appear to be of small size. There is an astrocytic gliosis in which the epileptic neurons are embedded; the epileptic neurons are characterized, in the Go'gi stain, by a striking loss of dendritic spines and other changes in dendritic structure.

Electrophysiologically, the focus is determined by the presence of *epileptic spikes* in the electrocorticogram. The activity of individual neurons in the focus is characterized by autonomous high frequency firing, often in bursts with special properties of timing. It is difficult to evoke such neurons in sensory cortex by peripheral sensory volleys.

The current data would suggest that complex mechanisms are operating and that there may be several varieties of neuronal behavior in the focus. The class of neurons whose behavior is most rigidly described are those which fire in stereotyped bursts where the timing pattern within bursts reveals an unusually long interval between the first and second spikes of each burst, with the later spikes time-locked to the second spike, not to the first spike. There are two general classes of burst mechanism which are well documented. With the first mechanism, firing frequency is proportional to the time course of synaptic depolarization; in the second, a regenerative spike mechanism keeps the cell firing even after removal of the stimulus. Thus the high-frequency-only character of the bursts in epileptic neurons could be due to an EPSP–IPSP sequence, which is the most common sequence of membrane potential behavior seen following stimulation of a mixed collection of afferent fibers [4]. A self-limiting regenerative mechanism, such as the summating depolarizing afterpotentials which Kandel and Spencer [37] considered to be the explanation of the bursts seen in hippocampal pyramidal cells, is at the opposite extreme. A pathological example of such a regenerative mechanism is the strychninized stretch receptor of the crayfish [87], where a single antidromic spike is followed by a long depolarization in the soma which, in turn, generates a long train of spikes.

However, the presence of the long first intervals in the stereotyped bursts of these particular epileptic neurons places certain constraints on hypotheses utilized to explain the genesis of such bursts. It is most difficult to see how ordinary synaptic input could account for them, either with regenerative firing mechanisms or ones which follow a synaptic depolarization. The bimodality and the extraordinarily precise timing properties of these bursts have led us to consider conduction time as one of the possible explanations, since conduction time is one of the most precise timing mechanisms in the nervous system. Furthermore, we have considered the possibility of an axonal recording site for the microelectrode as opposed to a site near the cell-body region. While this would normally make little difference in the spike timing patterns observed, it would make a great deal of difference if the first spike were antidromic. We would then see the first spike going away from the focus toward a distant cell body, then the rest of the burst returning from the cell body. This would produce a long first interval whose duration would depend upon conduction velocity and the distance from the cell body.

Such a model might be consistent with previous observations we obtained by intracellular recordings in a similar epileptic preparation [2]. All records from cells demonstrating firing-pattern characteristics previously documented by extracellular recordings also had waveform characteristics which would be consistent with a recording site in the axon. As noted in Fig. 10-11, no postsynaptic potentials are observed in such epileptic cells firing in the typical autonomous bursts, and there is no evidence of synaptic activity preceding the burst. The rising phase of individual spikes is rapid and does not contain an inflection point. The underlying membrane potential is unusually free of spontaneous fluctuations.

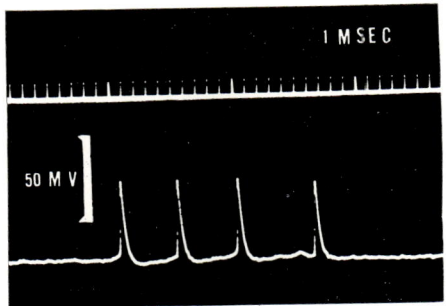

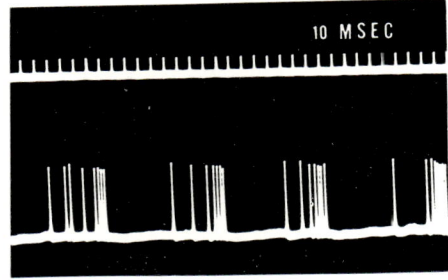

Fig. 10-11. Spontaneous action potentials in epileptic cortex of monkey obtained with intracellular microelectrode. Both traces from same cell. Time marks, 1 and 10 msec; vertical line, 50 mV. (From Atkinson and Ward [2].)

Such records were obtained from epileptic units for many minutes without evidence of deterioration. In none of the forty-four stable intracellular records obtained in epileptic preparations was there evidence of the electrical criteria customarily utilized to define soma membrane activity. In spite of diligent search, studies in chronic epileptic focus yielded records fulfilling the criteria of soma membrane firing on only three occasions and in these the patterns of firing were not typical of the high frequency burst activity usually characteristic of epileptogenic cortex. However, more recent studies by Prince and Futamachi [58] have demonstrated that it is possible to obtain intracellular recording from the soma of cells in the chronic alumina focus in which rhythmic membrane depolarizations are associated with bursts of spike discharges. However, patterns of firing were not characterized by stereotyped bursts with a long first interval between the first and second spikes of the burst.

If the first spike in such bursts is antidromically induced and the rest of the burst returns from the direction of the more distant cell body, many features of the data may be explained. Since most of the delay between the first spike and the rest of the burst is conduction time, the first interval would be rather precise. Two sites along the axon where the antidromic stimulus arose (such as two branches of the axon) could account for the bimodal behavior. The model also predicts that the cell body is probably located at some distance from the epileptogenic focus. Assuming the average conduction velocities to be between 1 and 20 meters per sec, a first interval 8.6 msec long would suggest a conduction distance of 4–80 mm (4.0 msec from recording site back to cell body; 0.6 msec delay; then 4.0 msec back again). If the cell bodies are indeed located at some distance, with their axons merely terminating in the epileptogenic region, they could be rather healthy cells with merely an abnormal input, which might be able to sustain such hyperactivity indefinitely. Once the antidromic spike reaches the cell body, the rest of the stereotyped burst could be generated by a variety of mechanisms. Such repetitive firing could be generated by summating depolarizing afterpotentials [37] or by recurrent excitation, which has been demonstrated in pyramidal cells [73] and spinal motoneurons [91].

Possible mechanisms for generating the first antidromic spike are less easy to formulate since antidromic spikes are usually thought of as being produced by an experimenter rather than by nature. Presynaptic inhibition is often thought to operate via synapses upon presynaptic terminals of an axon. These synapses depolarize terminals, somehow serving to reduce the average quantity of transmitter released when a spike arrives [27, 77]. When strong enough, however, it is possible for this presynaptic depolarization to actually cross threshold and set up a spike itself, which will then propagate antidromically back up the axon. Wall has considered this to be the basis of the dorsal-root reflex [77]. It is perhaps of interest that the dorsal-root reflex in the trigeminal system [76, 77], which is augmented by convulsant drugs applied to the spinal trigeminal complex or chronically by the injection of alumina, is also depressed by the anticonvulsant drug diphenylhydantoin [38]. Since spontaneous activity of neurons in the spinal complex in these circumstances is also characterized by hyperactivity, mechanisms may be operating which are similar to those proposed for the cortical epileptogenic focus.

Axon Stimuli. There are other mechanisms by which excitability at axon terminals may be modified. Subsequent to conditioning by a high frequency stimulus, mammalian [71] and invertebrate axons [52] respond to single stimuli with brief trains of repetitive action potentials. This posttetanic repetitive activity is associated with hyperpolarization of the terminal branches of the axon [52, 64] and accounts for the posttetanic potentiation (PTP) of muscle response. The PTP of the monosynaptic reflex in the spinal cord is also thought to be based on hyperpolarization of presynaptic terminals. Evidence has recently been presented which indicates that PTP is the result of activity of an electrogenic pump in these terminal membranes. The pump is stimulated by increases in internal sodium; is associated with an ATP-splitting enzyme that needs both sodium and potassium for its activation; and it depends on the presence of potassium ions in the external medium [64]. The amplitude of the potassium-activated response increases with increasing concentration of extracellular potassium. The role of potassium in determining neuronal excitability and the interaction of these mechanisms with the glia will be dealt with by Orkand (Chap. 26). However, it should be noted that there is evidence suggesting that ionic concentrations shift during seizure phenomena [20].

Matsumoto and Ajmone-Marsan [50] have presented evidence that cortical neurons swell reversibly during development of seizures induced by topical penicillin, suggesting an influx of sodium ions and water; and ionic shifts have been implicated by Pollen and Lux [57] during paroxysmal discharges induced by strychnine. These experimental studies may be relevant to the phenomena of epilepsy in the human as evidenced by the relation of salt retention to epilepsy reviewed by Glaser [32].

If mechanisms in the epileptic focus could induce hyperpolarization of the presynaptic terminals by activation of an electrogenic pump, then a single spike originating in a distant cell body would evoke a repetitive discharge in these terminals as in the case of posttetanic repetitive firing. If the monitoring extracellular microelectrode is located close to the distant cell body, one would record the initial spike and the returning burst it caused in the preterminal fibers. The first spike would be separated from the burst by an interval determined by the round-trip conduction velocity and could again account for the fine structure of the long first-interval bursts recorded in epileptic neurons. This model suffers from the observation that the long first-interval neurons tended to be recorded close to the focus; but this might only reflect problems of sampling since the relevant fibers converging on the focus will be most dense close to the focus and rapidly become harder to find as they disperse in the cortical volume away from the focus.

It may be more than coincidence that one of the known physiological actions of the common anticonvulsant drug, diphenylhydantoin, is to suppress posttetanic repetitive firing at motor nerve terminals [61] as well as the PTP of the monosynaptic reflex in the cord [29]. Furthermore, this drug also depresses the augmented dorsal-root reflex in the trigeminal system induced by application of convulsant drugs to the spinal trigeminal complex [38]. If the data dealing with the augmented dorsal-root reflex were reinterpreted to indicate that it was also generated by a repetitive discharge in presynaptic terminals hyperpolarized by an electrogenic pump, this would then form a homogeneous body of data. However diphenylhydantoin, unfortunately, appears to have no acute effect on the patterns of spontaneous firing of epileptic neurons in the epileptogenic focus [62]. But it should be noted that this study was carried out under experimental conditions where stereotyped burst firing was rarely encountered, and data are not available regarding the action of diphenylhydantoin specifically on the long first-interval epileptic neurons. However, it may also be that more than one type of neuronal behavior is operating in the epileptogenic focus.

Denervation. The final factor which must be considered in any model of the epileptic neuron is the role of denervation. We have presented evidence indicating that partial deafferentation in several specific neuronal circuits results in spontaneous hyperactivity and that the autonomously hyperactive neurons which characterize the epileptogenic focus also appear to have an altered synaptic input. Li [44] pointed out some years ago that epileptic discharges from pathological nerve cells in the cortex might be based on the same sequence of events which occurs in denervated muscle fibers. He reported that both denervated muscle and muscle fibers grown in tissue culture are characterized by unstable resting membrane potentials. Ware et al. [86] have studied the resting membrane potentials of mammalian muscle following denervation and demonstrated that the resting membrane potential falls from the neighborhood of 100 mV to 77 mV at 50 days after denervation. The time at which the muscle fiber begins to fibrillate is closely correlated with the drop in membrane potential and, as they point out, as this autonomous activity quickly becomes established, the resting potential falls rapidly.

Thesleff [75] has confirmed the drop in membrane potential of denervated muscle and the association of this with autonomous spike activity. He found that electrical input resistance of the denervated membrane was increased to about twice its innervated value. He proposed that the changes induced by denervation might be accounted for by the assumption that denervation reduces potassium conductance of the resting membrane but increases duration of the outward potassium current during the action potential. The former would enhance the influence of sodium and chloride ions on the membrane potential in the direction of depolarization; the increase in duration of potassium current during the action potential would cause an initial hyperpolarization followed by a relative depolarization. In a fiber whose membrane potential is close to threshold, these changes could induce rhythmic spike activity.

However, it is not legitimate to treat a denervated cell as a homogeneous membrane. In fact, more detailed studies by Belmar and Eyzaguirre [3] indicate that fibrillatory potentials in denervated muscle originate from the denervated end-plate zone and that this region represents the only areas from which the generation of rhythmic discharges can be influenced. In the denervated muscle, they propose that fibrillation is probably produced by a steady generator potential at the denervated subsynaptic sites and not by continuous membrane oscillation. It appears that the membrane in the vicinity of the denervated end-plate zone is both chemically and electrically excitable. As they point out,

It is interesting to note that in terms of fibrillary activity the membrane at the denervated end-plate zone seems to have properties different from the rest of the muscle fiber membrane. Thus cathodal currents and drugs (such as ACh and noradrenaline) increase the frequency of fibrillation only when applied to the denervated end-plate zone in spite of the fact that currents and ACh induce membrane potential changes wherever they are applied. Therefore, changes in fibrillation frequency cannot be ascribed only to membrane potential changes. The pacemaker site must have some special properties which make it different from the rest of the muscle membrane.

They go on to point out that a cholinergic mechanism does not seem to be a likely cause of fibrillation.

The data reported by Csillik [21] would be consistent with such a model since he describes marked changes in the structure of denervated postjunctional membrane and cytoplasm based on changes in birefringence with polarization optical examination. He concludes that the data indicate a change in the orientation of lipids from an original transverse to a longitudinal state (as regards the orientation of the polypeptide chains) and proposes that this may account for increase in potassium flux and increased sensitivity to acetylcholine.

Since we have no direct data dealing with the structural or functional properties of denervated postsynaptic membrane in central neurons, we can only speculate, utilizing the models generated by the studies on denervated postjunctional membrane in muscle. If the denervated subsynaptic sites in cortical neurons produce a steady generator potential which can induce spikes and if such sites were located in dendrites, intracellular recording from the soma would be expected to reveal action potentials rising abruptly from the baseline without any antecedent prepotential. Such was the case in the intracellular records reported by Atkinson and Ward [2] which they interpreted as indicating a recording site in the axon. This reinterpretation of the data is not too dissimilar from that suggested by Purpura et al. [59], who stated:

In view of the present results (in hippocampal neurons) and studies of immature neocortical neurons [60], it is possible that spikes without depolarizing prepotentials observed in chronic epileptogenic neurons were, in fact, recorded from cell bodies and that such discharges were initiated in dendrites as a consequence of pathophysiological and structural alterations associated with the development of chronic epileptogenic activity. The implication here is that mechanisms which suppress regenerative responses in dendrites of neocortical neurons during ontogenesis [60] may be susceptible to a variety of severe traumatic and metabolic disturbances.

No mention has thus far been made of the possible role of denervation hypersensitivity to transmitter compounds such as acetylcholine in the autonomous hyperactivity that characterizes the epileptic neuron. As Echlin and his collaborators have pointed out [26], the chronic, partially isolated human or monkey cortex has many properties characteristic of epileptogenic cortex. (See Chap. 12.) Such partially isolated cortex gradually develops an increased susceptibility to experimentally induced epileptiform activity, and there is a supersensitivity of neurons in the slab to topically applied acetylcholine, physostigmine, and electrical stimulation, and to intravenous injections of acetylcholine. Rosenberg and Echlin [67] have also reported a decrease in specific acetylcholinesterase but not of nonspecific butyrylcholinesterase associated with seizures in chronic, partially isolated cortex. These charges were also associated with an increased membrane permeability to acetylcholine. The role of these phenomena in the genesis of epileptic seizures is not yet clear, particularly since there is no conclusive evidence that such hypersensitivity plays a role in the genesis of the spontaneous repetitive discharge in denervated muscle although, again, a "supersensitivity" can be demonstrated. It is of some interest that raised potassium concentration augments the release of acetylcholine by nerve terminals [45], so that some of these mechanisms may be interacting in the alterations of behavior postulated to occur in preterminal fibers ending in the epileptogenic focus.

Certainly the concept that denervation may play a role in the genesis of epilepsy is not new. Walter Cannon, in his Hughlings Jackson Memorial Lecture at the Montreal Neurological Institute in 1939 [16] stated:

In discussing epilepsy, Jackson wrote of the "discharging" lesion as a "physiological fulminate," i.e., the normal cells of a center becoming a hyperfunctioning part of it. Thus, there may be an abrupt and excessive local discharge from some highly unstable part of the cerebral hemisphere. What produces the instability? As already noted, Jackson suggested that tumors or blocking of blood vessels might produce it. . . . Is it not possible that tumors, and such lesions of the motor area as are associated with the name of Hughlings Jackson, may induce instability of the neighboring cortical cells by destroying their connections with other cortical cells? If that should prove to be true, it would be another illustration of the law of sensitization of denervated structures which I have endeavored to illustrate. Here is work to be done—work in which the great neurologist whom we memorialize today would be deeply interested.

SUMMARY

The epileptogenic focus might be schematically represented by an aggregate of partially denervated neurons in cortex. In some of these, the generator potentials generated in the denervated subsynaptic sites in dendritic membrane may induce repetitive firing; in others, only mostly large slow waves. Axons from distant, healthy cell bodies terminating or traversing the area are stimulated either synaptically or by alterations in the local electrical field [54] or ionic gradients or both. The antidromic spike so induced causes a burst in such cells. Both the antidromic spike and the consequent burst propagate via axon collaterals to normal cells providing a potent input to them capable of disrupting their normal activity. In view of the fragmentary state of current knowledge of the details of the mechanisms operating at the epileptic focus, such a model does not provide a unique explanation for the current data. Since many components of the model are capable of experimental test, it is hoped that these speculations will stimulate the generation of data which will lead to the formulation of more precise and explicit descriptions of the epileptic neuron.

REFERENCES

1. Anderson, L. S., Black, R. G., Abraham, J., and Ward, A. A., Jr. Unpublished data, 1968.
2. Atkinson, J. R., and Ward, A. A., Jr. Intracellular studies of cortical neurons in chronic epileptogenic foci in the monkey. *Exp. Neurol.* 10:285, 1964.
3. Belmar, J., and Eyzaguirre, C. Pacemaker site of fibrillation potentials in denervated mammalian muscle. *J. Neurophysiol.* 29: 425, 1966.
4. Biedenbach, M. A., and Stevens, C. A. Intracellular postsynaptic potentials and location of synapses in pyramidal cells of the cat olfactory cortex. *Nature* (London) 212:361, 1966.

5. Black, R. G., and Atsev, E. Unpublished data, 1967.
6. Black, R. G., Abraham, J., and Ward, A. A., Jr. The preparation of tungstic acid gel and its use in the production of experimental epilepsy. *Epilepsia* (Amst.) 8: 56, 1967.
7. Black, R. G., Anderson, L. S., and Canfield, R. Unpublished data, 1968.
8. Blum, B., and Liban, E. Experimental basotemporal epilepsy in the cat. Discrete epileptogenic lesions produced in the hippocampus or amygdaloid by tungstic acid. *Neurology* (Minneap.) 10:546, 1960.
9. Blum, B., Majnes, J., Bental, E., and Liban, E. Electroencephalographic studies in cats with experimentally produced hippocampal epilepsy. *Electroenceph. Clin. Neurophysiol.* 13:340, 1961.
10. Bokri, F., Konya, L., and Boczan, G. Investigation of the denervation supersensitivity of cat's spinal neurons. *Acta Physiol. Acad. Sci. Hung.* Suppl. 26, 12, 1965.
11. Brooks, V. B., and Asanuma, H. Action of tetanus toxin in the cerebral cortex. *Science* 137:674, 1962.
12. Calvin, W. H. Evaluating membrane potential and spike patterns by experimenter-controlled computer displays. *Exp. Neurol.* 21:512, 1968.
13. Calvin, W. H., and Stevens, C. F. Synaptic noise as a source of variability in the interval between action potentials. *Science* 155:842, 1967.
14. Calvin, W. H., and Stevens, C. F. Synaptic noise and other sources of randomness in motoneuron interspike intervals. *J. Neurophysiol.* 31:574, 1968.
15. Calvin, W. H., Sypert, G. W., and Ward, A. A., Jr. Structured timing patterns within bursts from epileptic neurons in undrugged monkey cortex. *Exp. Neurol.* 21:535, 1968.
16. Cannon, W. B. A law of denervation. *Amer. J. Med. Sci.* 198:737, 1939.
17. Cannon, W. B., and Haimovici, H. The sensitization of motoneurones by partial "deafferentation." *Amer. J. Physiol.* 126: 731, 1939.
18. Carrea, R., and Lanari, A. Chronic effect of tetanus toxin applied locally to the cerebral cortex of the dog. *Science* 137: 342, 1962.
19. Chusid, J. G., and Kopeloff, L. M. Epileptogenic effects of pure metals implanted in motor cortex of monkeys. *J. Appl. Physiol.* 17:697, 1962.
20. Colfer, H. F., and Essex, H. E. Distribution of total electrolyte, potassium and sodium in cerebral cortex in relation to experimental convulsions. *Amer. J. Physiol.* 150:27, 1947.
21. Csillik, B. *Functional Structure of the Post-synaptic Membrane in the Myoneural Junction.* Budapest: Hungarian Acad. Sciences, 1965.
22. DeMoor, J. La plasticité morphologique des neurones cérébraux. *Inst. Solvay Brux. Trav. de Lab.* 2:3, 1896.
23. Dimov, S. D. Changes in the Cerebral Bioelectric Activity of Rabbits Following Application of Cobalt to the Brain Cortex. In Servit, A. (Ed.), *Comparative and Cellular Pathophysiology of Epilepsy.* Amsterdam: Excerpta Medica Int. Congr. Series 124:235, 1966.
24. Dow, R. S., Fernandez-Guardiola, A., and Manni, E. The production of cobalt experimental epilepsy in the rat. *Electroenceph. Clin. Neurophysiol.* 14:399, 1962.
25. Drake, C. C., and Stravraky, G. W. An extension of the "law of denervation" to afferent neurones. *J. Neurophysiol.* 11:229, 1948.
26. Echlin, F. A., and Battista, A. Epileptiform seizures from chronic isolated cortex. *Arch. Neurol.* (Chicago) 9:64, 1963.
27. Eccles, J. C. *The Physiology of Synapses.* New York: Academic, 1964.
28. Eccles, J. C., Eccles, R. M., and Shealy, C. N. An investigation into the effect of degenerating primary afferent fibers on the monosynaptic innervation of motoneurones. *J. Neurophysiol.* 25:544, 1962.
29. Esplin, D. W. Effects of diphenylhydantoin on synaptic transmission in cat spinal cord and stellate ganglion. *J. Pharmacol. Exp. Ther.* 120:301, 1957.
30. Fischer, J., Holubar, J., and Malik, V. A new method of producing chronic epileptogenic cortical foci in rats. *Physiol. Bohemoslov.* 16:272, 1967.
31. Gelfan, S., and Tarlow, I. M. Altered neuron population in L7 segment of dogs with experimental hind-limb rigidity. *Amer. J. Physiol.* 205:606, 1963.
32. Glaser, G. H. Sodium and seizures. *Epilepsia* (Amst.) 5:97, 1964.
33. Goldensohn, E. S., and Purpura, D. P. Intracellular potentials of cortical neurons

during focal epileptogenic discharges. *Science* 139:840, 1963.

34. Halpern, L. M., and Black, R. G. Flaxedil (gallamine triethiodide): Evidence for central action. *Science* 155:1685, 1967.

35. Henneman, E., Somjen, G., and Carpenter, D. O. Functional significance of cell size in spinal motoneurons. *J. Neurophysiol.* 28:560, 1965.

36. Holubar, J., and Fischer, J. Electrophysiological properties of the epileptogenic cortical foci produced by a new cobalt-gelatine method in rats. An attempt to correlate the electrophysiological, histological and histochemical data. *Physiol. Bohemoslov.* 16:278, 1967.

37. Kandel, E. R., and Spencer, W. A. Electrophysiology of hippocampal neurons. II. Afterpotentials and repetitive firing. *J. Neurophysiol.* 24:243, 1961.

38. King, R. B., and Barnett, J. C. Studies of trigeminal nerve potentials. Overreaction to tactile facial stimulation in acute laboratory preparations. *J. Neurosurg.* 14:617, 1957.

39. King, R. B., Meagher, J. N., and Barnett, J. C. Studies of trigeminal nerve potentials in normal compared with abnormal experimental preparations. *J. Neurosurg.* 13:176, 1956.

40. Kopeloff, L. M. Experimental epilepsy in the mouse. *Proc. Soc. Exp. Biol. Med.* 104:500, 1960.

41. Kopeloff, L. M., Barrera, S. E., and Kopeloff, N. Recurrent convulsive seizures in animals produced by immunologic and chemical means. *Amer. J. Psychiat.* 98:881, 1942.

42. Kopeloff, L. M., Chusid, J. C., and Kopeloff, N. Epilepsy in *Macaca mulatta* after cortical or intracerebral alumina. *A.M.A. Arch. Neurol. Psychiat.* 74:523, 1955.

43. Kostyuk, P. G. Functional Changes During Degeneration of Central Synapses. In Gutmann, E. (Ed.), *The Effects of Use and Disuse on Neuromuscular Function*. Amsterdam: Elsevier, 1963, p. 291.

44. Li, C-L. Mechanisms of fibrillation potentials in denervated mammalian skeletal muscle. *Science* 132:1889, 1960.

45. Liley, A. W., and North, K. A. K. An electrical investigation of effects of repetitive stimulation on mammalian neuromuscular junction. *J. Neurophysiol.* 16:509, 1953.

46. Lockard, J. S. Unpublished data, 1968.

47. Lockard, J. S., and Barensten, R. I. Behavioral experimental epilepsy in monkeys. I. Clinical seizure recording apparatus and initial data. *Electroenceph. Clin. Neurophysiol.* 22:482, 1967.

48. Loeser, J. D., and Ward, A. A., Jr. Some effects of deafferentation on neurons of the cat spinal cord. *Arch. Neurol.* (Chicago) 17:629, 1967.

49. Loeser, J. D., Ward, A. A., Jr., and White, L. E. Chronic deafferentation of human spinal cord neurons. *J. Neurosurg.* 29:48, 1968.

50. Matsumoto, H., and Ajmone-Marsan, C. Cellular mechanisms in experimental epileptic seizures. *Science* 144:193, 1964.

51. Meyers, R. The surgical treatment of focal epilepsy. An inquiry into current premises, their implementation and the criteria employed in reporting results. *Epilepsia* (Amst.) 3:9, 1954.

52. Morrell, F. Experimental focal epilepsy in animals. *A.M.A. Arch. Neurol. Psychiat.* 1:141, 1959.

53. Nakajima, S., and Takahashi, K. Post-tetanic hyperpolarization and electrogenic pump in stretch receptor neurone of crayfish. *J. Physiol.* (London) 187:105, 1966.

54. Nelson, P. G. Interaction between spinal motoneurons of the cat. *J. Neurophysiol.* 29:275, 1966.

55. Nims, L. F., Marshall, C., and Nielsen, A. Effect of local freezing on the electrical activity of the cerebral cortex. *Yale J. Biol. Med.* 13:477, 1941.

56. Openchowski, P. Sur l'action localisée du froid, appliqué à la surface de la région corticale du cerveau. *C. R. Soc. Biol.* (Paris) 5:38, 1883.

57. Pollen, D. A., and Lux, H. D. Intrinsic triggering mechanisms in focal paroxysmal discharges. *Epilepsia* (Amst.) 7:16, 1966.

58. Prince, D. A., and Futamachi, K. J. Intracellular recordings in chronic focal epilepsy. *Brain Res.* 11:681, 1968.

59. Purpura, D. P., McMurtry, J. G., Leonard, C. F., and Malliani, A. Evidence for dendritic origin of spikes without depolarizing prepotentials in hippocampal neurons during and after seizure. *J. Neurophysiol.* 29:954, 1966.

60. Purpura, D. P., Shofer, R. J., and Scarff, T. Properties of synaptic activities and spike

potentials of neurons in immature neocortex. *J. Neurophysiol.* 28:925, 1965.

61. Raines, A., and Standaert, F. G. Pre- and postjunctional effects of diphenylhydantoin at the cat soleus neuromuscular junction. *J. Pharmacol. Exper. Ther.* 153:361, 1966.

62. Rand, B. O., Kelly, W. A., and Ward, A. A., Jr. Electrophysiological studies of the action of intravenous diphenylhydantoin (Dilantin). *Neurology* (Minneap.) 16:1022, 1966.

63. Rand, B. O., and Ward, A. A., Jr. Unpublished data, 1966.

64. Rang, H. P., and Ritchie, J. M. On the electrogenic sodium pump in mammalian non-myelinated nerve fibers and its activation by various external cations. *J. Physiol.* (London) 196:183, 1968.

65. Rayport, M. The Jacksonian hypothesis: An appraisal in the light of single unit recording in focal epileptogenic grey matter of man. *Proc. Rudolf Virchow Med. Soc. N.Y.* Suppl. 26, 301, 1968.

66. Rayport, M., and Waller, H. J. Technique and results of micro-electrode recording in human epileptogenic foci. *Electroenceph. Clin. Neurophysiol.* Suppl. 25, 143, 1967.

67. Rosenberg, P., and Echlin, F. A. Cholinesterase activity of chronic partially isolated cortex. *Neurology* (Minneap.) 15:700, 1965.

68. Scheibel, M. E., and Scheibel, A. B. On the nature of dendritic spines—report of a workshop. *Communications in Behavioral Biol.* 1:231, 1968.

69. Schmidt, R. P., Thomas, L. B., and Ward, A. A., Jr. The hyperexcitable neuron: Microelectrode studies of chronic epileptic foci in monkey. *J. Neurophysiol.* 22:285, 1959.

70. Servit, Z. *Epilepsie. Grundlagen einer evolutionären Pathologie.* Berlin: Akademie, 1964.

71. Standaert, F. G. Post-tetanic repetitive activity in the cat soleus nerve. *J. Gen. Physiol.* 47:53, 1963.

72. Sypert, G. W., and Ward, A. A., Jr. The hyperexcitable neuron: Microelectrode studies of the chronic epileptic focus in the intact, awake monkey. *Exp. Neurol.* 19:104, 1967.

73. Takahashi, K., Kubota, K., and Uno, M. Recurrent facilitation in cat pyramidal tract. *J. Neurophysiol.* 30:22, 1967.

74. Teasdall, R. D., and Stavraky, G. W. Responses of deafferented spinal neurons to corticospinal impulses. *J. Neurophysiol.* 16:367, 1953.

75. Thesleff, S. Spontaneous Electrical Activity in Denervated Rat Skeletal Muscle. In Guttman, E., and Hnik, P. (Eds.), *The Effect of Use and Disuse on Neuromuscular Functions.* Amsterdam: Elsevier, 1963, p. 41.

76. Turnbull, I. M., Black, R. G., and Scott, J. W. Reflex efferent impulses in the trigeminal nerve. *J. Neurosurg.* 18:746, 1961.

77. Wall, P. D. The origin of a spinal cord slow potential. *J. Physiol.* (London) 164:508, 1962.

78. Ward, A. A., Jr. The epileptic spike. *Epilepsia* (Amst.) 1:600, 1960.

79. Ward, A. A., Jr. The epileptic neurone. *Epilepsia* (Amst.) 2:70, 1961.

80. Ward, A. A., Jr. Epilepsy. *Int. Rev. Neurobiol.* 3:137, 1961.

81. Ward, A. A., Jr. Autorhythmic Activity of Epileptic Neurons. In Servit, Z. (Ed.), *Comparative and Cellular Pathophysiology of Epilepsy.* Amsterdam: Excerpta Medica, 1966, p. 60.

82. Ward, A. A., Jr. The Seizure and Its Propagation. In Servit, Z. (Ed.), *Comparative and Cellular Pathophysiology of Epilepsy.* Amsterdam: Excerpta Medica, 1966, p. 171.

83. Ward, A. A., Jr., McCulloch, W. S., and Kopeloff, N. Temporal and spatial distribution of changes during spontaneous seizures in monkey brain. *J. Neurophysiol.* 11:377, 1948.

84. Ward, A. A., Jr., and Ojemann, G. A. Unpublished data, 1968.

85. Ward, A. A., Jr., and Schmidt, R. P. Some properties of single epileptic neurons. *Arch. Neurol.* (Chicago) 5:308, 1961.

86. Ware, F., Jr., Bennett, A. L., and McIntyre, A. R. Membrane resting potential of denervated mammalian skeletal muscle measured in vivo. *Amer. J. Physiol.* 177:115, 1954.

87. Washizu, Y., Bonewell, G. W., and Terzuolo, C. A. Effect of strychnine upon the

electrical activity of an isolated nerve cell. *Science* 133:333, 1961.

88. Westrum, L. E. Unpublished data, 1968.

89. Westrum, L. E., White, L. E., and Ward, A. A., Jr. Morphology of the experimental epileptic focus. *J. Neurosurg.* 21:1033, 1965.

90. Wiesendanger, M. Rigidity produced by deafferentation. *Acta Physiol. Scand.* 62:160, 1964.

91. Wilson, V. J., and Burgess, P. R. Intracellular study of recurrent facilitation. *Science* 134:337, 1961.

Discussion

EXPERIMENTAL SEIZURE MECHANISMS*

ELI S. GOLDENSOHN

In the previous part of this chapter, Ward's concept of the chronic epileptogenic focus as an aggregate of partially denervated cells has been extended. He suggests that a population of partially denervated neurons in the focus [37, 40, 41] may bring about excessive neuronal discharges in large part by antidromically stimulating axon terminals of relatively distant normal cell bodies. The concept is based both on his observations that intracellular potentials of neurons in the alumina focus show properties suggestive of axons [1, 34, 38] and on the pattern of firing of single neurons observed extracellularly [5]. The sequence of firing is characterized by longer latency between first and second discharges of the train than between second and subsequent discharges. The recording electrode is presumed to be on an axon which is antidromically activated within the focus. The relatively long interval is accounted for by the time elapsed between the antidromic firing and a subsequent orthodromic firing which is initiated in the distant healthy cell body by the antidromic impulse.

Ward raises a number of pertinent questions concerning the validity of this model. He reminds us that recent information on firing patterns supporting his hypothesis has been obtained so far from extracellular recordings and that the possible role of synaptic influences on both the first and subsequent spikes must still be explored. He also mentions that he has encountered other types of firing patterns. It will be important to analyze further and compare the discharge patterns obtained from the alumina focus with those from other experimental models, particularly because the interictal characteristics of neurons within an epileptogenic focus—whether the result of alumina, penicillin, or cold lesion—have many features in common.

FOCI, SPIKES, AND WAVES. In the chronic focus produced by alumina and in both acute and chronic foci produced by cortical freezing and penicillin, the essential electrocorticographic or electroencephalographic (EEG) abnormality in the interictal state is the intermittent appearance of focal spikes and sharp waves. Our intracellular recordings of the transmembranal shifts and firing patterns in the cold lesion with Purpura [11] established that EEG spikes and sharp waves are temporally related to depolarization and hyperpolarization occurring in neurons within the epileptogenic focus. Intracellular recordings by Matsumoto and Ajmone-Marsan in the acute penicillin focus [23] and recently by Prince and Futamachi in neurons in the chronic alumina focus [28] showed similar changes, each also indicating that spikes and sharp waves are reflections of membrane depolarization and hyperpolarization of neurons in the cortex.

The polarity of a focal EEG discharge appears to be the consequence of variations in magnitude of hyperpolarizing (inhibitory) and depolarizing (excitatory) synaptic potentials generated at different depths in the cortex by complex synaptic organizations. In the freezing lesion focus, in addition to acceleration of firing with depolarization (Fig. D10-1A) and inhibition of firing with hyperpolarization (Fig. D10-1B–E), sometimes there occur depolarizations of sufficient magnitude (paroxysmal depolarization shifts or PDSs) to result in soma-spike inactivation (Fig. D10-2A, B, C). Recording from the

---

* These studies supported by PHS Research Grants NB03359 and NB04613 from National Institute of Neurological Diseases and Stroke.

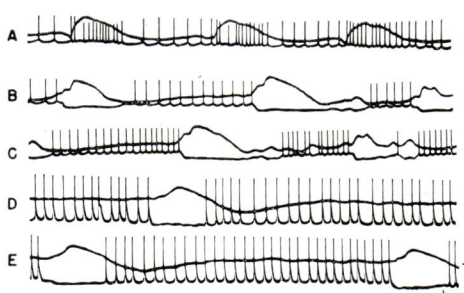
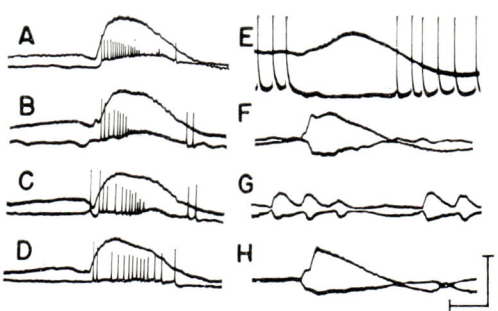

FIG. D10-1. Upper trace, monopolar recording of focal surface EEG discharge in an epileptogenic area following a small focal cortical freezing lesion involving motor cortex (negativity upward). Lower trace, intracellular recordings from three neurons impaled during a single penetration of the lesion site (negativity downward). (A) Neuron in the cortical depths exhibiting minimal depolarization and acceleration of firing during surface negativity. (B) and (C) Continuous recording from another cell approximately 50 μ above neuron shown in (A). Membrane hyperpolarization with inhibition of cell discharge is evident during all phases of EEG paroxysmal waves. (D) and (E) Continuous recording from cell superficial to that shown in (B) and (C). Inhibition of cell discharge occurs only during surface negativity of diphasic, low frequency EEG paroxysmal activity. Calibrations, horizontal bar, 0.1 sec, vertical bar, 50 μV for surface EEG trace and 50 mV for intracellular records. (From Goldensohn and Purpura [11].)

FIG. D10-2. (A) to (D) Examples of different characteristics of prolonged membrane depolarizations in the same cell during the course of continuous recording of EEG discharge shown in Fig. D10-1A. (E) through (H) Relationship of hyperpolarizations to membrane potential level in another cell. (E) Cell in condition similar to that shown in Fig. D10-1D. (F) Several seconds after loss of spike-generating mechanism subsequent to progressive deterioration. Cell depolarized 30 mV below level shown in (E). Despite severe depolarization, prominent repolarizing potentials are generated during focal EEG activity. Note in (G) and (H) the close correlation between characteristics of EEG discharge and membrane potential changes. Calibrations, same as in Fig. D10-1. (From Goldensohn and Purpura [11].)

same cell at another time (Fig. D10-2D) may show milder depolarizations sufficient only to increase the firing rate but not great enough to result in a PDS with depolarization inactivation. That these influences are synaptic is strongly supported by the fact that deteriorating cells (Fig. D10-2F, G, H) which have become depolarized to the level of spike inactivation exhibit augmented repolarizing potentials. In these neurons repolarizations during EEG spikes are augmented and exhibit a relationship to membrane potential expected for inhibitory postsynaptic potentials [6, 15]. The similarity of depolarizing and hyperpolarizing membranal shifts in firing patterns which occur in interictal discharges of alumina, freezing, and penicillin lesions suggests that a common mechanism for generation of interictal discharges in chronic focal lesions may be present. The theory of an aggregate of partially denervated neurons applies equally well to all three types. Alternative hypotheses include conductance change without alteration in resting potential and changes in the release of, or responsivity to, transmitter substances.

With Escueta [7] we have attempted to assess the role of inhibitory and excitatory synaptic influences in generating surface paroxysmal activity in the cold lesion focus, including observations on the interaction of local seizure discharges with thalamically evoked activity and the roles played by PDSs, EPSP-induced spikes, spikes without prepotentials, and spikes showing properties similar to potentials from axons.

Intracellular potentials were recorded from 57 units in the cold lesion focus in the cat during intermittent epileptogenic slow-wave, sharp-wave, and spike discharges which usually recurred about once per second. Cortical epileptogenic lesions were produced in the anterior and posterior sigmoid gyri by gently touching the pial surface for 45 sec with a tip of a 3-mm-diameter metal rod attached to a chamber containing dry ice. Focal discharges from the freezing lesion usually appeared within an hour. The site chosen as the "focus" [33] had the largest amplitude and earliest discharge and was found not more than 6 mm away from the lesion. The discharges are referred to as spikes, sharp waves, or slow waves, according to the recommendations of the terminology committee of the International Federation for EEG and Clinical Neurophysiology [2]. Intracellular recording was done with glass micropipettes with tip diameters of 0.5 to 1.5 μ filled with 2.7 molar potassium citrate. Recordings considered suitable for analysis had stable membrane potentials of at least 40 mV.

Neuronal firing patterns and transmembranal potential levels showed clear correlations with intermittent EEG sharp waves, slow waves, and spike discharges in 55 of 57 cells. EEG discharges at the focus showed an initial negative deflection in nearly all cases. In 37 of the 55 cells the major intracellular changes were membrane depolarization and increased firing rate during the surface negative phase of the EEG; this was followed in 28 of the 37 cells by membrane hyperpolarization and decrease or absence of firing during an ensuing surface positive phase of the EEG deflection. In 18 of the 55 cells, hyperpolarization and inhibition of firing were the main accompaniments of the initial surface negative phase. In an additional 16 cells, impaled 8 mm or more from the focus, the sequences of membrane shifts were similar, but the surface negative phase was more often associated with hyperpolarization and decreased firing of the cell. Out of a total of 71 cells (55 at the focus and 16 at 8 mm or more away) PDSs were seen in only 10 cells. PDSs in the freezing focus were more frequent, however, when seizure discharges became continuous (Fig. D10-8).

In nearly all cells in the freezing focus, whether the major membrane shifts were depolarizing or hyperpolarizing, minor shifts of opposite polarity were also present, demonstrating that most cells involved in the spike focus were subjected to both excitatory and inhibitory influences during a single paroxysmal discharge. Usually a sequence of rather small changes, including both depolarization and hyperpolarization phases, accompanied each EEG epileptiform discharge (Fig. D10-3A, B), and, as can be seen in Fig. D10-3C, even the injection of

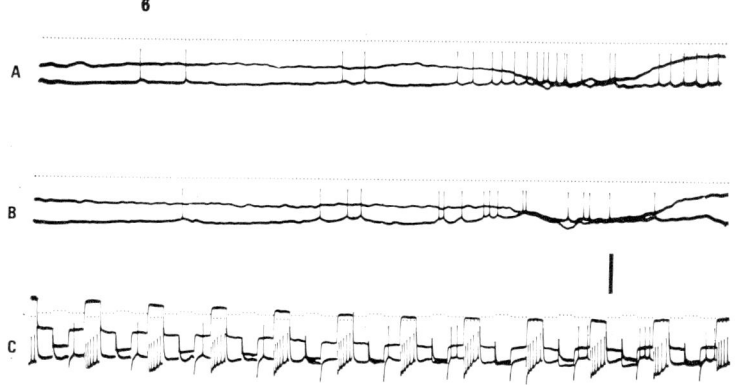

Fig. D10-3. (A) and (B) Upper traces (negative upward). Lower traces, intracellular recording (negative downward) EEG spike is associated with complex firing patterns and depolarization and hyperpolarization shifts of the impaled cell at the cold lesion focus. (C) Addition of injected hyperpolarizing and depolarizing currents (hyperpolarizing causes upward, depolarizing downward shifts of 10 msec time line) results in modification of firing patterns of cells, but the added depolarization influence does not activate PDS. Calibration bar: 50 mV for intracellular trace, and 100 μV for cortical activity. Time marker, 10 msec.

depolarizing current sufficient to increase the firing rate did not usually precipitate PDSs. It appears that in association with the interictal surface EEG spike or sharp wave the effect on most cells penetrated was toward grouping of the discharges into faster and slower sequences with the overall effect being an increase in the number. This effect on cell firing also appears to be the case in chronic alumina foci (Fig. D10-4, C1, 2, 3). In the acute penicillin focus, however, large PDSs are the most common pattern of the neurons involved [23]. PDSs do occur in interictal discharges from freezing lesions and from the chronic alumina focus, but they are seen far less often. As compared with the penicillin focus, there appears to be less synchronized excitatory synaptic bombardment in the relatively indolent freezing and alumina foci and perhaps also in the interictal discharges of the chronic cobalt lesion [5, 16, 26].

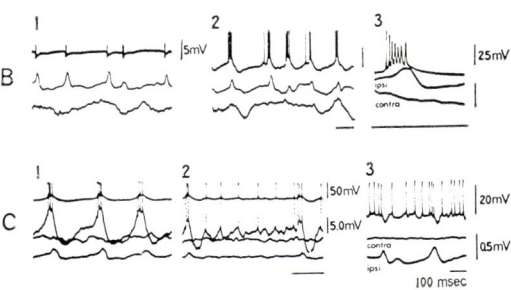

Fig. D10-4. Recordings from neurons of chronic alumina foci during interictal discharges. (B1, 2) Extracellular and intracellular records from the same neuron. (B3) Burst from another cell at a faster sweep. (C1, 2) Intracellular activities from a cell during rhythmic focal discharge (C1) and during a period of sporadic, low voltage surface waves (C2). (C3) Activities from a cell which generates IPSPs during each surface epileptiform event. Ipsi: Cortical surface activities at site of microelectrode penetration. Contra: Cortical activity from the homotopic point in opposite hemisphere. In (C1, 2) top trace, dc microelectrode recording; second trace, high-gain rc coupled recording with tops of spikes cut off. Calibrations: Lower vertical bar in (B3) for all surface traces. Vertical bars in (C2) for (C1) and (C2). Horizontal bars: 100 msec. Spikes in (B1, 2) retouched for clarity. (From Prince and Futamachi [28].)

When PDSs in the penicillin focus were first described [23], it was felt that paroxysmal depolarization shifts in the penicillin focus possibly were related to intrinsic changes in the neural membrane characteristic of the epileptic neuron. Although it is generally agreed that depolarization shifts are characteristic of epileptic activity, they are, as can be seen from our results, not a necessary concomitant of the interictal focus. Matsumoto [22] on the basis of further studies gave evidence that PDSs were graded responses which result from synaptic drive. Our data in the epileptogenic focus (Fig. D10-2A, B, C, D) also demonstrate the graded nature of the PDS. It is unlikely that the depolarization shift is related to chronic intrinsic changes in nerve membrane because we have seen the phenomenon to be readily reversible in nonepileptic cortex during spreading depression [13]. The major difference in behavior between the chronic and more indolent foci as compared to the acute penicillin focus appears to be quantitative rather than qualitative. Intermittent shifts toward depolarization characterize the neurons in the chronic as well as the acute epileptogenic focus.

Intensity of polarization shifts correlates with the magnitude and form of the surface paroxysmal events in freezing lesions. Slow waves are associated with the slowest and lowest amplitude intracellular shifts while sustained spikes and sharp waves have the most rapid and highest voltage polarization shifts. This is in accord with the finding of various sizes of ESPSs in thalamic neurons during periods of intensive synaptic drive by reticular activation [30]. Although a negative standing steady potential has been reported at the chronic focus [20], depolarization at the freezing-spike focus does not appear to last for more than 30 minutes after the lesion is produced [29].

THALAMIC STIMULATION. Because of the difficulty he encountered in influencing the firing pattern of neurons in the epileptic focus by thalamic stimulation, Ward raised the question of "busy line" by asking whether the same cortical neurons are involved in the epileptic process as those involved in evoked activity. We confirmed the difficulty to effect the firing pattern of the epileptic cells by thalamic stimulation, but our recordings from both the cat and man demonstrated that most single neurons studied were involved in both the epileptic focal discharge and in the evoked responses. The interaction between an interictal spike and a recruiting response in the cat is shown in Fig. D10-5. Both affect the neuron separately but when both effects act together the paroxysmal influence is clearly prepotent over the thalamic influence. This marked preponderance of paroxysmal activity over the thalamic- and surface-evoked responses was seen in every cell studied. The preponderance is also seen in the EEG record where recruiting waves are suppressed during sharp-wave discharge. A similar phenomenon involving interaction between the superficial cortical response (SCR) and seizure discharges in man is shown in Fig. D10-6. The data suggest that interaction among neurons in the interictal epileptogenic region utilizes the inherently complex synaptic organization which underlies the normal function of cortical neurons.

SPREADING DEPRESSION. The role of spreading depression (SD) in chronic seizure disorders in man is unknown, but SD profoundly influences experimentally produced seizure discharges. In a personal communication cited in Marshall's comprehensive review of SD [21], Leão, who originally described the phenomenon, remarked on the similarity of the velocity of the propagation of the Jacksonian march in clinical seizures to that of spreading depression. Pathological phenomena other than seizures including movement of scotomas across the visual field in migraine, also have a time course similar to SD [24]. In SD, the slowly moving depression of cortical activity travels across the surface of the brain at the rate of 2–3 mm per min and lasts about 3 minutes, at a given point on the cortex, before it moves on. The depression is associated with a sequence of slow variations in potential at the cortical surface measured in millivolts [19]. The main slow potential variation is negative, and the association of a negative slow potential change with depression of cortical activity is the most consistent part of the sequence.

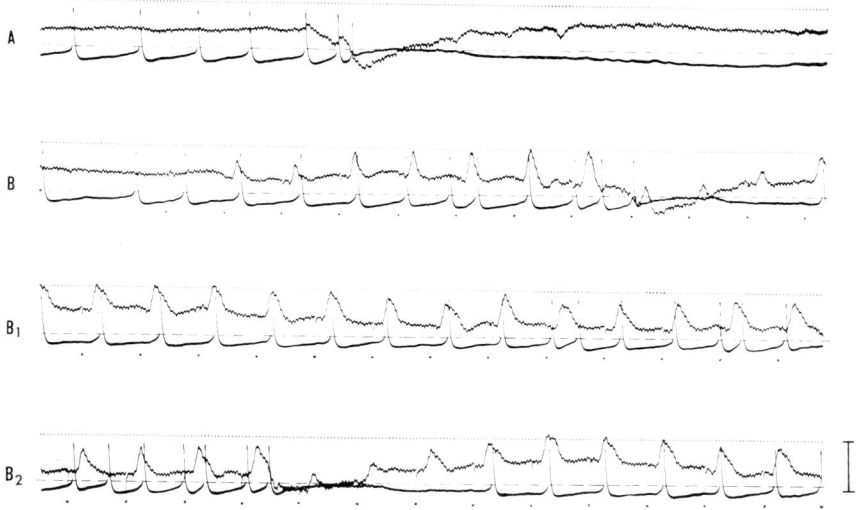

FIG. D10-5. Interaction of interictal cortical spike and recruiting response in cold lesion focus in cat. Upper traces, cortical activity; lower traces, intracellular recording. Dashed line is firing level of cell. Dots below indicate midline thalamic stimulation. (A) EEG spike associated with intracellular firing and membrane shift. (B) Interaction of recruiting response with cortical spike. Recruiting responses depressed. Effect on intracellular firing sequence related to EEG spike is essentially unchanged by thalamic stimulation. (B_1) shows thalamic stimulation modulating firing pattern. Calibration bar: 50 mV intracellular and 80 μV EEG. Time marker, 10 msec.

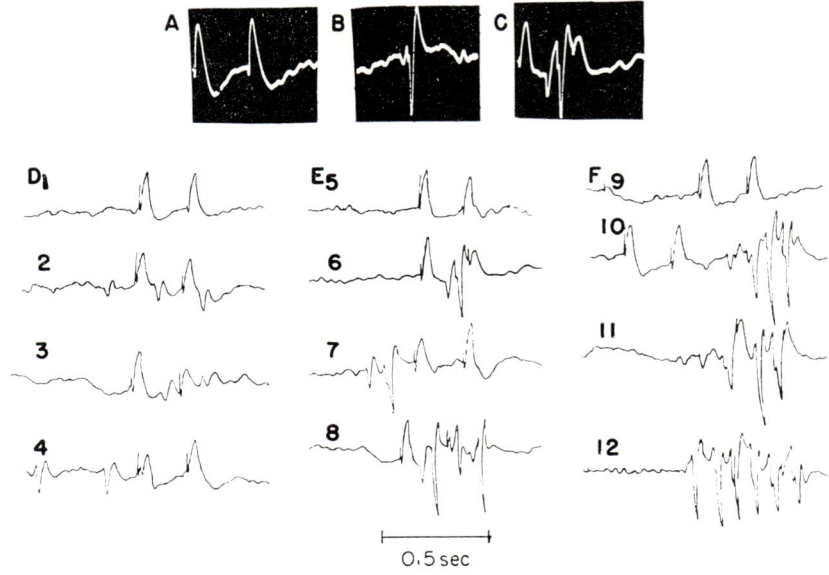

Fig. D10-6. Interaction of cortical discharges with superficial cortical responses in patient with epilepsy. (A) Pair of SCRs. (B) Interictal cortical spike. (C) Interaction of interictal spike with second pair of SCRs. Traces 1 through 12 show a variety of interactions between interictal spikes and pairs of SCRs which are often obliterated by paroxysmal discharges. Negative, up.

Graftstein [14] described paroxysmal discharges which occur as the slow potential wave front approaches. A number of other investigators including Bures, Leão, and O'Leary have called attention to the appearance of EEG paroxysmal activity as part of the SD, and spreading excitation can also be considered a characteristic part of the phenomenon.

In our studies on the ontogenesis of SD and focal-spike discharges in cats [12], it was found that spreading depression rarely occurs before the cat is 4 weeks old and that the capacity to generate regularly recurrent focal spikes over prolonged periods from a circumscribed freezing lesion does not appear until after the twelfth week of life. Of 8 animals, 6 developed SD between 4 and 8 weeks of age, and all animals after 8 weeks. Sustained regular spiking from freezing lesions failed to occur in 19 of 20 animals under 8 weeks old but occur regularly after the twelfth week. Both phenomena occur long after most other electrophysiological phenomena studied are fully developed. Superficial cortical responses, primary responses, and recruiting are all well developed by the fourteenth day. The conduction rate in axons and pyramidal neurons, however, increases markedly during the fifth week of life at about the same time that spreading depression makes its appearance. During roughly the same period, glial activity in the cortex is at its peak.

Morlock, Mori, and Ward [25] using extracellular recording postulated that spreading depression was accompanied by depolarization of nerve-cell membranes. Collewijn and Van Harreveld [4] with intracellular recording showed in the rabbit that the cell indeed was depolarized during spreading depression. We demonstrated this phenomenon independently in neurons of the cat [8], and Karahashi and Goldring [18] showed similar depolarization in so-called *idle* cells, which never showed action potentials. In a recent study with Walsh, which has appeared in preliminary form [13], adult cats were examined for changes in the behavior of single cells influenced by spreading depression and focal-seizure discharges.

Intracellular and extracellular potential changes during spreading depression are

TABLE D10-1. Potential Changes Measured with Microelectrodes during Spreading Depression

Conditions	Large Extracellular 1–20 mV N = 25	Intracellular RP 42–75 mV N = 13
Major dc shift		
Duration	52 sec	91 sec
Polarity	Negative	Positive
Amplitude	−24 mV	+23 mV
Increased firing at initiation of dc shift	21 (N = 25)	7 (N = 11)
Decrease in amplitude of spike during major shift	25 (N = 25)	12 (N = 12)
Average resting potential		61.5
Amplitude of spikes	6.1 mV (1–20 mV)	38 mV (33–55 mV)

given in Table D10-1. During SDs, 25 extracellular recordings were obtained. The SDs observed with extracellular electrodes had an average maximal shift of 24 mV with an average duration of 52 sec. In 8 of the 24 SDs, the negative shift was preceded by a positive shift (average 3.8 mV) lasting 29 sec. In 15 of 25 instances the negative wave was followed by a second positive shift (average 4.5 mV) lasting 76 sec. Extracellularly recorded single unit discharges gradually decreased in amplitude and increased in duration before firing stopped. In nearly all cases an increase in rate of firing occurred during the early negative phase. Diphasic unit discharges showed decreased size of both the positive and negative phases proportionately until the cell ceased firing as in the previous study by Morlock, Mori, and Ward [25]. Intracellular recordings were maintained for average duration of 34 min. With intracellular recordings the average depolarization was 23 mV with an average duration of 91 sec. In 7 of the 13 SDs recorded, a negative shift (average 7.1 mV) with an average duration of 16 sec preceded the major positive shift. In 2 cases negative shifts followed the positive shift.

In control periods, neural noise was seen [9] consisting of 100 to 200 μV potentials lasting 1–20 msec each. Spreading depression depressed and eliminated neural noise, which returned as the cell repolarized (Fig. D10-7). With intracellular recording during SD the duration of the spike potentials increased, sometimes by as much as 4 msec (Fig. D10-7).

Spreading depression causes the recruiting EEG negative wave to go through a sequence of depression, inversion, and elimination (Fig. D10-7), while the underlying

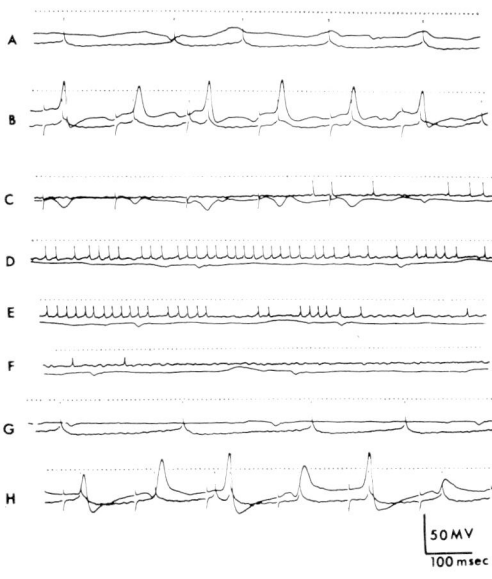

FIG. D10-7. Segments from a complete spreading depression. Upper traces, EEG (negative upward). Lower traces, intracellular (negative downward). (A) Resting. (B) Recruiting response before SD. (C) Reversal of recruiting wave with reduction in amplitude of membrane potential and action potential. (D) through (F) Further depolarization leading to loss of action potential. (G) and (H) Recovery.

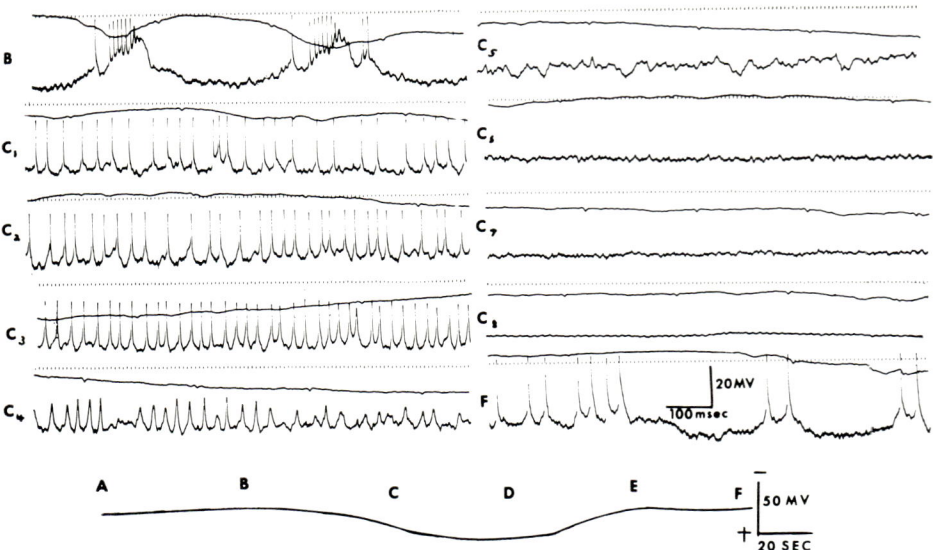

Fig. D10-8. Across bottom, (A) through (F) is continuous dc recording of SD from surface of anterior sigmoid gyrus. Above are epochs from (B) and (C) portion of SD. (B) Upper trace, EEG; lower trace, intracellular record using ac recording to show PDS before SD arrives. (C_1) through (C_8) Developing SD with elimination of PDSs and progressive increase in firing rate until complete absence of surface and intracellular activity. (F) Recovery.

single cell undergoes a sequence of progressive depolarization associated with diminished amplitude of action potential and increased rate of firing, until the point of depolarization inactivation.

The effect of spreading depression on PDSs occurring in the epileptogenic freezing lesion is seen in Fig. D10-8. The depolarization shift is eliminated as spreading depression invades the cell, but the firing rate increases early in the depolarization phase. No evidence of recurrent previous EEG spikes is noted while the cell action potentials gradually decrease in amplitude and increase in duration with suggestive AB breaks. Under these circumstances, previously sustained focal spiking can be suppressed for as long as 6 minutes.

Inasmuch as the extracellular shifts average 24 mV negative and the intracellular shifts average 23 mV positive at the height of the SD (see Table D10-1), the effective potential across the membrane is practically zero. At such times no evidence of membrane function can be seen as even neural noise is completely absent (Fig. D10-8, C_8). Although gradual decrease in amplitude and increase in duration of spikes was seen in almost all recordings in association with AB breaklike configurations, this finding must be confirmed using antidromic stimulation. Preservation of the firing capacity during early depolarization with decreasing amplitude and longer duration of discharges also suggests that the apical dendrites and soma may be depolarized before the initial segment. The complete loss of the PDS and epileptic firing pattern early in the SD (Fig. D10-8C) while rapid firing is still occurring also suggests that the PDSs and firing patterns are synaptically generated.

CONCLUSION. There appears to be a hierarchy among epileptogenic agents relating to the time of the appearance of focal seizures and the intensity of focal seizure discharges. Strychnine and penicillin cause very acute and powerful paroxysmal activity. Activity from alumina, freezing, and cobalt lesions somewhat more closely resembles the characteristics seen in human chronic, focal-seizure disorders. However, examination of intracellular events seems to indicate that, in spite of the difference in degrees of epileptogenicity, similar synaptic mechanisms are involved in both acute and chronic foci. Regardless of the intensity of epileptogenic discharge in any cell so far impaled, the epileptic process always overcomes physiologic or simulated physiologic influences. One cerebral mechanism which can initiate seizure discharges and abolish focal paroxysmal activity for periods of minutes is the spreading depression of Leão. Although much is known about the characteristics of neurons involved in an epileptic discharge, a unique characteristic is yet to be defined that differentiates the "epileptic neuron" from the other neurons involved in the area of the focus.

REFERENCES

1. Atkinson, J. R., and Ward, A. A., Jr. Intracellular studies of cortical neurons in chronic epileptogenic foci in the monkey. *Exp. Neurol.* 10:285, 1964.
2. Brazier, M. A. B., Cobb, W. A., Fischgold, H., Gastaut, H., Gloor, P., Hess, R., Jasper, H. H., Loeb, W., Magnus, O., Pampiglione, G., Remond, A., Storm van Leeuwen, W., and Walter, W. Grey. Proposal for an EEG terminology by the terminology committee of the International Federation for Electroencephalography and Clinical Neurophysiology. *Electroenceph. Clin. Neurophysiol.* 13:646, 1961.
3. Calvin, W. H., Sypert, G. W., and Ward, A. A., Jr. Structured timing patterns within bursts from epileptic neurons in undrugged monkey cortex. *Exp. Neurol.* 21:535, 1968.
4. Collewijn, H., and Van Harreveld, A. Membrane potential of cerebral cortical cells during spreading depression and asphyxia. *Exp. Neurol.* 15:425, 1966.
5. Dow, R. S., Fernandez-Guardiola, A., and Manni, E. The production of cobalt experimental epilepsy in the rat. *Electroenceph. Clin. Neurophysiol.* 14:399, 1962.
6. Eccles, J. C. The mechanism of synaptic transmission. *Ergebn. Physiol.* 51:299, 1961.
7. Escueta, A. V., and Goldensohn, E. S. Original and mirror foci in the epileptogenic focus of the frozen cortical lesion: Intracellular recordings, 1969. In preparation.
8. Goldensohn, E., Escueta, A., and Runk, L. Unit membrane shifts and firing patterns during spreading depression. *Electroenceph. Clin. Neurophysiol.* 23:84, 1967.
9. Goldensohn, E. S., and McLain, L. W. Extracellular field of low amplitude neural activity in cat cortex. *Electroenceph. Clin. Neurophysiol.* In press, 1969.
10. Goldensohn, E. S., Perez, M., and Feierman, J. Intracellular potentials and unit discharge patterns in primary and mirror epileptogenic foci. *Electroenceph. Clin. Neurophysiol.* 18:513, 1965.
11. Goldensohn, E. S., and Purpura, D. P. Intracellular potentials of cortical neurons during focal epileptogenic discharges. *Science* 139:840, 1963.
12. Goldensohn, E. S., Shofer, R., and Purpura, D. P. Ontogenesis of focal discharges in epileptogenic lesions of cat neocortex. *Electroenceph. Clin. Neurophysiol.* 15:153, 1963.
13. Goldensohn, E. S., and Walsh, G. Sequential changes in single cortical neurons during spreading depression. *Electroenceph. Clin. Neurophysiol.* 24:290, 1968.
14. Graftstein, B. Neuronal Release of Potassium during Spreading Depression. In Brazier, M. A. B. (Ed.), *Brain Function.* UCLA Forum in Medical Sciences, No. 1. Berkeley: University of California Press, 1963, pp. 87–122.
15. Grundfest, H. Synaptic and Ephaptic Transmission. In Field, J. (Ed.), *Handbook of Physiology, Neurophysiology,* vol. 1. Washington, D.C.: American Physiological Society, 1959, p. 147.
16. Henjyoji, E. Y., and Dow, R. S. Cobalt-induced seizures in the cat. *Electroenceph. Clin. Neurophysiol.* 19:152, 1965.
17. Kandel, E. R., and Spencer, W. A. Excitation and inhibition of single pyramidal cells during hippocampal seizure. *Exp. Neurol.* 4:162, 1961.
18. Karahashi, Y., and Goldring, S. Intracellular potentials from "idle" cells in cerebral cortex of cat. *Electroenceph. Clin. Neurophysiol.* 20:600, 1966.

19. Leão, A. A. P. The slow voltage variation of cortical spreading depression of activity. *Electroenceph. Clin. Neurophysiol.* 4:315, 1951.
20. Mahnke, J. H., and Ward, A. A., Jr. Standing potential characteristics of the epileptogenic focus. *Epilepsia* (Amst.) 2:161, 1961.
21. Marshall, W. H. Spreading cortical depression of Leão. *Physiol. Rev.* 39:239, 1959.
22. Matsumoto, H. Intracellular events during the activation of cortical epileptiform discharges. *Electroenceph. Clin. Neurophysiol.* 17:294, 1964.
23. Matsumoto, H., and Ajmone-Marsan, C. Cortical cellular phenomena in experimental epilepsy: "Inter-ictal" manifestation. *Exp. Neurol.* 9:286, 1964a.
24. Milner, P. M. A possible correspondence between the scotomas of migraine and spreading depression of Leão. *Electroenceph. Clin. Neurophysiol.* 10:705, 1958.
25. Morlock, N. L., Mori, K., and Ward, A. A., Jr. A study of single cortical neurons during spreading depression. *J. Neurophysiol.* 27:1192, 1964.
26. Mutani, R. Cobalt experimental hippocampal epilepsy in the cat. *Epilepsia* (Amst.) (Fourth Series) 8:223, 1967.
27. O'Leary, J. L., and Goldring, S. Slow cortical potentials—their origin and contribution to seizure discharge. *Epilepsia* (Amst.) 1:561, 1960.
28. Prince, D. A., and Futamachi, K. J. Intracellular recordings in chronic focal epilepsy. *Brain Res.* 11:681, 1968.
29. Purpura, D. P., Goldensohn, E. S., and Musgrave, F. S. Synaptic and non-synaptic processes in focal epileptogenic activity. *Electroenceph. Clin. Neurophysiol.* 15:1050, 1963.
30. Purpura, D. P., and Shofer, R. J. Intracellular recording from thalamic neurons during reticulocortical activation. *J. Neurophysiol.* 26:494, 1963.
31. Sano, K., Miyake, H., and Mayanagi, Y. Steady Potentials in Various Stress Conditions in Man. In Widen, L. (Ed.), *Recent Advances in Clinical Neurophysiology.* Amsterdam: Elsevier, 1967, p. 264.
32. Schadé, J. P. Maturational aspects of EEG and of spreading depression in rabbit. *J. Neurophysiol.* 22:245, 1959.
33. Smith, T. G., Jr., and Purpura, D. P. Electrophysiological studies on epileptogenic lesions of cat cortex. *Electroenceph. Clin. Neurophysiol.* 12:59, 1960.
34. Sypert, G. W., and Ward, A. A., Jr. The hyper-excitable neuron: Microelectrode studies of the chronic epileptic focus in the intact awake monkey. *Exp. Neurol.* 19:104, 1967.
35. Vanasupa, P., Goldring, S., and O'Leary, J. L. Seizure discharges effected by intravenously administered convulsant drugs. *Electroenceph. Clin. Neurophysiol.* 11:93, 1959.
36. Van Harreveld, A. Changes in diameter of apical dendrites during spreading depression. *Amer. J. Physiol.* 192:457, 1958.
37. Ward, A. A., Jr. The epileptic neurone. *Epilepsia* (Amst.) 2:70, 1961.
38. Ward, A. A., Jr. Autorhythmic Activity of Epileptic Neurons. In Servit, Z. (Ed.), *Comparative and Cellular Pathophysiology of Epilepsy.* Amsterdam: Excerpta Medica, 1966, p. 60.
39. Ward, A. A., Jr. The Hyper-Excitable Neuron—Epilepsy. In Rodahl, K., and Issekutz, B., Jr. (Eds.), *Nerve as a Tissue.* New York: Hoeber, 1966, p. 379.
40. Ward, A. A., Jr., and Schmidt, R. P. Some properties of single epileptic neurons. *Arch. Neurol.* (Chicago) 5:308, 1961.
41. Westrum, L. E., White, L. E., and Ward, A. A., Jr. Morphology of the experimental epileptic focus. *J. Neurosurg.* 21:1033, 1964.
42. Wilson, S., and Schmidt, R. Steady potential, the direct cortical response and the epileptic focus. *Electroenceph. Clin. Neurophysiol.* 17:579, 1964.

11
Acute Effects of Topical Epileptogenic Agents

COSIMO AJMONE-MARSAN

IN THE EXPERIMENTAL APPROACH to the study of focal epileptogenic lesions there are at our disposal a large number of agents, both physical and, in particular, chemical, which when topically applied possess the property of inducing characteristic alterations in the activity of the neuronal aggregates at the site of the application [see recent reviews in 6–9, 74].

Many chemical epileptogenic agents manifest their action within a few minutes after topical application; certain physical agents, such as repetitive electrical stimulation, display their epileptogenic properties immediately and in a reversible way. It is thus possible to study resulting electrographic manifestations in the acute experiment; their description, analysis, and tentative interpretation form the subject of this presentation.

The gap between such an experimental situation and the focal form of human epilepsy—a clinical entity characterized by exquisitely chronic features—is only apparent (see also [5]). In an investigation of the development of pathological changes and related electrical phenomena in the epileptogenic lesion (and its concomitant motor manifestations), other experimental approaches should be designed [144], and, for instance, the use of alumina cream [85, 146] or metal-pellets implantation [43, 58, 70, 115, 116] would be more appropriate. Once an epileptic process has become established, its sporadic electrical manifestations, at least in their main qualitative aspects, appear to be rather stereotyped, and there is no convincing evidence for the existence of important differences in their underlying basic mechanisms that might be related to its type of development [127]. Thus it should be obvious that use of local epileptogenic agents and analysis of their acute effects offer the great advantage of convenience of a relatively simple experimental design. The latter is more susceptible to control and to various manipulations than are other approaches (even though these might seem to reproduce more faithfully the clinical situation), and the findings one can derive from it should be of relatively easier and more reliable interpretation.

For the description and analysis of such findings, it is convenient to use those obtainable with typical epileptogenic agents, such as strychnine or penicillin, since with these two drugs we probably possess the largest amount of pertinent information.

In dealing with epilepsy it is important to maintain a conceptual distinction between the static state, or latent condition that can be vaguely defined as tendency or susceptibility to seizures on the one hand, and the seizures themselves which are the episodic, open manifestations on the other. In both human and experimental situations, the former condition is clinically silent, and its existence can be determined only by the occurrence of certain relatively brief changes in the electrical activity of the neuronal aggregates that are involved in the epileptic process. These changes (Fig. 11-1) have been termed *interictal* while those of longer duration and generally associated with peripheral epileptic mani-

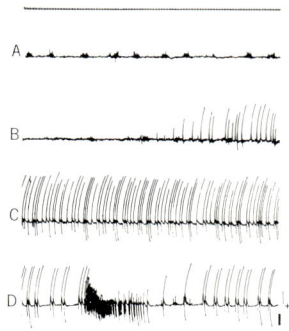

Fig. 11-1. Development of epileptiform activity in a penicillin focus. Gross electrode, surface recording from sigmoid gyrus of cat (light barbiturate anesthesia). (*A*) Before application of the drug. (*B*) A few minutes after application of penicillin (100,000 units per milliliter). (*C*) About 30 min later. (*D*) About 2 hours later. Note interictal changes in (*B*), (*C*), (*D*) and spontaneous ictal episode in (*D*). Calibrations: 1 sec (top line) and 1 mV. (From [112], unpublished.)

rowed from EEG nomenclature. Presence of these discharges is a convenient and technically easy way to demonstrate epileptogenic involvement of a neuronal population. Activity of individual elements in such a population undergoes typical and rather stereotyped changes [67, 105, 112, 120] characterized by (a) episodic nature, relatively brief duration, and full reversibility; (b) random recurrence in the absence of obvious causal factors; but also (c) great susceptibility to be triggered by a variety of stimuli; and (d) quasi-simultaneous involvement of most neuronal elements within the affected population.

The changes themselves reflect transitory alteration of membrane activity in otherwise normally behaving neurons. Specifically to be observed are recurrent paroxysmal shifts of depolarization (PDSs) much larger and of longer duration than normal EPSPs (Figs. 11-2, 11-3, 11-4). Such shifts in membrane festations are referred to as *ictal* [2, 131]. In practice, the two phenomena may often overlap or share some features, particularly in the transition from one to the other. Actually, they may occasionally lose or even reverse their characteristic relationship to peripheral manifestations, so that we have ictal episodes which remain clinically silent and the interictal which are accompanied by obvious motor effects. In principle, however, this is a valid distinction, particularly useful in the description and analysis of the two main types of electrical phenomena characteristic of the epileptic condition.

INTERICTAL PHASE

Acute electrographic effects of strychnine, following topical application over an area of the cortical surface have been repeatedly investigated since the pioneer work initiated more than thirty years ago [1, 15, 25, 62, 71, 81, 99]. As a rule, these effects are limited to changes of the interictal type. When monitored with gross electrodes, the changes consist of the well-known sporadic discharges labeled as *spikes*, a widely used but somewhat inappropriate term, bor-

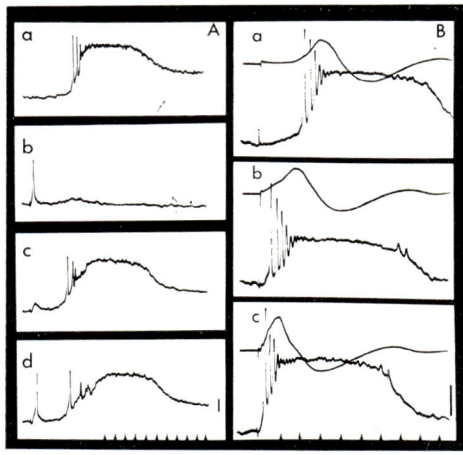

Fig. 11-2. Paroxysmal depolarization shifts (PDSs) induced by penicillin in two different neurons of the anterior (*A*) and posterior (*B*) sigmoid gyrus in cat. In (*B*) the upper tracing is from the corresponding surface activity. PDS occurs spontaneously (*Aa*) or is triggered by a brief electrical pulse applied locally to cortical surface. In (*Ab, c, d*) the same stimulation parameters, at barely above the threshold for elicitation of an EPSP, are used. In (*B*) stimulus strength is increased from (*a*) to (*c*). See also Fig. 11-3. Calibrations: 10 msec and 10 mV. (Modified from [111].)

potential, inasmuch as they quickly exceed the critical firing level, are accompanied by clusters of multiple spikes at a frequency grossly proportional to the level of depolarization and lasting until inactivating (cathodal block) phenomena intervene when the polarization has remained for some time at an excessively low level. The latter is a most common situation so that early and pronounced inactivation of action potentials actually becomes one of the characteristic features in the intracellular records of epileptic neurons (Figs. 11-2, 11-3). Other phenomena, either less constant and characteristic or requiring specific tests for demonstration, will be mentioned subsequently in connection with analysis of the nature and underlying mechanisms of PDS.

The paroxysmal depolarization shift (in close parallelism with surface discharges shown in Fig. 11-1) reaches full development within a few minutes after application of the epileptogenic agent, then keeps recurring for several hours with rather similar features. Such a pattern of neuronal activity, an obviously abnormal form of behavior of the membrane of elements involved in the epileptogenic process, may result from basic mechanisms of different nature. Specifically it might (a) reflect an intrinsic alteration of properties of the membrane itself, or (b) result from an alteration of synaptic mechanisms, or (c) be the expression of extrasynaptic (ephaptic) influences.

Some form of direct membrane involvement cannot be ruled out, but would not seem to be the exclusive or even primary factor. Data derived from different neuronal elements [51, 56, 76, 102, 107, 112, 120, 121, 126, 136] failed to demonstrate any consistent alteration of the membrane resting potential (and of its resistance and time constant) by the epileptogenic agent. The impulse-generating mechanism is similarly unaffected: EPSPs and action potentials, indistinguishable from those of normal neurons, can be observed in the paroxysmal-free intervals (Figs. 11-2, 11-3, 11-4). Such spikes, occurring either "spontaneously" or when induced by orthodromic or antidromic stimulation or by depolarizing currents, do not display any obviously abnormal feature: their amplitude and duration as well as their ability to display A and B breaks remain unaffected even when the spikes alternate, in very close temporal relationship, with the PDS.

The spike-firing threshold does not appear to be significantly altered. Indeed, in neurons involved in the epileptic process in the neocortex of adult animals, there are only a few reported examples [126] of rare spikes arising from slightly higher polarizing levels or without a slow prepotential, or both, or of diphasic negative-positive spikes coexisting with action potentials of normal amplitude and configuration. In spite of the fact that similar properties in other experimental situations (and in different elements) have been interpreted as indicative of a spike origin at some distance from the soma [130], it would appear premature to conclude from their sporadic occurrence, that the dendritic spike generation represents a characteristic property of the epileptic neuron. These rare findings remain an exception confirming the fact that action potentials from such neurons are indeed quite normal and that in intervals free of paroxysmal surface events, it is practically impossible to distinguish neurons of the epileptogenic focus from those in the intact cortex.

PDS: SYNAPTIC MECHANISMS. The preceding data, as well as observations [114, 125, 126] that a transmembrane injection of depolarizing current sufficient to decrease the potential beyond the firing level for isolated spikes is incapable of eliciting a PDS, suggest that the PDS is more likely the result of some alteration in synaptic mechanisms. This conclusion is reinforced by findings that (a) a PDS is not easily elicited by a purely antidromic stimulation ([114]; see, however, [55]), while (b) it is regularly activated by a variety of orthodromically generated volleys of impulses [111, 114, 124]. The latter, so-called triggering, phenomenon is actually one of the most characteristic features of PDS; it has been the primary object of a number of studies which might help in understanding, at least in part, the nature of PDS itself.

Since early investigations by means

of gross surface electrodes [31, 34, 36, 41, 42, 122, 123], the phenomenon of triggering epileptiform discharges has never been thoroughly elucidated. Critically dependent upon concentration of the epileptogenic agent, the first detectable effects of the latter (in subconvulsant doses) often consist of enhancement of late components of the normal evoked potential. With concentrations sufficient to elicit spontaneous paroxysmal discharges, findings tend to be less clear: late components of the evoked potential might increase further to reach the amplitude of spontaneous discharges and be practically indistinguishable from the latter, or show a clear-cut inflection separating the two (evoked and paroxysmal) events. Their close relationship and dependence of the latter upon the former represent the *triggering phenomenon*. This relationship, however, remains quite variable in its temporal characteristics, particularly with changes in the amount of afferent impingement.

Analogous findings are obtained when the same phenomenon is analyzed at the unitary level by means of intracellular electrodes [111, 114, 124–126]. With this technique, and by manipulating stimulation intensity, it is possible to reproduce any one of the following events in most neurons of the epileptic focus (Figs. 11-2, 11-3): (a) activation of an EPSP alone; (b) activation of an EPSP with action potential; (c) activation of a PDS alone; (d) activation of an EPSP with or without spike followed by a PDS; (e) modification, within a relatively wide range, of the latency of the PDS so that this may follow the EPSP-spike complex with delays of from less than one up to fifty or more milliseconds.

The PDS may develop either from a preceding depolarization of variable steepness or as an explosive change out of a stable resting membrane potential; if this occurs following a normal EPSP (with or without spike), the membrane may undergo a complete repolarization so that clear temporal separation is possible between the two events (Figs. 11-2Ac, d and 11-3A_3, B). Changes in stimulus intensity are a practical way of reproducing these various events and also exert differential effects on EPSP and PDS; a weaker stimulus might markedly increase latency of the latter without affecting that of the former; on the other hand, it might decrease slope and amplitude of the EPSP while the PDS is either absent (Figs. 11-2Ab, 11-3C) or appears in full development without appreciable alterations in its main configuration, amplitude, and duration (see other sections of Figs. 11-2, 11-3).

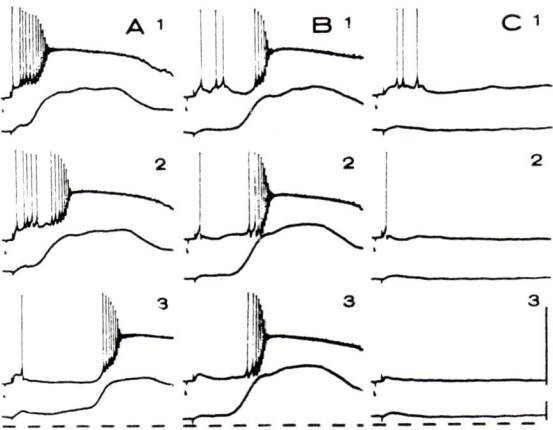

FIG. 11-3. Triggering of PDS. Records are from the same pyramidal tract cell (upper tracing) and from overlying cortical surface (lower tracing) following topical application of penicillin. Pulses of various intensity, decreasing in the order from (A_1) to (A_2), (B), (C), and (A_3), are applied to thalamic n. VL at 0.5 per sec. Calibrations: 1 and 50 mV, 10 msec. (Courtesy of Matsumoto et al. [114], unpublished.)

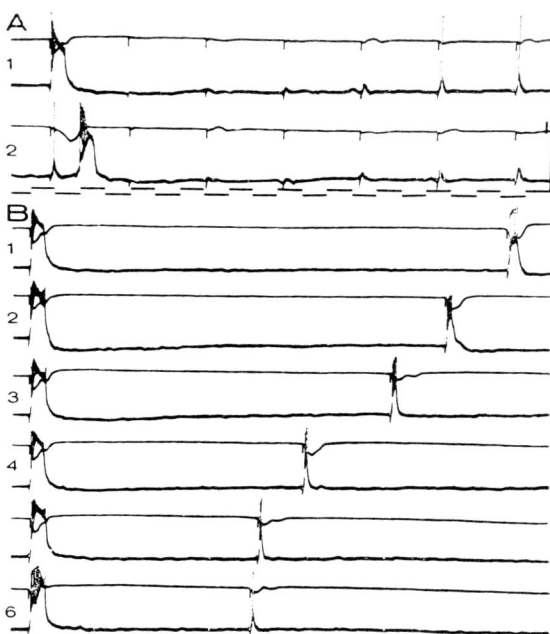

Fig. 11-4. Triggering of PDS. Same situation as in Fig. 11-3, surface record in upper tracings. (*A*) VL stimulation at 3.3 per sec. (1) and (2) are continuous. (*B*) Pairs of stimulating pulses applied to VL at different interstimuli intervals, from about 2 sec in (1) to 900 msec in (6). Calibration: 100 msec and 50 mV (Courtesy of Matsumoto et al. [114], unpublished.)

This observation, as well as that on the stereotyped uniformity of the PDSs that recur spontaneously after the epileptogenic agent has been applied for some time (10–15 minutes in the case of strychnine), would tend to support the concept of the all-or-nothing nature of the phenomenon in question. But by following from its very onset the development of PDS after application of the drug [112] or by repeating the triggering of stimulation pulses above the critical frequency of approximately 0.5 per sec (or applying twin pulses separated by critical interstimuli intervals [111, 114]), it is evident that PDS is actually a graded phenomenon (Fig. 11-4). This can be demonstrated even more convincingly when the epileptogenic agent is applied iontophoretically by means of an extracellular pipette in close proximity to a single neuron, while its activity is monitored with an intracellular microelectrode [89].

In such a situation, it has been possible to follow modifications undergone by the synaptically activated membrane potential (Figs. 11-5, 11-6). In the course of 5–15 minutes during injection of the drug, EPSPs elicited by stimuli of constant parameters become progressively larger and of longer duration to assume a configuration suggestively reminiscent of a typical PDS. These changes are reversible so that, upon interruption of the injection, EPSPs resume progressively their original form and size. Whereas this observation might suggest very close relationship between EPSP and PDS or even identity of the mechanisms at the basis of these two phenomena, the situation is actually more complex when the epileptogenic agent has affected an aggregate of neurons rather than a single or a few elements.

It has been pointed out how changes in stimulus strength affect EPSP and PDS in a different way. But changes in stimulation frequency or twin pulse experiments or both (Fig. 11-4) or even the critical timing of a stimulus after the spontaneous occurrence of a PDS also have different effects on the two phenomena: PDSs are clearly char-

TABLE 11-1. STRYCHNINE EFFECTS: CENTRAL NERVOUS SYSTEM (EXCEPT SPINAL CORD)

Structure	Phenomenon Tested	Effects[a]	Authors[b]
Cerebral cortex, gross activity	spontaneous activity amplitude, frequency	increase	25, 33
	interictal paroxysms ("spike")	present	1, 24, 33, 62, 81, 99, 103, 105
	ictal paroxysms	rare or absent	1, 24, 33, 62, 81, 99, 103, 105
	local evoked potential, component I	no effects	41
	local evoked potential, component II	increase	41
	local evoked potential, positive deflection	abolished	41
	evoked potential (sensory), late components	increase	31, 34, 36, 42, etc.
	evoked potential, inhib. (by basal ganglia)	block	100
	sensory afterdischarge	no effects	27
Cerebral cortex, dendrites	excitability	increase	44
	response, amplitude	decrease	44
Cerebral cortex, PT neurons	membrane, resting potential	no effects	107, 120, 136
	membrane, resistance	no effects	107
	membrane, conductance (during IPSP)	no effects	121
	membrane, polarizing deflections (spontaneous)	decrease	120, 136
	membrane, depolarizing deflections (spontaneous)	increase	120, 136
	spike frequency	increase	38
	spike threshold	increase	107
	spike duration	no effects	107
	recurrent inhib.	decrease	40
	IPSP	decrease or block	89, 121, 139
	IPSP	reverse	120, 136
	IPSP	no effects	38
Cerebellar cortex	interictal paroxysms	absent	57, 129
	ictal paroxysms	absent	57, 129
	Purkinje cell inhib. (from parallel fibers)	no effects	11, 48
Hippocampus	interictal paroxysms	present	14, 55, etc.
	ictal paroxysms	present	14, etc.
	pyramidal cell inhib. (from fimbria)	no effects	11, 48
Olfactory bulb	interictal paroxysms	absent	73
	ictal paroxysms	absent	73
	cell inhib. (from lat. olf. t. or ant. comm.)	no effects	82, 141
Thalamus	interictal paroxysms	absent	96
	interictal paroxysms	present	137
	ictal paroxysms	absent	96, 137
	evoked potential inhib. (by basal ganglia)	block	100
	VPL cell inhib. (by periph. stim.)	no effects	11
Inferior colliculus	interictal and ictal paroxysms	present	33

TABLE 11-1, CONTINUED

Structure	Phenomenon Tested	Effects[a]	Authors[b]
Oculomotor n.	interictal paroxysms	absent	142
Edinger-Westphal n.	interictal paroxysms	absent	142
Vagus nerve n.	interictal paroxysms	absent	73
Olivocochlear bundle	inhibitory action	depression	54

[a] Effects are for various dosages and different ways of administration.

[b] In this and following tables references are provided only as a guide or for historical reasons. No attempt was made to provide a complete survey of all the pertinent papers.

acterized by different recovery time than the EPSP [111, 114].

Most of the data reported so far have been derived from experiments utilizing either strychnine or penicillin, without important differences of effects between these two epileptogenic agents. Actually, there remains some question as to identity of their effects on other forms of cellular activity such as the various types of hyperpolarizing potentials.

STRYCHNINE AND PENICILLIN EFFECTS. Concerning strychnine, good evidence indicates that the drug has the property of reducing all postsynaptic "inhibitory" phenomena in neurons of the spinal cord (Table 11-2). Whether it possesses the same property at higher levels of the CNS remains controversial, although (Table 11-1) it is possible to demonstrate that the drug can affect various forms of hyperpolarizing potentials in cortical pyramidal cells [89, 120, 121, 136], particularly during development of the overt epileptiform manifestations described above. On the other hand, after these have become fully established, some of the PDSs might occasionally be

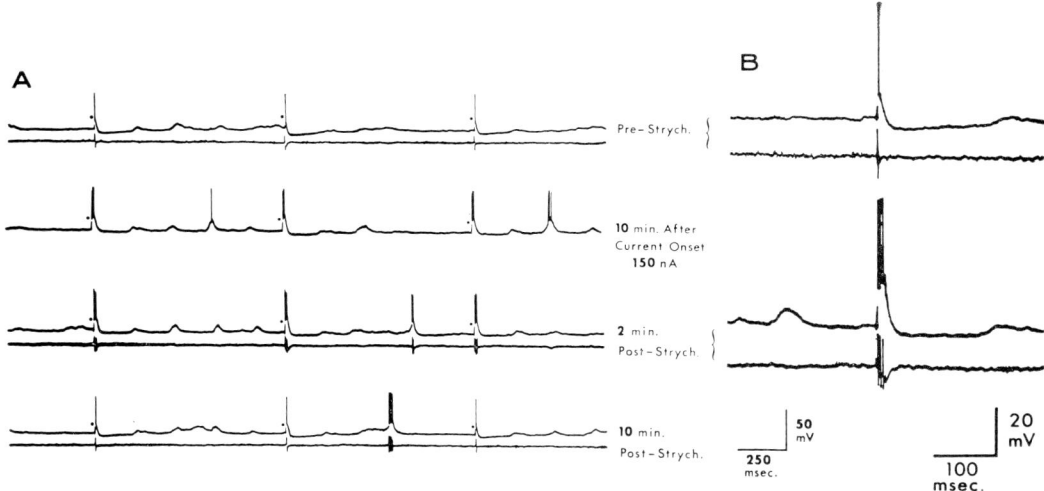

FIG. 11-5. Iontophoretic application of strychnine to a pyramidal tract cell. Double-barrel micropipette for intracellular dc recording (upper tracing) and, about 50 µ away, for drug injection and ac extracellular recording (lower tracing). (A) Response to stimuli applied to n. VL of thalamus (dots) at the four indicated stages of the experiment. (B) Detail of one response at two stages (note different calibrations). Some of the changes and their time-course relation to iontophoretic procedure are plotted in Fig. 11-6. (Courtesy of Humphrey [89].)

TABLE 11-2. Strychnine Effects: Spinal Cord

Element	Phenomenon Tested	Effects[a]	Authors[b]
Motoneurons	membrane potential	no effects	51, 76, 102
	membrane potential	steady depolarization	39
	membrane (postsynaptic)	no direct excitation	51
	excitability, to extracell. stimul.	no effects	143
	excitability, to intracell. stimul.	no effects	76
	spike firing threshold	no effects	102
	antidromic stimul., critical interval	no effects	76
	inhib. from peripheral n.	decrease	50, 93
	inhib. from cerebellum	decrease	50, 93
	inhib. from ret. format.	decrease	93, 108
	inhib. (α) from ret. format.	no effects	106
	IPSP (cat)	decrease or block	23, 45, 50, 51, 64, 95, 106
	IPSP (toad)	decrease and EPSP unmask.	102
	hyperpol., popliteal (by semitend. & tibialis stretch)	no effects	94, 95
	depression (by amino acids)	no effects	50, 52
	hyperpol. by GABA	no effects	53
	hyperpol. by glycine and β-alanine	block	53
Interneurons	potential generated on inhib. path	no effects	50
	Renshaw cell, cholinoreceptive	no effects or slight potentiation	37, 63
Relay cells	cuneate n., IPSP	decrease or block	22
Dorsal root	antidromic response (to ventr. horn stim.)	decrease	143
	potential, declining phase	prolongation	32, 60, 65, 66, 140
	potential, amplitude	increase	32, 59, 135
	potential, latency	increase	52
	terminals, excitability	decrease	143
	terminals, polarization level	increase	143
Ventral root	potential, amplitude	increase	32
	potential, amplitude	increase, then decrease	135
Ventral horn	fibers, affer. terminals, threshold	increase	143
Reflex	monosynaptic	no effects	17, 23, 45, 50, 51, 64, 95, 106
	monosynaptic, depression by dopamine	abolition	109
	monosynaptic, depression by factor I, fraction A	decrease	72, 88
	polysynaptic	increase	17, 28, 134
	inhibition	decrease	23, 50, 51, 64

TABLE 11-2, CONTINUED

Element	Phenomenon Tested	Effects[a]	Authors[b]
Synapses	antidromic trans-synaptic firing	absent	142
	transmission, one-way	"destroyed"	90
Ictal activity	(tetanus)	present	10, 26, 28, 32, 33, 39, 98
Ictal activity	(tetanus), inhibition (central)	possible	80

[a,b] See Table 11-1.

followed by hyperpolarization of long duration [105, 111–114, 124]. This last observation is relatively rare in the strychnine-induced epileptic foci but rather common when the foci have been elicited by application of penicillin. Indeed, with this agent, the most typical interictal manifestations do not consist so much of the simple PDS but rather of a PDS-hyperpolarization complex (Fig. 11-7A, H). The later component of this complex should probably be interpreted as an IPSP [114, 126], at least on the basis of its behavior to current injections and because it is accompanied by concomitant increase in membrane conductance. In any case, it is not a simple aftereffect of PDS inasmuch as it may start earlier than, or even be present in the absence of a PDS. It should be added that especially with penicillin [112], but to a lesser extent also with strychnine [105], it is possible to observe cells the membrane of which undergoes paroxysmal shifts that are only or predominantly in the *hyperpolarizing* direction —rather than the typical PDSs—in correspondence with the surface epileptiform discharges. This finding has been systematically studied by Prince and Wilder [128] at the neocortical level and by Dichter [55] in the hippocampal elements and will be elaborated upon by these investigators (see also [92]).

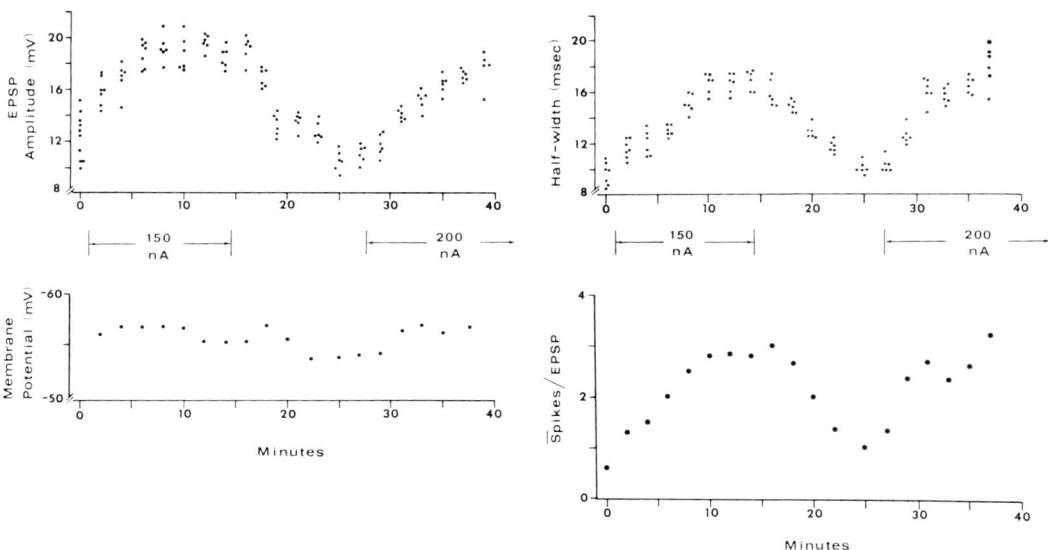

Fig. 11-6. Graphic display of changes in amplitude and duration of the EPSP (elicited by n. VL stimulation), in average number of spikes per each EPSP and in membrane potential level during a 40-min period when strychnine was iontophoretically injected twice. Duration and amounts of current indicated below the abscissa. (Courtesy of Humphrey [89].)

On the basis of preceding data, the PDS would not result primarily from an alteration of the properties of the neuronal membrane, as previously suggested [112, 120], but rather would reflect response of what could be considered an essentially normal membrane to an altered barrage of impulses. As such, it can be viewed as a form of greatly enhanced PSP of an excitatory nature. This interpretation raises several points which may be crucial in understanding the mechanism of action of drugs under consideration and the essence of the epileptogenic process itself. For instance, it might suggest that this experimental model and probably most other forms of focal epilepsy should be included in the broad category of "reflex" epilepsy [17]; all epileptiform manifestations, even when occurring apparently spontaneously, are indeed triggered and only the specific nature of the triggering factors may not always be obvious.

EXCITATORY PHENOMENA. Having established that predominant manifestations within the epileptic focus are the expression of excitatory phenomena, it still remains to be determined whether their marked enhancement is a direct effect of the epileptogenic agent or whether it results, indirectly, from interference with inhibitory mechanisms. In the case of strychnine, effects are commonly considered a typical example of inhibition of inhibitory synapses [52, 83], but (Table 11-1) this type of effect has not been definitely established as occurring at all levels of the CNS; it is even possible to challenge the common assumption that elimination of an IPSP, per se, might be functionally equivalent to elimination of "inhibition" [120, 121].

Since hyperpolarizing potentials may still be present in neocortical neurons directly involved in the epileptic process, it can be concluded that for the establishment of the latter, elimination of inhibitory mechanisms is not crucial, the enhancement of excitatory phenomena being the most important factor and probably representing a direct effect of the epileptogenic agents. On the other hand, if suppression of inhibitory mechanisms is deemphasized, there is still need to explain how the excitatory potentials are so dramatically increased, since it appears reasonable to assume that a topically applied epileptogenic agent will not alter substantially the degree of excitatory synaptic impingement that normally converges from various sources upon any given neuronal aggregate of the cerebral cortex. A clue is provided here by comparison between the PDS and normal EPSPs. These have been seen to coexist in the same neuronal element, but, with appropriate manipulations of the parameters of a triggering stimulus, they can be easily separated, the PDS undergoing considerable variations in its latency and displaying a much longer recovery rate ([111, 114] and Figs. 11-2, 11-3, 11-4). These findings suggest the polysynaptic nature of pathways responsible for PDS activation and could be explained by postulating existence of facilitatory interneurons, as in the hippocampus [55, 56, 92], and their selective sensitization by the epileptogenic agent. A recurrent facilitatory loop would also provide an ideal substratum and possible explanation for the other characteristic manifestation of the epileptic neuronal population: the prominent, explosivelike synchronization of activity of most elements of the population.

As to the role of inhibitory mechanisms, probably in general they are simply overcome and masked by the grossly enhanced excitatory phenomena, at least throughout the interictal phase. It is conceivable that persistence of these IPSPs is partly responsible for controlling the overall duration of PDS [112] or for contributing to its termination; their spatial and temporal characteristics could well account for such restraining effects and, at the same time, for their inability to prevent the PDS occurrence [114]. It has also been suggested [112] that their preservation plays some role in determining rate of incidence of PDS themselves or at least in setting the lowest limit of the interval at which two PDSs may follow each other.

ICTAL PHASE

The ictal phase, as previously defined, consists of a form of activity which differs in many respects from that described so far.

Changes which characterize it have much longer duration, often on the order of a minute or more. These changes have also been described as "self-sustained," because, when induced by some controllable stimulation, they develop into a pattern which is fully independent of that of the generating stimulus and are then maintained long after its termination.

These changes are easily induced by repetitive stimulation under the well known form of electrical afterdischarge [15, 20, 33, 49, 79, 97, 101, 117, 132, 133, 138]. In neocortical foci produced by topical application of the epileptogenic agents, ictal episodes can be elicited or facilitated by this same method, but may also take place spontaneously, if somewhat unpredictably. In the strychnine-induced focus, and in the absence of repetitive electrical or peripheral [81] stimulation, such episodes are rarely seen. Spontaneous ictal episodes which develop occasionally in the penicillin-induced focus ([113, 131] and Fig. 11-1) are briefly described and analyzed here.

In describing interictal phenomena, brief mention has been made about occasional observation of neurons in which the epileptogenic effects manifested themselves primarily or exclusively in the form of paroxysmal hyperpolarizing shifts. This type of behavior is observable also in the course of ictal episodes [13, 55, 113] but this will be provisionally ignored here and analysis left to others [92], in an attempt to simplify interpretation of a functional situation which, even in its more typical manifestations, is rather complex.

DEVELOPMENT AND COURSE OF ICTAL EPISODE. A typical ictal episode (analyzed at the single-cell level on the basis of changes of its membrane potential) appears to develop progressively from, and in suggestively close relationship with, the interictal events (see also [131]). The earliest detectable sign of an impending ictal episode is progressive

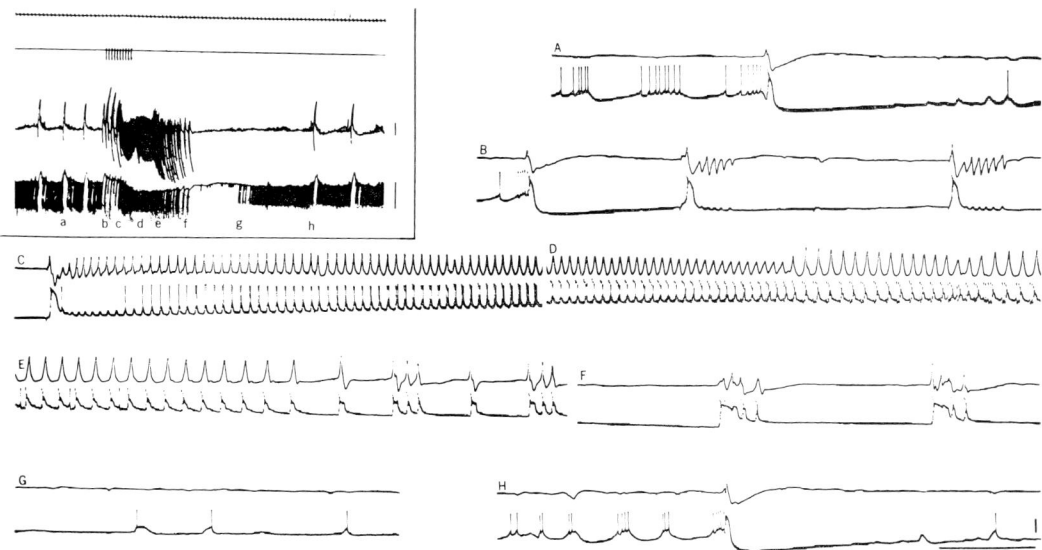

FIG. 11-7. Ictal episode in penicillin focus induced in postsigmoid gyrus of cat. Entire episode (including preceding interictal patterns, postictal stage, and its recovery) is shown in insert, consisting of ink-writing tracing of gross surface (above) and intracellular (below) activities. The ictal episode here is "facilitated" by a brief train of shocks at 1.5 per sec applied to contralateral homologous region. Calibrations: 1 sec, 2 mV for surface, and 20 mV for intracellular record. The eight portions (a)–(h) are displayed for greater detail in the CRO tracings identified by the corresponding letters (A–H). The first three stimuli are shown in (B). Note, in the postictal phase, the late recovery of PDS in comparison with that of "normal" action potentials (G) and (H). Calibrations: 500 msec and 10 mV, for intracellular record only. (From [113] unpublished.)

decrease and disappearance of hyperpolarization that follows each PDS (Fig 11-7*A*, *B*).

The original PDS-hyperpolarization complex is changed into a PDS followed by an afterdepolarization of progressively longer duration and higher degree, with rhythmical oscillations on its top, in increasingly longer trains; this phase is accompanied by increase in membrane conductance reflecting [13] increase in synaptic impingement. Eventually the membrane potential reaches and maintains a very low polarization level (Fig. 11-7*C*, *D*). The PDSs may persist for a time at a rate similar to that of the preictal condition or at increased frequency, their amplitude decreasing proportionally to the level of depolarization from which they arise. More often, however, typical PDSs disappear when the membrane reaches a critical level of depolarization, and at this point, cellular behavior reflects the *tonic phase*. During this phase, membrane polarization level keeps steadily decreasing while displaying rhythmical oscillations of increasing frequency and decreasing amplitude, up to the point where a plateau is reached and maintained for a variable period of time. The rhythmical oscillations reach and eventually exceed the firing level, often to the point of spike inactivation.

This first phase is followed by the *clonic phase*, the transition between these two phases being arbitrarily placed at the point where the membrane begins to repolarize (Fig. 11-7*D*, *E*). In the course of such process, frequency of the oscillations decreases, their amplitude and duration keep increasing, and as the membrane approaches the original polarization level, they lose their rhythmical character, occurring at longer and longer intervals and progressively resuming most features of preictal PDSs (Fig. 11-7*F*). Eventually the membrane potential reaches, and occasionally exceeds, the resting level of polarization at which point the ictal episode ends, to be followed by a period of neuronal inactivity of variable duration.

This description is valid for only certain types of neurons and for one of several forms of electrical behavior which may be displayed in the course of the ictal episode [13, 113]. Analysis of this form, however, should provide a clue to basic mechanisms subserving an ictal episode in general.

Excitatory Impingement and Polarization. The interictal event has been felt to result mainly from a greatly enhanced barrage of excitatory impulses; it has also been suggested that inhibitory phenomena are not significantly affected in this stage of the epileptogenic process and that through simultaneous activation, and because of their different temporal course, they might control the duration and be responsible for the termination of each interictal episode.

Enhancement of excitatory impingement appears to be also an important factor in determination of the ictal episode. Such enhancement alone, however, would not be sufficient, since development of the ictal episode would still be prevented by persistence of powerful hyperpolarizing potentials. It is therefore reasonable to assume that the episode could take place only if these were eliminated or greatly decreased.

It is not immediately obvious why a hypothetical, additional effect of the epileptogenic agent (depression of hyperpolarizing phenomena) should only become manifest sporadically to account for occurrence of an ictal episode. If depression of inhibition were an important component of direct effects of these agents, a series of ictal epsiodes would be expected; namely, the experimental correlate of a true status epilepticus. At the spinal cord level, where there is good evidence that strychnine eliminates IPSPs (see Table 11-2), it can be noted that epileptogenic action of this drug is characterized by the production of a tetanus, that is, an exceedingly longlasting episode of continuous ictal activity [10, 26, 32, 39, 98].

It could be suggested that interference with inhibitory mechanisms which permits development of a seizure is not due to a direct effect of the drugs, but probably reflects a secondary effect of an excessive impingement upon inhibitory interneurons of such intensity as to result in their temporary inactivation. (This interpretation implicitly deprives the drug of any specificity in genesis of the ictal episode, therefore fails to account for preferential occurrence of ictal episodes with penicillin and for their exceptional observation with strychnine—at least at the neocortical level.)

A similar mechanism was originally proposed by Dichter [55] to explain the genesis of ictal episodes in the hippocampal elements and will be elaborated upon by Kandel and Spencer [92]. Whether the falling-out of inhibitory mechanisms takes place in this or in some other undetermined way, combination of this phenomenon with enhanced excitation creates a favorable situation for development of the ictal episode. Once started, this appears to proceed through its various phases in an autonomous way, and the process becomes totally independent of whichever epileptogenic agent might have originally induced the focus [4].

Once the excitatory impingement has depolarized the neuronal membrane beyond a certain level at which rhythmical oscillations begin to appear, the depolarizing process continues, probably due to both a progressive recruitment of activated elements (and a consequent increase in the amount of synaptic bombardment) and parallel inactivation of inhibitory influences. Eventually, after the membrane has remained at excessively low levels of polarization for a relatively long time, inactivation processes are likely to set in, and will result in progressive dropping-out of active units, with progressive decrease in the synaptic excitatory drive to which the remaining active elements are subjected. In the meantime inhibitory neurons begin to recover, contributing more and more to the repolarization process of each element, by pulling its membrane toward the resting level and by diminishing the excitatory drive through inhibition of other elements. The combination of these various factors will eventually end the ictal episode.

These mechanisms appear compatible with many of the observed phenomena and could be provisionally accepted as the most likely to operate in determining the various phases of a typical ictal episode. It should be added that this interpretation is based on the reasonable assumption that we are dealing with a population phenomenon and carries with it the implication that an ictal episode could only take place in a neuronal aggregate where a complex synaptic network is potentially available among its various elements [2]. It is probable that a similar limitation may also be valid—though less crucial—for genesis of the PDS.

DISCUSSION AND ADDITIONAL CONSIDERATIONS

A first, additional consideration concerns the propriety of the term *epileptic neuron,* which obviously reflects close analogy between the cell and the entire organism, that is, the "epileptic" patient. Beside the fact that it is questionable whether it is justified to define a given neural element as epileptic simply on the basis of transient and reversible changes in its activity, it has been seen that such an element cannot be separated from the other members of the population and that changes of its activity are primarily the reflection of synaptic phenomena, so that, at most, the validity of the concept of *epileptic neuronal aggregate* could be defended, rather than that of the epileptic neuron. These arguments are applicable to the acute experimental situation under discussion and would be even more appropriate in the case of the ictal episodes which can be readily reproduced in normal neural structures with repetitive electrical stimulation.

Other considerations apply to the two types of abnormal cellular behavior: interictal and ictal episodes are not simply different degrees of the same phenomenon but reflect different forms of epileptic manifestations and different underlying mechanisms. But separation of these two forms of activity is useful also for the simple purpose of reproducing or confirming certain findings or for their interpretation. For instance, the statement that the elimination of inhibition is a crucial factor in the genesis of epileptiform activity is rather meaningless and may be both correct and incorrect since, as shown, it would apply to the genesis of ictal episodes but not necessarily to that of the interictal events. Likewise our interpretations are made firmer when effects of strychnine upon the membrane potential of spinal motoneurons are reviewed and reports are found of no appreciable changes [76, 102] on the one hand and of a steady depolarization [39] on the other. The conflicting nature of these reports is only apparent since the former would apply to the preictal or the interictal stage between paroxysms, whereas the latter refers to the long-lasting ictal (or tetanic) phase.

Another characteristic feature common to both types of epileptiform activity is represented by its massive, quasi-simultaneous occurrence in most elements of the neuronal population involved in the epileptogenic process. Synchronization of unitary activity is a phenomenon which, in a less prominent form, is normally observed at all levels of the CNS, where it is generally defined—rather than explained—as a characteristic property inherent to all neuronal aggregates [29, 30, 33]. A knowledge of the underlying mechanisms of this phenomenon in the normal situation (see [3]) would provide closer understanding of those responsible for the enhanced synchronization in the epileptic condition.

Of the two main types of potentially available mechanisms for synchronization, the one which could be involved in both normal and abnormal situations is that based on synaptic effects. In both cases, this would require existence of either a pacemaker system or a complex network of recurrent excitatory circuits with relatively widespread interconnections. It is less likely that the other, or ephaptic mechanisms, play an important role; such mechanisms could become operant only under a pathological condition since normally, in the CNS of vertebrates, neurons appear to possess only synaptic interconnections (see, however, [84]). In the epileptic focus it is possible to postulate the presence of various types of alterations which would permit ephaptic effects or—as recently suggested [87]—these might become evident by way of an intermediary action of glial elements [118].

The real nature of synchronizing mechanisms within the neural elements of an epileptic focus is not definitely established. It has been seen that (a) the PDS should very probably be considered a potential of the synaptic type (see also [55]), and (b) a recurrent excitatory circuit, such as the one postulated for genesis of each individual PDS, appears quite suitable also to account for the quasi-explosive and simultaneous activation of many elements within a focus.

CONCLUSIONS

To conclude on the most probable mode of action of topically applied epileptogenic agents, such as strychnine and penicillin, we may review the findings which have been obtained with the administration of these same compounds in subliminal doses, or just prior to the appearance of full-blown epileptiform manifestations, and look for those effects which may be critically important for, and could be considered as probable intermediary steps in the development of the latter. Table 11-1 summarizes some of these findings as well as others that have been reported for different cerebral structures following administration of strychnine in various ways. Tables 11-2 and 11-3 deal with similar data at the spinal cord and peripheral levels and with some of the findings obtained with the same drug from various structures in lower species. (Previous reviews on the mode of action of strychnine in the nervous system [28, 52, 61] should also be consulted.)

Most of the material included in Table 11-3, particularly that related to effects of strychnine on the peripheral nerve, has been derived from relatively old experiments. It might be of interest to repeat some of these experiments with more sophisticated techniques since it seems obvious that the drug is not entirely devoid of action upon conduction and related phenomena. It is curious that all the modern views on action of strychnine on the CNS seem to ignore any possible effect of this drug upon the axonal functions.

Some years ago it was suggested that the

TABLE 11-3. STRYCHNINE EFFECTS: PERIPHERAL NERVOUS SYSTEM AND MISCELLANEA

Structure	Phenomenon Tested	Concentration	Effects	Authors[a]
Peripheral nerve (in vitro)	excitability, oscillation amplitude	10^{-5}–10^{-3}	increase	68
	excitability, oscillation amplitude	10^{-7}–10^{-6}	increase	47, 86, 119
	excitability, oscillation amplitude	$>10^{-6}$	decrease	47, 86, 119
	excitability, oscillation amplitude	10^{-17}–10^{-5}	increase	110
	excitability, oscillation amplitude	10^{-6}–10^{-3}	decrease	110
	excitability, cycle	$<10^{-5}$	no effects	47, 119
	excitability, subnormal phase	$>10^{-5}$	increase	47, 119
	refractory period, absolute	$>10^{-5}$	increase	47, 119
	refractory period, relative	$>10^{-5}$	increase	47, 119
	recovery period	10^{-15}	decrease	110
	recovery period	10^{-5}	increase	110
	cronaxy	$>10^{-6}$	no effects or decrease	21, 47, 86, 119
	accommodation	$>10^{-6}$	decrease	86
	action potential, amplitude	$>10^{-6}$	decrease	86, 110
	action potential, negative after pot.	$>10^{-6}$	decrease	86, 110
	action potential, positive after pot.	$>10^{-6}$	increase	12, 47
	action potential, duration	$>10^{-5}$	increase	75, 110
	action potential, conduction	$6 \cdot 10^{-3}$	block	47
	autorhythmicity, tendency	10^{-5}–10^{-3}	increase	47, 110
	rhythmic activity (hypocalcemic)	10^{-5}–10^{-3}	no effects	47
Motor nerve (in situ)	cronaxy		decrease	35, 104
Neuromuscular preparation	transmission	$3 \cdot 10^{-3}$	block	21, 46
	ACh action on muscles	$5 \cdot 10^{-5}$	block	19
Sup. cervical ganglion	preganglionic fibers, threshold	$<10^{-6}$	decrease	86
	synaptic transmission	1–$5 \cdot 10^{-5}$	block	69
Dorsal root ganglion	interictal activity	10^{-2}	absent	142
Crayfish stretch receptor	membrane resting potential	$3 \cdot 10^{-4}$	no effects	145
	membrane resistance	$3 \cdot 10^{-4}$	no effects	145
	threshold to direct cathod. stim.	$3 \cdot 10^{-4}$	no effects	145
	spike, duration	$3 \cdot 10^{-4}$	increase	145
	inhibitory synaptic processes	$3 \cdot 10^{-4}$	no effects	145
	spike, repetitive firing, tendency	$3 \cdot 10^{-4}$	increase	145
Mauthner cell	inhibition, early		decrease, +	77, 78
	inhibition, late		decrease, ++	77, 78
Abdominal ganglion (Aplysia)	membrane resting potential	$3 \cdot 10^{-4}$–$4 \cdot 10^{-3}$	no consistent effects	91
	spike, amplitude	$3 \cdot 10^{-4}$–$4 \cdot 10^{-3}$	decrease	91
	spike, duration	$3 \cdot 10^{-4}$–$4 \cdot 10^{-3}$	increase	91
	spike, afterhyperpolarization	$3 \cdot 10^{-4}$–$4 \cdot 10^{-3}$	decrease	91
	spike, activation, latency	$3 \cdot 10^{-4}$–$4 \cdot 10^{-3}$	decrease then increase	91

[a] See Table 11-1.

epileptogenic agent might induce some changes in intrinsic properties of the neuronal membrane and that this change might contribute to genesis of the large depolarization shifts [112]. Negative findings in relation to a number of membrane characteristics in resting conditions (see Tables 11-1, 11-2) did not support the validity of this suggestion. The concept of a hypothetical membrane damage was subsequently modified to include (a) its limitation to the subsynaptic region and (b) the assumption that, electrically, it could manifest itself only during synaptic activity.

As far as cortical neurons are concerned, data pointing to possible interference with IPSPs could support the hypothesis of a subsynaptic membrane alteration [120, 121, 136] or, alternatively, reflect a purely synaptic effect, for instance, in the form of a blockade of inhibitory transmitter [23]. Regardless of actual mechanisms involved, the data themselves remain controversial. Evidence has been offered that "powerful inhibitory actions" are quite resistant to strychnine in hippocampal pyramidal cells [11, 55] as well as in Purkinje cells of the cerebellum [11, 48], yet the drug is known to have a prominent epileptiform effect on the former but not in the latter structure. Therefore, it seems reasonable to conclude that *development of typical PDSs* in a given cell does not depend on a preceding or concurrent IPSP elimination in that same element.

The theoretical possibility of disinhibitory mechanisms at a presynaptic level cannot be eliminated but has not been demonstrated with the drugs under consideration. If it is concluded that action of such epileptogenic drugs consists primarily of enhancement of excitatory mechanisms, it must also be recognized that the latter remains a rather vague concept. There is no experimental evidence to suggest a direct effect of the drug on the subsynaptic membrane at the excitatory receptor sites, resulting in alteration of its characteristics in response to the excitatory transmitter. The other, more likely hypothesis of facilitatory circuits, capable of providing a powerful positive feedback, rests on the assumptions that (a) such circuits do exist as part of the normal synaptic organization of the cerebral cortex (as well as of other, but not all, cerebral structures), and that (b) they become operant mainly under action of the epileptogenic agent. But the intimate nature of such an action would still escape us. It is also important to keep in mind that these conclusions, even if proven correct, should be valid only as far as they apply to the pathophysiology of only one type of cortical epileptiform activity: that which has been defined as *interictal*.

The development of typical *ictal* forms of activity, as discussed, would appear to depend on the synergistic combination of two mechanisms: enhancement of excitatory impingement and depression of inhibitory influences. At least at the cortical level there is no evidence to indicate that both mechanisms should be considered part of a direct action by the epileptogenic agent.

REFERENCES

1. Adrian, E. D., and Moruzzi, G. Impulses in the pyramidal tract. *J. Physiol.* (London) 97:153, 1939.
2. Ajmone-Marsan, C. Electrographic aspects of "epileptic" neuronal aggregates. *Epilepsia* (Amst.) 2:22, 1961.
3. Ajmone-Marsan, C. Electrical activity of the brain: Slow waves and neuronal activity. *Israel J. Med. Sci.* 1:104, 1965.
4. Ajmone-Marsan, C. A newly proposed classification of epileptic seizures. Neurophysiological basis. *Epilepsia* (Amst.) 6:275, 1965.
5. Ajmone-Marsan, C. Micro-Structural Mechanisms of Seizure Susceptibility. In Servit, Z. (Ed.), *Comparative and Cellular Pathophysiology of Epilepsy*. Amsterdam: Excerpta Medica, 1966.
6. Ajmone-Marsan, C. Epilepsy. In Spiegel, E. A. (Ed.), *Progress in Neurology and Psychiatry*, vol. 21. New York: Grune & Stratton, 1966, p. 195.

7. Ajmone-Marsan, C., and Abraham, K. Epilepsy. In Spiegel, E. A. (Ed.), *Progress in Neurology and Psychiatry*, vol. 18. New York: Grune & Stratton, 1963, p. 244.

8. Ajmone-Marsan, C., and Abraham, K. Epilepsy. In Spiegel, E. A. (Ed.), *Progress in Neurology and Psychiatry*, vol. 19. New York: Grune & Stratton, 1964, p. 261.

9. Ajmone-Marsan, C., and Abraham, K. Epilepsy. In Spiegel, E. A. (Ed.), *Progress in Neurology and Psychiatry*, vol. 20. New York: Grune & Stratton, 1965, p. 286.

10. Ajmone-Marsan, C., and Marossero, F. Studio sperimentale di attività elettriche provocate in livelli diversi del sistema nervoso. *Sist. Nerv.* 5:174, 1953.

11. Andersen, P., Eccles, J. C., Løyning, Y., and Voorhoeve, P. E. Strychnine-resistant central inhibition. *Nature* (London) 200:843, 1963.

12. Auger, D., and Fessard, A. Propagation et forme du potentiel d'action d'un nerf soumis à l'action de la strychnine. *C. R. Soc. Biol.* (Paris) 112:645, 1933.

13. Ayala, G. F., Matsumoto, H., and Gumnit, R. J. Inhibitory mechanisms during tonic-clonic seizures. *Electroenceph. Clin. Neurophysiol.*, 1969, in press.

14. Baker, W. W., Kratky, M., and Benedict, F. Electrographic response to intrahippocampal injections of convulsant drugs. *Exp. Neurol.* 12:136, 1965.

15. Baumgartner, G., and Jung, R. Hemmungsphänomene an einzelnen corticalen Neuronen und ihre Bedeutung für die Bremsung convulsiver Entladungen. *Arch. Sci. Biol.* 39:474, 1955.

16. Bernhard, C. G., Taverner, D., and Widén, L. Differences in the action of tubocurarine and strychnine on the spinal reflex excitability of the cat. *Brit. J. Pharmacol.* 6:551, 1951.

17. Bickford, R. G. Sensory Precipitation and Reflex Mechanisms. In Jasper, H. H., Ward, A. A., Jr., and Pope, A. (Eds.), *Basic Mechanisms of the Epilepsies*. Boston: Little, Brown, 1969.

18. Black, R. G., Abraham, J., and Ward, A. A., Jr. The preparation of tungstic acid gel and its use in the production of experimental epilepsy. *Epilepsia* (Amst.) 8:58, 1967.

19. Bolly, M. H., and Bacq, Z. M. Strychnine et contraction acetylcholinique du muscle strié. *C. R. Soc. Biol.* (Paris) 127:1459, 1938.

20. Bonnet, V., and Bremer, F. Analyse des modifications préconvulsives de la réaction de l'écorce cérébrale à un stimulus direct répété. *J. Physiol.* (Paris) 48:399, 1956.

21. Bouman, H. D. Experiments on the mechanism of strychnine "curarization." *J. Physiol.* (London) 88:328, 1936.

22. Boyd, E. S., Meritt, D. A., and Gardner, L. C. The effect of convulsant drugs on transmission through the cuneate nucleus. *J. Pharmacol. Exp. Ther.* 154:398, 1966.

23. Bradley, K., Easton, D. M., and Eccles, J. C. An investigation of primary or direct inhibition. *J. Physiol.* (London) 122:474, 1953.

24. Bremer, F. Quelques propriétés de l'activité électrique du cortex cérébral "isolé". *C. R. Soc. Biol.* (Paris) 118:1241, 1935.

25. Bremer, F. Action de la strychnine en application locale sur l'activité électrique du cortex cérébral. *C. R. Soc. Biol.* (Paris) 123:90, 1936.

26. Bremer, F. Le tétanos strychnique et le mécanisme de la synchronisation neuronique. *Arch. Int. Physiol.* 51:51, 1941.

27. Bremer, F. Étude oscillographique des réponses sensorielles de l'aire acoustique corticale chez le chat. *Arch. Int. Physiol.* 53:53, 1943.

28. Bremer, F. Le mode d'action de la strychnine à la lumière des travaux récents. *Arch. Int. Pharmacodyn.* 69:249, 1944.

29. Bremer, F. L'activité électrique spontanée des centres nerveux et l'électroencéphalogramme. Essai d'interprétation. *J. Belge Neurol. Psychiat.* 47:542, 1947.

30. Bremer, F. Considérations sur l'origine et la nature des ondes cérébrales. *Electroenceph. Clin. Neurophysiol.* 1:177, 1949.

31. Bremer, F. Analyse oscillographique des réponses sensorielles des écorces cérébrale et cérébelleuse. *Rev. Neurol.* (Paris) 87:65, 1952.

32. Bremer, F. Strychnine Tetanus of the Spinal Cord. In Wolstenholme, G. E. W., and Freeman, J. S. (Eds.), *The Spinal Cord. Ciba Foundation Symposium*. London: Churchill, 1953.

33. Bremer, F. Les processus d'excitation et d'inhibition dans les phénomènes épileptiques. In Th. Alajouanine (Ed.), *Bases Physiologiques et Aspects Cliniques de l'Epilepsie*. Paris: Masson, 1958.

34. Bremer, F., Bonnet, V., and Terzuolo, C. Etude électrophysiologique des aires audi-

tives corticales du chat. *Arch. Int. Physiol.* 62:390, 1954.

35. Bremer, F., and Rylant, P. L'action locale de la strychnine sur les nerfs et les centres. *C. R. Soc. Biol.* (Paris) 91:1329, 1924.

36. Bremer, F., and Stoupel, N. Interprétation de la réponse de l'aire visuelle corticale à une volée d'influx sensoriels. *Arch. Int. Physiol.* 64:234, 1956.

37. Biscoe, T. J., and Curtis, D. R. Noradrenaline and inhibition of Renshaw cells. *Science* 151:1230, 1966.

38. Biscoe, T. J., and Curtis, D. R. Strychnine and cortical inhibition. *Nature* (London) 214:914, 1967.

39. Brooks, C. McC., and Fuortes, M. G. F. Potential changes in spinal cord following administration of strychnine. *J. Neurophysiol.* 15:257, 1952.

40. Brooks, V. B., and Asanuma, H. Pharmacological studies of recurrent cortical inhibition and facilitation. *Amer. J. Physiol.* 208:674, 1965.

41. Chang, H. T. An observation on the effect of strychnine on local cortical potentials. *J. Neurophysiol.* 14:23, 1951.

42. Chang, H. T., and Kaada, B. An analysis of primary response of visual cortex to optic nerve stimulation in cats. *J. Neurophysiol.* 13:305, 1950.

43. Chusid, J. G., and Kopeloff, L. M. Epileptogenic effects of pure metals implanted in motor cortex of monkeys. *J. Appl. Physiol.* 17:697, 1962.

44. Clare, M. H., and Bishop, G. H. Action of strychnine on recruiting responses of dendrites of cat cortex. *J. Neurophysiol.* 20:255, 1957.

45. Coombs, J. S., Eccles, J. C., and Fatt, P. The specific ionic conductances and the ionic movements across the motoneuronal membrane that produce the inhibitory post-synaptic potential. *J. Physiol.* (London) 130:326, 1955.

46. Coppée, G. Les mécanismes de la décurarization. *Bull. Classe Sci. Acad. Roy. Belg.* 27:452, 1941.

47. Coppée, G., and Coppée-Bolly, M. H. Effets de la strychnine sur le nerf isolé. *Arch. Int. Physiol.* 51:97, 1941.

48. Crawford, J. M., Curtis, D. R., Voorhoeve, P. E., and Wilson, V. J. Strychnine and cortical inhibition. *Nature* (London) 200: 845, 1963.

49. Creutzfeldt, O., Baumgartner, G., and Schoen, L. Reactionen einzelner Neurone des senso-motorischen Cortex nach electrischen Reizen. 1. Hemmung und Erregung nach direkten und kontralateralen Einzelteizen. *Arch. Psychiat. Nervenkr.* 194:597, 1956.

50. Curtis, D. R. Pharmacological investigations upon inhibition of spinal neurones. *J. Physiol.* (London) 145:175, 1959.

51. Curtis, D. R. The depression of spinal inhibition by electrophoretically administered strychnine. *Int. J. Neuropharmacol.* 1:239, 1962.

52. Curtis, D. R. The pharmacology of central and peripheral inhibition. *Pharmacol. Rev.* 15:333, 1963.

53. Curtis, D. R., Hösli, L., Johnson, G. A. R., and Johnston, I. H. The hyperpolarization of spinal motoneurons by glycine and related amino acids. *Exp. Brain Res.* 5:235, 1968.

54. Desmedt, J. E., and Delwaide, P. J. Neural inhibition in a bird: Effect of strychnine and picrotoxin. *Nature* (London) 200:583, 1963.

55. Dichter, M. A. Experimental Penicillin Epilepsy in the Cat Hippocampus. Ph.D. thesis, New York University, 1968.

56. Dichter, M., and Spencer, W. A. Hippocampal penicillin "spike" discharge: Epileptic neuron or epileptic aggregate? *Neurology* (Minneap.) 18:282, 1968.

57. Dow, R. S. The electrical activity of the cerebellum and its functional significance. *J. Physiol.* (London) 94:67, 1938.

58. Dow, R. S., Fernández-Guardiola, A., and Manni, E. The production of cobalt experimental epilepsy in the rat. *Electroenceph. Clin. Neurophysiol.* 14:399, 1962.

59. Dun, F. T. Restoration of the dorsal root potential after strychnine. *Proc. Soc. Exp. Biol. Med.* 49:479, 1942.

60. Dun, F. T., and Feng, T. P. A note on the two components of the dorsal root potential. *J. Neurophysiol.* 7:327, 1944.

61. Dusser de Barenne, J. G. The mode and site of action of strychnine in the nervous system. *Physiol. Rev.* 13:325, 1933.

62. Dusser de Barenne, J. G., and McCulloch, W. S. Functional organization in the sensory cortex of the monkey (*Macaca mulatta*). *J. Neurophysiol.* 1:69, 1938.

63. Eccles, J. C., Eccles, R. M., and Fatt, P. Pharmacological investigations on a cen-

tral synapse operated by acetylcholine. *J. Physiol.* (London) 131:154, 1956.

64. Eccles, J. C., Fatt, P., and Koketsu, K. Cholinergic and inhibitory synapses in a pathway from motor-axon collaterals to motoneurones. *J. Physiol.* (London) 126:254, 1954.

65. Eccles, J. C., and Malcolm, J. L. Dorsal root potentials of the spinal cord. *J. Neurophysiol.* 9:139, 1946.

66. Eccles, J. C., Schmidt, R., and Willis, W. D. Pharmacological studies on presynaptic inhibition. *J. Physiol.* (London) 168:500, 1963.

67. Enomoto, T. F., and Ajmone-Marsan, C. Epileptic activation of single cortical neurons and their relationship with electroencephalographic discharges. *Electroenceph. Clin. Neurophysiol.* 11:199, 1959.

68. Erlanger, J., Blair, E. A., and Schoepfle, G. M. A study of the spontaneous oscillations in the excitability of nerve fibers with special reference to the action of strychnine. *Amer. J. Physiol.* 134:705, 1941.

69. Feldberg, W., and Vartiainen, A. Further observations on the physiology and pharmacology of a sympathetic ganglion. *J. Physiol.* (London) 83:103, 1934.

70. Fischer, J., Holubár, J., and Malik, V. A new method of producing chronic epileptogenic cortical foci in rats. *Physiol. Bohemoslov.* 16:272, 1967.

71. Fischer, M. H., and Löwenbach, H. Aktionsströme des Zentralnervensystems under der Einwirkung von Krampfgiften. II. Mit Cardiazol, Caffein und andere. *Arch. F. Exp. Path. U. Pharmakol.* 184:502, 1934.

72. Florey, E., and McLennan, H. Effect of an inhibitory factor (Factor I) from brain on central synaptic transmission. *J. Physiol.* (London) 130:446, 1955.

73. Frankenhaeuser, B. Limitations of method of strychnine neuronography. *J. Neurophysiol.* 14:73, 1951.

74. Friedlander, W. J. Epilepsy. In Spiegel, E. A. (Ed.), *Progress in Neurology and Psychiatry*, vol. 22. New York: Grune & Stratton, 1967, p. 217.

75. Fromherz, H. The action of veratrine, curare and strychnine on the response of medullated nerve. *J. Physiol.* (London) 79:67, 1933.

76. Fuortes, M. G. F., and Nelson, P. G. Strychnine: Its action on spinal motoneurons of cats. *Science* 140:806, 1963.

77. Furshpan, E. J., and Furukawa, T. The intracellular and extracellular responses of the several regions of the Mauthner cell of goldfish. *J. Neurophysiol.* 25:732, 1962.

78. Furukawa, T., Fukami, Y., and Asada, Y. Effects of strychnine and procaine on collateral inhibition of the Mauthner cell of goldfish. *Jap. J. Physiol.* 14:386, 1964.

79. Gerin, P. Microelectrode investigations on the mechanisms of the electrically induced epileptiform seizure ("afterdischarge"). *Arch. Ital. Biol.* 98:21, 1960.

80. Gernandt, B. E., and Terzuolo, C. A. Effect of vestibular stimulation on strychnine-induced activity of the spinal cord. *Amer. J. Physiol.* 183:1, 1955.

81. Gozzano, M. Ricerche sui fenomeni elettrici della corteccia cerebrale. *Riv. Neurol.* 8:212, 1935.

82. Green, J. D., Mancia, M., and von Baumgarten, R. Recurrent inhibition in the olfactory bulb. I. Effects of antidromic stimulation of the lateral olfactory tract. *J. Neurophysiol.* 25:467, 1962.

83. Grundfest, H. Synaptic and Ephaptic Transmission. In Field, J., et al. (Eds.), *Handbook of Physiology.* Washington, D.C.: Amer. Physiol. Soc., 1959, chap. V.

84. Grundfest, H. Some Determinants of Repetitive Electrogenesis and Their Role in the Electrical Activity of the Central Nervous System. In Servit, Z. (Ed.), *Comparative and Cellular Pathophysiology of Epilepsy.* Amsterdam: Excerpta Medica, 1966.

85. Guerrero-Figueroa, R., Barros, A., Heath, R. G., and Gonzales, G. Experimental subcortical epileptiform focus. *Epilepsia* (Amst.) 5:112, 1964.

86. Heinbecker, P., and Bartley, S. H. Mode of action of strychnine on the nervous system. *Amer. J. Physiol.* 125:172, 1939.

87. Hertz, L. Possible role of neuroglia: A potassium-mediated neuronal-neuroglial-neuronal impulse transmission system. *Nature* (London) 206:1091, 1965.

88. Honour, A. J., and McLennan, H. The effects of γ-aminobutyric acid and other compounds on structures of the mammalian nervous system which are inhibited by Factor I. *J. Physiol.* (London) 150:306, 1960.

89. Humphrey, D. R. Unpublished data, 1968.

90. Jalavisto, E. Reflex motor discharges in single nerve fibers of the frog in strychnine poisoning and in other convulsive states. *Acta Physiol. Scand.* 9:313, 1945.
91. Johnson, W. L., and O'Leary, J. L. Assay of convulsants using single unit activity. *Arch. Neurol.* (Chicago) 12:113, 1965.
92. Kandel, E., and Spencer, W. A. Synaptic Inhibition in Seizures. In Jasper, H. H., Ward, A. A., Jr., and Pope, A. (Eds.), *Basic Mechanisms of the Epilepsies.* Boston: Little, Brown, 1969.
93. Kawai, I., and Sasaki, K. Effects of strychnine upon supraspinal inhibition. *Jap. J. Physiol.* 14:309, 1964.
94. Kellerth, J. O. Strychnine-resistant postsynaptic inhibition in the spinal cord. *Acta Physiol. Scand.* 63:469, 1965.
95. Kellerth, J. O., and Szumski, A. J. Two types of stretch-activated post-synaptic inhibitions in spinal motoneurones as differentiated by strychnine. *Acta Physiol. Scand.* 66:133, 1966.
96. Kendrick, J. F., and Gibbs, F. A. Interrelations of mesial temporal and orbital areas of man revealed by strychnine spikes. *Arch. Neurol. Psychiat.* 79:518, 1958.
97. King, R. B., Schricker, J. L., and O'Leary, J. L. An experimental study of the transition from normal to convulsoid cortical activity. *J. Neurophysiol.* 16:286, 1953.
98. Koizumi, K. Tetanus and hyperresponsiveness of the mammalian spinal cord produced by strychnine, guanidine and cold. *Amer. J. Physiol.* 183:35, 1955.
99. Kornmüller, A. E. Der Mechanismus des epileptischen Anfalles auf Grund bioelektrischer Untersuchungen am Zentralnervensystem. *Fortschr. Neurol. Psychiat.* 7:414, 1935.
100. Krauthamer, G. M. Inhibition of evoked potentials by striatal stimulation and its blockage by strychnine. *Science* 142:1175, 1963.
101. Kreindler, A. *Experimental Epilepsy,* Progress in Brain Research, vol. 19. Amsterdam: Elsevier, 1965.
102. Kuno, M. Effects of strychnine on the intracellular potentials of spinal motoneurons of the toad. *Jap. J. Physiol.* 7:42, 1957.
103. Landau, W. M., Bishop, G. H., and Clare, M. H. Analysis of the form and distribution of evoked cortical potentials under the influence of polarizing currents. *J. Neurophysiol.* 27:788, 1964.
104. Lapique, L., and Lapique, M. Action locale de la strychnine sur le nerf; hétérochronisme non curarisant; poisons pseudocurarisants. *C. R. Soc. Biol.* (Paris) 74:1012, 1913.
105. Li, C.-L. Cortical intracellular potentials and their responses to strychnine. *J. Neurophysiol.* 22:436, 1959.
106. Llinas, R. Mechanisms of supraspinal actions upon spinal cord activities. Pharmacological studies on reticular inhibition of alpha extensor motoneurones. *J. Neurophysiol.* 27:1127, 1964.
107. Lux, H. D., and Pollen, D. A. Electrical constants of neurons in the motor cortex of the cat. *J. Neurophysiol.* 29:207, 1966.
108. McLennan, H. The effect of some catecholamines upon a monosynaptic reflex pathway in the spinal cord. *J. Physiol.* (London) 158:411, 1961.
109. McLennan, H. On the action of 3-hydroxytyramine and dichloroisopropyl-noradrenaline on spinal reflexes. *Experientia* 18:278, 1962.
110. Maruhashi, J., Otani, T., and Yamasa, M. On the effects of strychnine upon the myelinated nerve fibers of toads. *Jap. J. Physiol.* 6:175, 1956.
111. Matsumoto, H. Intracellular events during the activation of cortical epileptiform discharges. *Electroenceph. Clin. Neurophysiol.* 17:294, 1964.
112. Matsumoto, H., and Ajmone-Marsan, C. Cortical cellular phenomena in experimental epilepsy: Interictal manifestations. *Exp. Neurol.* 9:286, 1964.
113. Matsumoto, H., and Ajmone-Marsan, C. Cortical cellular phenomena in experimental epilepsy: Ictal manifestations. *Exp. Neurol.* 9:305, 1964.
114. Matsumoto, H., Ayala, G. F., and Gumnit, R. J. Neuronal behavior and triggering mechanism in cortical epileptic focus. In preparation.
115. Mutani, R. Cobalt experimental amygdaloid epilepsy in the cat. *Epilepsia* (Amst.) 8:73, 1967.
116. Mutani, R. Cobalt experimental hippocampal epilepsy in the cat. *Epilepsia* (Amst.) 8:223, 1967.
117. Noel, G. Etude oscillographique de l'épilepsie corticale chez le chat. *Arch. Int. Physiol.* 51:162, 1941.
118. Orkand, R. K. Neuroglial-Neuronal Interactions. In Jasper, H. H., Ward, A. A.,

Jr., and Pope, A. (Eds.), *Basic Mechanisms of the Epilepsies*. Boston: Little, Brown, 1969.

119. Peugnet, H. B., and Coppée, G. E. Effects of strychnine on peripheral nerve. *Amer. J. Physiol.* 116:120, 1936.

120. Pollen, D. A., and Ajmone-Marsan, C. Cortical inhibitory postsynaptic potentials and strychninization. *J. Neurophysiol.* 28:342, 1965.

121. Pollen, D. A., and Lux, H. D. Conductance changes during inhibitory postsynaptic potentials in normal and strychninized cortical neurons. *J. Neurophysiol.* 29:369, 1966.

122. Prince, D. A. Long duration periodic changes in excitability of penicillin spike foci: Cyclical spike driving. *Electroenceph. Clin. Neurophysiol.* 19:139, 1965.

123. Prince, D. A. Cyclical spike driving in chronically isolated cortex. *Epilepsia* (Amst.) 6:226, 1965.

124. Prince, D. A. Modification of focal cortical epileptogenic discharge by afferent influences. *Epilepsia* (Amst.) 7:181, 1966.

125. Prince, D. A. The depolarization shift in "epileptic" neurons. *Exp. Neurol.* 21:467, 1968.

126. Prince, D. A. Electrophysiology of "epileptic" neurons: Spike generation. *Electroenceph. Clin. Neurophysiol.* 26:476, 1969.

127. Prince, D. A., and Futamachi, K. Intracellular recordings in chronic focal epilepsy. *Brain Res.* 11:681, 1968.

128. Prince, D. A., and Wilder, B. J. Control mechanisms in cortical epileptogenic foci. *Arch. Neurol.* (Chicago) 16:194, 1967.

129. Purpura, D. P., and Grundfest, H. Physiological and pharmacological consequences of different synaptic organizations in cerebral and cerebellar cortex of cat. *J. Neurophysiol.* 20:494, 1957.

130. Purpura, D. P., McMurtry, J. G., Leonard, C. F., and Malliani, A. Evidence for dendritic origin of spikes without depolarizing prepotentials in hippocampal neurons during and after seizure. *J. Neurophysiol.* 29:954, 1966.

131. Ralston, B. L. The mechanism of transition of interictal spiking foci into ictal seizure discharges. *Electroenceph. Clin. Neurophysiol.* 10:217, 1958.

132. Rosenblueth, A. E., and Cannon, W. B. Cortical responses to electric stimulation. *Amer. J. Physiol.* 135:690, 1942.

133. Sawa, M., Maruyama, N., and Kaji, S. Intracellular potential during electrically induced seizures. *Electroenceph. Clin. Neurophysiol.* 15:209, 1963.

134. Scherrer, J. Action de la strychnine sur l'activité spinale réflexe. *J. Physiol. Pathol. Gen.* 44:29, 1952.

135. Schmidt, R. F. Pharmacological studies on the primary afferent depolarization of the toad spinal cord. *Pflueger Arch. Ges. Physiol.* 277:325, 1963.

136. Stefanis, C., and Jasper, H. Strychnine reversal of inhibitory potentials in pyramidal tract neurones. *Int. J. Neuropharmacol.* 4:125, 1965.

137. Stoll, J., Ajmone-Marsan, C., and Jasper, H. H. Electrophysiological studies of subcortical connections of anterior temporal region in cat. *J. Neurophysiol.* 14:305, 1951.

138. Sugaya, E., Goldring, S., and O'Leary, J. L. Intracellular potentials associated with direct cortical response and seizure discharge in cat. *Electroenceph. Clin. Neurophysiol.* 17:661, 1964.

139. Suzuki, H., and Tukahara, Y. Recurrent inhibition of the Betz cell. *Jap. J. Physiol.* 13:386, 1963.

140. Umrath, K. Der Erregungsvorgang in den Motoneuronen von Rana esculanta. *Pflueger Arch. Ges. Physiol.* 233:357, 1933.

141. von Baumgarten, R., Green, J. D., and Mancia, M. Recurrent inhibition in the olfactory bulb. II. Effects of antidromic stimulation of commissural fibers. *J. Neurophysiol.* 25:489, 1962.

142. Wall, P. D., and Horwitz, N. H. Observations on the physiological action of strychnine. *J. Neurophysiol.* 14:256, 1951.

143. Wall, P. D., McCulloch, W. S., Lettvin, J. Y., and Pitts, W. H. Effects of strychnine with special reference to spinal afferent fibers. *Epilepsia* (Amst.) 4:29, 1955.

144. Ward, A. A., Jr. The Epileptic Neuron: Chronic Foci in Animals and Man. In Jasper, H. H., Ward, A. A., Jr., and Pope, A. (Eds.), *Basic Mechanisms of the Epilepsies*. Boston: Little, Brown, 1969.

145. Washizu, Y., Bonewell, G. W., and Terzuolo, C. A. Effect of strychnine upon the electrical activity of an isolated nerve cell. *Science* 133:333, 1961.

146. Westrum, L. E., White, L. E., Jr., and Ward, A. A., Jr. Morphology of the experimental epileptogenic focus. *J. Neurosurg.* 21:1033, 1964.

Discussion

MICROELECTRODE STUDIES OF PENICILLIN FOCI*

DAVID A. PRINCE

Two crucial questions regarding the basic mechanisms of focal epileptogenesis are posed by clinical observations and studies in human epilepsy: (1) What are the pathophysiological alterations in the population of neurons within the focus which give rise to epileptiform discharges? (2) What are the relationships between this "epileptic" neuronal aggregate and cellular organizations outside of the epileptogenic focus? Ajmone-Marsan has reviewed the first of these questions [1]. The problem of the electrophysiological characteristics of epileptic neurons will be discussed here before considering some aspects of the relationships between epileptic and normal neuronal aggregates.

Epileptic Neurons

No unique set of functional abnormalities has been defined by which certain cells in experimental foci may be identified as epileptic neurons. Intracellular data which support this conclusion have been discussed in detail [1, 3, 6, 17, 21–24] and are summarized in the following sections.

The Depolarization Shift

The most obvious electrophysiological feature of focal epileptogenesis at a cortical cellular level is the development of paroxysmal depolarization shifts (DSs) in neurons of the focus, coincident with each interictal epileptiform discharge. DSs have been recorded in one form or another in every experimental focus studied with intracellular recording techniques [10, 15, 18, 24, 31]; however, we do not know the precise mechanisms responsible for their generation or whether these mechanisms are similar in the various foci. Potentials indistinguishable from DSs may be evoked in neurons of normal cortex during periods of intense excitatory synaptic drive (Fig. D11-6 and [26, 29]).

The differences between cellular activities in acute and chronic experimental foci discussed elsewhere [24] could be mainly quantitative, related to the concentrated nature of the chemical (penicillin) focus as opposed to the more diffuse area of the cortical abnormality in the chronic (alumina gel) focus. This would explain why a smaller number of neurons appear to be involved in epileptogenesis in the chronic focus and why surface epileptiform transients and associated cellular depolarizations are of much lower amplitude in chronic alumina foci than in acute, chemically induced foci. The possibility that different disturbances in cellular function contribute to DS generation in each experimental model cannot be excluded. The question of which particular experimental system most closely resembles human epilepsy is complex, because human epilepsy is a symptom produced by a number of structural and functional lesions. It is likely that there is no single "defect" which underlies all human epileptogenesis but rather a variety of alterations in neuronal function which can result in epilepsy.

Available data strongly suggest that the DS is a *giant* synaptic potential reflecting response of neurons to orthodromic activation [6, 22]. Results supporting this conclusion may be summarized: (1) DS amplitude may be increased by intracellular polarizing currents (Fig. D11-1*B*, 3–5 and [2, 22]), and the DS may be markedly decreased in amplitude or even inverted to a negative-going potential when it is evoked

---

* These studies supported by PHS Research Grant NB06477–03 from National Institute of Neurological Diseases and Stroke and Research Grant from Epilepsy Foundation of America.

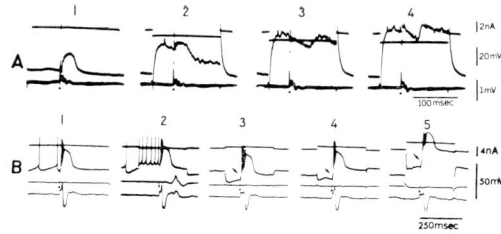

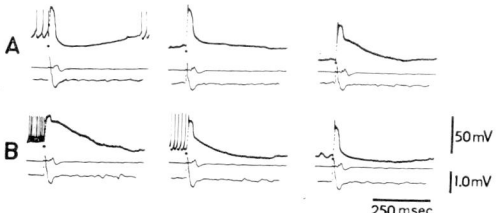

FIG. D11-1. Effects of intracellular current pulses on DS generation. In (*A*1) and (*B*1) stimulation of n. ventralis lateralis evokes DSs. DSs triggered during increasingly intense depolarizing current pulses in (*A*2–4) show decreased amplitude (*A*2) and become isoelectric or possibly inverted (*A*3–4). In (*B*2) depolarizing current initiates repetitive spiking and triggered DS is smaller in amplitude than in (*B*1). During hyperpolarizing pulses in (*B*3–5), DS amplitude increases; however, increment takes place in early depolarizing potential (arrows) preceding first spike. Positivity following DS (*B*3–5) may represent an inverted IPSP. Recordings from cortical surface near microelectrode penetration in third trace of (*A*) and fourth trace of (*B*). Third trace of (*B*) from contralateral cortical surface. (Modified from [22].)

FIG. D11-2. Effects of intracellular chloride injection on post-DS hyperpolarization. Dots: VL stimuli. During chloride injection, hyperpolarization inverts to a depolarizing potential which begins during DS (*A*2–3). In (*B*), immediately after current off, rebound firing occurs. Inverted IPSP reverts to hyperpolarization during recovery (*B*). Surface polarity: positivity up. Lowest trace: surface recording close to microelectrode penetration. Middle trace: contralateral homotopic cortex. (From [21].)

during an intense depolarizing current pulse (Fig. D11-1*A* and [2, 22]). These responses to current injections are similar to those of excitatory synaptic potentials. Several problems in interpreting these results have been discussed elsewhere [22]. (2) In some cells, DSs appear to be composed of a series of summated high-amplitude EPSPs; in other neurons held for long periods of time, it has been possible to observe transition stages from DSs to partial DSs which have the configuration of augmented EPSPs [22]. (3) DSs may be dissociated from spike electrogenesis in deteriorating neurons [18, 22]; the DS is not a type of summed spike afterpotential [22].

Synaptic Activity and Spike Potentials in DS Generating Neurons. Since DS generation is not unique to the cells of the focus, some other criterion of abnormality would be necessary to distinguish primarily involved cells from those which are passively driven by excitatory synaptic barrage. Neurons of the penicillin focus appear to have no remarkable properties, other than their capacity to generate DSs. When not involved in epileptogenesis they participate in normal, spontaneous and evoked, cortical activities and generate synaptic potentials which are indistinguishable from those of neurons in normal cortex [6, 17, 21, 22].

Inhibitory postsynaptic potentials (IPSPs) are not obviously altered during interictal epileptogenesis; in fact the large hyperpolarizations which usually follow DSs in these cells have been identified as IPSPs (Fig. D11-2 and [21]). Spike-generating mechanisms are likewise normal in most involved neurons [3, 6, 18, 23]. Dendritic spike generation may occur in some cells [23]; however, this phenomenon is not peculiar to penicillin-treated cortex and may occur reversibly during seizures in "normal" hippocampal neurons [28]. Responses of neurons in the penicillin focus to direct stimulation through the micropipette are not obviously different from normal neurons. Depolarizing currents up to 3×10^{-8} amp, which produce high frequency spike generation, have never elicited a DS (Fig. D11-1*B*2 and [22]).

EPILEPTIC NEURONS IN CHRONIC FOCI. In the chronic focus, similar uncertainties exist as to the definition of epileptic neurons. No direct evidence is available to support the hypothesis that cells in the alumina focus of monkey are *hyperexcitable*—that is, more responsive than normal to direct (intracellular) stimulation or orthodromic and antidromic activation. The characteristic rhythmic spike bursts which Ward and his collaborators have described in cells of the alumina focus [32, 33, 35] are not necessarily due to functional abnormalities in the involved neurons. Our intracellular data indicate that this bursting behavior may be synaptically driven [24]; however, the mechanisms which are responsible for these rhythmic sequences of synaptic potentials are unknown. "Bursting" neurons may generate normal-appearing spike and synaptic potentials when they are not involved in epileptogenesis [24].

MECHANISMS OF DS GENERATION. If DSs are synaptic potentials, then some disorder of synaptic function or some means of producing intense synchronization of synaptic drives must be present in the focus to account for large DS amplitudes. Attempts to define the nature of this disorder have been unsuccessful because of complexity of cortical organization and certain methodological limitations. Several general types of abnormality might be proposed.

Steady State Depolarization in the Epileptic Neuronal Aggregate. If epileptogenic agents produced a general disturbance in cellular function (decreased metabolic activity; blockade of electrogenic ionic pumps; or mechanical injury to the membrane), a decrease in membrane potential in a large group of cells might result without specific alterations in chemically excitable (subsynaptic) membrane. These neurons would be biased toward their firing level, and normal excitatory drives would tend to produce repetitive spike generation. Given the correct synaptic circuitry with recurrent facilitatory interactions, such a population might generate DSs and epileptiform discharge. The finding of steady potential negativity at the epileptogenic focus [16] might be relevant to this hypothesis (but see [27]). Because of variability in measurements of membrane potentials in cortical neurons, relative depolarization in the epileptic neuronal aggregate might be difficult to document; at least in the case of strychnine no effects on membrane potential have been reported [1].

Postsynaptic Membrane Abnormalities. Occurrence of normal PSPs in DS-generating neurons makes it unlikely that DSs result from a general abnormality of subsynaptic membrane. However, it might be possible for only portions of the membrane to be selectively affected by a convulsant agent as has been suggested for strychnine [1, 9, 19], either because of specific pharmacological sensitivity or exposure of only certain parts of the neuron to effective drug concentrations.

Presynaptic Abnormalities. Most of the available data are compatible with the hypothesis that differences between DSs and EPSPs depend upon characteristics of the presynaptic volley onto the impaled neuron [6, 17, 20, 22]. Intracellular recording techniques are of little value in assessing the function of portions of the cell membrane whose malfunction could produce presynaptic abnormalities. A number of defects in transmitter production, release, and inactivation could theoretically result in excessive postsynaptic depolarizations. For example, small degrees of alteration in function of axonal presynaptic terminals, not detectable by an intrasomatic electrode, might produce large changes in gain of the system because of resulting effects on excitation-secretion coupling [9].

It is well known that in certain preparations a variety of drugs selectively affect activities of presynaptic terminals so that repetitive firing may occur spontaneously or following a single orthodromic volley. These effects have been demonstrated with veratrine, barium, and guanidine in nerve-muscle preparations [7, 8] and with guanidine in dorsal-root afferent terminals of the cat spinal cord [4]. It is of interest that guanidine can produce rhythmic one-per-second discharges from dorsal roots without ventral-root discharge [4]. The possibility that such effects on presynaptic terminals might give rise to convulsive activity in any complex neuronal organization was suggested by Grundfest and Reuben [12] and recently discussed by Grundfest [11].

Examples of repetitive activity originating from the area of nerve terminals are

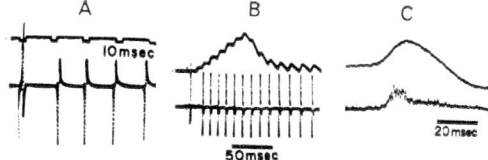

Fig. D11-3. (A) and (B) Repetitive antidromic activity following a single orthodromic impulse in lobster axon-muscle preparation, after application of drugs to presynaptic terminals. (A) After application of serotonin and picrotoxin. Orthodromic direction indicated by initial negativity (upward) of diphasic spike. Single orthodromic spike is followed by first four spikes of an antidromic burst. (B) Phenylethylamine and picrotoxin. Simultaneous recording from muscle fiber (upper trace, intracellular recording) and exciter axon (lower trace). Single orthodromic impulse is followed by a train of antidromic spikes which initiate summated EPSPs in the fiber. (C) Top: Single epileptiform transient recorded from nuclei gracilus cuneatus of cat after injection of strychnine directly into the nucleus. Bottom: Simultaneous recording from seventh lumbar dorsal root 2 cm from the cord. An antidromically running spike is seen in the root. (A) and (B) modified from Grundfest and Reuben [12]; (C) from Wall et al. [34].

shown in Fig. D11-3. (A) and (B) from Grundfest and Reuben [12] demonstrate that a single orthodromic volley in a lobster nerve-muscle preparation may be followed by repetitive antidromic spikes under conditions of drug application. Simultaneous intracellular recordings in the muscle fiber (B) show that bursts of spikes initiated summated EPSPs in the fiber. In Fig. D11-3C from Wall et al. [34], the upper trace shows an epileptiform potential recorded in the area of nucleus cuneatis gracilis after local strychnine injection. This local potential was followed by a burst of antidromic impulses which were conducted via the dorsal column into the cut lumbar dorsal root (lower trace). It was suggested that the antidromic volley originated in the terminal arborization of dorsal column fibers at the site of drug injection.

The hypothesis that presynaptic fiber terminals might fire repetitively (either autogenously or following a single ortho-dromic volley) during penicillin epileptogenesis might be examined experimentally in "simple" systems, but would be difficult to test directly in the cortex. It could be predicted that a microelectrode probing through penicillin-treated cortex would by chance encounter such bursting fibers if they were present. With this possibility in mind, we reviewed some of our penicillin focus data.

During surface epileptiform transients, two types of cortical spike bursts could be distinguished in extracellular records. One variety (Fig. D11-4A) had a maximum frequency of 400 per sec (usually less) with a burst duration usually less than 100 msec. These bursts most often began at the peak of the first positivity of the epileptiform transient and component spikes showed decremental amplitude suggesting cathodal block in the spike generator. Such elements were frequently penetrated successfully and typical soma potentials developed (Fig. D11-4B). The second type of spike burst which probably represents activity of axons or terminals often began at the earliest stage of interictal, surface-epileptiform wave (Fig. D11-4C1, D1). Component spikes had a much higher frequency, reaching rates of 800 per sec or more in some bursts without signs of cathodal blockade; burst duration was often much longer than 100 msec so that spiking continued during most of the surface-epileptiform transient. A few successful impalements of such elements were obtained, and in these instances no slow potentials were recorded and spikes had characteristics of axonal potentials.

Evidence suggests that this second type of spike burst originates from axons. However, sustained bursts of spikes at frequencies of 600–800 per sec without cathodal block were not seen in intracellular recordings from cell bodies. It is possible that such bursts are initiated at proximal axonal regions during periods of cathodal block in the soma [36]. These high frequency spike bursts could also represent discharge in axons of interneurons, perhaps those facilitatory interneurons selectively sensitized by an epileptogenic agent which Ajmone-Marsan mentioned [1].

A third possibility, relevant to the dis-

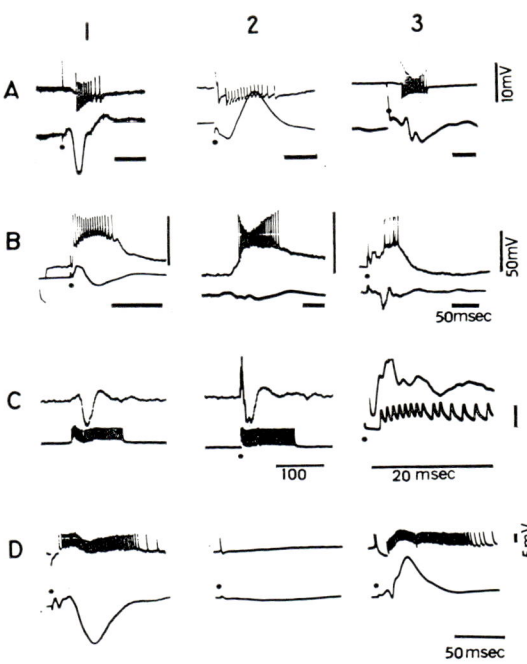

Fig. D11-4. Examples of spike bursts recorded from cell bodies (*A*) and (*B*) and axons (*C*) and (*D*) of penicillin-treated cortex. (*A*) and (*B*) Extracellular (*A*) and intracellular (*B*) recordings from DSs associated with spike frequencies of 500 per sec or less. Bursts are usually less than 100 msec in duration, and spike generator shows evidence of cathodal blockade at higher frequencies (*A*3) and (*B*3). (*C*) and (*D*) Extracellular records from three elements (*C*), (*D*1), and (*D*2–3), which generate spike bursts of much higher frequency and usually longer duration than (*A*) and (*B*) without signs of cathodal block. Dots: VL stimuli. Stimuli in (*D*2) and (*D*3) identical, but epileptiform activity triggered only in (*D*3). Surface polarity: positivity up in (*A*1), (*B*1), (*B*3), (*C*1–2), (*D*1), and down in other traces. Time cal. in (*B*3) for (*A*) and (*B*). Time cal. in (*C*2) for (*C*1) and (*C*2) and in (*D*3) for (*D*1–3).

cussion above and results illustrated in Fig. D11-3, is that these bursts are autogenous or orthodromically triggered discharges in axonal terminals which have been altered by the convulsant drug, so that they generate prolonged depolarizations and repetitive spikes. The observation that these rapid spike bursts may begin during the earliest portion of the surface-epileptiform event (Fig D11-4C1) is intriguing, for it suggests that neural elements involved may have pacemakerlike activities for other portions of the population. Bursts such as those shown in Fig. D11-4C, D would produce intense, prolonged synaptic-activation of other elements.

EPILEPTIFORM DISCHARGE AND NONEPILEPTIC NEURONAL AGGREGATES

Some aspects of the influences of acute interictal epileptiform discharge upon nonepileptic neuronal aggregates should be considered here, to emphasize that functional effects of even a seemingly small epileptiform focus are extremely widespread and that it would be unrealistic to neglect connectivity and consider *the epileptic focus* in isolation from the rest of the brain. The activities of two populations of cells outside the focus have been examined: those surrounding the focus on the same gyrus [26] and those at the site of the projected epileptiform discharge in the opposite hemisphere [25].

SURROUND INHIBITION. Although the large majority of neurons within foci in cat pericruciate cortex generate DSs [18], a number of neurons are primarily inhibited during each interictal discharge [10, 15, 18, 20]. When behavior of neurons at the center of the focus as opposed to that of neurons up to 8 mm distant on the same gyrus was analyzed [26], it was found that the large majority of cells in the surround were inhibited during surface discharge.

Figure D11-5 illustrates recordings from some of the neurons in the zone of *surround* inhibition. Each interictal epileptiform event was accompanied by a large amplitude long-duration IPSP in most of the neurons examined. Typical examples of this behavior are shown in the intracellular records of Fig. D11-5B. These IPSPs were of larger amplitude and longer duration than those which occurred spontaneously in the same neurons or even those triggered by stimulation of nucleus ventralis lateralis (Fig. D11-5B, first segment). In most cells the IPSP was preceded by a brief EPSP, which sometimes reached the firing level to trigger a single-unit spike. During pro-

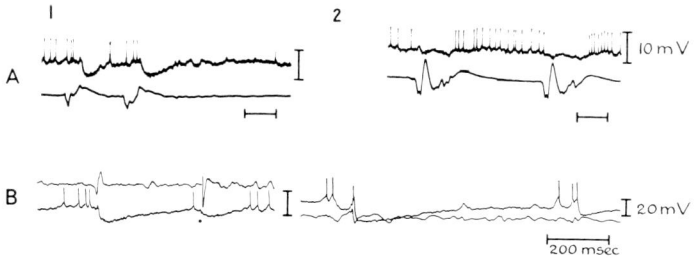

FIG. D11-5. Examples of extracellular (*A*) and intracellular activities (*B*) in neurons in zone of surround inhibition bordering a penicillin epileptogenic focus. Intracellular recordings (*B*) show that portions of each surface epileptiform event are associated with a small EPSP followed by a prolonged IPSP. Dot in (*B*): stimulus to VL. Surface polarity: positivity down. (Modified from [26].)

longed IPSPs, cells were less responsive to spontaneous or evoked excitatory drives; therefore their participation in normal activities was interrupted. These powerful inhibitory potentials had wide distribution and were recorded from neurons at all cortical depths. Similar zones of inhibitory activity surrounding an area of excitation have been described in normal neocortex [14] and in hippocampal penicillin foci [5]. When *ictal episodes* occurred in the focus, behavior of cells in the area of surround inhibition changed.

In Fig. D11-6 a cell which is primarily inhibited during interictal discharges (*A*) is gradually recruited into the epileptic neuronal aggregate, so that during the course of seizure it shows large depolarizations (Fig. D11-6*C–E*) identical to DSs which occur in cells of the focus. During the course of this conversion from an inhibited neuron to a DS-generating neuron,

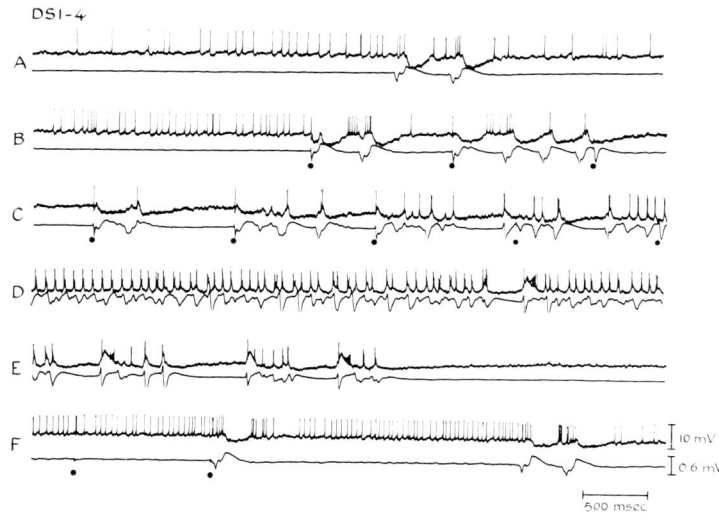

FIG. D11-6. "Partial" intracellular recording (upper trace) from neuron in zone of surround inhibition during spontaneous and triggered single-surface paroxysms (*A–B, F*) and sustained ictal discharge (*C–E*). Dots: VL stimuli. Cell inhibited during late negativity of surface discharges in (*A–B*). During "ictal" episode of (*C–E*), IPSP attenuated and EPSPs become prominent resulting in rhythmic spike discharges. Large depolarizations identical to DSs occur in (*D–E*). In (*F*), during recovery, cell reverts to behavior seen in (*A*). (From [26].)

IPSPs gradually disappear and EPSPs become more prominent. These changes in balance between excitation and inhibition have been discussed in connection with conversion from interictal to ictal discharge in cells of the focus [1]. Attenuation of inhibitory synaptic potentials occurs in normal cortical neurons during repetitive thalamic stimulation [30], also during development of seizure discharges from direct electrical stimulation of the cortex [31]. Elucidation of mechanisms which underlie this loss of inhibition with repetitive stimulation would be crucial to our understanding of focal epileptogenesis.

SYNAPTIC ACTIVITIES DURING PROJECTED EPILEPTIFORM DISCHARGES. Recordings have been obtained from a large number of cells in cat pericruciate cortex contralateral to the epileptogenic focus, at the site of projected epileptiform discharge [25]. In these units of the projected focus it was very rare to see an EPSP which was large enough to fire more than one or two spikes during the epileptiform transient. No DSs were seen. The usual pattern of synaptic activation coincident with projected, epileptiform discharges consisted of a brief EPSP, which might or might not reach the firing level, followed by a large-amplitude prolonged IPSP which interrupted spontaneous excitatory events and spike potentials for a long period (Fig. D11-7D, E). Patterns of synaptic activity of cells at the site of projected discharge were, therefore, quite similar to those observed in the majority of cells in cortex surrounding the epileptiform focus. During projected "ictal" discharge some cells of the homotopic contralateral cortex showed repetitive IPSP generation. In Fig. D11-7A (middle of segment), a neuron of the projected focus generates an IPSP during an isolated, projected epileptiform event. A sustained ictal episode produced by low frequency direct stimulation of the penicillin focus in the opposite hemisphere is associated with repetitive IPSPs and interruption of spike generation (Fig. D11-7B–C). This cell is

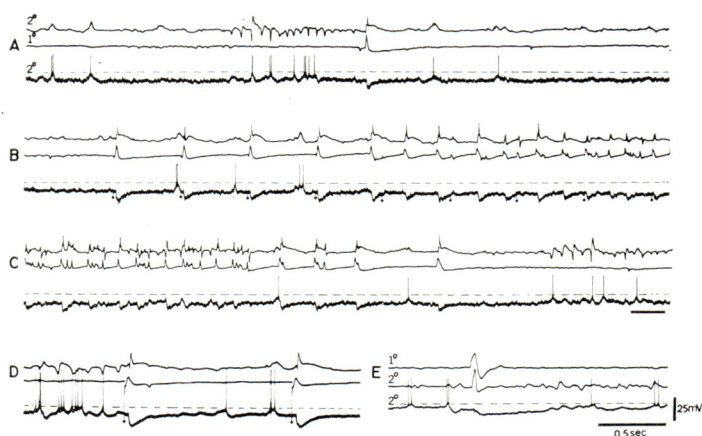

FIG. D11-7. "Partial" intracellular (A–C) and intracellular (D) recordings from neuron in area of projected epileptiform activity during a projected ictal discharge (B–C). In (A), cell generates PSPs and spikes during spontaneous surface waves and spindles. Spontaneous projected epileptiform wave immediately following spindle in (A) is associated with an IPSP. Repetitive stimulation of cortical surface at epileptogenic focus in opposite hemisphere (dots) triggers brief period of sustained epileptiform discharge in (B–C) during which repetitive IPSPs occur and neuron is tonically inhibited. (D) Intracellular recording from cell of (A–C) shortly after penetration. Stimuli to cortex of focus (dots) evoked projected epileptiform discharges and IPSPs. (E) IPSP in another cell during projected discharge. Dotted lines: approximate firing level. 1°: EEG activity for pial surface at site of penicillin focus. 2°: Recordings of EEG and cellular activity from site of projected epileptiform discharge contralateral and homotopic to 1°.

actually involved in an inhibitory seizure similar to those which occur under some conditions in hippocampal pyramidal cells [13].

Within cells of the focus, as well as those in surrounding and contralateral cortex, IPSPs are prominent during interictal discharge (Fig. D11-2 and [21]). In DS-generating neurons the IPSP begins during the preceding depolarization so that time of onset of inhibition cannot be precisely established (Fig. D11-2A3). It is probable that repetitive spike discharges which occur during DSs in most of the neurons of the focus activate the inhibitory circuitry responsible for large IPSPs in the population surrounding the focus, cells of the contralateral cortex, and cells of the focus itself. Although these widely distributed, powerful IPSPs may act to control spread of abnormal excitatory epileptogenic discharge into areas remote from the small focal area of excitation [5, 26], it should be pointed out that they are a form of *inhibitory epileptogenic discharge* which functionally disrupts activities of otherwise normal neuronal populations over large areas. In that sense, they are intimately associated with effects of the acute epileptogenic lesion. It has been suggested that widespread inhibitory activities may account for some of the disturbances in brain function which can occur with unilateral epileptogenic foci in man [26].

REFERENCES

1. Ajmone-Marsan, C. Acute Effects of Topical Epileptogenic Agents. In Jasper, H. H., Ward, A. A., Jr., and Pope, A. (Eds.), *Basic Mechanisms of the Epilepsies*. Boston: Little, Brown, 1969.
2. Ayala, G. F., Matsumoto, H., and Gumnit, R. J. Effect of transmembrane currents on the paroxysmal depolarizing shift in the epileptic focus. *Electroenceph. Clin. Neurophysiol.*, 1969, in press.
3. Ayala, G. F., Matsumoto, H., and Gumnit, R. J. Betz cell spike generating mechanisms during focal seizures. *Neurology* (Minneap.) 17:282, 1967.
4. Brooks, C. McC., and Koizumi, K. Origin of the dorsal root reflex. *J. Neurophysiol.* 19:61, 1956.
5. Dichter, M., and Spencer, W. A. Origin and inhibitory restriction of hippocampal epileptic spikes. *Physiologist* 10:155, 1967.
6. Dichter, M., and Spencer, W. A. Hippocampal penicillin "spike" discharge: Epileptic neuron or epileptic aggregate? *Neurology* (Minneap.) 18:282, 1968.
7. Dun, F. T., and Feng, T. P. Studies on the neuromuscular junction. XIX. Retrograde discharges from motor nerve endings in veratrinized muscle. *Chin. J. Physiol.* 15:405, 1940.
8. Dun, F. T., and Feng, T. P. Studies on the neuromuscular junction. XX. The site of origin of the junctional afterdischarge in muscles treated with guanidine, barium, or eserine. *Chin. J. Physiol.* 15:433, 1940.
9. Eccles, J. C. *The Physiology of Nerve Cells*. New York: Academic, 1964.
10. Goldensohn, E. S., and Purpura, D. P. Intracellular potentials of cortical neurons during focal epileptogenic discharges. *Science* 139:840, 1963.
11. Grundfest, H. Some Determinants of Repetitive Electrogenesis and their Role in the Electrical Activity of the Central Nervous System. In Servit, Z. (Ed.), *Comparative and Cellular Pathophysiology of Epilepsy*. New York: Excerpta Medica, 1966.
12. Grundfest, H., and Reuben, J. P. Neuromuscular Synaptic Activity in Lobster. In Florey, E. (Ed.), *Nervous Inhibition*. New York: Pergamon, 1961.
13. Kandel, E. R., and Spencer, W. A. Excitation and inhibition of single pyramidal cells during hippocampal seizure. *Exp. Neurol.* 4:162, 1961.
14. Krnjević, K., Randic, M., and Straughan, D. W. An inhibitory process in the cerebral cortex. *J. Physiol.* (London) 184:16, 1966.
15. Li, C.-L. Cortical intracellular potentials and their responses to strychnine. *J. Neurophysiol.* 22:436, 1959.
16. Mahnke, J. H., and Ward, A. A., Jr., Standing potential characteristics of the epileptogenic focus. *Epilepsia* (Amst.) 2:161, 1961.
17. Matsumoto, H. Intracellular events during the activation of cortical epileptiform

discharges. *Electroenceph. Clin. Neurophysiol.* 17:294, 1964.

18. Matsumoto, H., and Ajmone-Marsan, C. Cortical cellular phenomena in experimental epilepsy: Interictal manifestations. *Exp. Neurol.* 9:286, 1964.

19. Pollen, D. A., and Lux, H. D. Conductance changes during inhibitory postsynaptic potentials in normal and strychninized cortical neurons. *J. Neurophysiol.* 29:369, 1966.

20. Prince, D. A. Modification of cortical epileptiform discharge by afferent influences. *Epilepsia* (Amst.) 7:181, 1966.

21. Prince, D. A. Inhibition of "epileptic" neurons. *Exp. Neurol.* 21:307, 1968.

22. Prince, D. A. The depolarization shift in "epileptic" neurons. *Exp. Neurol.* 21:467, 1968.

23. Prince, D. A. Electrophysiology of "epileptic" neurons: Spike generation. *Electroenceph. Clin. Neurophysiol.* 26:476, 1969.

24. Prince, D. A., and Futamachi, K. J. Intracellular recordings in chronic focal epilepsy. *Brain Res.* 11:681, 1968.

25. Prince, D. A., Futamachi, K. J., and Gleason, C. Cortical synaptic activities during projected epileptiform discharges. Abstract *XXIV Int. Cong. Physiol. Sci.* 7:355, 1968.

26. Prince, D. A., and Wilder, B. J. Control mechanisms in cortical epileptogenic foci: "Surround" inhibition. *Arch. Neurol.* 16:194, 1967.

27. Purpura, D. P., Goldensohn, E. S., and Musgrave, F. S. Synaptic and non-synaptic processes in focal epileptogenic activity. *Electroenceph. Clin. Neurophysiol.* 15:1051, 1963.

28. Purpura, D. P., McMurtry, J. G., Leonard, C. F., and Malliani, A. Evidence for dendritic origin of spikes without depolarizing prepotentials in hippocampal neurons during and after seizure. *J. Neurophysiol.* 29:954, 1966.

29. Purpura, D. P., and Shofer, R. J. Intracellular recording from thalamic neurons during reticulocortical activation. *J. Neurophysiol.* 26:494, 1963.

30. Purpura, D. P., Shofer, R. J., and Musgrave, F. S. Cortical intracellular potentials during augmenting and recruiting responses. II. Patterns of synaptic activities in pyramidal and nonpyramidal tract neurons. *J. Neurophysiol.* 27:133, 1964.

31. Sawa, M., Maruyama, N., and Kaji, S. Intracellular potential during electrically induced seizures. *Electroenceph. Clin. Neurophysiol.* 15:209, 1963.

32. Schmidt, R. P., Thomas, L. B., Ward, A. A., Jr. The hyperactive neuron. Microelectrode studies of chronic epileptic foci in monkeys. *J. Neurophysiol.* 22:285, 1959.

33. Sypert, G. W., and Ward, A. A., Jr. The hyperexcitable neuron: Microelectrode studies of chronic epileptic focus in the intact, awake monkey. *Exp. Neurol.* 19:104, 1967.

34. Wall, P. D., McCulloch, W. S., Lettvin, J. Y., and Pitts, W. H. Effects of strychnine with special reference to spinal afferent fibers. *Epilepsia* (Amst.) 4:29, 1955.

35. Ward, A. A., Jr. The Hyperexcitable Neuron-Epilepsy. In Rodahl, K., and Issekutz, B., Jr. (Eds.), *Nerve as a Tissue*. New York: Hoeber, 1966.

36. Washizu, Y., Bonewell, G. W., and Terzuolo, C. A. Effect of strychnine upon the electrical activity of an isolated nerve cell. *Science* 133:333, 1961.

12

Isolated and Deafferented Neurons: Disuse Supersensitivity*

SETH K. SHARPLESS†

WALTER CANNON suggested, in the 1939 Hughlings Jackson Memorial Lecture, that those forms of epilepsy associated with the name of Jackson might be manifestations of denervation supersensitivity in the brain [14]. Ample evidence in this volume indicates that Cannon's hypothesis is still alive. In the quarter century that has elapsed since this hypothesis was introduced, the ubiquitous role of chemical transmission in the central nervous system has been established. Again and again, the chemical theory to which Cannon contributed has proved essential in elucidating central processes of excitation and inhibition. The concept of denervation supersensitivity developed alongside that of chemical transmission; the phenomenon was described in the paper where Elliott proved that epinephrine mimics the action of sympathetic nerve impulses [25]. This concept must be considered an important adjunct to the theory of chemical transmission.

Significant developments related to denervation supersensitivity have been made during the last decade, but there is an impression that information derived from research on denervation supersensitivity is less widely disseminated than information on other aspects of chemical transmission. Furthermore, the tendency has been for the field to be fractionated into subspecialties dependent on the tissue being studied: skeletal muscle [43, 45, 88], smooth muscle [89], glands [26], autonomic ganglia [90], or central nervous structures [80, 85], with less communication between these subspecialties than might have been desired. Part of Cannon's genius was his ability to extract some fundamental principle from a mass of detailed, seemingly disparate observations. It might be timely to reevaluate his suggestion about epilepsy in the light of new discoveries.

THE STATUS OF CANNON'S LAW TODAY

MEANING OF DENERVATION. One of the most remarkable features of denervation supersensitivity documented by Cannon and Rosenblueth in their 1949 monograph [15] was the apparent universality of the phenomenon. It occurred, apparently, in almost every excitable tissue investigated: smooth muscle, skeletal muscle, gland, neuron, and melanophore. This ubiquity led to formulation of Cannon's famous *law of denervation*. There is no advantage in dwelling on the precise wording of the various versions of the "law" [15]; both principal versions were vague in some respects and have turned out to be inaccurate in others. In essence, the law states simply that

---

* Includes research supported by PHS Research Grants NB04341 and NB02583 from National Institute of Neurological Diseases and Stroke.

† Recipient of PHS Research Career Development Award NB15–296 from National Institute of Neurological Diseases and Stroke.

denervation supersensitivity *is* a widespread phenomenon, that all excitable elements become supersensitive when denervated. Rather cumbersome formulas used to express the law represented attempts to extend the meanings of *denervation* and *supersensitivity* beyond the literal sense of these terms, to include phenomena that seemed to represent operation of the same principle but which did not, strictly speaking, involve either denervation or supersensitivity.

In a broad sense, the term *denervation* in the expression *denervation supersensitivity* has come to mean almost any weakening of nervous influence, whether produced by drugs, reduction of impulse traffic due to remote injury, or actual denervation, that is, degeneration of nerve fibers supplying the affected organ. The term *enervation* would have been more appropriate, but for its seventeenth-century sound.

A nerve ending impinging on an excitable structure can exert influence in two ways: as a source of signal or impulse input and as a structure that may influence the cell by its physical proximity and effects of its resting metabolism. Denervation—actual denervation—means loss of both influences; in this field, an important issue has been whether any given example of supersensitivity is caused by loss of impulse input per se (hereafter called *disuse*) or denervation (degeneration of the prejunctional element). In either case, a second issue arises: whether the agent maintaining the normal condition of the cell is (a) the transmitter itself (liberated both during impulse activity and in smaller quantities during rest so that the difference between disuse and denervation might be simply a quantitative one); (b) some trophic factor other than the transmitter; or (c) *removal* of some *sensitizing* factor from the vicinity of the cell, a factor which is allowed to accumulate after denervation or disuse.

Some progress has been made in solving these problems in peripheral structures. In certain autonomic effector organs, two kinds of supersensitivity are now known: one brought about by disuse and the other by denervation. Prolonged pharmacological blockade of impulse input to the effector organ will produce one form of supersensitivity, and degeneration of the motor nerve will add another. The form of supersensitivity caused by disuse per se can be reversed, or prevented from developing, by regular administration of agents which mimic the transmitter. This will be discussed in more detail.

Concerning skeletal muscle, it has not yet been possible to disentangle entirely the roles of disuse and destruction of the motor nerve. Spread of the ACh-sensitive membrane, which Thesleff believes to be the principal mechanism responsible for supersensitivity of skeletal muscle to ACh [88], is produced by botulin toxin [87]. Botulin toxin prevents neuromuscular transmission but also prevents release of ACh from the resting nerve ending; it may also prevent the release of some trophic factor other than ACh. An attempt to achieve disuse of the neuromuscular junction by decentralization of spinal motoneurons produced some expansion of the ACh-sensitive zone of the muscle membrane, but the effect was very slight compared with that produced by denervation or botulin toxin [56]. It is difficult to draw conclusions from experiments of this type; there is no assurance that the *decentralized* motoneurons are entirely silent. Nor is there any assurance that motor fibers do not undergo some shrinkage or other degenerative changes following spinal surgery. Thus, the possible effect of disuse on the size of the chemosensitive area of skeletal muscle is still uncertain.

Disuse affects profoundly the metabolism and structure of skeletal muscle, eventually causing atrophy [40, 43, 45]. It is not clear whether manifold effects of disuse on skeletal muscle include some form of supersensitivity other than that which can be attributed to spread of the ACh-sensitive membrane.

It is evident, then, that supersensitivity is caused by different factors in different structures and that several factors may be operating in the same structure. It has been suggested that the term *enervation* might be substituted for *denervation* in the expression *denervation supersensitivity* to indicate that supersensitivity is caused by weakening of nervous influence without specifying the nature of that influence. We might then distinguish between *disuse supersensitivity* and *denervation supersensitivity*. There would be some overlap between these categories, of course, since denervation can produce some forms of supersensitivity by removing a source of impulses, but there is evidence that it can produce other kinds of supersensitivity as well, due to withdrawal of influences exerted by prejunctional elements, even at rest.

The principal objectives here are to show that disuse supersensitivity occurs in the central as well as the peripheral nervous system, to explore its properties, and to indicate how it may be involved in the development of certain epileptic phenomena.

MEANING OF SUPERSENSITIVITY. The term *supersensitivity* has been overextended as much as *denervation*. Cannon and Rosenblueth used the term in reference not only to a condition in which the quantity of transmitter required to produce an effect was reduced, but to almost any exaggeration of the effect. The agents to which denervated elements were supposed to become supersensitive were identified vaguely as "chemical agents and nerve impulses," and it was claimed that inhibitory as well as excitatory actions would be exaggerated [15].

An apparent change in sensitivity of the disused postjunctional element to nerve impulses could result from any one of several changes in the transmission apparatus: (a) change in the postjunctional element so that it actually becomes more sensitive to the transmitter; (b) change in the mechanism inactivating the transmitter so that it is removed from its site of action more slowly; (c) increase in potency (capacity to deliver transmitter) of the disused prejunctional elements; or (d) some change in recovery processes in either prejunctional or postjunctional elements enabling them to better sustain a response to repetitive stimulation. Various experimental maneuvers might permit distinguishing between these mechanisms, but in many instances such distinction has not or cannot yet be made.

Literally, the term *supersensitivity* might appear applicable only to the first alternative: an actual increase in sensitivity of the disused postjunctional element. Cannon and Rosenblueth implicitly extended the meaning of the term to include the second alternative: retardation in transmitter inactivation. Moreover, although an increase in potency of disused presynaptic endings was not explicitly recognized as a form of supersensitivity, there is evidence that this occurs; classic examples of supersensitivity may involve potentiation of prejunctional transmitter processes as well as retardation of transmitter inactivation. An increase in the capacity of disused nerve endings to liberate transmitter is known to occur in at least one peripheral junction, and it may be a widespread mode of adjustment in the central nervous system (discussed below). Thus, we distinguish between disuse *potentiation* and disuse *sensitization*. The former implies that disused prejunctional elements become more effective in delivering transmitter, the latter that less transmitter must be delivered to elicit a given reaction in the postjunctional element.

It may be objected that use of the term supersensitivity to refer to both phenomena is contrary to Cannon's intention. Logically, the word probably should be abandoned in favor of a term with fewer mechanistic connotations. However, it has become too useful as a signpost to important and relevant literature to be thus lightly dismissed. It should be remembered that it signifies only an *apparent* change in sensitivity of the postjunctional element; the mechanism underlying this change may be quite different. In the broadest sense, supersensitivity signifies a change that tends to compensate for disuse or denervation, tending to restore input to the affected element. This is consistent with previous usage if not previous intent.

It may be that the seductive unifying power of Cannon's law, which brought many seemingly disparate phenomena under a single principle, was derived mainly from the teleological significance of these phenomena. Changes subsumed under the law were of such character that they would tend to reestablish neural (or humoral) control over excitable elements deprived of a dominant or controlling nervous influence. An excitable element isolated from the nervous system is either brought back under a form of nervous or humoral control or it is useless to the body's economy and will undergo degeneration. This principle of *compulsory nervous control* is the teleological residuum of Cannon's law, shorn of mechanistic connotations of the word supersensitivity. A tendency to reestablish control over enervated organs would be a valuable feature of nervous organization; it may be supposed that numerous and redundant mechanisms evolved to endow the nervous system with this property.

MECHANISMS OF COMPENSATION FOR DISUSE AND DENERVATION

After injury or disuse, an excitable tissue may undergo a number of changes with potential compensatory value. The following outline gives an idea of the scope and variety of such changes:

I. *Changes Affecting Sensitivity of Postjunctional Elements.*

(1) Gain of *active* receptors (that is, resulting in expansion of the ACh-sensitive zone of denervated skeletal muscle) [88].

(2) Changes in mechanism coupling receptor occupancy and depolarization (change in molecular structure of membrane affecting electrical properties or stability, that is, affecting calcium binding in membrane) [18, 62, 68].

(3) Changes in mechanism coupling depolarization and activation of contractile or secretory apparatus (that is, change in capacity of sarcoplasmic reticulum to sequester and release calcium) [44, 46, 50].

II. *Changes Affecting Transmitter Inactivation or Removal.*

(1) Loss of inactivating enzyme (that is, AChE) [40].

(2) Loss of neuronal or glial uptake mechanism (that is, catecholamine uptake mechanism in adrenergic nerve endings) [51].

(3) Loss of *silent* receptors (that is, binding sites that compete with active receptors for transmitter) [17].

(4) Change in diffusion barriers or rate of perfusion of denervated or disused tissue by blood.

III. *Changes Affecting Potency of Prejunctional Elements.*

(1) Change in quantity of transmitter released per nerve impulse due to increase in stores, redistribution into available pool, change in mechanism responsible for activating neurosecretory apparatus during impulse, and the like [10, 11].

(2) Growth in number of functional synaptic contacts (that is, brought about by branching of nerve endings and increased capacity of disused or partially denervated elements to accept new synaptic contacts) [19, 40, 41, 42, 67].

IV. *Changes Affecting Capacity for Repetitive Activity.*

Increased capacity for transmitter synthesis and storage or other metabolic changes affecting recovery functions in either prejunctional or postjunctional elements (for example, prolongation of posttetanic potentiation in injured nerve fibers [22]; changes in *slow* or *fast* characteristics of skeletal muscle [40]; capacity of denervated sympathetic ganglion cells to continue responding in the absence of normally essential metabolites [69, 74]; in CNS, capacity of disused optic nerve fibers to sustain repetitive transmitter action [12]; capacity of undercut cerebral cortex to sustain epileptiform afterdischarge, see below).

Many of the changes listed above are known to occur under certain conditions in disused or denervated peripheral structures. In denervated skeletal muscle, for example, there is loss of AChE [40], spread of ACh-sensitive area [88], increase in electrical resistance [68] and decrease in stability [62] of the membrane, increase in capacity of sarcoplasmic reticulum to sequester calcium [50], and increase in capacity of the muscle to accept new neural connections [40]. In skeletal muscle poisoned with botulin toxin, AChE is not lost, but the ACh-sensitive area expands, motor nerve endings branch and send out collaterals, and disused muscle reacts to these collaterals with aggregation of subsarcolemmal nuclei and formation of subneural AChE [19, 40]. These changes are of such a nature that they would tend, under certain conditions, to compensate for reduced input.

Supersensitivity in skeletal muscle has generally been measured by exposing most of the muscle surface to ACh, by close arterial injections. Thesleff has argued on quantitative grounds that this type of supersensitivity could be accounted for by the increased area of ACh-sensitive membrane, the absolute sensitivity of the end-plate region possibly remaining constant [88]. But there are other phenomena regarded as manifestations of supersensitivity in skeletal muscle which could not be thus explained, including increased susceptibility to the contracture-inducing properties of caffeine [44, 46]. Furthermore, the presumed constancy of end-plate sensitivity to ACh is not consistent with the recent observation by Frank and Inoue [30] that denervation of one of the two end-plates on frog sartorius fibers leads to increase in ACh-sensitivity of the remaining intact end-plate.

In autonomic effector organs there is also evidence that denervation supersensitivity involves more than one mechanism. The smooth muscle of the cat's nictitating membrane, innervated entirely by adrenergic fibers derived from the superior cervical ganglion, has been widely studied in this respect by pharmacologists, recently especially by Trendelenburg and associates [89].

It is known that adrenergic nerve endings take up norepinephrine from their immediate surroundings, this uptake mechanism being largely responsible for inactivating norepinephrine, both that which is released from nerve terminals and that diffusing into the neighborhood of the effector organs from the bloodstream [51]. It is now believed that loss of this uptake mechanism accounts for an important part of the supersensitivity that develops following denervation. After degeneration of adrenergic endings, the norepinephrine that diffuses into the region of adrenotropic receptors from the bloodstream attains higher concentration and persists for a longer time than it otherwise would, giving an appearance of increased sensitivity of the smooth muscle. This type of supersensitivity develops abruptly when nerve endings degenerate and is relatively specific for norepinephrine, affecting the response to epinephrine and related catecholamines to a smaller degree [51].

A second mechanism operates here, however, since even after nerve endings have degenerated, sensitivity of the smooth muscle continues to increase for several weeks [61]. This slowly developing change represents a form of *disuse* supersensitivity, because it is produced by any agent that interrupts the flow of excitatory impulses to the effector organ [89]. This includes: (1) decentralization (section of preganglionic fibers leaving the motor nerve intact); (2) long-acting ganglionic blocking agents; and (3) drugs that deplete adrenergic endings or otherwise prevent liberation of transmitter (reserpine, guanethidine, bretylium, and the like). Some of these drugs also produce rapid initial rise in sensitivity, presumably due to a direct effect on the uptake mechanism, but continued treatment results in the more slowly developing type of supersensitivity ascribed to disuse [8].

A form of disuse supersensitivity having similar characteristics can be produced in autonomic effector organs excited by cholinergic nerves (for example, salivary glands) by decentralization, long-acting ganglionic blocking agents, botulin toxin, and hemicholinium [26]. Salivary glands also become supersensitive during prolonged atropine treatment; however, in this case, supersensitivity to ACh may be masked by presence of the blocking agent itself, so that special techniques must be used to unmask the underlying change in the effector organ [26].

Properties of Disuse Supersensitivity in Autonomic Effectors

Certain features of disuse supersensitivity in autonomic effector organs are worthy of special consideration. In recent years, knowledge in this area has been greatly increased by the pharmacological investigations of Emmelin [26], Trendelenburg [89], and Fleming [29, 38] and associates. Supersensitivity produced by disuse has characteristics in common in many autonomic effectors, including cat salivary and sweat glands, smooth muscle of cat nictitating membrane and guinea pig ileum, which have been the objects of most study. There are five salient features:

(1) Disuse supersensitivity seems to be caused by inactivity of the effector organ itself; it is produced by any procedure that blocks the flow of impulses along a nerve that normally exerts a dominant excitatory influence on the effector organ. Its development has been prevented in denervated or decentralized glands simply by *exercising* these organs with daily injections of pilocarpine [26, 73].

(2) It develops slowly, about two-thirds of the maximum increment in sensitivity occurring during the first two or three weeks [80].

(3) It is relatively nonspecific, the effector organ becoming sensitized to any agent that is normally capable of exciting it. Thus, although the normal nictitating membrane does not receive cholinergic input, it reacts to ACh and, following a period of disuse, shows increased sensitivity to ACh as well as norepinephrine and all smooth-muscle stimulants [80, 89]. Similarly, the salivary gland, deprived of its cholinergic input, becomes supersensitive to epinephrine [26]. Because of this lack of specificity, Fleming [29] has used the expression *nonspecific supersensitivity* in referring to what we have called *disuse supersensitivity*.

(4) Disuse supersensitivity is caused by reduction of excitatory influences only. Pharmacological blockade of inhibitory, adrenergic input to guinea pig ileum does *not* produce supersensitivity [29, 38]. This is in contrast to denervation. Denervation would destroy the catecholamine uptake mechanism and thus prolong the action of epinephrine, whether the latter was excitatory or inhibitory.

(5) Disuse supersensitivity is reversible and declines when excitatory input is restored [80].

The cellular change responsible for disuse supersensitivity in autonomic effector organs is unknown. However, the nonspecific character of the sensitivity change makes it impossible to attribute it either to loss of a specific inactivating enzyme (such as AChE) or to proliferation of a specific membrane receptor (such as a cholinotropic or adrenotropic receptor). At present, the most probable site of the change seems to be in the mechanism that links receptor occupancy with activation of the contractile or secretory apparatus. That denervated effector organs exhibit disuse supersensitivity implies that the change must occur in the effector organ itself; however, this does not preclude the possibility that disused autonomic nerve endings also undergo changes affecting the efficacy of transmission.

The uniform character of disuse supersensitivity in structurally diverse autonomic effector organs raises some interesting questions. Superficially, changes wrought by disuse in skeletal muscle, autonomic effectors, and sympathetic ganglion cells (see below) appear to be different; however, exploring the cellular mechanics of these changes may yet reveal features in common. Disuse in autonomic effectors seems to affect excitation-contraction or excitation-secretion coupling. In some sympathetic nerve fibers, disuse causes an increase in the quantity of transmitter that the fiber is able to liberate during excitation. One thinks of the ubiquitous role of calcium in all these things, in neurosecretion as well as in excitation-contraction coupling. For what it is worth in this connection, denervated skeletal muscle becomes supersensitive to caffeine, which is believed to act directly on the sarcoplasmic reticulum, releasing calcium [44, 46]; moreover, the capacity of the sarcoplasmic reticulum to sequester calcium is increased by denervation [50]. These observations point to likely avenues of future research

DENERVATED AND DISUSED NEURONS

Formidable difficulties are associated with the study of supersensitivity in the central nervous system (CNS). Central neurons are relatively inaccessible to quantitative techniques for measuring chemosensitivity, and the transmitters are often unknown. Denervation supersensitivity must be distinguished from disinhibition (that is, release from inhibition due to selective damage to inhibitory pathways), direct injury to vascular system or diffusion barriers allowing more ready penetration of the agents used to test sensitivity. It is simply not possible to achieve partial denervation of central neurons by surgical means without causing other types of damage which might be responsible for the observed effects. Because of these difficulties, there is no single, unequivocal demonstration that partial denervation per se causes central neurons to become sensitized to excitatory agents; in every alleged demonstration there is some uncontrolled variable.

However, a great deal of research has been directed toward establishing the applicability of Cannon's law to the CNS; the weight of the evidence, en masse, indicates that central neurons conform in a general way to Cannon's law. George Stavraky, the Canadian physiologist, pioneered in this area and in his 1961 monograph made a persuasive case that partially denervated neurons in the CNS become supersensitive to various agents [85]; evidence collected elsewhere indicates that central neurons exhibit some form of disuse sensitization or potentiation [55, 80].

However, in illustrating changes that neurons are thought to undergo when wholly or partially denervated or otherwise deprived of input, it is somewhat easier to restrict attention to neurons of the outlying sympathetic ganglia, which are susceptible to a variety of controls that cannot be achieved in the CNS. In several instances, the phenomena could be illustrated equally well by experiments on a population of central neurons, but there are advantages in concentrating on this peripheral junction. It turns out that the effects of denervation and disuse on ganglion cells are complex and difficult enough. They indicate complexities and technical difficulties that are to be expected, and have indeed been encountered, in research on the CNS.

Do Denervated Ganglion Cells Become Supersensitive to ACh?

In earlier experiments on denervated ganglion cells [15], retraction of the nictitating membrane of the cat's eye was often used as an index of activity of superior cervical ganglion cells; elaborate controls were required to compensate for the effector organ itself becoming supersensitive after decentralization. In recent experiments in which electrical activity of postganglionic fibers or demarcation potentials of ganglion cells have been measured, earlier observations implying supersensitivity of denervated ganglion cells have not been confirmed [9, 91]. Denervated ganglion cells often appear to be *sub*sensitive to cholinergic agents.

There are difficulties in interpretation. For example, if ACh acts on presynaptic endings to cause liberation of more ACh, as proposed by Koelle [58], then it would be difficult to compare *direct postsynaptic* action of ACh on chronically and acutely denervated ganglia since, in the latter, nerve endings are intact [91]. Existence of heterogenous (*nicotinic* and *muscarinic*) cholinoceptive sites in ganglia creates another difficulty in interpreting the effects of denervation. Volle [90] cited some evidence suggesting that denervation may render nicotinic sites subsensitive and muscarinic sites supersensitive to ACh, but a recent effort to detect supersensitivity to the muscarinic action of ACh on ganglion cells failed [37].

On the whole, recent evidence, although not entirely unequivocal, fails to support earlier claims that denervated ganglion cells become sensitized to ACh. This is not to say that there are no changes in denervated neurons of sympathetic ganglia. There are striking changes: in metabolism, morphology, and the capacity to store and release neurohumor.

Disuse Potentiation in Sympathetic Nerve Endings

In early experiments on denervated sympathetic ganglia, various procedures were adopted to distinguish supersensitivity of decentralized effectors from supersensitivity of denervated ganglia. These procedures usually led to the conclusion that denervated ganglion cells had themselves become supersensitive to ACh. If this is not so, if ganglion cells do not become sensitized to direct action of ACh, then another interpretation of the earlier findings must be sought.

In a relatively recent and carefully executed experiment of this kind, Murray and Thompson measured intravenous doses of epinephrine and norepinephrine required to mimic effects on the nictitating membrane of ACh administered to the superior cervical ganglion by close arterial injection [67]. It was found that more intravenous norepinephrine was required to mimic the action of ACh on the chronically decentralized side than on the normal side. How is this to be explained if the ganglion cells do not become sensitized to ACh?

There are several possibilities. An increase in diffusion barriers surrounding nerve endings and tissue receptors, or a decrease in vascularity or perfusion rate of disused tissue, would cause the degree of supersensitivity to be underestimated by methods using intravenous injections of catecholamines. A more interesting hypothesis is that disused nerve endings liberate more transmitter per nerve impulse. This would account for the fact that the response of the nictitating membrane to ganglion cell stimulation changes more than its response to intravenous norepinephrine.

The research of Brown and associates [10, 11] on splenic nerve has provided independent evidence that the capacity of adrenergic endings to release transmitter is increased by a period of disuse. These investigators measured the overflow of sympathin in the venous effluent from spleen after using phenoxybenzamine to block catecholamine uptake by splenic nerve endings. Decentralization achieved by surgery or ganglionic blocking agents led to an increase in the quantity of norepinephrine released per nerve impulse. The store of norepinephrine in disused nerve endings was also increased [11]. The surplus store was not something that could be depleted by a few nerve impulses, provided the uptake mechanism was allowed to function, since efficacy of the uptake mechanism in disused endings was also improved. It was capable of maintaining a larger total store despite increased liberation. Disuse thus appeared to make the nerve ending capable of cycling larger total quantities of transmitter through the biophase comprising the ending and tissue receptors.

The effect of disuse on subsequent capacity of nerve endings to release transmitter has been investigated only in the splenic nerve. Increase in efficacy of impulse-induced neurosecretion in the spleen is associated with, and evidently proportional to, increase in the amount of norepinephrine stored in disused endings [11]. In other organs innervated by adrenergic nerves (for example, guinea pig vas deferens, smooth muscle of the cat's nictitating membrane), no increase in stores of norepinephrine following decentralization has been observed [5, 57, 84]. However, the quantity of neurohumor liberated by nerve impulses is not necessarily a constant fraction of the total amount stored; the fraction released could be affected by change in the process coupling arrival of nerve impulse with activation of secretory apparatus.

Collateral Growth in Denervated Sympathetic Ganglia

Following damage in the nervous system, there may be extensive sprouting and rearrangement of nerve terminals. Collateral growth and formation of new connections has been studied extensively in skeletal muscle, and recent work in this area has been reviewed by Guth [40]. It has been argued that neuromuscular connections are continuously undergoing renewal, that the motor nerve ending has a limited life span, after which it is replaced by a new sprout [2]. There must be powerful negative feedback influences at work in mammalian skeletal muscle, limiting formation of multiple connections, since at any one time most muscle fibers possess only a single end-plate innervated by a single motor-nerve fiber. Once a muscle fiber has been denervated, this negative feedback influence is removed, and the muscle fiber readily accepts new connections from sprouting or regenerating nerve fibers. Thus, denervation confers on skeletal muscle the capacity to form new connections; innervation at one site on the muscle fiber inhibits the formation of neuromuscular connections at other sites.

Guth and associates [41, 42] and Murray and Thompson [67] have investigated collateral sprouting in partially denervated sympathetic ganglia. Ganglion cells differ from mammalian muscle in receiving converging input from more than one nerve fiber, but preferential connections are formed with specific preganglionic terminals. Superior cervical ganglion cells controlling the cat's nictitating membrane and pupils receive most of their presynaptic supply from thoracic sympathetic rami, T1–T3. If these rami are sectioned, remaining intact preganglionic fibers from T4–T6 sprout and send out collaterals which form functional connections with denervated ganglion cells. Thus, as in the case of skeletal muscle, denervation confers on neurons of sympathetic ganglia a propensity to accept new presynaptic connections.

If the damaged preganglionic fibers which originally innervated ganglion cells are allowed to regenerate, original connections will be restored, and collateral sprouts will then become functionally inoperative [42]. It is not known whether collateral sprouts withdraw anatomically in favor of regenerated axons, but in skeletal muscle on which similar experiments have been performed, collateral sprouts may remain intact and functional after original connections have been reestablished; thus, denervation may lead to hyperneurotization in skeletal muscle [39]. A form of hyperneurotization of neurons in CNS has been postulated as accounting for increased susceptibility of chronically isolated cerebral cortex to paroxysmal activity (see below).

In sympathetic ganglia, collateral sprouting is not restricted to preganglionic fibers. Following damage to the preganglionic trunk, there is extensive branching and proliferation of catecholamine-bearing nerve fibers derived from ganglionic neurons [52, 72]. These catecholamine-containing fibers come into close apposition and appear to make contact with other ganglion cells and their processes. Since axons originating from cells in the superior cervical ganglion may project caudally through the sympathetic trunk, sprouting may be a reaction either to damage of axons originating in the ganglion or to denervation of ganglion cells or both. The functional role of these catecholamine-bearing intraganglionic collateral fibers is not known.

Changes in Metabolism and Surface Properties of Denervated Ganglion Cells

Profound changes in metabolism occur in skeletal muscle both as a result of denervation and altered patterns of use, as is well known [40, 43, 45]. In general, sustained, strenuous exercise results in increase in oxidative enzymes and decrease in glycolytic activity. Exercise involving short bursts of activity with intermittent rest results in increased glycolytic enzyme activity. Slow muscles subjected to continuous activity tend to rely on oxidative mechanisms for energy, whereas fast muscles rely more on glycolytic enzymes. After denervation, there is a preferential decrease in the predominant enzymes.

Possible effects of different patterns of usage on enzymes controlling energy-yielding reactions in neurons have been little studied, although this subject seems important in view of the energy demands of neurons involved in convulsive activity. In some experiments undertaken to investigate action of methonium compounds (for example, hexamethonium) on denervated sympathetic ganglion cells, Perry and Reinert [69, 74] made observations suggesting that denervation led to a fundamental derangement in the metabolism of sympathetic neurons. In these experiments, intact and chronically denervated superior cervical ganglia were perfused with Locke-Ringer's solution with drugs added to the perfusion fluid. The normal blocking action of hexamethonium was converted into stimulant action by chronic denervation; after denervation, hexamethonium potentiated the action of ACh on the perfused ganglion and often elicited discharge of ganglion cells itself. (This is somewhat reminiscent of the action of D-tubocurarine on denervated skeletal muscle [7].)

An interesting feature of this observation was that the addition of certain amino acids to the perfusion fluid abolished the effect of denervation and restored the blocking action of hexamethonium [74], suggesting derangement in metabolism. Moreover, when glucose and amino acids were omitted from the perfusion fluid, normally innervated ganglia showed rapid fatigue. Transmission failed and ganglion cells rapidly ceased to respond to ACh. In contrast, chronically denervated ganglion cells seemed relatively indefatigable, continuing to respond to ACh in the complete absence of glucose and amino acids.

DISUSE SUPERSENSITIVITY IN THE SPINAL CORD

There is evidence that spinal motoneurons become more reactive to a variety of stimuli following cord section [15, 85], destruction of sensory nerve fibers [15, 63, 85], and a short period of asphyxia (which causes extensive degeneration of interneurons) [16, 33]. In all this research, the usual difficulty is encountered of determining whether altered responsiveness is due to denervation per se or another effect of injury.

Until recently, the prevailing view regarding effects of disuse (in contrast to denervation) on spinal reflex pathways was that of Eccles [21]: that disuse weakens and use strengthens excitatory synapses involved in monosynaptic spinal reflexes and probably other excitatory synapses as well. The main experimental support for this view was the early study by Eccles and McIntyre [22], showing that monosynaptic reflex response to stimulation of Group I fibers in the dorsal root declined if the root was sectioned distal to the point of stimulation (and distal to spinal ganglia). It was acknowledged, however, that this effect could have been due to shrinkage of intraspinal projections of dorsal root fibers. Proponents of the idea that use strengthens excitatory synapses also drew support from analogies (for example, muscle being strengthened by exercise) and theoretical arguments (for example, attempts to apply Pavlovian conditioning paradigms directly to simple synaptic networks). Recently, a more satisfying addition to this subject has appeared in the literature, in which disuse has been achieved by sensory deprivation rather than injury to sensory nerve fibers.

The Effects of Tenotomy on Monosynaptic Spinal Reflexes

Tenotomy should relieve tension on muscle spindles and thus reduce the activity of Group Ia sensory fibers, which constitute the afferent limb of monosynaptic reflex pathways (Fig. 12-1). The experiment was performed independently by Beránek and Hník [3] in Prague and by Kozak and Westerman [59] in Canberra. In both cases, several weeks after tenotomy, monosynaptic discharge elicited by stimulating Group I fibers from the tenotomized muscle had greatly increased in strength. This was true of monosynaptic discharges recorded from the dorsal spinocerebellar tract as well as those recorded from ventral roots [59]. (Both motoneurons and the cells of origin

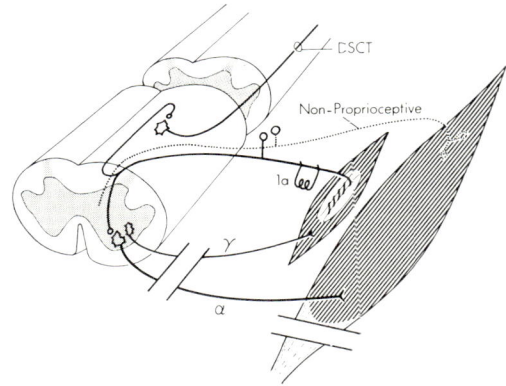

Fig. 12-1. Experimental procedures used to test effects of disuse on monosynaptic pathways in spinal cord. [1, 3, 59].

of the dorsal spinocerebellar tract in Clarke's column are supplied with monosynaptic afferent input from Group Ia fibers.)

Apparently this indicates that monosynaptic pathways had become stronger after a period of relative disuse; however, the Canberra group attempted to explain the results differently, consonant with Eccles' view regarding the effect of use on excitatory synapses. They suggested that increase in reflex strength was due to continuous use rather than disuse, the annulospiral endings in the tenotomized muscle being maintained in active state by increased gamma-efferent discharge, due to a kind of supraspinal adaptation. They cited two facts as evidence: (a) increase in reflex strength did not occur when the spinal cord was sectioned at the time of tenotomy, and (b) integrated spontaneous activity of the nerve from the chronically tenotomized muscle was greater than that from a nerve supplying an acutely tenotomized muscle [59].

It has since been shown by April and Spencer [1] that an increase in strength of monosynaptic discharge of the dorsal spinocerebellar tract occurs even if the ventral root is transected at the time of tenotomy (severing the gamma-efferent fibers to the tenotomized muscle). Thus, the explanation by the Canberra group is not tenable. Failure of the effect to occur in chronic spinal animals can probably be explained on grounds that any difference between the two sides produced by unilateral tenotomy would be masked by profound bilateral effects of spinal shock and subsequent degenerative changes.

The increased integrated activity of nerves supplying tenotomized muscle has yet to be explained. The Prague group subsequently showed that in rats, this activity originated in nonproprioceptive fibers (Fig. 12-1), possibly terminating in free nerve endings in the tenotomized muscle [49]. The possible role of this nonproprioceptive activity in strengthening the monosynaptic pathways is not known; however, it can be said that the synapse is strengthened during a period when presynaptic elements of the monosynaptic reflex are relatively quiescent. To that extent, at least, evidence supports the idea that monosynaptic spinal pathways are strengthened by disuse, contrary to the earlier view of Eccles. Unfortunately, the evidence is flawed by the uncontrolled increase in nonproprioceptive activity.

WITHDRAWAL SYMPTOMS AS DISUSE SUPERSENSITIVITY

Supersensitivity of Central Neurons after Cholinergic Blockade

It will be recalled that autonomic effector organs can be rendered supersensitive by prolonged treatment with agents that block transmission in autonomic ganglia or neuroeffector junctions. For example, the salivary gland can be rendered supersensitive by prolonged treatment with chlorisondamine or atropine. If the blocking agent could be withdrawn rapidly and input suddenly restored to the disused effector organ, an exaggerated reaction would be expected, a kind of *rebound* or *withdrawal* effect. Most of the blocking agents used for this purpose have long-duration action, and, since supersensitivity subsides pari passu with restoration of input, a significant (spontaneous) withdrawal reaction is not seen. However, this observation suggests that withdrawal phenomena following prolonged use of drugs that depress transmission in the CNS may be manifestations of disuse supersensitivity.

In our laboratory, Friedman and Jaffe [31, 32] have taken advantage of the existence of a group of cholinoceptive neurons in the anterior hypothalamus to study drug-induced disuse supersensitivity. Cholinoceptive elements are involved in thermoregulation; in the mouse, they respond to centrally acting cholinergic drugs (of the muscarinic type) by inhibiting certain thermogenic processes, thus producing a fall in body temperature [31, 64]. Hypothermic response to a drug such as pilocarpine is easily measured. It is readily blocked by scopolamine but not by methscopolamine. Since methscopolamine is a potent quaternary blocking agent, it can be used to block peripheral effects of pilocarpine while the centrally mediated effects are being measured. In this way, reaction of the central thermoregulatory mechanism to cholinergic drugs can be measured before and after various periods of scopolamine treatment. It is possible, therefore, to perform experiments on a cholinoceptive central nervous structure very similar to experiments that Emmelin and Muren performed on the salivary gland, which showed that the gland becomes supersensitive following prolonged atropine blockade [27]. Moreover, since scopolamine is rapidly metabolized in mice, responsiveness of the disused central elements to cholinergic agents can be tested during the withdrawal phase, before supersensitivity has subsided.

When scopolamine was administered to mice for various periods ranging from 5 days to 4 weeks and then withdrawn, it was possible to show exaggerated hypothermic response to pilocarpine and other centrally acting cholinergic drugs [31, 32]. An extensive and carefully designed series of control experiments ruled out possible changes in weight, water balance, diurnal cycles, baseline activity, and peripheral effects of the drugs as possible confounding factors. The use of these controls and the large number of animals provides, perhaps, the most convincing demonstration to date of drug-induced disuse supersensitivity in the CNS. It is closely analogous to experiments on autonomic effector organs.

In this experiment, as in others on disuse supersensitivity in the CNS, it has not been possible to distinguish between sensitization and potentiation. It is not known whether cholinoceptive elements themselves become more sensitive to cholinergic drugs or whether their action on other (possibly noncholinoceptive) neurons is potentiated, in the way that the transmitter-releasing capacity of the splenic nerve is potentiated by disuse.

The Disuse Theory of Physical Dependence

There is now reason to believe that many abstinence phenomena are manifestations of disuse supersensitivity in the brain. According to the *disuse theory* of physical dependence, presence of the drug entity is only indirectly responsible for development of dependence; the direct or proximal cause is depression of nervous activity for long periods of time. Any agent that depressed activity in the same pathways, regardless of its chemical structure and mode of action, would produce a similar pattern of withdrawal symptoms. With Jaffe, evidence in favor of the disuse theory has been discussed in some detail [55]. Since a significant prima facie case can be made for the theory on the basis of well-known facts, it is surprising that the connection between drug dependence and disuse phenomena is just being recognized. Perhaps the traditional view of the effects of use on nervous pathways (which goes back to Hartley and even Descartes) stood in the way of prior acceptance.

An adequate theory of physical dependence must account for three facts, which seem to make some form of disuse theory inevitable.

(1) *Patterns of Cross Dependence.* The drug user becomes dependent not on a specific chemical structure but always on a family of drugs, any one of which can be substituted for another, even though they are chemically disparate and follow entirely different metabolic routes in the body. Such drugs appear to have in common only some undetermined neuropharmacological action, that is, directly or indirectly, they depress activity in common central pathways.

(2) *Depressant and Stimulant Drugs.* Withdrawal phenomena characterized by hyperexcitability of central nervous pathways occur only when *depressant* drugs are withdrawn. Withdrawal phenomena associated with stimulants such as amphetamine or cocaine involve only depression, fatigue, and lassitude, with possibly some disturbance of REM sleep patterns, and are generally benign [53, 79]. This postulate has become accepted to such an extent that until recently, authorities were reluctant to consider amphetamine and cocaine as dependence-producing drugs. Thus, in their review, Seevers and Deneau state: "*It may be stated categorically that physical dependence is known to develop only to those drugs which produce overt depression*" ([79, p. 629] italics in original).

(3) *The Rebound Character of With-*

drawal Symptoms. Withdrawal phenomena generally seem to represent *rebound* effects, opposite in character to those produced by the drug itself, as if depressed pathways become hyperexcitable during withdrawal and stimulated pathways become depressed. Thus, morphine produces: miosis, analgesia, respiratory depression, and autonomic quiescence; withdrawal symptoms include: mydriasis, hyperalgesia, hyperventilation, and an autonomic *storm*. Barbiturates have soporific, hypothermic, and anticonvulsant actions; withdrawal produces insomnia, hyperthermia, and withdrawal seizures. Since an exact description cannot be given of the state of central nervous structures during drug action or withdrawal, such observations yield only prima facie validity to the concept of withdrawal phenomena as rebound effects; however, this concept is widely accepted [53].

The three facts just outlined would have been predicted by, and seem to compel acceptance of, some form of disuse theory.

It should be pointed out that Goldstein, Aronow, and Kalman have criticized the disuse theory in a recent textbook of pharmacology, contending that it is less explantory than descriptive. Goldstein and associates have proposed their own theory of physical dependence [34, 35], and they attribute physical dependence to an increase in an enzyme which catalyzes a reaction essential to synaptic transmission. It is supposed that the sole action of the narcotic is to inhibit this enzyme. In addition to impairing transmission, this brings about increased concentration of the enzyme, either due to derepression of enzyme synthesis as the concentration of the end product falls, or to stabilization of the enzyme by the narcotic drug, permitting its accumulation.

Cannon and Rosenblueth, discussing denervation supersensitivity, distinguish between mechanism and cause. A similar distinction is appropriate here. The disuse theory is a statement about *cause*: the necessary and sufficient conditions for development of physical dependence. As such, it is a stronger statement than Goldstein and associates contend, providing an accounting for the three useful generalizations on physical dependence mentioned.

Grounds are provided for predicting if a new drug will produce physical dependence, the nature of withdrawal symptoms, if any, and patterns of cross-tolerance and cross-dependence [55].

The enzyme *expansion* theory is a statement about mechanism, invoking a well-known biochemical mechanism to account for changes responsible for physical dependence. As such, it may be correct; probably many relatively long-lasting changes in neural function involve changes in synthesis or degradation of enzymes, and doubtless the enzyme concentration is often regulated by end product repression. However, much more needs to be said about the specific conditions of enzyme expansion. Which enzymes will be expanded by which drugs?

On this point, there may be some disagreement between the two theories. Goldstein and associates assume that the enzyme whose increase is responsible for dependence is the site of action of the drug, that the principal or sole action of the narcotic is inhibition of this enzyme [35]. This assumption seems gratuitous, considering the patterns of cross-dependence and cross-tolerance exhibited by compounds of entirely different structure which probably achieve their pharmacological effects by acting on different receptors. The difficulty could be obviated by invoking the disuse theory and assuming that an increase in enzyme level could be brought about by reduction in the level of transmitter or other byproducts of impulse activity due to a remote action of the drug (that is, by disuse) as well as by direct action on the enzyme involved. Considered this way, the two theories are complementary: the disuse theory specifies the cause of dependence; the enzyme expansion theory points to a possible biochemical mechanism.

WITHDRAWAL SEIZURES AS MANIFESTATIONS OF DISUSE SUPERSENSITIVITY

Increased susceptibility to seizures is characteristic of the withdrawal of general depressants: barbiturates, alcohol, and the like. The time course of development of physical dependence during chronic intoxication, and force of the analogy between this phenomenon and disuse supersensitivity, can be brought out by measuring susceptibility to pentylenetetrazol-induced seizures after various periods of drug intoxication. The procedure is feasible only with drugs that can be withdrawn rapidly, since with long-acting drugs, supersensitivity would subside pari passu with the fall in concentration of the drug. More dramatic signs of hyperexcitability would be masked by slowly declining concentrations of the drug. The experiment has been made with alcohol by McQuarrie and Fingl [65] and with a short-acting barbiturate by Jaffe and Sharpless [54].

In the latter study, cats were maintained in a state of deep barbiturate intoxication by injections of an anesthetizing dose of pentobarbital three or four times daily through a permanently implanted intravenous catheter. After various periods of intoxication, ranging from 1 day to 3 weeks, the barbiturate was withdrawn, and 18 hours later, the animal's seizure susceptibility was measured by infusing pentylenetetrazol through the catheter. Since the testing procedure itself would alter the time course of development of supersensitivity, different groups of animals were used for each period of intoxication, with considerable attention given to nursing care and controls for food and water intake. The results in Fig. 12-2 show steady emergence of an increased susceptibility to pentylenetetrazol-induced seizures, over a period of 2 or 3 weeks. Results are closely analogous with those obtained from studies of autonomic effector organs subjected to prolonged ganglionic or neuromuscular blockade [26, 89]. The time course of development is also similar.

An interesting feature of both the alcohol and barbiturate experiments was the rapidity with which first signs of supersensitivity appeared. Increased susceptibility to seizures could be demonstrated after only 8 hours of alcohol intoxication [65] and 26 hours of barbiturate intoxication [54]. Martin and Eades [66] demonstrated that characteristic withdrawal hyperexcitability can also be detected after short periods of morphine intoxication, if nalorphine is used to displace morphine from its receptors.

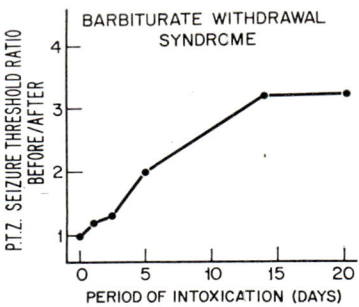

FIG. 12-2. Time course of development of disuse supersensitivity during depression produced by short-acting barbiturate. Each point represents a different group of eight or more cats. Periods of intoxication (26 hours to 20 days) were followed by 18-hour withdrawal period (not shown on the abscissa). Pentylenetetrazol was then infused intravenously and seizure threshold was compared with values obtained before period of intoxication. Significant ($p < 0.01$) increase in sensitivity appeared after only 26 hours of pentobarbital intoxication [54].

Again, in these studies it was not possible to determine whether nerve cells actually became more sensitive to pentylenetetrazol, or whether the cells excited by this substance were more potent in activating their neighbors after a period of relative disuse. Increased capacity for sustained repetitive activity might also play an important role here. Denervated sympathetic ganglion cells, as noted, are able to continue functioning in the absence of essential metabolites for much longer than normal cells. Burke and Hayhow [12], studying the effects of disuse on the lateral geniculate nucleus, observed that transmitter action of disused optic nerve fibers survived repetitive stimulation longer than did that of normal optic nerve fibers. Capacity to sustain repetitive activity might be an especially important determinant of susceptibility to convulsions.

CHRONICALLY ISOLATED CORTEX

According to the disuse theory of drug dependence, presence of the drug entity is only indirectly responsible for development of physical dependence; the direct or immediate cause is reduction of impulse traffic in certain central nervous pathways; any agent that reduces impulse activity in these same pathways should produce similar changes. Theoretically, if pathways depressed by a barbiturate could be rendered inactive by other means (such as by surgical deprivation of input or sensory deprivation), changes would be expected in excitability of the type occurring during development of physical dependence.

The principal change in excitability responsible for physical dependence on barbiturates occurs in subcortical structures rather than in cerebral cortex itself [28, 82]. It is doubtful whether the pattern of depression produced in these subcortical structures by barbiturates could be mimicked by surgical deafferentation without widespread damage to structures controlling vital functions. Whether a nervous network susceptible to paroxysmal activity can be rendered more susceptible by surgical deafferentation can be investigated using surgically isolated islands of cerebral cortex. An area of cortex, usually comprising the middle suprasylvian gyrus of the cat, is undercut and circumsected, using care to avoid damaging overlying meninges and superficial vessels. This technique, devised by Burns [13], has frequently been employed in the last decade to study the effect of partial denervation and isolation on cortical neurons. Slabs of cortex prepared in this manner become more susceptible to epileptiform activity over a period of several weeks [24, 36, 81].

The most conspicuous change is in the capacity of the isolated region to sustain paroxysmal activity initiated by a train of electrical pulses. In unanesthetized, unparalyzed preparations, acutely isolated cortex (isolated the same day) will rarely sustain an epileptiform afterdischarge for longer than 20 sec [70, 81, 82]. Epileptiform afterdischarges elicited in intact suprasylvian cortex are similarly limited, provided they do not spread. If afterdischarge initiated in the intact suprasylvian cortex spreads to adjacent regions, it may persist for minutes, possibly because of a shifting focus. Other factors may affect the duration of epileptiform afterdischarges. Thus, animals paralyzed with gallamine triethiodide tend to show longer afterdischarges in both intact and isolated cortex [47]. Changes in pCO_2 affect the duration of epileptiform afterdischarges in intact but apparently not in acutely isolated cortex [83, also unpublished studies by Sharpless and Jaffe]. However, in our experience, duration of electrically induced afterdischarges elicited in isolated suprasylvian cortex of unanesthetized, unparalyzed animals is strictly limited, the average value being about 10 seconds.

A few weeks after the operation, on the other hand, the isolated region is able to sustain an epileptiform afterdischarge for minutes, the average value increasing fivefold or tenfold (Fig. 12-3) [81, 82]. The change occurs gradually, over a period of several weeks. It is not due simply to recovery from traumatic effects of the isolation procedure, because reisolation, subjecting the isolated area to all the trauma of the original operation, does not prevent appearance of prolonged afterdischarges [82].

Echlin has suggested that increased susceptibility of isolated cortex to paroxysmal activity may be due to supersensitivity of

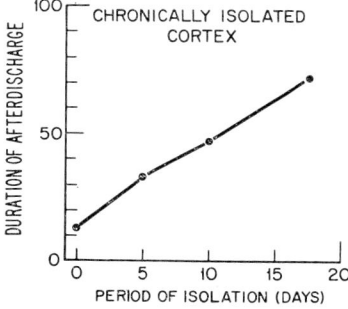

Fig. 12-3. Time course of development of increased capacity to sustain epileptiform activity in chronically isolated cortex. Ordinate represents mean duration in seconds of epileptiform afterdischarges produced by supramaximal electrical stimuli. Each point represents a different group of isolated cortical slabs prepared with aseptic procedures and subsequently studied in acute, cerveau isolé preparations. (Data from published [82] and unpublished experiments. Similar changes observed with implanted electrode techniques [81].)

partially denervated cortical neurons to ACh [24]. There is a marked fall in acetylcholinesterase content of isolated cortex [48, 75], and Rosenberg and Echlin [76] have shown that the time course of changes in acetylcholinesterase activity parallels the increase in susceptibility to epileptiform activity. It should be noted parenthetically that denervation supersensitivity in skeletal and smooth muscle cannot be attributed entirely to a fall in acetylcholinesterase, although this occurs. In effector organs, development of supersensitivity is not usually correlated with changes in cholinesterase content; denervated organs may become supersensitive to cholinomimetic agents that are resistant to cholinesterase [80]. In the central nervous system, however, the situation may be different. In view of these findings and those of Duncan, Rutledge, and Domino [20] described below, the effect of acetylcholinesterase activity on seizure susceptibility of cortex needs to be re-examined.

Numerous other changes occur in isolated cortex during the period when it begins to show increased susceptibility to paroxysmal activity:

(1) Pyramidal cells undergo retrograde chromatolytic changes. Spinal motoneurons undergoing similar changes following section of motor nerve fibers exhibit altered dendritic excitability [23].

(2) Extensive fiber degeneration is in the isolated region, of course, and there must be considerable rearrangement of endings on somadendritic membranes [86]. Purpura and Housepian [71] replicated Ramon y Cajal's observation of prolific growth of recurrent collaterals from severed axons in isolated cortex of kittens; they drew attention to the possible role of collateral proliferation in the development of seizure susceptibility.

(3) In degenerating and regenerating spinal and peripheral nerve fibers, there is a tendency for processes underlying post-tetanic potentiation to be greatly prolonged [22]. Prolongation of afterhyperpolarization in cortical fibers discharged by the electrical stimulus might also contribute to increased duration of afterdischarges.

(4) Biochemical changes in chronically isolated cortex are just beginning to be investigated. There is transient increase in glucose utilization and lactic acid production during the first week after isolation, but this subsequently returns to normal [60]. There are longer lasting changes in levels of amino acids, decrease in glutamic and aspartic acid beginning 4-6 hours after isolation, followed by decrease in gamma-aminobutyric acid and a concomitant rise in glutamine [4].

We are thus confronted with a variety of morphological and chemical changes, each of which might affect susceptibility of the isolated region to paroxysmal activity. Neurons of the isolated cortex are subjected to prolonged disuse, of course, but in view of the profound reaction to injury, there may be an inclination to discount the possible role of disuse in bringing about increased susceptibility to epileptiform activity. However, Sharpless and Halpern [81], using electrodes implanted over chronically isolated cortex, noted that the capacity of the isolated region to sustain long epileptiform afterdischarges declined to almost normal following experimental sessions in which afterdischarges were repeatedly elicited at 15-minute intervals; several days might then be required for the reemergence of increased susceptibility to epileptiform activity. This might be ascribed to some form of rather long-lasting postictal depression; however, Rutledge, Ranck, and Duncan [78], using the implanted electrode technique, found that daily stimulation at *subconvulsive* levels (20 applications of a 2-sec pulse-train daily) prevented development of increased susceptibility to epileptiform activity. Duncan, Rutledge, and Domino [20] subsequently reported that the fall in acetylcholinesterase could also be prevented by exercising the isolated area daily with electrical stimulation. These ingenious and difficult experiments provide the most convincing evidence to date that susceptibility of chronically isolated cortex to epileptiform activity may be a disuse phenomenon.

It is, of course, extremely difficult to apply highly analytic techniques, such as intracellular recording or iontophoretic application of drugs, to phenomena of this kind, involving slow, quantitative changes in sensitivity or potency of neurons. The sampling problem is formidable. Such studies are being undertaken, however, and may soon yield information about the character of changes occurring in isolated and disused cortical neurons. Because the cortex is regarded as the organ of learning, one is inclined to believe that in this organ at least, exercise will generally strengthen synapses. A recent study by Bliss, Burns, and Uttley [6] failed to support this prejudice. They used extracellular unit recording to investigate the effects of intermittent stimulation for various periods up to one hour on the *conductivity* of intracortical pathways in acutely isolated cortex. Changes in conductivity of cortical pathways were inferred from changes in the characteristic poststimulus histogram following a period of conditioning stimulation. The great majority of pathways examined showed decrease in conductivity with use, being less likely to transmit excitation to the unit being investigated the more often the pathway was used. Over three-quarters of the pathways examined behaved in this way; fewer than one-sixth conformed to the traditional formula that use strengthens neural pathways.

It may be that we have been blinded by tradition. It may be that in our preoccupation with learning, we have overlooked a much more primitive and pervasive neural process that enables the nervous system to compensate for the weakening of a pathway due to injury, disease, or poisons. It is likely that processes of this type are widespread in the brain, accounting for the remarkable functional constancy of this organ: constancy of personality, constancy of intellect, and perhaps even fixity of ideas in those over the age of 35, in whom neurons are daily deteriorating, dying, and being poisoned by alcohol. It has been claimed that during every day of adult life, one hundred thousand neurons die [13]. Man takes pride in the ability of his brain to learn, to be changed by experience. Far more impressive is its ability to stay the same.

REFERENCES

1. April, R. S., and Spencer, W. A. Enhanced ascending monosynaptic responses to activation of group I afferents from tenotomized, de-efferented muscles. *Physiologist* 10:111, 1967.
2. Barker, D., and Ip, M. C. Sprouting and degeneration of mammalian motor axons in normal and de-afferented skeletal muscle. *Proc. Roy. Soc. [Biol.]* 163:538, 1966.
3. Beránek, R., and Hník, P. Long-term effects of tenotomy on spinal monosynaptic response in the cat. *Science* 130:981, 1959.
4. Berl, S., and McMurtry, J. C. Isolated cerebral cortex: Changes in levels of glutamic acid, glutamine, aspartic acid and γ-aminobutyric acid. *Arch. Biochem.* 118:645, 1967.
5. Blakeley, A. G. H., and Harrison, V. Effect of decentralization on the noradrenaline content of the guinea pig vas deferens. *J. Physiol.* (London) 197:36P, 1968.
6. Bliss, T., Burns, B. D., and Uttley, A. Factors affecting the conductivity of pathways in the cerebral cortex. *J. Physiol.* (London) 195:339, 1968.
7. Bowman, W. C., and Raper, C. Spontaneous fibrillatory activity of denervated muscle. *Nature* (London) 201:160, 1964.
8. Boura, A. L. A., and Green, A. F. Adrenergic neurone blocking agents. *Ann. Rev. Pharmacol.* 5:183, 1965.
9. Brown, D. A. Depolarization of normal and preganglionically denervated superior cervical ganglia by stimulant drugs. *Brit. J. Pharmacol.* 26:511, 1966.
10. Brown, L. The release and fate of the transmitter liberated by adrenergic nerves. *Proc. Roy. Soc. [Biol.]* 162:1, 1965.
11. Brown, L., Dearnaley, D. P., and Geffen, L. B. Noradrenaline storage and release in the decentralized spleen. *Proc. Roy. Soc. [Biol.]* 168:48, 1967.
12. Burke, W., and Hayhow, W. R. Disuse in the lateral geniculate nucleus of the cat. *J. Physiol.* (London) 194:495, 1968.

13. Burns, B. D. *The Mammalian Cerebral Cortex*. London: Edward Arnold, 1958.
14. Cannon, W. B. A law of denervation. *Amer. J. Med. Sci.* 198:737, 1939.
15. Cannon, W. B., and Rosenblueth, A. *The Supersensitivity of Denervated Structures*. New York: Macmillan, 1949.
16. Collewijn, H., and Van Harreveld, A. Intracellular recording from spinal motoneurons in cats with post-asphyxial rigidity. *J. Physiol.* (London) 185:30, 1966.
17. Collier, H. O. J. Tolerance, physical dependence and receptors. *Advances Drug Res.* 3:171, 1966.
18. Csillik, B. *Functional Structure of the Post-Synaptic Membrane in the Myoneural Junction*. Budapest: Akadémiai Kiadó, 1967.
19. Duchen, L. W., and Strick, S. J. Changes in the pattern of motor innervation of skeletal muscle in the mouse after local injection of *Clostridium botulinum* toxin. *J. Physiol.* (London) 189:2P, 1967.
20. Duncan, J., Rutledge, L., and Domino, E. Acetylcholinesterase activity in partially isolated cerebral cortex after prolonged intermittent stimulation. *Exp. Neurol.* 20:268, 1968.
21. Eccles, J. C. The Effects of Use and Disuse on Synaptic Function. In Delafresnaye, J. (Ed.), *Brain Mechanisms and Learning*. Springfield, Ill.: Thomas, 1961.
22. Eccles, J. C., and McIntyre, A. K. The effects of disuse and of activity on mammalian spinal reflexes. *J. Physiol.* (London) 121:492, 1953.
23. Eccles, J. C., Libet, R., and Young, R. The behavior of chromatolysed motoneurones studied by intracellular recording. *J. Physiol.* (London) 143:11, 1958.
24. Echlin, F. A., and McDonald, J. The supersensitivity of chronically isolated and partially isolated cerebral cortex as a mechanism in focal cortical epilepsy. *Trans. Amer. Neurol. Ass.* 79:75, 1954.
25. Elliott, T. R. The action of adrenalin. *J. Physiol.* (London) 32:401, 1905.
26. Emmelin, N. Supersensitivity following "pharmacological denervation." *Pharmacol. Rev.* 13:16, 1961.
27. Emmelin, N., and Muren, A. The sensitivity of submaxillary glands to chemical agents studied in cats under various conditions over long periods. *Acta Physiol. Scand.* 26:221, 1952.
28. Essig, C. F., and Flanary, H. G. Convulsive aspects of barbital sodium withdrawal in the cat. *Exp. Neurol.* 3:149, 1961.
29. Fleming, W. W. Nonspecific supersensitivity of the guinea-pig ileum produced by chronic ganglion blockade. *J. Pharmacol. Exp. Ther.* 162:277, 1968.
30. Frank, G. B., and Inoue, F. Large miniature end plate potentials in partial denervated skeletal muscle. *Nature* (London) 212:596, 1966.
31. Friedman, M., and Jaffe, J. A central hypothermic response to pilocarpine in the mouse. *J. Pharmacol. Exp. Ther.* 167:34, 1969.
32. Friedman, M., Jaffe, J., and Sharpless, S. K. Central nervous system supersensitivity to pilocarpine after withdrawal of chronically administered scopolamine. *J. Pharmacol. Exp. Ther.* 167:45, 1969.
33. Gelfan, S., and Tarlov, I. M. Altered neuron population in L_7 segment of dogs with experimental hind-limb rigidity. *Amer. J. Physiol.* 205:606, 1963.
34. Goldstein, D. B., and Goldstein, A. Possible role of enzyme inhibition and repression in drug tolerance and addiction. *Biochem. Pharmacol.* 8:48, 1961.
35. Goldstein, A., Aranow, L., and Kalman, S. *Principles of Drug Action*. New York: Hoeber Med. Div., Harper & Row, 1968.
36. Grafstein, B., and Sastry, P. Some preliminary electrophysiological studies on chronically neuronally isolated cerebral cortex. *Electroenceph. Clin. Neurophysiol.* 9:723, 1957.
37. Green, R. D. The sensitivity of denervated superior cervical ganglion (SCG) to nicotinic and muscarinic stimulants. *Pharmacologist* 10:216, 1968.
38. Green, R. D., III, Fleming, W. W., and Schmidt, J. L. Sensitivity changes in the isolated ileum of the guinea pig after pretreatment with reserpine. *J. Pharmacol. Exp. Ther.* 162:270, 1968.
39. Guth, L. Neuromuscular function after regeneration of interrupted nerve fibers into partially denervated muscle. *Exp. Neurol.* 6:129, 1962.
40. Guth, L. "Trophic" influence of nerve on muscle. *Physiol. Rev.* 48:645, 1968.
41. Guth, L., and Bailey, C. J. Pupillary function after alteration of the preganglionic sympathetic innervation. *Exp. Neurol.* 3:325, 1961.

42. Guth, L., and Bernstein, J. J. Selectivity in the re-establishment of synapses in the superior cervical ganglion of the cat. *Exp. Neurol.* 4:59, 1961.
43. Gutmann, E. (Ed.), *The Denervated Muscle*. Prague: Czech. Acad. Sci., 1961.
44. Gutmann, E., and Hanzlíková, V. Contracture responses of fast and slow mammalian muscles. *Physiol. Bohemoslov.* 15:404, 1966.
45. Gutmann, E., and Hník, P. (Eds.), *The Effects of Use and Disuse upon Neuromuscular Functions*. Prague: Czech. Acad. Sci., 1963.
46. Gutmann, E., and Sandow, A. Caffeine-induced contractures and potentiation of contraction in normal and denervated rat muscle. *Life Sci.* 4:1149, 1965.
47. Halpern, L., and Black, R. Flaxedil (gallamine triethiodide): Evidence for a central action. *Science* 155:1685, 1967.
48. Hebb, C. O., Krnjević, K., and Silver, A. Effect of undercutting on the acetylcholinesterase and choline acetyltransferase activity in the cat's cerebral cortex. *Nature* (London) 198:692, 1963.
49. Hník, P., Beránek, L., Vyklický, L., and Zelená, J. Sensory outflow from chronically tenotomized muscles. *Physiol. Bohemoslov.* 12:23, 1963.
50. Howell, J. N., Fairhurst, A. S., and Jenden, D. J. Alterations of the calcium accumulating ability of striated muscle following denervation. *Life Sci.* 5:439, 1966.
51. Iversen, L. L. *The Uptake and Storage of Noradrenaline in Sympathetic Nerve*. London: Cambridge University Press, 1967.
52. Jacobowitz, D., and Woodward, J. K. Adrenergic neurons in the cat superior cervical ganglion and cervical sympathetic nerve trunk. A histochemical study. *J. Pharmacol. Exp. Ther.* 162:213, 1968.
53. Jaffe, J. Drug Addiction and Drug Abuse. In Goodman, L., and Gilman, A. (Eds.), *The Pharmacological Basis of Therapeutics* (3d ed.). New York: Macmillan, 1965.
54. Jaffe, J., and Sharpless, S. K. The rapid development of physical dependence on barbiturates. *J. Pharmacol. Exp. Ther.* 150:140, 1965.
55. Jaffe, J., and Sharpless, S. Pharmacological Denervation Supersensitivity in the CNS: A Theory of Physical Dependence. In Wickler, A. (Ed.), *The Addictive States. Res. Publ. Ass. Res. Nerv. Ment. Dis.* 47:226, 1967.
56. Johns, T. R., and Thesleff, S. Effects of motor inactivation on the chemical sensitivity of skeletal muscle. *Acta Physiol. Scand.* 51:136, 1961.
57. Kirpekar, S. M., Cervoni, P., and Furchgott, R. Catecholamine content of the cat nictitating membrane following procedures sensitizing it to norepinephrine. *J. Pharmacol. Exp. Ther.* 135:180, 1962.
58. Koelle, W., and Koelle, G. The localization of external or functional acetylcholinesterase at the synapses of autonomic ganglia. *J. Pharmacol. Exp. Ther.* 126:1, 1959.
59. Kozak, W., and Westerman, R. A. Plastic changes of spinal monosynaptic responses from tenotomized muscles in cats. *Nature* (London) 189:753, 1961.
60. Krass, M. E., Pinsky, C., and La Bella, F. S. Glucose metabolism in the neuronally isolated cerebral cortical slab of the cat. *J. Neurochem.* 15:1381, 1968.
61. Langer, S. Z., and Trendelenburg, U. The onset of denervation supersensitivity. *J. Pharmacol. Exp. Ther.* 151:73, 1966.
62. Li, C-L. Mechanism of fibrillation potentials in denervated mammalian skeletal muscle. *Science* 132:1889, 1960.
63. Loeser, J. D., and Ward, A. A., Jr. Some effects of deafferentation on neurons of the cat spinal cord. *Arch. Neurol.* (Chicago) 17:629, 1967.
64. Lomax, P., and Jenden, D. Hypothermia following systemic and intracerebral injection of oxotremorine in the rat. *Int. J. Neuropharmacol.* 5:353, 1966.
65. McQuarrie, D. G., and Fingl, E. Effects of single doses and chronic administration of ethanol on experimental seizures in mice. *J. Pharmacol. Exp. Ther.* 124:264, 1958.
66. Martin, W. R., and Eades, C. G. Demonstration of tolerance and physical dependence in the dog following a short-term infusion of morphine. *J. Pharmacol. Exp. Ther.* 133:262, 1961.
67. Murray, J. G., and Thompson, J. W. The occurrence and function of collateral sprouting in the sympathetic nervous system of the cat. *J. Physiol.* (London) 135:133, 1957.
68. Nicholls, J. G. The electrical properties of denervated skeletal muscle. *J. Physiol.* (London) 131:1, 1956.

69. Perry, W. L. M., and Reinert, H. The effects of preganglionic denervation on the reactions of ganglion cells. *J. Physiol.* (London) 126:101, 1954.

70. Pinsky, C., and Burns, B. D. Production of epileptiform afterdischarges in cat's cerebral cortex. *J. Neurophysiol.* 25:359, 1962.

71. Purpura, D. P., and Housepian, E. M. Morphological and physiological properties of chronically isolated immature neocortex. *Exp. Neurol.* 4:377, 1961.

72. Quilliam, J. P., and Tamarind, D. L. Ultrastructural changes in the superior cervical ganglion of the rat following preganglionic denervation. *J. Physiol.* (London) 189:13P, 1967.

73. Reas, H. W., and Trendelenburg, U. Changes in the sensitivity of the sweat glands after denervation. *J. Pharmacol. Exp. Ther.* 156:126, 1967.

74. Reinert, H. H. R., and Perry, W. L. M. On the metabolism of normal and denervated sympathetic ganglion cells. *J. Physiol.* (London) 130:603, 1955.

75. Rosenberg, P., and Echlin, F. Cholinesterase activity of chronic partially isolated cortex. *Neurology* (Minneap.) 15:700, 1965.

76. Rosenberg, P., and Echlin, F. Time course of changes in cholinesterase activity of chronically isolated cortex. *J. Nerv. Ment. Dis.* 147:56, 1968.

77. Rothballer, A. B., and Sharpless, S. K. Effects of intracranial stimulation on denervated nictitating membrane of the cat. *Amer. J. Physiol.* 200:901, 1961.

78. Rutledge, L., Ranck, J., and Duncan, J. Prevention of supersensitivity in partially isolated cerebral cortex. *Electroenceph. Clin. Neurophysiol.* 23:256, 1967.

79. Seevers, M. H., and Deneau, G. Physiological Aspects of Tolerance and Dependence. In Root, W., and Hofmann, F. (Eds.), *Physiological Pharmacology, Vol. I.* New York: Academic, 1963.

80. Sharpless, S. K. Reorganization of function in the nervous system—use and disuse. *Ann. Rev. Physiol.* 26:357, 1964.

81. Sharpless, S. K., and Halpern, L. The electrical excitability of chronically isolated cortex studied by means of permanently implanted electrodes. *Electroenceph. Clin. Neurophysiol.* 14:244, 1962.

82. Sharpless, S. K., and Jaffe, J. The electrical excitability of isolated cortex during barbiturate withdrawal. *J. Pharmacol. Exp. Ther.* 151:321, 1966.

83. Sherwin, I. Differential effects of hyperventilation on the excitability of intact and isolated cortex. *Electroenceph. Clin. Neurophysiol.* 18:599, 1965.

84. Smith, C. B., Trendelenburg, U., Langer, S. Z., and Tsai, T. H. The relation of retention of norepinephrine-H_3 to the norepinephrine content of the nictitating membrane of the spinal cat during development of denervation supersensitivity. *J. Pharmacol. Exp. Ther.* 151:87, 1966.

85. Stavraky, G. *Supersensitivity Following Lesions of the Nervous System.* Toronto: Univ. Toronto Press, 1961.

86. Szentágothai, J. (Ed.), Modern Trends in Neuromorphology. *Symposia Biologica Hungarica*, Vol. 5. Budapest: Akadémiai Kiadó, 1965, p. 251.

87. Thesleff, S. Supersensitivity of skeletal muscle produced by botulinum toxin. *J. Physiol.* (London) 151:598, 1960.

88. Thesleff, S. Effects of motor innervation on the chemical sensitivity of skeletal muscle. *Physiol. Rev.* 40:734, 1960.

89. Trendelenburg, U. Supersensitivity and subsensitivity to sympathomimetic amines. *Pharmacol. Rev.* 15:225, 1963.

90. Volle, R. L. Modification by drugs of synaptic mechanisms in autonomic ganglia. *Pharmacol. Rev.* 18:839, 1966.

91. Volle, R. L., and Koelle, G. B. The physiological role of acetylcholinesterase (AChE) in sympathetic ganglia. *J. Pharmacol. Exp. Ther.* 133:223, 1961.

Discussion

EFFECT OF STIMULATION ON ISOLATED CORTEX*

LESTER T. RUTLEDGE

In response to Sharpless' presentation, attention will be directed toward the mammalian cerebral cortex. It has been found difficult to translate and apply findings on denervated muscle and glands to explanations of epileptic foci or of supersensitivity in cerebral cortex. On the other hand, as discussed by Sharpless, certain techniques, concepts, and theories originating with work on denervated muscle and glands have been effective stimuli for our own sensitivity to cerebral cortical problems. Of prime concern are the related hypotheses of *use, disuse,* and *compensation.*

Compensatory Processes

In regard to compensation, it seems imperative to define for a denervated system *what* is compensated. Further, the *specific conditions* producing compensation must be identified and defined. These restrictions may be difficult to follow but some authors leave the wrong impression, it seems, that irritative lesions, injuries, denervations, and the like of the central nervous system will automatically produce an attempt by neurons to readjust, regrow, or effect new growths in order to establish normal conditions. For the mature cerebral cortex there is not much solid evidence that this kind of compensation occurs.

The most intriguing challenge is to attempt a definition, at the neuronal level, of compensatory processes caused by controlled experimental pathology. For the neuromuscular junction and some autonomic systems this has been done, but for the mature central nervous system, especially for the cerebral or cerebellar cortex, we know neither what is compensated nor the conditions promoting it.

A denervated neuron in the cerebral cortex undergoes a predictable course of degenerative change, as excellently described by Ramón y Cajal [2] and more recently by others [4, 23, 26]. In the mature denervated cerebral cortex little evidence can be found of a compensation in terms of structural or functional regeneration. A recent study [11] comes close to defining a true compensatory structural change in one sensory system following loss of another.

A persistent error relative to *what* is compensated, and *under what conditions,* has crept into the recent literature [10, 15, 21]. It has been stated that growth of axon collaterals following deefferentation of cortical pyramidal cells represents a type of compensatory mechanism, which leaves the impression that this is an established fact for all brains. For the record, a correction should be made. The technique of surgically undercutting the cerebral cortex in order to denervate it for systematic study was devised and used by Ramón y Cajal [2] near the turn of the century. His preparations were cats and dogs under 30 days of age, also adult animals. In the immature brain, *but not in the adult, mature brain,* axon collateral proliferation occurred. Contrary to more recent suggestions or implications, axon collateral proliferation as seen in the *immature* cortex cannot be used to explain supersensitivity in the partially or completely neuronally isolated *mature* cortex. Thus in this important instance a compensatory process is seen only if there is capacity for continued growth. In the studies by Rose et al. [16] on young rabbits, it is still unclear whether the fiber proliferation they observed following laminar lesions of cerebral cortex

---

* This work supported in part by PHS Research Grant NB04119 from National Institute of Neurological Diseases and Stroke.

was really an expression of continued growth potential. Further mention of axon collateral proliferation will be made subsequently.

Use, Disuse, and Degeneration Changes

The hypotheses of *use* and *disuse* are even stickier to handle than is *compensation*. As pointed out by Sharpless [21], it is virtually impossible to make a distinction between disuse and the degenerative effects of denervation. However, in definite instances, disuse has led to degeneration changes [3, 25]. Degenerative changes after a certain point has been reached are irreversible, at least until it is proven otherwise for a particular case. Perhaps a demonstration of reversibility of disuse changes might be a useful criterion for distinguishing between disuse and the better understood neuronal degeneration.

The hypothesis of excessive *use* in structures of the central nervous system probably fares somewhat better. The significant findings of Rosenzweig and colleagues [18] must be recognized. In their studies, carefully channeled experience led to both chemical and structural changes of cortical neurons. Persistent electrical changes in a multisynaptic, interhemispheric pathway as a result of excessive, but "meaningful," use has been reported recently [19].

The terms use, disuse, and compensation are, in a general sense, relevant to considerations of supersensitivity of experimentally isolated cerebral cortex. But with what has been said, it seems necessary that these terms serve as points of departure for investigation rather than as explanations. This caution must be kept in mind in looking at attempts to approach the problem of supersensitivity in partially neuronally isolated cerebral cortex. Some of our work has been published [6, 20], but in order to make these efforts familiar, the rationale, technique, and experimental results will be reviewed.

SUPERSENSITIVITY IN PARTIALLY ISOLATED CORTEX

The first observation was that we could interfere with the expected appearance of supersensitivity in partially isolated cat cortex. The time course of development of supersensitivity by measuring thresholds and durations of afterdischarges to electrical stimulation had been described previously [22]. Our findings indicated that if we applied daily electrical stimulation to undercut cortex, we could, in most preparations, prevent the appearance of afterdischarges upon later testing with stronger shocks. Daily stimulation consisted of twenty 2-sec trains of 1.0 msec pulses at 50 per sec spaced 1 min apart. Stimulation for the first 20 days was 0.6 mamp, for the next 20 days 0.8 mamp, and for the last 10 days 1.0 mamp. Presumably these intensities were below threshold for inducing afterdischarges, which was verified in later experiments with other animals (unpublished). Subsequent testing at weekly intervals after cessation of daily stimulation showed absence of afterdischarges as a persistent phenomenon. These results were puzzling since initially it had been assumed that degeneration produced by the undercutting would be progressive and this, plus the presence of indwelling, stimulating electrodes and daily stimulation, would enhance the appearance of supersensitivity. Obviously further study was imperative.

We were challenged by the finding [8, 17] that acetylcholinesterase was decreased about 50 percent in neuronally isolated cerebral cortex. Was it possible that this enzyme was involved in our preparations not showing supersensitivity after long-term electrical stimulation? It was fortunate to have had the collaboration of Domino in a new series of chemical studies [6]. It was found that in most, but not all undercut cortexes a significant reduction of AChE activity averaged 24 percent. In long-term electrically stimulated undercut cortex, AChE activity did not differ significantly from normal in the majority of animals. Thus, changes in neuronal chemistry and absence of electrical signs of supersensitivity seemed related.

It was reasoned that perhaps such profound electrical and chemical changes would be accompanied by neuronal morphological alterations. One possibility implicated the proliferation of pyramidal-cell axon collaterals in a recurrent inhibitory pathway. Using our own modification of the Golgi-Cox technique, adapted for adult brain, a study was begun of undercut, long-term stimulated undercut and intact cerebral cortex. Tentative results of these ongoing studies will be reported here.

Undercut Cortex, Procedures

Figure D12-1 is a Nissl-stained cross section of an adult cat brain and shows the type of undercut which we normally prepare. Entrance for the surgical procedure is through the lateral edge of suprasylvian gyrus at a midline depth in marginal gyrus of 3–4 mm and an anterior-posterior length of 18–22 mm. Although curvature of the brain in the posterior area means that the thickness of the slab is frequently somewhat less than 3–4 mm, an endeavor is made to maintain as much viable cortex as possible at the anterior and posterior extents.

Cortical tissues were prepared for the Golgi-Cox method as follows. A terminal acute experiment, on the chloralose-anesthetized cat with the cortex bilaterally exposed, was done on each cat with undercut or stimulated undercut cortex for the purpose of determining the presence or absence of supersensitivity to electrical stimulation. Finally the surface of the brain was thoroughly flushed with room-temperature physiological saline and the animal quickly given an overdose of sodium pentobarbital intravenously. As soon as the

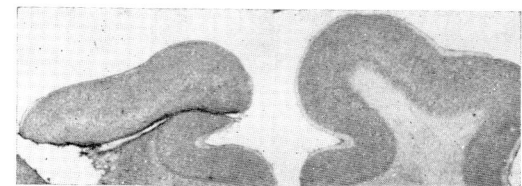

FIG. D12-1. Portion of cross section of undercut adult cat cortex, Nissl stain. Cut through mid-region of marginal gyri. (Adapted from Rutledge et al. [20].)

cortex blanched, four 2–4 mm pieces of cortex were cut from the marginal gyrus of each side and placed directly in freshly made fixative solution. Usually samples from suprasylvian gyri were also taken. Serial sections of 80–140 μ were cut, blackened, cleared, and mounted on special slides under optically high-grade cover slips. Sections were studied dry and under oil immersion with the light microscope.

First attention was directed toward preserved axons and axon collaterals. Impregnation of axons was sufficient to enable comparison to be made between undercut, stimulated undercut, and intact tissue. It became readily apparent that although many axons and their collaterals could be followed for several hundred micra, no evidence could be found for collateral proliferation in *any* preparation. Marked differences, though, were apparent elsewhere.

Figure D12-2 is of main apical dendritic

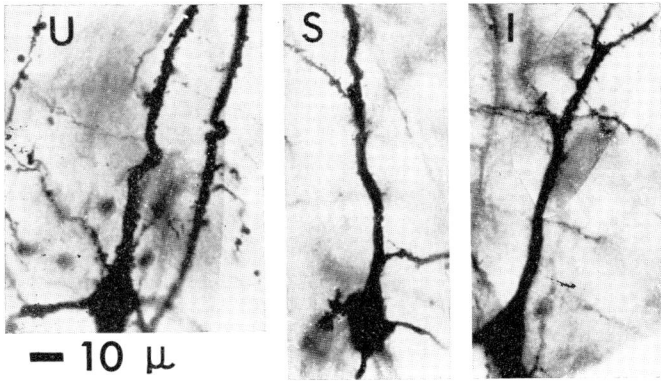

FIG. D12-2. Modified Golgi-Cox preparations from cortex of three adult cats. High-power enlargements of proximal portions of main dendritic shafts of layers II and III pyramidal neurons. U from undercut tissue; S from stimulated undercut tissue; and I from intact tissue.

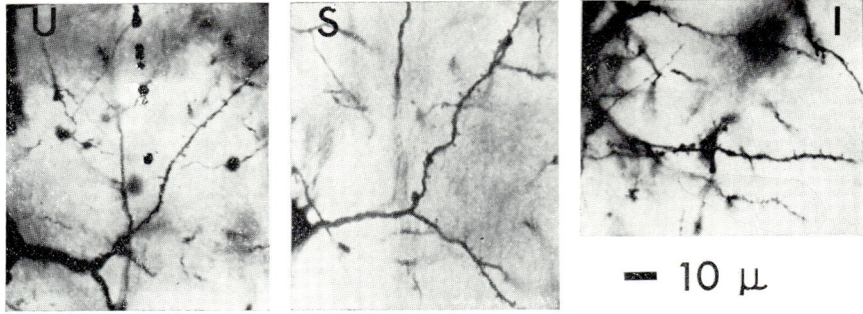

Fig. D12-3. Basal dendrites of layer II pyramidal cells. Preparation as Fig. D12-2.

shafts of cells from the three types of tissue. In all of the figures, representative photomicrographs have been selected. In the figures, U refers to the undercut cortex, S to the stimulated undercut, and I to the intact. In the undercut sections, cell bodies are in layers II and III. Degeneration pathology as previously described [2, 26] is seen. There is a marked beading or moniliform appearance of the shafts. Contortions of the shafts are abnormal and this, too, is characteristic of pyramidal cells in undercut cerebral cortex of the adult animal. Another marked change is the relative absence of dendritic spines on the more distal portions of the main dendritic shafts.

The cell in the center of Fig. D12-2 is also a layer II cell but from undercut cerebral cortex which was electrically stimulated, though not continuously, over a period of 36 weeks after undercutting. The animal did not show supersensitivity. This cell is different from the condition of the cells on the left; the shaft is less beady, and there is less contortion. More dendritic spines can be seen on this cell, especially on the branch in the upper part of the figure.

On the right is a layer II cell from intact cerebral cortex. Note the smoothness of the shaft, especially when compared with the undercut preparation. No contortions are seen, and dendritic spines show clearly.

Figure D12-3 is a comparison of layer II pyramidal cells' basal dendrites. Considerable difficulty was found in effecting good impregnation of basal dendritic spines even in intact tissues. This figure shows that the three types of tissue cannot be distinguished easily on the basis of possible differences in basal dendritic or spiny processes. The spines that do show in the stimulated undercut photomicrograph in this example are larger and darker than in the other two pictures. Caution prevails in drawing even tentative conclusions about possible differences in basal dendritic processes.

Figure D12-4 shows differences among the three conditions, at the level of a major branch point in the apical dendritic field. On the left, in the undercut, two major branch points on two different neurons can be seen. Both cell bodies are in layer II. The expected changes, the loss of dendritic spines and beading, are seen in the branchings. On the right cell, dendritic distortion and beady deposition can be seen. A few dendritic spines do show on these branches of the cell on the right.

For the stimulated undercut (S) virtually no beading can be seen on the apical dendritic branches of this layer II cell. There is also marked difference in the appearance of dendritic spines in contrast with the undercut tissue. Spines are very much in evidence. A photomicrograph of intact tissue is on the right. A count was made of spines, under 675 power magnification, just below major branch points, in over 100 samples in each of the three types of tissue. The average concentrations per 10 μ were: undercut, 3.6 ± 0.16; stimulated undercut, 4.2 ± 0.17; and intact, 6.2 ± 0.19 ($\pm$ = the standard error). Differences between any two are significant ($p = <0.02$ to >0.001).

Figure D12-5 shows comparisons made for terminal branches of apical dendrites,

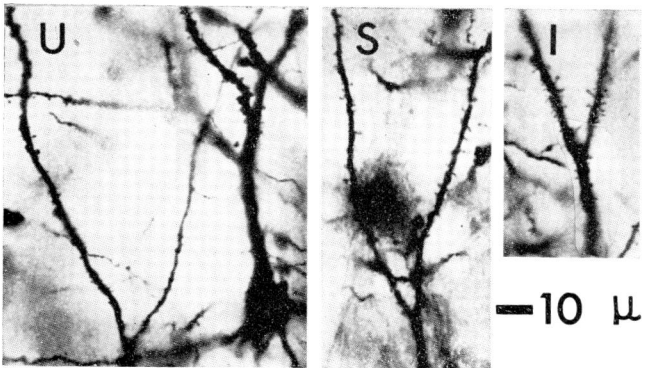

FIG. D12-4. Some principal branch points of apical dendrites of layer II pyramidal cells. Preparation as Fig. D12-2.

all layer II cells. It may be well to look first at the intact on the right. There is a nice concentration of dendritic spines in these two examples of intact tissue. The average for over one hundred 10-μ counts was 11.5 ± 0.18. This is considerably higher than counts recently made by other workers [9]. Compare this with undercut tissue on the left. In the examples here of two different cells, one shows a branching dendrite which has very marked beadiness and an absence of dendritic spines. The other example illustrates that in some instances, dendritic spines are to a certain extent preserved in the undercut cerebral cortex, but are usually sparse compared with intact tissue. A count of over 100 examples, selecting those branches that still had spines, averaged 6.9 ± 0.17 per 10 μ. Remaining spines appear distorted, and, under higher power, many seem to be shells of membranes.

In the middle of Fig. D12-5, two examples of dendritic terminations show the preservation of dendritic spines in stimulated undercut cortex. Some beadiness can be seen on the one illustration, but the preservation of dendritic spines is very apparent. An average of 10.7 ± 0.15 spines per 10 μ was found in over 100 examples. This is significantly different from undercut tissue ($p = \ll 0.001$) but also significantly less than for intact ($p = <0.001$).

The morphological changes seen are most readily described as the preservation of apical dendritic spines and relative absence of expected degenerative changes. These alterations permit the postulation that

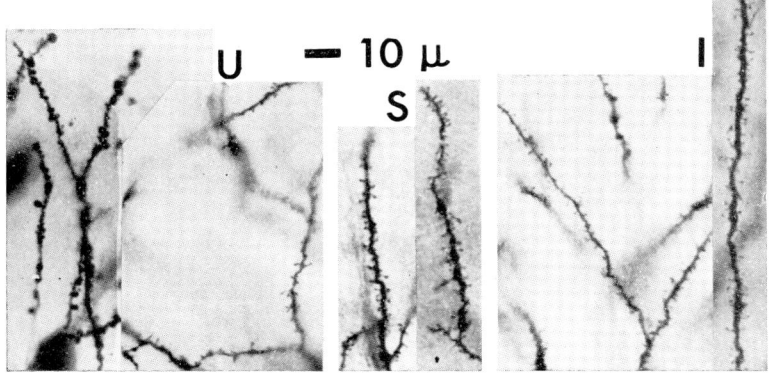

FIG. D12-5. Terminal twigs of apical dendrites of layer II pyramidal cells. Preparation as Fig. D12-2.

pyramidal neurons in stimulated undercut cortex resemble cells in intact cortex more than they resemble those in nonstimulated undercut cortex. We are faced with the likely conclusion that long-term electrical stimulation of undercut cortex is responsible for preservation of synaptic areas of cortical neurons. The preservation seems most strong for axodendritic synapses although it must be recognized that the limitations of the Golgi method do not rule out the possibility that there are unseen but significant changes elsewhere.

Axodendritic and Axosomatic Synapses

Axodendritic as compared with axosomatic synapses in cerebral cortex show an especially strong staining for acetylcholinesterase [14]. The finding of normal AChE activity in stimulated undercut tissue is probably explained by the fact that axodendritic synapses are preserved. These data lead to consideration of some tentative functional implications.

It is suggested that a critical feature in undercut, supersensitive cortex is deafferentation of stellate (short axon or Golgi type II) cells. It must be assumed that many if not most stellate cells are inhibitory. Such a role has been suggested [7] and recently strongly supported with experimental evidence [12]. Although afferent axons have endings on pyramidal cell shafts, basal and apical dendrites, there is an exceedingly rich pattern of afferent termination in layer IV, where stellate cells are most abundant [4, 13]. It is suggested that the stellate cells' normal strong bias of inhibition upon pyramidal cells is lost following deafferentation with undercutting. Thus, whatever process contributes to pyramidal cell excitability, such as electrical or chemical stimuli, it will shift the general activity level strongly toward persistent, uncontrolled excitation. The fact that there may be inhibition upon pyramidal cells via preserved axosomatic synapses [23], which are thought to be inhibitory [5], apparently is not sufficient to result in adequate inhibition of pyramidal cells. The excitatory endings of pyramidal-cell axon collaterals upon stellate cells may participate in this pathway with recurrent inhibition, but it is still inadequate. Also opposing inhibition are the excitatory synapses of pyramidal-cell axon collaterals upon neighboring pyramidal cells' basal dendrites. For total efferent discharge this would be a positive feedback, promoting more excitation.

What about the stimulated undercut, nonsupersensitive cortex? It is suggested here that the daily, long-term electrical stimulation has an excitatory effect upon presynaptic fibers leading to axodendritic synapses of pyramidal cells. Undoubtedly the stimulation also invades stellate cell bodies and their action-potential trigger zones. Such forced activity through the axodendritic synapses not only preserves the structures of presynaptic and postsynaptic membranes but also preserves essential metabolic machinery in the presynaptic cell. The paradoxical feature about our story is that axodendritic synapses are asymmetrical and the presynaptic terminal or bouton contains mostly spheroidal vesicles. These synapses are thought to be excitatory [1, 5, 24]. A further problem is to explain how the preserved and possibly enhanced postsynaptic dendritic activity of pyramidal neurons prevents the expression of supersensitivity as measured by electrical stimulation.

These results offer experimental challenges to studies of synaptic plasticity utilizing chemical, electrical, and histological methods. Even now, if preservation of synaptic areas produced by presynaptic activation can be equated with *excessive use,* then our data support the *use* hypothesis.

ACKNOWLEDGMENTS. I am especially indebted to my research assistant, Miss Joyce Duncan, who played an active role in many phases of the experiments. I owe grateful thanks to Miss Christine McBride for *her persistence* with the capricious Golgi technique.

REFERENCES

1. Bodian, D. Synaptic types on spinal motoneurons: An electron microscopic study. *Bull. Hopkins Hosp.* 119:16, 1966.
2. Cajal, S. Ramón y. *Degeneration and Regeneration of the Nervous System.* (Trans.), R. M. May. New York: Hafner, 1959.
3. Coleman, P. D., and Riesen, A. H. Environmental effects on cortical dendritic fields. I. Rearing in the dark. *J. Anat.* 102:363, 1968.
4. Colonnier, M. L. The Structural Design of the Neocortex. In Eccles, J. C. (Ed.), *Brain and Conscious Experience.* New York: Springer, 1966.
5. Colonnier, M. Synaptic patterns on different cell types in the different laminae of the cat visual cortex. An electron microscope study. *Brain Res.* 9:267, 1968.
6. Duncan, Joyce A., Rutledge, L. T., and Domino, E. F. Acetylcholinesterase activity in partially isolated cerebral cortex after prolonged intermittent stimulation. *Exp. Neurol.* 20:268, 1968.
7. Eccles, J. C. Conscious Experience and Memory. In Wortis, J. (Ed.), *Recent Advances in Biological Psychiatry.* New York: Plenum, 8:235, 1965.
8. Echlin, F. A., and Battista, A. Decreased cholinesterase activity in epileptogenic chronically "isolated" cerebral cortex. *Trans. Amer. Neurol. Ass.* 87:190, 1962.
9. Globus, A., and Scheibel, A. B. Synaptic loci on visual cortical neurons of the rabbit: The specific afferent radiations. *Exp. Neurol.* 18:116, 1967.
10. Grundfest, H. Some Determinants of Repetitive Electrogenesis and Their Role in the Electrical Activity of the Central Nervous System. In Servít, Z. (Ed.), *Comparative and Cellular Pathophysiology of Epilepsy.* New York: Excerpta Medica, 1966.
11. Gyllensten, L., Malmfors, T., and Norllin, M. L. Growth alteration in the auditory cortex of visually deprived mice. *J. Comp. Neurol.* 126:463, 1966.
12. Holubár, J., Hanke, B., and Malík, V. Intracellular recording from cortical pyramids and small interneurons as identified by subsequent staining with the recording microelectrode. *Exp. Neurol.* 19:257, 1967.
13. Lorente de Nó, R. La corteza cerebral del raton; primiera contribucion—la corteza acustica. *Trab. Lab. Invest. Biol., Univ. Madrid* 20:47, 1922.
14. de Lorenzo, A. J. Darin. Electron microscopy of the cerebral cortex. I. The ultrastructure and histochemistry of synaptic junctions. *Bull. Hopkins Hosp.* 108:258, 1961.
15. Purpura, D. P., and Housepian, E. M. Morphological and physiological properties of chronically isolated immature neocortex. *Exp. Neurol.* 4:377, 1961.
16. Rose, J. E., Malis, L. I., Kruger, L., and Baker, C. P. Effects of heavy, ionizing, monoenergetic particles on the cerebral cortex. II. Histological appearance of laminar lesions and growth of nerve fibers after laminar destructions. *J. Comp. Neurol.* 115:243, 1960.
17. Rosenberg, P., and Echlin, F. A. Cholinesterase activity of chronic partially isolated cortex. *Neurology* (Minneap.) 15:700, 1965.
18. Rosenzweig, M. R. Environmental complexity, cerebral change, and behavior. *Amer. Psychol.* 21:321, 1966.
19. Rutledge, L. T. Facilitation: Electrical response enhanced by conditional excitation of cerebral cortex. *Science* 148:1246, 1965.
20. Rutledge, L. T., Ranck, J. B., Jr., and Duncan, Joyce A. Prevention of supersensitivity in partially isolated cerebral cortex. *Electroenceph. Clin. Neurophysiol.* 23:256, 1967.
21. Sharpless, S. K. Reorganization of function in the nervous system—use and disuse. *Ann. Rev. Physiol.* 26:357, 1964.
22. Sharpless, S. K., and Halpern, L. M. The electrical excitability of chronically isolated cortex studied by means of permanently implanted electrodes. *Electroenceph. Clin. Neurophysiol.* 14:244, 1962.
23. Szentágothai, J. The synapses of short local neurons in the cerebral cortex. *Sympos. Biol. Hung.* 5:251, 1965.
24. Uchizono, K. Excitatory and inhibitory synapses in the cat spinal cord. *Jap. J. Physiol.* 16:570, 1966.
25. Valverde, F. Apical dendritic spines of the visual cortex and light deprivation in the mouse. *Exp. Brain Res.* 3:337, 1967.
26. Westrum, L. E., White, L. E., and Ward, A. A., Jr. Morphology of the experimental epileptic focus. *J. Neurosurg.* 21:1033, 1964.

13

Physiology and Histochemistry of the Mirror Focus[*]

FRANK MORRELL

ALMOST TEN YEARS have passed since the first systematic study of secondary epileptogenic lesions (SEL) was published [20]. At this time it might be well to review the phenomenon and what has been learned further about it.

Chronic epileptogenic lesions were induced by topical freezing of the cortical surface of one cerebral hemisphere [19] applied through a small (2 mm) burr hole. The opposite hemisphere was unexposed and untouched. A primary epileptogenic lesion developed at the site of ethyl chloride application. After a few days to weeks, depending on species and locus, paroxysmal discharge developed in the homotopic region of the untouched hemisphere. The secondary lesion always appeared in the region of callosal terminations of the cells involved in the primary focus, that is, homotopic, contralateral cortex.

Although the callosally mediated SEL is the most thoroughly studied, it is by no means the only pathway through which secondary epileptogenesis has been shown to occur. Thus, Wada and Cornelius [41] demonstrated a similar phenomenon in thalamic nuclei anatomically related to primary cortical focus. Guerrero-Figueroa et al. [11] confirmed the observation for limbic system nuclei. Morrell, Proctor, and Prince [26] and Proctor, Prince, and Morrell [31] showed that cryogenically induced primary foci in subcortical nuclei were also associated with development of secondary foci in anatomically connected nuclei. No foci were found in similarly implanted areas without anatomical connection to the zone of the primary focus. Therefore, a more general statement may now be made to the effect that the mirror focus or secondary epileptogenic lesion (SEL) is an electrophysiologically defined area of paroxysmal discharge, at least one synapse removed from a primary epileptogenic zone, connected with the latter by relatively massive neural pathways.

Development of SEL

There are two stages in the development of SEL. The secondary discharge is at first related spike-for-spike with that in the primary focus. It seems to be a mirror image and thus has earned the colloquial term, *mirror focus*. The secondary spike is actually an evoked potential—evoked by synchronous bombardment from the cellular discharge in the primary region. It is, in fact, *dependent* upon such discharge as evidenced by its cessation if the primary focus is ablated or isolated. Microelectrode investigations during the first or dependent stage of secondary epileptogenesis have not revealed any unusual or aberrant forms of cell discharge [2, 43, 44].

Eventually, however, the abnormal paroxysmal discharge at the secondary site becomes *independent* of that in the primary region. Epileptiform spikes occur spontaneously without triggering from the pri-

---

[*] This work supported in part by PHS Research Grants NB03543 and 1–F–11–NB1485–01 from National Institute of Neurological Diseases and Stroke.

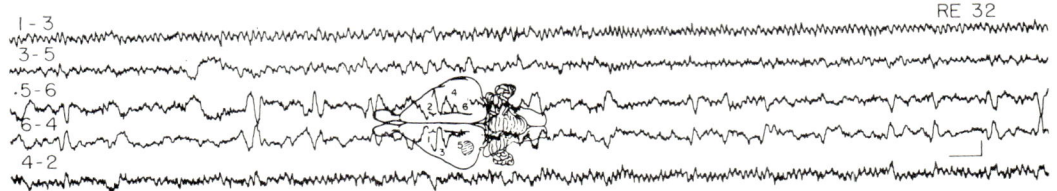

Fig. 13-1. Electroencephalogram, unanesthetized rabbit 3 weeks after production of ethyl chloride lesion. In this instance, there was only minimal abnormality at primary site (electrode 5), but active epileptiform discharge was present in mirror focus (electrode 6). Calibration: 50 μV and 1 sec. (From Morrell [20].)

mary focus. Indeed, long runs of secondary spikes may be seen at times when the primary focus appears quiescent (Fig. 13-1). Secondary discharge then persists indefinitely, despite complete ablation of all discharging tissue in the primary lesion. Microelectrode explorations during the second or independent stage of secondary epileptogenesis have shown abnormalities in cellular discharge [43, 44] entirely analogous with those observed in primary foci [10, 17, 18, 30]. These include the depolarization shift, giant EPSPs, fast prepotentials, and electrophysiological signs suggestive of dendritic spike initiation [43, 44]. These are all electrophysiological indexes of an autonomous epileptic lesion (Fig. 13-2).

Very early in the study of secondary epileptogenic lesions, it was discovered that the process was more complex than that of continuous, synchronous bombardment over a single internuncial pathway. Animals were prepared with subpial partial isolation of a large cortical slab in one hemisphere. The isolation deprived the

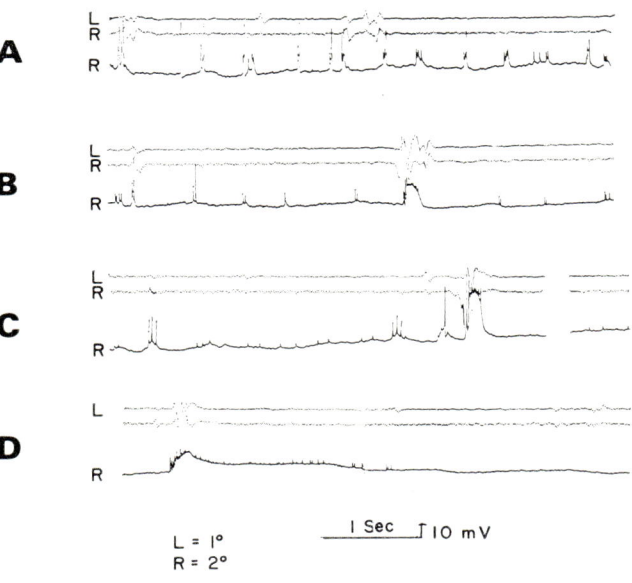

Fig. 13-2. Intracellular microelectrode record (channel 3) from independent mirror focus in unanesthetized frog. EEG tracings from primary epileptic lesion (channel 1) and from secondary focus (channel 2). Note characteristic depolarizing shift in intracellular tracing which coincides with paroxysmal discharge in EEG. Fast prepotentials and dendritic spikes. (From Wilder and Morrell [44].)

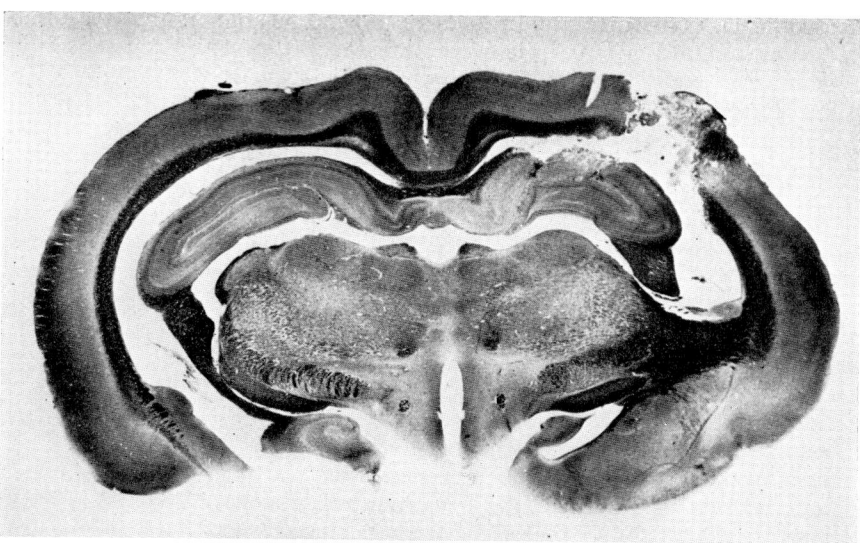

FIG. 13-3. A Weil-stained section of rabbit brain to illustrate integrity of callosal pathway in the extracallosal isolation preparation. (From Morrell [20].)

tissue of all subcortical and long intrahemispheric connections (Fig. 13-3) while preserving intact the callosal pathway relating the slab to the opposite hemisphere. At the end of the procedure, the bone flap was replaced and recording electrodes screwed into the bone over both hemispheres.

In a second operation several days later, a small burr hole was made over the opposite hemisphere at a site homotopic with the center of the partially denervated area. The dura was incised and viability of the cortical slab as well as integrity of the callosal pathway were checked by recording typical transcallosal responses elicited by electrical stimuli delivered to the cortical surface through the dural opening. In all cases, the slab proved to be viable and the callosal pathway sufficiently intact to mediate good transcallosal potentials. An ethyl chloride lesion was then produced through the burr hole used for stimulation. Although all of the animals developed electrographic signs of a dependent mirror focus, none showed the electrographic features of independent secondary discharge. This finding suggested that the establishment of an independent secondary focus requires that at least two forms of synaptic input be available to the cortical region concerned; the callosal pathway alone is necessary but is not sufficient to mediate this process.

HISTOCHEMISTRY AND
MICROSPECTROPHOTOMETRY

The area of the electrophysiologically defined mirror focus could be measured very precisely by plotting the field of the abnormal electric activity using multiple, closely spaced electrodes. Often the secondary discharge was limited to a zone 3–4 mm in diameter. After careful mapping of the fields for both primary and secondary foci, the animals were sacrificed and brains perfused in situ. Serial whole brain sections were prepared and stained with methyl green pyronine (or in later series with aqueous azure B bromide or gallocyanin at acid pH) [21–25]. Zones of primary and secondary foci were compared with electrically normal regions. In sections passing directly through the foci, comparisons between normal and epileptogenic areas could be made on the same slide.

Those areas exhibiting epileptogenic activity could be readily identified from the microscopic slide. They contained nests of pyronine-dense cells; that is, cells exhibited extreme basophilia. The increase in dye-binding was limited to neurons; glia were not altered.

It is important to point out that considerable care was taken with respect to techniques of fixation, staining, and sectioning of tissue, in order to minimize any possibility of technical artifact [3]. As mentioned above, the original findings have been replicated with two other histochemical methods for identification of RNA (azure B and gallocyanin). Staining specificity was routinely checked with ribonuclease extraction (crystalline, 1 mg per ml adjusted to pH 6.5 with NaOH, 60 min at 25°C), which invariably eliminated the dye-binding. On the other hand, pretreatment of slides with deoxyribonuclease (crystalline, 0.2 mg per ml in 0.003 M magnesium sulfate, pH 6.5) for 90 min at 25°C did not eliminate dye-binding. Removal of DNA was further checked by loss of Feulgen stainability.

The site of the primary lesion was systematically varied from animal to animal; location of the secondary focus varied accordingly, thus excluding the possibility that a particular cell type or grouping might have been inherently sensitive to basic dyes. Brains were perfused with fixative while animals were under deep anesthesia but still alive. This procedure minimized cell changes due to poor fixation. Moreover, it seems highly unlikely that fixation artifact would vary in location from animal to animal in a manner precisely concordant with variations in the site of electrical discharge. There remains one argument, which may be valid at least for the primary lesion, that the dark cells are simply partially chromatolyzed neurons. Yet the same sort of cells is seen in the mirror focus, an area untouched by the experimental procedure, the cortex remaining unexposed until the brain itself was removed. Nor can these findings be accounted for on the basis of retrograde degeneration, for such histochemical changes are not seen contralateral to a simple cortical excision.

The next step was to obtain a more quantitative estimate of the alteration in dye-binding by using microspectrophotometry and visible light. Measurements were made of the RNA–azure B binding with the two-wavelength method of Patau [28] and Ornstein [27]. Technical details are given by Morrell [24]. The essential finding was that neurons of the secondary focus showed an average increase (over control values in adjacent normal cortex) of 35–50 percent in azure B binding. Again, the specific staining procedures and RNAse digestion has identified the basophilic substance within these neurons as RNA.

Autoradiographic Studies of RNA Turnover in Cells of Secondary Epileptogenic Foci

Since the histological data available for neurons of mirror foci reveal only the binding characteristics of intracellular RNA, further investigation was carried out to study the turnover of RNA within neurons of such foci as compared with normal cortical neurons. Time course of RNA migration between various intracellular compartments was measured autoradiographically by the appearance of labeled material in nuclei, nucleoli, and cytoplasm of the cells studied at various time intervals following intravenous injection of uridine ^{3}H, a radioactive RNA precursor. This experiment provides means of evaluating and comparing metabolic activity of RNA in neurons of undamaged epileptic cortex and normal cortex, while simultaneously observing the histological appearance and staining properties of the cells involved.

The autoradiographic study was carried out by Dr. Jerome Engel, Jr., who prepared a new series of 23 rabbits. Fourteen of the animals had primary epileptogenic lesions induced by application of dry ice to the cortical surface of one hemisphere. All of these developed secondary foci in the appropriate regions of contralateral cortex. Nine animals served as controls: five completely normal animals and four implanted but nonlesioned animals. When secondary foci were considered fully developed and independent (this occurred between 14 and 30 days following the primary lesions), the animals were given a subconvulsant dose (35 mg) of pentylenetetrazol in order to activate any quiescent epileptogenic foci present. In animals with epileptogenic lesions, selective activation of those areas was observed. Exactly the same treatment was given to all the control animals, but no electrographic abnormalities were produced in any of them. Five days following pentylenetetrazol activation, the animals were sacrificed after intravenous injection of 500 microcuries (μc) of tritiated uridine (New England Nuclear) in 1 cc of sterile water. Two rabbits with secondary foci were injected with 500 μc of tritiated cytidine, two with 500 μc of tritiated adenosine, and two with 500 μc of tritiated guanosine. These latter groups were treated in the same manner as those of the uridine series. Groups of the injected animals were killed at four different time intervals after isotope injection: 15 minutes, 1 hour, 8 hours, 24 hours. Sacrifice was accomplished quickly by cardiac perfusion with Bouin's fixative after rapid administration of a large dose of pentobarbital.

Seventeen uridine-injected rabbits were partitioned into four groups depending on the time interval between isotope administration and sacrifice. The 1-hour, 8-hour, and 24-hour groups each contained one normal control rabbit, one implanted control rabbit, and two rabbits with secondary epileptogenic foci. The 15-minute group contained an extra normal control rabbit because of the greater chance for error in a short time interval.

Coronal sections were cut at 6 μ through the region of the primary epileptic lesion and secondary focus as well as through adjacent and distant regions exhibiting normal electrical activity. Equivalent sections were taken from brains of those rabbits which had no lesions with and without electrodes.

The sections were mounted on one-inch glass slides, cleared in xylol and dried by pretreatment with 100 percent alcohol and ether. Representative slides were hydrated, incubated for one hour at 37°C in a 0.4 mg per 100 ml solution of RNAse buffered to a pH of 7.6 and redried in the same manner.

The dried slides were coated with photographic emulsion according to the dipping technique described by Leblond, Kopriwa, and Messier [14], dried in air overnight, and exposed for 3, 5, and 7 weeks at 4°C in tightly sealed, black plastic slide boxes containing a small amount of calcium sulfate. This entire procedure was carried out in absolute darkness. Six slides from each of the three areas of each brain were coated and two from each area were exposed for 3 weeks, two for 5 weeks, and two for 7 weeks. After proper exposure time, slides were developed for 2 minutes in 1:2 Dektol (developer) and water at 17°C and stained with thionine. The RNAse-treated slides were coated, exposed, developed, and stained in the same fashion.

The course of RNA synthesis and movement from nucleus to cytoplasm was estimated by the amount of radioactivity found in nucleus, nucleolus, and cytoplasm at the various time intervals mentioned above. Radioactivity was seen as silver grains in the photographic emulsion directly above the tritiated compounds.

Silver grains in all of the slides were examined, but only those slides taken from the 17 uridine-injected rabbits exposed for 5 weeks were used in the quantitative experiment. The 3-week and 7-week exposures were used as checks on the reproducibility of these data, and the 6 cytidine, adenosine, and guanosine rabbits provided information which served to supplement some of the specific results obtained with uridine injection. Grain counts were always made in the same manner by the same observer. Grains observed over 100 neurons in the first three layers of the right motor cortex were counted and scored as being over nuclei, nucleoli, or cytoplasm. The percentage of labeled cells was also determined by counting 100 random cells. This same procedure was used for the three deep cortical layers. These counts were made on 100 cells from each of 6 different regions (layers 1–3 and layers 4–6 for sections 1, 2, and 3) on each of the 17 animals. The data were tabulated as percentage of cells labeled, total intracellular grains, and percentage of intracellular grains found over nuclei, nucleoli, and cytoplasm. Comparative observations were taken from the autoradiographs pretreated with RNAse.

There were clear differences among the groups related to time between the single pulse label and sacrifice of the animal. Thus, the total amount of label and the percentage of cells labeled increased steadily from 15 minutes to 8 hours. After that, the label reached its peak and then began to disappear from the cells. This pattern was most characteristic of the nucleus. The nucleolus, however, reached a peak more rapidly and demonstrated loss of labeled material before 8 hours. The cytoplasm showed a steady increase in label with time throughout the time-intervals studied (Fig. 13-4).

These systematic, time-dependent relationships delineate the migration of newly synthesized RNA between the various intracellular compartments. They also serve as a control for reliability of the scoring system and technical adequacy of the radioactive labeling. It is particularly significant, therefore, that there were no differences within groups that could be attributed to treatment of the animals (with the exception that animals demonstrating the lowest number of grains per cell were almost invariably rabbits which received no surgical manipulation). In other words, as measured by average absolute grain counts per 100 cells, there were no statistically significant differences between epileptic and nonepileptic animals or between electrically normal and electrically abnormal regions in the epileptic animals. Representative autoradiographs of normal-appearing cells from the mirror focus region are shown in Fig. 13-5. However, other kinds of cells were also found in mirror foci.

One or more of the sections from each of the epileptic animals and none of the control animals showed nests of *dense* cells when the autoradiographs were stained with thionine. This pattern was also found when adjacent sections were stained with azure B. The results of this histological observation were comparable to those of Morrell [22, 24]. These dense cells showed characteristic increase in dye-binding with basophilia extending into the apical dendritic tree, and many were elongated or fibrillar in appearance. They were easily distinguishable from other more normal-appearing cells with darker than average

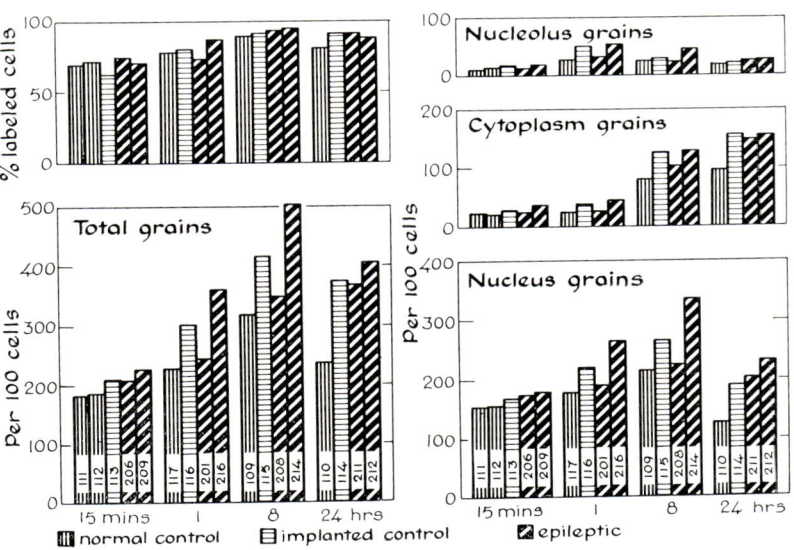

Fig. 13-4. Histograms show percentage of labeled cells observed for all epileptic, implanted control, and normal control animals in each of four time groups: average absolute grain counts per 100 cells; their nucleoli; cytoplasm; and nuclei for each of these animals. (Numbers on bars are numbers on animals from which cell counts were taken.) (From Jerome Engel, Jr., Ph.D. Thesis, Stanford University, 1965.)

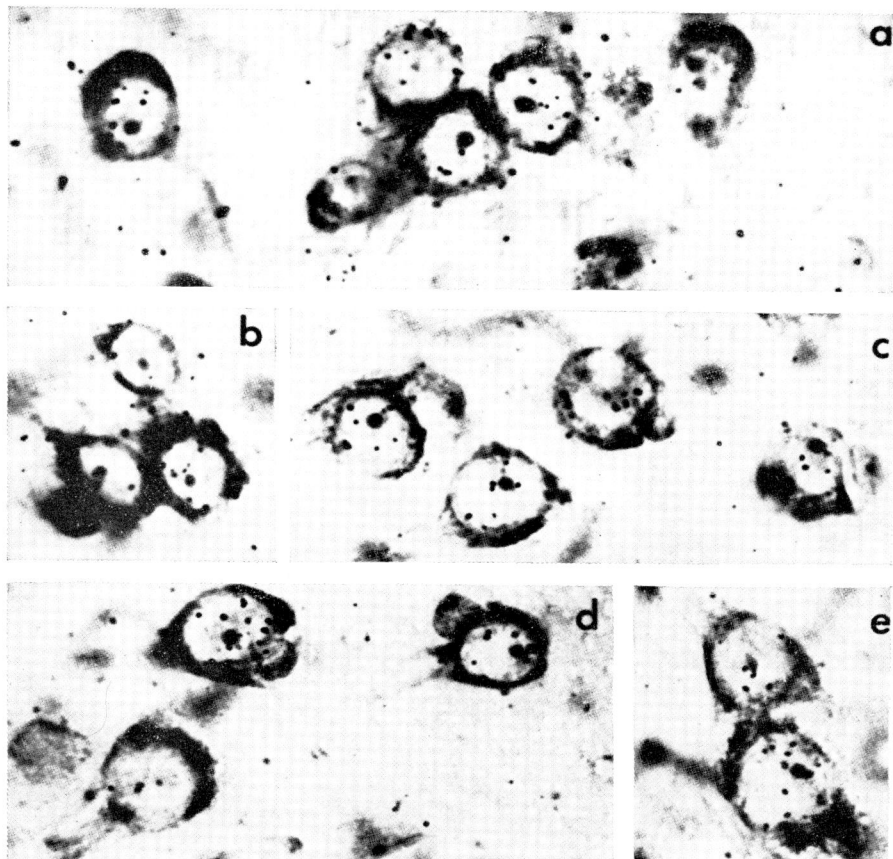

Fig. 13-5. Autoradiographs of normal-appearing cells from mirror focus region. (a) and (b) With long time intervals, some cells show labeling predominantly in cytoplasm, others still contain most or all grains in nucleus. (c), (d), and (e) At earlier time intervals almost all intracellular label is in nucleus. Note darkly stained cytoplasm of cells in (b) and (d). Compare with abnormal *dense* cells in Fig. 13-6. Thionine stain, ×400. (From Jerome Engel, Jr., Ph.D. Thesis, Stanford University, 1965.)

staining cytoplasm, but which were also found as frequently in sections taken from normal animals. Whereas the latter basophilic but normal-appearing cells characteristically showed an average or greater than average number of grains per cell, the former dense cells peculiar to the mirror focus regions showed very little or no radioactivity. Examples of *dense* cells are shown in Fig. 13-6. Because of the very low grain counts obtained from the dense cells, it was not possible to come to any valid conclusions regarding distribution of labeled material within various intracellular compartments.

Digestion of sections with RNAse prior to autoradiographic exposure and staining abolished the appearance of cell label, whereas incubation with buffer alone did not alter the characteristic grain patterns described above. The increased dye-binding properties of the dense cells of the mirror focus were also abolished by RNAse digestion. This indicates that both labeled material within normal cells and darkly stained but unlabeled material of dense cells were RNA.

Autoradiographic investigations of mirror foci in rabbits injected with tritiated cytidine, adenosine, and guanosine were car-

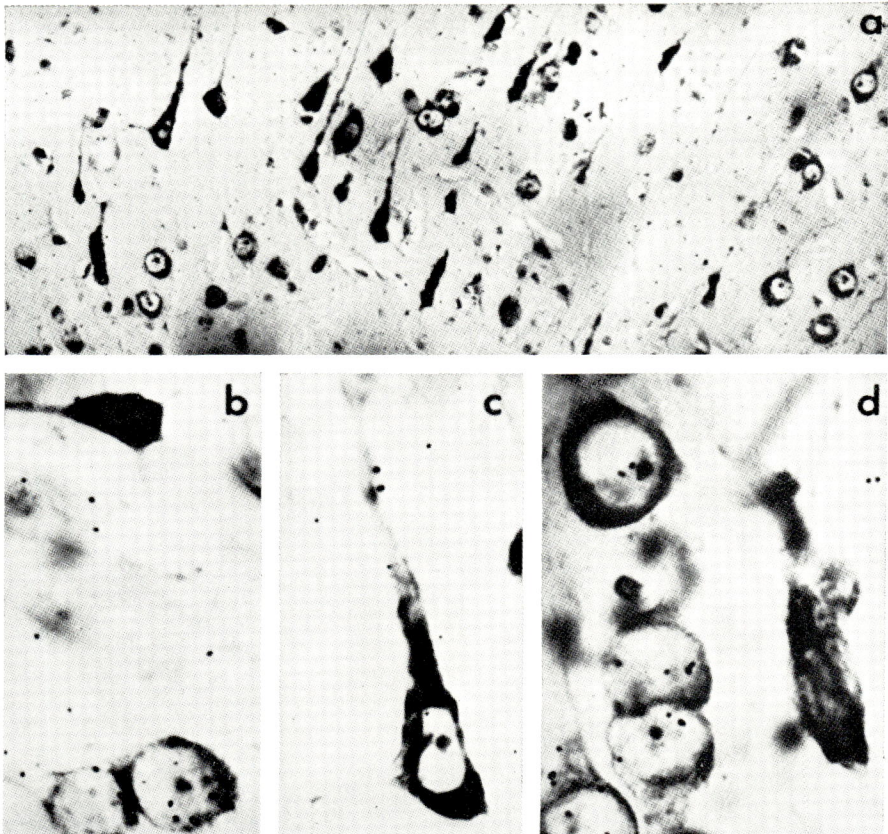

Fig. 13-6. Autoradiographs of dense cells from mirror focus region. (*a*) Low power (×250) field showing nest of dense cells with other more rounded, normal-appearing cells also in field. Note characteristic staining pattern of apical and some basilar dendrites of abnormal cells. Silver grains are not readily visible at this power. (*b*) and (*d*) Dense cells containing very little labeled material in same field with labeled, more normal-appearing neurons. (*c*) Higher power of dense cell seen in (*a*) showing dendritic staining properties and low grain content. Thionine stain, × 400. (From Jerome Engel, Jr., Ph.D. Thesis, Stanford University, 1965.)

ried out specifically to determine whether decrease in dense cell RNA uridine incorporation should be attributed to decrease in RNA synthesis in these cells or, rather, to a change in ratio. The incorporation of cytidine into normal cortical neurons at 8 hours resembled that for uridine at the same time interval; adenosine incorporation at 8 hours was considerably less, however, and guanosine incorporation at 8 hours was barely above background. Heavy labeling of dense cells in the mirror region was never observed for any of the three nucleotides, and, in the case of cytidine, grain density in normal neurons was great enough to discern a definite lack of label in the dense cells.

The appearance of intracellular label reported here is believed to represent RNA since the characteristic autoradiographic patterns were abolished by digestion with RNAse. The findings presented, therefore, provide information regarding intracellular positions of RNA molecules which were synthesized within given time periods. The amount of intracellular label and its location in the neuron at various time periods studied are believed to indicate the rate of RNA synthesis, its migration through the neuron, and its eventual breakdown.

The appearance of nests of dense cells in sections of mirror foci, the affinity of these cells for azure B (an RNA specific stain), and disappearance of this characteristic staining property with RNAse digestion are all in agreement with previous reports [22, 24]. These findings leave little doubt that the densely stained material within these cells is RNA. The decrease in tritiated uridine incorporation by the RNA of these cells indicates that at the times tested, RNA synthesis was suppressed. The possibility of a shift in base ratios was ruled out by absence of uptake for the other three nucleotide bases. Thus, there remains the paradox of increased concentrations of RNA in cells which show little or no sign of active RNA synthesis.

HYPOTHESES ABOUT RNA CONCENTRATION. *First.* The simplest explanation is that these cells might be dying, or at least dehydrated, and that the increased RNA concentration is a function of decreased cell size rather than increased RNA content. Many of these cells do, in fact, appear somewhat fibrillar or even pyknotic, although there are others which do not have the configuration of dying cells but still show extremely dense staining properties with few or no intracellular grains. If these cells are dying neurons, the reason for their death is not clear. It is unlikely that this would represent retrograde degeneration of cells secondary to destruction of axon terminals at the site of the primary lesion since these animals were sacrificed 3 to 5 weeks after the lesioning procedure. Transneuronal degeneration is a more likely possibility since cellular changes described in this phenomenon [38, 39] and the longer time course for these events are similar to those seen in the mirror focus. Such dense cells are not seen contralateral to nonepileptogenic cortical ablation or with callosal section, however [23]. The possibility exists that continuous bombardment from the primary focus, across the callosal pathways, is sufficient to cause damage and eventual death of neurons in the mirror focus region. All of the above forms of degeneration, however, should involve eventual cell destruction with neuronophagia and glial proliferation; this is not seen in the mirror focus.

Second. Another explanation might derive from the similarity of dense cells described here and inactive neurons described by Einarson [5, 6]. Einarson reported studies suggesting that physiological *inhibition* of activity in a neuron would cause decreased RNA consumption and result in extremely chromophilic cells due to the accumulation of this substance intracellularly. This explanation might be applied even more validly in the case of the dense cells of the mirror focus since decreased RNA turnover has been demonstrated here. Further, there is striking resemblance between pictures of Einarson's cells and the dense cells of the mirror focus. If inactive neurons accumulate RNA, the findings presented here might be considered the result of some mechanism within the epileptogenic focus which causes neuronal inactivation.

Third. If the RNA alterations reported here are to be considered responsible for, and not the result of, the epileptic behavior observed in these secondary foci, then the abnormal electrophysiological properties of epileptogenic activity should be explained by this biochemical alteration. Electrophysiologic investigations at the cellular level have revealed two phenomena which can be considered characteristic of neuronal activity within an epileptogenic focus: the abnormal hypersynchrony of graded or all-or-none membrane events of a great number of neurons, or both [2, 4, 10, 13, 15, 35, 40] and the abnormally rapid spike frequency of individual neurons within this cell population [1, 12, 33, 42].

A theory to explain how hypersynchrony and rapid unit discharges could result from intracellular alterations in RNA might be offered in terms of the fixed charge hypothesis of Ling [16], which attributes membrane potential to the selectivity of large intracellular anions for potassium. Since the hydrated potassium ion has a much smaller diameter than the hydrated sodium ion, this selectivity can be accounted for by spatial configurations. These anions are presumably largely proteins and lipoproteins either in or near the cell membrane, although RNA also has many anionic sites and can be found in the cytoplasm near the external membrane. Whether the observed dye-binding properties of the RNA molecules within the dense cells of epileptic foci are actually due to an increase in total RNA or merely an unfolding of the molecular structure, such increased dye-binding represents a total increase in closely spaced anionic charges since this is what determines the metachromasia of basic dyes [34]. Therefore, changes in the anionic sites of cytoplasmic RNA molecules could influence potassium concentrations near the membrane and consequently, the membrane potential. The effect of an increase in closely spaced anionic sites intracellularly would be, according to the fixed charge hypothesis, to increase intracellular potassium and cause membrane hyperpolarization. Although hyperpolarized cells would be less excitable than normal cells, rather than more excitable, as might be expected of neurons in an epileptic focus, such cells would also be less susceptible to random, continuous, asynchronous afferent input. Therefore, a larger population of neurons would be available for excitation by specific synchronizing input and would be expected to react hypersynchronously to such stimuli.

If the sodium current of the action potential were due to some mechanism which would destroy the anionic specificity for potassium [16], then an abnormally large sodium influx would be expected for these abnormally dense cells since the number of anionic sites is increased. Such increased amount of intracellular sodium might then prolong repolarization in the dendrites. Differential repolarization, with the dendritic structures drawing current from the already repolarized soma and axon hillock, has already been offered by some investigators to explain the rapid spike frequencies seen during electroshock afterdischarge [7, 29]. If such a fixed-charge mechanism exists with the RNA macromolecule significantly contributing to the total number of anionic sites available, it would appear likely that prolonged differential repolarization would occur in the dense cells described above since extreme basophilia was observed extending into their apical dendritic trees. Decreased RNA synthesis observed in these neurons might attest to their generally hyperpolarized and therefore less active state since decreased activity would decrease the demand for proteins and consequently, decrease RNA turnover.

KINDLING PHENOMENON. One of the implications of the entire mirror focus investigation is that untreated or inadequately treated epilepsy may be a progressive disease [25].

Dramatic support for this concept is provided by the experimental model developed by Goddard [9], who implanted bipolar electrodes chronically in various brain sites in a large series of rats. He found that minimal stimulation (50 µamp for 1 min per day) usually produced only minor alterations in behavior on the first few occasions. After many days of such stimulation, the same stimulus elicited unequivocal behavioral convulsions upon each subsequent stimulus presentation. He calls this a *kindling effect*. The following features of Goddard's model are pertinent to our discussion.

(1) Different brain regions differ with regard to epileptogenicity. Thus, stimulation of the amygdala required 15 days before convulsions were triggered. The caudate putamen required 74 days. In the reticular formation, there was no detectable kindling after 200 days of stimulation.

(2) Goddard has shown that intermittent rather than continuous stimulation is necessary. In the amygdala, the optimal interval between stimulations was found to be about 24 hours.

(3) The epileptogenic effect was permanent in the sense that once convulsions occurred, they could be triggered by the same stimulus even after a 3-month period during which no stimulation was given.

Goddard recently joined our laboratory at Stanford for collaborative work. His original observations have been extended by the experiment in the cat and by correlating electrophysiologic recordings with behavioral measurements.

Figure 13-7 shows a *learning curve* for epilepsy. The ordinate represents duration

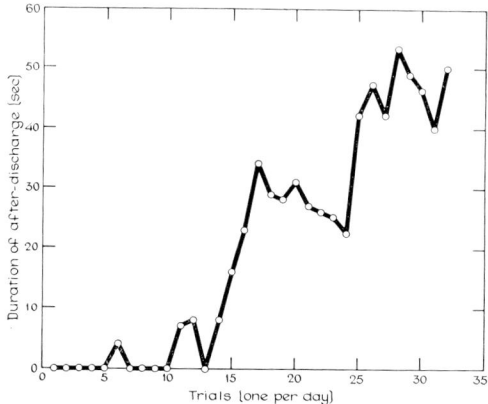

FIG. 13-7. Duration of epileptiform afterdischarge following each daily trial of electrical stimulation of amygdala in cat. (Goddard and Morrell, unpublished data.)

of epileptiform afterdischarge in seconds; trials (one per day) are plotted on the abscissa. Electrical stimulation was delivered through chronically implanted bipolar electrodes situated in the lateral nucleus of the amygdala. Stimulus parameters were 200 μamp, 5 sec, 62.5 pulses per second (pps).

Similar electrodes were placed in 12 other locations to monitor the electrical activity. Except for brief afterdischarge on the sixth day, there was no sign of epileptiform activity until the eleventh day of testing. Thereafter, duration of afterdischarge gradually increased (Fig. 13-7). On the sixth day, correlated with the brief afterdischarge, the cat was seen to arrest ongoing behavior, half crouch, and exhibit rhythmic facial twitching. On the eleventh day, the cat seemed to freeze suddenly; there was saliva drooling and rhythmic head bobbing. Succeeding stimulations elicited increasingly extensive and prolonged signs of local limbic system discharge. On the eighteenth day, these local signs extended to include clonic twitching of shoulders. Further progression was seen with each succeeding convulsion until on day 26 and every day thereafter there was full tonic-clonic seizure. These behavioral signs of progression were correlated both with increasing amplitude and duration of afterdischarge and with involvement of more and more structures in the epileptiform activity.

The discharge duration was all-or-nothing in character. Afterdischarges ceased

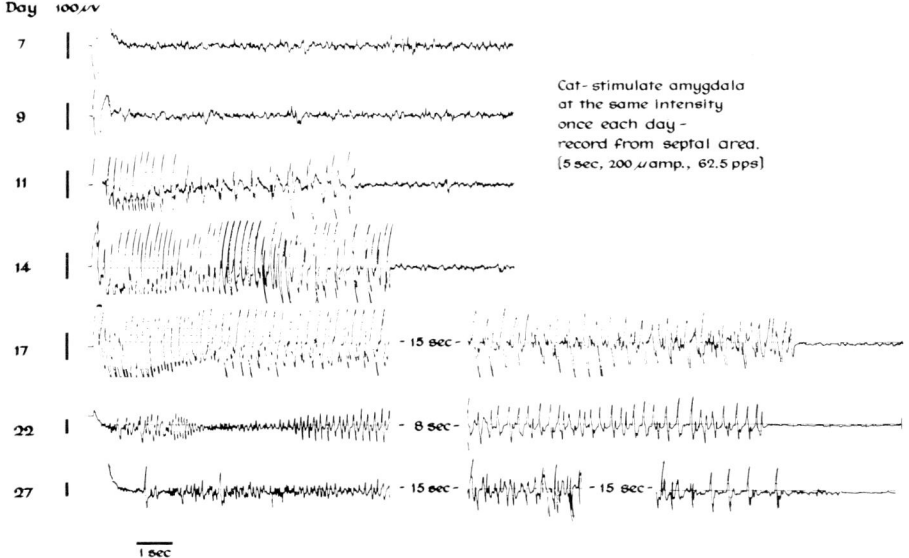

FIG. 13-8. Examples of afterdischarge activity showing progressive changes resulting from daily repetition. Each record begins at end of stimulation. Note absence of epileptiform activity in first two examples and change of amplifier gain in last two traces. (Goddard and Morrell, unpublished data.)

abruptly and simultaneously in all areas where they occurred. Structures which initially did not participate in epileptiform activity invariably responded with full-duration discharge on the first occasion of involvement. Hence, durations plotted in Fig. 13-7 represent duration of afterdischarge in all structures where any discharge occurred on that day.

Figure 13-8 illustrates representative EEG tracings from the septal nuclei taken on the days indicated. In each case, stimulus was applied to the amygdala. Afterdischarge patterns recorded in the amygdala itself were virtually identical with those of the septum implant. (Localizations mentioned are based upon Horsley-Clarke coordinates; we do not yet have histological verification of these sites.)

The Goddard model has been incompletely explored as yet. Nevertheless, there are certain obvious similarities to the more classical mirror focus paradigm. Thus, chronic stimulation of brain at subconvulsant levels gradually creates a state wherein convulsive responses not only occur, but result in a permanent, plastic change in neural excitability which transcends synaptic barriers. A crucial feature of the model is the discovery that intermittent stimulation is more effective than continuous afferent barrage. Indeed, continuous stimulation leads to elevation of the convulsive threshold as though a kind of adaptation or habituation were taking place. More obviously, the model substitutes a well controlled and defined electrical stimulus under precise experimenter control for the far more variable, chronic epileptogenic lesion which exerts its effect in its own good time and to its own individual degree.

The Goddard model should prove extremely valuable for further analysis of the pathophysiology of epilepsy, especially as a more realistic test situation for evaluation of potential anticonvulsant agents.

ACKNOWLEDGMENTS. I am indebted to Dr. Jerome Engel, Jr., for permission to use Figs. 13-4, 13-5, and 13-6 from his Ph.D. Thesis. His work is discussed in the section on autoradiography; I am responsible for any errors made in transcription.

REFERENCES

1. Adrian, E. D., and Moruzzi, G. Impulses in the pyramidal tract. *J. Physiol.* (London) 97:153, 1939.
2. Ajmone-Marsan, C. Unitary analysis of "projected" epileptiform discharges. *Electroenceph. Clin. Neurophysiol.* 15:197, 1963.
3. Cammermeyer, J. The post-mortem origin and mechanism of neuronal hyperchromatosis and nuclear pyknosis. *Exp. Neurol.* 2:379, 1960.
4. Creutzfeldt, O. D. Convulsive discharges of single cortical neurones. *Electroenceph. Clin. Neurophysiol.* 9:353, 1957.
5. Einarson, L. Notes on the morphology of the chromophil material of nerve cells and its relation to nuclear substances. *Amer. J. Anat.* 53:141, 1933.
6. Einarson, L. Nuclei Acids as Structural Constituents of Nerve Cells. In Cumings, J. N. (Ed.), *Modern Scientific Aspects of Neurology*. London: Edward Arnold, 1960, pp. 1–67.
7. Gerin, P. Microelectrode investigations on the mechanisms of the electrically induced epileptiform seizure ("after-discharge"). *Arch. Ital. Biol.* 98:21, 1960.
8. Glick, D., Engstrom, A., and Malmstrom, B. G. A critical evaluation of quantitative histo- and cytochemical microscopic techniques. *Science* 114:253, 1951.
9. Goddard, G. V. Development of epileptic seizures through brain stimulation at low intensity. *Nature* (London) 214:1020, 1967.
10. Goldensohn, E. S., and Purpura, D. P. Intracellular potentials of cortical neurons during focal epileptogenic discharges. *Science* 139:840, 1963.
11. Guerrero-Figueroa, R., Barros, A., Heath, R. G., and Gonzalez, G. Experimental subcortical epileptiform focus. *Epilepsia* (Amst.) 5:112, 1964.
12. Jung, R. Neuronal discharge. *Electroenceph. Clin. Neurophysiol.* Suppl. 4, 57, 1953.
13. Kandel, E. R., and Spencer, W. A. Excitation and inhibition of single pyramidal cells during hippocampal seizure. *Exp. Neurol.* 4:162, 1961.

14. Leblond, C. P., Kopriwa, B., and Messier, B. Radioautography as a Histochemical Tool. In Wegmann, R. (Ed.), *First International Congress of Histochemistry and Cytochemistry*. London: Pergamon, 1963, pp. 1–31.
15. Li, C-L. Synchronization of unit activity in cerebral cortex. *Science* 129:783, 1959.
16. Ling, G. N. *A Physical Theory of the Living State*. Waltham, Mass.: Blaisdell, 1962.
17. Matsumoto, H., and Ajmone-Marsan, C. Cortical cellular phenomena in experimental epilepsy: Interictal manifestations. *Exp. Neurol.* 9:286, 1964.
18. Matsumoto, H., and Ajmone-Marsan, C. Cortical cellular phenomena in experimental epilepsy: Ictal manifestations. *Exp. Neurol.* 9:305, 1964.
19. Morrell, F. Experimental focal epilepsy in animals. *Arch. Neurol.* (Chicago) 1:141, 1959.
20. Morrell, F. Secondary epileptogenic lesions. *Epilepsia* (Amst.) 1:538, 1960.
21. Morrell, F. Microelectrode studies in chronic epileptic foci. *Epilepsia* (Amst.) 2:81, 1961.
22. Morrell, F. Lasting Changes in Synaptic Organization Produced by Continuous Neuronal Bombardment. In Fessard, A. (Ed.), *CIOMS Symposium on Brain Mechanisms and Learning*. London: Blackwell, 1961, pp. 375–392.
23. Morrell, F. Information Storage in Nerve Cells. In Fields, W. S., and Abbott, W. (Eds.), *Information Storage and Neural Control*. Springfield, Ill.: Thomas, 1963, pp. 189–229.
24. Morrell F. Modification of RNA as a Result of Neural Activity. In Brazier, M. A. B. (Ed.), *Brain Function. II. RNA and Brain Function, Memory and Learning*. Los Angeles: Univ. of Calif. Press, 1964, pp. 183–202.
25. Morrell, F., and Baker, L. Effects of drugs on secondary epileptogenic lesions. *Neurology* (Minneap.) 11:651, 1961.
26. Morrell, F., Proctor, F., and Prince, D. A. Epileptogenic properties of subcortical freezing. *Neurology* (Minneap.) 15:744, 1965.
27. Ornstein, L. The distributional error in microspectrophotometry. *Lab. Invest.* 1:250, 1952.
28. Patau, K. Absorption microphotometry of irregular-shaped objects. *Chromosoma* 5:341, 1952.
29. Pinsky, C., and Burns, B. D. Production of epileptiform after-discharges in cat's cerebral cortex. *J. Neurophysiol.* 25:359, 1962.
30. Prince, D. A. The depolarization shift in "epileptic" neurons. *Exp. Neurol.* 21:467, 1968.
31. Proctor, F., Prince, D., and Morrell, F. Primary and secondary spike foci following depth lesions. *Arch. Neurol.* (Chicago) 15:151, 1966.
32. Sawa, M., Maruyama, N., and Kaji, S. Intracellular potential during electrically induced seizures. *Electroenceph. Clin. Neurophysiol.*, 15:209, 1963.
33. Schmidt, R. P., Thomas, L. B., and Ward, A. A., Jr. The hyperexcitable neurone: Microelectrode studies of chronic epileptic foci in monkey. *J. Neurophysiol.* 22:285, 1959.
34. Semmel, M. and Huppert, J. The interaction of basic dyes with ribonucleic acid. *Arch. Biochem.* 108:158, 1964.
35. Sugaya, E., Goldring, S., and O'Leary, J. L. Intracellular potentials associated with direct cortical response and seizure discharge in cat. *Electroenceph. Clin. Neurophysiol.* 17:661, 1964.
36. Swift, H. Quantitative aspects of nuclear nucleoproteins. *Int. Rev. Cytol.* 2:1, 1953.
37. Swift, H., and Rasch, E. Microphotometry with Visible Light. In Oster, G., and Pollister, A. W. (Eds.), *Physical Techniques in Biological Research. Vol. III. Cells and Tissues*. New York: Academic 1956, pp. 353–400.
38. Torvik, A. Transneuronal changes in the inferior olive and pontine nuclei in kittens. *J. Neuropath. Exp. Neurol.* 15:119, 1956.
39. Van Buren, J. M. Trans-synaptic retrograde degeneration in the visual system of primates. *J. Neurol. Neurosurg. Psychiat.* 26:402, 1963.
40. Von Baumgarten, R., and Schaefer, K. P. Synchronization phenomena of neighboring intracerebral nerve cells. *Electroenceph. Clin. Neurophysiol.* 9:353, 1957.
41. Wada, J. A., and Cornelius, L. R. Functional alteration of deep structures in cats with chronic focal cortical irritative lesions. *Arch. Neurol.* (Chicago) 3:425, 1960.
42. Ward, A. A., Jr. The epileptic neurone. *Epilepsia* (Amst.) 2:70, 1961.

43. Wilder, B. J., and Morrell, F. Secondary epileptogenesis in the frog forebrain. *Neurology* (Minneap.) 17:1041, 1967.

44. Wilder, B. J., and Morrell, F. Cellular behavior in secondary epileptogenic lesions. *Neurology* (Minneap.) 17:1193, 1967.

Discussion

THE MIRROR FOCUS AND LONG-TERM MEMORY STORAGE*

SAMUEL H. BARONDES

In the simplest sense, the establishment of a *mirror focus* is an expression of the more general tendency of both halves of the brain to behave in concert. This has been amply demonstrated in the study of interhemispheric transfer of memory in both birds [7] and mammals [9].

ESTABLISHMENT OF MIRROR FOCUS

The establishment of the mirror focus shares with *long-term memory* three other properties: (a) the time required for the establishment of both these processes is substantially greater than the milliseconds in which most neural events are measured; (b) macromolecular synthesis may play a critical role in both processes; and (c) both processes may persist for the life of the organism.

Because of these similarities, research on the biological basis of long-term memory storage may shed some light on the mechanism of establishment of the mirror focus. Indeed the mechanism by which memory is transferred to and stored in the hemisphere not directly involved in certain learning experiments may be particularly similar to the mechanism of establishment of the mirror focus. To illustrate the time required to establish long-term memory and the role of macromolecular synthesis in this process, a brief description will be given of some work from my laboratory on the effect of inhibitors of cerebral protein synthesis on learning and memory.

In a typical experiment, mice are injected either intracerebrally or subcutaneously with cycloheximide or acetoxycycloheximide in doses which inhibit up to about 95 percent of cerebral protein synthesis. Although their cerebral protein synthesis is inhibited to this extent, these mice trained in a variety of maze situations learn as well as controls [3]. When tested for retention 3 hours after training, their performance is quite normal. However, when tested 6 or more hours after training, their retention is found to be markedly impaired (Fig. D13-1). Similar impairment was found when acetoxycycloheximide-treated mice were tested 1 month after training [2]. These studies suggest that cerebral protein synthesis is not required for short-term memory storage (memory for at least 3 hours after training in the situation studied). However, cerebral protein synthesis is apparently required for long-term memory storage (memory for 6 or more hours after training in the situation studied).

Occurrence of Long-Term Memory Storage

To determine at what time during or after training the cerebral protein synthesis apparently required for long-term memory storage occurs, the effect of administration of the inhibitor of cerebral protein synthesis at various times was studied. For these studies, large doses of acetoxycycloheximide were administered subcutaneously. In contrast with the delayed onset of generalized inhibition after intracerebral injection, maximal inhibition of cerebral protein synthesis is established within 10 minutes of subcutaneous injection of acetoxycycloheximide [3]. It was found that administration prior to training (so that inhibition of cerebral protein synthesis was maximal during training and for minutes to hours thereafter) was most effective in preventing

---

* This work supported by PHS Career Development Award K3–MH18232 from National Institute of Mental Health. Research cited in this report supported by PHS Research Grant MH12773 from National Institute of Mental Health.

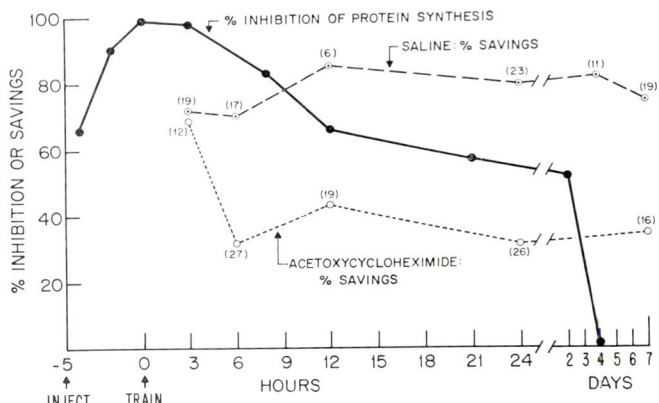

Fig. D13-1. Effect of intracerebral injection of acetoxycycloheximide on cerebral protein synthesis and memory. Mice were injected intracerebrally with 20 μg acetoxycycloheximide 5 hr before training to escape shock by choosing the left limb of a T maze to a criterion of 3 out of 4 consecutive correct responses. Groups were tested for retention at the indicated time after training. Number of mice in each group indicated in parentheses. (For details see Barondes and Cohen [2].)

the formation of long-term memory (Fig. D13-2). Administration immediately after training also impaired memory but to a significantly smaller extent. Administration of the drug 30 minutes after training in this situation had no significant effect. In a passive avoidance situation, a detectable amnesic effect remained if cycloheximide was given 30 minutes after training, but not 2 hours after [6].

These experiments suggest that the protein synthesis apparently required for long-term memory occurs during training or within minutes after training, or both. However, the effect of inhibition of protein synthesis during this period is not apparent until the short-term memory process has terminated. For this reason, amnesia does not become detectable until 6 hours after training.

It is presumed that neuronal activation, in some manner, directs the brain protein synthesis which mediates long-term memory. The nature of this activation and its relationship to the activation of neurons in the evolving mirror focus is not known. For the purpose of this discussion it may be speculated that in both situations activation mediates increased macromolecular synthesis which in turn may produce long-standing changes in neural function. This speculation is consistent with the few facts

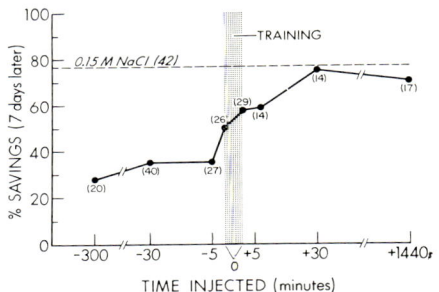

Fig. D13-2. Effect of subcutaneous administration of acetoxycycloheximide at times before and after training on memory. Mice were injected subcutaneously with 240 μg of acetoxycycloheximide at indicated time relative to training. Inhibition of about 90 percent of cerebral protein synthesis was established within about 10 min after injection. Training, designated as O, took an average of 8 min. Mice were tested for retention 7 days after training. Numbers in parentheses are number of mice in each group. Mice injected with acetoxycycloheximide before or within 5 min after training all had significantly less savings ($p < 0.05$ or less, Mann-Whitney U test) than saline controls. Mice injected 5 or more minutes before training had significantly less savings than those injected immediately after training. Injections of acetoxycycloheximide 30 min or more after training had no significant effect on memory. (For details see Barondes and Cohen [3].) (Copyright 1968 by the American Association for the Advancement of Science.)

we have but is by no means established.

If this is accepted, there are still differences between establishment of an identifiable mirror focus and the development of long-term memory. The time required to establish these processes, although relatively long in terms of usual neuronal events, differs. The former may be measured in units of days to months [8] whereas the latter seems to be measured in units of minutes. In addition, the neurons in the region of the mirror focus undergo gross morphological changes whereas there is no evidence that such striking changes occur in neurons involved in long-term memory storage.

Perhaps it is fruitful to speculate that the mirror focus is an *excessive* manifestation of a normal process. Presumably the cells destined to become involved in the mirror focus are stimulated by frequent activation in the cells of the primary focus with which they are connected. Alteration in these cells probably begins within minutes after the primary focus is established. However, the gross changes, including autonomous spike generation and morphological abnormalities, do not occur until there has been prolonged and marked activation. It seems likely that a large amount of stimulation is required before the mirror focus is established, possibly by processes which are dependent upon protein synthesis. In this view, the mirror focus is established by processes similar to those which mediate long-term memory, but there are quantitative differences due to unusually intense and persistent stimulation.

Cerebral RNA Synthesis

The possible participation of RNA synthesis in the establishment of the mirror focus, which Morrell has investigated [8], deserves special comment. On the basis of studies with actinomycin D, a potent inhibitor of RNA synthesis, there is evidence that cerebral RNA synthesis is not critical for short-term memory [5]. Because of the profound toxicity of the drug, we have thus far been unable to test the possibility that cerebral RNA synthesis is required for long-term memory, but studies in goldfish are consistent with this possibility [1]. The cerebral protein synthesis which is apparently required for long-term memory may well be directed by newly synthesized messenger RNA or require the synthesis of ribosomal RNA. There is indeed evidence for increased cerebral RNA synthesis in certain learning situations [10]. The marked increase in incorporation of radioactive uridine into RNA in these studies [10] may represent stimulation of neuronal RNA synthesis due to marked cellular activation.

The presence of what appears to be an increased quantity of RNA in the cells in the region of the mirror focus might be a manifestation of a similar process. The mirror focus cells may have undergone chronic and marked activation due to stimulation by the activity in the primary focus. In this regard it is important to be aware that the attempts made thus far to study cerebral RNA synthesis in the mirror focus [8] must be viewed as extremely incomplete. Since changes in a relatively small number of cells must be investigated, the audioradiographic method has been employed. This method permits studies of alterations in individual cells but produces results which are often difficult to interpret, since there is no way of determining whether the labeled precursors of RNA are present in the same concentration in the cells of interest as in control cells. Thus, increases in the incorporation of administered radioactive nucleosides might reflect either an increase in the specific activity of these substances and their products, the nucleoside triphosphates, in the involved cells (due, for example, to an increased uptake of the radioactive precursor) or a true increase in RNA synthesis. The decreased incorporation in the hyperchromatic cells, which Morrell describes in the established mirror focus [8], could likewise be due to changes in the uptake of the radioactive precursor. Furthermore the formation and utilization of nucleoside triphosphates from the precursor which was administered could well be altered in cells with bursts of excessive activity.

The interpretation of the results described is also difficult for another reason. When the mirror focus has already been established and when there is gross change in many cells in this region, many of the metabolic changes which were involved may have terminated. Thus, it is quite possible that RNA synthesis in the hyperchromatic cells in the mirror focus was indeed substantially increased in the period shortly after the primary focus was established. Such increases in RNA synthesis might have led to the "pathological" properties of the cells observed at this later time. However, these altered cells may no longer manifest the increases in RNA synthesis which may have predisposed to their altered properties. This could be resolved by studies of RNA synthesis in the region destined to become the mirror focus, made at a number of times after establishing the primary focus.

Despite the difficulties of such research, the mirror focus may well prove to be an important system for studying alterations in neuronal macromolecular metabolism with repetitive stimulation. It may also prove a useful, although exaggerated, model for studying the transfer of information from one side of the brain to the other.

REFERENCES

1. Agranoff, B. W., Davis, R. E., Casola, L., and Lim, R. Actinomycin-D blocks formation of memory of shock avoidance in goldfish. *Science* 158:1600, 1967.
2. Barondes, S. H., and Cohen, H. D. Delayed and sustained effect of acetoxycycloheximide on memory in mice. *Proc. Nat. Acad. Sci. USA* 58:157, 1967.
3. Barondes, S. H., and Cohen, H. D. Memory impairment after subcutaneous injection of acetoxycycloheximide. *Science* 160:556, 1968.
4. Cohen, H. D., and Barondes, S. H. Acetoxycycloheximide effect on learning and memory of a light-dark discrimination. *Nature* (London) 218:271, 1968.
5. Cohen, H. D., and Barondes, S. H. Further studies on learning and memory after intracerebral actinomycin-D. *J. Neurochem.* 13:207, 1966.
6. Geller, A., Robustelli, F., Barondes, S. H., Cohen, H. D., and Jarvik, M. E. Impaired performance by post-trial injections of cycloheximide in a passive avoidance task. *Psychopharmacologia* (Berlin) 14:371, 1969.
7. Mello, N. K. Concerning the interhemispheric transfer of mirror-image patterns in pigeons. *Physiology and Behavior* 1:293, 1967.
8. Morrell, F. Physiology and Histochemistry of the Mirror Focus. In Jasper, H. H., Ward, A. A., Jr., and Pope, A. (Eds.), *Basic Mechanisms of the Epilepsies*. Boston: Little, Brown, 1969.
9. Sperry, R. W. Split-brain Approach to Learning Problems. In Quarton, G. C., Melnechuk, T., and Schmitt, F. O. (Eds.), *The Neurosciences, A Study Program*. New York: Rockefeller Univ. Press, 1967.
10. Zemp, J. W., Wilson, J. E., Schlesinger, K., Boggan, W. D., and Glassman, E. Brain function and macromolecules. I. Incorporation of uridine into RNA of mouse brain during short-term training experience. *Proc. Nat. Acad. Sci. USA* 55:1423, 1966.

14
DC Potential Shifts in Paroxysmal States

HEINZ CASPERS AND ERWIN-JOSEF SPECKMANN

RECORDINGS made with suitable techniques of various brain areas indicate that the central nervous system produces a dc component besides the ac waves of the conventional EEG. This bioelectric phenomenon has been labeled as *steady potential*, but the term may be misleading, since the dc gradients by no means prove *steady*. They can be influenced by technical generators such as electrode potentials, and, in particular, depend on a variety of physiological test conditions. At first the dc level is clearly related to the sleep-wakeful cycle of the individual; at the transition from wakefulness to sleep, the cortical dc component undergoes a surface-positive shift, while an arousal reaction is associated with a surface-negative displacement [4, 5, 32, 48]. In the waking individual similar negative dc deflections can be elicited by sensory, reticular, and thalamic stimulations [1, 3, 4, 5, 31, 32, 37, 47]. The deflections have also been shown to occur in motor regions of the cerebral cortex preceding each voluntary movement [4, 5, 21].

All these physiological fluctuations of the dc component can be depressed or extinguished by anesthetics and a variety of drugs having sedative actions. Simultaneously, the basic level of the cortical dc potential shows a surface-positive shift and may finally reach a steady state [6, 32, 45]. However, considerable dc deviations can occur also in deeper stages of anesthesia. As a rule, they coincide very strictly with alterations of the respiratory rate and cerebral blood flow and can be attributed to changes of blood-gas tensions [6, 12, 41, 42, 45].

Distinct dc shifts are to be found during seizure activity, a particular subject which has been dealt with extensively [3, 7, 10, 11, 13, 14, 17, 24, 26, 29, 30, 32, 44, 46]. The results have added some new data to the analysis of convulsive discharges, but the question arises as to whether they have also contributed to a better understanding of the intimate mechanisms of seizure activity. Opinions are obviously conflicting. O'Leary and Goldring [32] query, as do the authors of this chapter, whether seizure mechanisms have been studied thoroughly if investigations of concomitant dc shifts have not been performed.

Objections concerning the reliability of dc recordings arise from the fact that they prove particularly sensitive to technical artifacts, but the main reason appears to be that generation of the steady potential is still poorly understood. Although neuronal structures are obviously involved in producing a dc component, a variety of other sources must be taken into account [10, 25, 33, 44, 45]. As long as the dc generation remains rather obscure, speculations continue about its functional significance.

More information on the origin and significance of dc displacements during seizure activity may be obtained by systematic comparison of the steady potential shifts with other bioelectric, motor, autonomic, and metabolic functions of the brain.

METHODS

In the majority of investigations performed on albino rats anesthetized with phenobarbital, the animals were ventilated artificially, although some comparative measurements were carried out with spontaneous respiration. In the latter cases, convulsive activity of the animal was recorded by means of an activity cage.

In most experiments, generalized convulsions induced by pentylenetetrazol served as a model. In anesthetized animals, repeated applications of the drug in doses of about 50 mg per kg finally evoke some degree of epileptic condition with periodic fits recurring spontaneously at intervals of 3–10 minutes [7].

The cortical steady potential was led from the surface of the intact sensorimotor cortex against a reference electrode in the front portion of the nose. Selected silver–silver chloride electrodes were employed in these experiments, and a special chopper-type dc amplifier with high gain and stability was used. Recording techniques have been described in detail [3, 4, 5, 6]. Besides the cortical dc potential, the conventional EEG and the direct cortical response were recorded in each case. Averaging of the electrically evoked responses was performed on a computer of average transients (CAT 400B), and the sequential interval histogram of single EEG spikes was determined by means of an amplitude discriminator (TMC 605) and the CAT 400B.

The effect of increasing pCO_2 in tissue on postsynaptic and action potentials of interneurons and motoneurons was investigated after lumbosacral laminectomy and preparation of ventral and dorsal roots as well as peripheral nerves. For intracellular recordings, glass micropipettes were used, filled with 3-M KCl; preferred resistance, 10–30 megohms (MΩ). Intracellular potentials were amplified by a high-impedance preamplifier and led in parallel to an oscilloscope (Tektronix 555; with plug-in unit 1-A-7) and to an inkwriter for recording the membrane potential. Frequency of spontaneously firing interneurons was analyzed off-line by using an FM tape recorder.

Arterial and venous pO_2, pCO_2, and pH were continuously recorded in the carotid artery and the jugular vein, respectively.

A polarographic pO_2 electrode, a pCO_2 electrode of Severinghaus type, as well as a conventional glass pH electrode, were arranged in a small, thermostabilized blood bypass. Arterial blood pressure was sufficient to propel blood through the bypass, while a small peristaltic pump was necessary for recordings in the venous blood. In both cases blood flow took about 5 sec to pass the device. Special latencies of the pO_2 and pH electrodes amounted to 15 sec, those of the pCO_2 electrode to 30 sec.

The pO_2 in cortical tissues was measured polarographically by means of an electropolished platinum microelectrode; this electrode was isolated by glass with the tip left free. The silver–silver chloride reference electrode was similarly manufactured. Both electrodes were fixed together at their tips by polystyrol. The tip diameter of this arrangement amounted to 5–20 μ. Marked steps in the polarogram of Pt microelectrodes are usually missing, proving it necessary to prevent changes of external dc potentials between the Pt and Ag–AgCl electrode. Therefore, the reference electrode is placed a few microns distant from the Pt tip; this special technique will be described in detail in another paper elsewhere.

Cortical pH was measured with a flat glass membrane electrode placed on the cortical surface and an Ag–AgCl ring contacting the cortex around the glass electrode. In this way the presence of dc potentials other than the pH component between the two electrodes could be prevented. The glass and reference electrodes were shunted for ac potentials by a capacitor to avoid rectification at the glass membrane. Changes of cortical blood flow were measured thermoelectrically in the majority of experiments.

Main Types of dc Shifts Associated with Seizure Activity

Development of seizure activity is always accompanied by distinct dc shifts, a survey of which is presented in Fig. 14-1. Tracings were recorded at a low paper speed from the intact cerebral cortex of rats with periodically recurring fits which were released by repeated applications of pentylenetetrazol. All dc displacements are surface-negative or negative-positive in polarity and not basically different in shape. A systematic study of their bioelectric, motor, autonomic, and metabolic correlates reveals, however, that two main types can be differentiated.

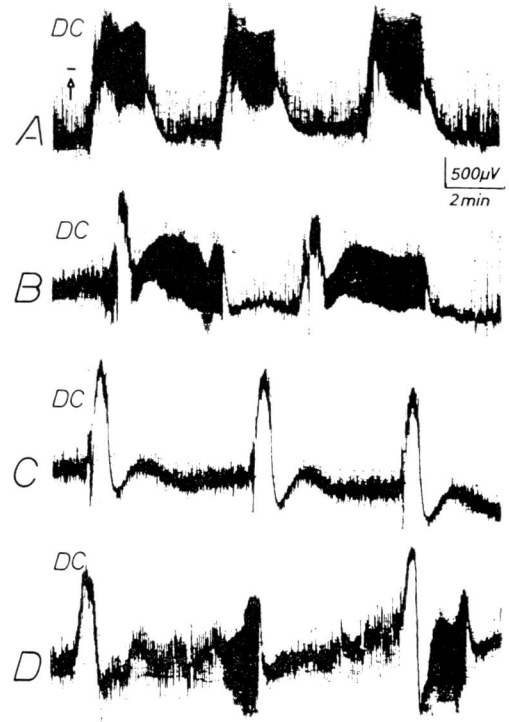

FIG. 14-1. Various types of cortical dc shifts during periodically recurring seizure attacks following repeated applications of pentylenetetrazol. (A) Seizure (S) type. (B) S type with delayed clonic phase. (C) Spreading depression (SD) type. (D) S and SD types occurring alternately.

One form of dc shifts, which is illustrated in Fig. 14-1A and B, coincides very strictly with manifest convulsions and therefore will be referred to as the *seizure type* (S). A second form of negative-positive dc deviations, which is represented in Fig. 14-1C, may also be initiated by a short series of spikes, but further development of the shift is characterized by a more-or-less complete extinction of both slow and sharp EEG waves. In accordance with this finding, some other criteria indicate that seizure susceptibility is diminished rather than increased. As a whole, this type of dc shift offers some of the essential properties of a spreading depression and will therefore, provisionally, be abbreviated as the SD type. Both groups of dc shifts may occur independently of each other (Fig. 14-1D). Occasionally they are linked in such a way that the SD shift rises from the peak or from the subsequent negative portions of the S type; an inversion of this sequence is not to be found.

THE SEIZURE (S) TYPE OF DC SHIFTS

Polarity, Time Course, and Distribution. Time course of the S type of dc shift is closely related to various stages of the epileptic fit. The onset of each single attack coincides with a steep surface-negative dc deviation which culminates in the tonic phase. At the transition to clonic convulsions, the shift tends to decay and turns to a rapid surface-positive deflection as soon as seizure activity passes over to the postictal silent period (Figs. 14-1, 14-2B, 14-7, 14-9, 14-10). With generalized seizures, dc displacements of the S-type occur synchronously on both hemispheres and show similar shapes in homotopic cortical fields. SD shifts, on the other hand, which sometimes emerge from an S type are usually restricted to one side.

With local seizures, form and polarity of observed dc shifts depend on the recording site. Within the immediate area of a unilateral focus, seizure activity is associated with the same negative-positive dc deflections as those which appear in generalized convulsions. At greater distance from this field, however, development of focal negativity leads to surface-positive dc reaction. Similar results are obtained with recordings from the homotopic point of the opposite hemisphere; an example of such an experiment is in Fig. 14-2. In this case, seizure susceptibility was elevated by pentylenetetrazol to an extent that periodic epileptic attacks failed to appear spontaneously but could be triggered by unilateral, continuous, weak stimulation of the cerebral cortex at a rate of 0.5 per sec [cf. 7]. Within the directly stimulated area, dc fluctuations associated with each single epileptic fit tend to be negative-positive in polarity as described above. Simultaneous recordings from the corresponding field of the other hemisphere, however, show an opposite sign (Fig. 14-2A). At this site, positive-negative dc deflections reverse in polarity as soon as the different recording electrode

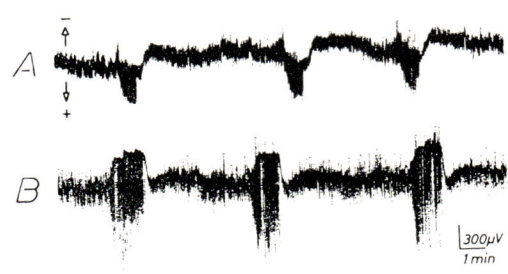

FIG. 14-2. Direct current recording from right motor cortex during continuous low frequency stimulation (0.5 per sec) of homotopic area in opposite hemisphere. (A) Weak stimuli evoke periodic surface-positive dc deflections. (B) The dc shifts reverse in polarity if stimulus strength is increased. Before stimulation, seizure susceptibility had been elevated by three applications of 30 mg pentylenetetrazol each.

penetrates the cortex from the surface to the fourth and fifth layers. A similar change in sign is found also in surface leads if stimulus strength is increased (Fig. 14-2B); in this condition, however, the above-mentioned differences between various cortical layers disappear. With stronger stimulations of the contralateral hemisphere, both time course and polarity of depth recordings of the dc component from the opposite side resemble those obtained in the surface leads.

These findings correspond, in principle, to observations reported by O'Leary and Goldring [30], Gumnit and Takahashi [14], and others. They suggest that this type of surface-positive dc displacement can be attributed to horizontally and vertically oriented dipoles or both which originate in the vicinity of more localized negative dc shifts in superficial and deeper cortical layers. Such positive dc deviations offer all the peculiarities of an increased seizure susceptibility and differ basically from positive displacements which occur in the postictal silent period. This postulate is supported by the various bioelectric, autonomic, and metabolic correlates of the dc shifts.

Relations between S Type of dc Shifts and EEG Waves. Previous investigations have already shown that S type of dc shifts is closely related to changes of ac potentials in the conventional EEG [7, 11, 13, 32].

This refers first to the spike discharge pattern reflected in the sequential interval histogram. Tracings in Fig. 14-3 indicate that both voltage and steepness of negative dc shifts increase whenever distance shortens between successive spikes within a train of convulsive discharges. Plotting the amplitude of negative dc deviation against spike intervals reveals an approximate linear relationship over a wide range. Considerable fluctuations of the sequential interval histogram which reflect clustering of seizure discharges in the clonic phase are usually associated with distinct decay of the surface-negative wave, even when the total number of spikes per second is not essentially diminished.

The findings can be reproduced by direct electrical stimulation of the cerebral cortex with various pulse patterns [7]. Strict coincidence between disappearance of EEG waves and positive dc deflection in the postictal silent period has already been mentioned. Recordings of the sequential interval histogram of EEG spikes during an epileptic attack allow prediction of the particular shape of the concomitant dc shift and vice versa.

Another relation between S type of dc shifts and EEG waves refers to polarity of single convulsive spikes. Such linkage can

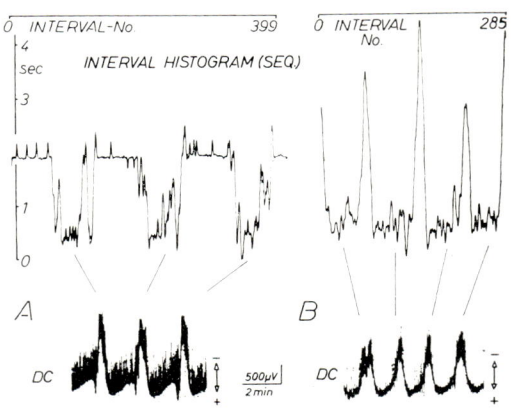

FIG. 14-3. Relations between cortical dc shifts and EEG spike intervals during periodical convulsions released by pentylenetetrazol. Amplitudes of negative dc shifts correspond to decrease of mean spike interval length in sequential histogram.

be shown to occur with spontaneous seizure discharges, but becomes more evident with superficially evoked cortical potentials, because their parameters are subject to more precise experimental control. Therefore, dc shifts will be compared with changes of direct cortical response to an electrical stimulus (DCR).

Numerous investigations have already shown that development of seizure activity by direct electrical excitations of the cerebral cortex is accompanied by striking alterations of the DCR. With continued stimulation, the primary negative response to each single electrical stimulus decreases in amplitude and finally reverses in polarity, provided that the local response is recorded within the directly stimulated area (Fig. 14-4, IIA). A critical voltage of the inversed DCR appears to be prerequisite for selfsustained afterdischarges. Comparative measurements with dc amplifiers show that reversal of direct cortical response is closely related to voltage of the concomitant dc shift (Fig. 14-4, I). This is substantiated by the fact that anticonvulsant drugs, such as hydantoins, reduce amplitude of the evoked negative dc shift which parallels changes of the DCR (Fig. 14-4). Correspondence between cortical dc displacements and locally evoked ac potentials is not confined to electrically induced convulsions, but can be shown to exist with a variety of other experimental procedures

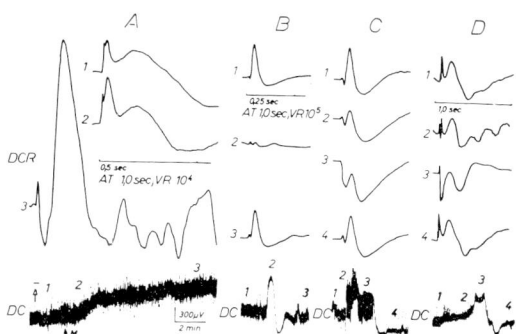

FIG. 14-5. Relation between cortical dc shifts (DC) and average direct cortical responses (DCR) during various seizure types. (A) Slow negative dc deviation and enhancement of DCR after first application of pentylenetetrazol. (B) Extinction of DCR during dc shift of SD type. (C) Reversal of normal DCR during steep surface-negative dc shift of S type. (D) Reversal of normal DCR during negative dc shift recorded from epileptogenic focus.

Technical data of DCR recordings: Number of sweeps: 26 (A), 38 (B), 36 (C), and 32 (D); analysis time 1.0 sec. Sweep speed identical in (A)–(C), diminished in (D). Amplification: note vertical range differences between (A) and (B)–(D). Voltage and time calibrations of dc recordings apply to all columns.

which initiate focal seizure activity, provided all recordings are taken from the immediate focal area.

Figure 14-5D demonstrates reversal of the

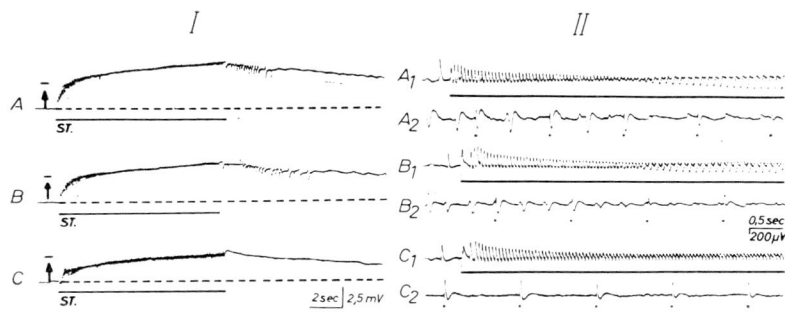

FIG. 14-4. Action of diphenylhydantoin (DH) on dc and ac responses of cerebral cortex to electrical stimuli. (IA) Negative dc shift during 20 per sec epicortical stimulation (St); (IIA₁) ac response to a 20 per sec stimulation; (IIA₂) ac responses to one per sec stimulation (dots) mixed with spontaneous afterdischarges immediately following (IIA₁). About 5 min (B) and 45 min (C) after application of 50 mg per kg DH, both reversal of ac responses and spontaneous afterdischarges gradually disappeared. Effect is associated with reduction of evoked negative dc shift.

normal DCR in the course of a negative dc deviation led from a chronic epileptogenic lesion during a focal attack; in generalized seizures, relations between dc shift and DCR prove more complex. Extensive increase of seizure susceptibility elicited by a single application of 50 mg per kg pentylenetetrazol is accompanied by a slowly rising negative dc displacement. This shift coincides with considerable enhancement of surface-negative components of the normal DCR (Fig. 14-5A). Progressive reduction and final reversal of direct cortical response occur only during additional and steep negative dc deviations which accompany a manifest convulsion (Fig. 14-5C). On the whole, relations between dc shifts and DCR during seizure activity resemble those obtained with cathodal polarization of cerebral cortex or after local application of GABA, which also gives rise to surface-negative dc displacement [3, 34].

Relations between Seizure (S) Type of dc Shifts and Changes of Local pO_2, pCO_2 and pH. Results of earlier studies indicate that the dc component is particularly sensitive to changes in oxygen and carbon dioxide tensions in blood and tissue [6, 12, 32, 41, 42]. Lowering of pO_2 as well as decrease of pCO_2 produce a surface-negative dc shift usually at threshold levels, at which the conventional EEG is scarcely altered. Rise of pCO_2 and corresponding change of pH, on the other hand, release a surface-positive dc deviation; examples are illustrated in Fig. 14-10, 14-13, and 14-14. These results raise the question as to whether, and to what extent, alterations of gas metabolism which occur during seizure activity [9, 19, 28] may contribute to observed dc shifts. Particular responsiveness of the dc component to changes of gas tensions and pH values has fostered the hypothesis that at least a major portion of evoked shifts originates across the blood-brain barrier and the meninges rather than in neuronal structures [25, 44, 45]. For further clarification of associated problems, it was felt necessary to study in greater detail relations between dc shifts and gas tensions during seizure activity.

In a first series of experiments, dc component and tissue pO_2 at the recording site were simultaneously traced, applying a platinum-silver double microelectrode with tip diameter of 5–20 µ (see METHODS). Results show that reactions of cortical pO_2 in the course of a generalized seizure vary considerably; both increases and decreases of local pO_2 are found. Actual change of oxygen tension in each single case (Fig. 14-6) is clearly related to simultaneous alterations of cortical blood flow (CBF). With stronger enhancement of CBF, due to concomitant rise of pCO_2, increase in oxygen consumption during seizure activity may even be overcompensated by increase of oxygen supply. In this condition, onset of convulsions is always associated with moderate rise of cortical pO_2, followed by a steep overshoot as soon as the clonic convulsive phase merges into the postictal silent period. Such findings are obtained particularly with animals in good circulatory condition and during the first convulsions within a series of epileptic fits (Fig. 14-7). With repeated attacks, the basic level of pCO_2 tends to increase, and reactivity of cortical vessels is consequently diminished. Finally, a stage may be reached in which CBF remains almost unaltered during an epileptic fit; in such experimental situations, the profile of cortical pO_2 shifts depends primarily on changes of oxygen consumption, provided that arterial pO_2 is kept constant by artificial ventilation. Under this condition, fluctuations of both the dc component and cortical pO_2

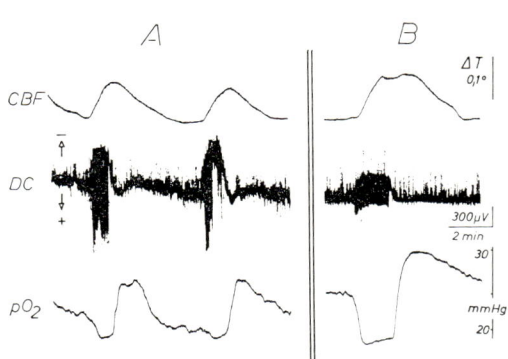

FIG. 14-6. Relations between negative dc shifts of S type, cortical blood flow (CBF), and cortical pO_2 during generalized seizure discharges in two experiments.

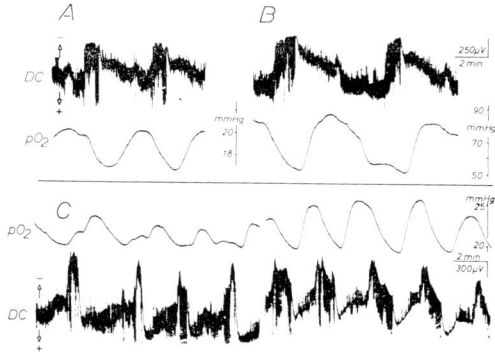

FIG. 14-7. Simultaneous recordings of cortical dc shifts and tissue pO_2 at recording site during generalized convulsions. Animal ventilated artificially with air (A) and 100% oxygen (B). Note different pO_2 calibrations. Tracing (C) demonstrates changes of local pO_2 reactions in the course of repeated seizure discharges.

run parallel. Each negative dc shift during seizure activity is accompanied by reduction of oxygen tension and vice versa. This finding, illustrated in Fig. 14-8, corresponds, in principal, with observations of Ingvar et al. [18].

Comparative measurements prove that the described variability of the cortical pO_2 during generalized convulsions is not reflected in concomitant dc shifts, which show a rather uniform time course (Fig. 14-8). This finding permits the conclusion that oxygen deficiency does not contribute measurably to initiation of typical dc dis-

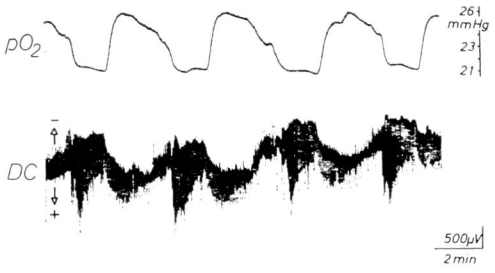

FIG. 14-8. Relations between cortical dc shifts of S type and tissue pO_2 at recording site during generalized seizure discharges. Recordings taken in epileptic status at stage when cortical blood flow had reached stable state; arterial pO_2 kept constant by artificial ventilation.

placements. Correspondence between dc reactions and cortical pO_2, shown to exist at a constant oxygen supply, suggests that S type of dc shifts is closely related to an increase in energy metabolism. In this respect, the S type differs basically from the SD type, as will be indicated later.

The above-mentioned results imply an answer to another question: it has often been suspected that cessation of epileptic discharge might be due to critical reduction of local pO_2. There is no doubt that oxygen deficiency can exert such an inhibitory influence, but the present findings indicate that it does not play a decisive role. A seizure discharge may cease independently whether local pO_2 is raised or diminished. This can be supported by other experimental evidence derived from Fig. 14-7, where tracings were obtained during an epileptic status in a stage when reactivity of CBF had already been reduced. Each convulsive attack is therefore accompanied by decay of local pO_2. A comparison of Fig. 14-7A and B demonstrates that duration of seizure discharge is only slightly increased if oxygen instead of air is applied. In this case, convulsions tend to stop, even when local pO_2 ranges far above the normal level.

Another series of experiments was devoted to the question of whether changes of carbon dioxide tension and of pH in cortical tissues might contribute to dc shifts during seizure activity. Continuous recordings in the venous blood usually show a rise of pCO_2 and lowering of pH concomitant with each single epileptic attack (Fig. 14-9). This suggests that surface-negative dc shifts are not essentially influenced by such metabolic effects, since an increase of pCO_2 regularly causes surface-positive deviations [5, 12, 41]. Measurements in the jugular vein, however, integrate metabolic processes in the whole brain and do not necessarily reflect changes in the cerebral cortex. Therefore, local determinations are required. Reliable microelectrodes for continuous direct measurements of the tissue pCO_2 are not yet available and for this reason, cortical pH was chosen to serve as an indicator.

Results show that changes of pH during

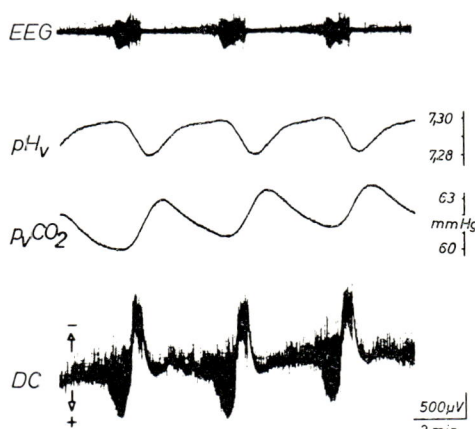

FIG. 14-9. Relations between cortical dc shifts of S type, pCO$_2$, and pH recorded in jugular vein. Conventional EEG was simultaneously traced from opposite hemisphere. As to latencies of pCO$_2$ and pH recordings, see METHODS.

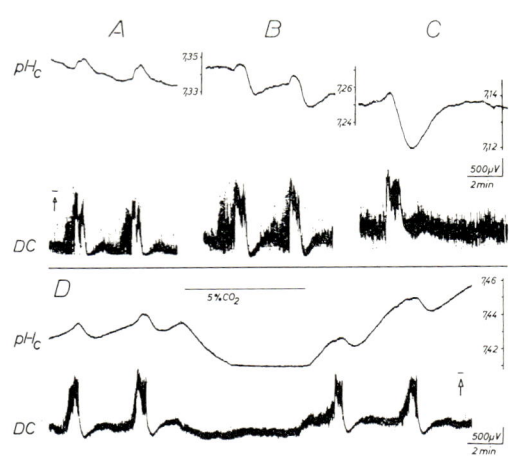

FIG. 14-10. (A), (B), and (C) Simultaneous recordings of cortical dc potential and cortical pH in the course of repeated epileptic attacks in one animal. (D) Demonstrates interruption of periodically recurring fits during decrease of local pH released by rise of inspiratory pCO$_2$. Extinction of seizure discharges was accompanied by surface-positive dc displacement.

an epileptic attack vary in the same way as those of local pO$_2$. In this case too, variability can be attributed preferentially to different reactions of CBF. With stronger increase in flow, metabolic acidosis which develops at the onset of seizure discharge may be rapidly overcompensated and thus turn to an "alkaline wave," which corresponds with earlier observations [19, 44] and is illustrated in Fig. 14-10A, D. After repeated convulsions, absolute level of pH tends to fall. Simultaneously, responsiveness of CBF to each single epileptic fit diminishes strongly. In this condition, the primary rise of pH passes over to a biphasic and finally to an "acidic wave" (Fig. 14-10B, C). Comparative evaluations of the concomitant dc displacements do not reveal any significant differences as to voltage and time course of shifts, whether pH changes turn out to be alkaline, acidic, or biphasic. This permits the conclusion that fluctuations of pH which occur during an epileptic attack do not exert an essential influence on dc generator structures. They are obviously limited to a subthreshold range.

The above-mentioned results touch upon another important problem concerning cessation of self-sustained seizure discharge. Critical lowering of tissue pO$_2$ has been discussed as a possible cause, but the pres-

ent findings indicate that such a mechanism does not play a decisive role. Complete inhibition of seizure discharges can be achieved by stronger rise of pCO$_2$ and by lowering the local pH. A typical example is presented in Figs. 14-10D and 14-13. Tracings show that extinction of seizure activity is accompanied by surface-positive dc displacement. This gives rise to the question of whether cessation of an epileptic attack which coincides with a steep surface-positive dc shift might be due to concomitant alterations of local pCO$_2$ and of pH or both. The present findings do not support such an assumption.

As soon as CBF reaches a steady state, all dc deviations during an epileptic fit run parallel to decrease of both local pO$_2$ and pH. These observations suggest that surface-negative dc shifts of the S type are closely related to increase in energy metabolism.

Spreading Depression (SD) Type of dc Shifts

Since the first observations of Leão, the SD type of dc shifts has been the subject of extensive studies (for literature, see [27]).

Although obviously related to seizure phenomena, SD type differs in many respects from the S type and is found only in exceptional cases to arise synchronously in both cerebral hemispheres.

Usually, the shift starts from a frontal or central area on one side and spreads at a rate of a few millimeters per minute. It may develop from the top of a preceding S type, but reversal of such sequence has not been observed. In further contrast, surface-negative dc deviations of SD form are usually associated with extinction of both spontaneous and evoked EEG waves. Comparative measurements are illustrated in Fig. 14-5. Striking differences emerge, moreover, from simultaneous recordings of local pO_2 and pH. As was already pointed out, dc shifts of the S type show a close relation to changes of tissue pO_2 as soon as cortical oxygen supply reaches a stable state.

The tracings in Fig. 14-11 indicate that transition from S type to SD form of dc deflections is accompanied by a sudden rise of cortical pO_2, although amplitude of the negative shift may even exceed the preceding level. This finding could be attributed to a rapid and strong increase in cortical blood flow. Controversial observations in the literature on this particular subject do not support such an interpretation [2, 15, 16, 19, 23], and we failed to detect any significant rise of blood flow during SD shifts, when an initial series of spike discharges was missing [7]. In this condition, enhancement of local pO_2 can be explained only by decrease of oxygen consumption; findings suggest that SD type of dc deviations during seizure activity reflects lowering of energy metabolism.

ORIGIN AND FUNCTIONAL SIGNIFICANCE OF DC SHIFTS ASSOCIATED WITH SEIZURE ACTIVITY

Direct current recordings from cerebral structures may be influenced, in principle, by a variety of sources. In the first place, technical generators such as electrode potentials must be considered which prove sensitive to changes of pH, of temperature, and of tissue impedance at the recording site. Various biological sources may contribute to observed dc shifts; in this context, potential differences across the blood-brain barrier and the meninges have been taken into account [25, 44, 45]. Present findings indicate that such possible generators are not involved essentially in producing the typical dc shift during seizure activity; they point more toward neuronal origin and in particular, toward summation of membrane potential changes. This interpretation is supported by results of intracellular recordings from single neurons [10, 20, 38, 43].

Many published data demonstrate similarity between fluctuations of neuronal membrane potentials and concomitant dc shifts in the course of an epileptic fit. Findings show, especially, a connection between SD type of dc shifts and excessive membrane depolarization, where the spike generating mechanism is blocked. The negative component of the S type, on the other hand, which tends to be smaller in amplitude, coincides with considerable increase of excitatory postsynaptic potentials (EPSPs) usually associated with rise of spike discharge rate. Such a finding is illustrated in Fig. 14-12.

If dc shifts during seizure activity do reflect membrane potential changes of neu-

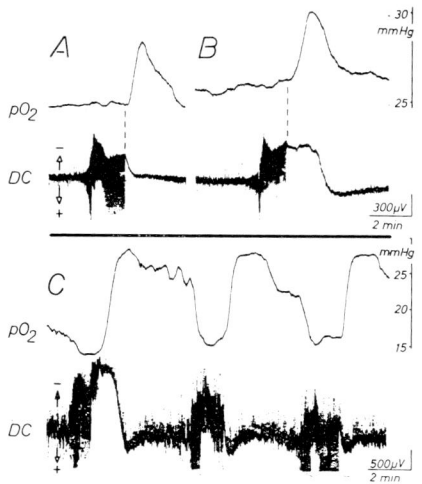

FIG. 14-11. Simultaneous recordings of cortical dc potential and tissue pO_2 at recording site during dc shifts of both the S and SD types (A)–(C). Transition from S type to SD form in (B) and (C) was associated with sudden increase of local pO_2.

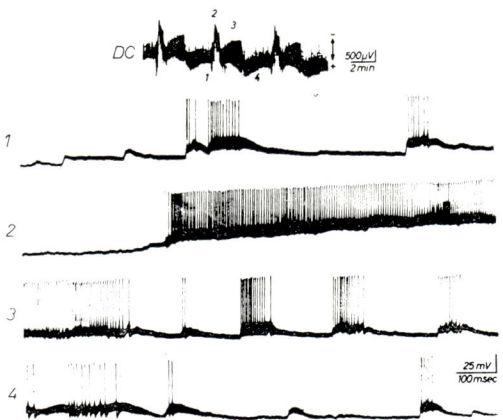

Fig. 14-12. Relations between cortical dc shifts (DC) and intracellularly recorded membrane potential changes of motoneuron during generalized epileptic attacks induced by repeated application of pentylenetetrazol. Unit recordings 1–4 taken during periods indicated by corresponding numbers in upper dc tracing. Membrane depolarizations of motoneuron are related to surface-negative dc deflections in various phases of fit.

rons, close relationship between the two phenomena has to be expected also with seizure inhibition. Figures 14-10 and 14-13 demonstrate complete extinction of convulsive discharges parallel to surface-positive dc displacement induced by increase of pCO_2. A neuronal interpretation of this effect would postulate membrane hyperpolarization with the EPSPs being simultaneously

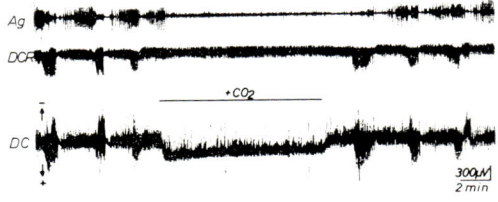

Fig. 14-13. Inhibition of periodically recurring seizure discharges by application of 10 percent CO_2 via inspired air. Ag: Motor activity of animal traced by means of activity cage. DCR: Direct cortical response; extinction of seizure activity coincides with surface-positive dc displacement. Inhibition of motor-seizure phenomena outlasts suppression of cortical convulsive discharges.

reduced, but a survey of pertinent literature indicates that such a mechanism cannot be readily predicted. Rise of pCO_2 causes different types of excitable structures to depolarize rather than the reverse [8]. Except for the respiratory system and the immediately adhering structures, very little is known about response of cortical and spinal neurons in mammals. For this reason we have studied actions of CO_2 on single cells in the lumbar region of the spinal cord and in the motor cortex of rats.

Previous investigations on the response patterns of spontaneously firing spinal interneurons had already shown [40, 42] that two types of cells can be differentiated. One, type I, becomes clearly inhibited by a rise of the pCO_2, while type II is activated. Meanwhile similar findings were obtained with motoneurons. Of the whole population studied in the upper lumbar region, about 85 percent proved to be type I neurons. Comparative measurements indicate that this type predominates at the cortical level to a still greater extent. For further clarification of the CO_2 actions, interneurons and motoneurons of type I have been recorded intracellularly. In these experiments, pCO_2 was raised in part via inspired air, but sometimes another procedure was preferred which avoids respiratory pulsations at the recording site. The animal was ventilated artificially with pure oxygen for some 30 minutes before breathing was stopped; in this condition, oxygen supply stays at a normal level for a rather long time, while pCO_2 shows continuous rise. An example is presented in Fig. 14-14.

The tracings demonstrate parallelism between surface-positive dc deflection and increase of pCO_2; both normal EEG waves and seizure discharges are gradually being depressed. At such a stage, type I neurons always show distinct hyperpolarization and simultaneously, voltage as well as steepness of EPSPs decrease until spike generation fails. This is illustrated in the upper part of Fig. 14-15. The lower part of the figure demonstrates gradual inhibition of a spontaneously firing interneuron during an apneic phase. Measurements by means of current injections show, moreover, considerable increase in membrane resistance.

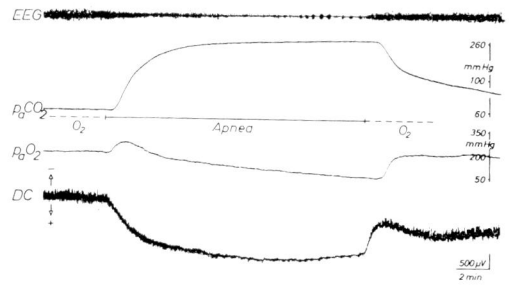

FIG. 14-14. Changes of conventional EEG, of the arterial pO_2 and pCO_2, and of the cortical steady potential (DC) during apnea following ventilation with 100 percent oxygen for about 30 min. In the course of the apnea, O_2 reservoir remained in contact with respiratory tract of the animal. Positive dc shift was related to increase of the pCO_2.

Summary

The present findings support the assumption that at least a major portion of dc deflections associated with seizure activity originates at neuronal membranes. The S type of dc shifts can more easily be attributed to a summation of postsynaptic potentials, while the SD form reflects excessive depolarization of generator structures, which appears to be due to local metabolic disorders rather than to synaptically induced excitations. Such differentiation between the two types of dc shifts is also substantiated by their various bioelectric and metabolic correlates.

So far, the term *neuronal membrane potentials* has been used in a wider sense, but the question may be raised as to whether all parts of a neuron contribute to generation of the dc component in a similar way. Computations by Rall et al. [35, 36] derived from original data have shown that time constants of both rise and decay of EPSPs in dendrites prove significantly longer than in the cell soma. For this reason, dendritic membrane potentials appear to be more effective in producing a dc component. According to observations by Smith et al. [39], EPSPs obviously predominate at dendritic membranes while inhibitory postsynaptic potentials (IPSPs) are restricted, more or less, to somatic regions. This finding might account for the fact that dc shifts associated

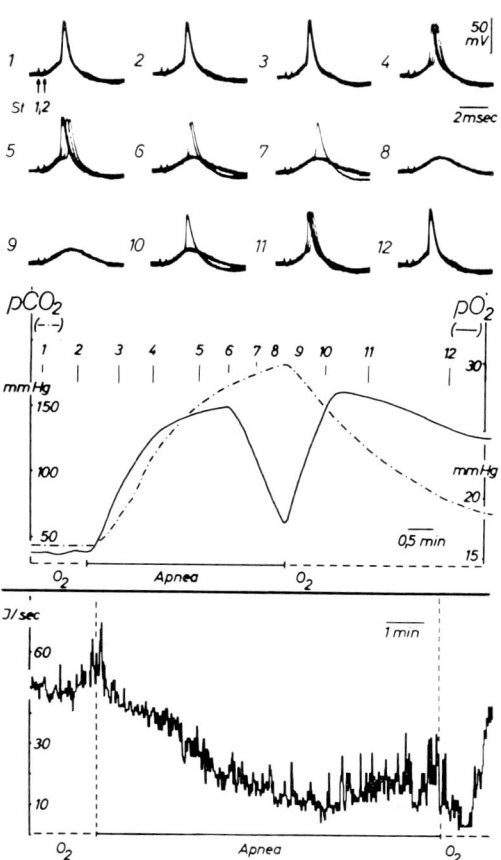

FIG. 14-15. Upper part: Intracellular recording of a rat motoneuron activated orthodromically by two stimuli (St. 1, 2). Simultaneously, tissue pO_2 and arterial pCO_2 were measured. During apnea following administration of pure oxygen, both pO_2 and pCO_2 increase (cf. Fig. 14-14). Due to rising pCO_2, EPSPs (4, 5, and 6) gradually decrease until spike generation fails (6, 7, and 8). Complete recovery of EPSPs occurs as soon as pCO_2 returns to normal level. About 20 sweeps are superimposed in each record. Lower part: Decrease of spontaneous firing rate of a spinal interneuron in lumbar region of spinal cord during apnea under the same conditions as described above.

with seizure activity used to be surface negative in polarity, although high voltage IPSPs can occur, especially in the clonic phase.

In this context, another possible source of dc potentials has to be considered.

Studies by Kuffler et al. [22, 33] permit a conclusion that membrane potential changes in glial cells run almost parallel to dc shifts in a variety of experimental situations. Therefore, glial potentials might contribute to observed dc shifts provided that dimensions of membrane and internal resistances permit sufficient summation. The work of the authors mentioned indicates that membrane potential fluctuations of glial cells are closely related changes in activity of adherent neuronal structures. Thus, dc recordings would reflect neuronal excitation processes even if the steady potential is generated in part by glial membranes.

If interpretation of origin of dc potentials proves correct, the question arises as to whether dc displacements not only reflect excitation processes but also exert an influence on origin and spread of seizure discharge. Experimental data are not yet sufficient to give a satisfactory answer, but some mechanisms may be mentioned. An excessive dendritic depolarization, for instance, reflected by surface-negative dc shift, could influence the membrane potential at pertinent soma and thus modulate the time course of seizure discharge. Another mechanism, frequently discussed, depends on development of dipoles preferentially during localized convulsive discharge. As already pointed out, negative dc shift in the immediate area of a focus is surrounded by a field of positive shift, which might have an inhibitory action.

REFERENCES

1. Brookhart, J. M., Arduini, A., Mancia, M., and Moruzzi, G. Thalamocortical relations as revealed by induced slow potential changes. *J. Neurophysiol.* 21:499, 1958.
2. Buresova, O. Changes in cerebral circulation in rats during spreading EEG depression. *Physiol. Bohemoslov.* 6:1, 1957.
3. Caspers, H. Über die Beziehungen zwischen Dendritenpotential und Gleichspannung an der Hirnrinde. *Pflueger Arch. Ges. Physiol.* 269:157, 1959.
4. Caspers, H. Die Veränderungen der corticalen Gleichspannung und ihre Beziehungen zur sensomotorischen Aktivität (Verhalten) bei Weckreizungen am freibeweglichen Tier. *Proc. XXII, Int. Physiol. Congr.*, Leiden, vol. 1. Amsterdam: Excerpta Medica, 1962.
5. Caspers, H. Relations of Steady Potential Shifts in the Cortex to the Wakefulness-Sleep Spectrum. In Brazier, M. A. (Ed.), *Brain Function*. Berkeley: Univ. of Calif. Press, 1963.
6. Caspers, H., Schütz, E., and Speckmann, E.-J. Gleichspannungsveränderungen an der Hirnrinde bei Sauerstoffmangel. *Z. Biol.* 114:112, 1963.
7. Caspers, H., and Simmich, W. Cortical DC shifts associated with seizure activity. *Excerpta Medica*, ICSU 124:151, 1966.
8. Chalazonitis, N. Chemopotentials in Giant Nerve Cells (*Aplysia fasciata*). In Florey, E. (Ed.), *Nervous Inhibition*. Oxford: Pergamon, 1961.
9. Gellhorn, E., and Heymans, C. Differential action of anoxia, asphyxia and carbon dioxide on normal and convulsive potentials. *J. Neurophysiol.* 11:261, 1948.
10. Glötzner, F., and Grüsser, O.-J. Membranpotential und Entladungsfolgen corticaler Zellen, EEG und corticales DC-Potential bei generalisierten Krampfanfällen. *Arch. Psychiat. Nervenkr.* 210:313, 1968.
11. Gloor, P., Vera, C. L., Sperti, L., and Ray, S. N. Investigations on the mechanisms of epileptic discharge in the hippocampus. *Epilepsia* (Amst.) 2:42, 1961.
12. Goldensohn, E. S., Schönfeld, R. L., and Höfer, P. F. A. The slowly changing voltage of the brain and the electrocorticogram. *Electroenceph. Clin. Neurophysiol.* 3:231, 1951.
13. Goldring, S. Negative Steady Potential Shifts which Lead to Seizure Discharge. In Brazier, M. A. (Ed.), *Brain Function*. Berkeley: Univ. of Calif. Press, 1963.
14. Gumnit, R. U., and Takahashi, T. Changes in direct current activity during experimental focal seizures. *Electroenceph. Clin. Neurophysiol.* 19:63, 1965.
15. Harreveld, A. van, and Ochs, S. Electrical and vascular concomitants of spreading depression. *Amer. J. Physiol.* 189:159, 1957.

16. Harreveld, A. van, and Stamm, J. S. Vascular concomitants of spreading cortical depression. *J. Neurophysiol.* 15:487, 1952.
17. Harreveld, A. van, and Stamm, J. S. Spreading cortical convulsions and depressions. *J. Neurophysiol.* 16:352, 1953.
18. Ingvar, D. H., Lübbers, D. W., and Siesjö, B. K. Normal and epileptic EEG patterns related to cortical oxygen tension in the cat. *Acta Physiol. Scand.* 55:210, 1962.
19. Jasper, H., and Erickson, T. C. Cerebral blood flow and pH in excessive cortical discharge induced by metrazol and electrical stimulation. *J. Neurophysiol.* 4:333, 1941.
20. Kandel, E. R., and Spencer, W. A. The pyramidal cell during hippocampal seizure. *Epilepsia* (Amst.) 2:63, 1961.
21. Kornhuber, H. H., and Deecke, L. Hirnpotentialänderungen bei Willkürbewegungen und passiven Bewegungen des Menschen: Bereitschaftspotential und reafferente Potentiale. *Pflueger Arch. Ges. Physiol.* 284:1, 1965.
22. Kuffler, S. W., Nicholls, J. G., and Orkand, R. K. Physiological properties of glial cells in the central nervous system of amphibia. *J. Neurophysiol.* 29:768, 1966.
23. Leão, A. A. P. Pial circulation and spreading depression of activity in cerebral cortex. *J. Neurophysiol.* 7:391, 1944.
24. Liberson, W. T., and Cadilhac, G. Further observations on DC potentials during electrically induced seizure discharge activity in guinea pig. *Electroenceph. Clin. Neurophysiol.* 5:320, 1953.
25. Loeschcke, H. H. Über den Einfluss von CO_2 auf die Bestandpotentiale der Hirnhäute. *Pflueger Arch. Ges. Physiol.* 262:532, 1956.
26. Mahnke, J. M., and Ward, A. A., Jr. Standing potential characteristics of epileptogenic focus. *Epilepsia* (Amst.) 2:161, 1961.
27. Marshall, W. H. Spreading cortical depression of Leão. *Physiol. Rev.* 39:239, 1959.
28. Meyer, J. S., Gotoh, F., and Favale, E. Cerebral metabolism during epileptic seizures in man. *Electroenceph. Clin. Neurophysiol.* 21:10, 1966.
29. Morrell, F. Microelectrode and steady potential studies suggesting a dendritic locus of closure. *Electroenceph. Clin. Neurophysiol.* Suppl. 13, 65, 1959.
30. O'Leary, J. L., and Goldring, S. Slow cortical potentials. Their origin and contribution to seizure discharge. *Epilepsia* (Amst.) 1:561, 1960.
31. O'Leary, J. L., and Goldring, S. Changes Associated with Forebrain Excitation Processes: D.C. Potentials of the Cerebral Cortex. In Field, J. (Ed.), *Handbook of Physiology*. Baltimore: Williams and Wilkins, 1960.
32. O'Leary, J. L., and Goldring, S. D-C potentials of the brain. *Physiol. Rev.* 44:91, 1964.
33. Orkand, R. K., Nicholls, J. G., and Kuffler, S. W. Effect of nerve impulses on the membrane potential of glial cells in the central nervous system of amphibia. *J. Neurophysiol.* 29:788, 1966.
34. Purpura, D. P., Girado, M., and Grundfest, H. Selective blockade of excitatory synapses in the cat brain by γ-aminobutyric acid (GABA). *Science* 125:1200, 1957.
35. Rall, W. Distinguishing theoretical synaptic potentials computed for different soma-dendritic distributions of synaptic input. *J. Neurophysiol.* 30:1138, 1967.
36. Rall, W., Burke, R. E., Smith, T. G., Nelson, P. G., and Frank, K. Dendritic location of synapses and possible mechanisms for the monosynaptic EPSP in motoneurons. *J. Neurophysiol.* 30:1169, 1967.
37. Rowland, V., and Goldstone, M. Appetitively conditioned and drive-related bioelectric baseline shift in cat cortex. *Electroenceph. Clin. Neurophysiol.* 15:474, 1963.
38. Sawa, M., Maruyama, N., and Kaji, S. Intracellular potential during electrically induced seizures. *Electroenceph. Clin. Neurophysiol.* 15:209, 1963.
39. Smith, T. G., Wuerker, R. B., and Frank, K. Membrane impedance changes during synaptic transmission in cat spinal motoneurons. *J. Neurophysiol.* 30:1072, 1967.
40. Sokolov, W., and Speckmann, E.-J. Aktivitätsänderungen spinaler Neurone während und nach einer Asphyxie. *Pflueger Arch. Ges. Physiol.* 300:85, 1968.
41. Speckmann, E.-J., and Caspers, H. Les modifications du potentiel continu cortical pendant l'arrêt respiratoire. *Rev. Neurol.* 117:5, 1967.
42. Speckmann, E.-J., and Caspers, H. Verschiebungen des corticalen DC-Potentials

und ihre Beziehungen zu den Änderungen der Blutgasdrucke bei Hypo- und Hyperventilation. *Proc. XXIV, Int. Physiol. Congr.* Washington, D.C., 7:411, 1968.

43. Sugaya, E., Goldring, S., and O'Leary, J. L. Intracellular potentials associated with direct cortical response and seizure discharge in cat. *Electroenceph. Clin. Neurophysiol.* 17:661, 1964.

44. Tschirgi, R. D., Inanaga, K., Taylor, J. L., Walker, R. M., and Sonnenschein, R. R. Changes in cortical pH and blood flow accompanying spreading cortical depression and convulsion. *Amer. J. Physiol.* 190:557, 1957.

45. Tschirgi, R. D., and Taylor, J. L. Slowly changing bioelectric potentials associated with the blood-brain barrier. *Amer. J. Physiol.* 195:7, 1958.

46. Vanasupa, P., Goldring, S., and O'Leary, J. L. Seizure discharges effected by intravenously administered convulsant drugs. *Electroenceph. Clin. Neurophysiol.* 11:93, 1959.

47. Walter, G. W. Slow potential waves in the human brain associated with expectancy, attention and decision. *Arch. Psychiat. Nervenkr.* 206:309, 1964.

48. Wurtz, R. H., and O'Flaherty, J. J. Physiological correlates of steady potential shifts during sleep and wakefulness. *Electroenceph. Clin. Neurophysiol.* 22:30, 1967.

Discussion

POLARIZATION OF GENICULATE AND CORTICAL NEURONS
JAMES L. O'LEARY

The notion of polarization of neurons is an old one. In 1881 Bubnoff and Heidenhain [6] showed that on closing a dc circuit having the negative pole in contact with motor cortex, contractions were produced at considerably lower intensity than with positive-pole contact. In other early studies with different emphases, Beck and Cybulski [1] noted that frontal was positive to occipital cortex and exterior of cortex to depth on a cut surface (Caton [7]). Kappers [11] developed the theory of neurobiotaxis which involves growth of cell dendrites toward a center of stimulation and shift of the somata in the same direction; the axon grows away from the center of stimulation. Herrick [10] also features polarization of neurons in his structural theories of nervous organization.

A mass of neurons of uniform orientation shares a potential field configuration which can be deduced from form and polarity of evoked potentials, recorded serially as an electrode is passed through a buried cell mass. Analysis is cleanest when presynaptic axons enter one surface of a cell sheet and postsynaptic axons emerge from the other, the electrode passing parallel to the soma-axon axes. These conditions are fulfilled in the lateral geniculate nucleus of the cat which has been studied intensively [3, 4]. Lorente de Nó [12] has conducted similar studies upon the hypoglossal nucleus, a cell mass of different configuration.

Lateral Geniculate Nucleus

In the lateral geniculate nucleus (Bishop and O'Leary [3]), the closely packed relay neurons are formed of several layers which receive their input from contralateral and ipsilateral eyes respectively (Fig. D14-1). A significant extent of cell layers produces a plane surface lying nearly horizontal to the long axis of the forebrain (Fig. D14-1A). The optic tract layer spreads out below, its presynaptic terminal axons passing perpendicularly upward to ramify between dendrites of the contained neurons. Postsynaptic axons issuing from cell layers follow an upward course to form the origin of optic radiation. Thus an appropriately oriented needle electrode passed vertically downward through cell layers will encounter (1) massed axons of the radiation, (2) the cell layer representing the contralateral retina, (3) that of the homolateral retina, and (4) the optic-tract fiber layer. It may be led appropriately against an electrode inserted into the optic-tract layer, (Fig. D14-1B, 1) and, alternately, (Fig. D14-1B, 2) to one situated at sufficient distance to render it relatively indifferent to visually induced activity.

This recording arrangement is nearly ideal for studying changes in configuration of the electrical record of response evoked by optic-nerve stimulation and has since been used by numerous other investigators to study various aspects of activity of the visual relay system. In the field potential record deriving from the cell layers, first, second, and even a third optic-tract spike may be recorded together with a postsynaptic potential signifying outward conduction along optic radiation axons.

It is important to recognize that when an impulse occupies a region between two such electrodes situated upon a linear path, existing differences in polarity are such that the active region becomes negative to positive regions in either direction from it. If such differences in potential are oppositely directed and the electrodes are at a distance, they tend to be affected equally, and no record will be obtained until impulses approach one or the other of the electrodes.

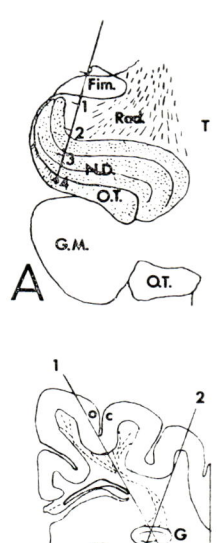

Fig. D14-1. Anatomical arrangements basic to polarization studies. (A) Parasagittal section through lateral geniculate nucleus and neighboring brain stem. Fim, fimbria; N.D., dorsal nucleus, lateral geniculate body with contained cell layer (stipple); OT, optic tract; Rad, radiation; G.M., medial geniculate nucleus. Superficial (dorsal) surface, up; inferior (ventral) surface, down. Unbroken line follows usual course of *critical* electrode through cell layers. Numerical series indicates depth in millimeters. (B) Cross section, dorsomedial quadrant, cerebral hemisphere, indicating position of lateral geniculate nucleus in a frontal section with regard to visual cortex. Lines 1 and 2 follow usual tracks of *reference* electrodes. G, lat. geniculate; Th, thalamus. Broken line, course of optic radiation.

On the other hand, when such nonuniformity exists between electrodes that activity on two sides of the transition zone has a different effective value, a potential difference between the active impulse as it arrives at the transition point and the inactive regions to either side of it is no longer equal. Then the overall difference between the two inactive regions on either side on the active point may be recorded as a simple monophasic deflection, even though neither electrode is at the locus of activity. The amplitude of such a record is higher the nearer the electrodes are to the active region and the larger the number of parallel elements involved.

Besides the nonuniformities in synaptic centers due to branching and termination of presynaptic axons, the other unique situation which affects the form of activity is the transition across the cell body from origin of the axon to the dendrites (Fig. D14-1A, Fig. D14-2). As the critical electrode passes through the geniculate nucleus, it records a positive postsynaptic spike in the optic radiation whether linked with one or the other of the reference electrodes, whereas below the cell layers the same electrode records a negative postsynaptic deflection.

Reversal from positive to negative takes place as the critical electrode enters the cell layers, the reversal taking place some-

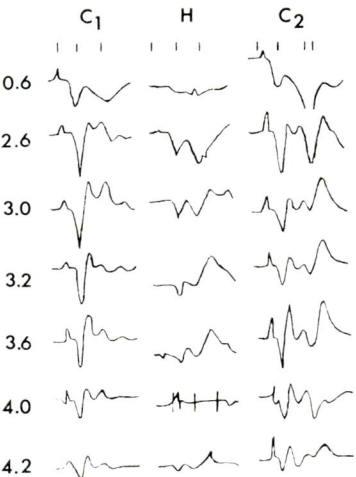

Fig. D14-2. Records from the lateral geniculate nucleus of cat. C_1, contralateral optic nerve stimulated, weak stimulus. H, ipsilateral optic nerve stimulated, weak. C_2, contralateral nerve, strong stimulus. Perpendicular lines above records indicate shock artifact and average positions of maxima for first tract spike (presynaptic) and its postsynaptic radiation response and for C_2, second tract spike preceding radiation response. As electrode penetrates cell layers (see numerical series, 0.6–4.2), the later part of the tract spike and all of the radiation spike reverse. Reversal for records of contralateral stimulation occurred at shallower position than for those of homolateral, corresponding to first and second layers respectively,

what deeper when the ipsilateral instead of the contralateral optic nerve is stimulated (Fig. D14-2). The reversal can be taken to indicate that there is a strongly negative region in the vicinity of the cell bodies and their dendrites and a positive region in the vicinity of the active optic radiation which rises from these cells. The paradox develops that during activity, cells become negative to their own axons, even as the latter are conducting "negative" impulses.

Applied Polarization. Interpretation becomes quite significant when one considers the cell bodies as constituents of a membrane so polarized during its activity that its radiation surface is positive to its tract surface. This led to investigation of the effect of applied polarization (using polarizing electrodes separate from those used for recording) upon this situation, in an effort to reverse usual polarities of the geniculate wave complex. Results were interesting enough to be extended to include similar studies upon visual cortex.

These studies (Bishop and O'Leary [4]) proceeded from deduction concerning polarization of linear axon arrangements in peripheral nerve (Blair and Erlanger [5]) and were based on the presumption that if a resting cell's surface were everywhere equally polarized, no potential difference would be detected, assignable to a potential between electrodes in its vicinity. Similarly, if a cell depolarizes with activity as does the fiber of peripheral nerve, and again equally over its surface, no action potential could be recorded unless depolarization occurred at different times on different parts of the exterior. It is almost certain that the different parts of a cell depolarize unequally during activity because of the magnitude of action potentials which can be recorded from active cells and the slight chance that depolarization would be so uniform as to be undetectable. This is upheld by the results quoted previously, is further strengthened by observations during applied polarization.

An element in an artificially induced field corresponds in activity to short segments of peripheral axons between electrodes. Polarizing currents passed through the geniculate region in the experimental model already described alter the amplitude and finally the sign of postsynaptic visual response recorded from surrounding brain tissue. With polarizing electrodes passed at different angles to the principal axes of orientation of postsynaptic neurons, the least current required for a given change is effective when direction of current flow in the main parallels the elements and is perpendicular to the plane of cell layers.

In the geniculate nucleus, when the dendritic side of this layer (next to the optic tract) is polarized positively by applied current, polarity of record remains the same as in the normal condition even though the record amplitude may be increased [13]. If, on the contrary, the dendritic aspect is made cathodal, amplitude of the trace is at first reduced and finally reversed.

In Fig. D14-3 the effects of polarization applied across the geniculate cell layers upon geniculate and cortical evoked responses

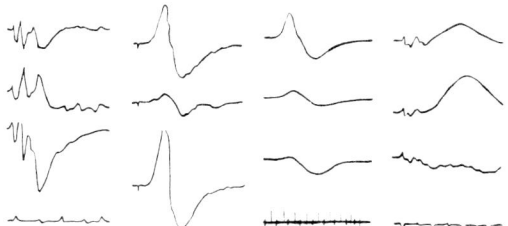

FIG. D14-3. Effects of polarization applied across cell layers of lateral geniculate while eliciting evoked response from geniculate and visual cortex. Far left column, lateral geniculate nucleus (cat), control record above compared with presynaptic positive polarization in middle and negative in lower trace. Second column shows (above) control cortical evoked potential (rabbit) compared with block created by polarization (middle trace) and postpolarization facilitation (lower trace). Third column (rabbit) shows that partial geniculate block can be produced without changing form of cortical record significantly. Fourth column (rabbit) shows the effect of cross-polarization of geniculate (presynaptic surface positive) in facilitating cortical record and in depressing it (presynaptic surface negative). Amplifications 50–200 mm per mV, depending on positions of electrodes and structures from which recorded. Oscillograph record reduced.

are illustrated. In the far left column, normal response from the lateral geniculate nucleus (upper trace) is compared with presynaptic positive polarization in the middle and with negative polarization in the lower trace. This only increases the positive (up) postsynaptic component in the middle trace while it reverses it in the lower trace.

In the second column (rabbit), cortical response from lateral gyrus (visual cortex) is largely blocked by polarization across the geniculate nucleus but shows postpolarization facilitation lasting more than one second in the lower trace. The third column is from rabbit visual cortex using polarization across the geniculate nucleus in opposite directions and recording leads across the cortex. This shows that partial geniculate block can be produced without changing the form of the cortical record.

In the fourth column, the cerebral cortical response was recorded from the rabbit during crosspolarization of the geniculate. In the middle record, the presynaptic geniculate surface is polarized positively, increasing the cortical response in the middle trace as compared with the control in the upper trace. In the lower trace, the cortical record is abolished upon applying oppositely directed polarization to the presynaptic surface. It is important that at the reversal point, as a critical recording electrode is passed through the geniculate nucleus and only a minimum record is obtained from postsynaptic neurons, conduction can still take place to complete activation of cortex. Under these circumstances, the minimal record is diphasic, and this response might be assigned to equalization of response in both amplitude and duration at the two ends of the conducting element.

Strong polarizing currents applied in either direction finally block geniculate conduction, as indicated by failure of cortical response, this complication being assignable to an effect on presynaptic terminals as much as upon postsynaptic dendrites. Under optimal conditions, 3 to 6 volts applied through a fixed 2000-ohm resistor plus electrode-tissue resistance up to 1000 ohms induce maximal effect on potential amplitude, and twice or more as much may induce complete block.

Transcortical Polarization. Changes of amplitude and reversal of polarity such as occur at the geniculate level can also be induced in cerebral cortex by transcortical polarization. The visual cortex response consists of several recognizable components with specific polarities, of which the most prominent consists in a diphasic or triphasic series the initial phase of which is surface positive; the second, surface negative; and a third, where it occurs, also surface positive. A series of fast spikes can also be identified riding upon the rising phase of the initiating surface-positive component.

Figure D14-4 illustrates the effect of surface-positive and of surface-negative polarization upon the evoked potential of visual cortex. In (*Aa*) compare the effect of weak surface-positive polarization during application of current (*Aa*2) with control responses recorded before (*Aa*1) and after (*Aa*3) applied polarization. The reduction of the positive phase and the augmentation

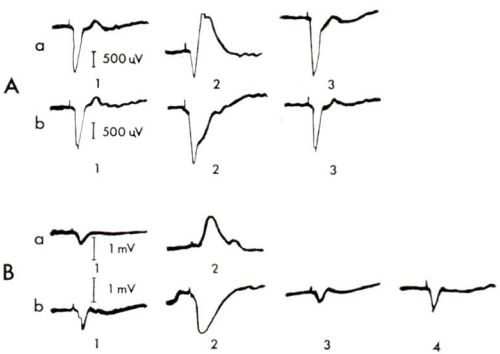

FIG. D14-4. Effect of surface-positive and surface-negative polarization upon primary visual response. (*Aa*1) Normal response before weak surface-positive polarization; (*Aa*2) during; and (*Aa*3) 1 sec after. (*Ab*1, 2, 3) Similar series, weak surface-negative polarization. (*Ba*1) Normal response before strong surface-positive polarization; (*Ba*2) during strong surface-positive polarization. Paroxysm developed, and postpolarization record is not illustrated for this sequence. (*Bb*1) Normal response before strong negative polarization; (*Bb*2) during; (*Bb*3) 1 sec after; (*Bb*4) 3 sec after.

of the negative phase during passage of the current are clearly evident. Contrast these traces with a similar series (Ab) relating to surface-negative polarization where the opposite effect was obtained. It can be seen in (Ab2) that this results in a marked exaggeration of the surface-positive deflection.

Records of surface-positive and surface-negative polarization are illustrated using significantly stronger current for polarization (Fig. D14-4B). The opposite augmenting effects are much exaggerated by comparison with the weak currents but of the same kind. (Note reduced sensitivity in Fig. D14-4B compared with Fig. D14-4A, indicated in the calibration signals.) Particularly with strong surface-positive polarization, a paroxysm may develop such as in the (Ba) sequence, where it developed as an afterpolarization discharge. With surface-negative polarization, cyclic spreading depressions can occur as an aftermath of the application of strong current and be detectable through the use of calomel-cell recording electrodes and dc amplification.

It would appear that wherever tested, the direction of change of response potential is opposite the direction of the polarizing current. Any wave which is negative toward an electrode is less negative, or changes in a positive direction, when that electrode is in a region of cells polarized cathodally and higher or more negative when that electrode is in a region polarized anodally. Both the specific responses and the slow aftereffects of evoked potentials follow this rule [9].

Spontaneous spikes and trains of spikes induced by strong strychnine are also affected by polarizing current in the manner described [9]. When strong surface-positive polarization effected the appearance of paroxysm, primary visual response disappeared completely during the spike series. Following strong negative polarization there might be a delayed change in steady potential during which the cortex becomes markedly negative, then shifts positive, a sequence of dc change similar to that seen in spreading depression. During such a period of postpolarization negativity, the surface-positive phase of the visual evoked response disappears gradually, the second negative phase persisting. Later, as the steady potential reverts to the resting level, the positive phase of the evoked response reappears.

DISCUSSION

Results indicate that polarization by externally applied currents affects the cell's discharge by altering the discharging source quite the same as functional activity itself does. Correspondences are also to be noted between effects of externally applied currents and certain spontaneous changes in steady potential. From this it may be deduced that any slowly developing biological potential from nervous or other sources should be looked upon as a factor which, perhaps, influences excitability of the neurons upon which it acts.

Besides the references quoted previously, units have also been studied during and after applied polarization. Bindman, Lippold, and Redfearn [2] have shown that unit cortical spikes recorded beneath the surface are increased in number and firing frequency by surface-positive polarization, suppressed by surface-negative polarization. Here the altered activity did not reverse immediately and effects lasting as long as one hour were produced. Enduring effects of intracellular stimulation of single neurons of frog's brain have also been observed by Strumwasser and Rosenthal [14], presumably the result there of positive or negative feedback from a small population of interconnected neurons whose activity can be modified by the one cell excited. Creutzfeldt, Fromm, and Kapp [8] produced similar immediate effects in studies on single cells of motor and visual cortexes of cat, neurons being activated by surface-positive and inhibited by surface-negative currents. Whatever the final interpretation of the phenomena under consideration here, these results upon units are consonant with results of our own studies upon field potentials.

Finally, results presented here suggest a mechanism for the action of strychnine, since the progressive effect of strychnine is almost identical with the progressive shift toward increased surface-positive polarization.

Summary

No potential at all need be recorded from the medium surrounding a cell which is uniformly and synchronously active over its entire surface; the potentials recorded always represent a difference in activity between apical (dendrites) and basal (cell) regions. Diphasic records are inferred to be summations of cell discharges, some of which, represented predominantly in one phase, have a difference of potential of one polarity; others, represented chiefly in the other phase, have a potential difference of opposite polarity.

Polarizing currents applied across the lateral geniculate nucleus, a thalamic synapse which can be used to illustrate the effects of polarization because of uniform orientation of dendrites toward the presynaptic optic tract terminals and of axons toward the oppositely emerging radiation, have the effect of facilitating synaptic transmission to visual cortex in the case of presynaptic positive polarization, blocking transmission with presynaptic negative polarization. The latter has the effect of equalizing the charges at the opposite poles of the geniculate neurons, the former of rendering them more disparate. With application of sufficiently strong polarizing currents, conduction is blocked indiscriminately in either direction.

The surface of cerebral cortex is comparable in effect to the presynaptic approach of the optic tract to the geniculate nucleus because pyramidal neurons are uniformly oriented with apical dendrites extending toward the surface and axons extending downward toward the white matter instead of (as in geniculate) into the optic radiation. In this instance, surface anodal polarization increases the negative component of the diphasic evoked potential, whereas surface cathodal polarization increases the amplitude of its initial positive component. These findings are believed to be in agreement with the general thesis supported here that applied polarization which increases the disparity between the two poles of the cortical neurons during their activity in a fashion so as to render their soma ends more negative to their principal dendritic arbors facilitates neuronal discharge; applied polarization which tends to equalize the charges between the two ends of the neuron tends to reduce discharge.

REFERENCES

1. Beck, A., and Cybulski, N. Weitere Untersuchunger über die Elektrischen Erscheinungen in der Hirnrinde der Affen und Hunde. *Zbl. Physiol.* 6:90, 1892.
2. Bindman, L. J., Lippold, O. C. J., and Redfearn, J. W. T. The prolonged afteraction of polarizing currents on the sensory cerebral cortex. *J. Physiol.* (London) 162:45P, 1962.
3. Bishop, G. H., and O'Leary, J. L. Factors determining the form of the potential record in the vicinity of the synapses of the dorsal nucleus of the lateral geniculate body. *J. Cell. Comp. Physiol.* 19:315, 1942.
4. Bishop, G. H., and O'Leary, J. L. The effects of polarizing currents on cell potentials and their significance in the interpretation of central nervous system activity. *Electroenceph. Clin. Neurophysiol.* 2:401, 1950.
5. Blair, E. A., and Erlanger, J. Effects of polarization of nerve fibers by extrinsic action potentials. *Proc. Amer. Physiol. Soc.* 1932, pp. 9–10.
6. Bubnoff, N., and Heidenhain, R. On Excitatory and Inhibitory Processes within the Motor Centers of the Brain (trans. by G. von Barin and R. Heindenhain). In Bucy, P. C. (Ed.), *Precentral Motor Cortex.* Illinois Monographs in the Medical Sciences, vol. IV. Urbana: Univ. of Illinois Press, 1944.
7. Caton, R. The electric currents of the brain. *Brit. Med. J.* 2:278, 1875.
8. Creutzfeldt, O. D., Fromm, G. H., and Kapp, H. Influence of transcortical D-C currents on cortical neuronal activity. *Exp. Neurol.* 5:436, 1962.

9. Goldring, S., and O'Leary, J. L. Experimentally derived correlates between ECG and steady cortical potential. *J. Neurophysiol.* 14:275, 1951.
10. Herrick, C. J. *The Evolution of Human Nature*. Austin: Univ. of Texas Press, 1956.
11. Kappers, C. V. A. Further contributions on neurobiotaxis. *J. Comp. Neurol.* 27:261, 1917.
12. Lorente de Nó, R. Action potential of the motoneurons of the hypoglossal nucleus. *J. Cell. Comp. Physiol.* 29:207, 1947.
13. O'Leary, J. L. The Role of Architectonics in Deciphering the Electrical Activity of the Cortex. In Bucy, P. C. (Ed.), *Precentral Motor Cortex*. Illinois Monographs in the Medical Sciences, vol. IV. Urbana: Univ. of Illinois Press, 1944.
14. Strumwasser, F., and Rosenthal, S. Prolonged and patterned direct extracellular stimulation of single neurons. *Amer. J. Physiol.* 198:405, 1960.

15
Neuronal Mechanisms Underlying the EEG

O. D. CREUTZFELDT

THE EEG WAVES recorded from the surface of the cortex or the skull result from the summation of potential transients of excitable neuronal elements within or just below the cortex. This hypothesis was put forward in 1935 by Adrian and Yamagiva [2] and has since been further elaborated. The hypothesis that evoked EEG potentials and probably also spontaneous EEG waves may be due to the summation of postsynaptic potentials (PSPs) is suggested by several authors [6, 14, 49], who also provided extensive, indirect experimental support. Direct experimental evidence was made known during the past 10 years, establishing that PSPs contribute essentially to the spontaneous and surface potentials of the EEG [8, 12, 13, 28]. Fiber activity may contribute to surface potential only if it is highly synchronized [12, 49].

Cortical Elements. There are still gaps in our exact knowledge of the actual contributions of different cortical elements to the surface potential. It remains to be determined if a certain EEG potential represents the summation of excitatory or inhibitory potentials, or both, elicited by a stimulus; how the potentials are distributed along the somadendritic membrane; and where the circumscribed sources and sinks should be localized along the vertically arranged neuronal elements within the different horizontal layers of the cortex.

In some epicortical phenomena, surface-negative potentials clearly coincide with depolarization and activation of the majority of cortical pyramidal cells, while in others a reversed relationship may be found, that is, surface negativity coinciding with cellular inhibition. Such variable relationships are demonstrated in Fig. 15-1.

Averaged cortical evoked potentials of the motor cortex and averaged cellular responses from the same area are shown in Fig. 15-1 after electrical stimulation of the bulbar pyramid, the VL nucleus of the thalamus, and the contralateral cortex. These different stimuli lead to different temporal excitation-inhibition patterns of the cortical cell population, possibly to involvement of different synapses at each individual cell and of different cell populations in the same cortical volume. This results in different surface evoked potentials and in different relations of surface polarities to cellular events.

Clearly, only limited conclusions can be drawn from the form of a surface potential in regard to the cellular activities causing it, without knowing the responses of individual cells contributing to this surface response. On the other hand, if the cellular basis of certain types of EEG potentials is known from experiments, these may serve in themselves as indicators of the activity of the neuronal population. Some correlations between the EEG and cellular activities revealed in recent years will be reviewed subsequently in order to facilitate interpretation of certain interictal and ictal EEG potentials.

SPONTANEOUS EEG WAVES IN ANIMALS WITHOUT EPILEPTIC LESIONS

Spindle Waves. Available material on the correlation between spontaneous EEG waves and membrane potential changes of cortical neurons was reviewed recently by

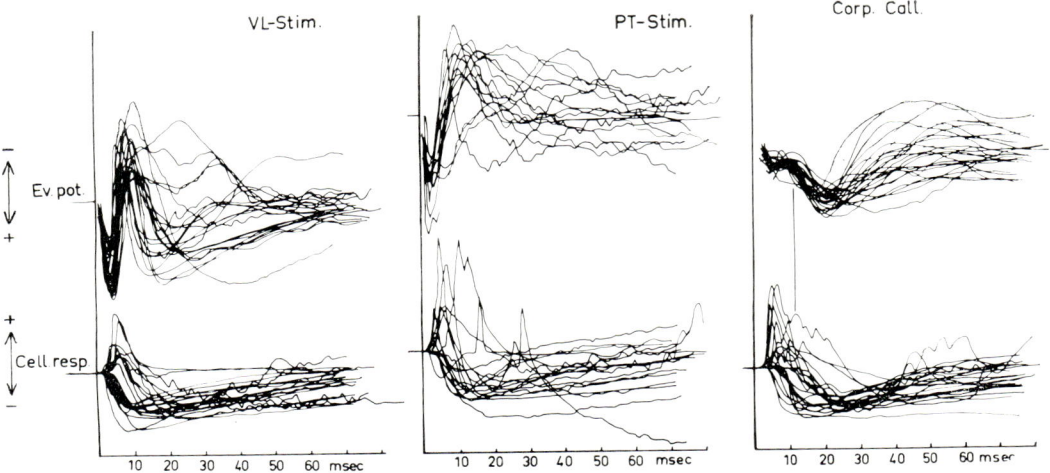

Fig. 15-1. Evoked potentials and cellular responses in the precruciate gyrus after electrical stimuli of nucleus VL thalami (left), the bulbar pyramidal tract (center, PT), and the homologous contralateral cortex (right, corp. call.). In the cat, under nembutal anesthesia, evoked potentials (upper traces) are averaged responses from different experiments; these were superimposed by hand. Cell responses (lower traces) are also averaged potentials (10 stimuli each) of intracellularly recorded responses. Cellular responses to different stimuli are from the same unselected cell population. Averaging of intracellular responses smears out excitatory reactions because of variable firing probability and latency; about 50 percent of the cells show a primary inhibition after VL stimulation with practically the same latency as primary excitation of remaining cells. After PT stimulation, inhibition is later than antidromic excitation (recurrent inhibition). After contralateral stimulation, early and late inhibition are observed; note variable relationship between polarities of surface potentials and intracellular events after the different stimulations. (From Creutzfeldt, Maekawa, and Hösli, in preparation.)

Andersen and Andersson [3]. These findings, summarized, are that the negative components of the surface waves during a spindle group are in phase with the depolarizing waves of cortical neurons. During barbiturate anesthesia, these rhythmical depolarizations involve practically all cortical neurons from which different investigators were able to record [4, 8, 12, 13, 28, 34]. Similar findings were reported in humans [41].

The exact phase relationship between the single neurons and the surface potential may vary slightly even during one spindle train, which indicates a somewhat loose *synchronization* of the neurons, the summation of which forms one EEG wave. Spindle waves in the nonanesthetized animal show principally the same relationship to the cellular membrane potential changes [15, 40]. An example is shown in Fig. 15-2, where it is also seen that the beginning and

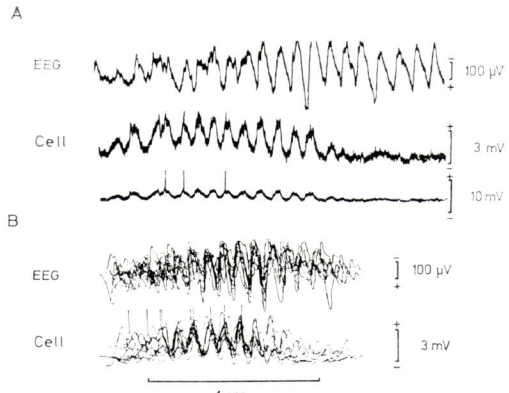

Fig. 15-2. Original recording of one (*A*) and superimposition of several (*B*) spindle groups in the cat. Insulin-induced hypoglycemia (25 mg per 100 ml blood sugar): dc recording of cellular activity with different amplification in (*A*). Amplitude of action potential 45 mV (not fully shown); ac recording of EEG. (From Mergenhagen et al. [40].)

end of the EEG spindle may run independently from the recorded cell. This indicates that not all the recorded cells here were necessarily involved in the whole spindling period.

The depolarizing waves of the cortical neurons during spindles were, as a rule, composed of well-discriminable single EPSPs, which implies that they were synaptically driven. Location and mechanism of this driving activity in the thalamus has been discussed extensively by Andersen and Andersson [3]. Rhythmical activity (except after trains of strong epicortical stimulation or spontaneous large EPSPs) were not seen in small slabs of isolated cortex [52], although occasional bursting activity may be present in some preparations.

The contribution of spontaneous IPSPs to spindle waves is minor since, under resting conditions and especially in the anesthetized animal, synchronized IPSPs are not regularly seen. If present, they coincide with the positive shift of the surface potential which follows the negative wave. Highly synchronized IPSPs (after electrical stimulations of afferent or efferent cortical pathways) may be accompanied by a surface negative wave [25, 44] or may lead to a surface positivity, mostly preceded by a short negativity [12, 51], as in the corpus callosum potential (Fig. 15-1, right).

Recently, it has been shown that the large surface positivity of the visual evoked potential in cats corresponds to the active inhibitory phase of the majority of the visual cortex neurons [54].

Slower Waves. Unitary neuronal correlates of slower waves such as ϑ-waves and δ-waves, which may also be found in the normal EEG (during sleep), have been investigated only during hypoglycemia with extracellular [10] and intracellular recordings [40]. This state leads to EEG phenomena which imitate most EEG potentials known from humans. Slower surface negative rhythmical waves of the ϑ-range are correlated to depolarizing neuronal potentials such as during normal spindle waves. Also, the smooth rhythmical δ-waves ("monomorphic δ-waves" of the EEG nomenclature) show a positive correlation between surface negativity and cellular depolarization (Fig. 15-3).

Sharp Waves. Of special interest to basic mechanisms of the epilepsies are the *sharp* waves observed during deeper hypoglycemia (below 25 mg per 100 ml). Fig. 15-4 shows examples of sharp waves with the simultaneous activity of one neuron recorded during an experiment. Relationship between sharp surface waves and unit activity is obviously different for the different waveforms; in IV, short activation of the unit coincides with sharp surface positivity whereas in I–III, main unit activation coincides with surface negativity. In I, II, and III, the broad surface positive potential coincides with a polarizing shift of the membrane potential. Results in these experiments indicated that surface positive sharp waves accompanied by cellular activation were always short (20–80 msec) while surface negative waves accompanied by cellular activation were broader (100 msec and more). Broad surface positive poten-

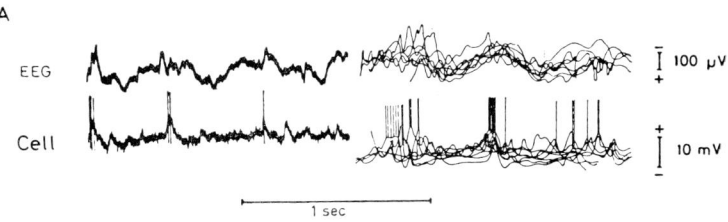

Fig. 15-3. Original recording and graphic superimposition of periodic δ-waves during hypoglycemia (25 mg per 100 ml blood sugar) in the cat after insulin injection. Quasi-cellular or juxtacellular recording of the cellular activity showing slow potentials and primary phase of action potentials as in intracellular recording; amplitude of action potential 25 mV. (From Mergenhagen et al. [40].)

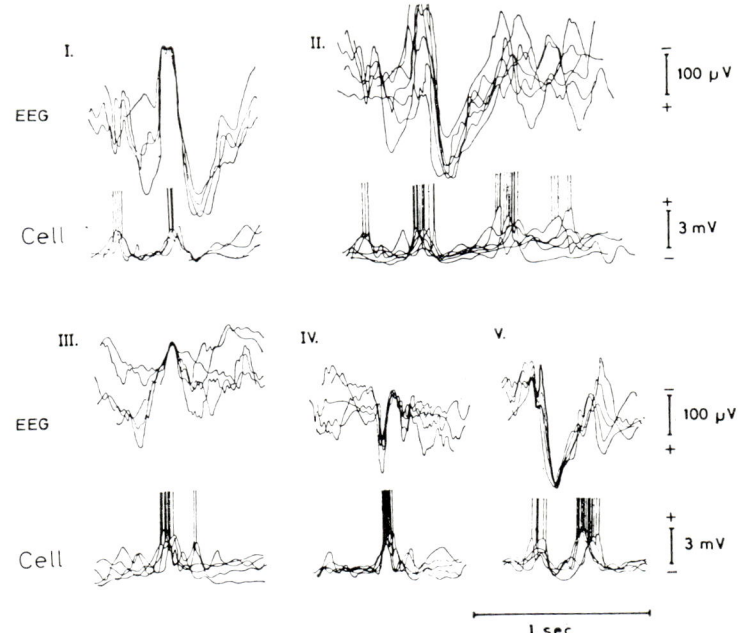

Fig. 15-4. Sharp waves recorded during hypoglycemia in the same experiment as in Fig. 15-3, with the same cell, in the cat, quasi-intracellular recording (action potential 30 mV). Waves of same configuration, selected and superimposed with simultaneous unit activity. Activation of unit during broad surface negative waves (I–III, duration of surface negativity 100 msec) and during short surface positive wave (IV, duration about 70 msec). Inhibition during broad surface positivity (V). (From Mergenhagen et al. [40].)

tials coincided with lack of excitation, or even inhibition, of neurons (Fig. 15-4, V).

In Fig. 15-5, records of a complex wave pattern observed frequently during deep hypoglycemia are shown together with activity of one representative unit. This complex wave sequence started with one or two sharp positive waves, followed about 200 msec later by one or several spindle waves, which was comparable to an evoked potential with afterdischarge following afferent stimulation. The unit was strongly activated with high-frequency bursts during the primary positive wave and showed a synaptic depolarization with some spike discharges during the negative waves of the afterdischarge.

INTERICTAL PAROXYSMAL DISCHARGES

Focal epileptogenic lesions due to intracortical injection of alumina cream or cobalt, after cortical cooling or after epicortical application of pentylenetetrazol, strychnine, or penicillin, produce characteristic polyphasic EEG potentials; these are related to synchronous neuronal events in a characteristic manner.

Interictal Paroxysmal Activity after Penicillin Poisoning

Characteristic interictal paroxysmal type of activity of cortical neurons after local application of penicillin is the *paroxysmal depolarization shift* (PDS) (Ajmone-Marsan, Chap. 11), which may appear either spontaneously or following an electrical stimulus of the afferent pathways or the cortical surface itself [38, 39, 46, 47, 48].

It is suggested that the main mechanism of the PDS is an increased excitatory action of EPSPs. But the temporal relation of PDS to thalamic stimulus as shown in the reports cited, as well as its dependence on stimulus strength and frequency [39], show the same characteristics as IPSPs elicited by thalamic stimulation in the

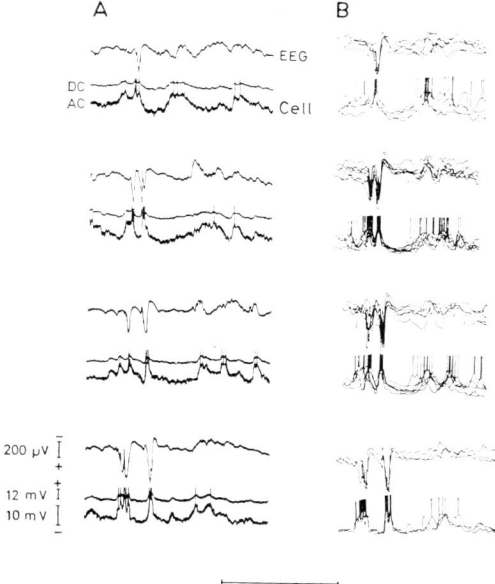

FIG. 15-5. Complex wave pattern during hypoglycemia in the cat, 20 mg per 100 ml blood sugar. (A) Original records; (B) superimposed records. Quasi-intracellular recording, action potential 35 mV. Single or double sharp surface positive EEG potentials are followed by a "silent period" and an afterdischarge with surface negative waves of spindle type. Activation of cell during surface positive sharp potential and less synchronized activity during negative spindle waves. (From Mergenhagen et al. [40].)

normal cortex [9]. This may suggest a relationship between PDS and inhibitory mechanisms and perhaps can best be explained by assuming that a disturbance of the inhibitory process was caused by penicillin. Polarization following PDS, comparable to polarization following an inactivation process in cerebellar [23] and hippocampal neurons [31, 32], may be due to an increased K permeability after excessive depolarization. Normally present inhibitory interaction between cortical neurons would thus be converted into abnormal excitation resulting in an avalanche-like population response, similar to the spinal strychnine convulsion. Inhibition in the surrounding unaffected cortex appears to limit spread of the discharge [48].

Paroxysmal EEG response above the focus consists mostly of a large surface negative wave inconsistently preceded by a sharp, and followed by a slower, positive potential. Between frequently appearing paroxysmal discharges, a positive dc shift was noted [24]. The cellular PDS is mostly associated with the large surface negative transient (Fig. 15-6A); the exact phase relationship may vary. The main spike activity may already start during the preceding positivity while, during the fully developed hyperdepolarization, the spike generator is already inactivated.

Relationship between evoked PDS and surface negative wave is more consistent (Fig. 15-6B). No explanation has been offered for the variable form of the spontaneously appearing EEG paroxysm and the corresponding variability of the exact relationship with the unitary events. However, a variable extent of surrounding inhibition,

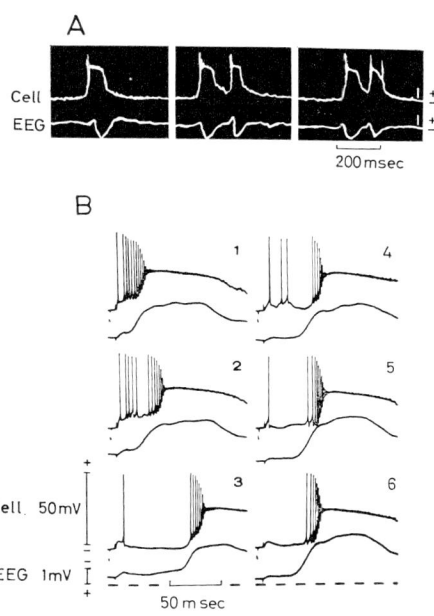

FIG. 15-6. Spontaneous (A) and evoked (B) PDS in a penicillin focus in the cat, anterior sigmoid gyrus. (A) Positivity up in surface EEG. (From Matsumoto and Ajmone-Marsan [38].) (B) VL stimulation every 2 sec. Different stimulus intensity (arbitrary units): 20 in 1, 15 in 2, 7 in 3, and 10 in 4–6. Variation of latency of PDS depends on stimulus intensity. (From Matsumoto et al. [39].)

around the focus [48], and the variable involvement of neurons within a focus [37], as well as different triggering mechanisms of PDSs, are bound to cause different surface potentials. Correspondingly different relationships between one member of the neuronal population and the average of all neuronal potentials (the EEG paroxysm) should be expected.

Pentylenetetrazol and Strychnine Potentials

The neuronal correlates of the biphasic or triphasic pentylenetetrazol and strychnine potentials after local and systemic application have been investigated with extracellular and intracellular recordings [13, 16, 35, 36]. The majority of units recorded extracellularly from within a focus showed a grouped discharge of variable length during paroxysmal discharge of the EEG. This discharge starts and reaches its maximum during the primary positive phase of a strychnine spike but continues in many neurons into the negative phase (Fig. 15-7). It is followed by a depression of activity; a few units are not affected at all and a few are inhibited. Whether these represented fibers of extracortical origin or from neighboring cortical areas, or both, was not determined; no consistent relationship between depth of a given neuron and its functional relationship to the surface potential was found [36].

Findings on strychnine potentials correspond well to those described for EEG spikes after local cooling of the cortex [22] and after intravenous injection of pentylenetetrazol [13]. In contrast to the phase relationship between increased spindle waves immediately after pentylenetetrazol injection and slow cellular depolarization (Fig. 15-8A), the well-developed pentylenetetrazol spike corresponds with its positive phase to the sharp depolarization and spike burst of the cell (Fig. 15-8B). At the end of the spiking period, in-phase relationships between the EEG and cellular potentials are seen again. At that time small negative-positive surface potentials may appear which are related to small isolated IPSPs of the cells.

The Spike-Wave (SW) Complex

In human epileptics, the spike-wave (SW) complex may appear either as an isolated potential or in regular sequence. As an isolated potential, it is an interictal phenomenon appearing either generalized over the whole cortex or restricted to certain areas; the form of this complex is variable. In the second case, the SW complexes follow each other in regular sequence (3 per sec), accompanied by loss of consciousness with or without minor motor manifestations (petit mal). This form is found mainly, but not exclusively, in children. Its self-sustained character and generalization over the whole cortex has always suggested that the SW complexes are triggered by some subcortical, *centrencephalic* structures. For the first, more variable form, a local cortical mechanism must be assumed.

Animal Experiments. For many years an attempt was made to imitate, experimentally, the SW complex in animals and thus simulate its mechanism. Complex waveforms such as the SW complex could be elicited by electrical stimulation of the mesencephalon [53], midline thalamic structures [27, 43], and the cortex itself [26]. In most of the experiments, special conditions of anesthesia were necessary [43]. In the baboon, SW complexes and other more complex paroxysmal interictal waveforms may appear over frontal areas without involvement of subcortical structures [17, 33]. These are involved only during generalization of discharges over the whole cortex (Naquet, Chap. 20).

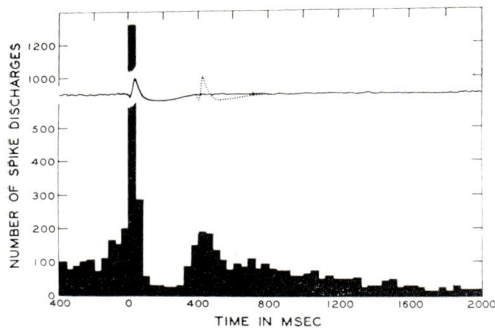

FIG. 15-7. Histogram showing number of spike discharges from 200 cells in relation to strychnine waves. (From Li [36].)

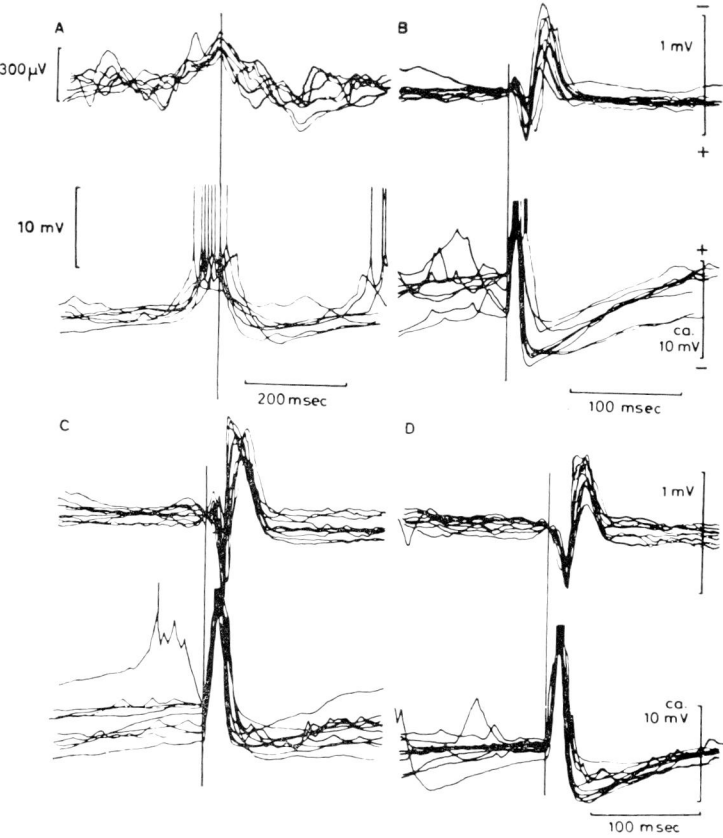

FIG. 15-8. Superimposition of pentylenetetrazol-induced convulsive potentials in the cat, nembutal anesthetized, a few seconds after injection of pentylenetetrazol. (*A*) Enhanced surface negative spindlelike wave shortly after injection. (*B*)–(*D*): Typical positive-negative pentylenetetrazol spikes. Note IPSPs in (*B*) and (*D*) following the excitation of the cell. (From Creutzfeldt et al. [9].)

The actual SW complex with a periodicity of about 300 msec suggested to several authors [18, 28, 30] that the wave may be the expression of an inhibitory phenomenon. Long duration of cortical IPSPs following synchronous excitation of the cortex (up to 150 msec) further supported this assumption. Experimental evidence for this interpretation was offered by Pollen [44] and Weir and Sie [53]. Pollen observed that in potentials like SW, evoked after thalamic 3-per-sec stimulation, primary excitation of cortical nerve cells coincided with the primary spike component and the subsequent IPSP with the "wave" (Fig. 15-9). Extracellular recordings of Weir and Sie [53] show, after mesencephalic electric stimulation, more complex relationship between extracellularly recorded discharges and surface transients. It was also suggested here that "the summated EPSPs or depolarizing shifts, alternating with IPSPs and hyperpolarization shifts, are the intracellular correlates of the initial positivity-spikes and the wave."

In spite of certain similarities between experimentally induced SW complexes with those found in human petit mal, it is still uncertain whether both phenomena are really comparable. The neuronal correlate of the human SW complex in petit mal must still be considered an open prob-

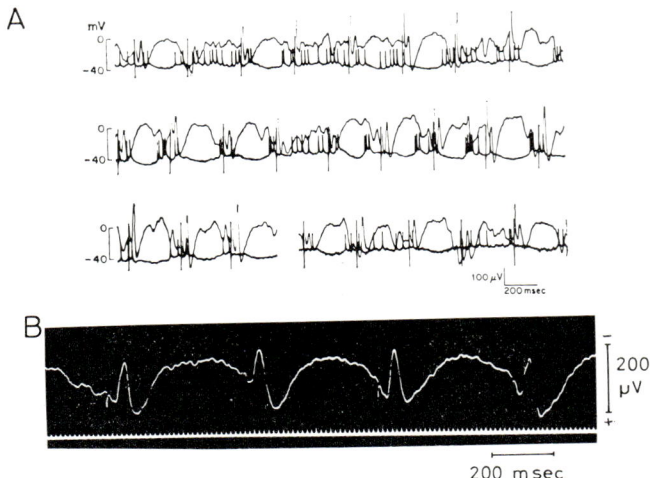

Fig. 15-9. Spike-wave complex elicited by stimulation in intralaminar thalamic nuclei. (A) SW complexes and intracellular records during intralaminar stimulation. Note stop of firing and polarization during surface negative wave. (From Pollen [42].) (B) Spike-wave complex 3.5 per sec in intralaminar thalamus. (From Pollen and Sie [45].)

lem although, from the functional point of view, the alternation of synchronous excitation and inhibition processes can be considered an interesting hypothesis.

It must also be realized that SW complexes after thalamic stimulation have been recorded in animal experiments in which the wave component was clearly related to a late, broad EPSP superimposed on the

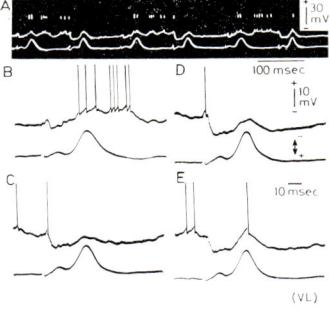

Fig. 15-10. Augmenting response to VL stimulation in the cat anesthetized with nembutal similar to spike-wave complex; 8 per sec stimulation. (A) Continuous record. (B)–(E) Selected sweeps. The SW-like response is shorter than the typical 3 per sec of the human petit mal. Note broad surface negativity in phase with large secondary EPSP. (From Creutzfeldt, Maekawa, and Hösli, in preparation.)

post-primary IPSP (Fig. 15-10) [12]. Since such patterns of late excitation superimposed on IPSPs are found only in some animals, it may also be argued that the SW complex may represent an atypical primary-secondary excitation cycle. Neither hypothesis explains the rhythmicity and self-sustained character of the petit mal discharge, which was always sought in a subcortical, triggering structure.

Ictal EEG Phenomena

The only models of epileptic seizures are those after electrical and chemical stimulation of the brain. Both types have some similarities with grand mal or focal seizures of the human epileptic patient, but their development is certainly different.

Self-Sustained Afterdischarge following Prolonged Epicortical Stimulation

This type of seizure activity has concerned many neurophysiologists and consequently has been studied extensively in the isocortex [29, 30, 55] and hippocampus [5, 7, 19, 21, 29]. Isocortical and hippocampal afterdischarges differ in quantitative aspects of threshold, length, and wave frequency. The fully developed seizures after direct electrical stimulation have in common: an initial flattening of the record immediately following the stimulus; a phase of regular oscillating waves (*tonic phase*); and the *clonic phase* with bursts of similar waveforms interrupted by increasingly longer pauses.

The whole sequence is followed by a postparoxysmal flattening of the EEG. In the isocortex (neurophysiology of hippocampal seizures is described by Spencer and Kandel, Chap. 21) a self-sustained afterdischarge develops only as a consequence of excessive depolarization of the cortical neurons during electrical surface stimulation (Fig. 15-11) [13, 50, 51], which may lead to inactivation of the spike generator in many cells. Following the stimulus period, the membrane potential slowly returns to its normal value, passing through a phase of regular oscillations which nearly duplicate the surface potentials. During the first phase of these oscillations, spike generation may still be blocked and fully developed spikes appear only after recovery of the membrane potential. Measurements of extracellularly recorded spike potentials gave comparable results [20]. The self-sustained afterdischarge following electrical stimulation may be interpreted as recovery of the cortical neurons following artificially induced hyperdepolarization.

Depolarization and Surface Positivity. Oscillations of the membrane potential are related to surface EEG potentials in a way so that depolarization coincides with surface positivity. This can also be observed in the small, chronically isolated cortical slab, where surface positive potentials are related to deep negative potentials accompanied by spike discharges [11]. Afterdischarge and phase reversal thus do not depend on vertically oriented afferent-fiber systems within the cortex, nor on the completely intact cortical-cell population. During the clonic phase, sudden depolarizations with superimposed oscillations are seen in neurons together with surface positive waves of cortical-clonic bursts. During postparoxysmal silence, relative hyperpolarization of neurons is often seen, which is due to lack of EPSPs.

Some neurons are always recorded which are driven only synaptically during self-sustained afterdischarge. Less strong or short electrical stimulation leads only to "abortive afterdischarges" with only a few bursts. In contrast to the relationship between cellular and EEG potentials during fast transients of self-sustained afterdischarge, slow dc potential changes of cortex accompanying electrical surface stimulation and seizure discharge are in phase with the intracellular potential variations. The increasing, negative dc shift during electrical stimulation parallels membrane depolarization; during afterdischarge the oscillating repolarization of cells goes together with a decrease of the negative surface dc potential to its normal value (Fig. 15-11).

Ictal Activity in Epileptogenic Cortex

Spontaneously developing seizures in a penicillin focus, after pentylenetetrazol injection, have been recorded. Seizure development in the penicillin focus [38] starts with increase of interictal phenomena or short clonic oscillations of the EEG, accompanied by paroxysmal depolarizations of neurons. Actual seizure may start from one such large group, leading into the tonic period characterized by regular surface posi-

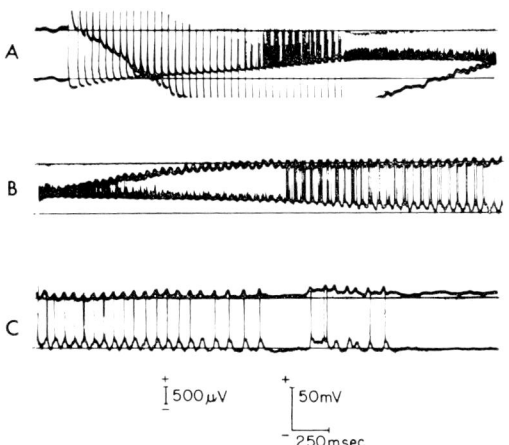

FIG. 15-11. Self-sustained afterdischarge following electrical stimulation of the cortical surface. Note negative shift of cortical dc potential, depolarization, and inactivation of cell during stimulation (*A*) and return of both potentials during the afterdischarge. (From Sugaya et al. [51].)

tive potentials similar to self-sustained afterdischarge following electrical stimulation. This regular activity is then followed by clonic bursts separated by increasingly longer pauses, finally leads into the postparoxysmal flat record. Comparable to the electrically induced afterdischarge, positive EEG waves are accompanied by large, depolarizing potentials of neurons which often show characteristics of PDSs (Fig. 15-12). Apart from these similarities between both types of seizures, progressive depolarization of active neurons during the first part of the penicillin seizure is different from electrically induced seizure. Only when maximal depolarization is reached, does the mechanism of repolarization appear comparable.

Seizure activity in the penicillin focus may be accompanied and sometimes even preceded by marked negative dc potential shift in the depth of the cortex [38]. Sudden negative intracortical dc shifts can be seen also during clonic bursts of a pentylenetetrazol seizure. Here they are accompanied by sudden, negative potential shifts (Fig. 15-13). In the hippocampus there is also increased negativity in the soma region, relative to apical dendritic structures [21].

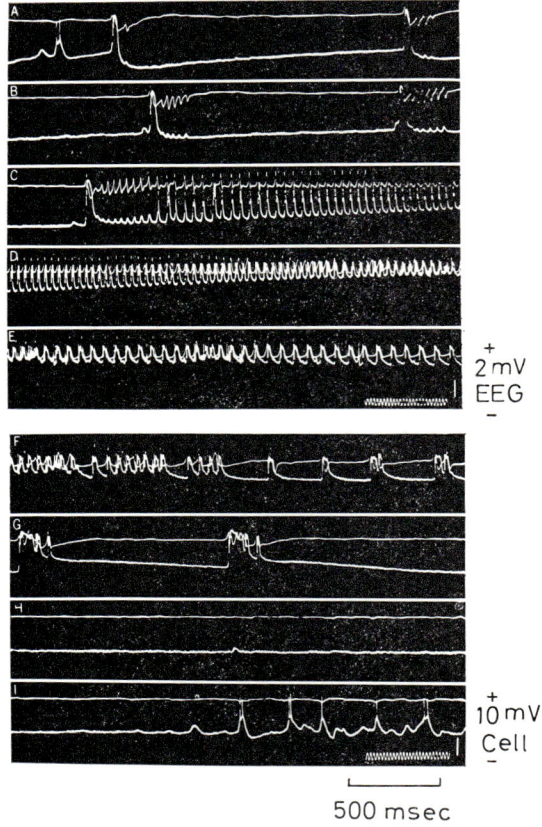

FIG. 15-12. Spontaneous ictal episode in one active neuron in a penicillin focus in the cat, anesthetized with light thiopental, cerveau isolé. (A)–(E) Continuous recording. (A), (B) Onset of ictal episode; (C)–(E) tonic phase; (F), (G) clonic phase; (H) end of ictal episode; (I) 6 sec after (H), recovery of spontaneous activity after seizure. Calibration, 2 mV for surface tracing, 10 mV for microelectrode; in both records positivity up; 50 cycles per sec. (From Matsumoto and Ajmone-Marsan [38].)

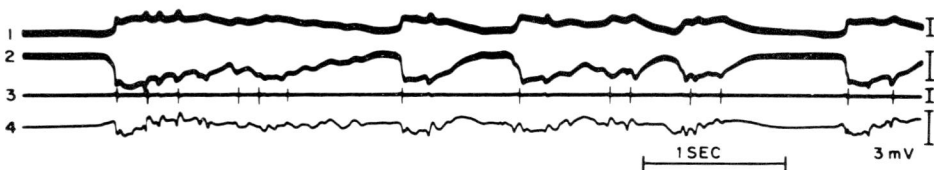

FIG. 15-13. Clonic phase from a pentylenetetrazol seizure in the cat, encéphale isolé, motor cortex. Records (1) and (3): Extracellular microelectrode recording from about 1200 μ below surface; dc recording in (1) and ac recording with short time constant in (3). (2) and (4): Surface EEG with dc recording (2) and ac recording ($t = 0.1$ sec) in (4). Negativity up in all records.

Conclusions

Observations on neuronal correlates of interictal and ictal EEG phenomena provide evidence that the latter are the expression of abnormally synchronized normal or abnormal membrane transients. These can be of self-sustained oscillatory character (self-sustained afterdischarge following electrical stimulation), or they may be due to disturbance of synaptic mechanisms (PDS). Slow membrane transients apparently contribute most significantly to the EEG and during ictal as well as interictal phenomena the spike generation may even be partially disturbed. The main contribution to surface potentials under conditions described come from excitatory, or depolarizing, membrane transients. These synchronized depolarizing transients may lead to a surface positive or negative potential: positive waves as a result of synchronized depolarizations are seen during seizure activity as well as during highly synchronized sharp waves, such as during hypoglycemia; negative waves accompany synchronized interictal PDSs in penicillin focus. Pentylenetetrazol and strychnine potentials are accompanied by activation mainly during the initial surface positivity.

A "classical" explanation of such differences would be that those phenomena which lead to a phase-reversed surface potential take place mainly in the deeper parts of the vertically oriented neurons, that is, in the soma region; those phenomena leading to in-phase surface potentials take place mainly in the apical dendritic structures of the pyramidal cells. Even if dendrites were partially invaded by depolarizations in the soma region, there would still be an apicobasal potential difference with a superficial source, as will be discussed by Pollen in the second part of this chapter.

Relationship between cortical surface potentials and cellular potentials during seizure activity is simpler than that observed during normal synaptic activity of the cortex. Synaptic depolarizations during spindling, recruiting, augmenting, and other types of evoked and spontaneous activity result in surface negative waves. Highly synchronized synaptic depolarizations after electrical stimulation of specific afferents or under certain pathological conditions lead to surface positivity. Synchronized IPSPs elicited by different modes of stimulation may result either in surface positivity or negativity (examples: [51] for epicortical stimulation; [12, 13] for thalamic and epicortical stimulation; [25] for antidromic stimulation; [54] for the visual evoked potential). Slowly developing potential changes (slow dc potentials) of the cortical surface are in phase with the intracellular potential change (a negative dc shift is accompanied by cellular depolarization [51], Caspers, Chap. 14), while abrupt dc changes during seizure activity show an inverse relationship.

The differences may be explained by assuming involvement of different synapses and, possibly, by different cell populations in a variable temporal sequence during different types of activity [12, 13, 25]. The degree of synchronization of the cortical-cell population also plays a role in the shape and polarity of the surface potential:

highly synchronized activation or inhibition leads to a reversed surface potential while more loosely synchronized events lead to in-phase surface potentials. This may indicate that at least in those neurons with short apical dendrites, only a slight apicobasal potential difference exists during slow and long-lasting synaptic actions. Careful measurements of field potentials around individual neurons are necessary to further substantiate this assumption. It was recently assumed by Humphrey [25] that in Betz cells of the motor cortex with mostly long dendrites, apical dendrites are invaded only a little by transients supposedly located in the soma area. But this would leave the difficulty that the apical dendrites could also not serve as sources or sinks for soma transients because of the high internal and relatively small membrane resistance.

From the practical point of view, empirical findings available so far are of great value in that they provide sufficient material to interpret many EEG phenomena in terms of activity of the cortical neuronal population. The surface positive potentials during self-sustained afterdischarge and during other seizures indicate that apical dendrites serve mainly as sources for such cellular phenomena, that they are only slightly involved directly in this pathological membrane phenomenon, which constitutes the basic electrophysiological mechanism of seizure activity. Close correlation between surface negative interictal paroxysmal discharges and PDS in penicillin foci suggests stronger involvement of apical dendritic structures. This may be relevant to the hypothesis that neurons in epileptic foci show mainly alterations on their apical dendrites (Ward, Chap. 10). Excessive depolarization of cortical neurons, necessary for a self-sustained seizure discharge and which can be artificially induced by strong electrical stimulation, may develop under certain conditions through such a "dendritic leak."

REFERENCES

1. Adrian, E. D., and Moruzzi, G. Impulses in the pyramidal tract. *J. Physiol.* (London) 97:153, 1939.
2. Adrian, E. D., and Yamagiva, K. The origin of Berger rhythm. *Brain* 58:323, 1935.
3. Andersen, P., and Andersson, S. A. *Physiological Basis of the Alpha Rhythm.* New York: Appleton-Century-Crofts, 1968.
4. Andersson, S. A., Lundberg, A., and Wolpow, E. R. Intracellular slow wave potentials in the somatosensory area of cat. *Acta Physiol. Scand.* 61:141, 1964.
5. Andy, O. J., and Akert, K. Electroencephalographic and behavioral changes during seizures induced by stimulation of Ammons formation in the cat and monkey. *Electroenceph. Clin. Neurophysiol.* Suppl. 3, 42, 1953.
6. Bremer, F. Cerebral and cerebellar potentials. *Physiol. Rev.* 38:357, 1958.
7. Creutzfeldt, O. D. Die Krampfausbreitung im Temporallappen der Katze. Die Krampfentladungen des Ammonshorns und ihre Beziehungen zum übrigen Rhinencephalon und Isocortex. *Schweiz. Arch. Neurol. Neurochir. Psychiat.* 77:163, 1956.
8. Creutzfeldt, O. D., Fuster, J. M., Lux, H. D., and Nacimiento, A. Experimenteller Nachweis zwischen EEG-Wellen und Aktivität corticaler Nervenzellen. *Naturwissenschaften* 51:166, 1964.
9. Creutzfeldt, O. D., Lux, H. D., and Watanabe, S. Electrophysiology of Cortical Nerve Cells. In Purpura, D. P., and Yahr, M. D. (Eds.), *The Thalamus.* New York: Columbia University Press, 1966, pp. 209–230.
10. Creutzfeldt, O. D., and Meisch, J. J. Changes of cortical neuronal activity and EEG during hypoglycemia. *Electroenceph. Clin. Neurophysiol.* Suppl. 24, 154, 1963.
11. Creutzfeldt, O. D., and Struck, G. Neurophysiologie und Morphologie der chronisch isolierten Cortexinsel der Katze: Hirnpotentiale und Neuronentätigkeit einer isolierten Nervenzelle population ohne afferente Fasern. *Arch. Psychiat. Nervenkr.* 203:708, 1962.
12. Creutzfeldt, O. D., Watanabe, S., and Lux,

H. D. Relations between EEG phenomena and potentials of single cortical cells. I. Evoked responses after thalamic and epicortical stimulation. *Electroenceph. Clin. Neurophysiol.* 20:1, 1966a.

13. Creutzfeldt, O. D., Watanabe, S., and Lux, H. D. Relations between EEG phenomena and potentials of single cortical cells. II. Spontaneous and convulsoid activity. *Electroenceph. Clin. Neurophysiol.* 20:19, 1966b.

14. Eccles, J. C. Interpretation of action potentials evoked in the cerebral cortex. *Electroenceph. Clin. Neurophysiol.* 3:449, 1951.

15. Elul, R. Brain waves: Intracellular recording and statistical analysis help clarify their physiological significance. *Data Acquis. and Proc. in Biol. and Med.* 5:93, 1968.

16. Enomoto, T. F., and Ajmone-Marsan, C. Epileptic activation of single cortical neurons and their relationship with electroencephalographic discharges. *Electroenceph. Clin. Neurophysiol.* 11:199, 1959.

17. Fischer-Williams, M., Poncet, M., Riche, D., and Naquet, R. Light-induced epilepsy in the baboon, *Papio papio*: Cortical and depth recordings. *Electroenceph. Clin. Neurophysiol.* 25:557, 1968.

18. Gastaut, H., and Fischer-Williams, M. The Physiopathology of Epileptic Seizures. In Field, J. (Ed.), *Handbook of Physiology,* vol. 1, sec. 1—Neurophysiol. Baltimore: Waverly, 1960, pp. 329–364.

19. Gastaut, H., Naquet, R., Vigouroux, R., and Corrieol, J. Provocation de comportements émotionnels divers par stimulation rhinencéphalique chez le chat avec électrodes à demeure. *Rev. Neurol.* 86:319, 1952.

20. Gerin, P. Microelectrode investigations on the mechanisms of the electrically induced epileptiform seizure. *Arch. Ital. Biol.* 98:21, 1960.

21. Gloor, P., Sperti, L., and Vera, C. L. A consideration of feedback mechanisms in the genesis and maintenance of hippocampal seizure activity. *Epilepsia* (Amst.) 5:213, 1964.

22. Goldensohn, E. S., and Purpura, D. P. Intracellular potentials of cortical neurons during focal epileptic discharges. *Science* 139:840, 1963.

23. Granit, R., and Phillips, C. G. Excitatory and inhibitory processes acting upon individual Purkinje cells of the cerebellum in cats. *J. Physiol.* (London) 133:520, 1956.

24. Gumnit, R. J., and Takahashi, T. Changes in direct current activity during experimental focal seizures. *Electroenceph. Clin. Neurophysiol.* 19:63, 1965.

25. Humphrey, D. R. Re-analysis of the antidromic cortical response. II. On the contribution of cell discharge and PSPs to the evoked potentials. *Electroenceph. Clin. Neurophysiol.* 25:421, 1968.

26. Ingvar, D. H. Electrical activity of isolated cortex in the unanesthetized cat with intact brain stem. *Acta Physiol. Scand.* 33:151, 1955.

27. Jasper, H. H., and Droogleever-Fortuyn, J. Experimental studies on functional anatomy of petit mal epilepsy. *Res. Publ. Ass. Res. Nerv. Ment. Dis.* 26:272, 1947.

28. Jasper, H., and Stefanis, G. Intracellular oscillatory rhythms in pyramidal tract neurones in the cat. *Electroenceph. Clin. Neurophysiol.* 18:541, 1965.

29. Jung, R. Hirnelektrische Untersuchungen über den Elektrokrampf. *Arch. Psychiat. Nervenkr.* 183:206, 1949.

30. Jung, R., and Tönnies, J. F. Hirnelektrische Untersuchungen über Entstehung und Erhaltung von Krampfentladungen: die Vorgänge am Reizort und die Bremsfähigkeit des Gehirns. *Arch. Psychiat. Nervenkr.* 185:701, 1950.

31. Kandel, E. R., and Spencer, W. A. Electrophysiology of hippocampal neurons. II. After-potentials and repetitive firing. *J. Neurophysiol.* 24:243, 1961a.

32. Kandel, E. R., and Spencer, W. A. Excitation and inhibition of single pyramidal cells during hippocampal seizure. *Exp. Neurol.* 4:163, 1961b.

33. Killam, K. F., Killam, E. K., and Naquet, R. An animal model of light sensitive epilepsy. *Electroenceph. Clin. Neurophysiol.* 22:497, 1967.

34. Klee, M. R., Offenloch, K., and Tigges, H. Cross-correlation of electroencephalographic potentials and slow membrane transients. *Science* 147:519, 1965.

35. Li, C-L. Functional properties of cortical neurones with particular reference to strychninization. *Electroenceph. Clin. Neurophysiol.* 7:475, 1955b.

36. Li, C-L. Some factors determining single cell discharges in cerebral cortex. In Servit, Z., and Blask, R. (Eds.), *Comparative*

and Cellular Pathophysiology of Epilepsy. Amsterdam: Excerpta Medica, 1966.

37. Matsumoto, H., and Ajmone-Marsan, C. Cortical cellular phenomena in experimental epilepsy: Interictal manifestations. *Exp. Neurol.* 9:286, 1964.

38. Matsumoto, H., and Ajmone-Marsan, C. Cortical cellular phenomena in experimental epilepsy: Ictal manifestations. *Exp. Neurol.* 9:305, 1964.

39. Matsumoto, H., Ayala, G. F., and Gumnit, R. J. Neuronal behavior and triggering mechanism in cortical epileptic focus. *J. Neurophysiol.* 1969, in press.

40. Mergenhagen, D., Creutzfeldt, O. D., and Neuweiler, G. Beziehungen zwischen Aktivität corticaler Neurone und EEG-Wellen des motorischen Cortex der Katze bei Hypoglykämie. *Arch. Psychiat. Nervenkr.* 211:43, 1968.

41. Morrell, F. Electrical Signs of Sensory Coding. In Quarton, G. C., Melnechuk, T., and Schmitt, F. O. (Eds.), *The Neurosciences.* New York: Rockefeller Univ. Press, 1967.

42. Pollen, D. A. Intracellular studies of cortical neurons during thalamic induced wave and spike. *Electroenceph. Clin. Neurophysiol.* 17:398, 1964.

43. Pollen, D. A., Perot, P., and Reid, K. H. Experimental bilateral wave and spike from thalamic stimulation in relation to level of arousal. *Electroenceph. Clin. Neurophysiol.* 15:1017, 1963.

44. Pollen, D. A., Reid, K. H., and Perot, P. Micro-electrode studies of experimental 3/sec wave and spike in the cat. *Electroenceph. Clin. Neurophysiol.* 17:57, 1964.

45. Pollen, D. A., and Sie, P.-G. Analysis of thalamic induced wave and spike by modifications in cortical excitability. *Electroenceph. Clin. Neurophysiol.* 17:154, 1964.

46. Prince, D. A. Inhibition in "epileptic" neurons. *Exp. Neurol.* 21:307, 1968.

47. Prince, D. A. The depolarization shift in "epileptic" neurons. *Exp. Neurol.* 21:467, 1968.

48. Prince, D. A., and Wilder, B. J. Control mechanisms in cortical epileptogenic foci. *Arch. Neurol.* (Chicago) 16:194, 1967.

49. Purpura, D. P. Nature of electrocortical potentials and synaptic organization in cerebral and cerebellar cortex. *Int. Rev. Neurobiol.* 1:47, 1959.

50. Sawa, M., Maruyama, N., and Kaji, S. Intracellular potential during electrically induced seizures. *Electroenceph. Clin. Neurophysiol.* 15:209, 1963.

51. Sugaya, E., Goldring, S., and O'Leary, J. L. Intracellular potentials associated with direct cortical response and seizure discharge in cat. *Electroenceph. Clin. Neurophysiol.* 17:661, 1964.

52. Watanabe, S., and Creutzfeldt, O. D. Spontane postsynaptische Potentiale von Nervenzellen des motorischen Cortex der Katze. *Exp. Brain. Res.* 1:48, 1966.

53. Weir, S., and Sie, P.-G. Extracellular unit activity in cat cortex during the spike-wave complex. *Epilepsia* (Amst.) 7:30, 1966.

54. Creutzfeldt, O., Rosina, A., Ito, M., and Probst, W. Visual evoked response of single cells and of the EEG in primary visual area of the cat. *J. Neurophysiol.* 32:127, 1969.

55. Rosenblueth, A., and Cannon, W. B. Cortical responses to electrical stimulation. *Amer. J. Physiol.* 135:690, 1942.

Discussion

ON THE GENERATION OF NEOCORTICAL POTENTIALS*

DANIEL A. POLLEN

The development of potential field theory culminating in the equations of Maxwell was one of the outstanding achievements of nineteenth-century classical physics [27]. By 1853 Helmholtz had considered the problem of the electric field set up in the medium outside cells and had made contributions, warmly praised by Lorente de Nó [22] and by Renshaw, Forbes, and Morison [43] in their own important studies in 1939.

In 1931 as Adrian [1] probed the central nervous system in search for generators of bioelectric potentials, he opened up a controversial problem area which was to witness numerous important contributions over the next three decades, resulting from the use of gross and extracellular microelectrode techniques by many workers whose studies have been well summarized by Purpura [38].

By 1965 the principal relationships between slow extracellular waves and intracellularly recorded potentials had been established in the neocortex [6, 16, 20, 23, 30, 39], the thalamus [2], and the hippocampus [3].

Evidence presented here, on the basis of potential theory, quantitatively establishes that one of the principal neocortical surface potentials is generated almost entirely by postsynaptic activity set up on vertically oriented neurons, with negligible contributions from action potentials and glia.

The general principles of potential theory applied to a volume conductor were well stated by Renshaw et al. [43], who noted that a reference electrode must be truly remote from a center of neural activity in order to be considered *indifferent* with regard to activity in that center. They realized that ". . . there is no external field set up and therefore no current flows in the medium about a cell as long as every part of the cell is at the same potential," and that external electric fields are set up only when potential differences occur between two or more regions of the cell's surface. An important corollary to this statement is that uniform synaptic activation of a neuron or uniform ionic change in the external environment or uniform intracellular metabolic change would fail to set up an external potential field even though the transmembrane potential would change uniformly. Renshaw et al. also appreciated that ". . . the density of current becomes rapidly greater as an active portion of a cell is approached, because of the decreasing volume through which the action current may flow."

Transcortical current densities can be derived from external potential field distribution and resistivity of the external medium [12, 48], and can be calculated for *spike and wave* responses, characteristic of petit mal epilepsy [15, 34]. Relation of these responses to certain problems of human petit mal has recently been considered in a journal article [31].

For present purposes, these potentials are *evoked* by electrical stimulation of the medial thalamus, although similar responses can occur spontaneously [4, 16, 30].

PRIMARY CURRENT GENERATORS

POSTSYNAPTIC POTENTIALS. The *spike and wave* responses are particularly useful as a tool for analysis of brain waves because the two principal components, the spike, identical with the recruiting response, and

---

* Research supported by PHS Career Development Award NB14353 from National Institute of Neurological Diseases and Stroke.

the long slow wave are both surface negative potentials but are generated by entirely different mechanisms (Fig. 15-1*A*). The initial positivity, which may precede recruiting response, and late depolarizing potentials, which may occur 100 msec or longer after the beginning of the slow wave, have been considered in published articles [30, 35].

The intracellular correlate of recruiting response is a depolarizing potential [20, 23, 30, 39], an EPSP, which may or may not reach firing level (Fig. D15-1*A*), and the intracellular correlate of the slow wave is an hyperpolarizing potential, an IPSP, whose generation is independent of occurrence of previous EPSPs, action potentials, and afterpotentials [30]. (See also [29, 34].)

It is of particular importance that action potentials from neurons subject to strong neocortical IPSPs cease very abruptly, for prolonged periods, after IPSP onset [23, 29, 32, 33, 44]. In studies utilizing microelectrodes suitable for extracellular [35, 36] and intracellular [30] recording, we have not found any neurons (or fine fibers) firing selectively during the first 100 msec of the slow negative wave. Therefore, no part of this surface potential during this interval can be attributed to *presence* of action potentials; nor can part of the surface counterpart of inhibitory potentials be at-

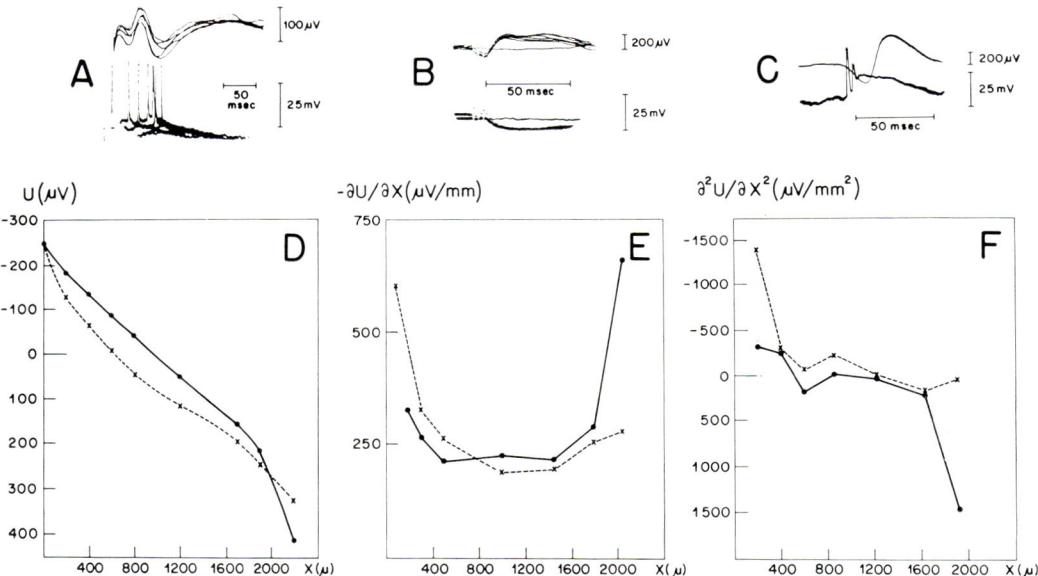

Fig. D15-1. In (*A*), (*B*), and (*C*), upper trace is surface activity (negative up) and lower trace is dc recording of intracellular activity (positive up) from precruciate cortex in cat. (*A*) Superimposed frames of first 225 msec of the *spike-wave* response following 3-per-sec stimulation in midline intralaminar system of thalamus. Beginning and end of intracellular trace partly cut off by circular scope screen; resting membrane level (-50 mV) indicated by small horizontal bar. (*B*) Surface and intracellular responses to antidromic stimulation of cerebral peduncles. Resting membrane level (-67 mV). (*C*) *Strychnine burst* with very large depolarization occurring after early *depolarizing inactivation* of action potential generator mechanism. Note diphasic slow fall of depolarizing potential. (*D*) Plot of laminar analysis of potential (*U*) for spike (broken line) and wave (solid line) measured at time of peak amplitude of surface responses in postcruciate cortex as a function of depth beneath cortical surface. Each point plotted represents average of five measurements. For computational convenience, data had been normalized with regard to comparable surface spike-wave amplitudes of 250 μV above the baseline. Decline of potentials below 2200 μ not shown. (*E*) Graphical differentiation of data in (*D*) for spike (broken line) and wave (solid line). (*F*) Graphical differentiation of data in (*E*) for spike (broken line) and wave (solid line).

tributed to consequences of *absence* of action potentials.

With strong *antidromic* IPSPs, virtually all action potentials cease well before the peak of IPSP action. The magnitude of the surface negative potentials occurring simultaneously with these IPSPs (Fig. D15-1B) varies according to the strength of the IPSPs [13, 32]; the surface potential does not exhibit any discontinuities during the period when generation of action potentials is first inhibited. Thus, action potentials do not make *any* contribution to the surface record during prolonged inhibitory potentials; the problem of identifying current generators producing the associated slow surface negative waves is thereby simplified.

Surface Negativity. Whenever superficial apical dendrites become depolarized with regard to the soma or when the soma becomes hyperpolarized with regard to apical dendrites, surface negativity results. Direction of extracellular current flow in the two cases is the same; however, intracellular potential shifts at the soma result respectively from an electrotonically propagated depolarizing potential and a predominantly locally generated hyperpolarizing response. The two surface potentials respond in opposite manner to application of certain pharmacological agents and surface dc polarizations [36].

Transcortical current densities attending the two surface potentials can be determined from the laminar potential distribution (Fig. D15-1D) [12]. With penetration of the cortex, we record from an *isoelectric* region (although at different depths for the two potentials) and finally record a polarity reversal for both potentials. (See also [4].) Determination of the isoelectric region alone does not specify where or how a potential is generated. Peak amplitudes in the cortical depths were usually obtained at 1.5–1.8 mm [35], although peak *depth reading* for the slow wave in Fig. D15-1D is somewhat greater, probably due to some obliquity of microelectrode penetration.

Because both surface and depth potentials involve rather large expanses of cortex and because dendritic arborizations are reasonably symmetrical, we can allow that average current along any line in a plane parallel to the cortical surface is effectively zero. (See also [12].) We must, therefore, be concerned only with the vertical field vector, **E**, and the areal current density, **I**, which can be derived from the scalar field potential, U, by the expressions [12, 25]

$$\mathbf{E} = -\mathbf{grad}\ U \quad \text{and} \quad \mathbf{I} = -G\ \mathbf{grad}\ U$$

where

$$\mathbf{grad}\ U = \mathbf{i}\frac{\partial U}{\partial x} + \mathbf{j}\frac{\partial U}{\partial y} + \mathbf{k}\frac{\partial U}{\partial z}$$

but

$$\frac{\partial U}{\partial y} = 0 \quad \text{and} \quad \frac{\partial U}{\partial z} = 0$$

Conductivity, G, is the reciprocal of cortical resistivity [8], which measures about 350 Ω cm at 5 cycles per sec [42]. Current density for recruiting response is highest at the active "sink" in the superficial cortical layers with a secondary rise near the passive *source* in the deep layers, and the converse profile of current density applies to the slow wave (Fig. D15-1E).

Net source (or sink) density, ρ, for each potential distribution taken at the time of peak amplitude when current flow is reasonably steady can be determined from the Poisson equation

$$\nabla^2 U = \rho$$

where

$$\nabla^2 U = \frac{\partial^2 U}{\partial x^2} + \frac{\partial^2 U}{\partial y^2} + \frac{\partial^2 U}{\partial z^2} = \rho$$

but

$$\frac{\partial^2 U}{\partial y^2} = 0 \quad \text{and} \quad \frac{\partial^2 U}{\partial z^2} = 0$$

(Time varying electric fields, unlike static charge distributions, give rise to magnetic fields and electromagnetic waves [27]. Frequency of even the fastest brain current oscillators, the action potentials, is so slow, 1–2 kilocycles per sec, and the dipole separations are so small that the power electromagnetically radiated by the nervous system is probably extremely low.)

The value of the charge or current density associated with recruiting response is of the greatest magnitude in superficial cortical layers and indicates a current sink, whereas density associated with the slow wave is of greatest magnitude in deep cortical layers and indicates a current source (Fig. D15-1F). Humphrey [12] has already demonstrated that the principal source for currents generated during antidromic neocortical IPSPs is also in the deep cortical layers; Andersen, Eccles, and Løyning [3], on the basis of laminar studies, have assigned the principal site of IPSP generation on hippocampal pyramidal cells to the somatic region.

Calculation of Wave. The number of current generators (neurons) required to produce any given peak amplitude of a surface negative slow wave, let us say 100 µV, can now be approximately calculated from extracellular current density estimates and intracellularly determined IPSP current strengths. Extracellular vertical current density at the site of IPSP generation, required for production of a surface negative wave of 100 µV peak amplitude, can be calculated from data of Fig. D15-1E and cortical conductivity, G, as 7.4 µamp per cm^2 or as 0.74 nanoamp per $(100\ \mu)^2$.

Under experimental conditions when the slow wave rose above the baseline by 100 µV, IPSPs of 3–4 mV were usually recorded in neurons with high resting potentials [30]. From related data [33], we know (now accepting that most, but not all [36], IPSP current is generated on or near the soma) that currents generated during 3–4 mV IPSPs in large deep pyramidal cells with comparable resting potentials would range 1–1.5 nanoamp. If, allowing generously for horizontal current spread to basilar dendrites [14], and for some vertical current return through proximal inactive segments of the apical shaft and axon, we assume that the deep, large neurons in the 100 µ cube subjected to IPSPs would distribute even one-tenth of their extracellular current vertically across a common plane, then we can estimate that 5–7 such neurons would be required to generate extracellular current density of 0.74 nanoamp per $(100\ \mu)^2$.

Ramon-Moliner [41] has estimated neuronal density in a 100 µ cube in the large, pyramidal cell layer as 20–25 neurons per $(100\ \mu)^3$ of which 5–8 neurons are large pyramidal cells.

Furthermore, we know that most cells recorded intracellularly from this depth are subject to IPSPs during the slow wave [30]; therefore, numbers and strength of the current generators are ample to produce extracellular potential distributions.

The above calculations, it should be emphasized, are based on experimental measurements and have shown that even comparatively weak IPSPs on an appropriate number of pyramidal cell somata can generate 100 µV of surface negativity. IPSPs of 3–5 times the strengths considered here can be recorded in normal and convulsive states and could therefore generate 500 µV of surface negativity, even if only about one-fourth the deep-lying large neurons were involved.

Direct comparison of intracellular and extracellular current has been possible for the slow wave because of available data on intracellular IPSP strengths at the principal site of generation. We cannot make a direct comparison for the EPSP currents because their origin is primarily dendritic; we have no intracellular data on magnitude of dendritic currents generated. However, considering dendritic receptive surfaces in superficial layers, there is no reason to doubt that currents calculable from Fig. D15-1E can be generated by postsynaptic activity.

Points to Consider. Before considering other cortical current generators, seven points should be briefly noted.

1. Analysis of the first and second spatial derivatives of the potential has helped localize the current generators. But, from extracellular studies alone, we cannot exclude secondary sites of current generation because any uniform synaptic change could theoretically be impressed upon the entire neuron without changing the extracellular field distribution. However, intracellular potential data from the soma and estimates of the extent of electrotonic spread from distant sites can help determine if secondary sites are required in a given case [14].

2. Distribution and sources of currents generating *dc potential shifts* can be determined by the above method. Change in a

transcortical dc potential could reflect change in the *resting potential* along certain neurons; such change could result from either steady synaptic activity at one or another region of a cell or from differing levels of metabolic activity (such as extrusion of Na^+) at different neuronal regions. Such dc changes would modify the magnitude of current generated for any given synaptic input, because current generated depends upon the difference between the resting potential and the PSP equilibrium potential as well as upon associated conductance change.

3. Methods outlined are also applicable to determine if field potentials in nonlaminated structures result from neural activity within or outside such structures by determining if potential distribution satisfies Poisson's equation, $\nabla^2 U = \rho$, or Laplace's equation, $\nabla^2 U = 0$. (See also [11].)

Theoretically, even in grossly nonlaminated structures, selective cells or certain dendritic branches could be nonrandomly oriented (functionally laminated) with regard to selective afferents.

4. Inhomogeneities in the intracortical conducting medium (both vertical and horizontal) require further study. Extracellular conductivity is provided by the electrolyte filling the 200-Å spaces around cells and their fine processes. Most of the space is provided by spaces around the small (1–2 μ) processes; if fewer of them are available in a volume where many or large cell bodies predominate, or both, such as in the layer of small and medium pyramidal cells and in layer V [41], then the associated conductivity must be accordingly decreased. Such changes must be known for accurate evaluation of current density from the field potential distribution.

Changes in intracortical conductivity may be of importance during seizures inasmuch as Matsumoto and Ajmone-Marsan [25] have shown that involved neurons probably swell during seizures, and this, at least theoretically, could lead to extracellular conductivity changes.

5. The problem of potential changes incurred by sequential synaptic activation over different neurons as well as over different branches of the same neuron is amenable to solution by sequential laminar analysis [12, 48].

6. While the potential at the active end of a neuron is selectively increasing, electrotonic spread to passive regions of the cell modifies the slope of the rising phase and the peak amplitude, but not the polarity of the extracellularly recorded potentials as shown in Fig. D15-1B. Here the surface negative wave [12, 13, 30], resulting from deep IPSPs generated by recurrent collaterals of pyramidal cells [29, 44], continues to rise with IPSP increase. In theory, a field potential polarity reversal could attend the late falling phase of such potentials if—let us suppose—the apical dendritic membrane of the neuron (electrotonically charged to a fraction of the somatic end [14]) had a markedly longer time constant and slower decay than the soma-basilar dendritic membrane. In practice, however, I have never seen diphasic surface potentials resulting from generation of deep and long-lasting IPSPs.

The problem of external field distribution would be more complicated in the case of a brief synaptic input to an intermediate region of a neuron (between soma and distal dendrites), wherein the pattern of dendritic and somatic electrotonic spread would be very complex. As a further note of caution, data thus far considered apply to fields generated by PSPs on larger pyramidal neurons of deep cortical layers; there are much fewer intracellular data on smaller neurons of middle cortical layers.

7. In interpreting surface potentials during convulsive disorders, it is important to realize that many different cells at different layers are involved; the surface potential form is probably never explainable simply on the basis of PSPs observed in a given neuron. Even for the simplest *strychnine spike*, Enomoto and Ajmone-Marsan [7] have shown significant participation by both middle and deep layered neurons. When recording from pyramidal cells during strychnine spikes, we usually find a very large depolarizing potential beginning about the time of initial surface positive

response; but from intracellular evidence alone, it cannot be determined whether surface positivity is caused by excitatory endings on pyramidal cells close to the soma or by excitatory endings on basilar dendrites of cells in middle cortical layers. The surface record shifts toward negativity, while the depolarizing potential recorded at the soma is increasing (Fig. D15-1C), indicating that significant apical dendritic depolarization must be occurring on the recorded neuron or on cells activating this neuron.

Much of the depolarization shown in Fig. D15-1C is probably generated on the dendritic tree of this cell, because the intracellularly recorded depolarizing potential is decaying very much slower than would be attributable to passive decay of the membrane charge and spread of current toward the dendrites had the site of generation been the soma. The slow fall-off probably represents a balance between passive decay and prolonged electrotonic spread from distant dendrites to soma [40].

ACTION POTENTIALS. That brief action potentials of cortical neurons contribute negligibly to potentials recorded from the surface is supported by much evidence. Li, McLennan, and Jasper [21] showed that neocortical slow potentials persisted after blocking of action potentials by barbiturate. (See also [1].) Furthermore, Renshaw et al. [43] showed that amplitude of the action potential from hippocampal pyramidal cells was largest close to the cell body and fell off very rapidly, vanishing with distance, away from the soma; similar experience holds for recording neocortical action potentials. (See also [47].)

Action potentials and their brief hyperpolarizing afterpotentials contribute negligibly to the surface record, according to convincing evidence recently provided by Humphrey [12, 13]. He showed that antidromic spikes of large Betz cells, which occur before any PSPs are generated, are associated extracellularly with a deep but localized field potential, which falls off very rapidly with distance away from the soma and does not reach the cortical surface. Humphrey notes the principal reason the action potential is not observed at the cortical surface: this potential change is extremely brief (rise time 0.3 msec) and surfaces of the cell adjacent to the site of impulse generation act, in effect, as a *low pass filter*. The field potential at points distant from the site of generation of the action potential is very small, because the very brief extracellular current largely returns to the cell interior through the large membrane capacity [24] of inactive regions adjacent to the site of impulse generation, making the sinks and sources very close together. (It is not simply the time constant of inactive membrane which determines distribution of the extracellular current, but values of both the membrane specific resistance and specific capacitance.) To a first approximation, the external field, at distances that are large compared to the charge separation, depends linearly upon the dipole moment (that is, separation of the charge as well as the charge magnitude) [27]. (See also [13].)

Values that Lux and Pollen [24] obtained for the electrical constants of the Betz-cell somatic membrane were used by Humphrey [13] in calculating the expected field potential distribution for the action potential; his experimental measurements showed excellent agreement. The action potentials, because of spatially restricted, extracellular current flows, contribute negligibly to the surface record. Current flows around small unmyelinated fibers traversing the cortical gray matter must also be very small and spatially restricted; for these reasons, in addition to whatever cancellations of these currents may occur, there is no significant contribution to the surface record. Humphrey [12, 13] also demonstrated that axonal activity can contribute slightly to the surface record, although the contribution is small compared to that of PSPs. Quantitative details have been carefully considered by Humphrey.

The principal primary current generators for the surface negative and surface positive potentials known to be associated with excitation in the superficial and middle (or deep) cortical layers, respectively, must thus be the EPSPs [6, 20, 22, 23, 30, 38, 39, 48]; negligible contributions come from somatic action potentials with only small contributions from afferent and efferent axonal activity.

Significant widening of duration of the action potential would have to occur before such potentials could contribute significantly to the surface record; it is doubtful that the action potentials of cleanly penetrated neurons widen enough, even during intense epileptiform activity, to contribute significantly to surface records.

SECONDARY CURRENT GENERATORS

In penetrations of the cortex with fine micropipettes, so-called *idle cells* with very stable resting potentials close to −80 to −90 mV are frequently encountered [19, 28, 45]. Potential changes may be observed, but only in the depolarizing direction in temporal association with either EPSPs and action potentials, or IPSPs generated in neighboring neurons [17, 45, 46]. In such respects, these cells behave similarly to the glial cells in the amphibian optic nerve, where Orkand, Nicholls, and Kuffler [26] showed that the resting potential is a K^+ equilibrium potential, and where glial depolarizations result from any increase in extracellular K^+ which, in brain, can occur as a consequence of either excitatory or inhibitory ionic exchanges from neighboring neurons.

Cell bodies of the idle cells are about 12–15 μ in widest dimension, distributed evenly throughout the cortical layers and are probably glia, according to recent evidence obtained by use of marking techniques [9]. During surface *spindle bursts*, glial depolarizations were slower than the surface oscillatory activity, and glial membrane potentials returned to resting level in 1–2 sec after the end of the spindle burst [9]. Microelectrodes just outside such cells failed to record any extracellular potential specifically attributable to idle cell depolarizations [9].

After 5–15 sec paroxysms of 3 per sec spike-wave activity accompanied by a surface negative dc shift in man, the dc level returns to, or very close to, control levels immediately after cessation of the last wave response [5]. In the few cases when slight postdischarge dc shifts occurred, they were of positive polarity, but the magnitude of the shift was less than a tenth of that of the negative shifts that occured during the spike-wave discharges [5]. Under these conditions, any prolonged effect of extracellular accumulation of K^+ on the generators of the potentials recordable at the cortical surface, either oscillatory or steady, seems very small.

Glial Cells. Extracellular potentials set up by glial cells may be very small in relation to their transmembrane potential changes for a number of reasons. Uniform ionic changes in the medium around a cell and its processes, uniform orientation of cell processes, and a close sink-source relationship between active and inactive regions all work to minimize the potential field at significant distances from a cell.

The problem of the extracellular field around glial cells may be more complex because processes from one glial cell may be connected to those of many other glial cells by low-resistance pathways [26]; there is an opportunity for greater separation of current sinks and sources than would be afforded subsequent to nonuniform depolarization on a similarly small but noncoupled cell. Membrane specific resistivity would be a principal determinant of the current spread between active and inactive boundaries of the coupled cell network; this value has not yet been determined for cortical glial cells in vivo.

In tissue cultures of cerebellar explants, Hild and Tasaki [10] found the glial specific resistance to range from 3 to 10 Ω cm^2 In our tissue culture studies of tumor cell lines of glial origin [18], established after tumor extirpation from cerebral cortexes of seven patients, input resistances ranged from less than 0.5 MΩ to 3 MΩ. In determining specific resistances of these cells, selection of cells was from the periphery of the cell colony where it could be confirmed by microscopic observation (×320) and photographic study that these cells and their processes did not make contact with any other cells. Specific resistances ranged from 8 to 15 Ω cm^2 [18]; these values would represent an underestimation if there were significant (but uncounted) infoldings of the surface membrane. However, Trachtenberg (by personal communication) reports that the time constant of both human fetal glial cells in tissue culture and idle cells in the intact cat cortex is not greater than 0.5–0.8 msec, which is only 1/10 to 1/20 of the pyramidal cell membrane time constant of 8.40 ± 1.41 msec [24]. Assuming that specific capacity of the glial membrane is not less than that of the pyramidal cell membrane, then the glial specific resistivity cannot be greater than 1/10 to 1/20 of that of the pyramidal cell. Even these values are so low that extracellular current spreads between active and inactive glial network boundaries would be spatially very restricted. Low resistivity does not appear to be a consequence of the tissue-culture technique, because resistivities of meningioma cells measured under similar conditions were very high [37]. It is possible that glial tumor cells have somewhat different membrane resistances than normal glial cells; however, the same range of specific resistance was found for all three grades of glial tumors studied: astrocytoma grades II and III and glioblastoma grade IV.

These resistance measurements, it must be emphasized, were obtained on glial tumor cells in tissue culture. Unless there are cortical glial cells with very much higher specific resistances and nonrandom process orientations, it is highly unlikely that transmembrane potential changes in such cells are associated with the widespread extracellular current distributions required to contribute significantly to the cortical surface record.

Inasmuch as currents associated with postsynaptic potentials, where they can be measured, are sufficient to generate oscillatory surface potentials, and because action potentials and glial potential changes do not contribute significantly to these surface waveforms, there is every reason to believe that all normal neocortical oscillatory potentials and interictal epileptiform discharges are almost entirely the consequence of excitatory and inhibitory postsynaptic activity, with minimal axonal contributions present only during excitatory activity. However, during prolonged and intense convulsive activity, a considerable accumulation of K^+ might be expected to occur extracellulary and modify the *standing* dc potentials around neurons as well as glia. Under these conditions, Na^+ extrusion and K^+ re-uptake mechanisms might preferentially act at one or another neuronal locus, further modifying the dc fields around such cells. Identification of current sinks and sources associated with dc shifts occurring during and after severe and prolonged convulsive activity remains to be solved.

SUMMARY

Certain pertinent principles of potential theory in a volume conductor have been discussed.

Extracellular current densities have been derived from transcortical potential distributions for two principal cortical waveforms. Currents generated by IPSPs in deep cortical layers are ample to explain the magnitude of the depth positive extracellular wave and surface negative wave.

The experimental and theoretical basis for the negligible contribution to the surface record from action potentials and for the small contributions of axonal activity has been indicated.

Glial cells probably do not contribute significantly to oscillatory surface potentials under normal conditions, possibly because current sinks and sources are very close together as a consequence of a very low specific resistance of these cells.

Gross oscillatory potentials recorded from the surface of the neocortex, spontaneous and evoked, normal and epileptiform, are almost entirely the consequence of postsynaptic activity set up on vertically oriented neurons. The polarity, form, and magnitude of the principal waveforms can be satisfactorily explained on the basis of potential theory and data obtainable from combined intracellular and extracellular microelectrode studies on definable cell populations.

ACKNOWLEDGMENT. It is a pleasure to thank Dr. D. R. Humphrey for many helpful suggestions.

REFERENCES

1. Adrian, E. D., and Buytendijk, F. J. J. Potential changes in the isolated brain stem of the goldfish. *J. Physiol.* (London) 71:121, 1931.
2. Andersen, P., and Eccles, J. C. Inhibitory phasing of neuronal discharge. *Nature* (London) 196:645, 1962.
3. Andersen, P., Eccles, J. C., and Løyning, Y. Location of postsynaptic inhibitory endings on hippocampal pyramids. *J. Neurophysiol.* 27:592, 1964.
4. Calvet, J., Calvet, M. C., and Scherrer, J. Étude stratigraphique corticale de l'activité EEG spontanée. *Electroenceph. Clin. Neurophysiol.* 17:109, 1964.
5. Chatrian, G. E., Somasundaram, M., and Tassinari, C. A. DC changes recorded transcranially during "typical" three per second spike and wave discharges in man. *Epilepsia* (Amst.) 9:185, 1968.
6. Creutzfeldt, O. D., Lux, H. D., and Watanabe, S. Electrophysiology of Cortical Neurons. In Purpura, D. P., and Yahr, M. D. (Eds.), *The Thalamus.* New York: Columbia University Press, 1966.
7. Enomoto, T. F., and Ajmone-Marsan, C. Epileptic activation of single cortical neurons and their relationship with electroencephalographic discharges. *Electroenceph. Clin. Neurophysiol.* 11:199, 1959.
8. Freygang, W. H., and Landau, W. M. Some relations between resistivity and electrical activity in the cerebral cortex of the cat. *J. Cell Comp. Physiol.* 45:377, 1955.
9. Grossman, R. G., and Hampton, T. Depolarization of cortical glial cells during electrocortical activity. *Brain Res.* 11:316, 1968.
10. Hild, W., and Tasaki, I. Morphological and physiological properties of neurones and glial cells in tissue culture. *J. Neurophysiol.* 25:277, 1962.
11. Howland, B., Lettvin, J. Y., McCulloch, W. S., Pitts, W., and Wall, P. D. Reflex inhibition by dorsal root interaction. *J. Neurophysiol.* 18:1, 1955.
12. Humphrey, D. R. Re-analysis of the antidromic cortical response. I. Potentials evoked by stimulation of the isolated pyramidal tract. *Electroenceph. Clin. Neurophysiol.* 24:116, 1968.
13. Humphrey, D. R. Re-analysis of the antidromic cortical response. II. On the contribution of cell discharge and PSPs to the evoked potentials. *Electroenceph. Clin. Neurophysiol.* 26:421, 1968.
14. Jacobson, S., and Pollen, D. A. Electrotonic spread of dendritic potentials in feline pyramidal cells. *Science* 161:1351, 1968.
15. Jasper, H. H., and Droogleever-Fortuyn, J. Experimental studies on the functional anatomy of petit mal epilepsy. *Res. Publ. Ass. Res. Nerv. Ment. Dis.* 26:272, 1946.
16. Jasper, H. H., and Stefanis, C. Intracellular oscillatory rhythms in pyramidal tract neurones in the cat. *Electroenceph. Clin. Neurophysiol.* 18:541, 1965.
17. Karahashi, Y., and Goldring, S. Intracellular potentials from "idle" cells in cerebral cortex of cat. *Electroenceph. Clin. Neurophysiol.* 20:600, 1966.
18. Kornblith, P., Prieto, A., and Pollen, D. A. Alterations in glial and mesenchymal tumor cell membrane resistance with heteroimmune and autologous sera. *Ann. N.Y. Acad. Sci.* 159:585, 1969.
19. Li, C-L. Cortical intracellular potentials and their responses to strychnine. *J. Neurophysiol.* 22:436, 1959.
20. Li, C-L. Cortical intracellular synaptic potentials in response to thalamic stimulation. *J. Cell. Comp. Physiol.* 61:165, 1963.
21. Li, C-L., McLennan, H., and Jasper, H. H. Brain waves and unit discharges in cerebral cortex. *Science* 116:656, 1952.
22. Lorente de Nó, R. Transmission of impulses through cranial motor nuclei. *J. Neurophysiol.* 2:402, 1939.
23. Lux, H. D., and Klee, M. R. Intracelluläre Untersuchungen über den Einfluss hemmender Potentiale im motorischen Cortex, I. Die Wirkung elektrischer Reizung unspecifischer Thalamuskerne. *Arch. Psychiat. Nervenkr.* 203:648, 1962.
24. Lux, H. D., and Pollen, D. A. Electrical constants of neurons in the motor cortex of the cat. *J. Neurophysiol.* 29:207, 1966.
25. Matsumoto, H., and Ajmone-Marsan, C. Cellular mechanisms in experimental epileptic seizures. *Science* 144:193, 1964.
26. Orkand, R. F., Nicholls, J. G., and Kuffler, S. W. Effect of nerve impulses on the membrane potential of glial cells in the

central nervous system of amphibia. *J. Neurophysiol.* 29:788, 1966.
27. Peck, E. R. *Electricity and Magnetism.* New York: McGraw-Hill, 1953.
28. Phillips, C. G. Intracellular records from Betz cells in cat. *Quart. J. Exp. Physiol.* 41:58, 1956.
29. Phillips, C. G. Action of antidromic pyramidal volleys on single Betz cells in the cat. *Quart. J. Exp. Physiol.* 44:1, 1959.
30. Pollen, D. A. Intracellular studies of cortical neurons during thalamic induced wave and spike. *Electroenceph. Clin. Neurophysiol.* 17:398, 1964.
31. Pollen, D. A. Experimental spike and wave responses and petit mal epilepsy. *Epilepsia* (Amst.) 9:221, 1968.
32. Pollen, D. A., and Ajmone-Marsan, C. Cortical inhibitory postsynaptic potentials and strychninization. *J. Neurophysiol.* 28:342, 1965.
33. Pollen, D. A., and Lux, H. D. Conductance changes during inhibitory postsynaptic potentials in normal and strychninized neurons. *J. Neurophysiol.* 29:369, 1966.
34. Pollen, D. A., Perot, P., and Reid, K. H. Experimental bilateral wave and spike from thalamic stimulation in relation to level of arousal. *Electroenceph. Clin. Neurophysiol.* 15:1017, 1963.
35. Pollen, D. A., Reid, K., and Perot, P. Micro-electrode studies of experimental 3/sec. wave and spike in the cat. *Electroenceph. Clin. Neurophysiol.* 17:57, 1964.
36. Pollen, D. A., and Sie, P.-G. Analysis of thalamic induced wave and spike by modifications in cortical excitability. *Electroenceph. Clin. Neurophysiol.* 17:154, 1964.
37. Prieto, A., Kornblith, P., and Pollen, D. A. Electrical recordings from meningioma cells during cytolytic action of antibody and complement. *Science* 157:1185, 1967.
38. Purpura, D. P. Nature of electrocortical potentials and synaptic organizations in cerebral and cerebellar cortex. *Int. Rev. Neurobiol.* 1:47, 1959.
39. Purpura, D. P., Shofer, R. J., and Musgrave, F. S. Cortical intracellular potentials during augmenting and recruiting responses. II. Patterns of synaptic activities in pyramidal and non-pyramidal tract neurons. *J. Neurophysiol.* 27:133, 1964.
40. Rall, W. Distinguishing theoretical synaptic potentials computed for different soma-dendritic distributions of synaptic input. *J. Neurophysiol.* 30:1138, 1967.
41. Ramon-Moliner, E. The histology of the post-cruciate gyrus in the cat. *J. Comp. Neurol.* 117:43, 1961.
42. Ranck, J. B. Specific impedance of rabbit cerebral cortex. *Exp. Neurol.* 7:144, 1963.
43. Renshaw, B., Forbes, A., and Morison, B. R. Activity of isocortex and hippocampus. Electrical studies with microelectrodes. *J. Neurophysiol.* 3:74, 1940.
44. Stefanis, C., and Jasper, H. H. Intracellular microelectrode studies of antidromic responses in cortical pyramidal tract neurons. *J. Physiol.* (London) 27:828, 1964.
45. Sugaya, E., and Goldring, S. Intracellular potentials associated with direct cortical response and seizure discharge in cat. *Electroenceph. Clin. Neurophysiol.* 17:661, 1964.
46. Tasaki, I., and Chang, J. J. Electric response of glia cells in cat brain. *Science* 128:1209, 1958.
47. Tasaki, I., Polley, E. H., and Orrego, F. Action potentials from individual elements in cat geniculate and striate cortex. *J. Neurophysiol.* 17:454, 1954.
48. Towe, A. L. On the nature of the primary evoked response. *Exp. Neurol.* 15:113, 1966.

16

Mechanisms of Propagation: Extracellular Studies*

HERBERT H. JASPER

AN UNDERSTANDING of basic mechanisms of the epilepsies can never be achieved by considering properties of single cells alone, for seizures are always the consequence of mass discharge of thousands or many millions of cells, usually in excessively synchronized rhythmic discharge. Many of the cells so involved may not be inherently abnormal. They may be driven to this abnormal group behavior by excessively strong and synchronous synaptic bombardment, breaking down the delicate mechanisms of control which operate in their normal integrative functions. Of course, the control systems themselves may be defective, facilitating their breakdown with excessive synaptic drive. Included in these control systems is the neuroglial and neurochemical environment of nerve cells which probably plays a role of importance equal to synaptic circuitry in normal resistance offered by neuronal aggregates to massive, synchronized, epileptiform discharge.

Self-sustained excessive synchronous discharge in neuronal ganglia seems to require interaction of a large number of single cells in a local neuronal aggregate, or mutual interactions between distant ganglionic centers. Consequently neuronal circuitry in local aggregates of neurons as well as functional relations between distant areas, cortical and subcortical, is a major problem in understanding the generation of epileptic seizures. Furthermore, local epileptic discharges in a very limited group of neurons may be manifest in the electrical activity of the brain as interictal spikes or even local, sustained afterdischarges without any obvious manifestation in behavior or obvious disturbance in cerebral functioning. It is when such local areas of minimal discharge increase or recruit sufficient neurons into their orbit to spread or be propagated from a focus into efferent pathways producing convulsive movements, or into other cortical or subcortical neuronal structures, that the clinical seizure becomes obvious. An understanding therefore of mechanisms of propagation and spread of epileptic seizures is of critical importance, first, in order to trace the development of clinical seizures from abnormal discharge in a local group of epileptic neurons, and second, for understanding of the form that such seizures take in different epileptic patients.

The speed of propagation of epileptic discharge varies widely. It may creep across the surface of the cerebral cortex, as in the slowly progressive Jacksonian motor seizure at rates of only a few millimeters per minute, or it may pass over the feltwork of the cortex at a more rapid rate, as in spread of local afterdischarge at rates of 10–40 cm per sec. In certain forms of clinical seizure, and in animals subjected to convulsant drugs, seizure discharge appears to spread, or to be propagated throughout the brain with almost explosive rapidity, involving both hemispheres simultaneously with massive tonic-clonic convulsive movements of

---

* Supported by Medical Research Council of Canada.

the entire body, followed by profound depression in the electrical activity of the brain and prolonged unconsciousness with generalized loss of muscle tone.

The pathophysiological mechanisms involved in sudden massive generalized seizures is a most complex problem. Equally difficult to explain are those attacks which, without significant convulsive movements, are characterized by sudden interruption of consciousness during bilaterally synchronous regular rhythmic 3-per-sec *wave-spike* electrical disturbances in the EEG, the classical *petit mal* attack.

It is necessary to distinguish clearly between three different forms of epileptic nerve tissue: *primary*, those with local chronic epileptogenic lesions (chemical or morphological or both); *secondary*, those with secondarily induced but self-sustained epileptic discharge periodically occurring in otherwise normal assemblies of neurons; and *projected*, those areas receiving a simple projection of epileptiform discharge, producing abnormal evoked potentials, but without inducing local self-sustained epileptic processes in the areas of projection. In this chapter the attempt will be made to distinguish between *spread* by contiguity and *propagation* over axonal pathways, both of which may establish *secondary* self-sustained paroxysmal discharge in distant normal ganglia.

It is apparent, however, that the three processes, primary, secondary, and projected, may be interrelated. Simple projection, if maintained, may lead to secondary activation. Secondary activation, if maintained over a longer period of time, may lead to a chronic, self-sustained epileptic process as discussed by Morrell in Chap. 13. There may also be other forms of chronic change in neuronal tissue resulting from repeated involvement in epileptic discharge, namely, establishment of preferential pathways of spread, a sort of learning process, since seizure patterns, although highly varied in different patients, are remarkably stereotyped in the same patient from time to time.

Since many details of microphysiological mechanisms involved in spread of epileptic paroxysm will be presented by other contributors in this volume, this chapter will be concerned chiefly with broader outlines of these problems. Purpura will review his microelectrode studies of this subject in the second half of this presentation.

We shall consider only those mechanisms which may operate in (1) the spread of epileptiform activity from one cell to another in a local aggregate of neurons, (2) the mode of spread from one local aggregate across the surface of the cortex by intracortical mechanisms, (3) projection of epileptic discharge over long transcortical and transcommissural fiber systems, (4) thalamocortical and corticothalamic circuits in the transmission of epileptic discharge, and (5) possible participation of the diffuse projection system of the mesial thalamus and brain stem.

INTRACORTICAL MECHANISMS

It has long been known that the cerebral cortex alone, independent of connections with extracortical structures, is capable of generating various forms of local self-sustained epileptiform discharge. Such local discharge will spread, if sufficiently intense and repetitive from a given point stimulated, to progressively involve all neurons in an undercut or completely isolated slab of cortical tissue. The synaptic circuitry of the cortex itself must, therefore, be capable of generating self-sustained rhythmic, neuronal discharge independent of synaptic drive or activation it normally receives from specific or nonspecific afferent input, providing initial activation is artificially provided by means of local electrical stimulation, or by the use of convulsant drugs.

Some twenty years ago, Kristiansen and Courtois [29] in our laboratories were able to show that rhythmic electrical activity, similar to spindle waves recorded from the cortex of the cat under barbiturate anesthesia, could be induced in completely isolated cerebral cortex by application of a solution of acetylcholine (0.1 percent) after treatment with an anticholinesterase. With a somewhat stronger concentration, applied for a longer time, long trains of remarkably regular rhythmic waves appeared, interrupted by periods of electrical silence, resembling a common form of epileptic discharge. Frequency of this exaggerated rhythm was very close to that which had been observed for spindle waves which appeared in the same area of cortex prior to undercutting. A few years later, MacIntosh and Oborin [34], using the superfusion chamber developed in our laboratories with Elliott, demonstrated that intact cortex liberated acetylcholine at measurable rates at rest, and at increased rates following sensory stimulation, but no measurable ACh was released from undercut cortex. These results were later confirmed, in collaboration with Sie and Wolfe [50] and with Celesia [11], and it was shown that in the unanesthetized animal aroused by natural stimulation or by electrical stimulation of the brain-stem reticular formation, acetylcholine accumulating in a local area of eserinized cortex would be sufficient to cause a local epileptiform discharge of a form similar to that previously observed by application of ACh to isolated cortex (Fig. 16-1). It was obvious, therefore, that even small concentrations of ACh liberated by physiological processes in the waking animal were sufficient to elicit epileptiform discharge when its destruction by enzymatic hydrolysis was reduced. Eserine or neostigmine alone, in the *cerveau isolé* preparation, did not produce epileptic activation unless allowed to act for several hours, consistent with the much reduced rate of ACh liberated in such preparations.

Cholinergic Mechanisms. These results suggest that cholinergic mechanisms within the cerebral cortex, depending upon certain activating afferent pathways from subcortical structures, might play a role not only in maintenance of rhythmic electrical activity in normal cortex, but could also be involved in activation of cortex to epileptic discharge. This form of activation could be

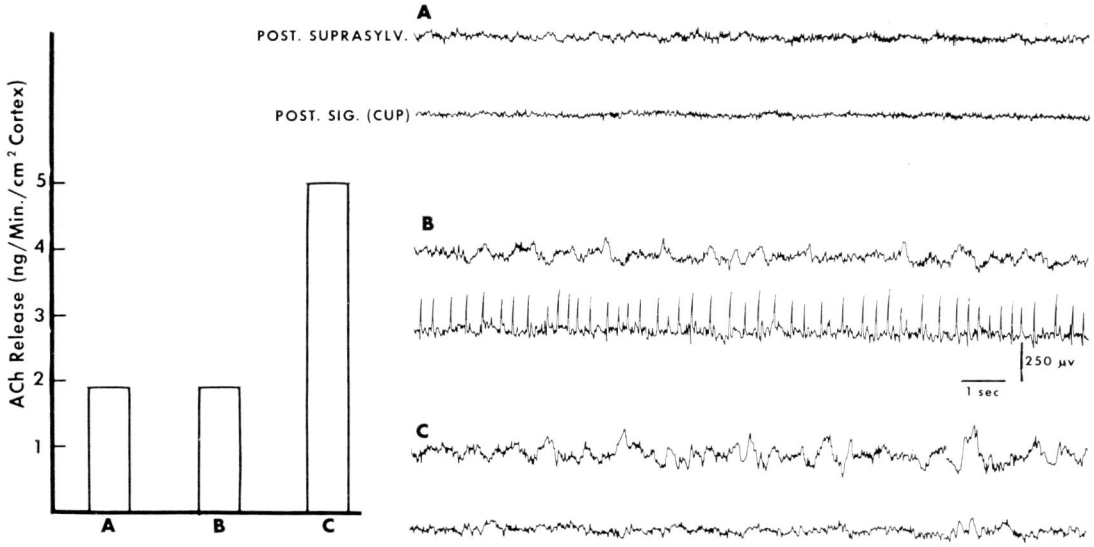

FIG. 16-1. Effect of local application of neostigmine solution (7.5×10^{-5} gm per ml) upon electrical activity of cerebral cortex in cat under local anesthesia immobilized with gallamine. In each of three pairs of tracings, upper one taken directly from surface of posterior suprasylvian gyrus as a control, second from cortical surface of postsigmoid gyrus within plastic cup through which was perfused neostigminized Elliott's solution, the perfusate collected at 10-min intervals for assay of acetylcholine. (A) Desynchronized activation occurred in 10 min, with ACh release rate of about 2 ng per min shown in graph at left. (B) Epileptiform spikes appeared without change in ACh release-rate. Spikes were abolished by intravenous atropine (1 mg per kg) shown in (B), rate of ACh release increasing to about 5 ng per min due presumably to blockade of ACh receptors. For further details, see Fig. 4 in Celesia and Jasper [11].

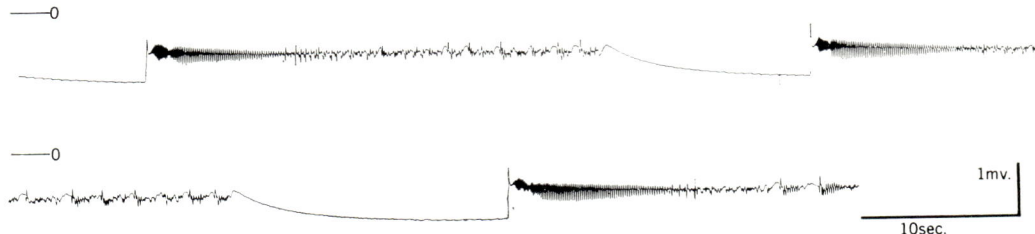

Fig. 16-2. Direct current records of ACh-induced paroxysms in isolated cortex of cat. Deflection up in surface negative relative to nonpolarizable electrode in white matter beneath cortex. Level of equilibrium between two recording electrodes is indicated by 0 lines above. See text for further description.

readily blocked with atropine or scopolamine, which also blocks desynchronized activation of the EEG in the normal *arousal* response mediated by the brain-stem reticular-activating system [27, 40]. However, electrical afterdischarge could still be induced by direct stimulation in atropinized cortex showing that no generalized cortical depression was present. Liberation of ACh from atropinized cortex was greatly increased, in spite of blocking of epileptic activation showing that specific ACh receptors must be involved in this process.

During the past year we have undertaken to reexamine mechanisms of ACh activation of isolated cortex, using dc recording with nonpolarizable electrodes, and microelectrodes for unit recording and plotting of electrical fields within the depths of cortex. Observations of Kristiansen and Courtois were readily confirmed. In addition, with Dr. John Ferguson, it was shown that each paroxysmal rhythmic discharge is associated with an abrupt negative shift in dc potential of the cortical surface which extended to the level of large pyramidal cells of the fifth layer of cortex beneath. The 8–10 per second rhythmic oscillations were always superimposed upon long-lasting negative shifts in dc (Fig. 16-2).

The sudden negative dc change of 1–5 mV was associated with rapid, continuous, repetitive discharge of deep-lying pyramidal cells, this discharge being interrupted by periodic inhibitory waves during the oscillating discharge (Fig. 16-3). The oscillations were apparently composed largely of periodic waves of inhibition gating the otherwise continuous excitatory drive imposed upon pyramidal cells by the prolonged depolarization. Although our intracellular and more complete extracellular unit studies have not been completed, these results would suggest that isolated cortex is capable of generating at least two forms of self-sustained rhythmic activity: one of very long duration appearing as a square wave relaxation-type of oscillation with a period of many seconds, and another at a frequency of 8–12 per sec induced by oscillating waves of inhibition superimposed upon the prolonged depolarization. A more rapid rhythm of 40–60 per sec was also occasionally observed and frequently preceded the 10–12 per sec rhythm at onset of paroxysm as shown in Fig. 16-2. Pyramidal cell activity was arrested during the positive dc change which occurred between paroxysms. However, a few unidentified cells,

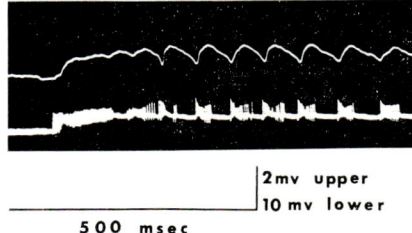

Fig. 16-3. Surface and extracellular microelectrode records of beginning of ACh-induced paroxysm in cerebral cortex of cat. Microelectrode situated at depth of 1.05 mm presumably recording from deep pyramidal cell which fires rapidly at onset of surface negative dc shift, is then interrupted rhythmically during superimposed oscillating surface waves. (Unpublished experiments with John Ferguson.)

presumably interneurons, were firing actively during the inhibition of pyramidal cells.

Gloor, Sperti, and Vera [18, 19] have described a similar "flip-flop" dc oscillation between pyramidal cells and dendritic layers of the hippocampus during epileptic paroxysms, the cell layer becoming relatively negative to the dendritic layer during excessive cellular discharge, the discharge ceasing abruptly with shift in the reverse direction. Burns and Grafstein [9] have described a "positive burst response" in isolated cortex of similar character which they suggest might be due to differential repolarization rates between dendrites and soma of radially oriented neurons lying about 1 mm beneath the cortical surface. Such a response was conducted throughout the slab of isolated cortex through a multisynaptic chain of deeper lying neurons, since a cut extending over 1 mm down from the surface was necessary to interrupt the spreading process [8].

The concept of differential rates of repolarization between dendrites and soma is supported by microelectrode studies of Tasaki, Polley, and Orrego [52] in the lateral geniculate body and visual cortex, and by Tasaki, Hagiwara, and Watanabe [51] in the giant Mauthner cell of the catfish showing that dendrites require about seven times longer to repolarize than do cell bodies. However, it is not proved that the more rapid repolarization of cell bodies is due to differential properties of somatic and dendritic cell membranes alone. The more rapid repolarization of the somatic membrane may be due to compensatory repolarizing by inhibitory synapses which are concentrated on somatic membranes [15]. The long time course of the dc changes, lasting 10–30 sec, raises additional problems, however, since a very long period of summation with gradual accumulation of inhibitory transmitter before overcoming the dendritic-somatic dipole would have to be postulated. Oscillating waves of inhibition which are superimposed upon the dc shift would suggest, however, that recurrent inhibition may well play a role in gradual repolarization of the soma membrane.

That synaptic mechanisms may well be involved in control of the oscillating dipole is suggested by the observation of Gloor et al. [18, 19] that it could be reset or controlled by a single afferent volley in the hippocampus. We have observed that the ACh dc oscillation in intact somatic cortex could be driven by weak afferent volleys such as light touch on the skin. The precise manner in which ACh acts, either when liberated normally by cholinergic nerve terminals in *eserinized* cortex or by direct application, remains obscure. That its action is readily blocked by atropine suggests that it must depend upon specific receptor sites on postsynaptic membranes which have been demonstrated for deep-lying pyramidal cells in the cortex.

Burns and Grafstein [9] were unable to demonstrate positive burst response in intact cortex. The ACh response is also altered somewhat in intact cortex, becoming somewhat less regular as might be expected from the influence of incoming afferent volleys. However, it occurs with equal amplitude in either intact or isolated cortex. Both responses are propagated without decrement through intracortical mechanisms in isolated cortex as well as in intact cortex. Propagation may be blocked by light barbiturate anesthesia, indicating that multisynaptic mechanisms are involved in the propagation process.

Anatomical and microphysiological studies have shown that the cerebral cortex is organized in columns of radially oriented cells with remarkably specific functional homogeneity, isolated from their neighbors with the aid of lateral or "surround" inhibition [36, 47]. Such columns of cells, with surface diameter of only about 0.5 mm or less, may also be the functional unit of local epileptic discharge, since the minimal dipole which will sustain a local, nonpropagated epileptic discharge appears to be of about the same dimensions [41]. Increased intensity and duration of repetitive local discharge is able to break down the inhibitory barriers afforded by deep-lying interneurons, permitting successive columns of cells to be driven by collaterals from axons of deep-lying cells which must terminate in excitatory synapses on adjacent columns. It has repeatedly been shown, since the original work of Adrian in 1936 [1], that intracortical propagation will not occur if excitation is limited to the more superficial layers, nor can self-sustaining afterdischarge be induced by surface stimulation producing only the simple surface-negative direct cortical response which appears to be confined to fibers of the molecular layer only.

There is some evidence to suggest that there is also a laminar-synaptic organization of importance to propagation of epileptic discharge from surface to depths of cortex. Local application of strychnine first induces surface-negative spikes which are not conducted over efferent projections from the cortex, apparently because deeply-lying pyramidal cells with corticofugal axonal projections are not involved. Under certain conditions, local rhythmic afterdischarge has also been oberved to be sustained in upper cortical layers without involving deep-lying pyramidal cells. Such discharges seem not to be propagated. Burns and Grafstein [9] have suggested from their microlaminar studies and sections at various depths that pyramidal cells responsible for more superficial response lie about 1 mm beneath the cortical surface, the type B neurons, while those with laterally extending axons lie deeper, the type A neurons.

With Olszewski, Burns and Grafstein [10] attempted to identify more precisely the A and B type neurons, but without success. There seemed to be considerable overlap. However, some of the A type neurons correspond to pyramidal cells of the fifth and sixth cortical layers, while the B type neurons corresponded mostly to the pyramidal cells of the second and third layers, prominent among which are the border cells of O'Leary, but with some recorded below this level. The potential functional independence of these two layers or classes of pyramidal cells, in spite of their synaptic interconnections and extension of apical dendrites of deep-lying cells to the cortical surface, remains a problem of considerable interest and importance for understanding the normal integrative function of cerebral cortex, as well as for generation of local paroxysm and their spread by intracortical conduction pathways.

SPREAD BY DIFFUSION. Another form of spread activity within the cortex itself has also been demonstrated in neuronally isolated cortical tissue, namely the spreading depression of Leão [30]. This phenomenon will not be discussed in detail since it has been extensively studied by many workers [35, 37, 55]. In the context of the present chapter, however, it should be included as a model of mechanisms of possible importance in slowly spreading, abnormal, excessive activation followed by depression of cortical cells. The profound generalized depolarization of all cortical cells during this process, with the associated slow wave of negative polarization of the cortical surface, represents a mechanism of spread which seems to involve mainly diffusion of chemical substances, probably potassium or glutamate or both. This chemically induced depolarization may well involve participation of glial cell networks within the cortex acting as bridges between neurons in the nonsynaptic propagation process.

On the leading wave front of spreading depression there may be an excessive discharge of nerve cells with accumulation of potassium (or glutamate or both) which acts to depolarize successive groups of nerve cells, which in turn liberate excessive potassium to continue the diffusion process throughout the cortex, at a rate of spread of only a few millimeters per minute. Such a process may not play a leading role in the more rapid propagation of epileptic discharge, but similar mechanisms cannot be ignored in the more slowly progressive spread across the cortex and in our understanding of some intercortical consequences of excessive neuronal discharge even when they do not reach the threshold of true spreading depression. Excessive discharge does, in fact, alter extracellular and glial environment of nerve cells, so that such a process may well play an important role in increased susceptibility of groups of neurons to paroxysmal discharge in response to a given synaptic drive. Thus the diffusion of chemical substances from hyperactive cells in abnormal amounts may serve to facilitate synaptic mechanisms which operate in more common forms of intracortical propagation of paroxysmal discharge.

POTENTIAL FIELDS AND "EPHAPTIC" EXCITATION. Extracellular potential fields which develop as radial dipoles in a local assembly of neurons during an epileptic paroxysm seldom reach over 1–2 mV in magnitude. They decrease rapidly by a sharp gradient to the field of contiguous columns of cells so that spread by ephaptic, nonsynaptic conduction would not be expected in normal cortical tissue. This is borne out by experiments in which intracortical spread can be interrupted by sharp transection of intracortical conducting pathways, leaving the edges in conjunction. Such observations do not prove, however, that ephaptic conduction may not play a role in facilitating synaptic propagation, or in triggering epileptic discharge in nerve tissue which is on the verge of spontaneous epileptic discharge, as can be produced experimentally by subconvulsive treatment with convulsant drugs.

Libet and Gerard [32, 33], in the isolated frog brain, were able to demonstrate propagation of caffeine-induced waves across a complete neuronal transection. Bremer [7] has shown that strychnine spikes remain synchronized in upper and lower segments of spinal cord even after complete transection with juxtaposition of the cut ends. If the cortex is in a subthreshold convulsive state even small electrical fields surrounding an actively discharging focus may be sufficient to trigger a self-sustained paroxysm in contiguous neuronal tissue. If two adjacent areas are engaged in self-sustained rhythmic epileptic discharge, as in the strychninized spinal cord of Bremer, ephaptic potential fields may well be sufficient to synchronize oscillations without benefit of synaptic mechanisms. However, in the intact brain, synaptic mechanisms appear to play a leading role in both triggering and synchronization of epileptic discharge, potential fields having probably only a facilitating action, though this may be of great importance for cells in the subliminal fringe, and in synchronizing discharges in large areas of activated nerve tissue.

PROJECTION AND PROPAGATION OVER LONG CONDUCTING PATHWAYS

Studies of projection and propagation of epileptic discharge over long conducting pathways, transcortical, transcommissural, or subcortical have been useful in mapping functional anatomical connections in the brain, as in original studies of Dusser de Barenne and McCulloch [14] with "strychnine neuronography." With implanted electrodes in experimental animals without anesthesia, relationships between location and propagation of seizure discharge to behavioral seizure patterns can be carried out. In such experiments it is important to differentiate between mechanisms of projection and true spread since it is possible for the area to which initial discharge is projected to become an independent focus of discharge and to successfully project to another area and continue the epileptic discharge in multiple steps eventually quite independent of focus of origin. A review of this extensive work is beyond the scope of this chapter. Reference will be made only briefly to a few studies and general conclusions which appear to be of importance in understanding some basic mechanisms involved. Some of these mechanisms will be discussed in greater detail by Purpura and others.

The pattern of impulses being projected over efferent pathways from a local assembly of neurons engaged in an epileptic paroxysm differ from the normal in four important respects.

1. Frequency of discharge in individual fibers is about ten times greater than that occurring during normal activity (50–500 or more per second).
2. Finely organized temporal patterning of impulses in single fibers is abolished.
3. Relative independence of firing in different fibers is also abolished, so that

sequential spatial patterns necessary for ongoing integrative function are obliterated.

4. Many more fibers become simultaneously activated. Both spatial and temporal summation become greatly enhanced. As Lennox has so well described it, "the harmony of the orchestra becomes a single note."

The effect of such a barrage of impulses upon the areas of projection depends upon synaptic organization of their terminal fibers as well as upon the state of ongoing activity and excitability of receiving areas. If the effect is predominately inhibitory the disturbed function of the receiving area should cease with discharge in the primary area, since development of a secondary area of self-sustained discharge would not occur. In many instances, however, the area of secondary projection receives sufficient excitatory drive, or inhibitory effects are suppressed, so that it becomes, at least for a time, capable of sustained epileptic discharge after epileptic activity of the primary area has ceased. It may then project its activity to other areas; the whole process repeats itself, even to complete the circle in some instances and return to reactivate the area of primary discharge.

In this manner epileptic discharge may spread sequentially throughout the brain, often being propagated back and forth between cortical and subcortical structures in the process. Some structures which become involved in this process may, however, have a dampening effect upon the spreading process, either because of presence of strong inhibitory control systems which are brought into play, or because certain ganglia are much less susceptible to sustained epileptic discharge than are others. In any case, integrative function in areas of projection would undergo serious disturbances, even though they did not become engaged in active generation of epileptic discharge. Insofar as they are only passively driven, they do not show postictal depression of function that characterizes the end of severe paroxysm in an area of primary discharge.

Experimental studies, as well as clinical observations, have shown great differences in the threshold for epileptic discharge in different parts of the brain. The hippocampus appears to be the most susceptible, while the cerebellum is the least so. In fact, Dow maintains that it is not possible to set up a self-sustained epileptic process in the cerebellum and the cerebellum may arrest seizure discharges in some areas of projection [12, 13]. This may well be due to predominance of strong inhibitory control systems within the cerebellum, and the fact that its projections to relay nuclei are predominantly inhibitory. However, it has been shown by others that epileptiform states may be induced in the cerebellum by systemic administration of certain convulsant drugs [54].

It has been proposed that the facility with which sustained rhythmic paroxysmal activity can be initiated in the hippocampus may be related to its simple laminar structure of closely packed pyramidal cells and deep layer of apical dendrites. The concentration of inhibitory synapses on somatic cell membranes should tend to attenuate excessive discharge of these cells, but perhaps it may also make possible the establishment of abnormal oscillating somatodendritic dipoles which Gloor et al. [18, 19] have shown to characterize sustained paroxysm in the hippocampus.

It has long been known that tonic-clonic convulsions can be induced in experimental animals by means of convulsant drugs or electrical stimulation even after decortication [46]. During recent years it has been shown that various forms of clinical and electrographic seizures can be induced in experimental animals by local injection of epileptogenic agents such as penicillin or aluminum hydroxide, or by local electrical stimulation of thalamus and midbrain, as well as amygdaloid and hippocampal structures [23, 28]. Such seizures are usually, but not always associated with projection to certain cortical areas where they may appear only as evoked potentials, or they may induce secondary self-sustained paroxysm in the cortex itself. Such projections may be to both hemispheres simultaneously, or they may be restricted to local areas of one hemisphere, depending upon the subcortical structure primarily involved, its interconnections with other subcortical structures, and upon density of direct projections to the cerebral cortex. Where reciprocal interconnections exist, such as between specific nuclei of thalamus and local areas of cortex, complex interactions occur in both directions. This may be complicated by interactions between subcortical systems, specific or nonspecific, as will be described by Purpura.

THALAMOCORTICAL INTERRELATIONSHIPS. Close interrelationships between local areas of cortex and specific nuclei of thalamus, first demonstrated by Dusser de Barenne and McCulloch [14] with local strychnine in the somatosensory system of monkey, have since been confirmed by other methods and in other experimental animals, and with other thalamic nuclei. It will be recalled that similar local hyperesthesia in the contralateral hand could be produced by application of local strychnine either to the postcentral hand area of the cortex or to the corresponding portion of nucleus ventralis posterior of the thalamus. Spontaneous or evoked strychnine spikes were recorded from both thalamus and cortex following local strychnine application to one or the other. Careful precautions were taken to avoid diffusion outside the immediate area of application. Spread to adjacent thalamocortical systems for leg and face did not occur. An example of such records in the cat, from our experiments with Knighton, is shown in Fig. 16-4.

Similar reciprocal interrelationships have been demonstrated by local repetitive electrical stimulation of sufficient intensity and duration to result in limited local afterdischarge. In collaboration with Hunter and Knighton [25] it was found that local afterdischarge in any given specific thalamic nucleus in monkey projected exclusively to those cortical areas known to receive their major afferent supply from these nuclei. This was not restricted to sensory relay nuclei, but was also true of association nuclei, such as from n. medialus dorsalis to Brodmann's areas 9 and 10 of the frontal lobe, as shown in Fig. 16-5.

With Stoll and Ajmone-Marsan [24], similar local projection of afterdischarge was found from local portions of n. lateralis posterior and pulvinar to temporal and parietal cortex. However, corticofugal projections also occurred to nonspecific structures such as n. centrum medianum of the

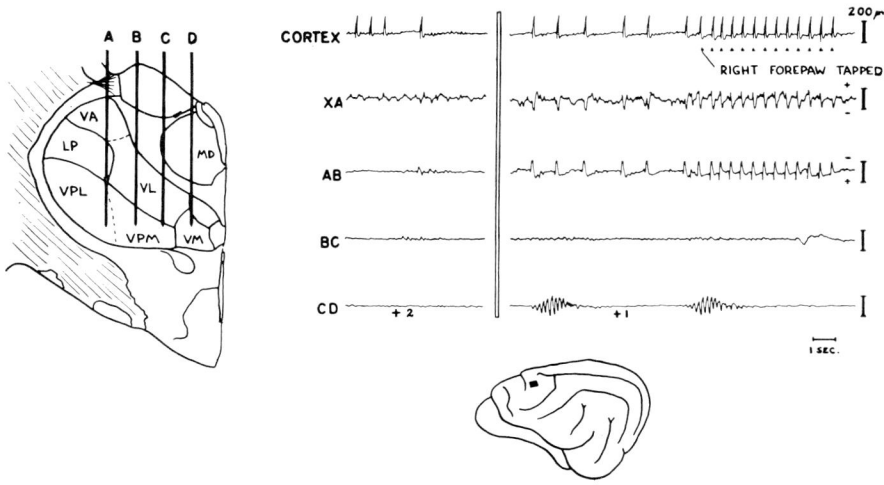

FIG. 16-4. Projection of cortical strychnine spikes from somatosensory forepaw area in cat to local area of VPL in thalamus (electrode A). Note that spikes were absent 1 mm above final position shown as illustrated in first set of tracings and present 1 mm below. Spikes could be triggered by light tactile stimulation of contralateral forepaw both in cortex and thalamus synchronously.

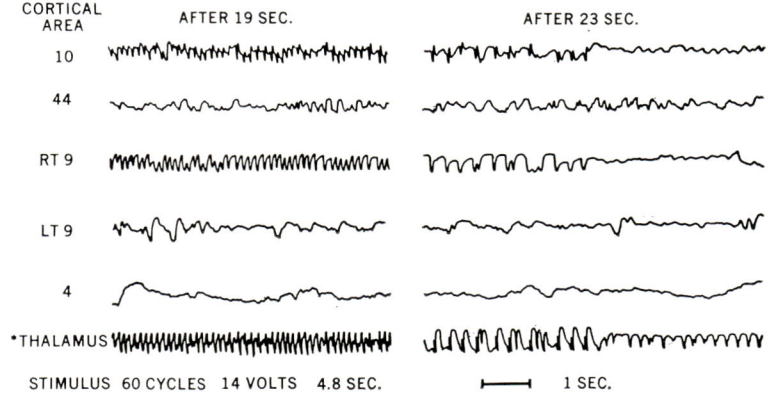

FIG. 16-5. Afterdischarge following local electrical stimulation of nucleus medialis dorsalis in monkey projected to Brodmann's areas 9 and 10 of frontal lobe. Note continuation of thalamic afterdischarge following cessation of cortical projection and change in form when cortical projection has ceased. (From Fig. V-12 of [38].)

thalamus and to the midbrain reticular formation as shown in Fig. 16-6. Reciprocal interaction also occurred, the form of the thalamic afterdischarge being suddenly changed with cessation of the cortical projection. In some instances, local cortical discharge continued after the primary thalamic discharge had ceased, or vice versa, as in Fig. 16-6B, which shows continued afterdischarge in n. centrum medianum after stimulation of the anterior cingulate gyrus in monkey. Similar results have been reported by Fields, King, and O'Leary [16] who studied projection of local afterdischarge from lateral geniculate to visual cortex and from ventralis-posterior to sensory cortex in cat.

Walker, in an extensive series of studies recently summarized with Udvarhelyi [53, 59], experienced considerable difficulty in eliciting sustained afterdischarge by local thalamic stimulation in monkey. They concluded that [the thalamus] "does not readily enter into spontaneous repetitive discharge. When such discharges are produced, they are focal or propagate mainly to other subcortical nuclei . . . the thalamus would be unlikely to originate or augment an epileptic cortical discharge. Its role might more appropriately be that of a modulator or inhibitor of convulsive activity passing through the thalamus or present in the cortex" [59, p. 361]. These authors also considered that basal ganglia as a whole, and particularly the striatum, appeared to inhibit rather than to facilitate or to propagate epileptic attacks.

This view is contrary to evidence provided by Aquino-Cías and Bureš [2, 3] who found in unanesthetized rats that thalamic spreading depression decreased activity of a pentylenetetrazol-induced cortical focus, as might be expected by deafferentation. Afterdischarges evoked by cortical or hippocampal stimulation were also reduced or abolished during thalamic spreading depression, and early manifestations of seizures induced by intravenous pentylenetetrazol were delayed. They concluded that the thalamus plays an important role in initiation of a generalized epileptic seizure, but that it is not indispensable in maintaining it, once it is fully developed. There is no assurance that such evidence for the facilitating action of thalamus upon cortically induced seizures holds true to an equal extent in higher mammals and primates, but it does cast some doubt upon the concept that the thalamus acts only in an inhibitory manner in genesis or elaboration of seizures.

The studies of Hayashi [21] and the recent work of Wilder and Schmidt [63], who recorded the subcortical propagation of seizures arising from chronic focal cortical, epileptogenic lesions (aluminum hy-

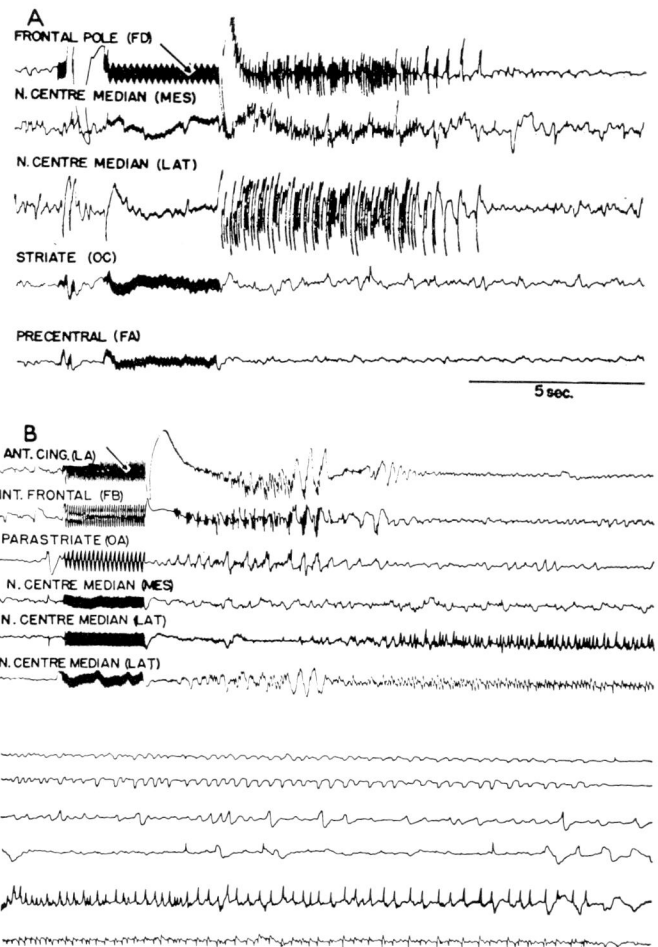

FIG. 16-6. (*A*) Corticofugal projection of local anterior frontal afterdischarge to lateral portion of n. centrum medianum in monkey. (From experiments with Ajmone-Marsan and Stoll [24].) (*B*) Corticofugal projection from anterior cingulate gyrus to n. centrum medianum in monkey [24]. Note persistence of thalamic afterdischarge from NCM in upper set of tracings with secondary projection to frontal lobe in lower set of tracings.

droxide) in monkeys, found a preferential spread to subcortical structures, including basal ganglia, thalamus, and midbrain reticular formation, and concluded that generalization of seizures of focal, cortical origin was primarily by means of these subcortical projection systems. Wilder and Schmidt did note, however, that cessation of some attacks was associated with the appearance of spike-wave formations in mesial thalamus and midbrain reticular formation and suggested that these structures may also play an inhibitory role in their interaction with cortical and subcortical structures in the arrest of generalized seizures. Wilder and Schmidt were so impressed with the preferential projection of cortical seizure discharge to subcortical structures that they raised considerable doubt as to the importance of corpus callosum in the generalization of seizures of unilateral focal cortical origin. These results, obtained with chronic cortical epileptogenic lesions in monkeys with implanted recording electrodes in subcortical and cortical structures, are in accord with previous more detailed studies in monkeys carried out in our laboratories [24].

The studies of Walker and associates with implanted electrodes in necessarily limited areas of subcortical regions, and with multiple sequential propagation of afterdischarge to many cerebral structures, cortical and subcortical, provide interesting relationships with behavioral changes observed in the unanesthetized animal, but cannot reveal the finely organized projection pathways between cortex and subcortical structures. In order to avoid these difficulties we have maintained monkeys in a stereotaxic instrument with local anesthesia, with only a quieting dose of thiopental, which served to minimize cortical spread of afterdischarge, thus making it possible to explore subcortical structures millimeter by millimeter to map more completely and in greater detail the preferential projection pathways from a cortical focus thus restricted to a few millimeters or less of cortical surface. We have called this the *limited afterdischarge* technique. With this method only the most direct projection pathways are revealed, and finer organization of corticofugal as well as transcortical pathways can be mapped out.

It was found that corticofugal projections to thalamus and brain stem occurred in a systematic manner, even in the absence of projection or spread to adjacent cortex, or, in many instances, in the absence of significant projection across the corpus callosum to the homologous area of cortex in the opposite hemisphere. In addition to specific reciprocal relationships with specific thalamic nuclei, there were strong convergent projections to intralaminar nuclei of thalamus and to tegmentum and reticular formation of the midbrain arising principally from frontal and temporoparietal association cortex, and the anterior cingulate cortex, but not from primary visual cortex unless the parastriate cortex became involved.

Samples of these results are shown in Fig. 16-6. They confirm many other studies indicating preferential propagation of epileptic discharge subcortically, though not ruling out, of course, the importance of intracortical and transcortical processes which undoubtedly play an important role in the intact unanesthetized brain. Such studies do not, however, provide evidence concerning the excitatory or inhibitory character of subcortical projections in the generalization of epileptic seizures.

The fact that generalized convulsive seizures, as well as attacks like petit mal with arrest of ongoing behavior, can be reproduced in experimental animals with stimulating electrodes or chronic epileptogenic lesions in mesial thalamus or midbrain structures, is strong evidence in favor of their importance in certain forms of generalized seizure, whether such seizures appear to be predominately of an inhibitory character or develop into a more generalized convulsive attack [5, 23, 28, 56]. To speak of solely inhibitory or facilitatory functions for either the so-called specific or nonspecific neuronal systems in thalamus or brain stem is obviously a gross oversimplification as will be pointed out by Purpura. Complex excitatory and inhibitory interactions between transcortical and subcortical projection systems, and between specific and nonspecific neuronal networks at both cortical and subcortical levels are probably involved in epileptic processes, as in all integrative functions of the brain.

The corpus callosum, for example, is not necessary for propagation of seizure discharge from one hemisphere to the other, although when present, propagation is facilitated between certain cortical areas with strong callosal interconnections, but not between others with weak or absent transcallosal interconnections. In the motor area, for example, transcortical spread from one segment to another along the motor strip may occur before a seizure is propagated to involve both sides of the body, providing a good example of the relatively greater functional importance of corticofugal projection systems, in spite of the fact that the presence of the corpus callosum seems necessary for development of a mirror focus and may facilitate bilateral propagation of focal motor seizures, although strong transcallosal inhibitory effects upon pyramidal tract neurons—via interneurons in motor cortex—have been demonstrated by Purpura and Girado [48] and by Berlin [6]. However, it has recently been shown that section of corpus callosum in patients with generalized seizures may improve their subsequent control by medication (see ADDENDUM by Bogen, Sperry and Vogel).

GENERALIZED SEIZURES OF SUDDEN BILATERAL ONSET

Physiopathological mechanisms responsible for generalized seizures of sudden bilateral onset have been the subject of much controversy during recent years [17]. Extensive clinical and experimental investigations pertaining to this problem were reviewed in a colloquium organized by Gastaut two years ago, material from which is soon to be published. Only a few of the many facets of this problem can be mentioned at this time.

Generalized seizures of simultaneous bilateral onset of various forms, including intermittent myoclonic jerks of the extremities, with more or less well-synchronized epileptiform discharges from homologous areas of both hemispheres in the EEG, occur in patients with diffuse diseases of the brain as a whole, or secondary to toxic states or enzyme deficiencies affecting brain metabolism. Experimentally such seizures may be induced with rapidly acting convulsant drugs such as pentylenetetrazol, by enzyme deficiencies such as of pyridoxal phosphate, or by means of enzyme poisons such as thiosemicarbazide or diisofluorophosphate. Under these conditions all cells and synaptic circuits in the brain become unstable, all control systems so defective that multiple pathways, both transcortical and subcortical, become rapidly involved in epileptic activation. In many patients, however, particularly those with classic petit mal seizures, or with combination of petit mal and grand mal attacks with sudden bilateral onset, no such metabolic disease and no local or diffuse brain pathology can be consistently demonstrated, except that which might result from the major seizures themselves.

In some of these patients, deep-lying epileptogenic lesions have been found in cerebral cortex, especially in parasaggital and orbital frontal regions, with local electric abnormality revealed only by implantation of deep electrodes. In most of these cases the electroencephalogram can readily be distinguished from that of patients with classic petit mal seizures if rigid criteria are employed. Some cannot be distinguished by clinical criteria alone, since both may be characterized by initial and sudden loss of consciousness without convulsive movements, and proceed to bilateral convulsive seizures without focal onset, though adversive movements of head and eyes often occur in those of origin in one frontal lobe.

By what neuronal pathways or mechanisms do such dramatic attacks occur: one in which mechanisms of consciousness are suddenly snuffed out for a few seconds, and suddenly turned on again, or one that may develop into a major convulsive seizure involving both sides of the body from the onset? During the past 30 years or more that Penfield and I have been concerned with this problem [38], in collaboration with many colleagues in neurophysiology, neuroanatomy, and neurochemistry, much new information has become available from many laboratories which has an important bearing upon this problem, some of which is being presented in this volume.

Penfield's proposal that there must be a *centrencephalic* system or systems of neurons with widespread reciprocal interconnections between the cortex of both hemispheres and the central core of diencephalon and brain stem subserving a specialized "highest level" integrative function in conscious experience, and in the regulation of states of consciousness, has received some strong support, but perhaps even stronger criticism. Much of this criticism has been misdirected to false concepts of the hypothesis itself, without offering satisfactory alternatives. This has been encouraged by the fact that the *centrencephalic system* has never been clearly identified in anatomical terms, except by exclusion of principal primary sensory and motor pathways. Insofar as the criticism has been constructive and well founded, it has served to sharpen our search with new and more precise techniques.

The multiplicity of mechanisms for spread and propagation of seizures throughout the brain and refinement of methods for study of only one at a time have led to overemphasis on some to the exclusion of all others. For example, Penfield and I have studied a number of patients with minor and major attacks initiated by sudden loss of consciousness, some resembling very much a form of petit mal *absence,* which were due to epileptogenic lesions involving the mesial surface of one frontal lobe. The EEG in these cases was characterized by bilaterally synchronous 2–2.5 per sec atypical spike-wave discharge with minor attacks resembling petit mal absence (Fig. 16-7). In major attacks this form of EEG was gradually changed to more rapid repetitive discharges, wthout the slow wave component, involving both frontal lobes simultaneously. There was no turning of the head as convulsive movements developed simultaneously on both sides of the body. Since there was no evidence for spread across the cortical surface and since experimental studies had shown that these areas of cortex have particularly prominent, strong corticofugal projections to mesial thalamus and midbrain, areas known to be involved in mechanisms of sleep and waking, as well as in bilateral control of cortical electric activity, it was proposed that sudden bilateral projection might be due to corticofugal activation of this system, designated the *centrencephalic system.*

Bancaud et al. [4] confirmed such findings with depth recording but have concluded that presence of an apparent cortical focus disproves participation of a subcortical projection system, and casts consider-

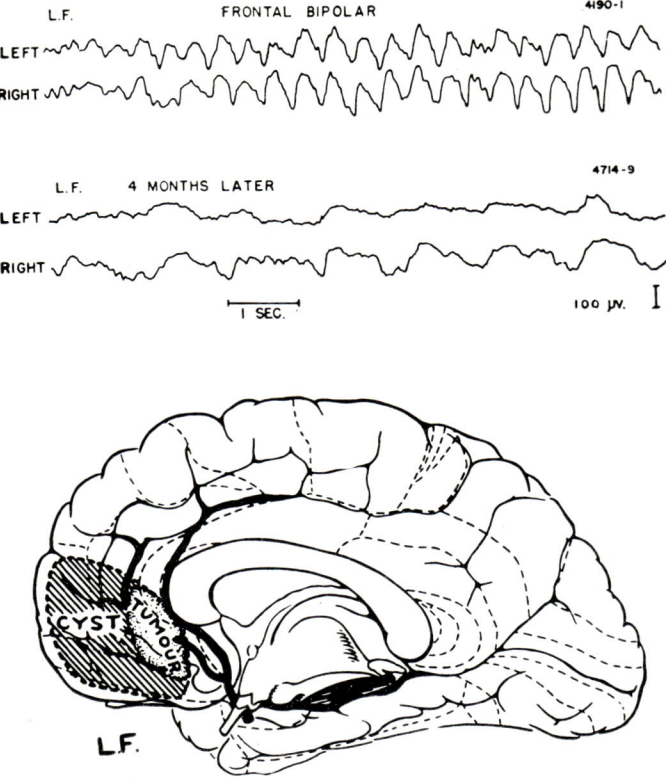

Fig. 16-7. Simulation of bilaterally synchronous rhythmic EEG abnormality at 2.5 per sec and clinical seizures resembling *petit mal absence* sometimes followed by generalized convulsions in patient with cystic tumor on inferior mesial frontal region of right hemisphere, as described by Penfield and Jasper [38].

able doubt on the whole concept of centrencephalic seizures, even in those cases without cortical lesions. Walker and Morello [58] reproduced a similar form of attack in monkeys by experimental epileptogenic lesions deep in the frontal lobe and called this a "model of petit mal epilepsy," with implication that all such seizures might be of similar nature. An equally convincing model of petit mal epilepsy has been reproduced in kittens by chronic epileptogenic lesions of the midbrain by Guerrero-Figueroa et al. [20], and by Hubel and Nauta [22] in the monkey. Reproduction of the cortical 3-per-second spike-wave pattern in the EEG by electrical stimulation of midbrain reticular formation and mesial thalamus has been confirmed, and interaction of the recruiting system of the intralaminar thalamus and mesencephalic reticular formation in the generation of cortical wave-spike complexes has been demonstrated [39, 43, 44, 45, 60, 61, 62].

However, Walker [57] has pointed out that these subcortical structures may not be primarily involved, or even necessary, for generalization of a convulsive seizure of cortical origin and proposes that loss of consciousness may result from involvement of a critical mass of brain tissue in the seizure discharge, rather than any specialized neuronal system, such as the centrencephalic system, which may be more especially related to regulation of states of consciousness. However, in the minimal petit mal seizure there is no evidence for massive involvement of the brain in true epileptic discharge, but rather a discrete arrest of conscious behavior, at times with preservation of automatic sensorimotor coordinations, and no period of depression following the brief attack, nor even following prolonged wave-spike discharge in the so-called *petit mal status*. There is now considerable evidence that inhibitory rather than excitatory mechanisms play a leading role in this form of seizure, as demonstrated experimentally by intracellular microelectrode studies of Pollen [42] and in a human patient with bilateral wave-spike EEG abnormalities by Perot [39] as illustrated in Fig. 16-8.

One of the greatest difficulties with the concept of the centrencephalic system is the question of its precise anatomical identity, and its functional relationship with major specific projection systems of the brain. There seems to be a persistent notion that it is a sort of seat of the soul, a separate localization of the mind, independent of more specialized sensory, motor, and associative systems of the brain. The fact that it gains its real significance by interaction with specific synaptic circuits throughout the neuraxis, cortical to spinal, has been thoroughly demonstrated by a variety of electrophysiological studies.

The clearest identification of anatomy and functional specificity of centrencephalic systems of neurons in diencephalon and brain stem capable of regulating or coordinating specific functions of both hemispheres has been provided by recent histochemical studies. The cholinergic system established by the splendid work of Shute and Lewis [31, 49] serves to demarcate very clearly the intralaminar system of the thalamus and a portion of the reticular system of the midbrain and their interconnections. Cholinergic connections with the limbic system, and with the striatum, were

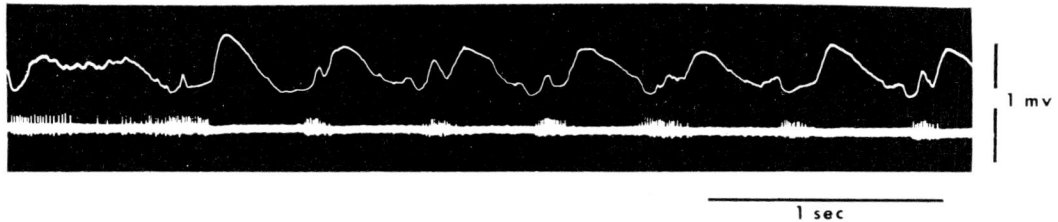

FIG. 16-8. Microelectrode recording of unit discharge together with surface cortical EEG in patient with bilaterally synchronous spike-wave EEG abnormality and generalized seizures (From Perot [39].) Note inhibition of unit discharge during slow-wave phase of the spike-wave complex.

also clearly demonstrated, corresponding to relationships previously demonstrated by anatomical and electrophysiological studies. Local electrical stimulation of this system increases the rate of liberation of ACh from cerebral cortex, and will induce epileptic discharge in an area of cortex pretreated with acetylcholinesterase [11]. The other two portions of the centrencephalic system appear to be noradrenergic and serotoninergic respectively, as described by Dahlström (Chap. 8), and appear to have antagonistic functional relationships in regulation of states of sleep and waking or arousal, according to the work of Jouvet [26].

The nature of the relationship between the cholinergic and noradrenergic activating systems has yet to be worked out, but there can be no doubt that these studies have considerable importance to our understanding of subcortical mechanisms, with functional properties different from those of the specific projection pathways, and which may play an important role in mechanisms of seizure propagation at least by means of their effect upon reactivity of many specific neuronal systems throughout the brain. Their reciprocal interrelations with cerebral cortex of both hemispheres has been clearly demonstrated as well as their special importance for regulation of sleep and wakefulness. Epileptiform discharges of cortical origin project strongly to these same areas so that they must be involved in the seizure process even though they may facilitate generalized convulsive attacks only by their activating influence upon other major, more specific neuronal systems of the brain, or they may have an inhibitory controlling action in some instances, contributing to the arrest of cortically induced seizures.

When considering a chemically distinct system or systems of neurons extending throughout the central core of the brain stem, into the intralaminar thalamus and hypothalamus with terminals diffusely projecting to the cerebral cortex, and with multiple *feedback* afferent fibers from widespread cortical areas, all of which have been clearly demonstrated by precise anatomical, histochemical, and electrophysiological studies, arguments based upon gross anatomical considerations of *cortical vs. subcortical* or *thalamic vs. cortical* lose their meaning. All of these systems are not necessarily equally involved in different forms of generalized attacks, as will be emphasized by Penfield in Chap. 29.

REFERENCES

1. Adrian, E. D. The spread of activity in the cerebral cortex. *J. Physiol.* (London) 88:127, 1936.
2. Aquino-Cías, J., and Bureš, J. The Effect of Thalamic Spreading Depression on the Epileptic Discharge in Rats. In Servit, Z. (Ed.), *Comparative and Cellular Pathophysiology of Epilepsy*. Amsterdam: Excerpta Medica, 1966.
3. Aquino-Cías, J., and Bureš, J. Seizure irradiation during functional elimination of the thalamus by spreading depression in the rat. *Epilepsia* (Amst.) 8:47, 1967.
4. Bancaud, J., Talairach, J., Bonis, A., Schaub, C., Szikla, G., Morel, P., Bordas-Ferer, M. *La stéréo-électroencéphalographic dans l'épilepsie*. Paris: Masson, 1965.
5. Bergmann, F., Costin, A., and Gutman, J. A low threshold convulsive area in the rabbit's mesencephalon. *Electroenceph. Clin. Neurophysiol.* 15:683, 1963.
6. Berlin, L. Increased synaptic excitability in the genesis of seizures. *Epilepsia* (Amst.) 7:1, 1966.
7. Bremer, F. Le tétanos strychnique et le mécanisme de la synchronisation neuronique. *Arch. Int. Physiol.* 51:211, 1941.
8. Burns, B. D. *The Mammalian Cerebral Cortex*. London: Edward Arnold, 1958.
9. Burns, B. D., and Grafstein, B. The function and structure of some neurones in the cat's cerebral cortex. *J. Physiol.* (London) 118:412, 1952.
10. Burns, B. D., Grafstein, B., and Olszewski, G. Identification of neurones giving burst response in isolated cerebral cortex. *J. Neurophysiol.* 20:200, 1957.
11. Celesia, G. G., and Jasper, H. H. Acetylcholine released from cerebral cortex in

relation to state of activation. *Neurology* (Minneap.) 16:1053, 1966.

12. Dow, R. S. Extrinsic regulatory mechanisms of seizure activity. *Epilepsia* (Amst.) 6:122, 1965.

13. Dow, R. S., Fernandez-Guardiola, A., and Manni, E. The influence of the cerebellum on experimental epilepsy. *Electroenceph. Clin. Neurophysiol.* 14:383, 1962.

14. Dusser de Barenne, J. G., and McCulloch, W. S. Functional interdependence of sensory cortex and thalamus. *J. Neurophysiol.* 4:304, 1941.

15. Eccles, J. C. Inhibition in thalamic and cortical neurones and its role in phasing neuronal discharges. *Epilepsia* (Amst.) 6:89, 1965.

16. Fields, W. S., King, R. B., and O'Leary, J. L. Study of multiplied cortical response to repetitive stimulation in thalamus. *J. Neurophysiol.* 12:117, 1949.

17. Gastaut, H., and Fischer-Williams, M. The physiopathology of epileptic seizures. In Field, J. (Ed.), *The Handbook of Physiology*, vol. 1. Baltimore: Williams and Wilkins, 1959.

18. Gloor, P., Sperti, L., and Vera, C. L. Electrophysiological studies of hippocampal neurons. II. Secondary postsynaptic events and single cell unit discharges. *Electroenceph. Clin. Neurophysiol.* 15:379, 1963.

19. Gloor, P., Vera, C. L., and Sperti, L. Electrophysiological studies of hippocampal neurons. I. Configuration and laminar analysis of the "resting" potential gradient, of the main-transient response to perforant path, fimbrial and mossy fiber volleys and of "spontaneous" activity. *Electroenceph. Clin. Neurophysiol.* 15:353, 1963.

20. Guerrero-Figueroa, R., Barros, A., Balbian Verster, F., and Heath, R. Experimental "petit mal" in kittens. *Arch. Neurol.* (Paris) 9:297, 1963.

21. Hayashi, T. A physiological study of epileptic seizures following cortical stimulation in animals and its application to human clinics. *Jap. J. Physiol.* 3:46, 1952.

22. Hubel, D., and Nauta, W. J. H. Electrocorticograms of cats with chronic lesions of rostral mesencephalic tegmentum. *Fed. Proc.* 19:287, 1960.

23. Hunter, J., and Jasper, H. H. Effects of thalamic stimulation in unanaesthetized animals. *Electroenceph. Clin. Neurophysiol.* 1:305, 1949.

24. Jasper, H. H., Ajmone-Marsan, C., and Stoll, J. Corticofugal projections to the brain stem. *A.M.A. Arch. Neurol. Psychiat.* 67:155, 1952.

25. Jasper, H. H., Hunter, J., and Knighton, R. Experimental studies of the thalamocortical systems. *Trans. Amer. Neurol. Ass.* (pp. 210–212), 1948.

26. Jouvet, M. Neurophysiology of the states of sleep. *Physiol. Rev.* 47:117, 1967.

27. Kanai, T., and Szerb, J. C. Mesencephalic reticular activating system and cortical acetylcholine output. *Nature* (London) 205:80, 1965.

28. Kreindler, A., Zuckermann, E., Steriade, M., and Chimion, D. Electroclinical features of convulsions induced by stimulation of the brain stem. *J. Neurophysiol.* 21:430, 1958.

29. Kristiansen, K., and Courtois, G. Rhythmic electrical activity from isolated cerebral cortex. *Electroenceph. Clin. Neurophysiol.* 1:265, 1949.

30. Leão, A. A. P. Spreading depression of activity in the cerebral cortex. *J. Neurophysiol.* 7:359, 1944.

31. Lewis, P. R., and Shute, C. C. D. The cholinergic limbic system: Projections to hippocampal formation, medial cortex, nuclei of the ascending cholinergic reticular system, and the subfornical organ and supra-optic crest. *Brain* 90:521, 1967.

32. Libet, B., and Gerard, R. W. Control of the potential rhythm of the isolated frog brain. *J. Neurophysiol.* 2:153, 1939.

33. Libet, B., and Gerard, R. W. Steady potential fields and neurone activity. *J. Neurophysiol.* 4:438, 1941.

34. MacIntosh, F. C., and Oborin, P. E. Release of acetylcholine from intact cerebral cortex. *Abs. XIX Int. Physiol. Congr.* 580-581, 1953.

35. Marshall, W. H. Spreading cortical depression of Leão. *Physiol. Rev.* 39:239, 1959.

36. Mountcastle, V. B. Modality and topographic properties of single neurons of cat's somatic sensory cortex. *J. Neurophysiol.* 20:408, 1957.

37. Ochs, S. The nature of spreading depression in neural networks. *Int. Rev. Neurobiol.* 4:1, 1962.

38. Penfield, W., and Jasper, H. H. *Epilepsy and the Functional Anatomy of the Human Brain.* Boston: Little, Brown, 1954.

39. Perot, P. Mesencephalic-Thalamic Relations in the Mechanisms of the Experimental Wave and Spike Complex in the Cat. Thesis, Montreal Neurological Institute and McGill University, Montreal, 1963.

40. Phillis, J. W., and Chong, G. C. Acetylcholine release from the cerebral and cerebellar cortices: Its role in cortical arousal. *Nature* (London) 207:1253, 1965.

41. Pinsky, C., and Burns, B. D. Production of epileptiform afterdischarges in cat's cerebral cortex. *J. Neurophysiol.* 25:359, 1962.

42. Pollen, D. A. Intracellular studies of cortical neurons during thalamic induced wave and spike. *Electroenceph. Clin. Neurophysiol.* 17:398, 1964.

43. Pollen, D. A., Perot, P., and Reid, K. H. Experimental bilateral wave and spike from thalamic stimulation in relation to level of arousal. *Electroenceph. Clin. Neurophysiol.* 15:1017, 1963.

44. Pollen, D. A., Reid, K., and Perot, P. Microelectrode studies of experimental 3/sec wave and spike in the cat. *Electroenceph. Clin. Neurophysiol.* 16:57, 1964.

45. Pollen, D. A., and Sie, P.-G. Analysis of thalamic induced wave and spike in cortical excitability. *Electroenceph. Clin. Neurophysiol.* 17:154, 1964.

46. Pollock, L. J., and Davis, L. Experimental Convulsions. In *Epilepsy and the Convulsive State,* Part I. Baltimore: Williams & Wilkins, 1931, pp. 158–175.

47. Prince, D. A., and Wilder, B. J. Control mechanisms in cortical epileptogenic foci. "Surround" inhibition. *Arch. Neurol.* (Chicago) 16:194, 1967.

48. Purpura, D. P., and Girado, M. Synaptic mechanisms involved in transcallosal activation of corticospinal neurons. *Arch. Ital. Biol.* 97:111, 1959.

49. Shute, C. C. D., and Lewis, P. R. The ascending cholinergic reticular system: Neocortical, olfactory, and subcortical projections. *Brain* 90:497, 1967.

50. Sie, P.-G., Jasper, H. H., and Wolfe, L. Rate of ACh release from cortical surface in "encephale" and "cerveau isolé" cat preparations in relation to arousal and epileptic activation of the ECoG. *Electroenceph. Clin. Neurophysiol.* 18:206, 1965.

51. Tasaki, I., Hagiwara, S., and Watanabe, A. Action potentials recorded from inside a Mauthner cell of the catfish. *Jap. J. Physiol.* 4:79, 1954.

52. Tasaki, I., Polley, E. D., and Orrego, F. Action potentials from individual elements in cat geniculate and striate cortex. *J. Neurophysiol.* 17:454, 1954.

53. Udvarhelyi, G. B., and Walker, A. E. Dissemination of acute focal seizures in the monkey. 1. From cortical foci. *Arch. Neurol.* (Chicago) 12:333, 1965.

54. Vanasupa, P., Goldring, S., and O'Leary, J. L. Seizure discharges effected by intravenously administered convulsant drugs, EEG and dc changes in cerebrum and cerebellum of the rabbit. *Electroenceph. Clin. Neurophysiol.* 11:93, 1958.

55. van Harreveld, A., and Stamm, J. S. Spreading cortical convulsions and depressions. *J. Neurophysiol.* 16:352, 1953.

56. Voinescu, I., Voiculescu, V., and Kreindler, A. Spreading of Discharges Generated by a Penicillin Focus in the Midbrain Reticular Formation. In Servit, Z. (Ed.), *Comparative and Cellular Pathophysiology of Epilepsy.* Amsterdam: Excerpta Medica, 1966, pp. 200–203.

57. Walker, A. E. The state of consciousness in focal motor convulsions. *Epilepsia* (Amst.) 1:592, 1959/60.

58. Walker, A. E., and Morello, G. Experimental Petit-Mal. *Proc. Amer. Neurol. Ass.,* 1967.

59. Walker, A. E., and Udvarhelyi, G. B. Dissemination of acute focal seizures in the monkey. II. From subcortical foci. *Arch. Neurol.* (Chicago) 12:357, 1965.

60. Weir, B. Spikes-wave from stimulation of reticular core. *Arch. Neurol.* (Chicago) 11:209, 1964.

61. Weir, B. The morphology of the spike-wave complex. *Electroenceph. Clin. Neurophysiol.* 19:284, 1965.

62. Weir, B., and Sie, P.-G. Extracellular unit activity in cat cortex during the spike-wave complex. *Epilepsia* (Amst.) 7:30, 1966.

63. Wilder, B. J., and Schmidt, R. P. Propagation of epileptic discharge from chronic neocortical foci in monkey. *Epilepsia* (Amst.) 6:297, 1965.

ADDENDUM: COMMISSURAL SECTION AND PROPAGATION OF SEIZURES

J. E. BOGEN*, R. W. SPERRY**, AND P. J. VOGEL*

The number and distribution of forebrain commissural fibers suggests a significant role in the spread of seizure activity. Furthermore, disease of the corpus callosum has occasionally ameliorated a preexisting seizure disorder. These considerations led Van Wagenen and Herren [11] to divide the corpus callosum to treat epilepsy. Most of their bisections were incomplete and only one, done seriatim, included the entire corpus callosum and anterior commissure; nevertheless, twelve patients had postoperative convulsions restricted to one side [1]. Since then, experiments by Frost et al. [5] and Poblete et al. [8] showed the importance of the anterior commissure for interhemispheric spread from temporal lobe foci. Meanwhile, split-brain studies showed an absence of disabling symptoms in ordinary behavior [9]; the occasional postsurgical seizures in monkeys were largely unilateral.

Importance of forebrain commissures for generation, maintenance, and transmission of epileptic seizures is further indicated in our recent experience with a group of patients having intractable epilepsy [2, 3]. Complete transection of corpus callosum and anterior commissure was done in a single operation. The hippocampal commissure, though not separately visualized, was presumed to have been divided along with the corpus callosum in all cases. The massa intermedia was also cut in three individuals. In a total of ten patients for whom seizure status can now be evaluated for a 2-year follow-up period or longer, only one has not shown improvement. Generalized convulsions that before surgery had been occurring with high and increasing frequency have been largely abolished for 7, 6, 5, 5, 4, 4, 3, 3, and 2 years in 9 cases. A few generalized convulsions have occurred when medication was reduced. Improvement is apparent in focal as well as generalized seizures, although most of the patients have continued to have at least an occasional brief focal episode. It thus appears that the combination of cerebral commissurotomy plus postoperative medication has limited propagation of seizure activity from a cortical focus.

Although we cannot review here all the experimental contributions, it can be said that they generally confirm participation of forebrain commissures in interhemispheric propagation of seizure activity, while at the same time demonstrating the importance of lower level pathways. It was suggested by Hoefer and Pool [6] and Straw and Mitchell [10] that interhemispheric spread following callosal section might be attributable to the anterior commissure. We also note that the latter authors as well as Marcus and Watson [7] used gallamine for immobilization whereas Erickson [4] used ether. Spread from a cortical focus via brain-stem circuits probably depends on the excitatory level of these circuits. All of our patients have been maintained on drugs following operation although in reduced amounts in most cases. The success of cerebral commissurotomy in largely eliminating generalized convulsions we tentatively interpret as being dependent upon concurrent suppression of subcerebral circuits by postoperative medication.

*Ross-Loos Medical Group, Los Angeles, California.
**California Institute of Technology, Pasadena, California.

REFERENCES

1. Akelaitis, A. J. A study of gnosis, praxis and language following section of the corpus callosum and anterior commissure. *J. Neurosurg.* 1:94, 1944.
2. Bogen, J. E., and Vogel, P. J. Treatment of generalized seizures by cerebral commissurotomy. *Surg. Forum* 14:431, 1963.
3. Bogen, J. E., Fisher, E. D., and Vogel, P. J. Cerebral commissurotomy: A second case report. *J.A.M.A.* 194:1328, 1965.
4. Erickson, T. C. Spread of the epileptic discharge. *Arch. Neurol. Psychiat.* 43:429, 1940.
5. Frost, L. L., Baldwin, M., and Wood, C. D. Investigation of the primate amygdala: Movements of the face and jaw. Afterdischarge and the anterior commissure. *Neurology* (Minneap.) 8:543, 1958.
6. Hoefer, P. F. A., and Pool, J. L. Conduction of cortical impulses and motor management of convulsive seizures. *Arch. Neurol. Psychiat.* 50:381, 1943.
7. Marcus, E. M., and Watson, C. W. Symmetrical epileptogenic foci in monkey cerebral cortex. *Arch. Neurol.* (Chicago) 19:99, 1968.
8. Poblete, R., Ruben, R. J., and Walker, A. E. Propagation of afterdischarge between temporal lobes. *J. Neurophysiol.* 22:538, 1959.
9. Sperry, R. W. Cerebral organization and behavior. *Science* 133:1749, 1961.
10. Straw, R. N., and Mitchell, C. L. Effect of section of the corpus callosum on cortical after-discharge patterns in the cat. *Proc. Soc. Exp. Biol. Med.* 125:128, 1967.
11. Van Wagenen, W. P., and Herren, R. Y. Surgical division of commissural pathways in the corpus callosum. *Arch. Neurol. Psychiat.* 44:740, 1940.

Discussion

MECHANISMS OF PROPAGATION: INTRACELLULAR STUDIES*

DOMINICK P. PURPURA

Neurons engaged in epileptic activity may exhibit various sequences of rhythmically recurring bursts of high frequency discharges and prolonged phases of membrane hyperpolarization. Such types of activity are also frequently observed in the normal operation of neurons under different experimental conditions. For even the so-called paroxysmal depolarizing shift of the epileptic neuron [16] has its counterpart in physiological responses that are not considered epileptogenic in nature. Examples of these include responses of pyramidal neurons to stimulation of specific thalamocortical projections [30] and responses of thalamic neurons to stimulation of nonspecific thalamic nuclei [28].

The epileptic process is not readily characterized in terms of the type of excitatory or inhibitory activities neurons display but the mode of generation and consequences of these activities. Several of the reports in this volume have been concerned with attempts to elucidate the possible cellular basis for production of these activities. The present discussion considers various mechanisms whereby abnormal excitatory activities in neurons influence other neurons locally and at a distance. The problem of local spread of paroxysmal activity is basically one of defining the extent to which ephaptic and synaptic mechanisms contribute to the progressive involvement of neurons in a particular synaptic organization during the seizure process. The problem of seizure propagation is multifaceted and requires consideration of preferential modes of transmission along projection pathways, specification of infiltration routes in and out of different neuronal organizations, and examination of the origin and nature of facilitatory and inhibitory influences on spread and propagation of seizure discharges [12].

ROLE OF EPHAPTIC MECHANISMS IN LOCAL SEIZURE SPREAD

Steep potential gradients and strong electrical fields generated by synchronously discharging neurons have long been viewed as important factors contributing to the local spread of paroxysmal discharges in different neuraxial sites as indicated in the report by Jasper. Distinctions are necessary between ephaptic effects produced by current flows in extracellular spaces and across contiguous neural membranes [3] and interactions mediated at specialized sites of membrane fusion, that is, electrotonic junctions between neural elements [4]. In the latter, prejunctional and postjunctional elements are essentially part of the same core conductor due to the low resistance of electrotonic or tight junctions. Consequently electrotonic transmission represents a variant of impulse conduction, although properties of the fused junctional membrane may introduce rectification and delay in the transmission process [4]. Morphologically distinct, tight junctions may not be an essential requirement for effective electrotonic transmission, since geometrical relations and properties of opposing electrically excitable membranes may be such as to restrict shunting effects of currents in the extracellular space [4, 5].

Although electrotonic junctions between neurons are extremely rare in the mam-

---

* Supported in part by PHS Research Grant NB07512 from National Institute of Neurological Diseases and Stroke and grant from United Cerebral Palsy Educational and Research Foundation.

malian brain, it has been suggested that a pathological condition involving a population of neurons might in some obscure fashion lead to development of membrane fusion between adjacent neurons with a resultant tendency to synchronized activity of electrotonically interconnected cells [10]. Alternatively, narrowing of extracellular spaces produced by inward Na^+, Cl^-, and water movement and extracellular K^+ accumulation during seizure activity [6] could augment the efficacy of ephaptic interactions between neurons with relatively large areas of membrane apposition [7]. Clearly, absence of electrotonic junctions does not preclude significant electrical interactions between central neural elements. Earlier studies on cat dorsal root interactions [11] and more recent investigations on excitability changes induced in cat spinal motoneurons by field effects of antidromic volleys [17] are relevant to this point. However, even in the latter studies electrotonic interactions across tight junctions, as proposed for frog spinal motoneurons [9], cannot be excluded as a possible basis for the observed effects.

The unusual spread of electrically included afterdischarges into, but not out of, an area of isolated neocortex has been cited as evidence for an extrasynaptic or ephaptic route of seizure spread [12]. A series of experiments carried out in our laboratory several years ago produced results which did not support the view that afterdischarges developing outside a slab of isolated neocortex could consistently invade the slab [19]. A more significant experiment to test for possible ephaptic influence of elements involved in focal epileptogenic discharges is illustrated in Fig. D16-1. In this experiment, focal discharges

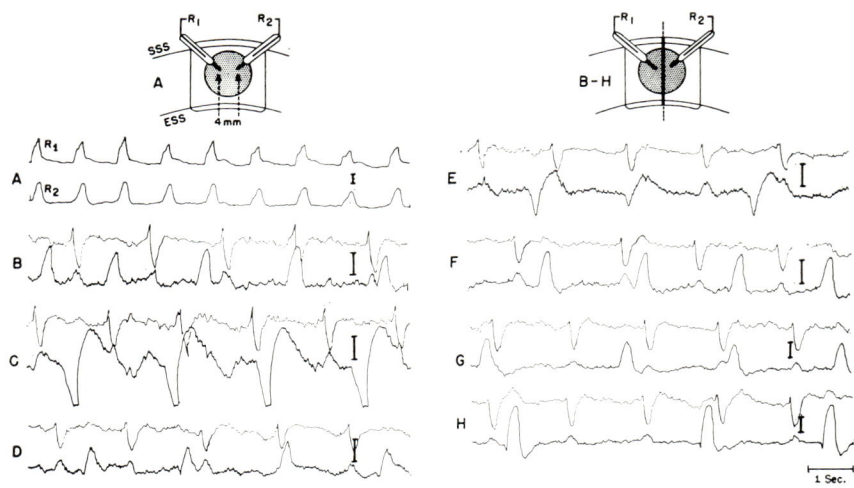

FIG. D16-1. Independence of focal paroxysmal discharges in an isolated and split epileptogenic lesion of cat neocortex. (A) Two recording electrodes (R_1 and R_2) are located in region of a freezing lesion of neocortex. Cortical area containing the lesion was isolated and undercut after development of low frequency paroxysmal activity, recorded synchronously by R_1 and R_2 as in records (A). (B) Several minutes after lesion site has been split and electrodes returned to their original position. Independent discharges are detected. (C) through (H) Examples of changes produced by various pharmacological agents on daughter-focus R_2 without significant effects on R_1 site. (C) Effects of topical GABA applied to R_2; marked augmentation and inversion of R_2-focal discharge is not reflected in recording across the cut at R_1. (D) Recovery of R_2-response after removal of GABA. (E) Effect of topical 2 percent KCl applied to R_2 site; note difference in effects of KCl and GABA. (F) Recovery following removal of KCl. (G) Topical procaine is relatively ineffective in altering activity at R_2. Data indicate that independent focal discharges in split, isolated epileptogenic lesions do not influence each other through ephaptic interactions. Amplitude calibrations 0.5 mV. (From Purpura [19].)

were produced in a freezing lesion of cortex which was subsequently completely isolated subpially and undercut. Careful mapping of the lesion site disclosed only one region that gave rise to the low frequency focal-spike discharge, typical of cortical freezing lesions. It is obvious from the fact that such discharges are essentially unaltered in frequency in the isolated slab that subcortical and intracortical influences do not contribute to the *basic rhythm* of the discharge [23]. Nevertheless a variety of pathways can be shown to modulate this frequency [32].

At a stage when the basic rhythm of the epileptogenic discharges is well established, splitting the lesion site will usually result in production of two independent foci which can be detected by recording electrodes a few millimeters apart, one on each side of the subpial incision [19]. Furthermore, it is possible to produce a variety of changes in one of the resulting *daughter-foci* without altering the electrographic characteristics of the other. It is thus clear from these studies that the field effects of synchronously discharging neurons in one daughter-focus of a freezing lesion of neocortex do not significantly influence adjacent neurons in another part of the lesion when neuronal connections within the focal site have been severed. Evidently a population of elements in the lesion site exerts considerable inhibitory control over less active elements in the lesion. Splitting the lesion effectively allows nondominant elements to express themselves in the form of a daughter-focus of epileptiform activity.

Studies more to the point of the effects of cortical steady potential gradients on neuronal excitability have attempted to replicate experimental designs that have revealed rather dramatic effects of extracellular potential fields on isolated neurons [33]. In our investigations, intracellular recording from neocortical [26] and hippocampal pyramidal neurons [24] was utilized to determine the effects of transcortical- and transhippocampal-applied steady currents. In the case of neocortical pyramidal neurons, it has been found that strong surface anodal or cathodal polarizing currents (100–400 μamp per mm^2) are required to produce significant alterations in transmembrane potentials of pyramidal neurons (Fig. D16-2). This is not true for changes in surface-evoked potentials which may be altered in polarity by relatively low-level applied currents (20–80 μamp per mm^2).

In the neocortical studies from which the data shown in Fig. D16-2 were taken it was rare that such polarizing currents initiated seizure activity. On the other hand, such currents could induce prolonged changes in dendritic excitability as indicated by the development of fast prepotentials in cells which did not exhibit these partial responses prior to cortical polarization [26]. Additionally polarizing currents produced persisting change in patterns of synaptic activation of nonpyramidal tract neurons (interneurons) at current levels which did not influence soma transmembrane potentials of pyramidal tract neurons.

Ephaptic Mechanisms in Hippocampus. The hippocampus has long been considered a favorable structure for studying the possible role of ephaptic mechanisms in the local spread of seizures. Two lines of inquiry have provided data consistent with the view that at some stage in the development of hippocampal paroxysmal activity, synchronized discharges of hippocampal neurons generate extracellular currents that may activate large populations of neuronal elements. Earlier studies of extracellular activities of hippocampal neurons during seizures disclosed large amplitude (10 mV) negative potentials (*pips*) maximal just below the stratum pyramidale [8]. These have been confirmed in extracellular and intracellular studies of hippocampal neurons during seizures initiated by subiculum stimulation [27]. Such large field potentials (10–20 mV) developing during postactivation facilitation phases are detectable intracellularly, though somewhat attenuated and altered in time course.

A point of major importance is that intracellular spikes are generally associated with these field potentials. When the latter undergo attenuation, spikes may be observed which arise directly from the baseline without depolarizing prepotentials (Fig. D16-3). Similar types of responses can be readily initiated by application of transhippocampal polarizing currents that estab-

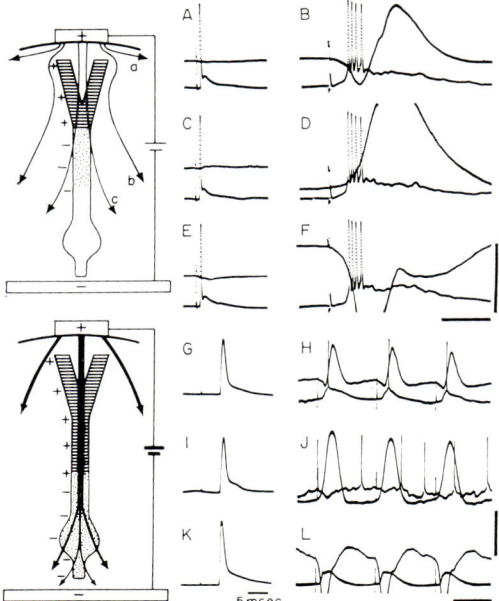

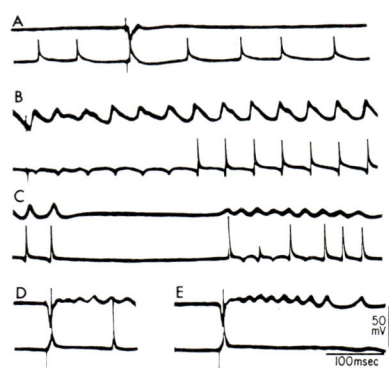

Fig. D16-2. (A) through (F) Dissociation of effects of weak surface polarizing currents (50 μamp per mm²) on evoked cortical responses and intracellular activities of a pyramidal tract neuron. Upper channel records are surface responses to stimulation of ventrolateral thalamus. (A) Antidromic spike with prominent delayed depolarization; (B) pattern of synaptic drive during stabilization phase of augmenting response; (C) and (D) during weak surface anodal polarization; (E) and (F) during surface cathodal polarization. Patterns of intracellularly recorded activities are uninfluenced during dramatic changes in surface-evoked responses. Calibrations 50 mV, 20 msec. Diagram, upper left, shows probable distribution of currents during weak anodal polarization: (a) fraction of current flowing along surface; (b) extraneuronal current flow; (c) proportion of current inward at terminals of apical dendrite, outward across proximal dendritic regions. No effect of this current is observed at the soma level with weak intensities as indicated in (D). (G) through (L) Effects of strong cortical surface polarization on a pyramidal tract neuron. (G), (I), (K) Antidromic responses; (H), (J), (L) activities evoked by repetitive ventrolateral thalamic stimulation; (G) and (H) controls; (I) and (J) during strong surface anodal polarization (150 μamp per mm²); (K) and (L) during strong surface cathodal polarization. Note changes in delayed depolarizing potential and amplitude of antidromic spikes. Anodal polarization produces depolarization of soma regions and increase in cell discharge. Cathodal polar-

Fig. D16-3. Initiation of intracellular spikes without depolarizing prepotentials in a hippocampal pyramidal neuron during postactivation facilitation state induced by prior repetitive, subiculum stimulation. (A) through (E) Examples of spontaneous and subiculum-evoked responses. Upper channel records, responses recorded from hippocampal surface, CA2–CA3 region. Note intermittent 2-per-sec negative waves in different records. (A) Subiculum stimulus evokes a short latency EPSP, spike potential and repetitive sequence of spikes initiated by negative potentials. The latter represents field activity of synchronously discharging hippocampal neurons. Failure of spike invasion from dendrites to soma occurs with second response of spontaneous repetitive train. (B) through (D) Examples of different interactions of spontaneous and evoked responses. Each surface negative wave is associated with a negative extracellular potential at level of soma-dendritic region that is detectable intracellularly. (E) Burst of repetitive spikes initiated by discharge lacking prepotential. (F) Subsidence of postactivation facilitation period. Subiculum stimulation elicits an EPSP and spike potential of larger amplitude than during phase of maximum facilitation; spontaneous spike follows, which arises from an attenuated prenegativity. Differences in firing levels of evoked and spontaneous spikes indicate that the latter have propagated from remote sites in dendrites subjected to intense axodendritic synaptic activation during phase of repetitive subiculum stimulation.

ization of surface hyperpolarizes soma and prevents EPSPs from attaining firing level. Diagram lower left: probable distribution of strong anodal currents. Increase in inward current through apical dendritic terminals of pyramidal neuron is associated with outward depolarizing currents through soma-initial axonal segment region. Calibrations at right: 50 mV; 100 msec. (From Purpura and McMurtry [26].)

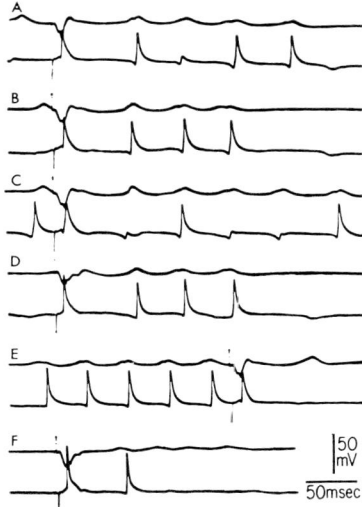

FIG. D16-4. Development of hippocampal neuron synchronization and associated negative field spikes recorded intracellularly during transhippocampal polarization. Upper channel records from surface of hippocampus. (A) Spontaneous activity and subiculum-evoked response prior to polarization. (B) Late phase of transhippocampal polarization, cathode on ventricular surface of hippocampus. Seizure induction is associated with brief negative potentials. Spikes superimposed on these as shown in latter part of record. (C) Variations in spikes without depolarizing prepotentials. Note first spike of train at right arises directly from the baseline. Spikes of different amplitude reflect variations in degree of dendrite-soma invasion. (D) Early stage of recovery after induced seizure activity. Spike amplitude markedly increased during membrane hyperpolarization accompanying recovery process; spontaneous spike after subiculum-evoked discharge arises from fast prepotential. (E) Later stage of recovery. Repetitive responses observed at hippocampal surface are not associated with discharges of impaled neuron. (From Purpura and Malliani, unpublished.)

lish potential gradients of 20–30 mV per mm as in Figs. D16-4 and D16-5 [24]. It is interesting to recall here that this is the same order of magnitude of extracellular potential gradient required to fire silent, isolated stretch receptors in the experiments of Terzuolo and Bullock [33]. Suffice it to say that marked differences in the effectiveness of transcortical polarizing currents have been found in studies of neocortex and hippocampus. And while it

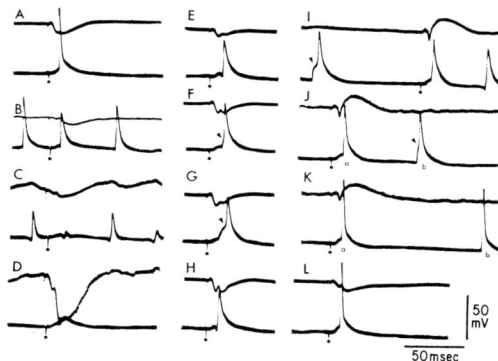

FIG. D16-5. Examples of changes in spike potentials of a hippocampal pyramidal neuron following transhippocampal polarization. (A) Control subiculum-evoked response initiated by an EPSP. (B), (C), and (D) During cathodal polarization of hippocampal-ventricular surface. (E) through (H) Stages of recovery following cathodal polarization. Arrow heads indicate inflections on rising phase of spike and reflect discontinuities produced by variable invasion of spikes from dendrites. Discontinuities clearly shown in (I) and (J), during surface anodal polarization which increases soma-membrane potential of hippocampal pyramidal cell. Note differences in firing level of subiculum-evoked response (a) and spontaneous discharge (b) in (K) and (L). In (K) spontaneous spike (b) arises directly from the baseline without a depolarizing prepotential. (L) Recovery. Residual membrane hyperpolarization is evident in increased spike amplitude. Data illustrate ease with which spike generation and propagation occur in dendrites of hippocampal pyramidal neurons during application of transhippocampal polarizing currents. (From Purpura and Malliani, unpublished.)

seems unlikely that field effects contribute significantly to the spread of convulsant activity in neocortical neuronal networks, this is not the case for hippocampal neurons. A considerable portion of the dendritic tree of hippocampal neurons can participate in the process of spike generation and potent excitatory synaptic actions may be initiated in dendritic elements [27]. Thus discharges initiated in dendrites by synaptic activities may ephaptically influence contiguous elements in such a fashion as to give rise to explosive involvement of hippocampal pyramidal neurons in seizure activity. It must not be inferred from this that ephaptic mechanisms are predominant in the *initiation* of seizure activity in the hippocampus. For even during the maximum phase of synchronized activity of hippocampal neurons, it is likely that synaptic events control the basic rhythmicity of neuron discharges [27].

SYNAPTIC INFLUENCES ON FOCAL EPILEPTOGENIC DISCHARGES OF NEOCORTEX

Focal discharges developing in acute freezing lesions of neocortex have been shown to be influenced in many different ways by stimulation of a variety of projection pathways to the lesion site [32]. Extensive studies of these effects clearly indicate that overt alterations in discharge characteristics of focal epileptogenic lesions are related to the manner in which different projection pathways engage neuronal organizations involved in the focal discharge and the degree to which these projections synaptically activate excitatory and inhibitory elements within the focus.

Different effects produced by activation of different modes of synaptic input to elements involved in focal epileptogenic discharges are appropriately illustrated in contrasting influences exerted by specific and nonspecific thalamocortical projections. In the case of focal lesions initiated in postcruciate cortex, stimulation of specific thalamocortical projections regularly alters discharge frequency. Low frequency stimulation may abruptly reset the rhythm of spontaneous discharges so that driving of the latter becomes apparent with the first or after several stimuli. On the other hand, high frequency specific thalamic stimulation often suppresses focal discharges. Paroxysmal discharges developing in an epileptogenic lesion may be modified in several ways even in preparations exhibiting sustained convulsant activity [32].

In contrast to the potent effects of specific thalamocortical projection activity on focal epileptogenic lesions, low frequency stimulation of nonspecific thalamic nuclei, which gives rise to typical long-latency recruiting responses, generally does not affect discharge characteristics of epileptogenic lesions [32]. This is true irrespective of the site of cortical location of the lesion. On the other hand, discharging lesions of cortex produce dramatic changes in the *waxing* and *waning* cycles of recruiting responses evoked by prolonged, low frequency stimulation of medial and intralaminar thalamic nuclei.

Since the demonstration of these contrasting effects of specific and nonspecific thalamocortical activation on focal epileptogenic lesions, a number of intracellular studies have been carried out which have provided a firm basis for interpretation of the effects. Thus, it is now established that specific thalamocortical projections exert powerful excitatory synaptic drives on cortical pyramidal neurons, whereas stimulation of nonspecific thalamocortical projections elicits relatively weak synaptic effects on cortical neurons (Fig. D16-6) [30]. It has also been shown that these different syn-

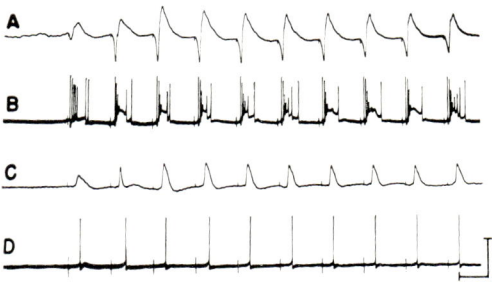

Fig. D16-6. Comparison of intracellular synaptic activities evoked in a pyramidal tract neuron by low frequency (7 per sec) repetitive stimulation in n. ventralis lateralis (VL) and medial thalamic nuclear complex. (*A*) Cortical surface augmenting response to VL stimulation (negativity upward). (*B*) Intracellular activities associated with augmenting sequence. (*C*) and (*D*) Cortical surface negative recruiting response and related intracellular activities, respectively. Buildup of augmenting sequence reflected in marked enhancement of EPSPs, repetitive firing, and "inactivation responses." In contrast, long-latency single discharges superimposed on low amplitude short-duration EPSPs are observed during recruitment. Examples shown indicate fundamentally different synaptic effects initiated in pyramidal neurons by specific and nonspecific thalamocortical projection pathways. Calibrations: 50 mV and 0.1 sec. (From Purpura, Shofer, and Musgrave [30].)

aptic effects are referable to differences in the nature of the intracortical interneuronal organization activated by specific and nonspecific projections, as well as differences in the mode of synaptic engagement of cortical neurons by these projections [29, 30].

EPSPs evoked in pyramidal neurons during specific thalamic stimulation presumably result from activation of excitatory synapses distributed on the soma as well as dendrites. In contrast, EPSPs associated with recruiting responses appear to be preferentially but not exclusively distributed on dendrites [20]. In view of the findings that both pyramidal neurons and interneurons of cortex exhibit many different patterns of PSPs during specific as opposed to nonspecific thalamocortical activation, it is not surprising that such differences will be reflected in the overt effects which these pathways exert on neurons involved in focal epileptogenic lesions of cortex [15, 32].

Synaptic influences on focal epileptogenic lesions have also been examined in respect to local cortical surface, transcallosal, and brain stem reticular-formation stimulation [32]. In each case complex interactions have invariably been observed. Such effects are dependent upon characteristics of focal discharge and parameters of stimulation of the pathway and organization activated. It is evident from such findings that while there may be intrinsic, pacemaker or pacemaker-like processes that determine basic discharge characteristics of neurons in focal epileptogenic lesions [23], such neurons may be markedly influenced by a variety of synaptic organizations. At some stage a "critical mass" of synchronously discharging neurons is activated and spread of seizure is facilitated with propagation along synaptic routes. EEG studies of propagation of afterdischarges within cortex and into subcortical structures have been particularly valuable in defining preferential invasion pathways as well as in characterizing the potentiality for seizure involvement in these structures [34]. Little is known, however, concerning factors which influence seizure propagation to different structures or the basis for varying participation of different subcortical organizations in the epileptic process. Projection via well-established anatomical pathways is only one such factor since activation of a synaptically related organization could conceivably result in sufficient involvement of inhibitory elements to suppress concomitant activity in that structure.

Involvement of neural systems with widespread and diverse synaptic influences on many structures seems likely to be a major factor in propagation and generalization of seizure, albeit the time course and intensity of the induced seizure in a particular structure will be functions of the intrinsic synaptic organization and properties of neurons in that structure. Although factors underlying preferential propagation and differential seizure susceptibility of different subcortical structures have not been examined in detail, a number of intracellular studies of subcortical organizations have been carried out in recent years which are immediately relevant to this problem.

Subcortical Pacemaker Systems. Central to the issue of the role of subcortical structures in the initiation and propagation of generalized seizure activity has been the problem of defining the nature and possible neural substrate of subcortical *pacemaker* systems. The pioneering studies of Jasper and his associates sought such pacemaker systems in the neuronal organizations of the thalamic reticular system (TRS) whose characteristics had been examined in another context by Morison and Dempsey (cf. [18]). Intracellular studies of thalamic neurons during stimulation of medial and intralaminar nuclei of the thalamus [22] have provided a firm basis for Jasper's hypothesis concerning the importance of TRS in synchronizing activity of neurons in widespread parts of the rostral thalamus. It has been shown that such synchronization is effected by complex internuclear interneuronal pathways, which generate powerful temporal sequences of EPSPs and IPSPs in thalamic neurons, some of which have direct projections to cortex (Fig. D16-7). Essentially similar PSP sequences have been studied in specific relay nuclei of the ventrobasal complex [2] following orthodromic and antidromic activation of thalamocortical relay cells. Results obtained in the lat-

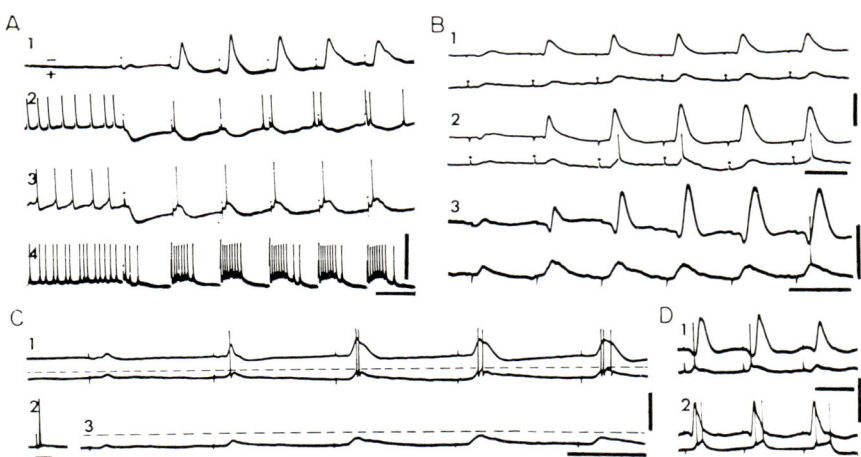

Fig. D16-7. Patterns of evoked synaptic activities observed in intracellular recordings from neurons in different structures during thalamocortical synchronization induced by low frequency (7–10 per sec) stimulation of medial nonspecific thalamic nuclei. Calibrations throughout, 50 mV for intracellular records; 100 msec. (*A*1) Example of surface negative cortical recruiting response. (2–4) EPSP-IPSP sequences recorded in thalamic neurons in different nuclei during recruiting responses. IPSPs prominent in thalamic elements during this type of activity play a major role in synchronizing thalamic neuronal discharges. (From Purpura and Shofer [28].) (*B*) Upper channel records, recruiting responses from motor cortex; lower channel records, intracellular activities of caudate neurons. (1) Threshold stimulation elicits prominent EPSPs in caudate neurons. (2) Increase in stimulus strength produces cell discharges. (3) Cell discharges are rare in caudate neurons despite large amplitude EPSPs during recruiting responses. IPSPs are not common in contrast to findings in thalamic neurons. (From Purpura and Malliani [25].) (*C*) Characteristics of EPSPs elicited in a pyramidal neuron of motor cortex during recruiting response. (1) EPSP builds up with repetitive stimulation. (2) Antidromically evoked response (calibration, 10 msec). (3) Slow increase in membrane potential reduces effectiveness of EPSPs. Dashed line through *firing level* as indicated in (1). (*D*) PSP patterns and associated cell discharges in two cortical interneurons. These elements generally exhibit a larger number of spike discharges than large pyramidal cells during recruiting responses. (From Purpura, Shofer, and Musgrave [30].)

ter studies have been extended to include an analysis of organization of intrinsic mechanisms involved in local synchronizing activities in different thalamic nuclei and within different parts of the same nucleus [1].

The data obtained in these studies have been interpreted as evidence for many different pacemakers for local cortical-synchronizing activities. These may be temporally and spatially quite distinct in operation, especially under experimental conditions, in which isolation or separation of intrathalamic pathways is achieved. It need hardly be pointed out that the concept of a thalamic pacemaker system was never meant to negate the operation of local semi-independent mechanisms for restricted synchronization of neuronal discharge. In fact, such is implied in the well-known repetitive sensory response which is usually confined to specific thalamic nuclei and their cortical projections. What is to be understood from the thalamic pacemaker concept is the notion that there exists within the nonspecific thalamus a complex neuronal system which distributes to other thalamic nuclei. Low frequency stimulation in this system activates EPSP-IPSP sequences whose specific characteristics are determined by the intrinsic organization of excitatory and inhibitory elements in different thalamic nuclei as well as other structures synaptically related to the nonspecific thalamic projection system (Fig. D16-7). So effective is the action of nonspecific nuclei on other thalamic nuclei in the intact thalamus of the locally unanesthetized encéphale isolé preparation that it is rare indeed to find neurons which do not exhibit EPSP-IPSP sequences time locked to the nonspecific thalamic stimuli.

Demonstration of nonspecific-specific internuclear interactions in the thalamus has considerable relevancy to mechanisms whereby strong activation of nonspecific nuclei may produce generalized involvement of the thalamus in a seizure process. However, it should not be inferred from this that such interactions are exclusively unidirectional. On the contrary, recent intracellular studies have provided information indicating that similar interactions may occur in the "reverse" directions, for example, specific-to-nonspecific. It is also clear that the latter interactions may develop with a shorter latency and be associated with more powerful inhibitory and excitatory effects than have heretofore been suspected (Fig. D16-8). Thus it is conceivable that involvement of a specific nucleus, such as VL, in a seizure initiated in the specific cortico-VL-cortical projection pathway may exert profound effects on nonspecific thalamic nuclei, thereby functionally inactivating integrative operations of the "thalamic reticular system."

Thalamic Activity. Effects of thalamic reticular activation are not confined to thalamocortical projection systems but are equally impressive in synaptic organizations of the corpus striatum [25] and mesencephalic reticular system [13, 21]. In these structures, evoked synaptic events exhibit some characteristics which are dependent upon the relative proportion of excitatory and inhibitory elements activated by nonspecific thalamic stimulation and intrinsic properties of neurons in different structures. EPSPs are generally well developed in caudate neurons but these seldom evoke repetitive discharges (Fig. D16-7). A unique feature of caudate-evoked activity is the rarity of IPSPs observed in responses to nonspecific thalamic stimulation. In contrast to this, neurons of the putamen exhibit relatively strong synaptic drives whereas pallidal neurons show both ex-

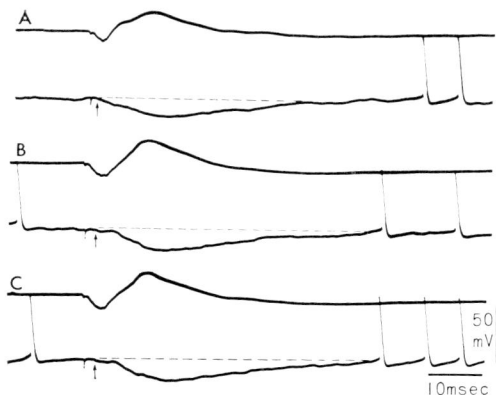

Fig. D16-8. Inhibitory effects of low frequency (7 per sec) repetitive stimulation of n. ventralis lateralis (VL) on a neuron in medial thalamus, region of n. centralis medialis. Upper channel records, primary and augmenting sequence, recorded from motor cortex. (*A*) First stimulus of repetitive train in VL elicits a 1.5–2.0 msec latency IPSP. (*B*) and (*C*) Second and third stimuli in VL, respectively. Note slight latency shift of initial IPSP and some depression of short latency IPSP. A longer latency and more prominent IPSP is initiated in the medial thalamic nucleus during augmenting response. Data illustrate powerful inhibitory effects exerted on medial nonspecific thalamic neurons during stimulation of VL and VL–VA specific thalamocortical projections. (From Purpura, Desiraju, and Broggi, unpublished.)

citatory and inhibitory PSPs following nonspecific thalamus stimulation [14]. Intracellular data obtained in recent investigations of caudate-amygdaloid and thalamoamygdaloid evoked activities have also indicated potent effects of convergent caudate and nonspecific thalamic projections on elements in the amygdaloid nuclear complex [31].

Intracellular data summarized above and reviewed in detail elsewhere [21] provide evidence for the operation of a potent system of complexly organized projections from medial and intralaminar nuclei to other thalamic nuclei, neocortex, corpus striatum, mesencephalic reticular formation and amygdaloid nucleus. These studies indicate that Jasper's thalamic reticular system does indeed exhibit properties required for a system capable of distributing synaptic input to a variety of different telencephalic and diencephalic structures. It does not follow from this that overt effects observed in different structures will be similar since these will be determined by differences in the intrinsic synaptic organization of each target site as well as additional interactions between such sites.

Several of the properties of synaptic organizations in subcortical structures may serve to explain a number of findings on the mode of propagation of seizures in these structures and their variable potentiality for seizure. Thus relatively strong electrical stimulation is required to induce minimal and brief afterdischarge in the thalamus and for this reason it has been suggested that the thalamus would be unlikely to originate epileptic discharge [34]. This observation may not be surprising when it is recalled that electrical stimulation of the thalamus activates inhibitory as well as excitatory pathways in both specific and nonspecific nuclei [21]. However, since activity initiated in the thalamus is likely to produce stronger excitatory drives in putamen than caudate, there will be a greater tendency for the former rather than the latter component of the corpus striatum to exhibit afterdischarge in response to thalamic stimulation [34].

It is beyond the scope of this discussion to review available data on spread and propagation of seizures in the mammalian brain in terms of properties of projection pathways and probable types of synaptic events which are generated in different structures. It is sufficient to indicate that critical factors in predisposing a particular region to seizure involvement are to be found in differences in degree of local excitatory and inhibitory interactions and capacity of intrinsic elements to exhibit high frequency repetitive discharges in response to repetitive excitatory inputs. These properties have been defined for neocortical and hippocampal pyramidal cells and are also now known for neurons in different thalamic nuclei, the corpus striatum, amygdaloid nuclear complex, and mesencephalic reticular system. It need hardly be pointed out that intracellular data at hand concerning normal operation of these synaptic organizations will serve as a useful basis for future intracellular studies of seizure propagation in the mammalian brain.

REFERENCES

1. Andersen, P., and Andersson, S. A. *Physiological Basis of the Alpha Rhythm.* New York: Appleton-Century-Crofts, 1968, p. 235.
2. Andersen, P., Eccles, J. C., and Sears, T. A. The ventro-basal complex of the thalamus: Types of cells, their responses and their functional organization. *J. Physiol.* (London) 174:370, 1964.
3. Arvanitaki, A. Effects in an axon by the activity of a contiguous one. *J. Neurophysiol.* 5:89, 1942.
4. Bennett, M. V. L. Physiology of electrotonic junctions. *Ann. N.Y. Acad. Sci.* 137:509, 1966.
5. Bennett, M. V. L., Pappas, G. D., Giménez, M., and Nakajima, Y. Physiology and ultrastructure of electrotonic junctions. IV. Medullary electromotor nuclei in gymnotid fish. *J. Neurophysiol.* 30:236, 1967.
6. Fertziger, A. P., and Ranck, J. R., Jr. Increase in brain interstitial potassium during three types of epileptiform activity as measured by K^{42} efflux. *Fed. Proc.* 27: 388, 1968.
7. Green, J. D., and Maxwell, D. S. Hippocampal electrical activity. I. Morphological aspects. *Electroenceph. Clin. Neurophysiol.* 13:837, 1961.
8. Green, J. D., and Petsche, H. Hippocampal electrical activity. IV. Abnormal electrical activity. *Electroenceph. Clin. Neurophysiol.* 13:868, 1961.
9. Grinnell, A. D. A study of the interaction between motoneurones in the frog spinal cord. *J. Physiol.* (London) 182:612, 1966.
10. Grundfest, H. Some Determinants of Repetitive Electrogenesis and Their Role in the Electrical Activity of the Central Nervous System. In Servit, Z. (Ed.), *Proc. Int. Sympos. Comparative and Cellular Pathophysiology of Epilepsy.* Prague:

Czech. Academy of Sciences, 1966, pp. 19–46.

11. Grundfest, H., and Magnes, J. Excitability changes in dorsal roots produced by electrotonic effects from adjacent afferent activity. *Amer. J. Physiol.* 164:502, 1951.

12. Kreindler, A. *Experimental Epilepsy. Progress in Brain Research*, vol. 19. Amsterdam: Elsevier, 1965, p. 213.

13. Maekawa, K., and Purpura, D. P. Excitatory processes and spike potential variations in reticular neurons. *Fed. Proc.* 26:434, 1967.

14. Malliani, A., and Purpura, D. P. Intracellular studies of the corpus striatum. II. Patterns of synaptic activities in lenticular and entopeduncular neurons. *Brain Res.* 6:325, 1967.

15. Matsumoto, H. Intracellular events during the activation of cortical epileptiform discharges. *Electroenceph. Clin. Neurophysiol.* 17:294, 1964.

16. Matsumoto, H., and Ajmone-Marsan, C. Cortical cellular phenomena in experimental epilepsy. *Exp. Neurol.* 9:286, 1964.

17. Nelson, P. G. Interaction between spinal motoneurons in the cat. *J. Neurophysiol.* 29:275, 1966.

18. Purpura, D. P. An historical study of neurophysiologic concepts in epilepsy. *Epilepsia* (Amst.) 2:115, 1953, III Series.

19. Purpura, D. P. Review and Critique. In Brazier, M. A. B. (Ed.), *Brain Function: Cortical Excitability and Steady Potentials; Relations of Basic Research to Space Biology*. Los Angeles: U.C.L.A. Forum in Medical Sciences, 1963, pp. 281–320.

20. Purpura, D. P. Comparative Physiology of Dendrites. In Quarton, G. C., Melnechuk, T., and Schmitt, F. O., (Eds.), *The Neurosciences: A Study Program*. New York: Rockefeller Univ. Press, 1967, pp. 372–393.

21. Purpura, D. P. Interneuronal Mechanisms in Synchronization and Desynchronization of Thalamic Activity. In Brazier, M. A. B. (Ed.), *The Interneuron*. Los Angeles: U.C.L.A. Forum in Medical Sciences, 1969, in press.

22. Purpura, D. P., and Cohen, B. Intracellular recording from thalamic neurons during recruiting responses. *J. Neurophysiol.* 25:621, 1962.

23. Purpura, D. P., Goldensohn, E. S., and Musgrave, F. S. Synaptic and non-synaptic processes in focal epileptogenic activity. *Electroenceph. Clin. Neurophysiol.* 15:1051, 1963.

24. Purpura, D. P., and Malliani, A. Spike generation and propagation initiated in dendrites by transhippocampal polarization. *Brain Res.* 1:403, 1966.

25. Purpura, D. P., and Malliani, A. Intracellular studies of the corpus striatum. I. Synaptic potentials and discharge characteristics of caudate neurons activated by thalamic stimulation. *Brain Res.* 6:325, 1967.

26. Purpura, D. P., and McMurtry, J. G. Intracellular activities and evoked potential changes during polarization of motor cortex. *J. Neurophysiol.* 28:166, 1965.

27. Purpura, D. P., McMurtry, J. G., Leonard, C. F., and Malliani, A. Evidence for dendritic origin of spikes without depolarizing prepotentials in hippocampal neurons during and after seizure. *J. Neurophysiol.* 29:954, 1966.

28. Purpura, D. P., and Shofer, R. J. Intracellular recording from thalamic neurons during reticulocortical activation. *J. Neurophysiol.* 26:494, 1963.

29. Purpura, D. P., and Shofer, R. J. Cortical intracellular potentials during augmenting and recruiting responses. I. Effects of injected hyperpolarizing currents on evoked membrane potential changes. *J. Neurophysiol.* 27:117, 1964.

30. Purpura, D. P., Shofer, R. J., and Musgrave, F. S. Cortical intracellular potentials during augmenting and recruiting responses. II. Patterns of synaptic activities in pyramidal and nonpyramidal tract neurons. *J. Neurophysiol.* 27:133, 1964.

31. Santini, M., and Purpura, D. P. Intracellular studies of amygdaloid neurons: Synaptic events initiated by caudate and thalamic stimulation. *Electroenceph. Clin. Neurophysiol.* 1969, in press.

32. Smith, T. G., Jr., and Purpura, D. P. Electrophysiological studies on epileptogenic lesions of cat cortex. *Electroenceph. Clin. Neurophysiol.* 12:59, 1960.

33. Terzuolo, C. A., and Bullock, T. H. Measurement of imposed voltage gradient adequate to modulate neuronal firing. *Proc. Nat. Acad. Sci. USA* 42:687, 1956.

34. Walker, A. E., and Udvarhelyi, G. B. Dissemination of acute focal seizures in the monkey. II. From subcortical foci. *Arch. Neurol.* (Chicago) 12:357, 1965.

17
Sleep Mechanisms*

OTTAVIO POMPEIANO

INTRODUCTION of the standard EEG technique to the study of epileptic patients [60] indicates that at least in some instances physiological sleep is a very efficient means of activating epileptic disturbances. This conclusion was reached at the time when our knowledge of sleep was rather phenomenologic and restricted to that phase of sleep characterized by large-amplitude slow, cortical waves, which in man has been divided into several stages [38]; in animal experiments it is commonly referred to as *synchronized sleep*.

More recently the thalamic [129] and brain stem [98, 99, 139] mechanisms responsible for this phase of sleep have been throughly investigated, and a new phase of sleep has been described, characterized by desynchronization of the electroencephalogram. During this phase of *desynchronized sleep,* two groups of phenomena occur: the tonic and the phasic. The main tonic events, which last throughout the episode, are characterized by the appearance of low voltage, fast cortical activity [33] and abolition of postural activity in the posterior cervical muscles [75]. Superimposed on these tonic events is the sudden eruption of phasic events, classified under: (a) rhythmic pontogeniculo-occipital activity characterized by large amplitude waves, which appear in the pons, lateral geniculate nucleus, and visual cortex [75]; and (b) bursts of rapid eye movements (REM) [33, 35].

During bursts of REM, rapid muscular contractions of facial and limb musculature also occur, which resemble myoclonic twitches induced by epileptic discharges [48]. Moreover, phasic inhibitory events affect transmission of somatic afferent volleys at the first relay station of several sensory pathways [121–124].

The result is that just at the time in which both spinal and ocular motoneurons are excited, transmission of sensory volleys along different somatosensory pathways is partially depressed by active processes, which may operate at both presynaptic or postsynaptic levels or both. Conversely, facilitation of sensory-evoked responses occurs at the level of both specific thalamic nuclei and sensory cortexes during bursts of REM. Reduced transmission of sensory volleys at the first relay station of different sensory pathways and facilitation of responses at the level of the specific thalamic nuclei are phenomena associated in time with bursts of REM. These phenomena are of particular importance in man [7, 8, 35, 37, 38], where striking relationship has been found between REM and dream activity.

SLEEP AND EPILEPSY

Two aspects of the problem should be considered: the first deals with modifications of abnormal EEG discharges as a function of different states of sleep; the second is concerned with changes in regular occurrence of the normal sleep-waking pattern as a function of epileptic discharges.

While in some instances sleep facilitates the occurrence of epileptic discharges, in

---

* This study supported by PHS Research Grants NB02990 and NB05695 from National Institute of Neurological Diseases and Stroke.

other instances sleep exerts just the opposite effect [6]. These clinical observations are reflected by a classification of the epilepsies which takes care of behavior of the crisis during the sleep-waking cycle [71, 76, 77, 79]. According to this classification, forms of epilepsies occur exclusively during sleep, or *sleep epilepsies*; during wakefulness, or *awakening epilepsies*; and finally forms occur both during sleep and waking, or *diffuse epilepsies*. Evidence also suggests that the location of either anatomical or electrical epileptogenic abnormality may determine occurrence of the spontaneous crisis during sleep or wakefulness [79, 80; cf. 71].

Effects of sleep on epileptic discharges have been reported recently in a group of papers dealing with complete recordings during the night of both synchronized and desynchronized phases of sleep [6, 10–14, 19–21, 29–32, 52–56, 62, 81, 83, 89, 101, 103, 107, 108, 110–113, 115, 138, 140, 142, 143]. Sleep activates mainly the interictal discharges; ictal discharges occur during generalized or partial epilepsies and are quite rare in both synchronized and desynchronized sleep.

During synchronized sleep, diffuse synchronous epileptic activity is well represented [61, 115, 140, 143, 144]; there is evidence that symmetrical and bilateral epileptic discharges can be facilitated during synchronized sleep [11, 19, 21, 30–32, 53, 54, 81, 103, 107, 108, 111, 138, 140, 144]. Forms of unilateral or partial, focal epilepsies can still be detected and even activated during synchronized sleep [6, 19, 21, 27, 31, 32, 53, 54, 56, 108, 111, 115, 142, 144]; the maximum amount and concentration of generalized and focal epileptic activity occurs during the light stages of synchronized sleep [6, 60, 115, 143].

Relation between desynchronized sleep and epilepsy is characterized by reduction of epileptic activity, which generally occurs during this phase of sleep regarding the synchronized phase; bilateral and symmetrical synchronous discharges are greatly reduced during desynchronized sleep [6, 10, 11, 19, 21, 32, 53, 55, 56, 103, 107, 108, 111, 138, 140]. Further suppression of the discharge rate of bilateral, synchronous paroxysmal activity actually occurs at the time of rapid eye movements [138]. Mechanisms responsible for both tonic and phasic events typical of desynchronized sleep are probably responsible for suppression of the epileptic discharges described above. Abolition of bilateral and symmetrical synchronous discharges during desynchronized sleep is not an absolute phenomenon, as assumed by Delange et al. [31], since it is possible to observe some generalized discharges during this phase of sleep [11, 52, 56, 140].

Focal discharges, it has been reported, are reduced or abolished during desynchronized sleep [142], although less constantly than are the bilateral synchronous discharges [14, 19, 31, 32]. But most investigators found that contrary to generalized epilepsies, focal discharges (particularly frontal or temporal) persist [54, 115] or can actually be activated during the desynchronized phase of sleep [14, 19, 21, 30, 32, 39, 47, 53, 55, 56, 103, 107, 109, 113].

Mean values of the epileptic activity, determined by counting the single elements in the nocturnal records independently upon their morphology and distribution, appear higher during synchronized than during desynchronized sleep [6, 22]. Waking from the last phase of sleep increases the occurrence of epileptic discharges.

In addition to differences in rates of occurrence of epileptic discharges among the various sleep stages, morphologic changes also affect interictal discharges of both generalized and focal epilepsies. As the patient passes from one stage to another not only the frequency but also the form, amplitude, and pattern of the discharges changes [19, 21, 53, 56, 140].

Most of the patients who had symmetric bilateral and constantly synchronous discharges during wakefulness showed generalized interictal discharges which still affected the two hemispheres during sleep [53, 115]. Sometimes these discharges appeared concentrated in more restricted regions of the two hemispheres; they could also be substituted by focal abnormalities, particularly during the deepest stages of synchronized sleep and during desynchronized sleep [6, 11, 19, 21, 53, 55, 56, 60, 61, 106, 115, 144]. On the other hand, interictal discharges due to focal epilepsies extend over a wider area during synchronized sleep than during wakefulness and may spread to the homotopic region of the contralateral side. Conversely, during desynchronized sleep, interictal discharges of partial epilepsies tend to show maximal localization.

Effects of Sleep on Generalized Epileptic Discharges

Synchronized sleep with slower rhythms originating from the thalamus actually acts as a convulsant, thus facilitating appearance of generalized bilateral hypersynchronism [19, 21, 29, 32, 53, 55, 57, 64, 72, 89, 114, 115, 149]. The possibility that mechanisms of intracortical diffusion may facilitate occurrence of bilateral and synchronous EEG convulsions should also be considered [9, 91, 146]. On the other hand, great reduction or abolition of generalized bilateral synchronous epileptic discharges during desynchronized sleep can be related to depression of synchronizing, sleep-inducing mechanisms, shown by the fact that during this phase of sleep, cortical "recruiting" responses produced by low frequency, electric stimulation of nonspecific thalamic nuclei are depressed or even abolished (Fig. 17-1*A*, *B*) [4, 44, 58, 102, 104, 141, 151].

Contrary to the recruiting responses, *augmenting* responses still persisted during desynchronized sleep [44, 102]. Since these responses were recorded from the same points where recruiting responses appeared to be depressed, it is not understood why the same cortical areas respond highly to specific and scarcely at all to nonspecific thalamic stimulation, unless depression is postulated in the nonspecific thalamic structures [141].

Thalamic mechanisms involved during desynchronized sleep may be comparable to those responsible for the shift from EEG

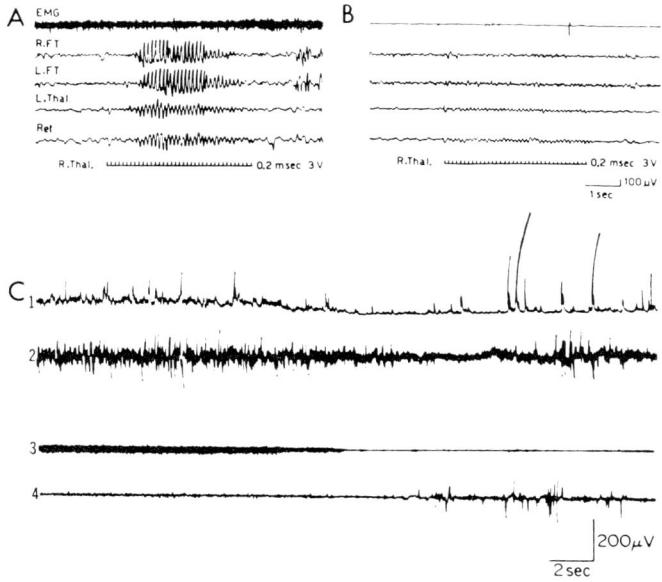

FIG. 17-1. (*A*) and (*B*) Cortical and subcortical effects of low rate electrical stimulation of midline thalamic nuclei during synchronized and desynchronized sleep. Stimulation of the right thalamic nucleus centralis lateralis (R. Thal.) with 0.2 msec, 3 V, 9 per sec pulses. Bipolar records from posterior neck muscles (EMG), right and left frontotemporal (RFT and LFT), left thalamic nucleus centralis lateralis (L. Thal.), mesencephalic reticular formation (Ret.). (*A*) Generalized synchronization (recruiting response) induced during synchronized sleep. (*B*) Depression of response during desynchronized sleep.

(*C*) Decrease of callosal activity at the beginning of a desynchronized phase of sleep. (1) integrated callosal activity; (2) electroencephalogram; (3) electromyogram from the posterior neck muscles; (4) electro oculogram. (From [15, 141].)

synchronization to the desynchronized EEG pattern typical of the waking state [128, 129]. In this instance, the effectiveness of the ascending reticular volleys in antagonizing evoked thalamocortical synchronization [100] has been related to blockade of inhibitory postsynaptic potentials, which are responsible for the phasing activity of thalamic cells during the synchronization process, possibly also to production of high frequency, excitatory, postsynaptic potentials in thalamic neurons. It seems likely that even during desynchronized sleep there are factors which can depress, also totally inhibit the periodicity tendency of nonspecific thalamic neurons to discharge in bursts.

The observation made by Huttenlocher [69] is relevant in this connection. He found that during desynchronized sleep, mesencephalic reticular units show high frequency discharges, thus indicating that at this time there is increase in excitability of many reticular units. It might be that the reticular activating system is really a modifying factor in the production of desynchronized sleep. The difference between the two behavioral stages of wakefulness and desynchronized sleep would be mainly the result of a refined distribution of dynamics in the cellular network of the ascending reticular system, rather than merely the result of changes in mean frequency of cell discharge within that system.

On the basis of this conclusion, it may be explained, at least in part, why depression of thalamocortical recruiting responses occurs not only during wakefulness but also during desynchronized sleep. Yet generalized epileptic discharges can still be detected during wakefulness [140], while they are greatly reduced or abolished during desynchronized sleep.

Depression of the generalized epileptic discharge during desynchronized sleep may also be due to tonic reduction in the traffic of interhemispheric impulses coursing through the corpus callosum, which occurs during desynchronized sleep (Fig. 17-1C) [15] and may therefore contribute to limiting occurrence and propagation of the epileptiform discharge.

Effects of Sleep on Focal Epileptic Discharges

Persistence, or even activation of focal discharges during both synchronized and desynchronized sleep indicates that to a certain extent they are independent of the functional activity of the synchronizing systems. On the other hand, occurrence of focal convulsive activities during sleep can be related with changes in cortical excitability.

In order to evaluate changes in cortical excitability during different phases of sleep, the postsynaptic components of cortical-evoked potentials have been investigated in primary areas following single-shock stimulation of specific thalamocortical radiations (cf. [122]). Cortical excitability is higher during sleep than during wakefulness, although no striking difference was found for it between synchronized and desynchronized sleep. These elements favor the cortical genesis and development of these epileptic manifestations [21].

Inhibitory mechanisms doubtless play an important role in limiting the buildup of excitability of cortical neurons, which would otherwise result in convulsions. Regularity in spike discharges of pyramidal-tract neurons depends upon activity of a recurrent inhibitory mechanism, which might act to prevent occurrence of high frequency bursts in pyramidal tract cells [116, 117]. Postspike hyperpolarization and afferent inhibition are prominent among additional mechanisms which might act to limit discharge frequency in pyramidal neurons. During sleep, one or more of these inhibitory mechanisms may be less effective [40–43]. Particularly during desynchronized sleep, the reduced excitability of intercalated, inhibitory interneurons may lead to reduction of inhibitory control on pyramidal cells, which would then facilitate the occurrence of high frequency bursts.

During synchronized sleep these bursts are short lasting and triggered by ascending volleys originating from the thalamic nuclei. During desynchronized sleep, bursts are longer lasting and can be related to the arrival in the cerebral cortex of ascending volleys originating from or triggered by the pontine structures and vestibular nuclei.

It has already been mentioned that two different types of phasic events occur during desynchronized sleep. The first type of activity is characterized by monophasic sharp waves which affect the pontine reticular formation, lateral geniculate nucleus (LGN), and visual cortex [75], particularly at the time of isolated ocular movements (cf. [97]). Lesion experiments indicate that the pontine activity is responsible for production of rhythmic potentials recorded from the lateral geniculate nucleus and visual cortex [68].

In addition to these events, the episode of desynchronized sleep is also characterized by sudden occurrence from time to time of bursts of high frequency, ocular movements (REM). Experiments of microelectrode recording of single neurons from the vestibular nuclei, performed during natural sleep [17], as well as lesion experiments [125], indicate that medial and descending vestibular nuclei are critically responsible for REM. Evidence also indicates that the same pontine structures which trigger the lateral geniculate nucleus and visual cortex are also responsible for phasic rhythmic discharge in medial and descending vestibular nuclei [97].

While ascending volleys related with rhythmic pontogeniculate activity impinge mainly upon the visual cortex, ascending volleys originating from vestibular nuclei impinge upon a wider cortical area including the sensorimotor cortex. It may well be concluded that gradients of electrical activity due to arrival of these ascending volleys during sleep are of critical importance in precipitating focal discharge in epileptic patients.

The traffic of impulses recorded from the corpus callosum is tonically depressed during desynchronized sleep. This activity, however, increases phasically during large bursts of REM (Fig. 17-1C) [15]. Whether this activity may actually facilitate spread of focal epileptiform discharge from a restricted cortical area to the homotopic region of the contralateral cortex is still unknown.

The detection of focal discharges in the scalp EEG of epileptic patients does not necessarily mean that in the underlying cortex there is a group of neurons whose altered function is primarily responsible for epileptic manifestations [3, 64, 114]. Abnormal activity may well be due to focal discharges originating from or triggered by subcortical structures. Some of these foci may well be localized within the thalamus. The view that thalamic nuclei serve as a single pacemaker or funnel for thalamo-cortical rhythmic impulses producing slow cortical waves is not entirely correct. In fact, local alteration of thalamic activity by injection of penicillin does not change the corticogram in general but only affects certain restricted areas of the cortex [132].

Recent experiments indicate that thalamocortical connections are arranged in precise point-to-point fashion, so that close relationship exists between a group of thalamic cells and a small cortical area to which these cells project [5]. The possibility therefore exists that restricted cortical regions are individually controlled by a thalamic rhythmic entity. This point-to-point relation was found in all major sensory projection systems and in one thalamic "association" nucleus and its corresponding "association" cortex. Small groups of thalamic neurons, particularly if deprived of their inhibitory control system, may well have the ability to generate paroxysmal activity, thereby affecting certain restricted areas of the cortex only. Paroxysmal activity in a group of thalamic cells can thus be faithfully reproduced in that part of the cortex to which these thalamic cells project.

It has already been mentioned that evoked potentials due to activity in the nonspecific thalamic system (the recruiting responses) are tonically depressed during desynchronized sleep [4, 44, 58, 102, 104, 141, 151]. Moreover, phasic suppression of responses occurs during bursts of REM [58]. Present evidence indicates that responses of specific thalamic nuclei, far from being depressed, are actually facilitated, probably due to reciprocal interaction which occurs during this phase of sleep between nonspecific and specific thalamic nuclei (cf.

[122]). In particular, excitability of the specific thalamic neurons, which is tonically increased during desynchronized sleep, shows further phasic enhancements during REM bursts, due to ascending volleys originating from the pontine and vestibular structures. This activity may well precipitate occurrence of focal epileptic discharge, particularly when the epileptic focus is endowed within specific thalamic structures or corresponding cortical areas.

Sensory Precipitation of Epilepsy

That convulsant effects can be induced reflexly is well known. Since transmission of afferent volleys at different relay stations of several sensory pathways is greatly modified during sleep, particularly during REM bursts of desynchronized sleep (cf. [121–124]), it may be expected that even the ability of sensory stimuli to elicit reflex epilepsy will be modified at that time. Changes, however, may occur even independently from these phasic events of desynchronized sleep, which is actually the case for epileptiform discharges elicited by intermittent photic stimulation. Ability of this photic stimulation to produce bisynchronous convulsive discharges decreases during synchronized sleep [28, 92, 136] and is virtually abolished during desynchronized sleep [28, 92, 145, cf. 67]. Mechanisms responsible for these depressions may actually differ during the two phases of sleep. In particular, reduced effectiveness of the rhythmic photic discharges during synchronized sleep may well be attributed to reduced transmission of orthodromic volleys through the LGN, which apparently occurs at this time (cf. [87, 88]). On the contrary, abolition of reflexly induced epileptiform discharge during desynchronized sleep is not due to mechanisms involving specific thalamic nuclei (LGN), since their excitability, far from being depressed, is actually tonically increased during this phase of sleep. Reduction of photo-induced epilepsy during desynchronized sleep has therefore been related to reduced excitability of the nonspecific thalamic nuclei [28].

The results of clinical observations indicate that changes in epileptic discharges may occur during different phases of sleep, but the possibility should be considered that epileptic attacks may alter regular occurrence of the normal sleep-waking pattern [30]. The sleep pattern of all adult mammals is characterized by regular alternation of synchronized and desynchronized phases of sleep [35, 82, 137]; this physiological periodicity is probably under neurohumoral control. In both adult humans or cats there is great stability in regard to the amount of time spent awake or in various stages of sleep [75, 137]. It would be interesting to determine whether in epileptic patients the percentage of time spent in each stage of sleep differs from that of nonepileptic subjects and whether seizure activity results in alterations in the regular shifts from one stage of sleep to another. Insufficient available data prohibit any conclusion being drawn on this subject. An important contribution to the problem was given in recent studies where relationships between sleep deprivation and epilepsy were investigated.

SLEEP DEPRIVATION AND EPILEPSY

The great similarity between myoclonic jerks due to convulsive activity and muscular twitches occurring during REM suggests that some mechanisms are involved in common.

The pathways responsible for motor events related in time with the REM course along the dorsolateral funiculi (Fig. 17-2A, B) [48] where both the corticospinal and rubrospinal tracts are located. It has already been mentioned that the temporal pattern of discharge of single, pyramidal-tract neurons is greatly modified during sleep [40–43]. In particular, bursts of activity separated by long intervals of complete inactivity occur during desynchronized sleep. Similar findings have also been obtained by recording unit activity in the red nucleus of the cat during this phase of sleep [51]. Recent experiments indicate that increase in unitary activity as well as in the integrated discharge of the pyramidal tract (Fig. 17-2C, D) [90, 95] and the red nucleus (Fig. 17-2E, F) [51] is strikingly related in time with outbursts of REM and

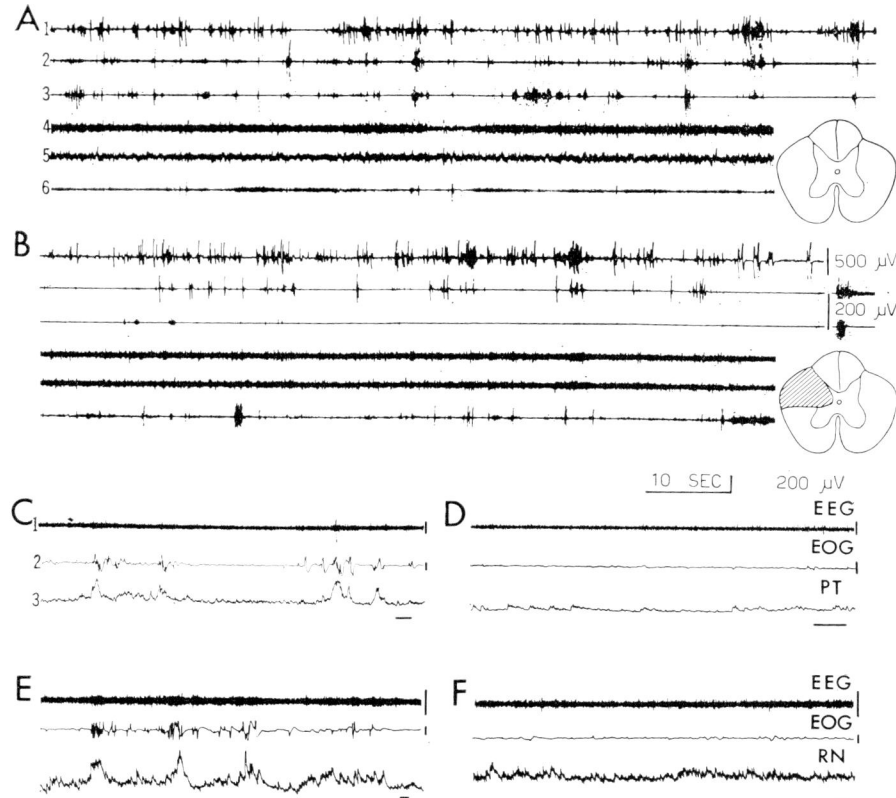

FIG. 17-2. (A) and (B) Myoclonic twitches during desynchronized sleep and their abolition after unilateral section of the dorsolateral funiculus. Unrestrained, unanesthetized cat. Bipolar records. (1) ocular movements; (2) left tibialis anterior; (3) right tibialis anterior; (4) left parieto-occipital; (5) right parieto-occipital; (6) EMG of the posterior cervical muscles. (A) Experiment made 8 days after implantation of electrodes. Bilateral and symmetrical twitches during an episode of desynchronized sleep. Soon afterward, right dorsolateral funiculus was sectioned at T12. (B) Records taken 2 days after the section. Note great reduction of myoclonic twitches on right side during an episode of desynchronized sleep.

(C) and (D) Phasic increase in pyramidal discharge during the REM of desynchronized sleep, its abolition after bilateral destruction of vestibular nuclei. (C) Unrestrained, unanesthetized cat. Experiment made 4 days after operation. Bipolar records. (1) right parieto-occipital; (2) ocular movements; (3) integrated activity of pyramidal tract. Note large phasic enhancement in pyramidal discharge during REM periods of desynchronized sleep. (D) Another experiment made 2 days after chronic implantation of electrodes and complete bilateral destruction of medial and descending vestibular nuclei. Large bursts of REM and related phasic enhancements of pyramidal discharge are absent. Time calibration: 5 sec. Voltage calibration: 0.2 mV (EEG), 0.5 mV (EOG).

(E) and (F) Phasic increase in rubral activity during REM of desynchronized sleep, its abolition following vestibular lesion. Unrestrained, unanesthetized cat. Bipolar records. EEG, left parieto-occipital; EOG, ocular movements; RN, integrated red-nucleus activity. (E) Experiment made 3 days after chronic implantation of electrodes. During desynchronized sleep, large phasic increases in rubral discharge are strikingly related in time with bursts of REM. (F) Same animal as in (E). Experiment made 7 days after chronic implantation of electrodes and 2 days after bilateral lesion of medial and descending vestibular nuclei. Absence during desynchronized sleep of large bursts of REM with related phasic enhancements of rubral discharge. Time calibration: 1 sec. Voltage calibration: 0.5 mV. (From [48, 96, 126].)

depends upon ascending vestibular volleys [96, 126]. Just at the time of REM bursts, monosynaptic and polysynaptic spinal reflexes are basically depressed (Fig. 17-3) [49] due to mechanisms of presynaptic inhibition [94, 95]. This effect is mediated by supraspinal volleys, originated from or triggered by vestibular nuclei, which descend along the ventral quadrants [119, 120]. Presynaptic depolarization of primary afferents may lead to a striking depression of spinal reflexes when REM bursts are not accompanied by muscular twitches. Simultaneous occurrence of myoclonic twitches in the same muscle reduces the extent of reflex depression brought about during bursts of REM. Indeed, the reflex response may be enhanced when strong twitches occur during large bursts of REM.

Similar to muscular twitches occurring during REM sleep, myoclonic jerks elicited by hypersynchronous discharges are due to pyramidal and extrapyramidal volleys [63]. It also appears that both facilitation and inhibition of the monosynaptic reflex occur during attacks in epileptic patients [130, 131] and that the synchronous cortical discharges produced by epileptogenic substances, such as pentylenetetrazol, are associated not only with motoneuronal activity [2] but also with presynaptic depolarization of the primary afferents [1].

In spite of all the experiments mentioned above, there is no doubt that the spinal mechanisms responsible for the myoclonic twitches are still unknown. For this reason we recorded the activity of single interneurons in the spinal cord of unrestrained, unanesthetized cats. This made possible the study of the effects of sleep and wakefulness on interneuronal discharge elicited by single-shock stimulation of hindlimb nerves [84]. Identification of these spinal cord neurons was made on the basis of the well-known characteristics of their spontaneous and induced unitary discharges [46]. The activity of 48 spinal interneurons was recorded. Significant changes of unitary responses did not occur during quiet wakefulness and synchronized sleep. On the contrary, during desynchronized sleep there was a remarkable increase in number and frequency of discharge of single units induced by somatic afferent volleys. These changes were strikingly related in time with bursts of REM (Fig. 17-4). Increase of interneuronal discharge appeared in spite of presynaptic depolarization of primary afferents, which reduces effectiveness of the orthodromic volley. Units recorded during sleep were located in layers V to VIII of Rexed [135], that is, in that region of the spinal cord where several supraspinal descending pathways, including the corticospinal and rubrospinal tracts, terminate. Unfortunately an analysis of interneuronal activity in the spinal cord during myoclonic jerks induced experimentally by hypersynchronous epileptic discharges is still lacking.

The conclusion that a striking relationship exists between epilepsy and the REM bursts of desynchronized sleep is supported in particular by experiments of sleep deprivation.

Interruption of REM Sleep

Dement [34] was the first to find that artificial interruption of REM sleep in humans is followed by a compensatory, striking increase in amount and percentage of the REM phase, if subjects are allowed uninterrupted sleep. This finding, with the observation that sometimes the subject went directly from wakefulness into REM sleep without passing through the synchronized phase of sleep, was regarded as evidence of a physiological *need* for REM sleep. The REM mechanism may be triggered by a neurochemical substance, probably a monoamine, which accumulates to a critical threshold level within a pontine center and is then released [74]. The deprivation-compensation effect has been experimentally validated in man as well as in other mammals. Selective deprivation of REM sleep can be accomplished not only by arousal at the onset of each REM period, but also by drugs [73–75]. In this instance, a major consequence of selective deprivation of REM sleep is an abrupt rise in the amount of this phase during recovery.

In addition to these compensatory changes in the REMs fraction, there were obvious changes in the intensity of REM sleep. Vigor of muscular twitching and

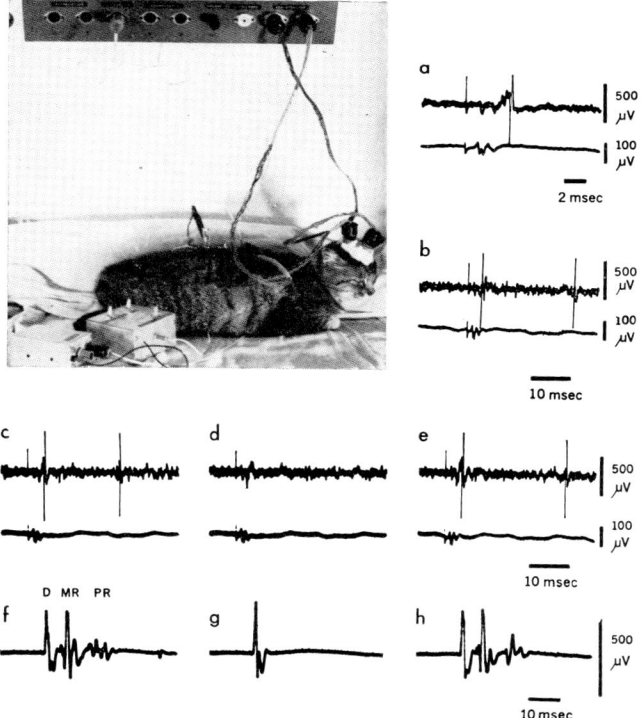

Fig. 17-3. Phasic inhibition of monosynaptic and polysynaptic reflexes involving α motoneurons during REM bursts of desynchronized sleep. (a) through (e) Unrestrained, unanesthetized cat. Experiment made 2 days after chronic implantation of electrodes. A stimulating bipolar electrode was placed on the left tibial nerve, tied distally to the electrode while the remaining hindlimb nerves were cut. A micromanipulator was also fixed rigidly to vestibular arcs, previous exposure of spinal cord at lumbar level. Extracellular recordings from single α motoneurons in layer IX of Rexed [135] were made with 0.75–1.5 MΩ tungsten electrodes attached to micromanipulator. Penetration of these electrodes through pia-arachnoid was generally made under light ether anesthesia, previous to a small opening of dura. A miniature emitter follower was mounted directly on micromanipulator, as shown in illustration of cat. Microelectrode advanced by a turning screw placed on top of the system. Indifferent electrode placed into back muscles. Volleys in dorsal roots produced by single-shock stimulation of tibial nerve, recorded from cord dorsum by ball-tipped silver electrode placed near entry point of microelectrode, against indifferent electrode in muscle.

(a) Monosynaptic response of tibial motoneuron to single-shock stimulation of homonymous nerve with 0.02 msec pulse duration, 2.67 times the threshold (T) for group I ingoing volley. (b) Record taken at slower sweep speed to show both monosynaptic and polysynaptic discharges of same motoneuron to tibial volley; same parameters of stimulation as in (a). (c), (d), and (e) Records taken with slightly higher stimulus intensity (2.87 T) before (c), during (d), and after (e) a REM burst of desynchronized sleep.

(f) through (h) Another experiment made in unrestrained, unanesthetized cat, 4 days after chronic implantation of electrodes. Electromyographic recording from intrinsic plantar muscles of both monosynaptic (MR) and polysynaptic (PR) reflexes elicited by single-shock stimulation of ipsilateral tibial nerve; 0.07 msec duration, 1.25 times the threshold for direct motor response (D). Responses recorded during desynchronized sleep before (f), during (g), and after (h) a large burst of REM. Note in (d) and (g) the phasic inhibition of both monosynaptic and polysynaptic reflexes during the bursts of REM. (From Lenzi, G. L., Pompeiano, O., and Rabin, B., unpublished observations.)

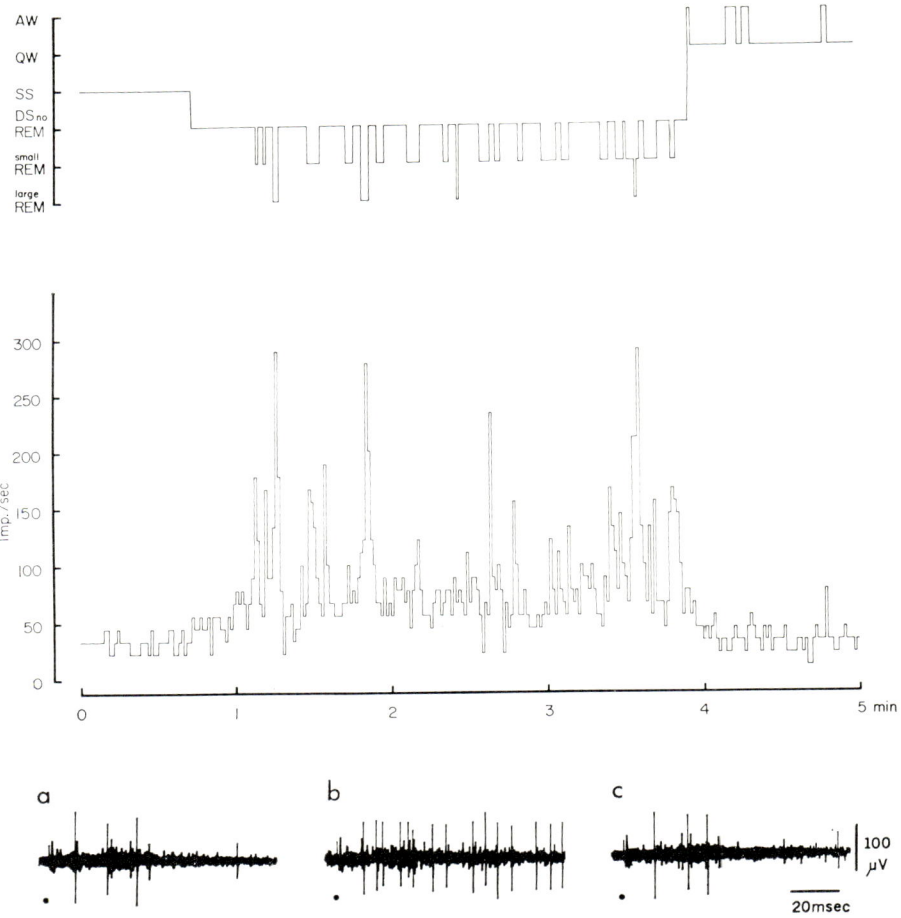

FIG. 17-4. Reflex responses of single interneurons in spinal cord during different backgrounds of sleep and wakefulness. Unrestrained, unanesthetized cat. Experiment made 2 days after chronic implantation of electrodes as illustrated in Fig. 17-3. Responses of single neuron located in layer VII of Rexed [135] to single-shock stimulation of ipsilateral sciatic nerve (0.02 msec pulse duration, 3.33 times the threshold for group I ingoing volley) recorded during different backgrounds of sleep and wakefulness. Characterized by burst of spikes which occurred with relatively long latency thus indicating its polysynaptic origin. Upper diagram shows progressive shift of EEG activity from synchronized sleep (SS) to desynchronized sleep (DS), active wakefulness (AW), and quiet wakefulness (QW). Note occurrence during desynchronized sleep of periods without REM (DS no REM) and periods with REM (small REM and large REM).

Lower diagram shows changes in frequency of discharge of single unit as a function of EEG background. In each record, frequency (impulses per second) was evaluated on basis of number of spikes which occurred during 90-msec period following shock artifact. Note regular occurrence of large increases in unit discharge at time of rapid eye movements, occasional appearance in awake-preparation of slight increase in reflex discharge during short-lasting episode of active wakefulness.

(a) through (c) Responses of same unit, recorded just before (a), during (b), and after (c) a REM burst of desynchronized sleep. (From Lenzi, G. L., Pompeiano, O., and Rabin, B., unpublished observations.)

frequency of eye movements increased greatly during recovery sleep after REM deprivation [23, 45]; severity of these spasms increased as the animal was increasingly deprived. In these instances, as soon as the animals became completely flaccid, they showed, against the background of muscular atonia, episodes of violent facial and limb twitches interspersed with convulsive movements of the entire body.

In these deprived animals, it appeared that REM sleep became a sort of convulsive state with muscular contractions resembling myoclonic twitches. This led to the speculation that REM sleep, at least in the deprived state, might have something in common with convulsive seizures, and that an effect of selective deprivation of REM sleep is a generalized increase in neuronal excitability [23, 36].

Effects of Deprivation of REM Sleep on Convulsive Threshold

This hypothesis was tested in a study using the threshold for electroconvulsive shock as a gross measure of change in excitability. Rats were deprived of desynchronized sleep for a 6-day period but were allowed substantial synchronized sleep [23, 36]. Thresholds for electroconvulsive shock dropped significantly (from 5 to 50 percent, mean 22 percent) in all these animals during the period of sleep deprivation, but threshold in control animals treated in a similar manner, but allowed REM sleep, exhibited no change (cf. also [18]).

In summary, results demonstrate a drop in threshold to electroconvulsive shock during REM sleep deprivation, which is reversed when the animals are allowed to recover lost REM-sleep time. This deprivation seems to heighten neural excitability, which is supported by observation [16, 36, 105, 127] of epileptic patients showing an increase in number of bursts of seizure discharges in the EEG as a result of sleep deprivation. Possibly REM deprivation directly produces certain neurochemical changes and the cumulative effects of these changes may be responsible for neurophysiological and behavioral changes observed in animals selectively deprived of REM sleep [23].

Effects of Convulsive Activity on REM Sleep

In the rat [23] it was found that convulsed animals tended to spend less time in the REM phase than their nonconvulsed controls, which led to speculation that the intense activity of convulsion could in some manner substitute for or interfere with REM sleep. Later studies were designed to explore this hypothesis [24, 36]. One electroconvulsive shock per day, administered for 5–7 days, reduced daily REM sleep time in cats to as little as 28 percent of the baseline level. Besides a drop in REM, a remarkable fall in frequency of eye movements during desynchronized sleep became evident by the fourth day. Tracking eye movements in the waking animal did not appear to be altered. Although partially deprived of REM for as long as 7 days, the cats showed no compensatory rise in REM time during the recovery period, but controls equally deprived gave significant rebound. Similar results were also obtained after convulsions induced by intravenous injection of pentylenetetrazol. These findings supported the hypothesis that seizures in some way substituted for REM sleep; the observations were confirmed not only in cats [78] but also in a group of patients receiving electroconvulsive therapy [24, 152]. The patients showed reduction in REM-sleep time, drop in the frequency of eye movements, and absence of compensatory rebound after shock.

It was concluded that electroconvulsive shock suppresses REM sleep. More surprising was the finding that when REM sleep was depressed after electroconvulsion, compensatory REM rebounds did not occur.

It is likely that intense activity accompanying the seizure in some manner alters brain levels of substances, or their precursors, that induce REM sleep. The amount of time spent in REM sleep is higher in the first days of life than in adult life [75, 82, 137]. Frequency and intensity of phasic muscular contractions in the newborn is comparable to that of adults after REM deprivation [45]. Conversely, the tendency toward epileptic discharge is poorly developed at birth and increases as maturation proceeds.

Observations made by Cohen et al. [25, 36] also disclosed that in cats a reduced compensatory rebound followed selective REM deprivation if electroconvulsive shocks were administered during the deprivation period. After REM deprivation, the phasic components of REM sleep increase in intensity [23, 45], most strikingly and easily observed in the intensification of muscle twitches and increased frequency and amplitude of individual eye movements. Apparently during recovery REM sleep, convulsed cats did not display exaggerated bursts of eye movements and body twitches seen in nonconvulsive controls. Data indicate that development of the REM deprivation-compensation effect is retarded by occurrence of convulsions during the deprivation period.

Anticonvulsant Experiments

For further clarification of possible specific interaction between REM sleep and convulsions, an independent study of sleep patterns in normal experimental animals treated with a major anticonvulsant, diphenylhydantoin (DPH), was carried out in cats [26]. During DPH treatment there was significant reduction in the daily amount of REM-sleep time, but waking and synchronized sleep were not significantly affected. Most surprising in this study was the complete absence of compensatory REM rebounds following long periods of partial REM-sleep loss after drug administration.

The actual pattern of DPH effect is similar to the response pattern in cats after a period of daily electroconvulsive shock administration, where pronounced reduction in REM time was followed only by an asymptomatic return to baseline which took at least several days [24]. In addition to suppressing, DPH apparently also prevents accumulation of factors responsible for deprivation effects and compensatory rebounds. Assuming that epileptic convulsions may "use up" the same substances which are also responsible for REM sleep, it would appear that anticonvulsants may interfere with the metabolism of catecholamines, since this metabolic system is currently the favored candidate for the job of regulating REM sleep [74, 75].

Another important phenomenon which occurred after DPH injection was the persistence of rhythmic pontogeniculate activity typical of the desynchronized phase of sleep. In the light of the known ability of DPH to limit repetitive neural discharge, probably by stabilizing sodium excretion at the cell membrane [147, 150], it could be expected to exert a suppressive effect on monophasic sharp waves. However, no change in this sharp-wave activity was evident, so it is unlikely that the REM suppressive effect of DPH was mediated via this system. It has been suggested that DPH affects REM sleep by interfering with the ability of pontine waves to trigger full-blown REM episodes, that is, the pontogeniculate spikes cannot spread [26]. Since REM bursts as well as all related motor events depend on vestibular activity [17, 96, 125], it would be of interest to know if DPH affects interaction between pontine and vestibular mechanisms which is required for the occurrence of typical bursts of REM.

Finally it may be assumed that DPH has a similar effect on REM sleep in humans. It is not unlikely that all-night sleep patterns will be abnormal in patients who have received the drug for long periods of time in relatively high dosage, and that the most likely abnormality will be excessively small amounts of REM sleep. Cohen et al. [26] have already made this observation in epileptic patients being treated with DPH at the time of recording. These authors point out a preclusion to attributing low REM times solely to a prior history of repeated seizures, even though the possibility that seizures might have this action as an independent effect is also supported by experimental evidence [24, 25]. Demonstrated relationship between REM sleep, REM deprivation, and seizure susceptibility [23] requires sorting out ways in which DPH or other anticonvulsants might permanently alter the course of the illness, via the mechanism of permanently altering the nature of REM sleep. Further studies are obviously indicated.

SLEEP AND NARCOLEPSY

Narcolepsy is a disorder characterized by sudden, recurring attacks of sleep. Narcoleptic patients have been divided into two groups [133]: those who show only the sleep attacks, and those who experience in addition one or more of the following auxiliary symptoms: cataplexy, sleep paralysis, or hypnagogic hallucinations.

Cataplexy. This is a sudden, dramatic decrement of muscle tone and loss of certain reflexes. It is well known that spontaneous muscular activity not only of posterior cervical muscles [75] but also of extensor and flexor muscles of hindlimbs is abolished during desynchronized sleep [48]. Moreover, monosynaptic reflexes recorded electromyographically from both extensor and flexor muscles, as well as polysynaptic reflexes, are tonically depressed throughout this phase of sleep [48, 59, cf. 118–120].

The hypothesis that this effect is due to postsynaptic inhibition of the α motoneurons to both extensor and flexor muscles is supported by the finding that response of deafferented motoneuronal pools to antidromic [50] or direct stimulation [93] is tonically depressed during desynchronized sleep (Fig. 17-5A–C).

This effect is likely due to reticulospinal volleys originating from medial reticular formation. Stimulation of this structure produces increase in membrane potential, attributable to postsynaptic inhibition of the α motoneurons, since it is reversed by passing hyperpolarizing currents through the membrane and is associated with conductance changes typical of inhibitory postsynaptic potentials [70, 85, 86]. These inhibitory potentials decrease reflex excitation of motoneurons as well as their response to antidromic and direct stimulation [50, 70, 85, 86, 93]. Both extensor and flexor motoneurons are equally inhibited (Fig. 17-5D–I) [70]. This finding explains depression of spinal cord activities occurring during desynchronized sleep as a generalized phenomenon; it affects both extensor and flexor motoneurons and their responses to stimulation of corresponding monosynaptic reflex pathways [49, 59].

Atonic manifestations and reflex inhibition of the spinal reflexes, occurring throughout the episode of desynchronized sleep (cf. [118–120]), are paralleled by decrement of muscle tone and reflex inhibition of cataplexy and sleep paralysis [66].

Sleep Paralysis. This involves episodes of inability to move which occur in the process of falling asleep. Postdormital paralysis, also observed in narcoleptics, is considered a variant of sleep paralysis, except that it occurs upon awakening.

It has been shown that motoneuronal responses produced by electrical stimulation of the pyramidal [90] and extrapyramidal (rubrospinal) pathways [51] are tonically depressed during desynchronized sleep. This effect can also be attributed to postsynaptic inhibition of the α motoneurons. Blockade of pyramidal discharges may well explain the terrifying experience of being unable to perform voluntary movements, an event occurring during sleep or postdormital paralysis.

Hypnagogic Hallucinations. These are vivid, sensory experiences during the transition between wakefulness and sleep. Hypnopompic hallucinations, instead, occur upon awakening. The hypnagogic hallucinations, which occur in narcoleptic patients, find their counterpart in dreams which are characteristic of desynchronized sleep [7, 37, 38].

There is reason to believe that all these aspects of narcoleptic pathology, as well as the sleep attacks, are related to the desynchronized phase of sleep. Characteristics of the narcoleptic syndrome fit well with characteristics of the desynchronized phase of sleep.

An association of narcolepsy itself and desynchronized sleep has also been established recently [133]. The EEG pattern of narcoleptics, usually observed at sleep onset, is characterized by a low voltage pattern, similar to that which occurs during desynchronized sleep. While the first episode of desynchronized sleep at onset of nocturnal sleep normally does not occur until after about one hour or more of synchronized sleep, a prominent characteristic of narco-

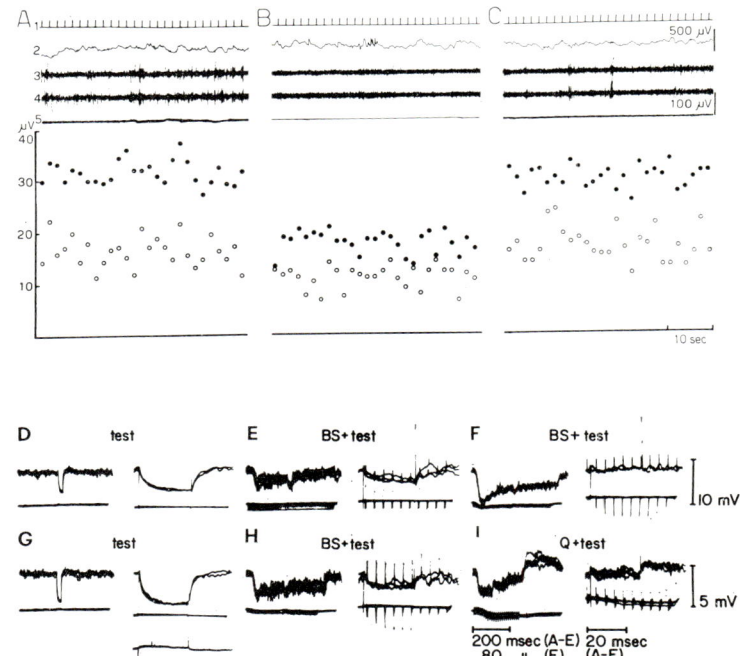

FIG. 17-5. (A) through (C) Tonic depression of α volleys elicited by direct stimulation of antagonistic motoneuronal pools during desynchronized sleep. Unrestrained, unanesthetized cat. Experiment made 2 days after section of left dorsal roots L6–S2. Obturator, quadriceps, and hamstring nerves cut, left tibial and deep peroneal nerves tied distally to bipolar recording electrodes. Stainless steel microelectrode (300 kΩ) chronically inserted into left ventral horn at upper level of S1. Responses elicited by direct stimulation of α motoneurons, recorded simultaneously from both tibial (circles) and deep peroneal nerve (dots) and plotted in diagrams.

(1) Signals of electrical shocks applied to left ventral horn (rectangular pulses: 1 every 1.7 sec, 0.05 msec pulse duration, 1.70 times threshold for direct α volleys); (2) eye movements; (3) left parieto-occipital; (4) right parieto-occipital; (5) EMG of posterior cervical muscles. (A) Synchronized sleep. (B) Tonic depression of α responses during desynchronized sleep. Note absence of phasic depression of motoneuronal responses during burst of REM. (C) Recovery of responses after end of desynchronized sleep episode.

(D) through (I) Conductance changes in flexor and extensor motoneurons due to stimulation of brain stem. Unanesthetized, decerebrate cat. Upper traces are intracellular records from two motoneurons, posterior biceps-semitendinosus in (D)–(F) and gastrocnemius-soleus in (G)–(I). Lower traces from dorsal-root entry zone. Lowermost trace in (G) is extracellular record taken after withdrawal of microelectrode from cell. (D), (G) Pulses of current applied through recording electrode. (E), (F), (H) Same pulses on background of an IPSP evoked from brain stem and (I) during IPSP produced by train of volleys in quadriceps nerve. In (F) and (H), same strength of brain-stem stimulation. In (E), stimulation weaker. All records taken simultaneously with two different sweep-speeds with time calibrations for slow and fast records in (I). Voltage calibrations are for microelectrode recording. (From [70, 93].)

leptics is special susceptibility to precocious occurrence of desynchronized periods and REM bursts at the beginning of nocturnal sleep [65, 134, 148].

Why should the narcoleptic show precocious triggering of brain stem centers responsible for desynchronized sleep? An attempt to answer this question is necessarily speculative, since not enough is known about the mechanism which regulates triggering in normals to know in what way this mechanism might be impaired in narcoleptics. It is possible that the source of pathology could be biochemical rather than neuroanatomical. Since narcoleptics are awake during cataplexy attacks, it is suggested that auxiliary symptoms of narcolepsy result from functional impairment of the mechanism whereby wakefulness normally prevents occurrence of the desynchronized phase of sleep [133].

It must be mentioned that narcolepsy and cataplexy may also occur in epileptic patients.

REFERENCES

1. Abdelmoumène, M., Besson, J. M., Aléonard, P., and Rivot, J. P. Corrélations entre les variations de l'électrocorticogramme et du potentiel de racine dorsale au cours de la crise d'épilepsie cardiazolique chez le chat. *J. Physiol.* (Paris) Suppl. 60, 207, 1968.
2. Ajmone-Marsan, C., and Marossero, F. Electrocorticographic and electrochordographic study of the convulsions induced by cardiazol. *Electroenceph. Clin. Neurophysiol.* 2:133, 1950.
3. Ajmone-Marsan, C., and Ralston, B. L. *The Epileptic Seizure. Its Functional Morphology and Diagnostic Significance.* Springfield, Ill.: Thomas, 1957.
4. Allison, T. Cortical and subcortical evoked responses to central stimuli during wakefulness and sleep. *Electroenceph. Clin. Neurophysiol.* 18:131, 1965.
5. Andersen, P., Andersson, S. A., and Lømo, T. Nature of thalamo-cortical relations during spontaneous barbiturate spindle activity. *J. Physiol.* (London) 192:283, 1967.
6. Andrioli, G., Angeleri, F., Bergonzi, F., Cantore, P., Ferroni, A., Gentilomo, A., Mingrino, S., Ricci, G. B., Rosadini, G., and Rossi, G. F. Inquadramento diagnostico dell'epilettico in neurochirurgia. *Minerva Neurochir.* 10:49, 1966.
7. Aserinsky, E., and Kleitman, N. Regularly occurring periods of eye motility and concomitant phenomena during sleep. *Science* 118:273, 1953.
8. Aserinsky, E., and Kleitman, N. Two types of ocular motility occurring in sleep. *J. Appl. Physiol.* 8:1, 1955.
9. Bancaud, J., and Talairach, J. *La stéréoélectroencéphalographie dans l'épilepsie.* Paris: Masson, 1965.
10. Bancaud, J., Talairach, J., Bordas-Ferrer, M., Auber, J. L., and Marchand, H. Les accès épileptiques au cours du sommeil de nuit. Étude stéréo-électroencéphalographique: In *Le sommeil de nuit normal et pathologique. Études électroencéphalographiques.* Électroencéphalographie et Neurophysiologie clinique (Nouvelle Série). Paris: Masson, 1965, vol. 2, p. 255.
11. Batini, C., Criticos, A., Fressy, J., and Gastaut, H. À propos du sommeil nocturne chez les sujets présentant une épilepsie à expression E.E.G. bisynchrone. *Rev. Neurol.* (Paris) 106:221, 1962.
12. Batini, C., Fressy, J., and Coquery, J. M. Critères polygraphiques du sommeil lent et du sommeil rapide. In *Le sommeil de nuit normal et pathologique. Études électroencéphalographiques.* Électroencéphalographie et Neurophysiologie clinique (Nouvelle Série). Paris: Masson, 1965, vol. 2, p. 156.
13. Batini, C., Fressy, J., and Gastaut, H. À propos du sommeil nocturne chez le sujet normal. *Rev. Neurol.* (Paris) 106: 218, 1962.
14. Batini, C., Fressy, J., Naquet, R., Orfanos, A., and Saint-Laurent, J. Étude du sommeil nocturne chez 20 sujets présentant des décharges irritatives localisées. *Rev. Neurol.* (Paris) 108:172, 1963.
15. Berlucchi, G. Callosal activity in unrestrained, unanesthetized cats. *Arch. Ital. Biol.* 103:623, 1965.
16. Berti Ceroni, G., Sabbatini, L., Gambi, D., and Lugaresi, E. Effetti della "sleep deprivation" in epilettici. *Riv. Neurol.* 37: 305, 1967.
17. Bizzi, E., Pompeiano, O., and Somogyi, I. Spontaneous activity of single vestibular neurons of unrestrained cats during sleep and wakefulness. *Arch. Ital. Biol.* 102: 308, 1964.
18. Bliss, E. L. Sleep in schizophrenia and depression. Studies of sleep loss in man and animals. *Res. Publ. Ass. Res. Nerv. Ment. Dis.* 45:195, 1967.
19. Cadilhac, J., and Passouant, P. L'influence des différentes phases du sommeil

nocturne sur les décharges épileptiques chez l'homme. In *Aspects anatomo-fonctionnels de la physiologie du sommeil.* Paris: Éditions du Centre National de la Recherche Scientifique, 1965.

20. Cadilhac, J., and Passouant-Fontaine, Th. Décharges épileptiques et activité électrique de veille et de sommeil dans l'hippocampe au cours de l'ontogénèse. In *Physiologie de l'hippocampe.* Paris: Éditions du Centre National de la Recherche Scientifique, 1962.

21. Cadilhac, J., Vlahovitch, B., and Mme. Delange-Walter. Considérations sur les modifications des décharges épileptiques au cours de la période des mouvements oculaires. In *Le sommeil de nuit normal et pathologique. Études électroencéphalographiques.* Électroencéphalographie et Neurophysiologie clinique (Nouvelle Série). Paris: Masson, 1965, vol. 2, p. 275.

22. Candia, O., Minobe, K., and Rossi, G. F. Epilessia e sonno: frequenza di manifestazioni elettroencefalografiche di tipo epilettico durante il ciclo sonno-veglia del gatto. *Boll. Soc. Ital. Biol. Sper.* 40:847, 1964.

23. Cohen, H. B., and Dement, W. C. Sleep: changes in threshold to electroconvulsive shock in rats after deprivation of "paradoxical" phase. *Science* 150:1318, 1965.

24. Cohen, H. B., and Dement, W. C. Sleep: suppression of rapid eye movement phase in the cat after electroconvulsive shock. *Science* 154:396, 1966.

25. Cohen, H. B., Duncan, R. F., II, and Dement, W. C. Sleep: the effect of electroconvulsive shock in cats deprived of REM sleep. *Science* 156:1646, 1967.

26. Cohen, H. B., Duncan, R. F., II, and Dement, W. C. The effect of diphenylhydantoin on sleep in the cat. *Electroenceph. Clin. Neurophysiol.* 24:401, 1968.

27. Corletto, F., Gentilomo, A., and Rosadini, G. Confronto tra andamento dell'attività EEG epilettica nel sonno farmacologico e nel sonno spontaneo. *Minerva Neurochir.* 10:313, 1966.

28. Corletto, F., Gentilomo, A., Rosadini, G., and Rossi, G. F. Comportamento durante il sonno delle scariche EEG epilettiche provocate dalla stimolazione luminosa intermittente. *Riv. Neurol.* 37:107, 1967.

29. Delange, M., Baldy, M., Cadilhac, J., and Passouant, P. Études d'épilepsies avec décharges électroencéphalographiques bilatérales. Influence du sommeil de nuit sur les crises et les décharges. *Rev. Neurol.* (Paris) 109:337, 1963.

30. Delange, M., Cadilhac, J. C., El Kassabgui, M., Cadilhac, J., and Passouant, P. The organization of night sleep to epileptics. *Electroenceph. Clin. Neurophysiol.* 23:289, 1967.

31. Delange, M., Castan, Ph., Cadilhac, J., and Passouant, P. A study of night sleep during centrencephalic and temporal epilepsies. *Electroenceph. Clin. Neurophysiol.* 14:777, 1962.

32. Delange, M., Castan, Ph., Cadilhac, J., and Passouant, P. Étude du sommeil de nuit au cours d'épilepsies centrencéphaliques et temporales. *Rev. Neurol.* (Paris) 106:106, 1962.

33. Dement, W. The occurrence of low voltage, fast electroencephalogram patterns during behavioral sleep in the cat. *Electroenceph. Clin. Neurophysiol.* 10:291, 1958.

34. Dement, W. The effect of dream deprivation. *Science* 131:1705, 1960.

35. Dement, W.C. Eye Movements during Sleep. In Bender, M. B. (Ed.), *The Oculomotor System.* New York: Hoeber Med. Div., Harper & Row, 1964.

36. Dement, W., Henry, P., Cohen, H., and Ferguson, J. Studies on the effect of REM deprivation in humans and in animals. *Res. Publ. Ass. Res. Nerv. Ment. Dis.* 45:456, 1967.

37. Dement, W. C., and Kleitman, N. The relation of eye movements during sleep to dream activity: an objective method for the study of dreaming. *J. Exp. Psychol.* 53:339, 1957.

38. Dement, W., and Kleitman, N. Cyclic variations in EEG during sleep and their relation to eye movements, body motility and dreaming. *Electroenceph. Clin. Neurophysiol.* 9:673, 1957.

39. Epstein, A. W., and Hill, W. Total phenomena during REM sleep of a temporal epileptic. *Arch. Neurol.* (Chicago) 15:367, 1966.

40. Evarts, E. V. Temporal patterns of discharge of pyramidal tract neurons during sleep and waking in the monkey. *J. Neurophysiol.* 27:152, 1964.

41. Evarts, E. V. Neuronal Activity in Visual and Motor Cortex during Sleep and Waking. In *Aspects anatomo-fonctionnels de la physiologie du sommeil.* Paris: Éditions

42. Evarts, E. V. Relation of Cell Size to Effects of Sleep in Pyramidal Tract Neurons. In Akert, K., Bally, C., and Schadé, J. P. (Eds.), *Sleep Mechanisms. Progress in Brain Research*, Vol. 18. Amsterdam: Elsevier, 1965.

43. Evarts, E. V. Activity of individual cerebral neurons during sleep and arousal. *Res. Publ. Ass. Res. Nerv. Ment. Dis.* 45:319, 1967.

44. Favale, E. Differente comportamento delle risposte talamo-corticali a reclutamento e ad aumento durante lo stadio più profondo del sonno. *Boll. Soc. Ital. Biol. Sper.* 37:1060, 1961.

45. Ferguson, J. M., and Dement, W. C. The effect of variations in total sleep time on the occurrence of rapid eye movement sleep in cats. *Electroenceph. Clin. Neurophysiol.* 22:2, 1967.

46. Frank, K., and Fuortes, M. G. F. Unitary activity of spinal interneurones of cats. *J. Physiol.* (London) 131:424, 1956.

47. Fujimori, M. Electroencephalographic study on the focal seizure discharges during nocturnal sleep of epileptics. II. Studies on nocturnal sleep of epileptics. *Psychiat. Neurol. Jap.* 68:330, 1966.

48. Gassel, M. M., Marchiafava, P. L., and Pompeiano, O. Phasic changes in muscular activity during desynchronized sleep in unrestrained cats. An analysis of the pattern and organization of myoclonic twitches. *Arch. Ital. Biol.* 102:449, 1964.

49. Gassel, M. M., Marchiafava, P. L., and Pompeiano, O. Tonic and phasic inhibition of spinal reflexes during deep, desynchronized sleep in unrestrained cats. *Arch. Ital. Biol.* 102:471, 1964.

50. Gassel, M. M., Marchiafava, P. L., and Pompeiano, O. An analysis of the supraspinal influences acting on motoneurons during sleep in the unrestrained cat. Modification of the recurrent discharge of the alpha motoneurons during sleep. *Arch. Ital. Biol.* 103:25, 1965.

51. Gassel, M. M., Marchiafava, P. L., and Pompeiano, O. Activity of the red nucleus during deep, desynchronized sleep in unrestrained cats. *Arch. Ital. Biol.* 103:369, 1965.

52. Gastaut, H., Balletto, M., Rhodes, J., Batini, C., and Fressy, J. Étude du sommeil nocturne de 9 sujets présentant un état de mal épileptique généralisé ou focalisé. *Rev. Neurol.* (Paris) 108:173, 1963.

53. Gastaut, H., Batini, C., Broughton, R., Fressy, J., and Tassinari, C. A. Étude électrographique des manifestations paroxystiques, non-épileptiques au cours du sommeil nocturne. *Rev. Neurol.* (Paris) 110:309, 1964.

54. Gastaut, H., Batini, C., and Fressy, J. À propos des crises épileptiques enregistrées au cours du sommeil nocturne chez l'enfant. *Rev. Neurol.* (Paris) 107:276, 1962.

55. Gastaut, H., Batini, C., Fressy, J., Broughton, R., and Tassinari, C. A. Étude électrographique du sommeil nocturne chez les épileptiques. *Rev. Neurol.* (Paris) 110:311, 1964.

56. Gastaut, H., Batini, C., Fressy, J., Broughton, R., Tassinari, C. A., and Vittini, F. Étude électroencéphalographique des phénomènes épisodiques épileptiques au cours du sommeil. In *Le sommeil de nuit normal et pathologique. Études électroencéphalographiques.* Électroencéphalographie et Neurophysiologie clinique (Nouvelle Série) Paris: Masson, 1965, vol. 2, p. 239.

57. Gellhorn, E. *Physiological Foundations of Neurology and Psychiatry*. Minneapolis: University of Minnesota Press, 1953.

58. Giaquinto, S. Changes in the threshold of the recruiting responses during sleep and wakefulness: a quantitative study. *Arch. Ital. Biol.* 106:364, 1968.

59. Giaquinto, S., Pompeiano, O., and Somogyi, I. Supraspinal modulation of monosynaptic and polysynaptic spinal reflexes during natural sleep and wakefulness. *Arch. Ital. Biol.* 102:245, 1964.

60. Gibbs, E. L., and Gibbs, F. A. Diagnostic and localizing value of electroencephalographic studies in sleep. *Res. Publ. Ass. Res. Nerv. Ment. Dis.* 26:366, 1947.

61. Gibbs, F. A., and Gibbs, E. L. *Atlas of Electroencephalography*. II. *Epilepsy*. Reading, Mass.: Addison-Wesley, 1952.

62. Gloor, P., Tsai, C., and Haddad, F. An assessment of the value of sleep electroencephalography for the diagnosis of temporal lobe epilepsy. *Electroenceph. Clin. Neurophysiol.* 10:633, 1958.

63. Halliday, A. M. The electrophysiological study of myoclonus in man. *Brain* 90:241, 1967.

64. Hill, D., and Parr, G. *Electroencephalography*. London: MacDonald, 1963.

65. Hishikawa, Y., Nan'no, H., Tachibana, M., Furuya, E., Koida, H., and Kaneko, Z. The nature of sleep attack and other symptoms of narcolepsy. *Electroenceph. Clin. Neurophysiol.* 24:1, 1968.

66. Hishikawa, Y., Sumitsuji, N., Matsumoto, K., and Kaneko, Z. H-reflex and EMG of the mental and hyoid muscles during sleep, with special reference to narcolepsy. *Electroenceph. Clin. Neurophysiol.* 18:487, 1965.

67. Hishikawa, Y., Yamamoto, J., Furuya, E., Yamada, Y., Migazaki, K., and Kaneko, Z. Photosensitive epilepsy: relationships between the visual evoked responses and the epileptiform discharges induced by intermittent photic stimulation. *Electroenceph. Clin. Neurophysiol.* 23:320, 1967.

68. Hobson, J. A. The effects of chronic brain-stem lesions on cortical and muscular activity during sleep and waking in the cat. *Electroenceph. Clin. Neurophysiol.* 19:41, 1965.

69. Huttenlocher, P. R. Evoked and spontaneous activity in single units of medial brain stem during natural sleep and waking. *J. Neurophysiol.* 24:451, 1961.

70. Jankowska, E., Lund, S., Lundberg, A., and Pompeiano, O. Inhibitory effects evoked through ventral reticulospinal pathways. *Arch. Ital. Biol.* 106:124, 1968.

71. Janz, D. The grand mal epilepsies and the sleeping-waking cycle. *Epilepsia* (Amst.) 3:69, 1962.

72. Jasper, H. H., and Drogleever-Fortuyn, J. Experimental studies on the functional anatomy of petit mal epilepsy. *Res. Publ. Ass. Res. Nerv. Ment. Dis.* 26:272, 1947.

73. Jouvet, M. Behavioural and EEG effects of paradoxical sleep deprivation in the cat. *Proc. XXIII Int. Congr. Physiol. Sci.* (Tokyo), 1965, p. 344.

74. Jouvet, M. Mechanisms of the states of sleep: a neuropharmacological approach. *Res. Publ. Ass. Res. Nerv. Ment. Dis.* 45:86, 1967.

75. Jouvet, M. Neurophysiology of the states of sleep. *Physiol. Rev.* 47:117, 1967.

76. Jovanović, U. J. Das Schlafverhalten der Epileptiker. I. Schlafdauer, Schlaftiefe und Besonderheiten der Schlafperiodik. *Deutsch Z. Nervenheilk.* 190:159, 1967.

77. Jovanović, U. J. Das Schlafverhalten der Epileptiker. II. Elemente des EEG, Vegetativum und Motorik. *Deutsch Z. Nervenheilk.* 191:257, 1967.

78. Kaelbling, R., Koski, E. G., and Hartwig, C. D. Reduction of rapid-eye-movement sleep phase in cats after electroconvulsions. *Psychophysiology* 4:381, 1968.

79. Kajtor, F. Some anatomo-functional factors which may predispose to epileptic seizures occurring during sleep. *Electroenceph. Clin. Neurophysiol.* 13:400, 1961.

80. Kajtor, F. The influence of sleep and the waking state on the epileptic activity of different cerebral structures. *Epilepsia* (Amst.) 3:274, 1962.

81. Kazamatsuri, H. Electroencephalographic study of petit mal epilepsy during natural sleep. I. Studies on nocturnal sleep of epileptics. *Psychiat. Neurol. Jap.* 66:650, 1964.

82. Kleitman, N. Phylogenetic, ontogenetic and environmental determinants in the evolution of sleep-wakefulness cycles. *Res. Publ. Ass. Res. Nerv. Ment. Dis.* 45:30, 1967.

83. Kruse, R. Sleep epilepsy in childhood. Grand mal and focal seizures. Clinical and EEG. *Nervenarzt* 35:200, 1964.

84. Lenzi, G. L., Pompeiano, O., and Rabin, B. Modificazioni ipniche dell'attività unitaria di interneuroni spinali nel gatto non anestetizzato. *Boll. Soc. Ital. Biol. Sper.* Fasc. 20 bis, 44:44, 1968.

85. Llinás, R., and Terzuolo, C. A. Mechanisms of supraspinal actions upon spinal cord activities. Reticular inhibitory mechanisms on alpha extensor motoneurons. *J. Neurophysiol.* 27: 579, 1964.

86. Llinás, R., and Terzuolo, C. A. Mechanisms of supraspinal actions upon spinal cord activities. Reticular inhibitory mechanisms upon flexor motoneurons. *J. Neurophysiol.* 28:413, 1965.

87. Maffei, L., Moruzzi, G., and Rizzolatti, G. Influence of sleep and wakefulness on the response of lateral geniculate units to sinewave photic stimulation. *Arch. Ital. Biol.* 103:596, 1965.

88. Maffei, L., and Rizzolatti, G. Effect of synchronized sleep on the response of lateral geniculate units to flashes of light. *Arch. Ital. Biol.* 103:609, 1965.

89. Mancia, M., and Torrigiani, G. Sonno "rapido" elettroencefalografico e suoi rapporti con l'attività convulsiva. *Riv. Neurol.* 33:475, 1963.

90. Marchiafava, P. L., and Pompeiano, O. Pyramidal influences on spinal cord

during desynchronized sleep. *Arch. Ital. Biol.* 102:500, 1964.

91. Marcus, C. M., and Watson, C. W. Bilateral synchronous spike wave electrographic patterns in the cat. *Arch. Neurol.* (Chicago) 14:601, 1966.

92. Meier-Ewert, K., and Broughton, R. J. Photomyoclonic response of epileptic and non-epileptic subjects during wakefulness, sleep and arousal. *Electroenceph. Clin. Neurophysiol.* 23:142, 1967.

93. Morrison, A. R., and Pompeiano, O. An analysis of the supraspinal influences acting on motoneurons during sleep in the unrestrained cat. Responses of the alpha motoneurons to direct electrical stimulation during sleep. *Arch. Ital. Biol.* 103:497, 1965.

94. Morrison, A. R., and Pompeiano, O. Central depolarization of group Ia afferent fibers during desynchronized sleep. *Arch. Ital. Biol.* 103:517, 1965.

95. Morrison, A. R., and Pompeiano, O. Pyramidal discharge from somatosensory cortex and cortical control of primary afferents during sleep. *Arch. Ital. Biol.* 103:538, 1965.

96. Morrison, A. R., and Pompeiano, O. Vestibular influences during sleep. II. Effects of vestibular lesions on the pyramidal discharge during desynchronized sleep. *Arch. Ital. Biol.* 104:214, 1966.

97. Morrison, A. R., and Pompeiano, O. Vestibular influences during sleep. IV. Functional relations between vestibular nuclei and lateral geniculate nucleus during desynchronized sleep. *Arch. Ital. Biol.* 104:425, 1966.

98. Moruzzi, G. Synchronizing influences of the brain stem and the inhibitory mechanisms underlying the production of sleep by sensory stimulation. *Electroenceph. Clin. Neurophysiol.* Suppl. 13, 231, 1960.

99. Moruzzi, G. The historical development of the deafferentation hypothesis of sleep. *Proc. Amer. Phil. Soc.* 108:19, 1964.

100. Moruzzi, G., and Magoun, H. W. Brain stem reticular formation and activation of the EEG. *Electroenceph. Clin. Neurophysiol.* 1:455, 1949.

101. Niedermeyer, E. The generalized multiple spike discharge. An electroclinical study. *Electroenceph. Clin. Neurophysiol.* 20:133, 1966.

102. Okuma, T., and Fujimori, M. Electrographic and evoked potential studies during sleep in the cat. I. The study on sleep. *Folia Psychiat. Neurol. Jap.* 17:25, 1963.

103. Okuma, T., Kuba, K., Tatsushita, T., Nakao, T., Fujii, S., and Shimoda, Y. Study on 14 and 6 per second positive spikes during nocturnal sleep. *Electroenceph. Clin. Neurophysiol.* 25:140, 1968.

104. Okuma, T., and Sekiguchi, M. Neurophysiology of sleep. *Clin. Psychiat.* 4:807, 1962.

105. Oller-Daurella, L. Deprivation of sleep as a method of activating epileptic attacks. *Electroenceph. Clin. Neurophysiol.* 23:288, 1967.

106. Passouant, P. Séméiologie EEG du sommeil normal et pathologique. *Rev. Neurol.* (Paris) 83:545, 1950.

107. Passouant, P. Epilepsie temporale et sommeil. *Rev. Roum. Neurol.* 4:151, 1963.

108. Passouant, P., and Cadilhac, J. Influence des differentes phases du sommeil nocturne sur les décharges épileptiques chez l'homme. In *Aspects anatomo-fonctionnels de la physiologie du sommeil.* Paris: Éditions du Centre National de la Recherche Scientifique, 1965.

109. Passouant, J., Cadilhac, J., and Delange, M. Indications apportées par l'étude du sommeil de nuit sur la physiopathologie des épilepsies. *Int. J. Neurol.* 5:207, 1965.

110. Passouant, P., Cadilhac, J., Delange, M., and Castan, Ph. Indications apportées par l'étude des divers stades du sommeil sur la physiopathologie du Petit Mal. *Arch. Franç. Pédiat.* 19:1389, 1962.

111. Passouant, P., Cadilhac, J., and Philippot, M. Rythmicité du petit-mal au cours du sommeil. Decharges rhythmiques généralisées et localisées. *Rev. Neurol.* (Paris) 84:659, 1951.

112. Passouant, P., Gros, C., Cadilhac, J., Delange, M., Baldy-Moulinier, M., and Billet, M. Accès en série dûs à une cicatrice de l'aire supplémentaire motrice. Effet du sommeil de nuit sur les décharges épileptiques. *Rev. Neurol.* (Paris) 109:360, 1963.

113. Passouant, P., Gros, C., Cadilhac, J., and El Kassabgui, M. Frontal epilepsy and night sleep: effects of the rapid eye movement phase. *Electroenceph. Clin. Neurophysiol.* 22:279, 1967.

114. Penfield, W., and Jasper, H. *Epilepsy and the Functional Anatomy of the Human Brain.* Boston: Little, Brown, 1954.
115. Perria, L., Rosadini, G., Rossi, G. F., and Gentilomo, A. Neurosurgical aspects of epilepsy: physiological sleep as a means of focalizing EEG epileptic discharge. *Acta Neurochir.* 14:1, 1966.
116. Phillips. C. G. Intracellular records from Betz cells in the cat. *Quart. J. Exp. Physiol.* 41:58, 1956.
117. Phillips, C. G. Action of antidromic pyramidal volleys on single Betz cells in the cat. *Quart. J. Exp. Physiol.* 44:1, 1959.
118. Pompeiano, O. Ascending and Descending Influences of Somatic Afferent Volleys in Unrestrained Cats: Supraspinal Inhibitory Control of Spinal Reflexes during Natural and Reflexly Induced Sleep. In *Aspects anatomo-fonctionnels de la physiologie du sommeil.* Paris: Éditions du Centre National de la Recherche Scientifique, 1965.
119. Pompeiano, O. Muscular Afferents and Motor Control during Sleep. In Granit, R. (Ed.), Nobel Symposium I. *Muscular Afferents and Motor Control.* Stockholm: Almqvist and Wiksell, 1966.
120. Pompeiano, O. The neurophysiological mechanisms of the postural and motor events during desynchronized sleep. *Res. Publ. Ass. Res. Nerv. Ment. Dis.* 45:351, 1967.
121. Pompeiano, O. Sensory Inhibition during Motor Activity in Sleep. In Yahr, M. D., and Purpura, D. P. (Eds.), *Neurophysiological Basis of Normal and Abnormal Motor Activities.* Hewlett, New York: Raven Press, 1967.
122. Pompeiano, O. Mechanisms of Sensory-Motor Integration During Sleep. In Stellar, E., and Sprague, J. M. (Eds.), *Progress in Physiological Psychology.* New York: Academic, in press.
123. Pompeiano, O. Vestibular Influences during Sleep. In *Handbook of Sensory Physiology.* VI. *Vestibular System.* Berlin, Heidelberg, New York: Springer, in press.
124. Pompeiano, O. Interaction between Vestibular and Nonvestibular Sensory Inputs. In Fourth Symposium on *The Role of the Vestibular Organs in Space Exploration.* NASA SP, in press.
125. Pompeiano, O., and Morrison, A. R. Vestibular influences during sleep. I. Abolition of the rapid eye movements during desynchronized sleep following vestibular lesions. *Arch. Ital. Biol.* 103:569, 1965.
126. Pompeiano, O., and Satoh, T. Vestibular influences on the red nucleus during sleep. *Pflueger Arch. Ges. Physiol.* 298:159, 1967.
127. Pratt, K. L., Mattson, R. H., Weikers, N. J., and Williams, R. EEG activation of epileptics following sleep deprivation: a prospective study of 114 cases. *Electroenceph. Clin. Neurophysiol.* 24:11, 1968.
128. Purpura, D. P., McMurtry, J. G., and Maekawa, K. Synaptic events in ventrolateral thalamic neurons during suppression of recruiting responses by brain stem reticular formation. *Brain Res.* 1:63, 1966.
129. Purpura, D. P., and Yahr, M. D. (Eds.). *The Thalamus.* New York: Columbia University Press, 1966.
130. Rabending, G. Les variations de l'excitabilité réflexe proprioceptive pendant les absences cliniques et au début du Grand Mal centrencéphalique photosensible. *Rev. Neurol.* (Paris) 117:168, 1967.
131. Rabending, G. Variations of proprioceptive reflex excitability during clinical absence and at the beginning of photosensitive centrencephalic grand mal. *Electroenceph. Clin. Neurophysiol.* 23:387, 1967.
132. Ralston, B., and Ajmone-Marsan, C. Thalamic control of certain normal and abnormal cortical rhythms. *Electroenceph. Clin. Neurophysiol.* 8:559, 1956.
133. Rechtschaffen, A., and Dement, W. Studies on the relation of narcolepsy, cataplexy, and sleep with low voltage random EEG activity. *Res. Publ. Ass. Res. Nerv. Ment. Dis.* 45:488, 1967.
134. Rechtschaffen, A., Wolpert, E. A., Dement, W. C., Mitchell, S. A., and Fisher, C. Nocturnal sleep of narcoleptics. *Electroenceph. Clin. Neurophysiol.* 15:599, 1963.
135. Rexed, B. A cytoarchitectonic atlas of the spinal cord in the cat. *J. Comp. Neurol.* 100:297, 1954.
136. Rodin, E. A., Daly, D. D., and Bickford, R. G. Effects of photic stimulation during sleep: study of normal subjects and epileptic patients. *Neurology* (Minneap.) 5:149, 1955.
137. Roffwarg, H. P., Muzio, J. N., and

Dement, W. C. Ontogenetic development of the human sleep-dream cycle. *Science* 152:604, 1966.

138. Ross, J. J., Johnson, L. C., and Walter, R. D. Spike and wave discharges during stages of sleep. *Arch. Neurol.* (Chicago) 14:399, 1966.

139. Rossi, G. F. Sleep inducing mechanisms in the brain stem. *Electroenceph. Clin. Neurophysiol.* Suppl. 24, 113, 1963.

140. Rossi, G. F., Corletto, F., Gentilomo, A., and Rosadini, G. Essai d'interprétation sur une base neurophysiologique des mécanismes de production de décharges convulsives bilatérales et synchrones. *Neurochirurgie* (Paris) 13:547, 1967.

141. Rossi, G. F., Favale, E., Hara, T., Giussani, A., and Sacco, G. Researches on the nervous mechanisms underlying deep sleep in the cat. *Arch. Ital. Biol.* 99:270, 1961.

142. Schwartz, B. A., and Guilbaud, G. Étude électroclinique de crisés B.-J.: enregistrement d'une nuit de sommeil. *Rev. Neurol.* (Paris) 106:126, 1962.

143. Schwartz, B. A., Guilbaud, G., and Fischgold, H. Études électroencéphalographiques sur le sommeil de nuit. II. L'épilepsie. *Presse Med.* 71:1978, 1963.

144. Schwartz, B. A., Guilbaud, G., and Fischgold, H. Single and multiple spikes in the night sleep of epileptics. *Electroenceph. Clin. Neurophysiol.* 16:56, 1964.

145. Scollo-Lavizzari, G., and Hess, R. Photic stimulation during paradoxical sleep in photosensitive subjects. *Neurology* (Minneap.) 17:604, 1967.

146. Shimizu, K., Refsum, S., and Gibbs, F. A. Effects on the electrical activity of the brain of intra-arterially and intracerebrally injected convulsant and sedative drugs (metrazol and nembutal). *Electroenceph. Clin. Neurophysiol.* 4:141, 1952.

147. Toman, J. E. P. Drugs Effective in Convulsive Disorders. In Goodman, L. S., and Gilman, A. (Eds.), *The Pharmacological Basis of Therapeutics*. New York: Macmillan, 1965.

148. Vogel, G. Studies in psychophysiology of dreams. III. The dream of narcolepsy. *Arch. Gen. Psychiat.* (Chicago) 3:421, 1960.

149. Walter, G. W. The functions of electrical rhythms in the brain. *J. Ment. Sci.* 96:1, 1950.

150. Woodbury, D. M. Effect of diphenylhydantoin on electrolytes and radiosodium turnover in brain and other tissues of normal, hyponatremic and postictal rats. *J. Pharmacol. Exp. Ther.* 115:74, 1955.

151. Yamaguchi, N., Ling, G. M., and Marczynski, T. J. Recruiting responses observed during wakefulness and sleep in unanesthetized chronic cats. *Electroenceph. Clin. Neurophysiol.* 17:246, 1964.

152. Zarcone, V., Gulevich, G., and Dement, W. Sleep and electroconvulsive therapy. *Arch. Gen. Psychiat.* 16:567, 1967.

Discussion

BASAL FOREBRAIN INHIBITION*

CARMINE D. CLEMENTE

Importance of the synchronized stages of sleep in reference to epilepsy was stressed by Pompeiano, since frequently there is observed in man a marked increase in epileptiform discharge when a waking patient becomes drowsy or falls asleep. For the past 9 years our research interests at the University of California at Los Angeles have dealt with brain mechanisms related to states of behavioral suppression. Interest, most specifically, was in those physiological states which, either during wakefulness or sleep, were accompanied by a synchronized electroencephalogram. Studies focused on two groups of behaviors: the slow-wave stages of sleep, where the synchronized EEG is generalized over widespread cortical regions; and the group of behaviors in which EEG synchronization is observed in alert cats performing a task which requires the withholding of some class of somatomotor response. This latter type of behavior was described as internal inhibition by Pavlov [8] and is accompanied by more localized cortical synchronization, especially over the sensory motor cortex [1, 6, 15]. The former of these two groups will be stressed—those related to forebrain structures which appear to be involved in the onset of slow-wave sleep.

With Sterman [14] it has been reported that low voltage electrical stimulation bilaterally of basal forebrain structures (especially the preoptic zones) had the behavioral effect of inducing onset of sleep. It was found that this behavior was accompanied by electrocortical correlates of sleep, a slowing of the EEG to synchronous patterns characteristic of the initial, slow-wave stages of sleep. Both the EEG synchronization and the induction of sleep could be conditioned by pairing an indifferent tone with brain stimulation [5]. We also found that the orbital gyrus of the frontal lobe was functionally related to these basal forebrain sites [13] and that in addition to influencing the EEG, electrical stimulation of these same areas profoundly affected reflexes in the brain stem and in the spinal cord [11, 12]. For the most part, the nature of this effect is a suppression of activity out the final common pathways to the musculature of the face, neck, and limbs and those muscles which close the jaw and move the eyes. Thus, it has been found that an inhibition of reflex activity can be induced by stimulation of the orbital gyrus along final pathways involving the oculomotor, trigeminal, and facial cranial nerves as well as monosynaptic and polysynaptic reflexes in the cervical, lumbar, and sacral regions of the spinal cord.

STUDIES INVOLVING CRANIAL NERVES

Evidence has been obtained that orbital gyrus stimulation induces suppression of activity reflexly initiated along the oculomotor, trigeminal, and facial nerves. Figure D17-1 shows the most recent of experiments in this series of studies. A response has been elicited along the oculomotor nerve by an electrical stimulus applied to the medial vestibular nucleus. It is well known, of course, that the vestibular nuclei transmit incoming signals along the medial longitudinal fasciculus to the motor nuclei innervating the extraocular muscles. This pathway is supposedly responsible for vestibulo-ocular reflexes [2] and presumably

---

* This research supported by PHS Research Grant MH10083 from National Institute of Mental Health.

DISCUSSION: BASAL FOREBRAIN INHIBITION 475

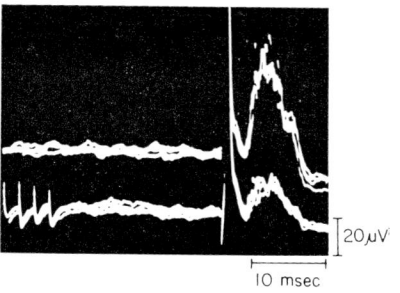

FIG. D17-1. Top trace shows four superimposed evoked potentials recorded along a branch of left oculomotor nerve which was dissected free within the orbit of adult cat. Stimuli delivered to ipsilateral medial vestibular nucleus at rate of 1 per sec (0.1 msec duration, 10 V). Lower trace shows five superimposed sweeps under same conditions except that each stimulus to vestibular nucleus was preceded by 4 pulses (0.1 msec duration, 7 V) applied to ipsilateral orbital gyrus commencing about 45 msec before test shocks. Note orbital gyrus stimulations suppressed activity along oculomotor nerve by about 70 percent.

is also the pathway regarded important in elicitation of eye movements during the paradoxical phase of sleep [10]. Although most investigators have wondered why the eyes move during the paradoxical phase of sleep (a phenomenon also existent during wakefulness), we have asked the question conversely. By which mechanisms do the eyes virtually stop moving and the eyelids relax during the initial slow-wave phases of sleep? It can be seen in Fig. D17-1 that four shocks applied to orbital gyrus 20–40 msec prior to stimulating the vestibular nucleus result in diminution of the evoked potential recorded along the oculomotor nerve by almost 70 percent. Other experiments involving the oculomotor, trochlear, and abducens nerves are in progress.

When stimulating electrodes are placed in the *trigeminal* mesencephalic nucleus and recording electrodes placed on the masseteric branch of the mandibular nerve, low voltage stimulation will give rise to a two-component peripheral, trigeminal nerve

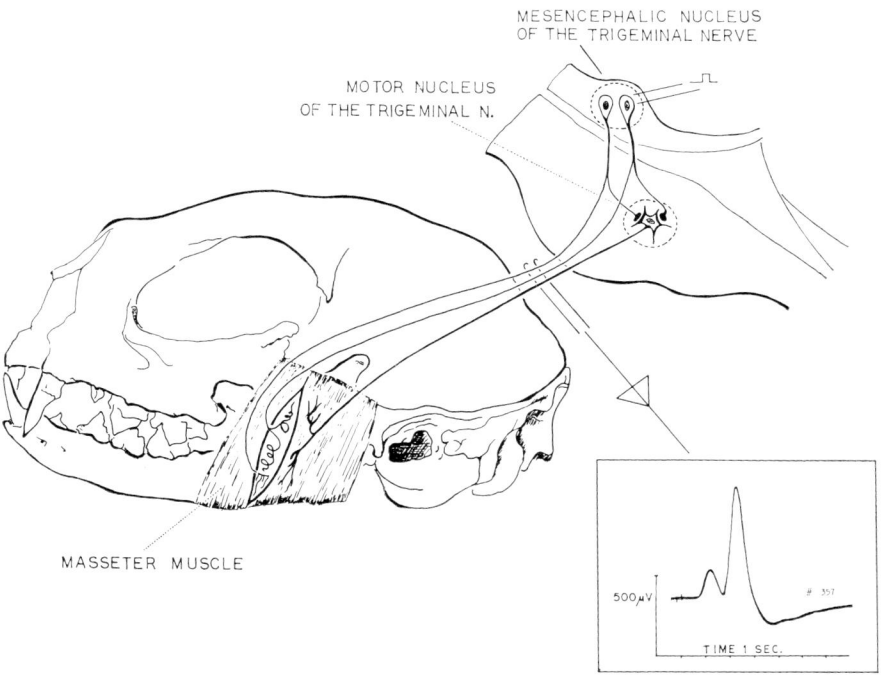

FIG. D17-2. Anatomical elements comprising masseteric reflex. Stimuli delivered to cells in mesencephalic nucleus and recordings made on masseteric nerve. Two-component response at lower right composed of initial antidromic potential and secondary reflex potential.

response (Fig. D17-2, insert). The first component of this masseteric nerve response is an antidromic volley mediated peripherally directly by axons of sensory neurons of the mesencephalic nucleus, while the second component is the orthodromic monosynaptic reflex potential through motoneurons in the motor nucleus of V. Axon collaterals from mesencephalic neurons act as the presynaptic elements of this reflex, while motor neurons are the postsynaptic elements (Fig. D17-2). Consistent inhibition of the masseteric reflex was observed by stimulation of anterior-lateral preoptic and other basal forebrain sites and by stimulation of the orbital gyrus of the frontal cerebral cortex (Fig. D17-5A).

Intracellular potentials were then recorded within masseteric motor neurons. These cells were identified by the antidromic spike-potential evoked by stimulation of the masseteric nerve as illustrated in Fig. D17-3A. When the intracellular recording had been identified as coming from a masseteric motor neuron by recording of the antidromic potential, stimulation in the mesencephalic nucleus of the trigeminal nerve evoked an orthodromic-masseteric reflex such as the potential illustrated in Fig. D17-3B. At this point

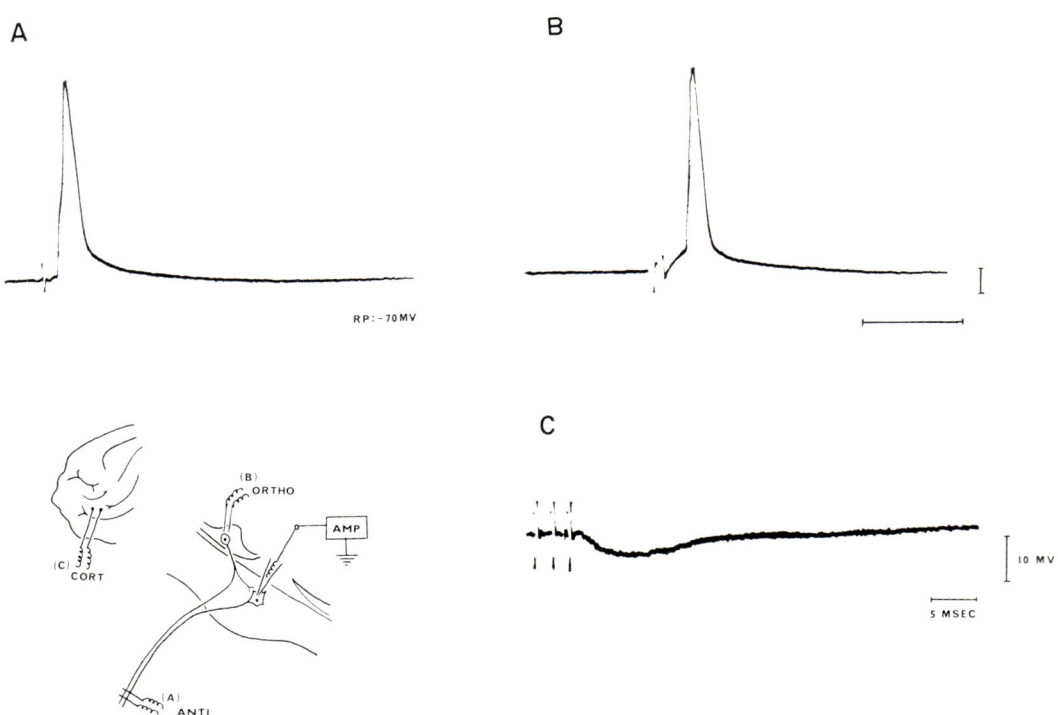

FIG. D17-3. Intracellular microelectrode (3M KCl-filled glass capillary electrode) recordings within motoneuron of trigeminal motor nucleus. (A) Antidromic spike potential recorded within a fifth motoneuron by stimulation antidromically along masseteric nerve (see diagram). This potential identifies motoneuron, consists of initial segment spike (IS), a somadendritic spike (SD), an afterdepolarization and an afterhyperpolarization. (B) Orthodromic intracellular spike-potential induced through stimulation of mesencephalic nucleus of trigeminal nerve (see diagram). This potential consists of an EPSP, IS, SD, an afterdepolarization, and an afterhyperpolarization. (C) Hyperpolarization induced within a fifth motoneuron by three shocks delivered to orbital gyrus of frontal lobe (see diagram). There is marked early hyperpolarization followed by later prolonged hyperpolarization. (Nakamura, Goldberg, Clemente, unpublished.)

DISCUSSION: BASAL FOREBRAIN INHIBITION

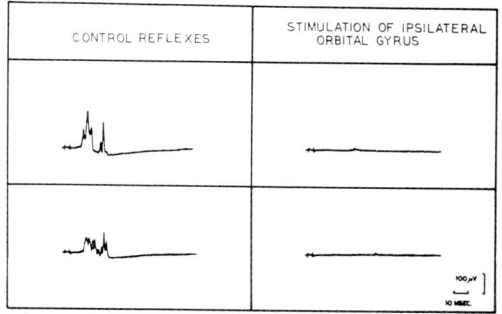

FIG. D17-4. Corneal reflexes and their inhibition. Control reflexes (left) obtained by electrically stimulating surface of cornea with silver ball electrodes (4 V, 2 msec duration) and recording along fibers of branch of facial nerve which innervates orbicularis oculi muscle. Upon stimulation of orbital gyrus with 6 pulses (frequency of pulses 300 per sec; 6 V; 0.75 msec) it can be observed that complete inhibition of reflex resulted. (Sauerland and Clemente, unpublished observations.)

stimulation of the orbital gyrus, using the same parameters found effective in reflexive inhibition, resulted in the induction of hyperpolarizing potentials within previously identified, masseteric motor neurons (Fig. D17-3C). These studies have been reported in more detail [7].

Electrical stimulation on the surface of the cornea will give rise to a reflexive closing of the eye. This muscular response is accompanied by evoked potentials which can be recorded along that branch of the *facial nerve* which innervates the orbicularis oculi muscle (Fig. D17-4). Once again such an evoked cranial nerve reflexive discharge could be completely inhibited if the orbital gyrus of the cerebral cortex was stimulated with pulses prior to the elicitation of the reflex.

STUDIES INVOLVING SPINAL NERVES

In addition to reflexes involving cranial nerves, a systematic exploration of spinal reflexes was performed in a series of acute experiments. Electrical stimulation applied to the orbital gyrus resulted in immediate and consistent inhibition of electrically elicited reflexes at cervical (Fig. D17-5B, C, and D), lumbar (Fig. D17-5E), and sacral levels (Fig. D17-5F). To achieve these results the most effective cortical stimulation pattern consisted of a train of 4–7 square-wave pulses with pulse intervals of 10–15 msec (individual pulse duration 0.7–2.0 msec; pulse amplitude 5–8 V). Optimal inhibition was obtained when the cortical pulses preceded the test reflex by intervals of 5–20 msec.

Initial stages of sleep behavior might best be described as consisting of a series of reactions involving various segments of the neuraxis. At the highest levels, the EEG becomes synchronized while postural adjustments are observed simultaneously at brain stem and spinal levels. In almost all higher animals, EEG synchronization is accompanied by reduction in extraocular eye movements, closure of eyelids, relaxation of unsupported lower jaw, and gradual diminution in tonic neck muscular activity along with reduced tone in muscles of extremities. Most animals assume some characteristic position, although this need not be the case.

Under all circumstances it has been our intention to analyze individual components of the total initial sleep behavioral pattern by studying relevant individual neuronal circuits separately in acute experiments and collectively in behaving animals. Each question which has been put to test has reinforced the notion that onset of sleep is an active process involving basal medial forebrain structures including the orbital surface of the frontal lobe [4]. It is also felt that these same forebrain sites can markedly suppress activity within pools of final common motoneurons in the direction expected with onset of sleep. It is of particular interest that certain observations in man have similarly implicated basal medial forebrain structures with synchronization of the EEG. Penfield and Jasper [9] have described bilateral synchronization of the EEG in patients in which these areas are the sites of parasagittal epileptogenic lesions resulting from basal medial frontal-lobe tumors.

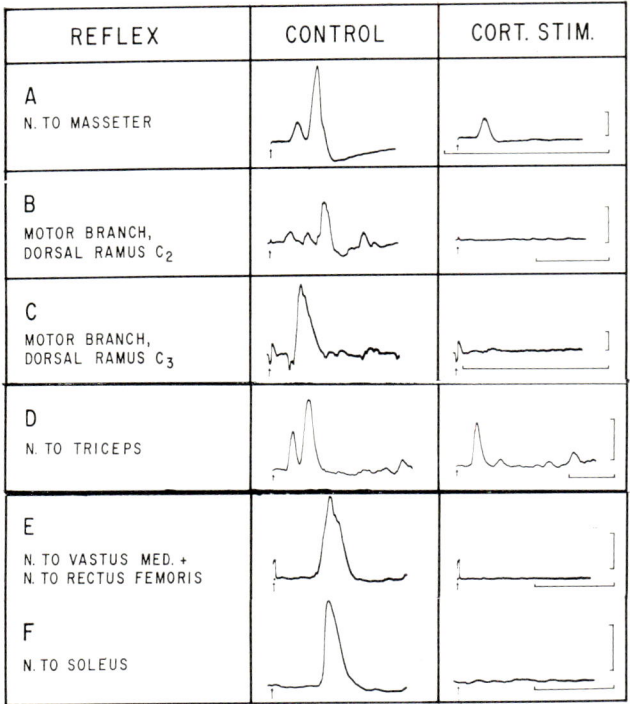

Fig. D17-5. Cortically induced inhibition of reflexes mediated in motor nerves of the face (A), neck (B) and (C), forelimb (D), and hindlimb (E) and (F) of the cat. Reflexes were recorded from the proximal portion of the severed motor nerve (A), (B), (C), and (D) or from the ventral root of L-5 (E) or L-7 (F). Reflex elicitation: (A) Stimulation of mesencephalic nucleus of trigeminal nerve by stereotaxically placed bipolar electrode. (B) and (C) Stimulation of proximal end of cut dorsal roots C_2 and C_3 respectively. (D) Stimulation of dorsal root of C_7. (E) and (F) Stimulation of proximal end of cut motor nerve. In all cases inhibition was achieved by applying 4–7 square-wave pulses to orbital gyrus with pulse intervals of 10–15 msec (individual pulse duration 0.7–2.0 msec; 5–8 V). Time line, (A), (B), and (C) 10 msec; (D), (E), and (F) 5 msec. Amplitude (A), (B), and (C) 200μV; (D), (E), and (F) 500 μV.

REFERENCES

1. Anokhin, P. K. Electroencephalographic analysis of cortico-subcortical relations in positive and negative conditioned reactions. *Ann. N. Y. Acad. Sci.* 92:899, 1961.
2. Brodal, A., Pompeiano, O., and Walberg, F. *The Vestibular Nuclei and Their Connections.* Edinburgh: Oliver and Boyd, 1962.
3. Clemente, C. D., Chase, M. H., Knauss, T. K., Sauerland, E. K., and Sterman, M. B. Inhibition of a monosynaptic reflex by electrical stimulation of the basal forebrain or the orbital gyrus in the cat. *Experientia* 22:844, 1966.
4. Clemente, C. D., and Sterman, M. B. Basal Forebrain Mechanisms for Internal Inhibition and Sleep. In Kety, S., Evarts, E., and Williams, H. (Eds.), *Sleep and Altered States of Consciousness*, Ass. Res. Nerv. Ment. Dis. Baltimore: Williams & Wilkins, 45:127, 1967.
5. Clemente, C. D., Sterman, M. B., and Wyrwicka, W. Forebrain inhibitory mechanisms: Conditioning of basal forebrain induced EEG synchronization and sleep. *Exp. Neurol.* 7:404, 1963.
6. Gastaut, H. Some Aspects of Neurophysiological Basis of Conditioned Reflexes and Behavior. In Wolstenholme, G. E. W., and O'Conner, C. M. (Eds.), *Ciba Founda-*

tion Symposium on the Neurological Basis of Behavior. London: Churchill, 1958.

7. Nakamura, Y., Goldberg, L. J., and Clemente, C. D. Nature of suppression of the masseteric monosynaptic reflex induced by stimulation of the orbital gyrus of the cat. Brain Res. 6:184, 1967.

8. Pavlov, I. P. Conditioned Reflexes. New York and London: Oxford University Press, 1928.

9. Penfield, W., and Jasper, H. Epilepsy and the Functional Anatomy of the Human Brain. Boston: Little, Brown, 1954.

10. Pompeiano, O., and Morrison, A. R. Vestibular origin of the rapid eye movements during desynchronized sleep. Experientia 22:60, 1966.

11. Sauerland, E. K., Knauss, T., Nakamura, Y., and Clemente, C. D. Inhibition of monosynaptic and polysynaptic reflexes and muscle tone by electrical stimulation of the cerebral cortex. Exp. Neurol. 17: 159, 1967.

12. Sauerland, E. K., Nakamura, Y., and Clemente, C. D. The role of the lower brain stem in cortically induced inhibition of somatic reflexes in the cat. Brain Res. 6:164, 1967.

13. Sterman, M. B., Chase, M. H., Knauss, T., and Clemente, C. D. Cortical, limbic and visceral connections of the basal forebrain area in the cat. Physiologist 7:264, 1964.

14. Sterman, M. B., and Clemente, C. D. Forebrain inhibitory mechanisms: Sleep patterns induced by basal forebrain stimulation. Exp. Neurol. 6:103, 1962.

15. Sterman, M. B., and Wyrwicka, W. EEG correlates of sleep: Evidence for separate forebrain substrates. Brain Res. 6:143, 1967.

18
Stability and Seizure Susceptibility of Immature Brain*

DOMINICK P. PURPURA

CLINICAL and electrographic manifestations of convulsions in the newborn human infant exhibit a number of characteristics that are distinctly different from those observed in later childhood or in adults [35]. In the neonatal infant, dissociations between EEG patterns and clinical events are prominent, and absence of generalization and restricted seizure propagation are frequently evident [15, 40]. Similar observations have been made in immature born animals of different species following paroxysmal activity induced by topically applied convulsants [4, 6, 12, 36, 75], cortical lesions [22], or electric stimulation [4, 10, 11, 24, 32, 33, 36, 41, 69]. It has long been established from these studies that maturation of seizure susceptibility parallels an ontogenetic decrease in threshold for seizure induction, increase in frequency, duration, and spread of afterdischarges, and augmentation in the capacity for seizure generalization. While such studies highlight complexities of the maturational processes in brain they have contributed little to the analysis of important details of physiological and pathophysiological mechanisms which underlie development of seizure susceptibility, or, for that matter, factors which limit the convulsant potentiality of the immature brain.

Attempts to understand seizure phenomena in the immature brain require consideration of the developmental patterns of immature neurons and their synaptic organizations at different postnatal periods. Suffice it to say that such analyses should be concerned with biophysical properties of immature neurons, nature and function of their synaptic relations, and the unique morphophysiological features of immature neurons that may contribute to stability or instability of neuronal-network operations.

The present report surveys a number of ontogenetic studies relevant to the foregoing problem. For the most part, these studies have utilized intracellular recording techniques to provide information on properties of immature cortical neurons that could not be obtained solely from studies of surface-evoked potentials. The author's decision to restrict the scope of this inquiry into the intimate behavior of immature neurons and neuronal organizations reflects his view that significant advances in understanding normal and abnormal functions of the immature brain are more likely to be forthcoming from studies of basic properties of immature neurons and their synaptic relations than from analyses of evoked potentials. This is not to infer that appropriately designed, evoked-potential studies are of little value. On the contrary, ontogenetic studies of evoked potentials have been extremely productive in elucidating, in a broad brush-stroke fashion, general features of functional development of the brain [19, 20, 27, 61, 63, 65, 67].

* Supported in part by PHS Research Grant NB07512 from National Institute of Neurological Diseases and Stroke and grants from United Cerebral Palsy Educational and Research Foundation and Given Foundation.

Evoked-potential studies combined with morphological investigations have provided data of considerable importance from the standpoint of structure-function correlations [3, 5, 12, 21, 23, 37, 38, 43, 44, 45, 47, 49, 66]. The point of emphasis is that such correlations must now be examined in greater detail to obtain necessary data on basic mechanisms. To achieve this requires a major effort in applying more refined experimental methods to the study of the immature brain [26, 28, 54, 58]. Several intracellular and electron microscopic studies which will be described may be considered initial steps in this direction. These and other studies bear on the general problem of designing adequate experiments to examine morphogenetic and pathophysiological factors underlying seizure susceptibility of the immature brain.

Relationship of Properties of Immature Cortical Neurons to Characteristics of Seizure Discharges in Neonatal Period

Analysis of the electrographic characteristics of focal epileptiform *spikes* in immature cortex has indicated that such discharges are generally longer in overall duration than discharges observed in adult animals [6, 11, 12, 22, 75]. These observations conform to numerous findings on evoked potentials recorded from the scalp or cortical surface in the newborn human infant and immature born animals [3, 5, 20, 21, 27, 37, 38, 44, 61, 67]. The changing characteristics of epileptiform spikes or evoked potentials during postnatal development undoubtedly reflect dramatic organizational changes in the morphology and functional properties of immature neurons and their synaptic relations. Evidence bearing on the nature of these changes has been obtained in several types of morphological studies of immature mammalian brain [7, 12, 13, 16, 21, 37, 38, 39, 56, 64, 66, 74, 76].

Examination of Golgi-Cox preparations of neonatal kitten neocortex discloses that pyramidal neurons have well-developed apical dendrites but poorly developed or absent basilar dendrites (Fig. 18-1). Apical dendrites at this developmental stage exhibit tuberosities and occasional tangential branches but lack typical spines until the end of the first postnatal week. Axons of pyramidal neurons are of small caliber (<2 μ) and generally lack axon collaterals in the immediate neonatal period. In contrast to most pyramidal neurons, stellate cells and granule cells exhibit extreme variability in maturational status in the newborn kitten [39, 66].

Only with electron microscopy [74] is it possible to obtain a more complete picture of the extraordinary packing density of apical dendrites in neuropil regions of cortex (Fig. 18-1B). Extensive dendrodendritic membrane appositions are common and relatively large dendritic and axonal processes are detectable in the neuropil. In view of current interest in the possible contribution of glial activities to cortical electrogenesis, it is noteworthy that in the immediate neonatal period glial cells are poorly developed [7]; interposition of glial processes between neural elements is seldom encountered unlike the situation in the kitten that is 1–2 weeks old. Accordingly, it is reasonable to refer to the neonatal kitten cortex as a *neural*, rather than a *neuralglial* brain, which more appropriately describes cellular relations in cortex of older kittens and adult animals [7].

It is likely that neuronal, particularly dendritic, packing density observed in the neonatal kitten cortex plays an important role in determining the long duration of evoked potentials and presumably cortical, epileptiform spikes. Since it has been shown that axodendritic synapses are differentially well developed in respect to axosomatic synapses in the neonatal kitten neocortex

Fig. 18-1. (*A*) Golgi-Cox preparation of pyramidal neurons in neocortex of newborn kitten. Note well-developed apical dendrites and absence of basilar dendrites. Dendritic spines are not observed at this stage, and tangential spread of apical dendrites in molecular layer is less than 50 μ. Apical dendrites are about 0.3 mm in length in this microphotograph. (From Purpura, Carmichael, and Housepian [49].) (*B*) Electron micrograph of elements in superficial regions of neocortex of fetal kitten. N, two neuron cell bodies with 4–6 dendrites packed between them. Note absence of glial

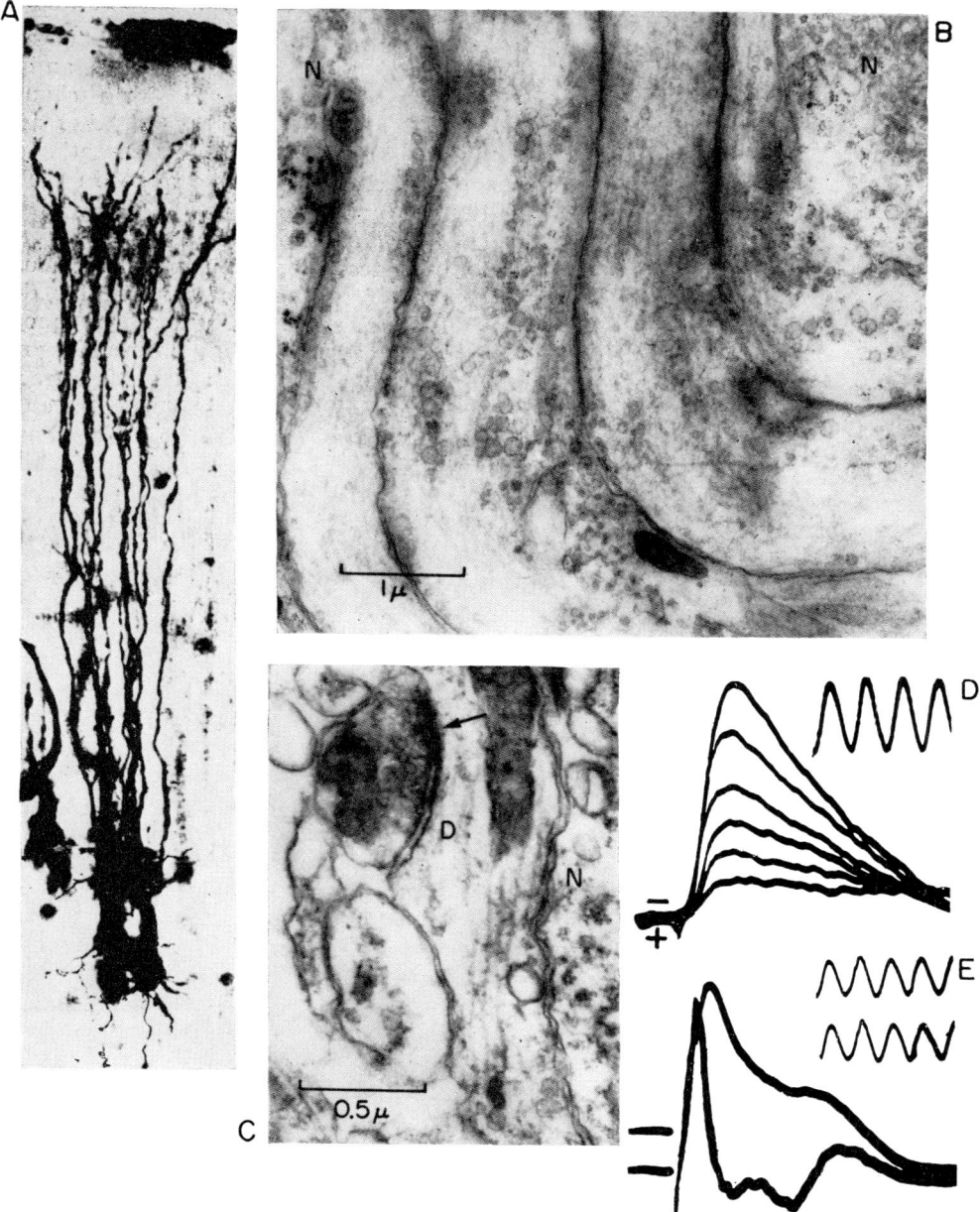

processes between neural elements at this developmental stage and indistinct appearance of dendritic tubules. (From Voeller, Pappas, and Purpura [74].) (C) Axodendritic synapse from the superficial neuropil of newborn kitten neocortex. D, dendrites. N, neuron cell body. Arrow indicates region of postsynaptic thickening. Presynaptic axon terminal exhibits clusters of synaptic vesicles and mitochondria. (From Purpura [45].) (D) Characteristics of long-duration graded superficial cortical responses recorded 1.5 mm from stimulating electrodes on suprasylvian gyrus of a near-term fetal kitten. Stimulus frequency 0.5 per sec. Six superimposed responses at different stimulus strengths. Calibrations, 100 cps; 0.1 mV. (E) Comparison of superficial cortical responses recorded at 1.5 mm with a large (0.5 mm) ball-tipped electrode (upper channel) and response recorded at site of stimulation with a 0.1 mm wire electrode in a newborn kitten, calibration 100 cps; 0.1 mV. (D and E from Purpura, Carmichael, and Housepian [49].)

[74], it follows that much of the electrical activity recorded during the neonatal period is referable to axodendritic synapses, both excitatory and inhibitory. In this context it may be noted that the superficial cortical response (SCR) evoked by local cortical-surface stimulation is similar in all respects (except in duration) when recorded several millimeters away from the site of stimulation in neonatal and near-term fetal kittens [49].

The substrate for SCR production must comprise the system of superficial axodendritic synapses since these are the only elements capable of being activated by conductile pathways over relatively long distances in immature cortex [49]. Duration of the SCR in immature cortex is similar to that observed in adult animals only when the recording electrode is placed as close as possible to the site of stimulation (Fig. 18-1D). Thus the long duration of the SCR, when recorded in immature cortex in a manner similar to that in adult animals, reflects: (a) the temporal dispersion in small caliber axons which constitute the presynaptic pathway, and (b) the summation of PSPs generated in a relatively large population of densely packed dendritic elements. Progressive decrease in duration of most components of evoked potentials and the shorter duration and more *hypersynchronous* nature of the focal epileptiform spike [75] occurs pari passu with decrease in packing density of cortical neurons. This is occasioned by elaboration of fine processes of the neuropil and interposition of glial elements [74].

Striking changes also occur in number and distribution of synapses on cortical neurons during the later postnatal period. Elaboration of axosomatic and dendritic spine synapses as well as decrease in temporal dispersion in presynaptic pathways contribute significantly to changes in duration, amplitude, and polarity characteristics of cortical surface potentials during postnatal development [56]. In addition, maturation of specific and nonspecific projection systems over different time periods also contributes to alterations in evoked activities [3, 61]. Inasmuch as electrocortical potentials are largely extracellular reflections of complex summations of axodendritic and axosomatic EPSPs and IPSPs [42], emphasis is placed on changes in properties of synapses in further assessing the basis for relatively long-duration evoked potentials and seizure spikes in the immature brain.

Defining PSP Characteristics. Intracellular recording from immature neurons is the most effective technique for defining PSP characteristics. It is also the most frustrating and frequently unrewarding method available. Interpretation of intracellular data from immature cortex is especially hazardous in view of the extraordinary fragility of immature neurons particularly in the immediate neonatal period. Thus, it is not uncommon to encounter very few elements in the neocortex of neonatal kittens in which significant (40–60 mV) membrane potentials and spike potential amplitudes in excess of 40–50 mV are recorded. On the other hand, numerous relatively small (10–20 mV) potential fluctuations are noted in excursions with ultrafine micropipettes through immature cortex. Some workers have considered these recordings indicative of relatively low resting membrane potentials of immature cortical neurons [8, 14]. Such findings have been interpreted as evidence for correlation between the membrane potential level in immature neurons and onset of spreading depression in the rat [8, 14]. Similar correlations have been made between low membrane potential of immature neurons in the rat and maturation of the cortical steady potential and superficial cortical response [14].

Studies from the author's laboratory have indicated the difficulty in eliciting spreading depression in the neonatal and young kitten [46]. However, there is little reason to suspect that this is due to the low membrane potential of immature cortical neurons since such *low* membrane potentials are probably entirely attributable to traumatic effects of impalement, which in many instances may develop so rapidly as to obscure registration of the *normal* membrane potential level. In the overall analysis, positive evidence is far more significant than the negative. In fact, the positive evidence strongly suggests that membrane potentials of cortical neurons in the neonatal period are not significantly different from those recorded in adult animals [58]. Most important, however, is the "fragility" difference between immature and mature neurons. This is most likely related to neuron size but also appears to reflect a significant difference in structural as well as physiological properties of the excitable membrane of immature neurons.

Postsynaptic potentials evoked in immature neocortical neurons by thalamic stimulation differ in several respects from those observed in adult animals. EPSPs generally have a slow rise time and may be extremely prolonged in duration (Fig. 18-2). Latency for EPSPs evoked by stimulation of specific thalamocortical projections is generally much longer than latency observed in adult animals [57]. There is no reason to suspect factors other than delayed conduction time in poorly myelinated or unmyelinated thalamocortical afferents and intracortical pathways as the major factor in the prolonged latency of most evoked PSPs in immature neurons [23, 25, 34, 37, 56, 73, 76]. IPSPs like EPSPs are also of very long duration in immature neocortical neurons. Such durations of PSPs evoked in immature neocortical neurons in response to stimulation of specific thalamic nuclei have rarely been observed in neocortical neurons of adult animals under essentially similar experimental conditions [57].

The intracellular data from immature cortical neurons are consistent with the view that an important factor in determining the time course of evoked potentials and seizure spikes in immature cortex is the relatively slow time course and duration of PSPs which underlie production of surface potentials. However, mechanisms responsible for these PSP characteristics have not been specified. The relatively large amplitude of PSPs in immature neurons has been noted in respect to spinal motoneurons in the kitten [18] and has been commented upon in findings from immature cortex [58]. The large amplitude of PSPs is probably related to the high in-

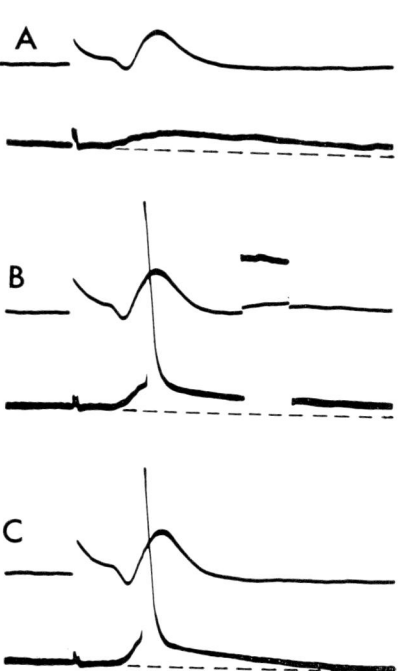

FIG. 18-2. Prolonged EPSPs (80–100 msec) evoked by ventrolateral thalamic stimulation in a sensorimotor-cortex neuron from a 6-day-old kitten. Upper channel records indicate cortical surface activity, negativity upward. Amplitude of cortical evoked responses, 200 μV. (A) Weak stimulation elicits an 18–20 msec latency EPSP with slow rise time and prolonged declining phase. (B) and (C) Stronger stimulation decreases rise time and increases amplitude of EPSP. Cell discharge secured at crest of EPSP. Note duration of spike potential and failure of discharge to alter time course of EPSP. Calibration in (B), 50 mV; 20 msec. (From Purpura, Shofer, and Scarff [58].)

put resistance of immature neurons but this may also be attributable to factors determining the quantal content of transmitter released by presynaptic activity. The long duration of PSPs in immature neocortical neurons may be due to delayed enzymatic inactivation of transmitter or continuing release of transmitter by repetitive presynaptic volleys. It must be emphasized that since repetitive discharges are rarely observed, it is unlikely that continuing activity in presynaptic pathways plays a major role in the production of prolonged PSPs in immature cortical neurons [58].

Factors Contributing to Stability of Immature Cerebral Cortex

Rapid depression of repetitively evoked cortical responses is characteristically observed in the immature brain [38, 44, 67]; the same has been noted in regard to frequency of focal epileptiform discharges [75]. Low-level excitability of immature cortical neurons has been commented upon above and is illustrated in Fig. 18-2, showing that even relatively large EPSPs fail to elicit more than one spike potential in most cortical elements in the neonatal period. This low-level excitability of immature cortical neurons is also reflected in the rarity of *spontaneous* unit discharges observed in extracellular unit studies in very young kittens [28, 29]. Similar observations have been made in newborn and young rats [14].

Lack of repetitive responses of immature cortical neurons may be related to differences in the ionic kinetics of the spike-generating mechanism or postspike recovery processes in immature as opposed to mature cortical neurons. Some support for this view has come from studies of relationship between sodium-potassium ATPase and development of spontaneous discharges in kitten cortex [29]. It was observed that intracellular spikes in cortical neurons from neonatal or very young kittens generally exhibit a longer duration than spikes in neurons of mature cortex. This is particularly clearly revealed in hippocampal pyramidal neurons activated by antidromic stimulation. In these elements prolongation of the spike potential may be induced by low frequency repetitive fornix stimulation. One of the most extreme examples of this is shown in Fig. 18-3, which illustrates progressive development of a plateau of delayed depolarization on the falling phase of the antidromic spike. While such examples of spike potentials lasting 150–200 msec are rare findings, they do serve to emphasize unusual membrane reactions and properties of immature cortical neurons. Unfortunately very little is known concerning the nature of these membrane properties due, in part, to experimental difficulties in studying immature neurons with intracellularly applied depolarizing and hyperpolarizing current pulses. It is thus not possible as yet

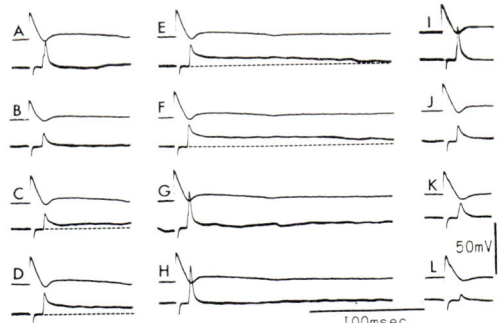

FIG. 18-3. Intracellularly recorded antidromic spike potentials of hippocampal neuron from 8-day-old kitten. Upper channel: Monopolar recordings from ventricular surface of hippocampus at fimbrial-hippocampal junction. Lower channel: Intracellular records obtained with a micropipette filled with 2M potassium citrate. (*A*) through (*F*) Consecutive responses to a 1-per-sec fimbrial stimulation. The second or somadendritic component of the antidromic response fails in (*B*). Initial component exhibits increase in amplitude and prolonged depolarizing plateau on its falling phase. (*G*) and (*H*) Responses at 1 per sec, 20 sec after (*F*). Antidromic response is fully recovered and somewhat facilitated. (*I*) through (*L*) Examples of decomposition of antidromic responses during 15-per-sec fimbrial stimulation. Amplitude calibration applies to intracellular records only.

to define mechanisms responsible for prolonged spikes of immature neurons or the basis for low-level excitability of these elements.

Prior to the application of intracellular recording techniques to the study of immature brain it was generally inferred that rapid depression of surface-evoked responses seen during repetitive stimulation of afferent pathways was attributable solely to prolonged relative refractoriness or fatigability of immature neurons [44, 47]. It was also suggested from pharmacological studies of evoked potentials that inhibitory synaptic activities were poorly developed relative to excitatory events in immature cortex [43]. Intracellular data on IPSPs of immature cortical neurons compel rejection of these hypotheses. While it cannot be denied that immature neurons exhibit decreased excitability as compared to mature neurons, it is now clear that the "depression" ob-

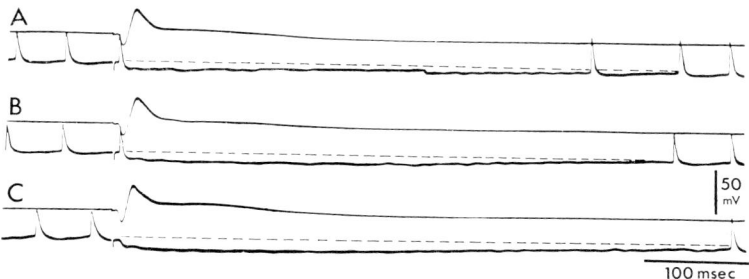

Fig. 18-4. Prolonged IPSPs recorded from sensorimotor cortex neuron in a 24-day-old kitten. (A) and (B) Single-shock stimulation of ventrolateral thalamus evokes positive-negative specific evoked response from cortical surface and a short-latency discharge succeeded by prolonged IPSP. (C) Same stimulus does not evoke early cell discharge but IPSP is still produced which suppresses "spontaneous" discharges for about 600 msec. Broken horizontal lines are drawn through baselines to facilitate estimation of IPSP duration. (From Purpura, Shofer, and Scarff [58].)

served in repetitively evoked responses reflects the operation of prolonged 100–600 msec IPSPs generated in the population of elements activated by afferent pathways (Fig. 18-4). Some effects of these prolonged IPSPs in conditioning variable modes of impulse initiation in immature neocortical neurons are considered below.

Inhibition in the Immature Hippocampus

The precocious development of inhibitory synaptic pathways in the cerebral cortex is perhaps best illustrated in hippocampal neuronal organizations. Intracellular recording from hippocampal pyramidal neurons in neonatal kittens has revealed prolonged IPSPs in response to fimbria or fornix stimulation [54]. These IPSPs resemble in all respects the IPSPs observed in adult animals [1, 2, 31]. It has also been noted that in the immediate neonatal period, repetitive fornix stimulation results in summation of IPSPs along with some attenuation of individually evoked IPSPs (Fig. 18-5).

IPSPs in hippocampal neurons of neonatal kittens are frequently preceded by EPSPs but these are often relatively small and ineffective in triggering cell discharges.

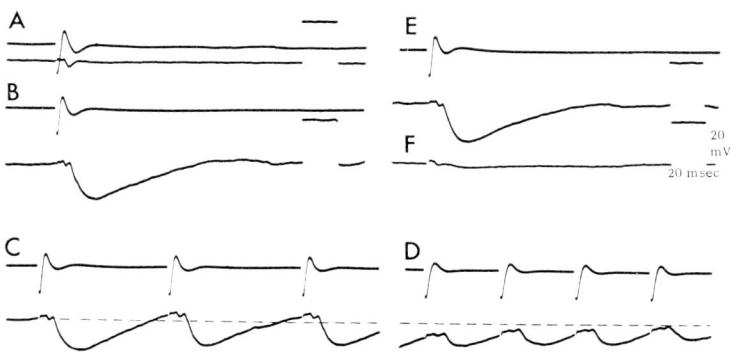

Fig. 18-5. Characteristics of IPSP summation in hippocampal pyramidal neuron from 2-day-old kitten during repetitive fornix stimulation. (A) Surface (upper channel) and intrahippocampal field activity (lower channel). (B) Impalement of neuron is achieved. Fornix stimulation evokes prominent 80 msec duration IPSP. (C) Attenuation of successively evoked IPSPs during 12-per-sec fornix stimulation. (D) Attenuation of successively evoked IPSPs during 25-per-sec fornix stimulation. Note increase in membrane polarization over that in (C). (E) Recovery of IPSP following (D). (F) Small negative field potential is recorded in extracellular position after a 10 μ displacement of the microelectrode. (From Purpura, Prelevic, and Santini [54].)

This situation does not obtain in kittens that are 1–2 weeks old in which fornix-evoked EPSPs are generally associated with cell discharge unless rapidly curtailed by development of IPSPs [54]. At this time it is commonly observed that repetitive fornix stimulation results in rapid *attenuation* of IPSPs (cf. below, Fig. 18-10) and increase in polysynaptic EPSPs as in the case of adult animals [30, 52, 62].

Examination of the morphological features of hippocampal neuronal and synaptic organizations in the neonatal period has been particularly rewarding in disclosing an important role of axodendritic synaptic pathways in production of IPSPs at this developmental stage. Electron microscope studies [68] indicate that in newborn kittens cell bodies of hippocampal pyramidal neurons are virtually devoid of synaptic contacts. Soma-to-soma appositions over a large extent of the surface membrane of neurons are common as are glial-soma appositions (Fig. 18-6). In contrast to the paucity of axosomatic synapses on hippocampal pyramidal neurons in the neonatal period, axodendritic synapses are abundant. The latter occurs on dendritic trunks, spines, and small dendritic processes in the neuropil. Elaboration of axosomatic synapses on hippocampal pyramidal neurons is essentially a postnatal event as has been

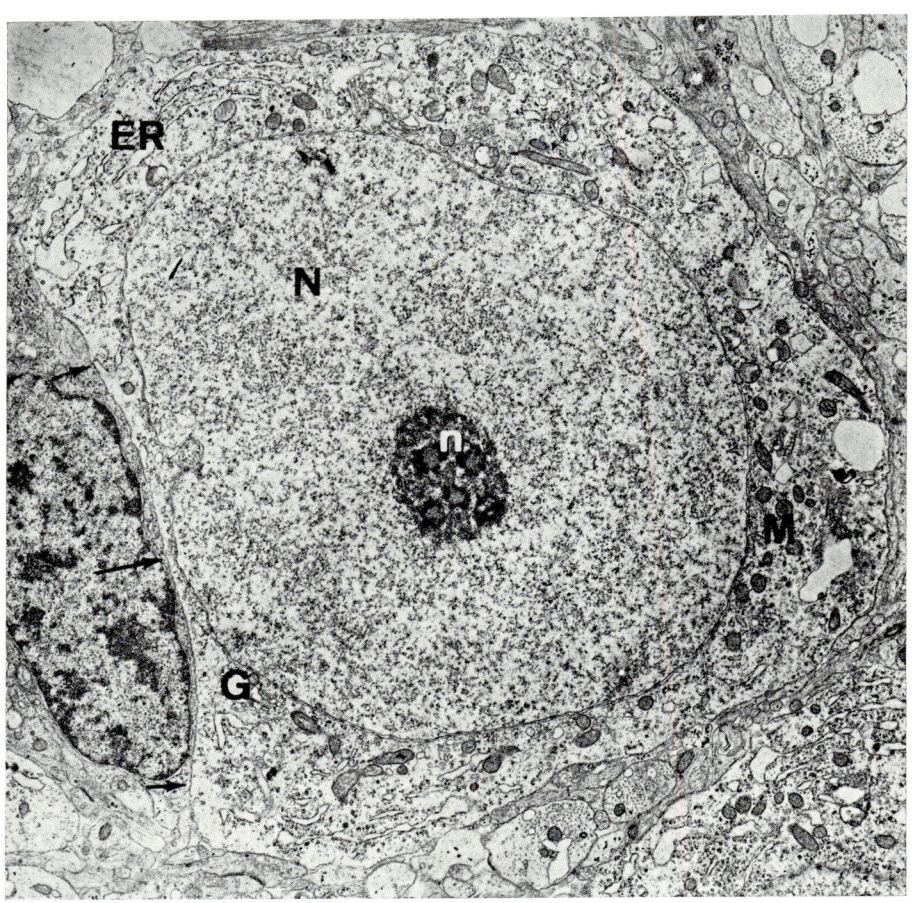

FIG. 18-6. A cross section through cell body of hippocampal neuron in 5-day-old kitten showing Golgi complex (G), extensive endoplasmic reticulum (ER), mitochondria (M), nucleus (N), and nucleolus (n). Note absence of axosomatic synapses and large extent of glial-soma apposition (arrows). Kitten perfused with 3 percent glutaraldehyde in M/15 Sorensen's buffer, pH 7.3. ×5800. (From Schwartz, Pappas, and Purpura [68].)

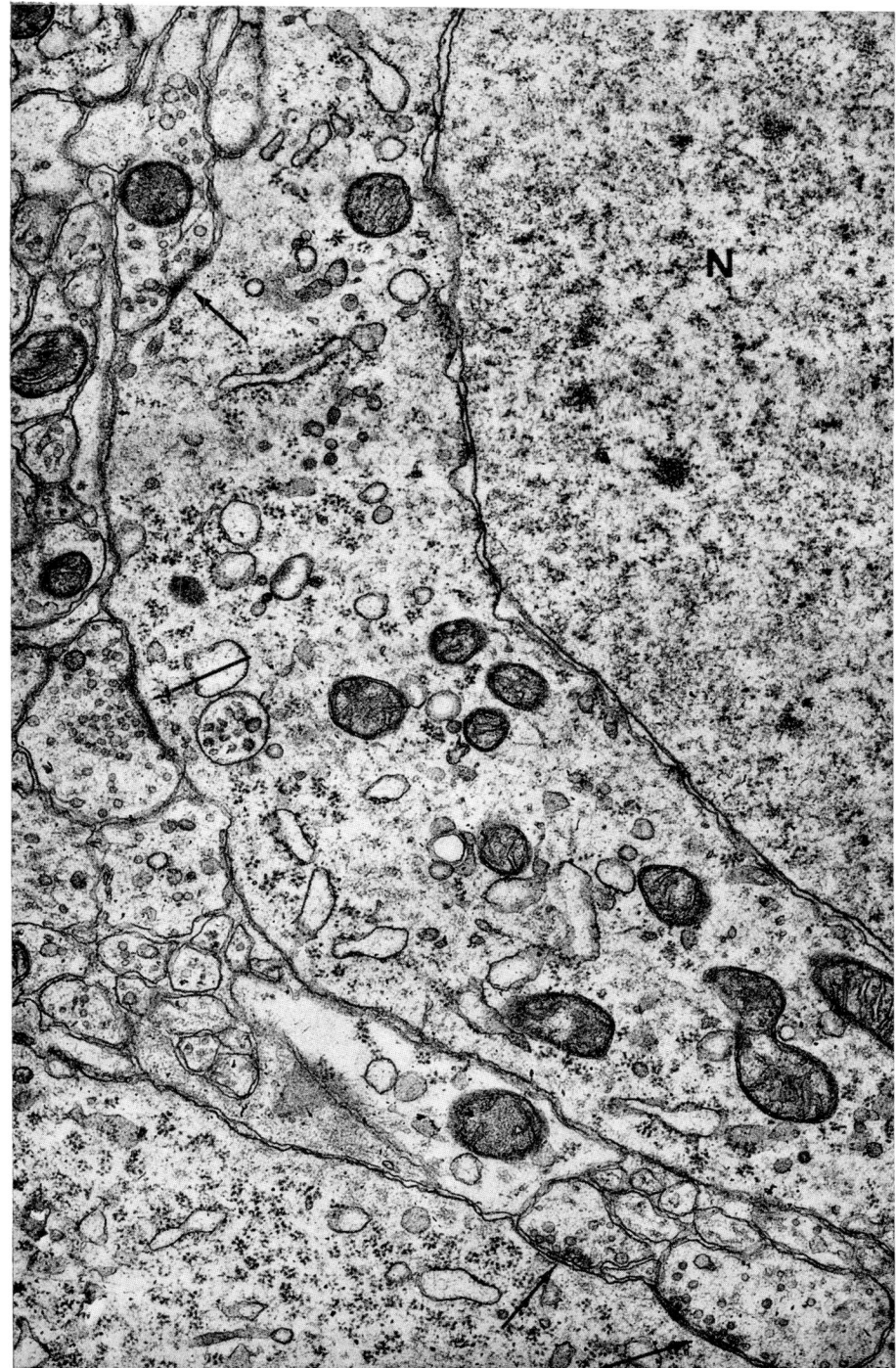

Fig. 18-7. Presence of a large number of axosomatic synapses (arrows) on two pyramidal cells of hippocampus in 21-day-old kitten. Note numerous small processes which occupy space between adjacent neurons. Ribosomal clusters are present in large numbers but amount of endoplasmic reticulum is slightly reduced compared to findings in younger kitten. Nucleus, N. Tissue immersed in 2 percent osmium tetroxide in veronal acetate buffer, pH 8.2. ×27,900. (From Schwartz, Pappas, and Purpura [68].)

described for immature neocortical neurons [74]. By the end of the third week at least a twentyfold increase in the number of axosomatic synapses can be estimated from electron micrographs (Fig. 18-7). This is paralleled by further increase in the number and variety of axodendritic synapses [68].

IPSPs evoked in hippocampal pyramidal neurons of adult animals by fimbria or fornix stimulation have been considered due to axon-collateral activation of basket cells of the stratum oriens which effect axosomatic synapses with many pyramidal neurons [1, 2]. The fact that axosomatic synapses are rarely observed on hippocampal neurons in neonatal kittens, at a time when IPSPs are well developed in these elements, strongly suggests that the hypothesis proposed to account for IPSPs in mature hippocampus is not generally applicable to the newborn kitten. Actually the electron microscope data obtained from neonatal kittens are consistent with the view that inhibitory neurons activated by axon-collateral pathways in the immature hippocampus are distributed largely in relation to dendrites of hippocampal pyramidal neurons. This has prompted an inquiry into the morphological characteristics of interneurons in the neonatal kitten hippocampus. Suffice it to say that Golgi-Cox studies [53] have indicated the existence of remarkably well-developed, modified basket-pyramidal neurons in the neonatal kitten hippocampus (Fig. 18-8). These elements have dendrites which subtend all layers of the hippocampus and are therefore admirably situated to receive inputs from many sources. Their dendrites are covered with prominent spines which are also present on the soma. Axons of these interneurons descend to the pyramidal cell layer and divide. Collaterals ascend along the apical dendrites and downward into the basilar dendritic plexuses of pyramidal neurons. It is not unreasonable to propose that these modified basket-pyramidal neurons may play an important role in generating IPSPs axodendritically in hippocampal pyramidal neurons in the neonatal and young kitten.

Axosomatic Synapses. If, as suggested,

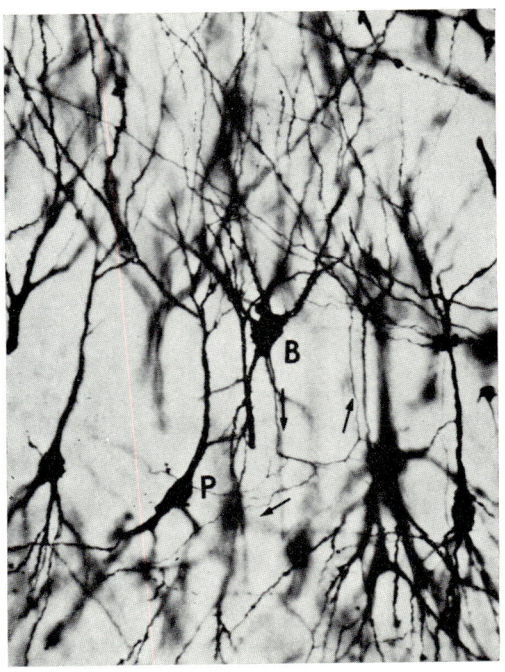

FIG. 18-8. Golgi-Cox preparation showing pyramidal and nonpyramidal neuron relations in hippocampus of 3-day-old kitten. P: Pyramidal neurons in superficial parts of stratum pyramidale; basilar dendrites and spines on apical and basilar dendrites are detectable. B: A modified basket-pyramid neuron of the stratum radiatum can be seen. Dendrites from superior pole of this neuron are thick, covered with prominent spines, and distributed in stratum moleculare. Dendrites from inferior pole course downward. Cell body of neuron also exhibits prominent spines. The main-stem axon, clearly visible, descends to stratum pyramidale and bifurcates. One branch ascends along apical-dendritic shafts of hippocampal neurons; the other descends along basilar dendrites of pyramidal neurons. ×250. (From Purpura and Pappas [53].)

IPSPs in the neonatal kitten are generated largely at axodendritic synapses, what functions are subserved by the later elaboration of axosomatic synapses? At least two hypotheses may be considered. During postnatal development inhibitory synapses at proximal dendritic loci may undergo progressive translocation to the soma. Alternatively, inhibitory axosomatic synapses may develop later along with an overall increase in excitatory synapses. In connection with the latter hypothesis, it is to be noted that a significant increase in EPSP effectiveness occurs in the postnatal period as already indicated. Since these EPSPs appear to be a consequence of activation of afferents in the fornix [30, 72], it is likely that in the early postnatal period responses to fornix stimulation resemble those elicited by stimulation of the deafferented fornix in adult animals [72]. It may be concluded from these studies that (a) inhibition is the most prominent synaptic event elicited in hippocampal neurons in the neonatal period, and (b) only in the later postnatal period do hippocampal neurons acquire their full complement of excitatory synapses, some of which are derived from fornix afferents.

The operation of potent inhibitory synaptic pathways in neocortex and hippocampus of neonatal and young kittens may contribute to the stability of neuronal pathways at this developmental stage. Additionally, recurrent-collateral inhibition in the immature hippocampus could serve to limit spread of convulsant activity in this structure as in the case of adult animals (cf. Spencer and Kandel, Chap. 21). This would be particularly effective in view of the relatively poor development of excitatory synaptic pathways in the neonatal animal.

One consequence of the differential development of inhibitory synaptic pathways in the hippocampus is of considerable interest from the standpoint of genesis of rhythmically recurring paroxysmal activity evoked by repetitive fornix stimulation in immature animals. Thus it is pertinent to recall here that stimulation of the deafferented fornix in adult animals may lead to seizure activity characterized by prolonged phases of membrane hyperpolarization of pyramidal neurons [30, 72]. At some stages of this seizure activity, rhythmically recurring IPSPs in hippocampal pyramidal neurons are well correlated with surface electrocortical potentials. Inhibitory synaptic events observed in hippocampal pyramidal neurons of adult animals with chronically deafferented fornix are in marked contrast to the predominately excitatory synaptic activities recorded during seizures evoked by repetitive stimulation of the intact fornix [30, 62].

Summation of IPSPs. Attention has been directed above to the observation that repetitive stimulation of the intact fornix in neonatal kittens results in summation of IPSPs (Fig. 18-5) rather than the depolarizing shifts detectable in adult animals. In kittens 1–2 weeks old, such stimulation may also lead to development of widespread rhythmically recurring IPSPs in pyramidal neurons (Fig. 18-9). Such IPSPs, recurring at frequencies of from 15–18 per sec, persist for several seconds following a brief fornix tetanus. This remarkably regular IPSP frequency can be interrupted by an evoked IPSP which is of longer duration than the IPSPs observed in the posttetanic period. Such an interpolated evoked IPSP effectively resets the timing and to a lesser extent the rhythm of shorter duration IPSPs. Two conclusions may be drawn from these observations: (a) the type of synaptic

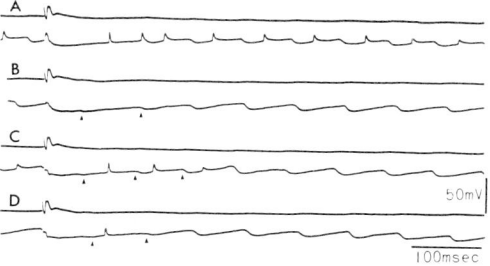

Fig. 18-9. Development of rhythmically recurring IPSPs in hippocampal neuron from 14-day-old kitten following repetitive fornix stimulation. Examples shown from 3 different cells in the same preparation but during different microelectrode penetrations of hippocampus. Upper channel records show surface responses to fornix stimulation. Gain is low and barely reveals small surface oscillations that coincide with intracellularly recorded rhythmical IPSPs. (*A*) Attenuated spikes occur on late phases of IPSPs in partially depolarized neuron. Evoked IPSP is longer in duration than spontaneously occurring IPSPs. (*B*) Another cell. Arrowheads indicate breakthrough of spontaneous IPSPs on long duration evoked IPSPs. Stimulus has reset timing of IPSPs. (*C*) and (*D*) Recordings from same cell further illustrate breakthrough of spontaneous IPSPs and resetting of timing of IPSPs after stimulus to fornix. Note throughout the remarkably regular rhythm of IPSPs.

event (inhibitory) initiated in pyramidal neurons of immature hippocampus by stimulation of the *intact fornix* is similar to that observed in pyramidal neurons of the adult animal following stimulation of the *deafferented fornix,* and (b) the rhythmical and synchronized discharge of inhibitory interneurons in immature hippocampus is initiated by a pacemakerlike process, which can be reset by interpolation of a stimulus that interjects a prolonged IPSP in the train of recurring IPSPs in pyramidal neurons. It follows from this that the mode of development of excitatory and inhibitory synapses on pyramidal neurons in the immature hippocampus can be an important factor in determining the type of paroxysmal activity generated in these elements at different developmental stages.

Little can be said concerning the mechanism by which brief fornix stimulation induces the rhythmical and synchronized discharge of inhibitory interneurons that results in 15–18-per-sec IPSPs in pyramidal neurons. The fact that the rhythm of spontaneously occurring IPSPs is reset but not interrupted during prolonged, evoked IPSPs indicates that the discharge of pyramidal neurons and subsequent recurrent-collateral activation of inhibitory neurons probably do not contribute to the basic mechanism of the rhythmicity. It seems reasonable to consider the possibility of an intrinsic pacemakerlike alteration in inhibitory interneurons which results in their synchronized, rhythmical activity. Further work is required to clarify the role of ephaptic and synaptic factors in facilitating synchronization of inhibitory interneuron discharge in immature hippocampus.

Spike Generation in Dendrites of Immature Cortical Neurons

Intracellular studies of immature neocortical neurons have disclosed characteristics of spike potentials in these elements which are rarely, if ever, observed in normal mature neocortical neurons. Spike generation in the vast majority of immature neocortical neurons is effected by EPSPs which are detectable with an intrasomatically located microelectrode. The mode of spike generation in these elements does not differ from that described for mature neurons in which impulse initiation is triggered at a low threshold region in the initial segment soma membrane. However, under appropriate conditions of activation or during spontaneously occurring increases in membrane polarization, variations in the mode of activation of orthodromically evoked spikes may be detectable in immature neurons. Two types of variations have been noted.

The first type is similar to that originally observed in chromatolyzed motoneurons [17] and some hippocampal pyramidal neurons in adult animals [52, 71]. This variation is characterized by development of an all-or-none rapid depolarizing prepotential or fast prepotential (FPP) [71] which may be superimposed on a small EPSP or may arise directly from the baseline, usually during a phase of increased membrane polarization. Evidence bearing on the presumed dendritic origin of these FPPs has been summarized elsewhere [48]. A point of major importance is that whereas FPPs are rarely observed in normal mature neocortical neurons [51, 55], they are encountered in a relatively large proportion of immature neocortical neurons [58]. Such FPPs may also be revealed in immature neocortical neurons by induced increases in membrane polarization which effectively displace EPSPs from the firing level. FPPs are more commonly observed in mature hippocampal [71] neurons than in mature neocortical neurons. However, they are observed with equal frequency in immature neocortical and hippocampal elements. Examples of the characteristics of FPPs in immature hippocampal neurons are shown in Figs. 18-10 and 18-11. In the case of some mature neocortical neurons, FPPs have been observed only during and after application of transcortical polarizing currents [51].

A second type of spike variation, that is, spikes which arise directly from the baseline (Fig. 18-12*B*), may be observed during surface application of similar polarizing currents which *activates* FPPs in immature neocortical neurons, as shown in Fig. 18-12*A*. Considerable interest has been attached to these spikes without depolarizing

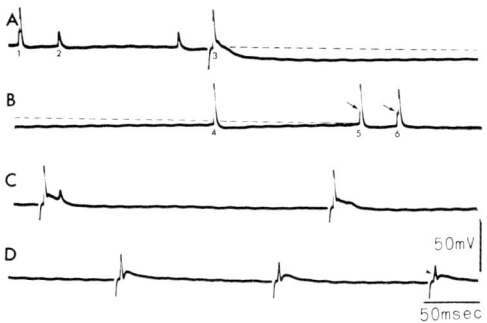

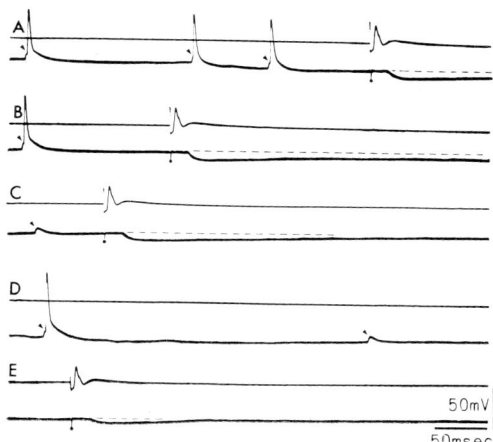

FIG. 18-10. Different characteristics of spike potentials recorded from hippocampal pyramidal neuron in 8-day-old kitten. (A) Spontaneous spike (1) with a distinct fast prepotential. This is succeeded by two FPPs that lack a second spike component (2). Fornix stimulation elicits an antidromic spike (3) which lacks the FPP. This difference in antidromic and orthodromically evoked spikes indicates that the prepotential (1 and 2) is not an initial axonal segment component since it is not evoked by antidromic stimulation. Antidromic spike is followed by small EPSP and very prolonged IPSP. (B) Continuation of (A). First spike elicited on late phase of IPSP arises from level of relative membrane hyperpolarization and does not show the FPP (4). The latter is revealed in successive spikes (5 and 6). (C) and (D) During low frequency fornix stimulation, IPSPs attenuate and EPSPs become more prominent. At higher fornix-stimulation frequencies there is progressive reduction in antidromic spikes and eventual appearance of small inflection, shown by arrowhead in (D), probably indicating initial segment component.

FIG. 18-11. Some consequences of spontaneously developing increase in membrane potential in hippocampal pyramidal neuron in 9-day-old kitten. (A) through (E) From continuous record. Arrowheads indicate inflection between fast prepotential (FPP) and spike in this element. (A) Fornix-evoked IPSP is prominent at a time when spike potential is about 40 mV. (B) and (C) Evoked IPSP becomes "smaller" as membrane potential increases and spike potential augments in amplitude. FPPs dissociated from spikes shown in (C) and (D). (E) IPSP is attenuated as membrane potential increases further. (From Purpura, Prelevic, and Santini [54].)

prepotentials in providing evidence for impulse origin and spike propagation in dendrites [58]. It is therefore of some importance to note the factors which may condition the appearance of dendritic spikes in immature neocortical neurons.

An example of an orthodromic spike initiated by an EPSP evoked by specific ventrolateral thalamic stimulation is shown in Fig. 18-13A. In this cell the EPSP was succeeded by a prolonged IPSP. A spontaneous spike preceding the stimulus might be followed by an IPSP during which stimulation elicited a smaller spike that was initiated at a much lower firing level (Fig. 18-13B). It was emphasized above that long-duration IPSPs in immature neocortical neurons exhibit a capacity for summation during repetitive stimulation. During this IPSP summation, spike potentials may be observed that arise directly from the baseline of membrane hyperpolarization. Such spikes exhibit rapid rise times (Fig. 18-13C) and second components or partial responses, which become more obvious with increasing stimulus frequency (Fig. 18-13D and E).

The diagrams of Fig. 18-13 illustrate the possible sequence of events underlying alterations in synaptically evoked spikes. Initially, EPSPs are generated in the soma-dendritic membrane and these trigger cell discharge presumably at the primary spike generating site in the soma initial axonal segment region, Fig. 18-13(1). During the IPSP there may be a tendency for secondary (or tertiary) sites of impulse initiation, Fig. 18-13(2). The buildup of IPSPs and depression of primary impulse trigger sites occur

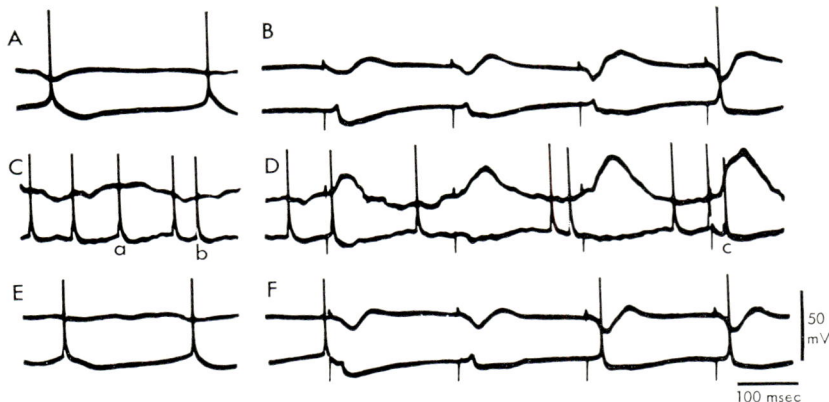

Fig. 18-12. Induction of fast prepotentials and spikes without depolarizing prepotentials in neocortical neuron from 3-week-old kitten during surface anodal polarization. Upper channel responses recorded from surface of sensorimotor cortex. (A) Appearance of spontaneous spikes prior to transcortical polarization. Spikes arise from *slow* depolarizing prepotentials (EPSPs). (B) Characteristics of EPSP-IPSP sequences evoked by repetitive ventrolateral thalamic stimulation. (C) and (D) During application of transcortical polarization, anode on cortical surface. Note in (C) increase in discharge frequency. Spikes exhibit FPPs (a) and occasionally arise directly from baseline (b). (D) Similar types of spikes are also noted during thalamic stimulation. Prepotential (c) is dissociated from spike during IPSP. Second component is attenuated. (E) and (F) Recovery, after termination of transcortical polarization.

along with increasing axodendritic EPSPs and development of active spike generating foci in dendrites. Spikes initiated in dendrites propagate into the soma in an all-or-none fashion. Consequently they lack the usual depolarizing prepotentials, Fig. 18-13(3).

A stage may be reached when partial dendritic responses are generated which fail to propagate into the soma. Thus the data on immature neocortical neurons suggest two factors that may condition the appearance of orthodromic spikes without prepotentials: the suppression of primary impulse trigger sites by IPSPs or spontaneously developing increases in membrane polarization; and the sustained excitatory bombardment by axodendritic synaptic pathways that leads to impulse initiation in dendrites.

The potentiality for impulse initiation in dendrites of immature neocortical neurons suggests a model of neuronal soma-dendritic relations that is vastly different from that recently proposed for the mature spinal motoneuron [59]. Importance is to be attached to the fact that although immature cortical neurons may have fewer synapses than mature neurons, excitatory synapses on dendrites in the neonatal and young kitten may have an augmented effectiveness in initiating cell discharge, by virtue of their capacity to elicit partial or full spikes at local dendritic sites.

A corollary of this is also of interest. Inasmuch as mature neocortical neurons do not ordinarily exhibit FPPs or evidence for impulse initiation and conduction in dendrites [48], it follows that absence of spike generation in dendrites of normal mature neocortical neurons must be an acquired property during postnatal ontogenesis. The implication here is that postnatal ontogenetic processes which transform cortical neurons from relatively simple bipolar elements to cells with complex dendritic systems, which function largely as receptor surfaces for a wide variety of synaptic inputs, also operate to *suppress* impulse initiation in dendrites, thereby restricting spike generation to the soma initial segment region and perhaps a variable portion of the juxtasomatic dendritic tree [48]. Whether this ontogenetic change in the membrane properties of dendrites of neocortical neurons is related to overall in-

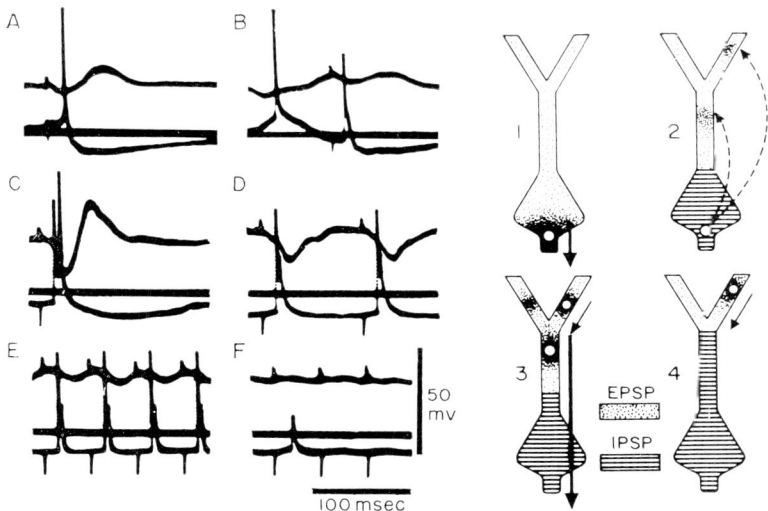

Fig. 18-13. Impulse initiation and propagation in dendrites of a neuron from 21-day-old kitten. Upper channel record, cortical surface evoked response to ventrolateral thalamic stimulation. Third beam of oscilloscope was placed at resting membrane potential level established in absence of stimulation. (A) Single-shock thalamic stimulus evokes small EPSP which triggers "normal" spike potential. Latter is succeeded by an IPSP. (B) Spontaneous discharge initiated by slow EPSP precedes stimulus. When stimulus occurs on small succeeding IPSP, evoked spike is smaller in amplitude and arises from a lower firing level. (C) Early phase of 5-per-sec thalamic stimulation during which IPSP-summation leads to sustained membrane hyperpolarization. Spike potential is evoked with shorter latency than in (A). Spike arises directly from baseline and exhibits rapid rise time. Note second component on shoulder of first spike. (D) and (E) Increase in stimulus frequency results in reduction of second component and finally in (F) failure of all-or-none spikes and appearance of partial response whose latency is similar to second component of spikes in (E). Diagrams to the right show (1) Original conditions similar to those in (A) when EPSPs trigger impulse at normal spike initiation sites (white dot). (2) IPSPs produce transitory shift in impulse trigger sites to dendrites. (3) Repetitive stimulation as in (C) through (E) leads to depression of primary impulse trigger site by IPSPs and activation of dendritic loci by axodendritic EPSPs. Large arrow indicates all-or-none propagating spike. Small arrow represents partial spike. (4) Conditions such as those in (F) at a stage when partial response arising in distal dendritic site is incapable of initiating conducted dendritic spike. (Modified from Purpura, Shofer, and Scarff [58].)

crease in the area of dendritic membrane occupied by axodendritic synapses, or to some *trophic* change mediated by such synapses, is not known. However, if synaptogenesis is a major factor in suppressing the spike-generating capacity of dendrites, it is not difficult to envision a number of pathological conditions developing in the antenatal or postnatal period that could interfere with synaptogenesis and thereby permit preservation of spike generation in dendrites with its attendant increase in overall neuronal excitability. Conceivably, this mechanism for producing augmented excitability in immature cortical neurons may be of importance in the development of seizure activity in immature neuronal organizations subjected to various traumatic and metabolic insults [47].

Comparative Excitability of Immature Neocortex and Hippocampus

The well-known difference in seizure susceptibility of neocortex and hippocampus in adult animals is well established at birth in immature born animals [11, 47]. Whereas strong electrical stimulation of the neocortical surface in neonatal kittens rarely elicits more than a brief local afterdischarge, stimulation of the fornix or subiculum in the same preparation generally produces a well-organized, prolonged afterdischarge, which may spread to the contralateral hippocampus via commissural pathways. The morphophysiological basis for this difference in seizure susceptibility of immature neocortex and hippocampus is evident in differences in the maturational status of neurons and synaptic organizations in the two different types of cerebral cortex [47, 68, 74].

Neuron cell bodies in the neocortex of neonatal kittens have poorly developed cytoplasmic organelles [74], whereas cell bodies of hippocampal neurons exhibit an extremely *busy* appearance particularly in regard to development of Golgi complex and other elements of the endoplasmic reticulum (Fig. 18-6). Striking differences in the development of dendritic systems of pyramidal neurons in neocortex and hippocampus are also evident. Apical dendrites are generally well developed on pyramidal neurons in both types of cortex in the neonatal kitten, but basilar dendrites are far more prominent and advanced in their morphological characteristics in the hippocampus (Fig. 18-8). Neocortical and hippocampal neurons possess rare axosomatic synapses in newborn kittens, but neurons in both types of cortex are well endowed with axodendritic synapses. There is, however, a significant difference in the number of dendritic spine synapses on hippocampal and neonatal pyramidal neurons in the neonatal animal. Whereas spines are ordinarily not observed on pyramidal neurons in the neocortex until the end of the first postnatal week [39, 66, 74], dendritic spines are prominent on all types of hippocampal neurons, pyramidal and nonpyramidal, in the newborn kitten (Fig. 18-8) [68].

The difference in excitability properties of neocortex and hippocampus in the newborn kitten is related, in part, to the relatively advanced maturational status of the latter type of cortex. However, it is clear that additional factors must contribute to this difference in seizure susceptibility which persists after maturation of the brain. The facility with which spike generation in dendrites of hippocampal neurons can be induced in the adult animal [52] indicates that many hippocampal neurons do not undergo the postnatal alteration in dendritic excitability that characterizes the maturational process in neocortical neurons. Fast prepotentials (FPPs), considered to be reflections of dendritic partial responses, are common in both neocortical and hippocampal neurons in newborn and young kittens as already indicated. But only in the hippocampus of adult animals are FPPs observed in a significant proportion of cells as apparently normal variations of the mode of impulse initiation in these elements [72].

Emphasis has been placed in the foregoing on finding IPSP summation in both neocortical and hippocampal neurons of neonatal kittens during repetitive stimulation of afferent or antidromic pathways or both. In the case of neocortex the tendency for IPSP summation during stimulation of mixed excitatory and inhibitory synaptic pathways appears to persist into the late postnatal period, although rare examples of attenuation of IPSPs and enhancement of EPSPs during and after repetitive stimulation have been noted [58]. The rapid development of excitatory synaptic pathways in the hippocampus in animals 1–2 weeks old contrasts sharply with the finding in immature neocortex. As a consequence of this rapid development of excitatory pathways, low frequency stimulation of the fornix in kittens that are 1–2 weeks old not uncommonly results in rapid attenuation of IPSPs and marked enhancement of EPSPs. Such alterations in evoked PSPs during fornix stimulation are reminiscent of the PSP changes observed as a prelude to the development of seizure activity in adult animals with intact fornix [30].

The correlation of relatively advanced structural and functional development in the hippocampus of newborn kittens is of interest from the standpoint of the well-known susceptibility of archicortex to various birth injuries and antenatal-neonatal hypoxemia. The fine structural characteristics of hippocampal neurons in the neonatal kitten are suggestive of a high metabolic activity critically dependent upon a relatively high tissue oxygen tension. It may be inferred from this that alterations in oxygenation secondary to disturbances in intracranial hemodynamics, pulmonary exchange, or minor asphyxial episodes may produce selective damage to hippocampal neurons by virtue of their relatively advanced differentiation and high metabolic activity. Thus, differences in the rate of maturation of neocortex and archicortex may not only explain the increased susceptibility of hippocampal neurons to these hypoxemic disturbances in the neonatal period, but may also account for the dominant role of hippocampal organizations in the electrographic expression of generalized abnormalities involving the immature brain [10].

Enhancement of Seizure Susceptibility of Immature Brain Following Alterations in Neuronal Maturation Patterns

It is evident from the foregoing considerations that progressive increase in seizure susceptibility of brain during postnatal development reflects alterations in the intrinsic excitability of neurons as well as an increasing capacity for neuronal interactions. Factors which may accelerate these ontogenetic alterations can be expected to lead to precocious enhancement in seizure susceptibility or the appearance of spontaneous epileptiform activity in the immature brain. Several mechanisms may be envisioned whereby these effects could be achieved. A rapid and abnormal increase in the number of synaptic relations of excitatory neurons or relative loss of inhibitory neurons could result in dramatic enhancement of seizure susceptibility in developing cortex. Additionally, changes in dendritic properties such as those described above might also serve to augment excitability in some neuronal organizations.

Two experimental procedures have been found to be particularly effective in providing model systems for elucidating the consequences of changes in maturational patterns in cortical neurons. One experimental design is undercutting immature neocortex in the neonatal period [50]. The other makes use of the well-known destructive effect of x-irradiation on external granular layer cells of the immature cerebellar cortex to produce a marked morphological and physiological change in Purkinje cell dendrites [70].

Stimulation of the intact neocortex in kittens less than one week old with stimuli that elicit a well-developed superficial cortical response does not evoke long-latency repetitive responses [50]. Acute subpial isolation of a slab of neocortex in young kittens generally results in some depression of evoked activities with gradual recovery in suitable preparations over 1–2 hours. On the other hand, an entirely different situation is encountered several days after cortical isolation is carried out on neonatal kittens. In preparations exhibiting adequate vascularization in the region of cortical isolation, weak surface stimulation elicits a prominent superficial negative response which is often succeeded by repetitive surface positive bursts (Fig. 18-14) not unlike those observed in chronically isolated mature cortex [9]. Spontaneous complex discharges are also detectable in different sites in the isolated slab of immature neocortex. A feature which distinguishes the burstlike responses in immature isolated neocortex from those noted in adult isolated preparations is the stereotyped configuration of evoked activities in immature animals.

Attempts to identify the elements in isolated cortex giving rise to the surface positive repetitive discharges have indicated that major generators for this activity are located at depths corresponding to the cell bodies and proximal portions of apical dendrites of the largest pyramidal neurons. Examination of Golgi-Cox preparations from animals utilized in electrophysiological studies has revealed several findings relevant to interpretation of the hyperexcitability of isolated immature neocortex. Pyramidal neurons in regions of hyperexcitability exhibit a precocious development of intracortical axon-collaterals of elements whose main stem axons were interrupted in the process of preparing the cortical slab (Fig. 18-15). Several days after damage to the parent axon, these axon-collaterals acquire developmental features

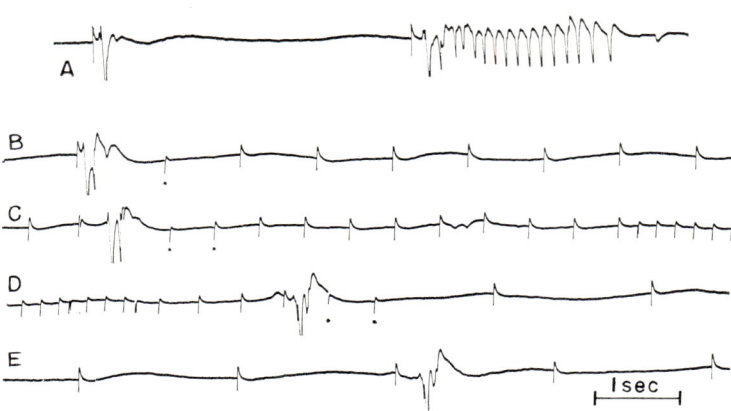

Fig. 18-14. Superficial cortical responses (SCRs) and repetitive activity evoked in isolated cortical slab in a 5-day-old kitten, 3 days after cortical isolation; recording electrode 1 mm from site of stimulation. (A) Stimulus to cortical surface evokes SCR and a multiphasic, predominantly surface-positive discharge, whereas a second stimulus delivered 3 sec later elicits SCR and a repetitive 8–10-per-sec train of positive-negative responses. (B) through (E) Continuous record in which surface stimulus frequency is increased from 0.5 to 5 per sec, then decreased to 0.5 per sec. Multiphasic discharges appear randomly, but when stimuli (indicated by black dots under stimulus artifacts) are superimposed on descending phases of surface-negative components of paroxysmal discharges, or 0.5 to 1 sec thereafter, evoked SCRs are markedly attenuated. (From Purpura and Housepian [50].)

which are not ordinarily seen in neocortical pyramidal neurons until after the third to fourth weeks [39].

The extraordinary development of axon-collaterals of traumatized pyramidal neurons results in conversion of large Type I neurons into Type II cells with axons ramifying completely in cortex [50]. The physiological consequence of this alteration in morphogenetic pattern is seen in the development of increased excitatory synaptic drives. Presumably these are initiated by recurrent axon-collaterals which effect synaptic relations with adjacent pyramidal neurons via their cell bodies as well as basilar dendrites and proximal portions of apical dendrites. These studies, which essentially confirm and extend the original morphological observations of Ramón y Cajal [60] on the effect of trauma to pyramidal neurons in newborn animals, provide an understanding of the substrate for development of paroxysmal activities in traumatized immature neocortex. It should be noted that the mechanism proposed above to account for the hyperexcitability of undercut or isolated immature neocortex is fundamentally different from the *denervation hypersensitivity* hypothesis. Whether some features of denervation hypersensitivity are evident in the development of hyperexcitability in traumatized immature neocortex cannot be evaluated. This problem is treated elsewhere in this volume (cf. Sharpless, Rutledge, Chap. 12).

The second experimental model for assessing the effects of altering maturational patterns derives from studies of the normal development of cerebellar cortex, particularly the relationship of changes in external granular layer cells to growth and elaboration of Purkinje cell dendrites [56, 70]. Purkinje cells in newborn kittens are extremely immature in appearance and exhibit many perisomatic protoplasmic processes. Their small dendrites terminate at the lower border of the external granular layer, which is approximately 10–12 cell layers thick in the neonatal period. Postnatal development of Purkinje cell dendrites in the kitten requires a minimum of 4–6 weeks. During this period progressive thinning of the external granular layer and inward migration of external granular layer cells occurs. The latter elements leave behind axons in the molecular layer, the

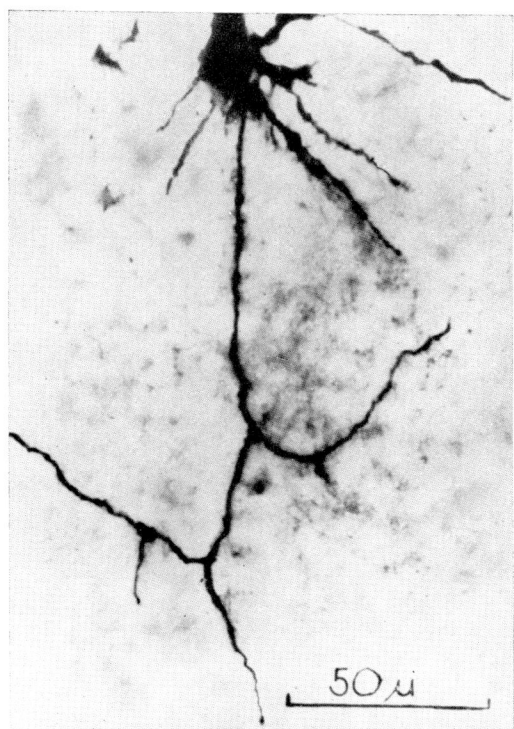

FIG. 18-15. Golgi-Cox preparation of a deep-lying arciform pyramidal neuron in a region of isolated neocortex from 5-day-old kitten, 2 days after cortical isolation. Microphotograph was retouched to emphasize some portions of basilar dendrites and initial axonal segment that were out of the plane of focus. Note extensive axon-collateral development. Such collaterals are never observed in 5-day-old intact immature feline neocortex. (From Purpura and Housepian [50].)

parallel fiber system, which constitutes the main afferent pathway to the spiny branchlets of Purkinje cell dendrites (Fig. 18-16).

The superficial negative response to local folial stimulation of immature cerebellar cortex follows a developmental sequence that parallels the elaboration of Purkinje cell dendrites and their presynaptic elements, that is, the parallel fibers which are derived for the most part from differentiation and inward migration of external granular layer cells (Fig. 18-16). The ontogenetic data thus indicate that the superficial negative response of cerebellar cortex is dependent upon development of a morphological substrate consisting of parallel fibers and Purkinje cell axodendritic synapses in the molecular layer [56].

Purkinje Cell Dendrites. Dramatic changes in the morphological characteristics of Purkinje cell dendrites and in their responses to local surface stimulation are detectable within a few days to several weeks after irradiation of the cerebellum in the neonatal period. Such irradiation destroys virtually all cells of the external granular layer, thus eliminating the major source of parallel fibers and axodendritic synapses on developing Purkinje cells. The morphological consequence of this is seen in the bizarre and pleomorphic appearance of Purkinje cells with main stem dendrites in contact with the pial surface of the molecular layer. Not uncommonly these dendrites course along the pia and direct smaller branches with a few spiny branchlets into deeper regions of the molecular layer (Fig. 18-17). For the most part, however, Purkinje cell dendrites have failed to elaborate their tertiary branches and spiny branchlets.

In kittens that are 2–3 weeks old, surface stimulation of the postirradiated cerebellum evokes fundamentally different types of responses from those observed in normal kittens. The smoothly graded, 10–20-msec, superficial negative response is no longer observed. Rather, surface stimulation evokes complex multiphasic responses, some of which have a distinct all-or-none character and multispikelike configurations (Fig. 18-18). It has been inferred that such responses to local stimulation reflect the directly excitable conductile responses of underlying main stem dendrites of Purkinje cells *stripped* of their parallel fiber-axodendritic synapses [70]. It should also be pointed out that in addition to changes in responses to surface folial stimulation, pronounced excitability increases are observed in evoked responses to motor-cortex stimulation in kittens exposed to cerebellar irradiation in the neonatal period [70]. Thus, while the loss of external granular layer cells results in marked *retardation* in Purkinje cell dendritic growth secondary to the absence of parallel fiber input, it is likely that other cells, some probably inhibitory, but as yet unidentified as to type,

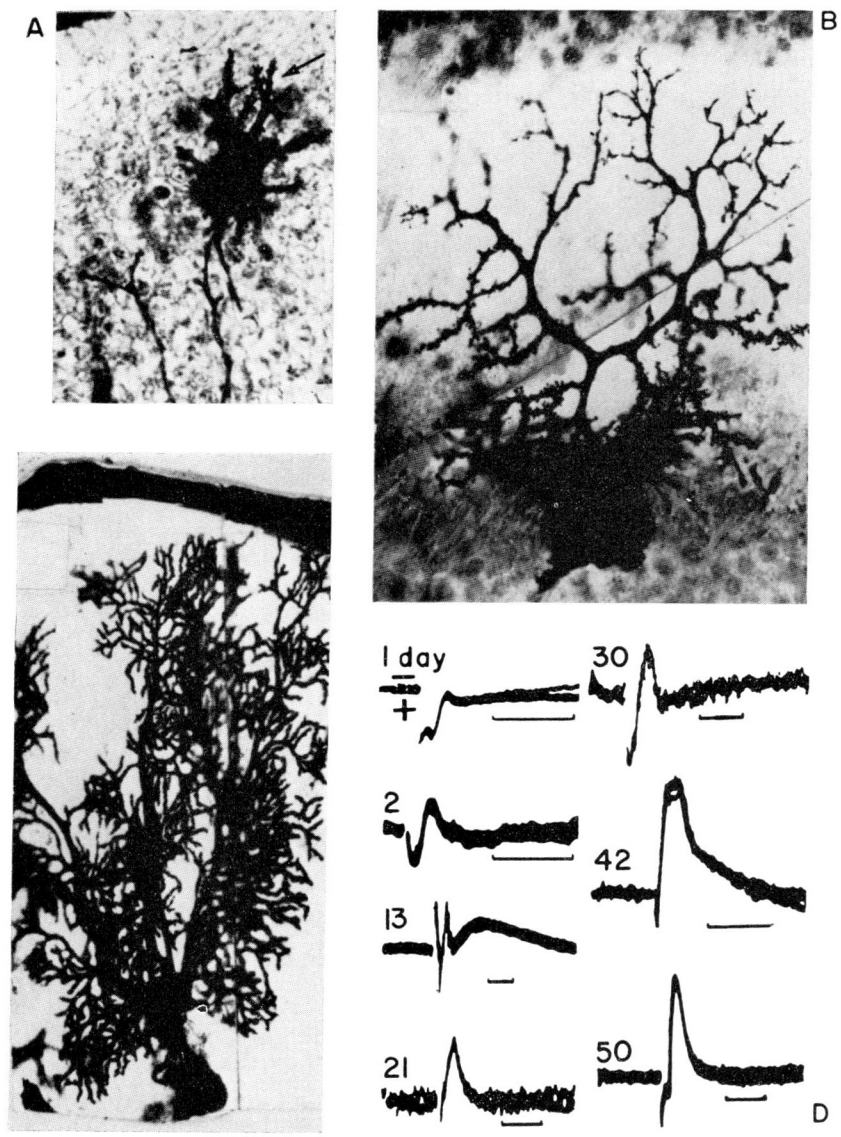

Fig. 18-16. (A) through (C) Microphotographs of Purkinje cells revealed in 200 μ-thick Golgi-Cox sections of cerebellum in kittens of various ages. (A) Two-day-old kitten. Main stem dendrites are short, occasionally branched, and have several protuberances. Dendritelike ramifications are seen emerging from cell body. (B) Appearance of Purkinje cell in 3-day-old kitten. (C) Characteristics of dendritic growth of Purkinje cell by the sixth postnatal week. In (A) and (B), superficial portions of dendrites do not penetrate into lower border of external granular layer. (D) Development of superficial cerebellar responses to local folial stimulation in kittens of various ages as shown. Recording electrode placed 1–3 mm from site of stimulation and parallel to long axis of folium. Spikelike responses seen in first week are succeeded by *transitional* responses with minimal negativity and late surface positivity. Superficial negative responses are clearly detectable by end of third postnatal week. Evoked responses in second month are similar to those recorded in adult animals. Time calibrations: 20 msec. (From Purpura et al. [56].)

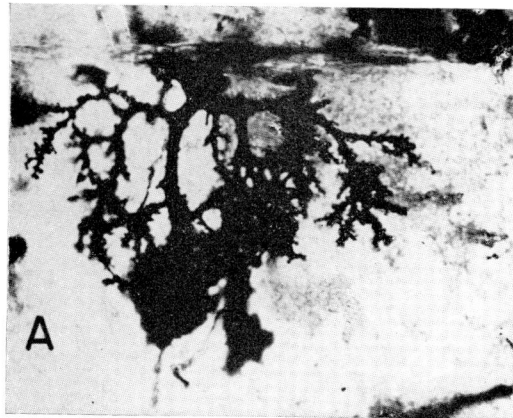

FIG. 18-17. Characteristics of Purkinje cell from irradiated cerebellum of 12-day-old kitten, Golgi-Cox preparation. Cerebellar irradiation was produced in neonatal period. Large main stem dendrites attain pial surface and are deflected laterally and downward during their attempted maturation. This bizarre pattern of dendritic growth is related to loss of external granular layer cells. Some of smaller dendritic branchlets in depths of molecular layer have a few spines. (From Shofer, Pappas, and Purpura [70].)

are also severely affected by cerebellar irradiation in the neonatal period.

The lines of inquiry illustrated in the foregoing two experimental models of pathophysiological changes in immature cerebral and cerebellar cortical neurons serve to characterize the range of correlated structure-function investigations that can be expected to provide new insights into basic mechanisms of epilepsy in the immature brain. There can be little doubt that continued application of refined morphophysiological studies to the analysis of such experimental model systems will permit more complete understanding of pathophysiological processes which underlie abnormal activity in the immature nervous system.

SUMMARY

Morphophysiological and electrophysiological studies of neurons in immature cortex have been considered in attempts to define properties of developing neuronal systems that contribute to the stability and excitability characteristics of immature

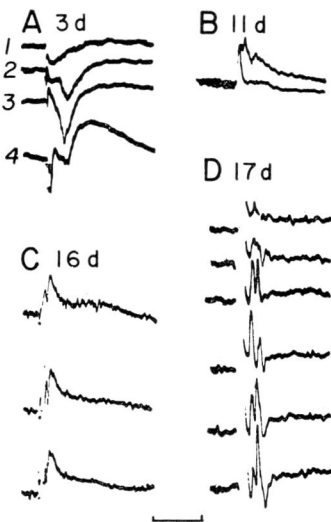

FIG. 18-18. Local responses to surface folial stimulation in irradiated kittens (ages as indicated). (A) Weak stimulation elicits prominent positivity and barely detectable spike (1), whereas stronger stimulation (2) through (4) evokes additional complex positive-negative components and large-amplitude early multiphasic spike. (B) and (C) Examples of spikes superimposed on slow negativities. (D) Stimulus-increment series illustrating reciprocal changes in magnitude of early and late components of multiphasic spikes. Contrast these complex responses evoked by stimulation of irradiated immature cerebellar cortex with those elicited in normal immature cerebellum (Fig. 18-16). (From Shofer, Pappas, and Purpura [70].)

brain at different postnatal ontogenetic stages. Emphasis has been placed on observations from intracellular recordings and light and electron microscope correlation studies.

Many of the electrographic features of evoked potentials and seizure discharges of immature brain are referable to the distinctive morphology of immature cortical neurons, their synaptic relations, and their responsiveness to excitatory and inhibitory inputs. Inhibitory activities are prominent and well developed in evoked responses of neocortex and hippocampus in the neonatal period, whereas excitatory synaptic activities exhibit relatively delayed maturation. Morphological correlations of this differential development of inhibitory synaptic activities are evident in the extraordinary development of axodendritic as opposed to axosomatic synapses in the neonatal period.

The low-level excitability of immature cortical neurons is, in part, a consequence of their lack of repetitive responsiveness to excitatory inputs and the disproportionate effectiveness of inhibitory synaptic drives. These factors operate to induce stability in immature neuronal networks. Stability is further enhanced by the slow rate of propagation, reduced neuronal interaction, and greater temporal dispersion of activity between different immature neuronal organizations. These stability-inducing factors are partially counterbalanced by the variable potentiality for impulse initiation and propagation in dendrites of immature cortical neurons. This property may be revealed under conditions of augmented excitatory axodendritic activation and concomitant IPSP-induced suppression of primary impulse initiation sites.

Experimentally produced alterations in morphogenetic patterns in cortex can exert profound effects on excitability characteristics of immature neuronal organizations. Two examples of such induced alterations are described. In one, a net increase in excitatory synaptic drive is shown to occur secondary to the growth of extensive axon-collaterals of excitatory neurons in traumatized immature cortex. In another, a loss of presynaptic excitatory synaptic pathways conditions changes in the morphophysiology of dendrites of cerebellar Purkinje cells. Both types of experimental models of pathophysiological processes are discussed in the context of possible mechanisms contributing to the seizure susceptibility of immature brain.

REFERENCES

1. Andersen, P., Eccles, J. C., and Løyning, Y. Location of postsynaptic inhibitory synapses on hippocampal pyramids. *J. Neurophysiol.* 27:592, 1964.
2. Andersen, P., Eccles, J. C., and Løyning, Y. Pathways of postsynaptic inhibition in the hippocampus. *J. Neurophysiol.* 27: 608, 1964.
3. Anokhin, P. K. Systemogenesis as a General Regulator of Brain Development. In Himwich, W. A., and Himwich, H. E. (Eds.), *The Developing Brain. Progress in Brain Research.* Amsterdam: Elsevier, 9:54, 1964.
4. Bernhard, C. G., Kaiser, I. H., and Kolmodin, G. M. On the epileptogenic properties of the fetal brain. An electrophysiological study on the electrically and chemically induced convulsive brain activity in sheep fetuses. *Acta Paediat.* (Upps.) 51:81, 1962.
5. Bernhard, C. G., Kolmodin, G. M., and Meyerson, B. A. On the Prenatal Development of Function and Structure in the Somesthetic Cortex of the Sheep. In Bernhard, C. G., and Schadé, J. P., (Eds.), *Developmental Neurology. Progress in Brain Research.* Amsterdam: Elsevier, 26: 60, 1967.
6. Bishop, E. J. The strychnine spike as a physiological indicator of cortical maturation in the postnatal rabbit. *Electroenceph. Clin. Neurophysiol.* 2:309, 1950.
7. Brizzee, K. E., Vogt, J., and Kharetchko, X. Postnatal Changes in Glia Neuron Index with a Comparison of Methods of Cell Enumeration in the White Rat. In Purpura, D. P. and Schadé, J. P. *Growth and Maturation of the Brain. Progress in Brain Research.* Amsterdam: Elsevier, 4: 136, 1964.
8. Bureš, J., Fifkova, E., and Mares, P. Spreading Depression and Maturation of Some Forebrain Structures in Rats. In Kellaway, P., and Petersén, I. (Eds.), *Neurological and Electroencephalographic Correlative Studies in Infancy.* New York: Grune and Stratton, 1964, pp. 27–36.
9. Burns, B. D. *The Mammalian Cerebral Cortex,* London: Arnold, 1958.
10. Cadilhac, J., and Passouant-Fontaine, Th. Décharges épileptiques et activité électrique de veille et de sommeil dans l'hippocampe au cours de l'ontogénèse. In *Physiologie de l'hippocampe.* Paris: C.N.R.S., 1962, pp. 429–442.
11. Cadilhac, J., Passouant-Fontaine, Th., Mihailovic, L., and Passouant, P. L'épilepsie expérimentale du chaton en fonc-

tion de l'âge. Etude corticale et sous-corticale. *Path. Biol.* (Paris) 8:1571, 1960.

12. Caveness, W. F., Nielsen, K. C., Yakovlev, P. I., and Adams, R. D. Electroencephalographic and clinical studies of epilepsy during the maturation of the monkey. *Epilepsia* (Amst.) 3:137, 1962.

13. Conel, J. L. *The Postnatal Development of the Human Cerebral Cortex*, vols. I–VI. Cambridge, Mass.: Harvard University Press, 1939, 1941, 1947, 1951, 1955, 1959.

14. Deza, L., and Eidelberg, E. Development of cortical electrical activity in the rat. *Exp. Neurol.* 17:425, 1967.

15. Dreyfus-Brisac, C., and Monod, N. Electroclinical Studies of Status Epilepticus and Convulsions in the Newborn. In Kellaway, P., and Petersén, I. (Eds.), *Neurological and Electroencephalographic Correlative Studies in Infancy*. New York: Grune and Stratton, 1964, pp. 250–271.

16. Eayrs, S. T., and Goodhead, B. Postnatal development of the cerebral cortex in the rat. *J. Anat.* 93:385, 1959.

17. Eccles, J. C., Libet, B., and Young, R. R. The behavior of chromatolysed motoneurons studied by intracellular recording. *J. Physiol.* (London) 143:11, 1958.

18. Eccles, R. M., Shealy, C. N., and Willis, W. D. Patterns of innervation of kitten motoneurons. *J. Physiol.* (London) 165:392, 1963.

19. Eidelberg, E., Kolmodin, G. M., and Meyerson, B. A. Ontogenesis of steady potential and direct cortical response in fetal sheep brain. *Exp. Neurol.* 12:198, 1965.

20. Ellingson, R. J., and Wilcott, R. C. Development of evoked responses in visual and auditory cortices of kittens. *J. Neurophysiol.* 23:363, 1960.

21. Fox, M. W. Neuronal development and ontogeny of evoked potentials in auditory and visual cortex of the dog. *Electroenceph. Clin. Neurophysiol.* 24:213, 1968.

22. Goldensohn, E. S., Shofer, R. J., and Purpura, D. P. Ontogenesis of focal discharges in epileptogenic lesions of cat neocortex. *Electroenceph. Clin. Neurophysiol.* 15: 163, 1963.

23. Grafstein, B. Postnatal development of the transcallosal evoked response in the cerebral cortex. *J. Neurophysiol.* 24:79, 1963.

24. Grossman, C. G. Electro-ontogenesis of cerebral activity. Forms of neonatal responses and their recurrence in epileptic discharges. *Arch. Neurol. Psychiat.* 74:186, 1955.

25. Hess, A. Post-natal development and maturation of nerve fibers of the central nervous system. *J. Comp. Neurol.* 100:461, 1954.

26. Hubel, D. H., and Wiesel, T. N. Receptive fields of cells in striate cortex of very young, visually inexperienced kittens. *J. Neurophysiol.* 26:994, 1963.

27. Hunt, W. E., and Goldring, S. Maturation of evoked response of the visual cortex in the postnatal rabbit. *Electroenceph. Clin. Neurophysiol.* 3:465, 1951.

28. Huttenlocher, P. R. Development of cortical neuronal activity in the neonatal cat. *Exp. Neurol.* 17:247, 1967.

29. Huttenlocher, P. R., and Rawson, M. D. Neuronal activity and adenosine triphosphatase in immature cortex. *Exp. Neurol.* 22:118, 1968.

30. Kandel, E. R., and Spencer, W. A. Excitation and inhibition of single pyramidal cells during hippocampal seizure. *Exp. Neurol.* 4:162, 1961.

31. Kandel, E. R., Spencer, W. A., and Brinley, F. J., Jr. Electrophysiology of hippocampal neurons. I. Sequential invasion and synaptic organization. *J. Neurophysiol.* 24:225, 1961.

32. Kling, A., and Coustan, D. Electrical stimulation of the amygdala and hypothalamus in the kitten. *Exp. Neurol.* 15:989, 1963.

33. Kolmodin, G. M., and Meyerson, B. A. Ontogenesis of paroxysmal cortical activity in fetal sheep. *Electroenceph. Clin. Neurophysiol.* 21:589, 1966.

34. Langworthy, O. R. A correlated study of the development of reflex activity in fetal and young kittens and the myelinization of tracts in the nervous system. *Contr. Embryol.* (Carneg. Inst.) 20:127, 1929.

35. Lennox, W. G. *Epilepsy and Related Disorders.* Boston: Little, Brown, 1960.

36. Libet, B., Fazekas, J. F., and Himwich, H. E. The electrical response of the kitten and adult cat brain to cerebral anemia and analeptics. *Amer. J. Physiol.* 132:232, 1941.

37. Marty, R., and Scherrer, J. Critères de maturation des systèmes afférentes corticaux. In Purpura, D. P., and Schadé, J. P. (Eds.), *Growth and Maturation of the*

Brain. *Progress in Brain Research.* Amsterdam: Elsevier, 4:222, 1964.

38. Meyerson, B. A. Ontogeny of interhemispheric functions. *Acta Physiol. Scand.* Suppl. 312, 1968.

39. Noback, C. R., and Purpura, D. P. Postnatal ontogenesis of cat neocortex. *J. Comp. Neurol.* 117:291, 1961.

40. Passouant, P., and Cadilhac, J. EEG and clinical study of epilepsy during maturation in man. *Epilepsia* (Amst.) 3:14, 1962.

41. Peeler, D. F., Jr., and Andy, O. J. Limbic system seizures in the kitten. *Electroenceph. Clin. Neurophysiol.* 23:1, 1967.

42. Purpura, D. P. Nature of electrocortical potentials and synaptic organizations in cerebral and cerebellar cortex. *Int. Rev. Neurobiol.* 1:47, 1959.

43. Purpura, D. P. Ontogenetic Analysis of Some Evoked Synaptic Activities in Superficial Neocortical Neuropil. In Florey, E. (Ed.), *International Symposium on Nervous Inhibition.* New York: Pergamon, 1961, pp. 424-446.

44. Purpura, D. P. Analysis of axodendritic synaptic organizations in immature cerebral cortex. *Ann. N.Y. Acad. Sci.* 94:604, 1961.

45. Purpura, D. P. Synaptic organization of immature cerebral cortex. *World Neurol.* 3:275, 1962.

46. Purpura, D. P. Critique and Review. In Brazier, M. A. B. (Ed.), *Brain Function. Cortical Excitability and Steady Potentials.* Los Angeles: Univ. of Calif. Press, 1963, pp. 281–320.

47. Purpura, D. P. Relationship of Seizure Susceptibility to Morphologic and Physiologic Properties of Normal and Abnormal Immature Cortex. In Kellaway, P., and Petersén, I. (Eds.), *Neurologic and Electroencephalographic Correlative Studies in Infancy.* New York: Grune and Stratton, 1964, pp. 117–154.

48. Purpura, D. P. Comparative Physiology of Dendrites. In Quarton, G. C., Melnechuk, T., Schmitt, F. O. (Eds.), *The Neurosciences. A Study Program.* New York: Rockefeller Univ. Press, 1967, pp. 372–392.

49. Purpura, D. P., Carmichael, M. W., and Housepian, E. M. Physiological and anatomical studies of development of superficial axodendritic synaptic pathways in neocortex. *Exp. Neurol.* 2:324, 1960.

50. Purpura, D. P., and Housepian, E. M. Morphological and physiological properties of chronically isolated immature neocortex. *Exp. Neurol.* 4:377, 1961.

51. Purpura, D. P., and McMurtry, J. G. Intracellular activities and evoked potential changes during polarization of motor cortex. *J. Neurophysiol.* 28:166, 1965.

52. Purpura, D. P., McMurtry, J. G., Leonard, C. F., and Malliani, A. Evidence for dendritic origin of spikes without depolarizing prepotentials in hippocampal neurons during and after seizure. *J. Neurophysiol.* 29:954, 1966.

53. Purpura, D. P., and Pappas, G. D. Structural characteristics of neurons in the feline hippocampus during postnatal ontogenesis. *Exp. Neurol.* 22:379, 1968.

54. Purpura, D. P., Prelevic, S., and Santini, M. Postsynaptic potentials and spike variations in the feline hippocampus during postnatal ontogenesis. *Exp. Neurol.* 22:408, 1968.

55. Purpura, D. P., and Shofer, R. J. Cortical intracellular potentials during augmenting and recruiting responses. I. Effects of injected hyperpolarizing currents on evoked membrane potential changes. *J. Neurophysiol.* 27:117, 1964.

56. Purpura, D. P., Shofer, R. J., Housepian, E. M., and Noback, C. R. Comparative Ontogenesis of Structure-Function Relations in Cerebral and Cerebellar Cortex. In Purpura, D. P., and Schadé, J. P., (Eds.), *Growth and Maturation of the Brain. Progress in Brain Research.* Amsterdam: Elsevier, 4:187, 1964.

57. Purpura, D. P., Shofer, R. J., Musgrave, F. S. Cortical intracellular potentials during augmenting and recruiting responses. II. Patterns of synaptic activities in pyramidal and nonpyramidal tract neurons. *J. Neurophysiol.* 27:133, 1964.

58. Purpura, D. P., Shofer, R. J. and Scarff, T. Properties of synaptic activities and spike potentials of neurons in immature neocortex. *J. Neurophysiol.* 28:925, 1965.

59. Rall, W. Distinguishing theoretical synaptic potentials computed for different soma-dendritic distributions of synaptic input. *J. Neurophysiol.* 30:1138, 1967.

60. Ramón y Cajal, S. *Studies in Vertebrate Neurogenesis.* Springfield, Ill.: Thomas, 1959.

61. Rose, G. H., and Lindsley, D. B. Visu-

ally evoked electrocortical responses in kitten: development of specific and nonspecific systems. *Science* 148:1244, 1965.

62. Sawa, M., Maruyama, N., and Kaji, S. Intracellular potential during electrically induced seizures. *Electroenceph. Clin. Neurophysiol* 15:209, 1963.

63. Schadé, J. P. Maturational aspects of EEG and of spreading depression in rabbit. *J. Neurophysiol.* 22:245, 1959.

64. Schadé, J. P., and Baxter, C. F. Changes during growth in the volume and surface area of cortical neurons in the rabbit. *Exp. Neurol.* 2:158, 1960.

65. Schadé, J. P., and Pascoe, E. G. Maturational Changes in Cerebral Cortex III. In Himwich, W. A., and Himwich, H. E. (Eds.), *The Developing Brain. Progress in Brain Research*. Amsterdam: Elsevier, 9: 132, 1964.

66. Scheibel, M., and Scheibel, A. Some Structural and Functional Substrates of Development in Young Cats. In Himwich, W. A., and Himwich, H. E. (Eds.), *The Developing Brain. Progress in Brain Research*. Amsterdam: Elsevier, 9:6, 1964.

67. Scherrer, J., and Oeconomos, D. Réponses évoquées corticales somesthésiques des mammifères adulte et nouveau né. In *Les grandes activités du lobe temporal*. Paris: Masson, 1955.

68. Schwartz, I. R., Pappas, G. D., and Purpura, D. P. Fine structure of neurons and synapses in the feline hippocampus during postnatal ontogenesis. *Exp. Neurol.* 22:394, 1968.

69. Servit, Z. Phylogenesis and ontogenesis of epileptic seizures. A comparative study. *World Neurol.* 3:259, 1962.

70. Shofer, R. J., Pappas, G. D., and Purpura, D. P. Radiation-Induced Changes in Morphological and Physiological Properties of Immature Cerebellar Cortex. In Haley, T. J., and Snider, R. S. (Eds.), *Response of the Nervous System to Ionizing Radiation*. Boston: Little, Brown, 1964, pp. 476–508.

71. Spencer, W. A., and Kandel, E. R. Electrophysiology of hippocampal neurons. IV. Fast prepotentials. *J. Neurophysiol.* 24:272, 1961.

72. Spencer, W. A., and Kandel, E. R. Hippocampal neuron responses to selective activation of recurrent collaterals of hippocampofugal axons. *Exp. Neurol.* 4:149, 1961.

73. Ulett, G., Dow, R. S., and Larsell, O. Inception of conduction in the corpus callosum and the corticoponto-cerebellar pathway in young rabbits with reference to myelinization. *J. Comp. Neurol.* 80:1, 1944.

74. Voeller, K., Pappas, G. D., and Purpura, D. P. Electron microscopic study of development of cat superficial neocortex. *Exp. Neurol.* 7:107, 1963.

75. Wright, F. S., and Bradley, W. E. Maturation of epileptiform activity. *Electroenceph. Clin. Neurophysiol.* 25:259, 1968.

76. Yakovlev, P. I. Maturation of cortical substrate of epileptic events. *World Neurol.* 3:299, 1962.

Discussion

ELECTRICAL ACTIVITY OF BRAIN TISSUE DEVELOPING IN CULTURE*

STANLEY M. CRAIN†

A variety of elegant experimental methods utilized to study the physiological properties of immature brain has been reviewed by Purpura. Emphasis was placed on intracellular recordings which provided extremely valuable data for analysis of cellular mechanisms underlying cerebral functions during maturation. His demonstration of well-developed inhibitory postsynaptic potentials in neonatal hippocampal cortex *prior* to the formation of axosomatic synapses offers dramatic illustration of the analytic power of the experimental ontogenetic method. Further reduction of cerebral complexity has been attempted by surgical isolation of small regions of the brain.

Purpura's studies of chronically isolated cerebral slabs in neonatal animals [21] indicate the potentialities of a combined ontogenetic and microsurgical approach. A more extreme application of this method consists of reduction 100 times in the size of in situ isolated cerebral slabs, down to the order of 1 mm³, and explantation of these fragments from the fetal or neonatal brain (Fig. D18-1X) into tissue culture vessels [2, 19]. Capillary circulation is no longer essential in such small pieces of brain tissue and simple diffusion of nutrients permits metabolic activities to proceed for long periods in vitro.

NEURAL NETWORKS ACTIVATED IN CNS TISSUES

Electrophysiologic study of mammalian cerebral explants during maturation in culture has demonstrated the *intrinsic* capacity of these CNS tissues to organize complex organotypic neural networks after complete isolation from the fetal or neonatal animal [7, 8, 9, 10]. Although the experimental techniques applied to cultured CNS tissues have been limited so far to extracellular recordings, they have demonstrated—in "broad brush-stroke fashion"—the remarkable degree to which an isolated cluster of a few thousand immature neurons and glial cells can develop sufficient cellular interrelationships to permit generation of long-lasting, rhythmic, highly synchronized bioelectric activities with strong mimicry of mammalian EEG patterns [8]. Development and maintenance of these complex, yet organotypic, bioelectric activities in such small cultured fragments of CNS tissue sets limits to the anatomical organization and to the critical functional components required to account for similar bioelectric phenomena when recorded from the CNS in situ.

Explantation of CNS tissues at suitably early stages of embryonic development permits study of these cultured fragments prior to and during the formation of cellular structures which may be essential for maturation of specific functions. Explants of fetal or newborn mouse cerebral neocortex, for example, show no signs of complex bioelectric activities during the first few days in vitro. Simple spike potentials can be evoked with electric stimuli (Fig. D18-1A), but no evidence of transmission of impulses from one neuron to another has been detected in these immature tissues. Extracellular recordings were made with 5 μ saline-filled, or 25 μ Ag-core, pipettes and electric stimuli (0.1–0.3 msec) were applied

---

* Supported in part by PHS Research Grant NB06545 from National Institute of Neurological Diseases and Stroke.

† Kennedy Scholar at the R. F. Kennedy Center for Research in Mental Retardation and Human Development, Albert Einstein College of Medicine.

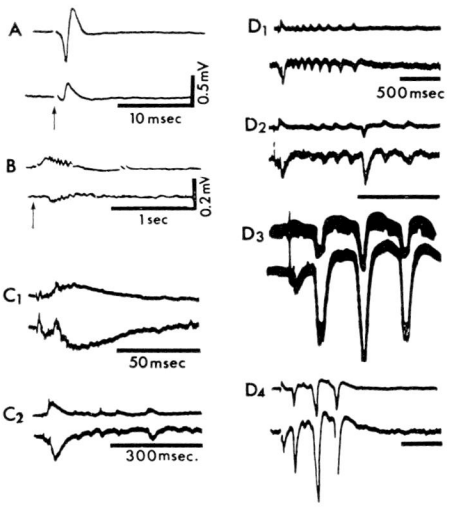
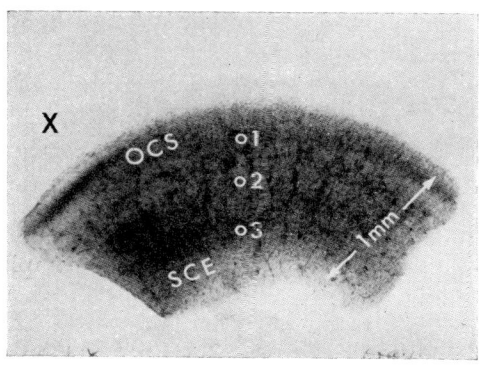

FIG. D18-1. Transition from simple to complex evoked responses in explants of newborn mouse cerebral cortex tissue (X), during first 2 weeks in vitro. OCS, original cortical surface; SCE, subcortical edge. (A) Simultaneous records showing simple spikes evoked in 3-day culture, at "cortical depths" of 200 μ (site 1 in X, upper sweep) and 400 μ (site 2) by stimulus applied near subcortical edge of explant (site 3). (B) Early signs of complex response patterns recorded, at much slower sweep rate, at same loci as in (A). Long-duration negativity appears with long latency after early superficial spike (upper sweep), and long-duration positivity develops with still longer latency after early deep spike. Arrow indicates onset of dual stimuli (spaced 50 msec apart). Note that the second pair of stimuli, applied 1 sec after first pair, is ineffective. (C_1) Simultaneous records of characteristic evoked potentials in 10-day culture at cortical depths of 250 μ (upper sweep) and 650 μ following stimulus applied at deeper site. Note 60 msec negative evoked response in superficial region and deep positive response of longer duration and greater latency. (C_2) Same as (C_1) at slower sweep rate. Small-amplitude repetitive potentials (10–20 per sec) follow primary responses at both sites and are also of opposite polarities. (D_1) After introduction of D-tubocurarine (100 μg per ml), repetitive afterdischarge becomes more pronounced. (D_2) Sudden increase in amplitude of *one* of the positive potentials in deep response (lower sweep) and reversal of polarity of corresponding potential in superficial response. (D_3) Large increase in amplitude of *all* positive potentials in deep response and reversal of polarity of *all* corresponding potentials in superficial response. Note marked decrease in frequency of repetitive discharge. (D_4) Subsequent decrease in amplitude of the large paroxysmal waves. Note: In this and subsequent figures, time and amplitude calibrations apply to all succeeding records until otherwise noted; upward deflection indicates negativity at active recording electrode. (From Crain [7].)

via 10 μ saline-filled pipettes. Indifferent electrodes were located near each active electrode, in fluid just below tissue.

By 3–5 days in culture, however, evoked potentials with durations of the order of 400 msec may occur (Fig. D18-1B), with latencies of as much as 100 msec following early spike response to a single stimulus. These long-lasting potentials increase in amplitude and regularity during the following week in vitro, and their durations generally decrease below 100 msec (Fig. D18-1C). They often show characteristic negative polarity (Fig. D18-1B, C, upper sweeps) when recorded with a microelectrode located near the original pial surface of the cortex (Fig. D18-1X), whereas potentials recorded simultaneously from *deep* loci tend to be positive and even longer in latency and duration. Facilitation of these complex evoked responses can be demonstrated with paired stimuli spaced at long test intervals. Small oscillatory (15–20 per sec) potentials appear, at times, during the long-duration evoked response (Fig. D18-1B), and both components of the afterdischarge may occur spontaneously. Strychnine, moreover, produces characteristic enhancement of these discharges [7].

EVOKED RESPONSES. Although intracellularly recorded postsynaptic potentials have not yet been obtained from cerebral tissue cultures, analysis of the extracellular data leaves little doubt that the complex bioelectric activities described above are mediated through synaptic networks. The characteristic negative and positive slow waves recorded from superficial and deep regions of the cerebral explants appear to be due to summated postsynaptic potentials that are predominantly excitatory and inhibitory, respectively [7, 10].

The negative evoked response recorded from superficial sites in cerebral explants shows marked similarities in temporal pattern to the prolonged EPSPs evoked in cortical neurons of the neonatal kitten in situ (cf. Fig. D18-1B, C, upper sweeps with Fig. 18-2A in Purpura's presentation). Furthermore, the positive evoked response recorded from deeper regions in young cerebral explants shows striking resemblance to the extraordinary long-lasting IPSPs characteristic of immature neocortical neurons in situ. Duration of evoked responses in many of the cerebral explants also decreases during maturation in culture (cf. Fig. D18-1C with 1B), as occurs in situ. Extracellular microelectrode recordings from cerebral explants appear, then, to provide at least a crude monitor of neuronal PSP activities, but these data must be interpreted with extreme caution pending closely correlated studies with intracellular electrodes [6, 17]. Recent analyses by Pollen (Chap. 15) provide additional theoretical support to these PSP interpretations of extracellular slow waves in the cultured tissues, especially in view of the relatively two-dimensional simplicity of these explants.

It is of interest that the capacity of cerebral explants to generate these complex discharges after 3–5 days in vitro (cf. Fig. D18-1B with 1A) coincides with the sudden development of abundant axodendritic synapses in this tissue [18]. As in Purpura's analysis of neonatal hippocampal cortex in situ, the paucity of axosomatic synapses in the newborn cerebral explants during the first week in vitro is not at all incompatible with generation of prominent IPSPs. A still closer correlation between the onset of complex bioelectric activity and the first appearance of synaptic junctions has been obtained during the maturation of 14-day embryonic rat spinal cord in vitro [4, 12]. In this case, too, roughly concomitant onset of function of inhibitory as well as excitatory synapses is suggested by the fact that strychnine could elicit long-lasting afterdischarges within one day after the first signs of complex (synaptically mediated) cord activity were detected.

The factors suggested by Purpura to account for the gradual decrease in duration of cerebral discharges during maturation in situ are all applicable to the tissue culture model. The cerebral explant shows a similar progressive decrease in neuronal packing density, during maturation in vitro, concomitant with elaboration of a dense neural and glial network throughout the tissue [2, 18]. Delayed enzymatic inactivation of transmitter in immature neurons appears to be a good working hypothesis to account for the prolonged PSPs both in situ and in vitro, but critical data are not yet available (for example, Fig. D18-5).

The rapid depression of surface evoked responses seen during repetitive stimulation of immature brain, in situ, is also characteristic of cerebral explants during the first week or two in vitro. Whereas stimulus rates greater than 1 per 5 sec often produce rapid block in young cultures (Fig. D18-1B), rates of 1–10 per sec become effective in older explants (Fig. D18-2A) and prolonged facilitation may occur [10]. As Purpura has emphasized, precocious development of inhibitory synaptic pathways may, indeed, be an important factor underlying the stability of immature cerebral cortex. Summation of the long-lasting IPSPs which appear so prominently in his recordings from these neonatal cortical neurons could easily account for much of the apparent fatigability and stability of the young brain.

The characteristic positive evoked potentials observed especially in the central and deep regions of the cerebral explants (Fig.

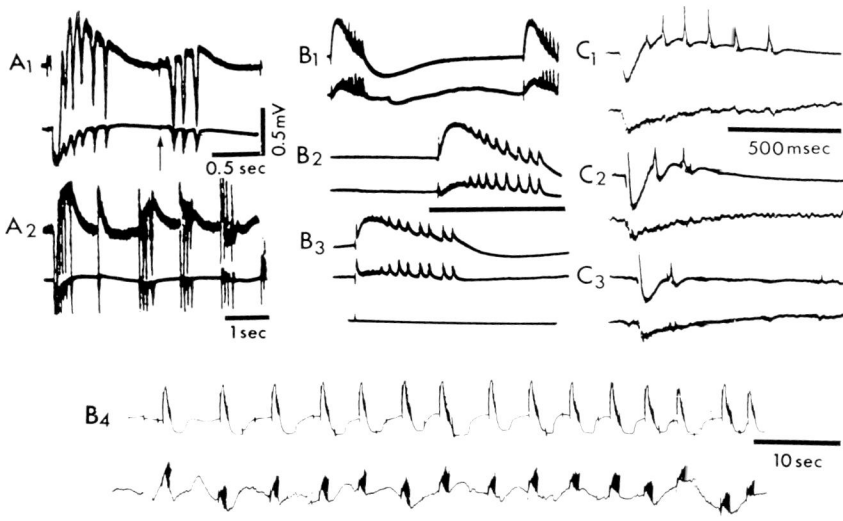

Fig. D18-2. Evoked and spontaneous oscillatory discharges recorded in long-term cultures of mouse cerebral cortex (1–2 months in vitro). (A_1) Repetitive afterdischarge evoked in two regions of explant by single stimuli applied several hundred micra away from both recording sites. Note decreased amplitude and increased latency of primary evoked response following stimulus applied (at arrow) 1 sec after onset of first afterdischarge. (A_2) Similar to (A_1) at slower sweep rate. Note marked variations in response pattern to successive stimuli at 1 per sec. ($B_{1,2,4}$) Simultaneous recordings of spontaneous activity, in another cerebral explant, at two sites 150 μ apart. Note extremely slow sweep in (B_4). (B_3) Similar discharges evoked, at same recording sites, by single stimulus. (C_1) Repetitive discharge evoked in another region of same cerebral explant. Note graded decrease in total duration of response sequence as temperature is lowered from 34°C to 29°C (C_2) and then to 27°C (C_3). (From Crain [7, 8].)

D18-1B, 1C, lower sweeps) may indicate the existence of similar inhibitory systems in vitro. The positive potentials can be greatly enhanced by D-tubocurarine (cf. Fig. D18-1$D_{3,4}$ with C_2) and, moreover, the polarity of characteristic negative potentials evoked in superficial regions of the cerebral explant may be inverted (cf. Fig. D18-1$D_{2,3}$ with D_1). At the same time, the threshold for evoked responses increases markedly. Appearance of paroxysmal (3–4 per sec) positive waves of unusually large amplitude, occurring synchronously over widespread regions of the explant (Fig. D18-1$D_{3,4}$), may represent unmasking of powerful IPSPs in the cultured tissue, following selective block of excitatory synapses by D-tubocurarine. This postulated action of D-tubocurarine on excitatory synapses in cerebral cortex may be due to the same mechanism by which this drug blocks ACh-mediated neuromuscular transmission (see Esplin and Stone, Chap. 7). Purpura's suggestion regarding the possibility of "an intrinsic pacemakerlike alteration in inhibitory interneurons" as the basis for the rhythmic IPSPs recorded in immature hippocampal cortex in situ may also apply to the rhythmic positive waves generated in cerebral cultures, especially if curare blocks excitatory synapses to recurrent inhibitory interneurons (vide infra). Correlative intracellular recordings in the isolated explants should help to clarify this problem. Strychnine, on the other hand, often causes polarity inversion of *positive* evoked potentials in cerebral explants, and may lead to appearance of characteristic negative sharp waves of large amplitude and long duration [10], as occurs in neonatal rat cortex in situ [5, 9]. These effects can be interpreted as a shift toward EPSP-dominance in the cultured tissue

Stimuli-Evoked Discharges. Purpura has discussed the hyperexcitability properties that develop in slabs of neonatal kitten neocortex several days after chronic neuronal isolation. Under these conditions, single surface stimuli can elicit a rather stereotyped sequence of repetitive surface-positive (or diphasic) discharges. Remarkably similar oscillatory afterdischarges have been evoked by single stimuli in many cerebral explants [7, 8]. The repetitive sequence generally consists of 3–12 large, diphasic potentials each lasting 25–50 msec, and occurring at a rate of about 10 per sec (Figs. D18-1D_1, 2, 3A, 4C, 6C_1). A large, early evoked potential is often followed by a long delay prior to appearance of a repetitive series of predominantly positive potentials of gradually increasing amplitude, which then terminates abruptly (Figs. D18-2A, 3A, 6C_1; see, however, Fig. D18-2B, 2C). In many cases, the positive sharp-waves appear to be superimposed on a much longer lasting negativity, of the order of 1 sec in duration.

Recordings at multiple sites indicate that these repetitive discharges are highly synchronized over large areas of the explant, and they may occur spontaneously (Fig. D18-2$B_{1,2,4}$) as in isolated cerebral slabs in neonatal kitten, in situ. They are quite prominent in cerebral explants after 1 to 2 weeks in culture, but they have been detected as early as 4 days in vitro, with much smaller amplitude (Fig. D18-1B). Comparable oscillatory discharges also occur in some explants of rat spinal cord after several weeks in culture, and a strikingly similar response sequence has been evoked in cultured human embryo spinal-cord tissue, after 3 months in vitro (Fig. D18-3A_2). Development of these complex, yet stereotyped, repetitive discharges which can be triggered by single, brief, electric stimuli in such diverse CNS tissues, neuronally isolated under such widely different environmental conditions in situ and in vitro (cf.

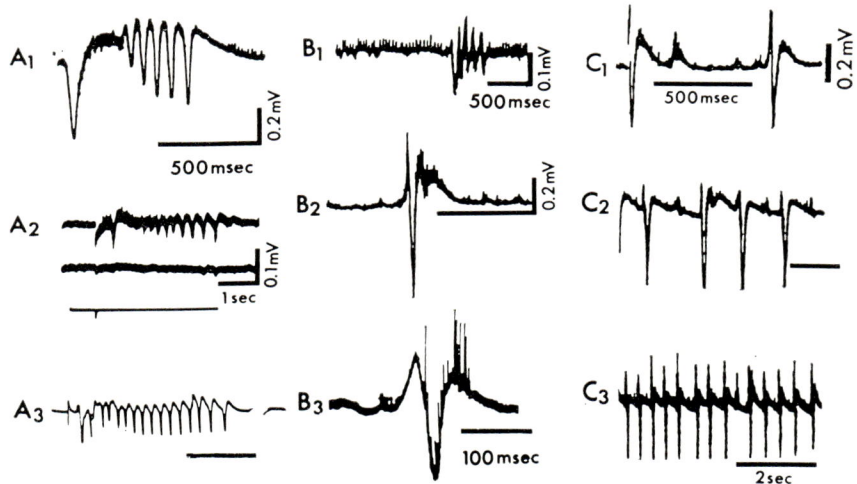

FIG. D18-3. Resemblance of repetitive afterdischarges in some CNS explants to abnormal hyperexcitability patterns in situ. (A_1) Oscillatory afterdischarge evoked by single stimulus in neonatal mouse cerebral explant (1 month in vitro; see also Fig. D18-2). (A_2) Afterdischarge evoked by single stimulus in human spinal cord explant (6-week embryo, 4 months in vitro). (A_3) Characteristic afterdischarge evoked in cerebral cortical slab in 5-day-old kitten, in situ, 3 days after neuronal isolation. Note remarkable similarity of these complex, yet stereotyped, repetitive discharge patterns in vitro and in situ. ($B_{1,2}$) Spontaneous discharges recorded in mouse cerebral explant (2 weeks in vitro). (B_3) Characteristic paroxysmal abnormal wave recorded in epileptic cortex of adult monkey, in situ. Note similarity of the triphasic, initially negative, complexes in (B_2) and (B_3), with superimposed bursts of unit spikes. (C_{1-3}) Long-lasting sequence of triphasic discharges (as in B_2) evoked by single stimulus applied at beginning of record (C_1). Note decreased sweep rate in C_2 and C_3. (A_1, $B_{1,2}$, C_{1-3} from Crain [7]; A_2 from Crain [8]; A_3 from Purpura and Housepian [21]; B_3 from Schmidt et al. [24].)

Fig. D18-3$A_{1,2,3}$), suggests that a basic type of neural network underlies generation of this common pattern of bioelectric activity [8]. Analysis of this network may be of significance for clarifying mechanisms underlying generation of complex rhythmic activities of the CNS, not only under pathologic conditions of isolation, but also in the normal state.

On the basis of correlative electrophysiologic and histologic analyses of chronically isolated neonatal cerebral slabs in situ, Purpura has concluded that extensive axon-collateral sprouting of the regenerating pyramidal neurons may be "the major factor responsible for the increase in excitatory synaptic drives that are reflected in evoked repetitive bursts" [21]. Moreover, the "major generators for . . . the surface positive repetitive discharges . . . [appear to be] . . . located at depths corresponding to the cell bodies and proximal portions of apical dendrites of the largest pyramidal neurons . . ." where repetitive focal negativities were recorded concomitantly. However, since these studies have been limited so far to extracellular recordings, the data do not exclude the possibility that generation of IPSPs in superficial cortical regions may play a major role in development of the surface positive discharges.

Axon-Collaterals and Synaptic Connections. It is, of course, quite reasonable to associate the increased excitability of chronically isolated immature cerebral tissues with growth of larger numbers of excitatory synapses on pyramidal neurons. Since, however, the evidence rests primarily upon histological analysis of a relatively small fraction of the cells (in Golgi sections), it does not constitute a compelling argument against the alternative concept of "denervation or disuse hypersensitivity," which has been demonstrated in many adult tissues under conditions where substantial growth of additional axon-collaterals and synapses appears to be precluded (see Sharpless and Rutledge, Chap. 12; Ward, Chap. 10; and [15, 25, 26]).

Some form of hypersensitivity may also occur in these immature cerebral tissues after neuronal isolation, thereby increasing the potency of *existing* excitatory synaptic connections. The axon-collaterals which sprout profusely from the regenerating pyramidal cells might actually be making most of their synaptic connections with *inhibitory* interneurons. Growth of new collaterals terminating directly in excitatory synapses on neighboring efferent neurons may be characteristic only of *localized* lesions where, as Ramón y Cajal [22] has suggested, "the nervous impulse that reaches the mutilated neuron is not absolutely lost, since it is now diverted, through the enlarged channel of the collaterals, towards other congenerous neurones . . . thus increasing the energy of the efferent currents."

In *completely* isolated CNS tissue, on the other hand, there are no such normal "congenerous neurones," since not only are *all* efferent neurons surgically severed, but they are also partly *deafferented*. Under these extreme conditions, increased numbers of *inhibitory* collaterals may develop as a major compensatory (homeostatic) reaction which would neutralize the "supersensitivity" of the partly denervated (and totally sensory-deprived) efferent neurons, and thereby tend to restore the injured CNS tissue toward a more stable state compatible with continued function [8]. Such hypertrophic recurrent innervation of inhibitory interneurons—which ramify profusely and, in turn, trigger IPSPs in hundreds of neighboring efferent neurons—would greatly enhance the synchronization and regularity of rhythmic waves generated by these cells (in accordance with the inhibitory "phasing" mechanism elaborated by Andersen and Eccles [1] and others), and would account for the unusually stereotyped character of the oscillatory afterdischarges in chronically isolated immature cerebral tissues.

From this point of view, duration of the repetitive oscillatory sequences and amplitude of the periodic sharp-wave components would depend on strength of the long-lasting excitatory drive impinging upon the efferent neurons (for example, summated EPSPs or other graded depolarizing potentials or both—note ca. 1-sec negativities in Figs. D18-1*B*; 2*A*, 2*B*; 3*A*) relative to strength of the summated, shorter duration, recurrent inhibitory discharges. If the latter are sufficiently powerful, the discharge sequence may be quenched rapidly following initial triggering of the system (Fig. D18-4A, B, C_1 vs. $4C_2$). The large positive monophasic evoked potentials observed in many of the older cerebral explants may be due to such inhibitory dominance (Fig. D18-4A); the latent hyperexcitability and capacity for generation of oscillatory afterdischarges can be revealed, by selective enhancement of EPSPs or depression of IPSPs, with drugs such as strychnine or bromophenol blue (Fig. D18-4C vs. 4A, 4B; cf. [16]) or by repetitive electric stimuli (Fig. 4 in [13]). These interpretations of extracellularly recorded repetitive discharge patterns in cerebral explants are, of course, highly speculative; correlative intracellular recordings (and more quantitative histological studies) will be required to provide a firmer foundation for analysis of the special excitability properties of isolated immature cerebral tissues, both in situ and in vitro. The above discussion simply raises the possibility that these isolated immature tissues may be valuable preparations for study of organized *inhibitory* systems associated with stabilization of hyperexcitable CNS networks (see, for example, [20]) in addition to their more obvious applicability to problems focused on *excitatory* processes.

Enhancement and Prolongation of Evoked Potentials. Relatively low concentrations of acetylcholine and eserine (about 0.1 μg per ml) may produce enhancement and unusual prolongation of evoked potentials in cerebral explants (Fig. D18-5B vs. 5A; see also Fig. D18-1B); also generation of long series of rhythmic sharp-waves of gradually increasing repetition rate (Fig. D18-5B_3, $C_{1,2}$; cf. Fig. D18-3$C_{2,3}$). Systematic studies of ACh sensitivity during maturation of cerebral tissues in culture may provide a useful model to supplement comparable studies in slabs of adult cerebral cortex in situ, where marked supersensitivity to ACh appears to develop within 1–3 weeks after neuronal isolation ([15, 23]; see, however, Krnjevic, Chap. 6). On the other hand, many cerebral explants appear to be in a more overtly hyperexcitable state even without introduction of pharmaco-

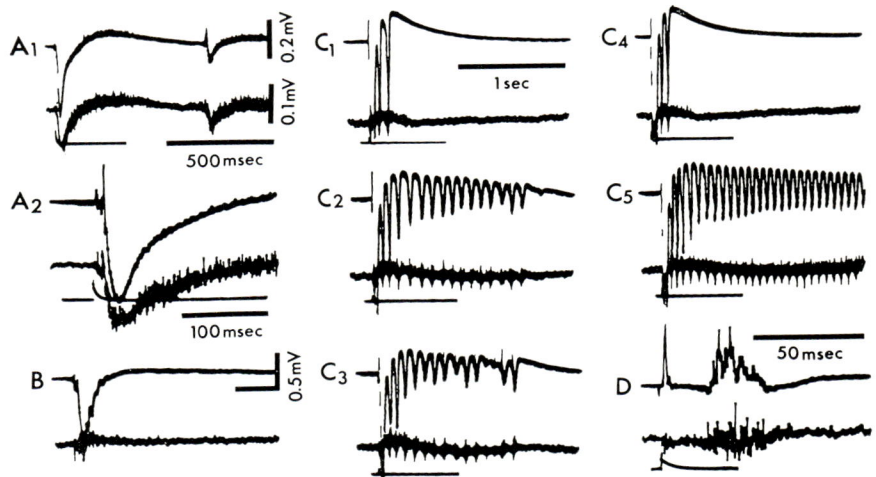

Fig. D18-4. Enhancement of oscillatory afterdischarges in cerebral explant after application of bromophenol blue (6 weeks in vitro). ($A_{1,2}$) Characteristic positive responses evoked at two cortical sites (300 μ apart) by single stimulus applied to subcortical tissue (1 mm deeper). (B) Simultaneous recordings of cortical evoked response, upper sweep as in (A), and smaller discharge elicited in subcortical region near same stimulus site as in (A). (C_{1-5}) Repetitive oscillatory afterdischarges evoked after introduction of bromophenol blue (100 μg per ml). Note unusually long duration of repetitive sequence in (C_5). (D) Disappearance of oscillatory afterdischarges after return to control medium. Note faster sweep. (From Crain [8] and unpublished observations.)

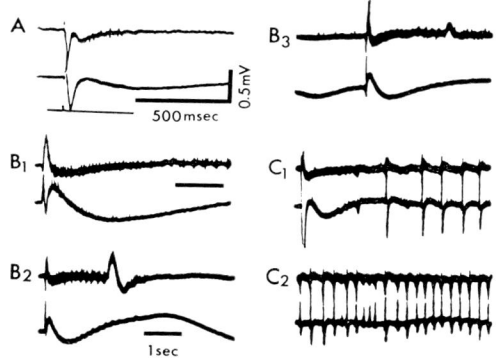

FIG. D18-5. Paroxysmal repetitive discharges in cultured mouse cerebral tissue after application of acetylcholine and eserine. (A) Complex, predominantly positive, evoked responses at superficial (upper sweep) and deep cortical sites (2 weeks in vitro). ($B_{1,2}$) Increased complexity and duration of discharges evoked after brief exposure to acetylcholine and eserine (each at 0.5 μg per ml) and then return to control medium. Note prominent long-lasting negative potentials elicited at both cerebral sites, with long latencies following single stimulus. (B_3) Onset of spontaneous discharges. ($C_{1,2}$) Repetitive afterdischarges occur at higher rates (3–5 per sec) following sustained exposure to these agents at lower concentration (0.05 μg per ml). (From Crain, unpublished observations.)

logic agents or electric stimuli. In some cases, spontaneous activities resemble the repetitive oscillatory (10 per sec) afterdischarges discussed above (Fig. D18-$2B_{1,2,4}$); in other explants, there has been remarkable mimicry of "paroxysmal abnormal waves" recorded with microelectrodes in epileptic cortex [24] in situ (cf. Fig. D18-$3B_2$ and B_3). The latter type of discharges often occur at relatively high repetition rates of about 1–3 per sec (Fig. D18-$3C_{2,3}$), whereas the longer lasting oscillatory sequences tend to be spaced by silent periods of about 3–15 sec (Fig. D18-$2B_{1,4}$).

Occurrence of epileptiform and other types of sustained paroxysmal activities in some of the cerebral explants may be related to uncontrolled parameters in the tissue culture environment. Depending upon the thickness, age, and other variables, the central zone of many of these (freehand dissected) explants becomes necrotic due to relatively poor diffusion of nutrients and waste products to and from this region [3, 19]. Although healthy, organized tissue surrounding this necrotic core may be maintained for months in vitro, neurons at the edge of the degenerated zone may be in a state resembling conditions at an epileptogenic focus near a cortical glial scar in situ. More controlled production of miniature epileptogenic foci in cerebral explants by localized chemical or physical alterations may provide a valuable model system to supplement studies of epileptic cortex in situ.

Patterns of Activity. A start has been made in studying the effects of brain-stem and other subcortical tissues on the properties of cerebral explants after growth in vitro of neural connections between the two closely apposed fragments [14]. In cultures of "coupled" medulla and cerebral tissues, characteristic repetitive oscillatory afterdischarges may be evoked in the cerebral explant by stimuli applied locally in either fragment, whereas simultaneous recording in the medulla explant often shows radically different patterns of activity—generally high frequency bursts of spikes (Fig. D18-6A, 6B). Spontaneous activities have been seen more regularly in these medulla-coupled as compared to isolated cerebral explants (cf. Fig. D18-6C through J with 6K), and the discharges often show complex, highly synchronized relationships between the explants, suggesting both excitatory and inhibitory interactions (Fig. D18-6B through F). Large positive cerebral slow waves tend to occur regularly after each prominent spike burst in the medulla explant (although the cerebral discharge can, at times, lead the medulla). Moreover, silent periods in the medulla spike-burst patterns appear to correlate with occurrence of negative cerebral slow waves. During intervals when spontaneous cerebral activity is absent, spike bursts in medulla appear to be longer lasting and less sharply interrupted by silent periods (Fig. D18-6G). In other cases, however, repetitive sequences of medulla spike bursts alternate with silent periods even in the absence of cerebral activity (or in completely isolated medulla explants).

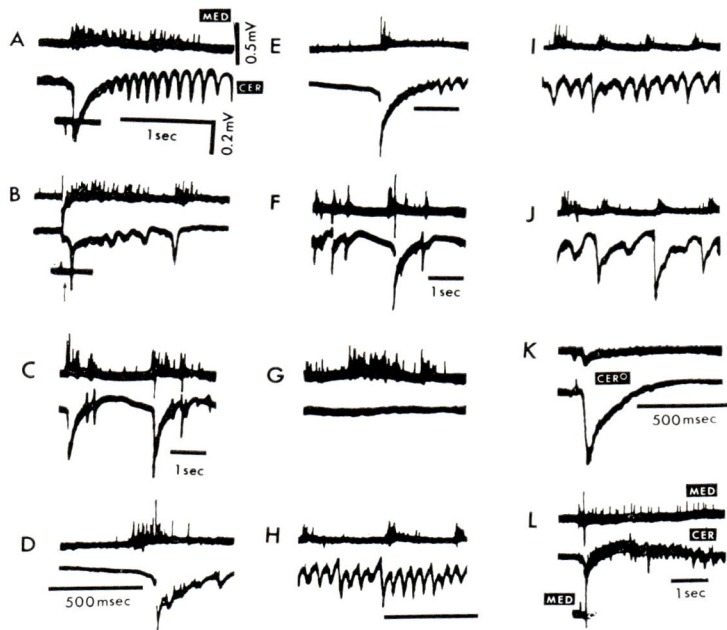

Fig. D18-6. Interactions between separate explants of fetal mouse cerebrum and medulla after formation of functional connections in culture (14-day fetus; 3 weeks in vitro). (A) Simultaneous recordings of afterdischarges evoked in cerebral (CER) and medulla (MED) explants by single cerebral stimulus (after brief exposure to strychnine at 10 μg per ml). Note characteristic long-lasting oscillatory (10 per sec) repetitive sequence triggered in the cerebral tissue (lower sweep), in contrast to the high frequency spike barrage elicited in the medulla explant. (B) Similar discharges evoked by paired medulla and cerebral stimuli. Note that medulla spikes occur in bursts which tend to be synchronized with positive phases of cerebral oscillatory sequences. (C) through (F) Rhythmic spontaneous discharges occurring synchronously in medulla and cerebrum explants. (G) Medulla spike-burst patterns appear less well defined during period of cerebral quiescence. (H) through (J) Development of *sustained* oscillatory discharges in cerebrum concomitant with appearance of more rhythmic spike bursts in medulla. (K) Only simple positive evoked potentials are evoked in another cerebral explant (CER°) in same culture but *not* coupled to a medulla explant. (L) After return to coupled cerebrum-medulla explants, long-lasting cerebral oscillatory afterdischarge is still evoked by single stimulus to medulla (or may occur spontaneously). (From Crain et al. [14].)

Repetitive stimulation of the medulla explant may produce a *sustained* increase in the excitability of the cerebral explant [14], resembling the triggering of a mild seizure in situ. At times, unusually well-sustained, rhythmic, oscillatory (10 per sec) cerebral activity occurs *concomitantly* with the appearance of rhythmic (1–2 per sec) spike bursts in the medulla explant (Fig. D18-6H through J), in contrast to the more typical occurrence of periodic *damping* of cerebral oscillatory discharges (Fig. D18-6C through F; note transition in Fig. D18-6J). Analysis of brain-stem pacemaker discharges which may control the bioelectric activities of cortical explants should be of great interest.

Many spinal cord and some cerebral explants show signs of hyperexcitability characterized by low thresholds for triggering long-lasting, asynchronous barrages of spike potentials and by sporadic occurrence of spontaneous discharges. Although the presence of inhibitory synapses is suggested by the marked sensitivity of these explants to strychnine [8, 11], no signs of repetitive oscillatory afterdischarges have been detected in these explants. It would be interesting to determine whether the capacity for generation of the stereotyped, synchronized, rhythmic slow-wave discharges in CNS explants correlates with development of the postulated inhibitory interneurons with profusely ramifying collaterals to pyramidal neurons. In addition to the hyperexcitability which would be expected in the absence of widespread innervation by recurrent-inhibitory interneurons, more bizarre types of instabilities may appear if a substantial area of *any* type of postsynaptic dendritic membrane loses its specialized chemoreceptor properties.

As Purpura has pointed out, the membrane in such denuded regions of the dendritic tree may then become conductile: capable of initiating and propagating spikes, which occurs normally in immature, cortical dendrites. This mechanism for producing augmented neuronal excitability by interference with dendritic synaptogenesis, or by degeneration of existing axodendritic synapses, can be viewed as a special type of "denervation hypersensitivity." In this regard, concentration of synapses on dendritic spines of adult cerebral cortical neurons (Szentágothai and Colonnier, Chap. 2) may be a *normal* mechanism which facilitates spike propagation in some types of dendritic branches by minimizing the area occupied by patches of nonconductile postsynaptic membrane in the dendritic "mainline." In addition to the elegant evidence of spike propagation in dendrites of immature cortical neurons which Purpura has obtained with intracellular recordings, similar conclusions have been reached on the basis of extracellular stimulation and recording with microelectrodes, positioned under direct visual control, on noninnervated dendrites of neurons in neonatal cerebellar [17] and cerebral [10] cultures. The latter experiments demonstrate the rather unique potentialities of CNS tissue cultures for close correlations of mammalian nerve (and glial) cell structure and function [8, 9].

In conclusion, it is hoped that these complementary bioelectric and morphologic studies of the brain during maturation in vitro as well as in situ, will lead to fresh insights into some of the baffling problems which are being brought into focus in this monograph.

ACKNOWLEDGMENT. Parts of Figs. D18-1 through 3 have been reproduced by permission from Grune and Stratton, Inc., New York.

REFERENCES

1. Andersen, P., and Eccles, J. C. Inhibitory phasing of neuronal discharge. *Nature* (London) 196:645, 1962.
2. Bornstein, M. B. Morphological Development of Neonatal Mouse Cerebral Cortex in Tissue Culture. In Kellaway, P., and Petersén, I. (Eds.), *Neurological and Electroencephalographic Correlative Studies in Infancy*. New York: Grune and Stratton, 1964, pp. 1–11.
3. Bunge, R. P., Bunge, M. B., and Peterson, E. R. An electron-microscope study of cultured rat spinal cord. *J. Cell Biol.* 24:163, 1965.
4. Bunge, M. B., Bunge, R. P., and Peterson, E. R. The onset of synapse formation in spinal cord cultures as studied by electron microscopy. *Brain Res.* 6:728, 1967.
5. Crain, S. M. Development of electrical activity in the cerebral cortex of the albino rat. *Proc. Soc. Exp. Biol. Med.* 81:49, 1952.
6. Crain, S. M. Resting and action potentials of cultured chick embryo spinal ganglion cells. *J. Comp. Neurol.* 104:285, 1956.
7. Crain, S. M. Development of Bioelectric Activity during Growth of Neonatal Mouse Cerebral Cortex in Tissue Culture. In Kellaway, P., and Petersén, I. (Eds.), *Neurological and Electroencephalographic Correlative Studies in Infancy*. New York: Grune and Stratton, 1964, pp. 12–26.
8. Crain, S. M. Development of "organotypic" bioelectric activities in central nervous tissues during maturation in culture. *Int. Rev. Neurobiol.* 9:1, 1966.

9. Crain, S. M. Tissue Culture Studies of Developing Brain Function. In Himwich, W. A. and Himwich, H. E. (Eds.), *Developmental Neurobiology*. Springfield, Ill.: Thomas, 1969, in press.

10. Crain, S. M., and Bornstein, M. B. Bioelectric activity of neonatal mouse cerebral cortex during growth and differentiation in tissue culture. *Exp. Neurol.* 10:425, 1964.

11. Crain, S. M., and Peterson, E. R. Complex bioelectric activity in organized tissue cultures of spinal cord (human, rat and chick). *J. Cell. Comp. Physiol.* 64:1, 1964.

12. Crain, S. M., and Peterson, E. R. Onset and development of functional interneuronal connections in explants of rat spinal cord-ganglia during maturation in culture. *Brain Res.* 6:750, 1967.

13. Crain, S. M., Bornstein, M. B., and Peterson, E. R. Maturation of cultured embryonic CNS tissues during chronic exposure to agents which prevent bioelectric activity. *Brain Res.* 8:363, 1968.

14. Crain, S. M., Peterson, E. R., and Bornstein, M. B. Formation of Functional Interneuronal Connections between Explants of Various Mammalian Central Nervous Tissues during Development In Vitro. In Wolstenholme, G. E. W., and O'Connor, M. (Eds.), *Growth of the Nervous System*. London: Churchill, 1968, pp. 13–31.

15. Echlin, F. A. The supersensitivity of chronically "isolated" cerebral cortex as a mechanism in focal epilepsy. *Electroenceph. Clin. Neurophysiol.* 11:697, 1959.

16. Feldberg, W., and Fleischhauer, K. The site of origin of the seizure discharge produced by tubocurarine acting from the cerebral ventricles. *J. Physiol.* (London) 160:258, 1962.

17. Hild, W., and Tasaki, I. Morphological and physiological properties of neurons and glial cells in tissue culture. *J. Neurophysiol.* 25:277, 1962.

18. Pappas, G. D. Electron Microscopy of Neuronal Junctions Involved in Transmission in the Central Nervous System. In Rodahl, K., and Issekutz, B., Jr. (Eds.), *Nerve as a Tissue*. New York: Hoeber, 1966, pp. 49–87.

19. Peterson, E. R., Crain, S. M., and Murray, M. R. Differentiation and prolonged maintenance of bioelectrically active spinal cord cultures (rat, chick and human). *Z. Zellforsch.* 66:130, 1965.

20. Prince, D. A., and Wilder, B. J. Control mechanisms in cortical epileptogenic foci. *Arch. Neurol.* (Chicago) 16:194, 1967.

21. Purpura, D. P., and Housepian, E. M. Morphological and physiological properties of chronically isolated immature neocortex. *Exp. Neurol.* 4:377, 1961.

22. Ramón y Cajal, S. *Degeneration and Regeneration of the Nervous System*. May, R. M. (Ed. and Transl.), London and New York: Oxford University Press, vol. 2, 1928, pp. 616–669.

23. Rosenberg, P., and Echlin, F. A. Time course of changes in cholinesterase activity of chronic partially isolated cortex. *J. Nerv. Ment. Dis.* 147:56, 1968.

24. Schmidt, R. P., Thomas, L. B., and Ward, A. A., Jr. The hyperexcitable neurone. Microelectrode studies of chronic epileptic foci in monkey. *J. Neurophysiol.* 22:285, 1959.

25. Sharpless, S. K. Reorganization of function in the nervous system—Use and disuse. *Ann. Rev. Physiol.* 26:357, 1964.

26. Stavraky, G. W. *Supersensitivity Following Lesions of the Nervous System*. Toronto: University of Toronto Press, 1961.

19
Ontogeny of Focal Seizures*

WILLIAM F. CAVENESS

WITH THE PHYLOGENETIC DEVELOPMENT of the central nervous system, there is an increase in seizure susceptibility, an elaboration of fit pattern, and greater consistency in the clinical expression. Servit has demonstrated this progression in seizure phenomena, as elicited by electroshock and pentylenetetrazol, from cyclostomata through amphibia and reptiles to mammals [11]. An ontogenetic recapitulation, in principle, is to be expected in the higher primates.

In an effort to better understand the developing seizure patterns in man, a study was begun with Nielsen, Yakovlev, and Adams on this phenomenon in the *Macaca mulatta* some eight years ago. Particular interest was centered in *Jacksonian seizures,* meaning rhythmic motor phenomena beginning in one part and progressing with an orderly march to involve successively adjacent parts of the body in the attack [3, 14]. The present report represents the conclusion of the first phase of this investigation.

The monkey was chosen because of its relatively high rank in the primate scale, not only in regard to the central nervous system but also the skeletomuscular system that make the unfolding clinical fit pattern easier to observe than one in lower animals. The selection of focal seizures for study permitted control of the origin of the discharge and some facility in following its spread. The hand-face area of the motor cortex was chosen because of its known susceptibility to seizure activation [5] and the known subcortical preferential pathways that subserve this area [13]. Penicillin was selected because we found this agent capable of producing seizures in monkeys at one day of age. Attempts to create focal seizures by single or multiple injection of alumina cream gave inconstant and disappointing results below three months of age. Electroshock was equally ineffective in the very young animal and brought to mind Fulton's comment, "During the first few weeks of life, it is generally difficult in the infant macaque to evoke isolated motor responses, even with strong stimulation of the cortex" [6].

MATERIAL. Twenty monkeys were selected that represented successive stages in development from birth to adulthood. Six were between 1 and 10 days of age, three between 2 and 24 weeks, eight between 7 and 24 months, and three between 4 and 6 years at the time of seizure induction.

At the outset let us consider the newborn monkey (Fig. 19-1A) and its central nervous system capabilities. While its brain weight is 70 percent of what will be achieved in

---

* The experimental observations were made in the neurological laboratories at Columbia University, College of Physicians and Surgeons, New York City, and the Warren Anatomical Museum of Harvard Medical School, Boston. Analyses of clinical and EEG patterns were facilitated by animation techniques afforded by William Hanna and Hanna-Barbera Productions, Hollywood, Calif.

These studies were supported by Association for the Aid to Crippled Children, National Institute of Neurological Diseases and Stroke, and United Cerebral Palsy Research and Educational Foundation.

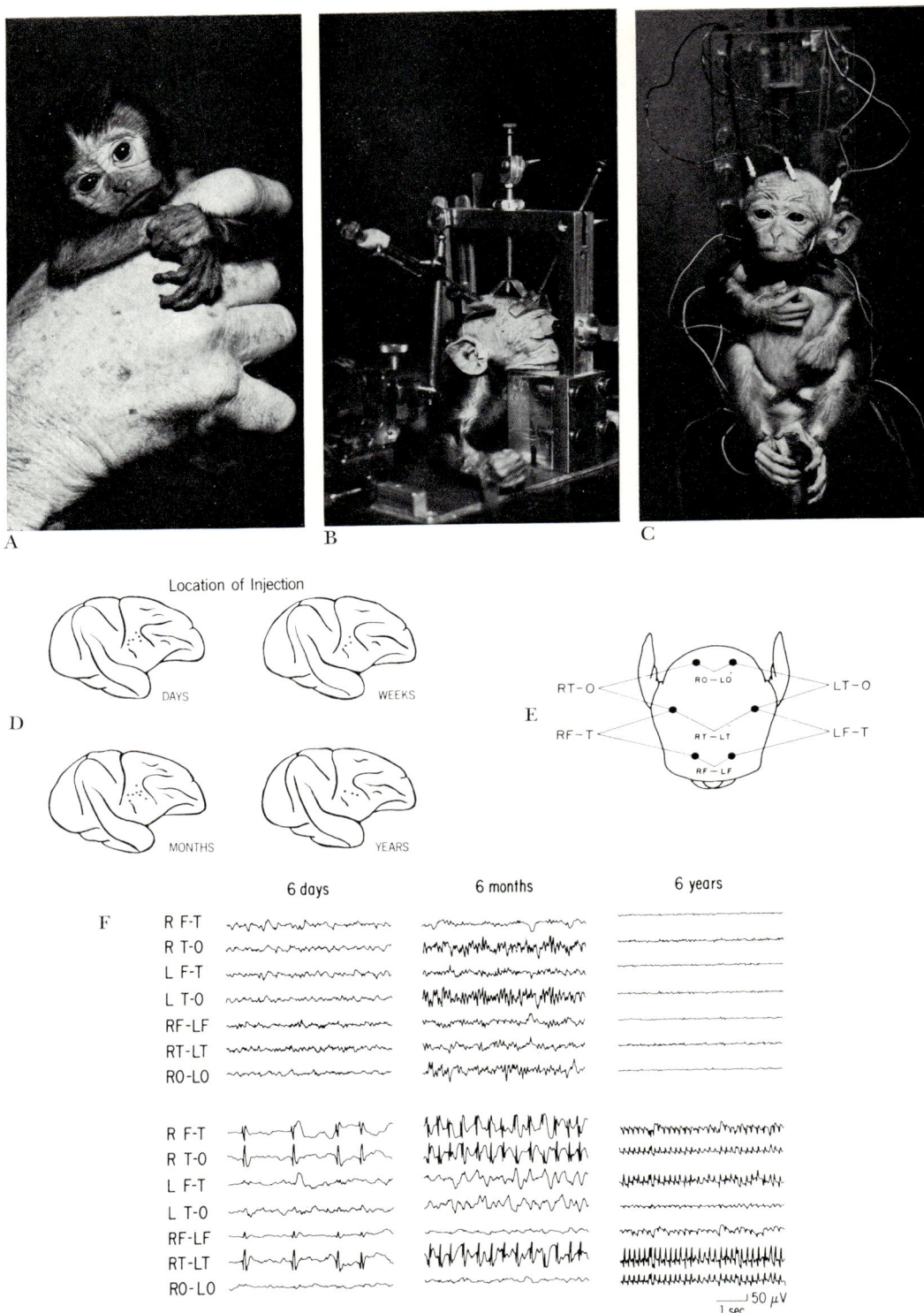

Fig. 19-1. (A) *Macaca mulatta*, age 1 day. (B) Semistereotactic injection of penicillin. (C) Position for clinical (cine-photographic and EMG) and electroencephalographic observations. (D) Injection sites in right sensorimotor cortex. (E) Electrode placement for bipolar recording. (F) Alpha activity, upper tracings, and focal paroxysmal activity, lower tracings, at different stages in brain development.

adulthood, there is still considerable maturation in structure and function yet to be accomplished. Some idea of primary sensorimotor development is gained from the observations of Hines [7]. She noted eye-following at 1 week, placing in reference to touch at 2 weeks, digital manipulation at 3 weeks, sitting at 1 to 2 weeks, standing at 3 months, and progression (adult form) at 3 to 4 months. Movements proximally initiated begin at 1 day with coordinated fine distal manipulation not taking place for 2 to 3 months. The maturation of the cortex is reflected, in part, by developing alpha activity in the electroencephalogram. Only rudimentary forms are present in the first weeks with well-modulated regular waking rhythms not becoming apparent for several months [4].

METHOD. Twenty-five thousand U crystalline penicillin in 0.025 cc of aqueous solution were injected 2–3 mm into the hand-face area of the right motor cortex (Fig. 19-1B). The agent was introduced with a 22-gauge needle that passed through the scalp, a previously created skull defect, the dura, and into the superficial brain substance. In effect the penicillin was *brought into contact with all layers of the cortex* as the excess solution escaped along the needle track. In every other respect, the animal was intact, alert, and without anesthesia. While some variation in the site and depth of the injection was inevitable, placement of the activating agent was found to be reasonably consistent (Fig. 19-1D).

Onset and elaboration of the attack pattern was simultaneously recorded by motion picture photography, electromyography, and electroencephalography (Fig. 19-1C). This permitted a detailed analysis of the evolving clinical phenomena, and the electrical reflexion of the discharging lesion and its spread as reflected from the scalp recording.

The EEG was obtained with six scalp electrodes, 27-gauge tungsten alloy needles, arrayed in three bilaterally symmetrical pairs over the frontal, temporal, and occipital regions. Laterally, the frontal and occipital placements were equidistant from that of the temporal electrode (Fig. 19-1E). From these, and accessory electrode placements, bipolar recordings were obtained in multiple combinations with a standard 16-channel Grass electroencephalograph.

Figure 19-1F provides examples of the focal abnormality at different stages in brain development. The upper tracings indicate the normal waking EEG at 6 days, 6 months, and 6 years. The lower tracings indicate the character of the paroxysmal activity following penicillin injection in the right motor cortex. From the newborn to the fully adult brain there is a pronounced increase in regularity and rate with a marked reduction in amplitude.

RESULTS. For clarity, representative observations from the neonatal period (1–10 days), puberty (24 months) and young adulthood (4–6 years) will be presented, with generalizations from the remainder of the material, when pertinent.

NEWBORN

Clinical Expression

Monkey number 81 received an induced seizure at 2 days of age. No abnormal movements were apparent for fifty minutes following the intracortical injection of penicillin in the right motor cortex (Fig. 19-2). At 50'30" a twitch was noted in the left face, with lateral extension of the lips every 1–2 seconds. At 64'00" the clinical activity extended to *wavelike* excursions of the left hand, coincident with the lateral extension of the left mouth. At 67'00" the movements increased in rate and definition. With each contraction there was flexion of the fingers, wrist, and elbow with slight supination of the forearm. At 77'00" the left fist clinched and the arm lifted and abducted at the shoulder. In addition to the rhythmic face and limb contractions that occurred every second or two, the head slowly turned to the left and remained in this position. At 80'00" the left leg extended from the hip and knee, with the toes spreading on a slightly dorsiflexed foot. At 82'00" the movements progressed to the opposite side of the body, and at 92'14" the

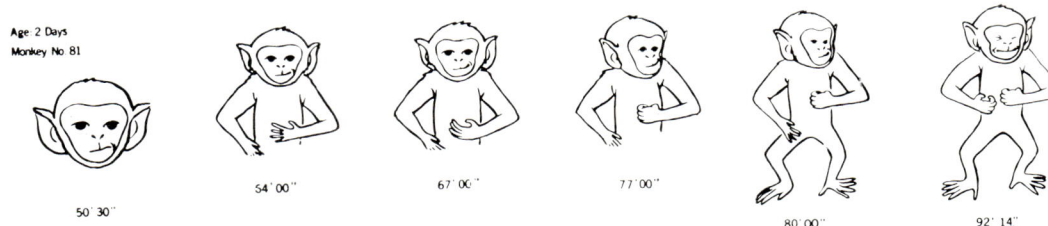

FIG. 19-2. Development of clinical expression in the newborn. Note the delayed onset, involvement of distal large joints before distal small joints, late and sustained head turning, and extension rather than flexion in lower extremities. Maximum activity was accompanied by minimum loss in responsiveness. See text for full description.

peak of the seizure was achieved, with each constellation of convulsive movements occurring at one second or less. Although all movements started at the same time, the right upper extremity lagged behind the left in full excursion and both lower extremities relaxed more slowly than the uppers.

There was considerable salivation and occasional micturition, but no other autonomic dysfunction was observed during this attack. Response to external stimuli was absent for short periods during the maximum expressions of these movements. Over the next two hours there was a gradual and irregular recession in all movements.

Electroencephalographic Expression

Development of the *focal abnormality*, as it is reflected in the right frontotemporal leads will be described first, then its spread to the ipsilateral and contralateral leads will be considered.

In monkey number 81 the first abnormality was noted at 4'23" after the injection of penicillin, *some 45 minutes prior to the first clinical expression* (Fig. 19-3). This abnormality was from the right frontotemporal leads and consisted of single sharp waves approximately a fifth of a second in duration, occurring every 3–5 sec. The peak-to-peak amplitude did not exceed 40 μV. At 4'43", the mean amplitude had increased to 80 μV, and the waves occurred at intervals of 1–2 sec. At 5'00", spikes of one-eighth second duration and of a mean amplitude of 90 μV appeared at intervals of 1–1.5 sec. At 7'00" these were one-tenth second in duration and 80 μV in amplitude, along with spike and sharp wave complexes lasting one-half second and 130 μV in amplitude. This mixture of waveforms occurred every 1–1.5 sec. At 17'45" there was further progression of the abnormal electrical activity, with a change in character. The spike and irregular wave complexes were continuous at 210 μV and were three-fourths to one second in duration. At 25'42" the spike component of the right frontal activity was single, double, or even triple. At 32'00" the complexes included single and double spikes 230 μV in amplitude and up to one-half second in duration. These occurred irregularly at 1–1.5 sec intervals. At 50'30" there was a dramatic increase in amplitude and complexity of the recorded activity from the right anterior region. There were double spikes with associated slow wave components of a mean amplitude of 960 μV and a duration of three-fourths second. These occurred fairly regularly at intervals of one-half to one second. Accompanying this enhanced electrical activity was the first clinical expression: rhythmic movements at the left corner of the mouth, concomitant with the bursts of paroxysmal activity. At 92'14", accompanying the bilateral clinical activity, there were very high voltage complexes consisting of multiple spikes, sharp waves, and slower components, 1680 μV in amplitude and lasting almost one second, that occurred irregularly at 1–1.5 sec intervals.

The *spread of the electroencephalographic abnormality* from the right frontal region to other regions in monkey number 81 may be described as follows.

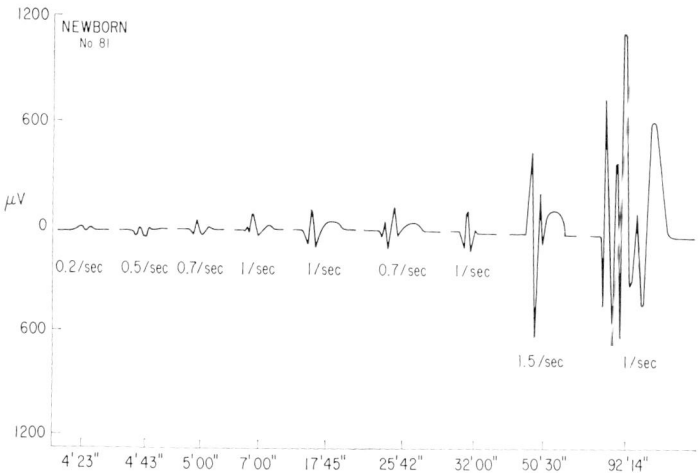

FIG. 19-3. Development of focal EEG abnormality, from the right frontotemporal leads, in the newborn. Microvolts are represented on the ordinate and selected time intervals, after penicillin injection, on the abscissa. From first appearance of paroxysmal activity at 4′32″ until first clinical activity, there was gradual and uneven progression in rate, amplitude, and complexity of waveforms. At 50′30″, concomitant with beginning of facial contractions, there was a fourfold increase in amplitude and an increase in rate from 1–1.5 complexes per second. With the advance of clinical activity to both sides of the body, 92′14″, there was further dramatic increase in amplitude and complexity of waveforms.

At 4′43″, twenty seconds after appearance of the first focal abnormality, low amplitude sharp waves, of no more than 40 μV, were seen over the left hemisphere from both anterior and posterior leads. These occurred independently, at intervals of 1–4 sec and out of phase with the abnormality on the right. Of special interest was the spread to the contralateral hemisphere, anterior and posterior, prior to spread to the ipsilateral posterior leads. At 5′00″ there was representation in the right temporo-occipital leads of less frequent, low voltage sharp waves. From the left anterior and posterior regions were less frequent, though occasionally synchronous, sharp waves of medium voltage. At 7′00″ from the right posterior leads and from the left side were low voltage sharp waves which were synchronous with the more prominent activity from the right anterior leads. At 17′45″ the activity from the right posterior leads was similar to that from the anterior leads though opposite in phase and less in degree. From the left side were lower voltage sharp waves, synchronous with the spike components of the more complex waveforms on the right. At 25′42″ the right posterior forms were similar to the anterior patterns though lower in voltage and reversed in phase. The left side showed synchronous, low voltage, sharp waves of less complex form. At 32′00″ the right posterior complexes were the same in form as the anterior but of lower potential and shorter in duration. On the left were single, sharp, 100 μV waves, one-fourth second in duration, appearing in synchrony with the complexes on the right. At 50′30″, with the dramatic increase in amplitude and complexity of the right anterior abnormality, there was a comparable enhancement of the right posterior abnormality. From the left there were single and double slow spike and waves at 400 μV, synchronous with, but of less complex form and not quite half the voltage of, the paroxysmal activity on the right.

Concomitant with this overall increase in surface electrical activity was the first clinical expression of the seizure. At 92′14″, at the height of the bilateral clinical activity, there were very high voltage multiple spike and slow wave complexes in all leads.

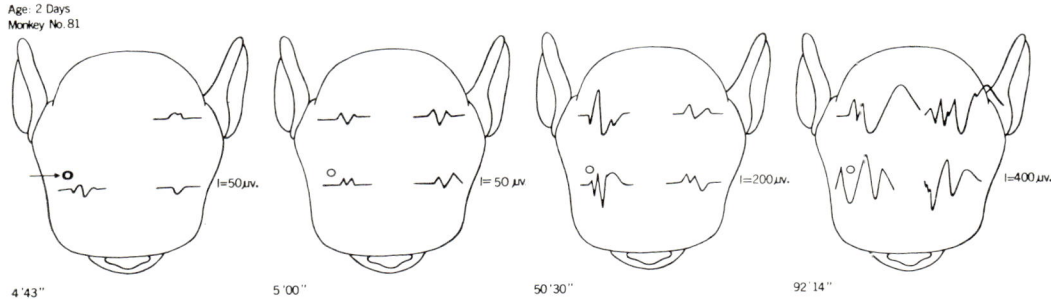

FIG. 19-4. Spread of EEG abnormality in the newborn. Arrow in figure on left points to site of penicillin injection. Note spread to opposite hemisphere at 4'43", prior to spread to posterior ipsilateral hemisphere at 5'00". With the first clinical activity at 50'30", paroxysmal activity was pronounced in both right anterior and posterior regions. With bilateral clinical activity at 92'14", there was greater uniformity in amplitude and waveform between the two hemispheres.

Though not exactly similar in form, the bursts were bilaterally synchronous (Fig. 19-4).

Of the six monkeys below 10 days of age with induced seizures, four had some bilateral expression, two did not. In one of the latter, 4 days of age at the time of injection, while there was a relatively early onset of movements in the left face, there was a protracted course in the involvement of the left upper extremity with no further extension of the clinical pattern and no loss in responsiveness. In the EEG there was an increase in complexity of the paroxysmal activity with the first clinical expression and with the progression from the left face to the left arm there was a marked increase in amplitude, 1280 μV, with the abnormal complexes appearing at roughly one each second.

Histology

In seeking a structural corollary for the seizure events in the newborn, the cerebra of the experimental, and a control series of animals, were examined for the level of development in cells, neuropil, and myelin with attention to the motor cortex and subcortical tracts that were deemed relevant (Fig. 19-5).

In the Nissl preparations (Fig. 19-5A), six cortical layers with well differentiated outer and inner granular lamina are apparent. The cortical cells are arranged in columns with a high density of cell bodies. Betz's pyramids in the fifth layer are very small, ovoid in shape, and poorly stained.

In the Golgi-Cox preparations (Fig. 19-5B through G), the neuropil is found to be sparse. While the apical dendrites are far better developed than the basilar process, few reach the molecular layer, but those that do may be of considerable significance (Fig. 19-5B). Shown in this figure is a discrete number of fine processes that reach the surface of the outer layer to form a rudimentary plexus. The neuronal assemblies, in the form of vertical columns, coaxial with the pyramids, appear almost in isolation (Fig. 19-5C). Endogenous and exogenous fibers are vertically aligned (Fig. 19-5D). While the pyramidal cells in the third and fifth layers are relatively immature as to size, shape, and number of pedunculated bulbs (Fig. 19-5C, E), there are a fair number of large pyramidal cells in the fifth layer that show a greater development in all parameters (Fig. 19-5F). Further, there are star cells in the fourth and fifth layers that show more extensive arborization and spines than those found in other layers (Fig. 19-5G). These findings are in accord with those of Poliakov [9] and others in studies of the newborn human. Of pertinence to the present discussion is the early development of a two-way corticosubcortical projection system, coupled on the level of layer five. The means of local organization within the cortex is limited, but exists in ramifications

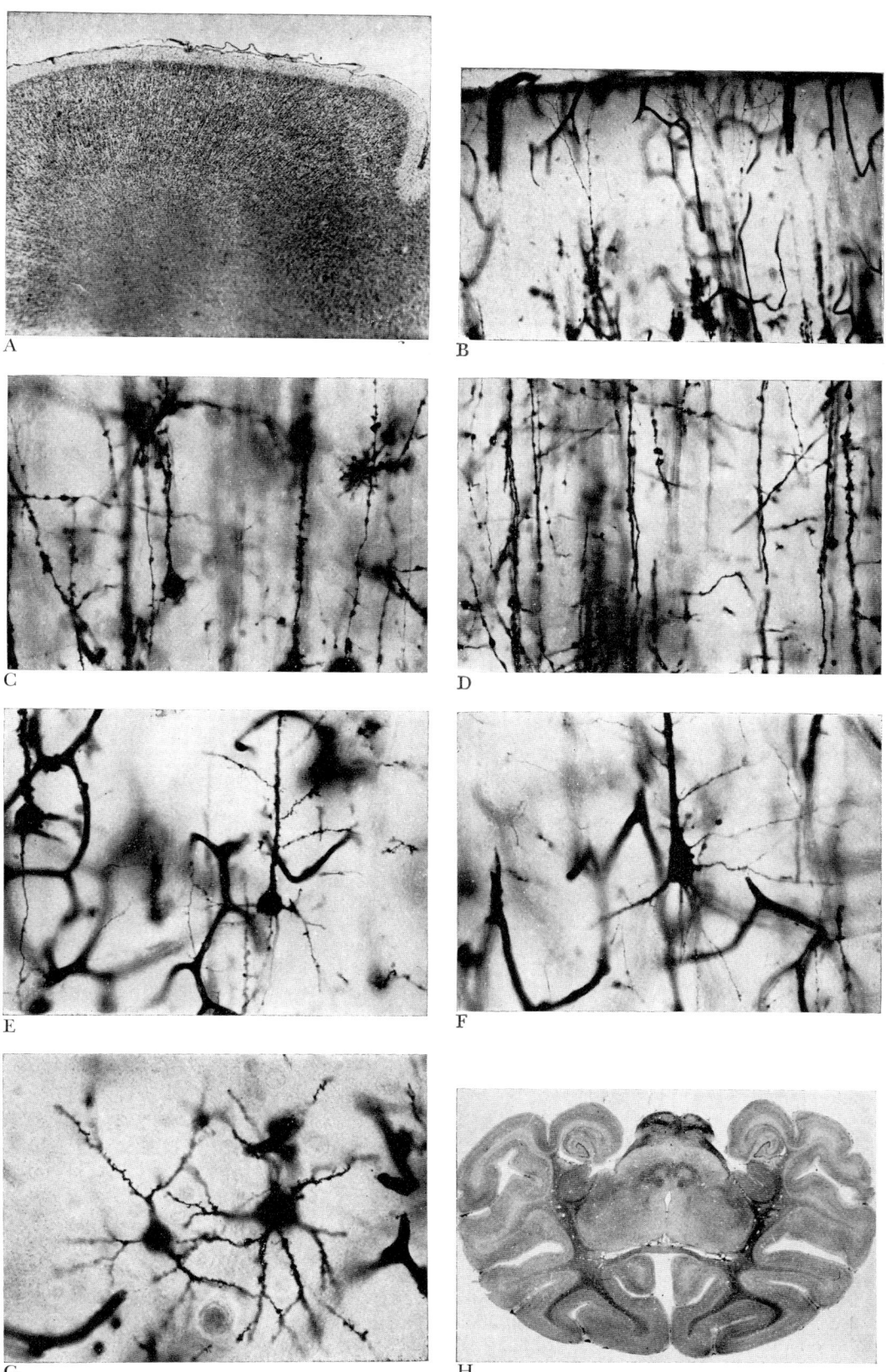

FIG. 19-5. Anatomical substrate in the newborn as exemplified by (*A*) Nissl stains; (*B*) through (*G*) Golgi-Cox preparations; and (*H*) myelin stains. Full description in text.

of the apical dendrites (Fig. 19-5B) and in axonal collaterals (Fig. 19-5E).

In the Loyez preparations (Fig. 19-5H), the subcortical structures show varying degrees of myelinization. The corpus callosum is almost devoid of myelin, while the internal capsule is much better supplied with well-myelinated fibers, most of which are in the thalamocortical projection systems. However, the pyramidal tracts are still pale and contain few myelinated fibers.

PUBERTY

Clinical Expression

Five monkeys received an induced seizure at 24 months of age. Representative of these is number 29, who showed no abnormal movements for 19 min following the penicillin injection (Fig. 19-6).

At 19'11" contractions began in the contralateral face, occurring once or twice each second. One minute later, at 20'11", these were accompanied by rotatory movements of the head, occurring together three times each second. At 20'44" there was flexion of the left thumb and index finger, each contraction forming a circle with these digits. At 21'50" the movements in the left hand included all digits in rhythmic flexion at 3 per sec. At 22'00" the wrist flexed with each tight closure of the fingers. At 24'13" the forearm supinated, the elbow flexed, and the arm lifted and retracted at the shoulder. These contractions were accompanied by less extensive excursions in the *right face and upper extremity,* all movements taking place at an uneven rate, two to four times each second. At 29'52" there was further extension of the seizure with involvement of the left lower extremity. The ankle flexed with internal rotation of the foot and curling of the toes. Contractions in the left upper extremity remained greater than those in the right. The left fist was tightly closed; the right had curled digits. The excursion of the lips to the right had increased. Both eyes blinked, the left more than the right. Head turning was less. At 38'15" the seizure progressed to include the right lower extremity, the combined movements occurring 1.5–2.5 per sec, during which the animal was unresponsive. At

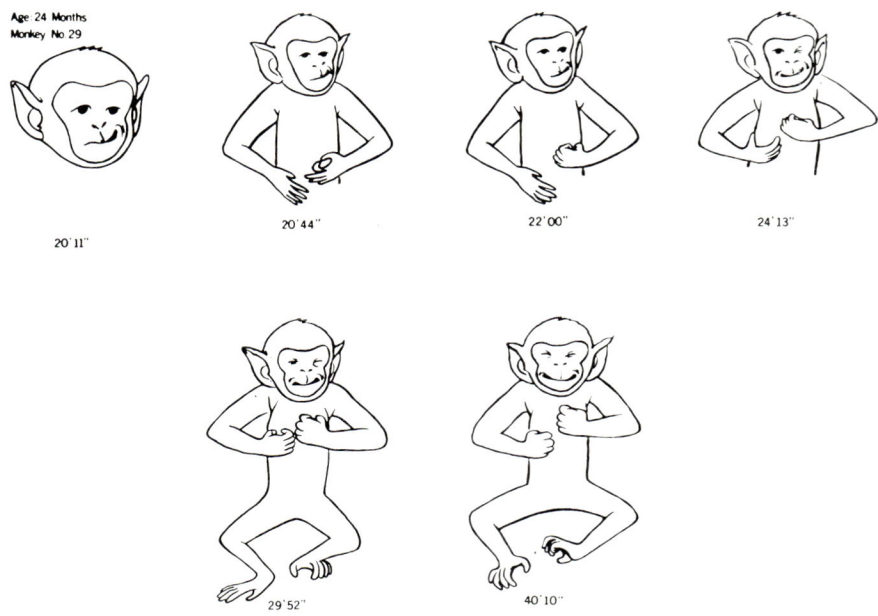

FIG. 19-6. Development of clinical expression at puberty. Note early rotatory movements of head and early fine movements of digits of left hand. With bilateral activity, greatest involvement remains on the contralateral side. Loss in responsiveness was transient. Full description in text.

39'00" the movements receded, and there was a recovery in responsiveness. At 40'10" the peak of the seizure activity was achieved with greater progression on the right side. There was minimal head turning. Facial contractions caused the eyes to blink equally, though the excursion of the mouth remained greater on the left. The contractions at shoulder and elbow were greater on the left, but both wrists remained flexed and both fists clinched. In both uppers there was less relaxation between the contractions that varied the starting position of each movement. In the left lower extremity there was flexion at hip, knee, and ankle, the foot rotating inward and the toes curling. The movement on the right was similar though less in degree. The rate was 3 per sec. The animal was again unresponsive with considerable salivation and micturition. Further seizure activity was prevented with sodium phenobarbital.

Electroencephalographic Expression

At 2'54" following the injection, some 16 min prior to the first clinical expression, there appeared in monkey number 29 a single spike complex from the right frontotemporal leads with a peak amplitude of 80 μV, a duration of one-tenth second, and a frequency of one to two spikes in 10 sec (Fig. 19-7). At 16'12" the frequency increased to three to five complexes in each 10 sec. At 18'23" spikes and sharp waves continued at a mean amplitude of 70 μV, a duration of one-eighth to one-tenth second, and at a faster, though still uneven rate. At 19'11" there were single spikes 60 μV in amplitude and one-eleventh second in duration and 100 μV spike and wave complexes of one-fourth second duration. These abnormalities occurred in bursts of 4 per sec and at intervals of one every 2 sec. The first clinical sign, twitching of the left side of the face, accompanied this EEG expression. At 20'44" multiple spike and wave activity had become rhythmic at a mean amplitude of 120 μV, each complex taking one-fifth second and occurring about three times per second. The clinical activity now included flexion of the left thumb and forefinger at the rate of 3 per sec. At 24'13" waveforms were more elaborate and included single, double, and triple spikes and spike and wave complexes with a mean amplitude of 130 μV and a frequency of 2–4 per sec. Clinically, there was the first ipsilateral activity: rhythmic movements of the right arm. At 40'10" there were multispike and wave complexes with an average amplitude of 170 μV. These occurred rhythmically, at 3 per sec. The clinical corollary was a generalized seizure.

The *spread* of the EEG abnormality at puberty is quite different from that in the newborn (Fig. 19-8). In monkey number 29, at 5'54" the first abnormality appeared

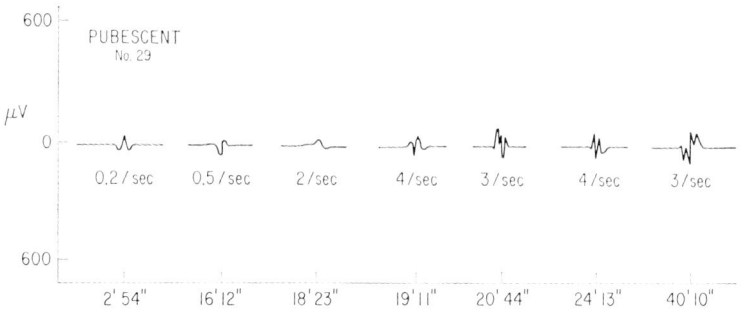

FIG. 19-7. Development of focal EEG abnormality, from right frontotemporal leads, at puberty. Microvolts represented on ordinate and selected time intervals after penicillin injection on abscissa. From first paroxysmal activity at 2'54" to maximal clinical expression at 40'10" there was only modest increase in amplitude; however, there was distinct increase in rate and complexity of waveforms with first clinical activity at 19'11". With progression to bilateral clinical activity at 24'13" and generalized seizure at 40'10", there was further increase in spike components of the paroxysmal complexes.

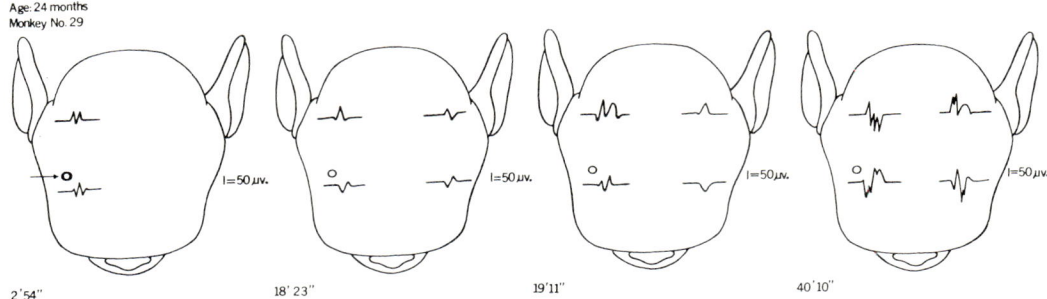

FIG. 19-8. Spread of EEG abnormality at puberty. Arrow in figure on left indicates site of penicillin injection. First abnormality, at 2′54″, appeared simultaneously in anterior and posterior leads. Spread to opposite hemisphere at 18′23″ was also simultaneously registered in anterior and posterior leads. With onset of clinical activity at 19′11″ and generalized seizure at 40′10″, abnormalities showed synchrony of spike components with greater complexity remaining on right side.

concomitantly from the anterior and posterior leads. About equal in amplitude and similar in waveform, the posterior abnormality was synchronous but in reversed phase. At 18′23″, when the right-sided activity had achieved a faster though still uneven rate, the first abnormality was seen on the left side. In both anterior and posterior leads, the complexes were similar in form, but less frequent in rate. When seen they were coincident with the right-sided activity. At 19′11″ the left-sided abnormality, though simpler in form (single spikes at less than 100 μV and one-eleventh second), was synchronous with the right-sided activity. Accompanying this expression was the first clinical sign. At 20′44″, from the left hemisphere there were single 100 μV spikes of one-fifteenth second duration and synchronous with the spike components from the right hemisphere. The clinical activity at that time included flexion of the left thumb and forefinger at 3 per sec. At 40′10″, following a brief recession in rate and complexity of the paroxysmal abnormalities, there were bilaterally synchronous multispike and wave complexes with an average amplitude of 170 μV occurring rhythmically at 3 per sec. The clinical corollary was a generalized seizure. It should be noted that at the peak of this seizure the abnormal bursts on the left were not quite as complex as those on the right.

Four out of the five monkeys that received penicillin injections at 24 months of age developed bilateral clinical seizures. In each of these, the most pronounced expression was on the contralateral side. The attack in the fifth monkey never progressed beyond the contralateral side. In all, the EEG abnormality remained relatively low in voltage with an increase in rate and complexity of waveform as the seizure advanced to its maximum expression.

Anatomical Substrate

When the Nissl preparations, from cortical area 4, were compared with those from the newborn, the pyramidal cells appeared larger in size with better staining characteristics, and stratification of cortical layers was less pronounced (Fig. 19-9).

The Golgi preparations demonstrated a marked increase in the dendritic plexus at the surface (Fig. 19-9B) and in endogenous and exogenous, horizontal, and tangential fibers (Fig. 19-9C) throughout the cortex. The pyramidal cells of layer three are better developed (Fig. 19-9D) and, along with the Betz cells of layer five (Fig. 19-9E), have a greater arborization of the basilar dendrites than was observed in the newborn.

In the Loyez preparations many of the cortical radiating and transverse fibers are seen to be myelinated, along with fairly dense bundles of vertical fibers that reach the molecular layer (Fig. 19-9F). In the sub-

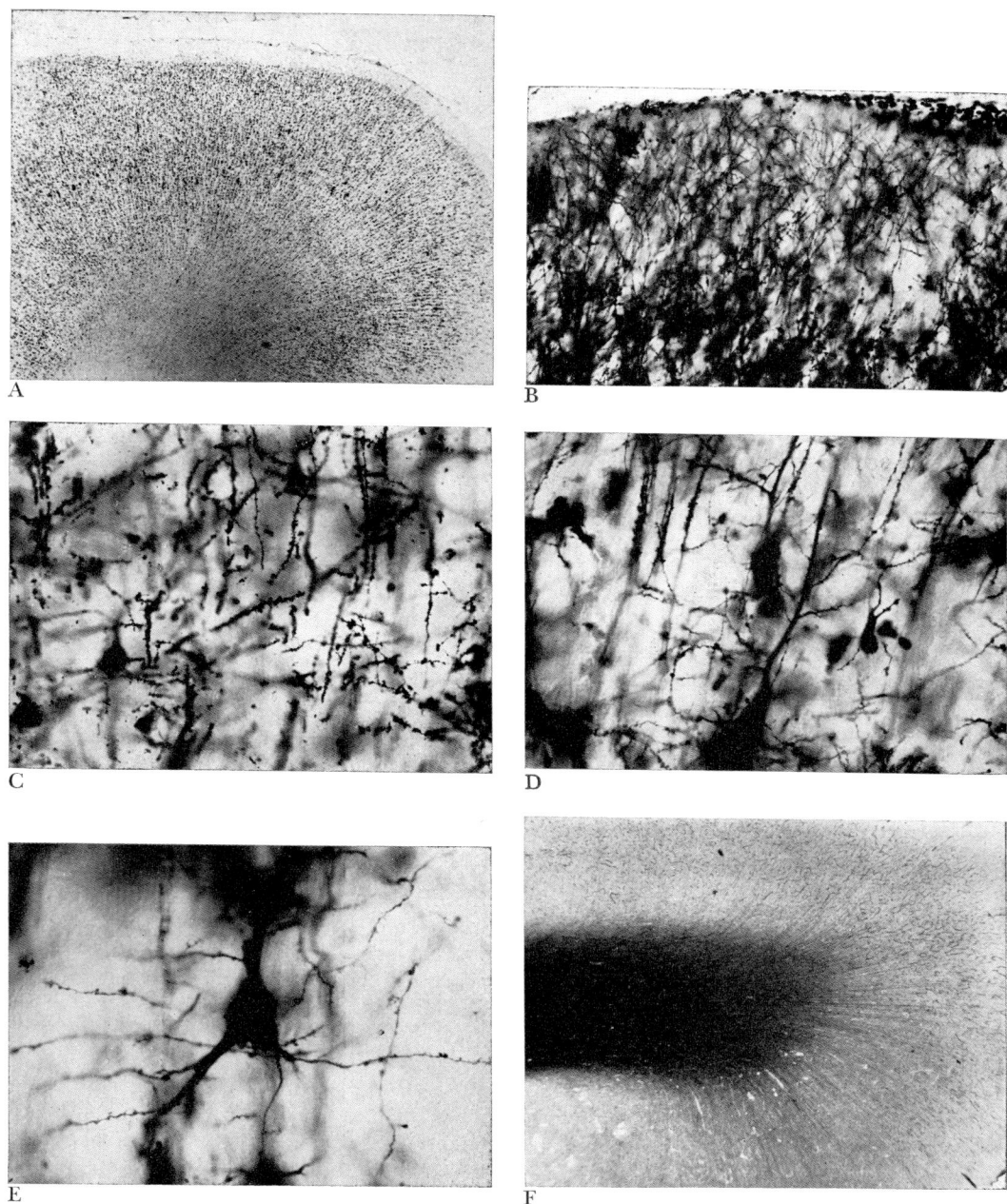

FIG. 19-9. Anatomical substrate at puberty as exemplified by (A) Nissl stains; (B) through (E) Golgi-Cox preparations; and (F) myelin stains. Full description in text.

cortical structures, the internal capsule is more deeply stained and the pyramidal tracts are well myelinated throughout their course. The myelinization of the arcuate subcortical fibers and of the corpus callosum has advanced in that order.

ADULT

Clinical Expression

Monkey number 131, representative of the adult group, received an induced seizure at 4 years of age (Fig. 19-10).

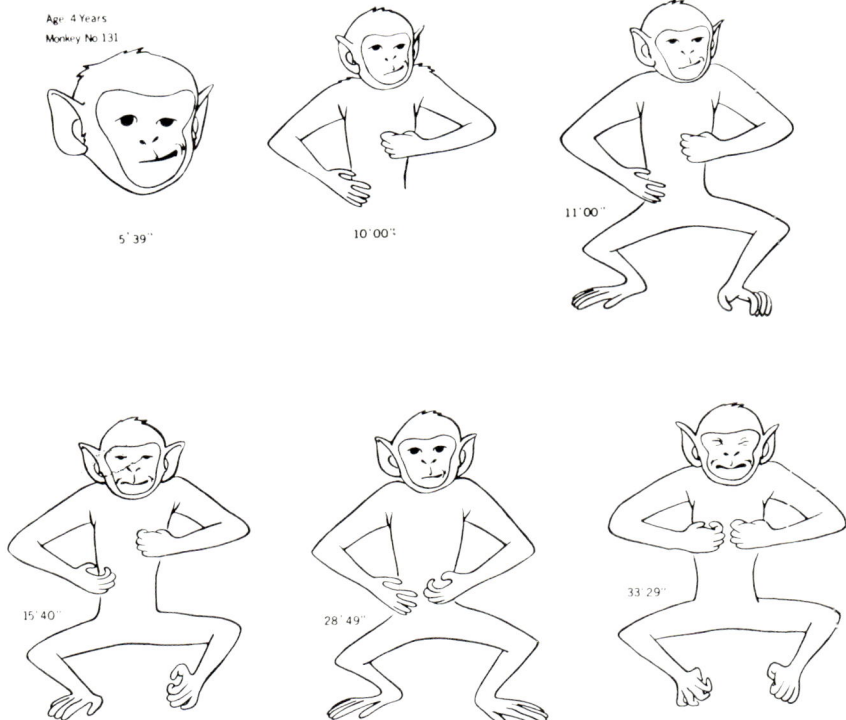

FIG. 19-10. Development of clinical expression in the adult. Note rapid, orderly progression from focal to unilateral to bilateral seizure phenomena, its reduction to limited focal activity, followed by generalized convulsion. In the latter, loss in responsiveness was sustained. Full description in text.

At 5′39″ there were left facial movements that, almost at once, increased in rate and excursion. With this advance there began short rotatory movements of the head to the left. At 10′00″ the clinical activity had progressed to the left upper extremity. The fingers were flexed rhythmically, as was the wrist, with slight supination of the arm. Beginning at one to one and one-half times per second, the movements quickened to two to three times per second with flexion at the elbow and elevation and retraction of the arm at the shoulder. At 11′00″ there was progression to the left lower extremity with flexion at the ankle, hip, and knee. The toes curled, and there was internal rotation of the foot. At 15′40″, as the contractions on the left increased in degree with a rate of 3 per sec, the right side of the body was implicated in movements similar in kind though smaller in degree. Responsiveness was retained.

At 17′29″ there was an abrupt reduction in all abnormal movements with the animal demonstrating alertness to changes in his environment. After a gradual, sequential buildup, there was a generalized seizure at 26′19″, the activity, however, remaining greater on the left than on the right.

At 28′49″ the animal again responded promptly to stimuli, including visual signals, and the only clinical expression of the seizure state was a contraction of the left side of the mouth with flexion of the fingers occurring every 1–2 sec. This was followed by an even stronger seizure that became generalized at 33′29″. Head movements were less; facial contractions appeared equal. Both hands remained closed, the left more tightly than the right. In both lower extremities, hips, knees, and ankles flexed. Both feet rotated internally with curling of the toes, more noticeable on the left. Bilateral movements were less in extent and regularity of excursion, by reason of the *increased tonic components*. Although all started in unison, there was unequal relaxation between the various parts. The rate of these contractions was 3–4 per sec. Autonomic activity, salivation, micturition, defecation, and dilation of the pupils were prevalent. Consciousness, as indicated by response to stimuli, was lost for two and one-half minutes during this major attack. With recovery of awareness and reduction in movements, further seizures were prevented by sodium phenobarbital.

Electroencephalographic Expression

In monkey number 131, the first abnormality was noted at 2′16″ following the penicillin injection, some 3 min prior to the first clinical expression. Single and multiple bursts of sharp waves occurred concomitantly from both the right anterior and posterior leads, 45 μV and 80 μV respectively. The development in the right frontotemporal leads is indicated in Fig. 19-11. At 5′39″ there were single and double spike and wave complexes of 60 μV occurring every 1–2 sec. *Coincident with this was the first clinical activity in the left face.* At 10′00″, accompanying the clinical progression, there was higher voltage and a modest increase in frequency. At 11′00″ there were multispike and wave complexes of 140 μV occurring about three times in each second. At 15′40″ with little change in waveform or frequency, *there was an advance in amplitude during the first extension of the clinical activity to both sides of the body.*

At 17′29″ there was a distinct lull in the EEG as well as in clinical activity. Simpler spike and wave complexes occurred irregularly at 0.5–2 sec intervals. At 26′19″, during the height of a bilateral seizure, there was multispike activity occurring in bursts of 3–4 per sec. At 28′49″ there was a second recession in aberrant activity. At 33′29″, reflecting a major seizure, there were multispike bursts, 125 μV, occurring three to four times each second.

The *spread* of the electroencephalographic abnormality in the adult during the onset of focal seizure and its progression to a major, generalized convulsion was characterized by several features which were not seen in the newborn, but were partially or completely evident in the animals at puberty. First was the concomitant appearance of the paroxysmal activity in both the right anterior and posterior leads. Second was the dominance of wave amplitude in the posterior leads that persisted

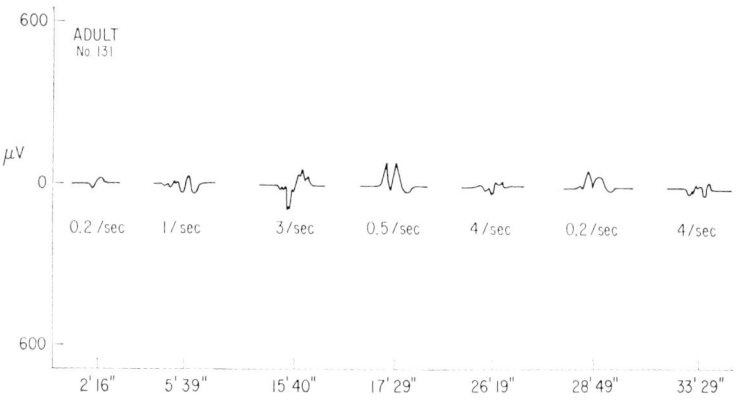

FIG. 19-11. Development of focal EEG abnormality, from right frontotemporal leads, in the adult. Microvolts represented on ordinate and selected time intervals, after penicillin injection on the abscissa. From onset at 2′16″ to first clinical expression at 5′39″ there was rapid increase in complexity of waveforms. With extension of clinical activity to both sides of the body at 15′40″ there was increase in amplitude and rate, as well as complexity of waveform. With recessions in clinical activity at 17′29″ and 28′49″ between generalized seizures, paroxysmal activity assumed a simpler form, slower rate, and higher amplitude.

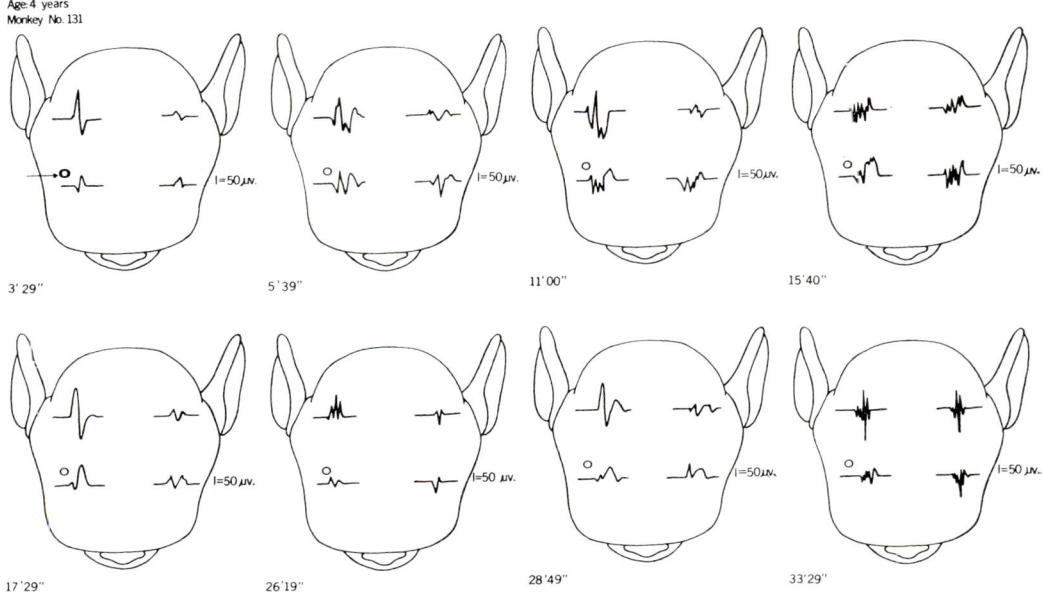

FIG. 19-12. Spread of EEG abnormality in the adult. Arrow in figure on left indicates site of penicillin injection. First abnormality, at 2'16", appeared simultaneously in anterior and posterior leads and at 3'29" was registered in opposite hemisphere in both anterior and posterior leads. From outset the amplitude dominance was in posterior leads. With onset of clinical activity at 5'39", there was increase in spike components throughout, with the two sides appearing almost equal during the first bilateral clinical activity at 15'40" and quite similar during the third and most severe generalized seizure at 33'29". Markedly reduced paroxysmal activity at 17'29" and 28'49" remained bilaterally synchronous.

throughout the course of the fit. The first expression of this in monkey number 131 was at 2'16".

At 3'29" the abnormality spread to the opposite (left) side. Though less prominent, the sharp components were synchronous with those from the right. The greater voltage on both sides was in the posterior leads (Fig. 19-12). At 5'39", following onset of the clinical seizure activity, there were single and double spike and wave components in all leads with the greater complexity of waveform and higher voltage remaining on the right. At 11'00", with progression in the unilateral clinical activity, the multispike and wave activity, occurring three times per second, was 250 μV in the right posterior leads and 140 μV in the right anterior leads. There was lower voltage activity from the left hemisphere in apparent synchrony with that from the right. At 15'40" there was an overall increase in amplitude and less difference between the two sides as the clinical activity extended to both sides of the body.

At 17'29", during the lull in clinical and electrical phenomena, the waveforms were simpler, slower in rate, and, while synchronous, they were dominant on the right side. At 26'19", with another progression from a focal to a bilateral seizure, there was another buildup to multispike complexes occurring three to four times per second in all leads. At 28'49" with the second, more pronounced recession in clinical seizure phenomena, the sparse, ictal complexes continued in bilateral synchrony. At 33'29" during the height of the generalized seizure there was a generalized electroencephalographic abnormality with bilateral posterior dominant, multispike bursts of 250 μV occurring three to four times each second.

The entire adult group showed a rapid and orderly progression in development of

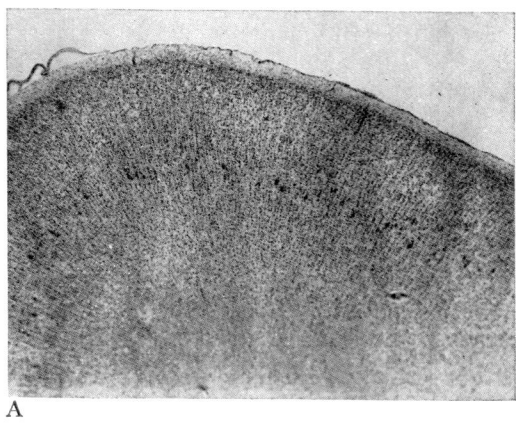 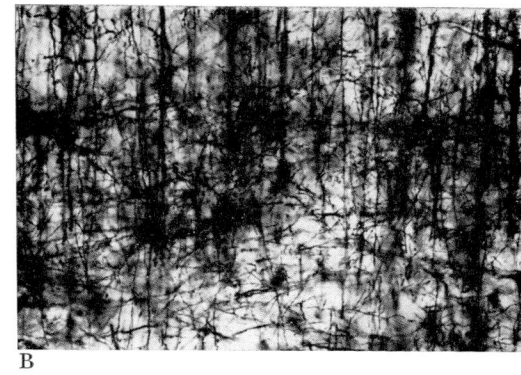
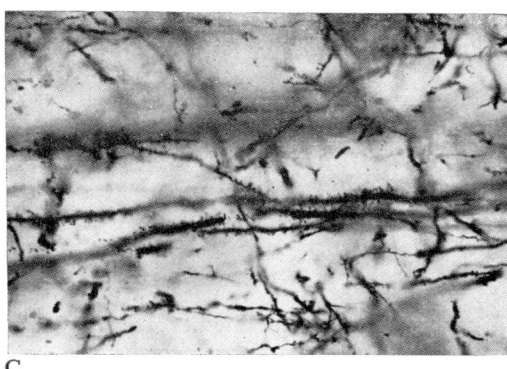 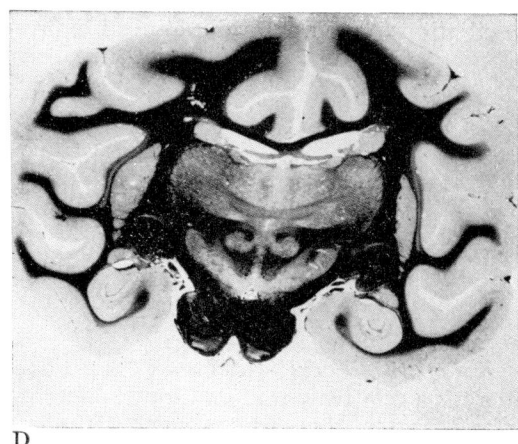

FIG. 19-13. Anatomical substrate in the adult as exemplified by (A) Nissl stains; (B) and (C) Golgi-Cox preparations; and (D) myelin stains. Full description in text.

the clinical seizure. The bilateral expression was accompanied by profound loss in responsiveness and excessive autonomic activity. The EEG abnormality appeared concomitantly in the anterior and posterior leads, with a synchronous expression over the opposite hemisphere shortly thereafter. There was a posterior dominance in amplitude throughout, with the two sides appearing equal at the height of the seizure.

Anatomical Substrate

In the Nissl preparations, from cortical area 4, there is less stratification in number and differentiation of layers. The columnar arrangement of cells is less distinct and their separation more evident. Though relatively unchanged in number, pyramidal and other cells are greatly increased in size, definition, and cytoplasmic chromatin (Fig. 19-13A).

In the Golgi-Cox preparations the neuropil forms a dense pattern of thick vertical and horizontal fibers and thin random fibers, the greatest contrast to the newborn being in the increased density of the superficial layers of the cortex (Fig. 19-13B). The apical dendrites of the pyramids extend to the surface and branch; the basilar dendrites, markedly increased in number and size, branch horizontally. Adding to the profusion of neuropil are star cells, their processes, and other endogenous and exogenous fibers. Many of the neurons have a vast number of argentophilic particles on the surface of the dendrites and cells that indicate an augmented synaptic surface (Fig. 19-13C).

In the Loyez preparations the subcortical projection systems of the forebrain are well myelinated (Fig. 19-13D).

DISCUSSION

The monkey at birth has an immature cortex and imperfectly developed subcortical projection systems. However, when a high concentration of penicillin is brought into contact with all layers of the motor cortex, the organization at hand is capable of supporting a repetitive focal discharge, its propagation, establishment of secondary oscillations, and finally the clinical expression of a focal motor seizure with unilateral or bilateral extension of the attack pattern.

Activating Agent. Ajmone-Marsan has discussed the action of penicillin [1] and concludes that its effect is an enhancement of neuronal excitatory influences as well as a blocking of inhibitory influences. Purpura has pointed out the paucity of both in the newborn kitten with somewhat better development of the inhibitory influences [10].

Repetitive Focal Discharge. At birth there is a relatively well developed afferent-efferent system that ensures elemental reflex activity. Within the cortex the sensory afferents, from the thalamus, are coupled via star cells in layers IV and V with large pyramidal cells in layer V. This basic switching circuit is likely to be the first involved in the oscillations evoked by the penicillin. The importance of the large pyramidal cells, with their vertical neuronal assembly, in the paroxysmal discharge has been emphasized by Jasper [8], and the significance of internuncial neurons preserving excitatory, as well as affording inhibitory, influences has been indicated by Beritov [2]. The early lack of rhythmicity and slow oscillations, one per second or less, reflect not only the immaturity in cellular development and paucity in synaptic connections, but the limited number of neurons involved.

The recruitment of adjacent cortical elements, that takes place with difficulty over a protracted period, probably comes about through the collateral connections that are particularly sparse in the newborn but do exist in the rudimentary plexus of apical dendrites in the molecular layer at the surface of the cortex and in the axon collaterals of the pyramidal cells. In this manner, the local hypersynchrony increases gradually in rate and amplitude until there is enough efferent discharge to set off subcortical neuronal assemblies.

Propagation. Available is the two-way projection system, indicated above, that is in working order at or before birth in all primates [9]. It may be assumed that the first propagation of the abnormal discharge takes place *vertically* in cortico-thalamo-cortical circuits, with involvement of specific and nonspecific thalamic nuclei. Critical to this argument is the gradual establishment of secondary oscillations in subcortical systems with augmentation of existing cortical activity and the recruitment of additional cortical elements through associational afferents. The projection to the opposite hemisphere probably takes place through midline integrative mechanisms, for example, the intralaminar system and upper brain stem reticular formation. The corpus callosum is poorly myelinated and probably plays little part in this transmission. The fact that the first contralateral expression in the surface recording is simpler in form, lower in amplitude, and not always in synchrony suggests an inconstant drive in multisynaptic pathways as well as in the inability of the contralateral cortex to sustain a paroxysmal discharge.

Of significance is the appearance of the abnormal electrical activity in the anterior and posterior leads of the opposite hemisphere before its appearance in the posterior leads on the side of the injection. This lag in homolateral propagation is probably related to the inadequate myelinization in the short arcuate fibers and in the long association bundles. The better developed cingulum may play an important part in the homolateral, as well as the contralateral, transmission when it takes place [15].

Clinical Expression. Minor to moderate increments in the interaction between the focal neuronal aggregates and subcortical structures is reflected in the scalp recording over a period of some thirty to forty minutes. There is then a dramatic increase in amplitude and complexity of waveform. Coincident with this enhanced electrical activity is the appearance of the first clinical contractions in the contralateral face. This dual expression of augmented paroxysmal activity must indicate the addition of subcortical elements within the thalamus, the striatum, and other components of the extrapyramidal system. Mediation of the clinical movements is most likely over the phylogenetically older extrapyramidal system and only in part over the imperfectly developed pyramidal tracts. The slow progression and movement pattern are evidence for the multisynaptic route. As the movements spread unilaterally and bilaterally there is progressive increase in amplitude and complexity of the surface recording implying progressive involvement of subcortical and cortical structures in independently sustained oscillations that are not perfectly synchronized. Contributing to the complexity of waveforms is the inadequacy of the inhibitory *gating* mechanism of the cortex to handle input from multiple subcortical structures. The very high voltage in the surface recording reflects not only the powerful augmenting influences but also the cortical circuitry that can only provide a slow cycling of the paroxysmal discharge.

As the process continues there is greater involvement of bilateral projections that now have the power to activate self-sustained secondary oscillations in both hemispheres. While the expression from the surface recording appears almost equal on the two sides, the clinical expression never achieves a bilateral symmetry, suggesting that the extrapyramidal and pyramidal systems never have quite the full input for the ipsilateral expression that they have for the contralateral expression. Other evidence for the lack of an unrestricted, diffuse spread of the paroxysmal discharge is the lack of any but the most transient loss in responsiveness. Whatever the mechanism, in cells or circuitry, that is necessary for the interruption in consciousness, it is imperfectly invoked in the newborn even when convulsive movements extend to both sides of the body.

Maturation. The continued development of cells and their processes after birth vastly increases synaptic organization within the cortex. Especially noticeable are: increase in the dendritic plexus at the surface, more abundant arborization of basilar dendrites, increase in number of axon collaterals of pyramidal cells, elaboration of internuncial neurons, and multiplicity of spines on cells and processes. Exogenous as well as endogenous fibers add to the density of the neuropil.

Szentágothai has provided us with a fascinating scheme for functional organization of cortical components [12], and Purpura has demonstrated the effect of development on some of these [10]. Poliakov stressed the importance of the sequential availability of *lateral* associational pathways originating in the upper layers of the cortex [9]. With these changes the focal paroxysmal discharge undergoes an increase in rate and regularity, a decrease in amplitude, and a more rapid spread from the site of origin. With advancing maturation of the subcortical projection systems, their capability of transmission and the establishment of secondary, self-sustained, synchronous oscillations are enhanced. In addition to the vertical systems, the transcallosal and homolateral associational systems now play a significant role. Evidence for the latter is the simultaneous appearance of paroxysmal discharge in the posterior as well as the anterior leads on the side of the injection, with the highest amplitude being in the posterior leads. This is followed by rapid, synchronous spread to both anterior and posterior leads over the opposite hemisphere. The spread anteriorly is evidenced by early, adversive movements of the head.

As the attack proceeds there are stronger contractions on both sides of the body, loss in responsiveness, and manifest autonomic activity. This development in seizure pattern is well along at puberty but still is not complete. In the young adult, further advance in central nervous system organization is reflected in the faster and more orderly progression of the attack pattern. Extent of propagation at the height of the seizure is indicated by the bilateral symmetry in the surface recording and the muscular contractions, with a profound loss in responsiveness. The recessions that follow each bilateral attack, in series, suggest an active inhibitory process rather than merely fatigue factors. Apparent at puberty, this aspect of the seizure pattern is well developed in the adult.

CONCLUSION

The interpretations offered in this discussion are based upon clinical phenomena, scalp recording of electrical activity, and routine histology that includes Golgi-Cox preparations. Their validity in detail must await the use of more precise techniques in electrophysiology and anatomical studies at an ultrastructural level.

While three epochs have been emphasized, neonatal, puberty, and young adulthood, additional material will be needed to better understand the rapid ontogenetic changes in the first few months after birth and the continued, though modest, development between puberty and young adulthood.

REFERENCES

1. Ajmone-Marsan, C. Acute Effects of Topical Epileptogenic Agents. In Jasper, H. H., Ward, A. A., Jr., and Pope, A. (Eds.), *Basic Mechanisms of the Epilepsies*. Boston: Little, Brown, 1969.
2. Beritov, I. S. Physiological significance of cerebral cortex nerve elements. *Arch. Anat.* (Strasb.) 39:3, 1960.
3. Caveness, W. F. Electroencephalography and clinical studies of epilepsy during the maturation of the monkey. *Epilepsia* (Amst.) 3:137, 1962.
4. Caveness, W. F. *Atlas of Electroencephalography in the Developing Monkey, Macaca mulatta*. Reading, Mass.: Addison-Wesley, 1962.
5. French, J. D., Gernandt, B. E., and Livingston, R. B. Regional differences in seizure susceptibility in monkey cortex. *A.M.A. Arch. Neurol. Psychiat.* 75:260, 1956.
6. Fulton, J. E. *Physiology of the Nervous System*. (3d ed.). New York: Oxford Univ. Press, 1949, p. 396.
7. Hines, M. The development and regression of reflexes, postures, and progression in the young macaque. *Contr. Embryol.* (Carneg. Inst.) 30:154, 1962.
8. Jasper, H. H. Mechanisms of Propagation: Extracellular Studies. In Jasper, H. H., Ward, A. A., Jr., and Pope, A. (Eds.), *Basic Mechanisms of the Epilepsies*. Boston: Little, Brown, 1969.
9. Poliakov, G. I. Some results of research into the development of the neuronal structure of the cortical ends of the analyzers in man. *J. Comp. Neurol.* 117:197, 1961.
10. Purpura, D. P. Stability and Seizure Susceptibility of Immature Brain. In Jasper, H. H., Ward, A. A., Jr., and Pope, A. (Eds.), *Basic Mechanisms of the Epilepsies*. Boston: Little, Brown, 1969.
11. Servit, Z. Phylogenesis and ontogenesis of the epileptic seizure. *World Neurol.* 3:259, 1962.
12. Szentágothai, J. Architecture of the Cerebral Cortex. In Jasper, H. H., Ward, A. A., Jr., and Pope, A. (Eds.), *Basic Mechanisms of the Epilepsies*. Boston: Little, Brown, 1969.
13. Udvarhelyi, G. B., and Walker, A. E. Dissemination of acute focal seizures in the monkey. I. From cortical foci. *Arch. Neurol.* (Chicago) 12:333, 1965.
14. Yakovlev, P. I. Maturation of cortical substrata of epileptic events. *World Neurol.* 3:299, 1962.
15. Yakovlev, P. I., and Lecours, A. R. The Myelogenetic Cycles of the Regional Maturation of the Brain. In Minkowski, A. (Ed.), *Symposium on Regional Development of the Brain in Early Life*. Oxford: Blackwell, 1967, pp. 3–70.

Discussion

MATURATIONAL FACTORS IN DEVELOPMENT OF SEIZURES
ANTONIA VERNADAKIS AND DIXON M. WOODBURY

A wide selection of classical and newer methods through which information has been gained on the structure and function of the adult central nervous system (CNS) has also been adopted, with modifications, in the study of developmental properties of neural activity.

Characteristics of single neurons during prenatal and postnatal development have been studied with intracellular electrodes and with microelectrodes (summarized in [14]). The activity evoked by sensory or local stimulation has been recorded in small populations of neurons with macroelectrodes (summarized in [14]). Spontaneous electrical activity has been used to localize developmental properties of cell population activity. Inducing functional changes by ablation or isolation of small neural areas has offered the further opportunity of observing regional relationships during maturation (summarized in [14]).

Basic aspects of CNS development and activity have been clarified by the use of drugs. The work of Caveness and co-workers (see first part of this chapter) has demonstrated that drugs can be used to investigate developmental properties of neural activity and has contributed in further elucidating neurophysiological and structural factors involved in seizure activity in the developing animal.

The present discussion will cover some developmental properties of seizure activity assessed by responses of the developing CNS to brain electroshock stimulation and direct stimulation of the spinal cord. Moreover, evidence will be presented to support the view that responses of the developing CNS to neurotropic drugs can be used as indices of the degree of neural organization which is a function of maturation of both facilitatory and inhibitory systems.

GROSS CNS DEVELOPMENT

Responses to Brain Electroshock Stimulation and Direct Stimulation of the Spinal Cord

Responses to electroshock stimulation and to direct stimulation of the spinal cord are used as indices of gross regional sequence of CNS development and activity. The developmental pattern of electrically induced brain seizures provides indirect evidence of gross maturation of higher CNS systems involved in minimal and maximal seizures, whereas the developmental pattern of spinal cord convulsions provides evidence of the maturation of lower CNS centers.

DEVELOPMENT OF MINIMAL ELECTROSHOCK SEIZURE PATTERNS

There are two types of electroshock seizure threshold (EST) tests: the threshold for 60 cycles per sec alternating current stimulation (ac EST) and the threshold for low frequency stimulation with unidirectional pulses at 6 cycles per sec for 3 sec (lf EST). The EST tests are measures of the threshold for evoking clonic discharge characterized by facial clonus and rhythmic movements of the vibrissae, jaws, and ears. Seizure threshold involves more than simply the threshold for initial excitation of the individual neurons involved. In order for the full minimal seizure (for example, 5 sec of sustained clonus) to occur, it is necessary for a substantial number of neurons to discharge for a considerable period of time. This collection of neurons, the discharge of which maintains minimal seizure activity, has been termed the *oscillator* to distinguish it from the seizure focus which ordinarily serves to trigger the oscillator. The lf stimulus excites the oscillator with maximum efficiency. The discharge elicited by the ac EST method is more intense and spreads over a wider area. Evidence indicates that the anatomical substratum of the oscillator may be that portion of the upper brain stem designated as the *centrencephalic system* by Penfield and Jasper [12]. Numerous investigations (summarized in [25]) clearly show the role of specific components of this region (reticular activating system and thalamus) in the initiation and maintenance of minimal seizure discharge, for example, petit mal. Thus, manifestations of minimal seizure activity, namely, loss of consciousness and slight clonus, can be related to activity in the centrencephalic system, including some involvement in the cortex.

In maturing rats and mice, the ac EST for clonus exhibited only after 8 days of age progressively and markedly decreases until 16 days of age in rats [22] and 18 days in mice and slowly increases somewhat thereafter [22]. Similarly, the lf threshold for clonus decreases markedly until 30 days of age in mice and remains relatively constant thereafter [22].

The progressive decreases in thresholds are interpreted to be a result of development of the oscillator and discharge of more excitatory neuronal elements. At early periods the lf threshold is very high, probably because the neuronal elements representing the oscillator have not fully matured and a self-sustained discharge cannot occur. As the oscillator develops and more neuronal elements respond to stimulation, a lower voltage can elicit repetitive neuronal discharge. With ac stimulation, both the oscillator and other developing excitatory and inhibitory systems are stimulated. If there is merit to the proposal that the decrease in the lf threshold during maturation is probably associated with development of the oscillator, then it is likely that the progressive decrease in ac threshold is a measure of the extent to which neuronal elements other than the oscillator participate in the seizure discharge.

Development of Maximal Electroshock Seizure Patterns

With electrical stimuli substantially above threshold, a tonic-clonic seizure (maximal electroshock seizure, MES) replaces the purely clonic minimal seizure. This convulsion has a characteristic stereotyped pattern consisting of tonic hindlimb flexion, tonic hindlimb extension, and clonus. A distinctive qualitative difference between this maximal seizure and a threshold convulsion concerns the extent of spread of seizure discharge, which in the maximal seizure involves the entire cerebrospinal axis.

In the *maturing rat* the maximal electroshock pattern develops in phases which appear in the following sequence first described by Millichap [11]: 1–8 days of age, hyperkinesia (paddling and running movement, shaking and hyperextension of the head); 13–15 days of age, forelimb flexion followed by forelimb extension and hindlimb flexion; 16 days of age and older, full tonic-clonic seizure pattern, including hindlimb extension [24].

This progressive increase in the intensity of seizure elicited by brain electroshock stimulation is in agreement with the findings of Caveness and co-workers. They showed that the complexity of EEG waveforms, particularly in number of sharp components, of penicillin-induced epileptiform activity in developing monkeys becomes progressively more pronounced with CNS maturation.

Development of Spinal Cord Convulsions

Spinal reflex systems play a substantial role in integrating maximal seizure discharge into the motor pattern. Stimulation of the cervical spinal cord in adult spinal animals can duplicate all the hindlimb motor patterns seen during generalized seizure activity in intact animals [3]. Flexor-extensor spinal cord convulsions can be elicited by electrical stimulation of the cord in 1-day-old rats [15]. The flexion-versus-frequency curve obtained in 12-day-old rats is similar to the response observed in adult rats, which indicates that the spinal cord convulsive pattern has developed by 12 days. The inability, therefore, of intact rats to exhibit a flexor-extensor convulsion with brain stimulation before 16 days of age is due to lack of maturation of the brain rather than of the spinal cord.

BIOCHEMICAL CORRELATIONS

Neurotransmission. Acetylcholinesterase (AChE) activity in various CNS areas has been used as evidence for the presence of acetylcholine, which has been implicated in the chemical transmission of nerve impulses at some synapses in the CNS.

The increase in AChE activity with age varies with different species and depends upon the degree of maturity at birth for a given species. In rats, AChE activity reaches adult levels in the spinal cord at birth [9], in the cerebellum, brain stem, and hypothalamus at 23 days after birth, and in the sensorimotor cortex at about 40 days after birth [10]. In the spinal cord the progressive increase of AChE activity during fetal development correlates with the appearance of bioelectric activity and synaptic vesicles [2] and the ability to exhibit spinal cord convulsions [15].

In the chick, AChE reaches peak activity in the spinal cord at 14 days of incubation and corresponds with the functional development of the spinal cord in chick embryos [16].

Myelination. The earlier functional development of the spinal cord in contrast to that of the brain can also be related to the process of myelination already progressing in the spinal cord at a time when no myelin can be found in the brain. Studies in 6-day-old rats have shown the concentration of cerebrosides to be 3.2 mg per 100 mg of lipids in the spinal cord, whereas it is only 0.8 mg in the cerebrum and 0.5 mg in the cerebellum [1]. It is known that myelination confers upon a nerve fiber the properties of lowered threshold, increased conduction velocity, and greater ability to carry repetitive impulses.

Rapid increases in conduction velocity and decreases in threshold occur during the period of rapid myelination. For example, in the corpus callosum of the rat, the greatest decrease in latency and, presumably, increase in conduction velocity occurs at 10–15 days of age with slower decrease from 15–30 days, when extensive myelination of the corpus callosum occurs [7].

Electrolytes. The ability of rats to exhibit full seizure activity by 21 days of age correlates well with the cerebral cortical concentrations of sodium, chloride, and potassium, which in the developing rat reach adult levels around 21 days after birth [19]. Furthermore, electrolyte distribution in the neuronal, glial, and interstitial compartments in the developing rat reaches adult patterns around 21 days [23].

DEVELOPMENT OF SPECIFIC NEURAL SYSTEMS

Responses to Convulsant and Anticonvulsant Drugs

Responses of the developing CNS to neurotropic drugs have been used as indices of the degree of neural organization which is a function of maturation of both facilitatory and inhibitory systems.

CHEMICALLY INDUCED SEIZURES

Pentylenetetrazol, strychnine, and picrotoxin are frequently used as test agents for assessing and evaluating CNS activity under a variety of conditions and as tools for elucidating patterns of neuronal organization during development. These convulsant drugs are used because the mechanisms, from a neuropharmacological standpoint, by which they produce seizures is at least partly understood; hence, they are useful in studying the development of specific neuronal systems.

Strychnine selectively blocks postsynaptic inhibition presumably by competing with the inhibitory transmitter at some postsynaptic site. It can serve, therefore, as a research tool to study mechanisms of inhibition and to investigate the nature of inhibitory transmitters. Although evidence has been accumulating that postsynaptic inhibition at some CNS sites is not blocked by strychnine, changes in the convulsive dose (CD_{50}) of strychnine with age is used as a measure of maturation of postsynaptic inhibitory pathways, provided that other factors such as development of the blood-CNS barrier do not obscure the results. Picrotoxin selectively blocks presynaptic inhibition without affecting postsynaptic inhibition. There is a question, however, as to whether the blockade of presynaptic inhibition plays an important role in convulsions produced by the drug.

The combination of picrotoxin and strychnine blocks most inhibitory pathways in the CNS. Some of the effects of picrotoxin, therefore, must be concerned with some type of inhibition, presumably presynaptic inhibition. This selective blockade of presynaptic inhibition must be involved in the seizure process, but other effects are probably also present.

Pentylenetetrazol blocks neither presynaptic nor postsynaptic inhibition, but activates all pathways. Pentylenetetrazol-induced convulsions are probably a result of activation of excitatory pathways that are unopposed by inhibition [8]. Since this drug freely distributes in total body water, its penetration into the brain is rapid and not restricted by the blood-CNS barrier. Consequently, changes in the CD_{50} of pentylenetetrazol with age represent neurophysiological rather than blood-CNS barrier changes.

In the *maturing* rat, the pattern of convulsions induced by strychnine, pentylenetetrazol, and picrotoxin develops in phases, as does the pattern of electrically induced seizures. Full flexor-extensor convulsions are exhibited between 13–16 days of age [24].

The dose of strychnine required to elicit the characteristic seizure pattern does not vary significantly in rats from 4–8 days of age. Beginning with the eighth day, the CD_{50} of strychnine continuously increases with age. Increase in the CD_{50} of strychnine until 17 days of age is interpreted to be due to an increase in strychnine-sensitive postsynaptic inhibitory synapses during this period, since the drug competes with the transmitter mediating this type of inhibition. The further increase in the CD_{50} of strychnine after 17 days of age may be attributed to two factors: additional maturation of inhibitory elements and development of the blood-CNS barrier to strychnine. Our other studies have shown that in rats, the blood-CNS barrier is present after 17 days of age [23]. That postsynaptic inhibition does develop most rapidly during the period from 8–21 days of age is indicated by the fact that the ability to exhibit clonus and tonic flexor-extensor convulsions develops during this period; these seizure responses require postsynaptic inhibition.

The CD_{50} of picrotoxin increases until the twelfth day, decreases slightly until the fourteenth day, then increases more rapidly thereafter. The latency for onset of seizures produced by picrotoxin is long and increases markedly after 16 days. It is suggested that the long latency for onset of picrotoxin seizures after 16 days of age, as well as the progressive increase in the CD_{50}, is due to slow penetration of the drug into the brain as a result of the blood-CNS barrier which develops after this time. However, the increase in CD_{50} of picrotoxin prior to 16 days represents changes in the functional activity of the CNS. It is concluded from these data that the presynaptic inhibition develops rapidly during the first 12 days after birth.

The CD_{50} of pentylenetetrazol increases to a peak at 12 days of age, then declines to the value of that of 8-day-old animals and remains at this level thereafter. The similarity of the CD_{50} of pentylenetetrazol in the early postnatal period and at 56 days of age is interpreted to mean that the excitatory systems activated by this drug achieve maturity at an early stage of development. The progressive rise of CD_{50} of pentylenetetrazol until the twelfth day of age may represent development of an inhibitory system activated by pentylenetetrazol at this period, thus raising the threshold at which the excitatory effects of pentylenetetrazol can be produced. That this developing inhibitory system is presynaptic is suggested by the fact that the CD_{50} for picrotoxin also reaches a peak at this time.

Studies of the electrical characteristics of single neurons during maturation also show that excitatory systems develop earlier than some inhibitory systems. In the kitten, excitation is established at the spinal level 2–3 weeks before birth (total gestation is 9 weeks) and in the cortical cells during the first week after birth; supraspinal inhibition of motoneurons occurs sometime after birth—20 days postnatally—and full expression of inhibitory activity in the cortex is not seen until 3–4 weeks postnatally (summarized in [14]).

RESPONSES TO ANTICONVULSANT DRUGS

Effects of Diphenylhydantoin on Electrically Induced Seizures during Development. Diphenylhydantoin in adult animals abolishes the extensor component of MES, elevates the EST for lf stimulation, but does not affect the threshold for high-frequency stimulation.

In *developing* mice diphenylhydantoin (20 mg per kg body weight) administered acutely does not significantly influence the lf EST prior to 17 days of age, but it markedly increases the threshold in the older age groups studied [22]. Lack of effect of diphenylhydantoin on lf EST in mice prior to 17 days of age is due to the fact that the lf EST is already very high; the neuronal system on which this threshold depends is not mature, and therefore, it cannot be further elevated by the anticonvulsant drug.

Diphenylhydantoin increases the ac EST up to 13 days of age in rats and does not change the threshold thereafter [22]. When diphenylhydantoin is given daily to developing rats [20] from 8–11 days after birth, the ac EST is lowered. This result and the lack of effect of diphenylhydantoin in rats older than 13 days of age are attributed to the depressant effect of diphenylhydantoin on a central inhibitory system which is developing during this age period.

In contrast to its effects on the thresholds for minimal seizures, diphenylhydantoin markedly raises the threshold for evoking the tonic flexor component of maximal electroshock seizures at all age periods [22]. Moreover, diphenylhydantoin administered acutely in rats who are 4, 8, and 12 days old significantly reduces the duration of tonic hindlimb extension of spinal cord convulsions [21]. These results illustrate the remarkable ability of diphenylhydantoin to modify the pattern of maximal seizures by preventing spread of seizure activity. In addition, the data illustrate the effects of diphenylhydantoin to reduce the degree of discharge during intense neuronal activity at many levels of the cerebrospinal axis.

Effects of Diphenylhydantoin on Chemically Induced Seizures. Diphenylhydantoin lowers the CD_{50} for picrotoxin at all age periods [24]. Hence, diphenylhydantoin appears to act like picrotoxin in that it blocks presynaptic inhibition. When tested against pentylenetetrazol-induced seizures, diphenylhydantoin has a biphasic effect [24]. Prior to 14 days of age it lowers the CD_{50} of pentylenetetrazol, and the peak that occurs at 12 days in the animals given only pentylenetetrazol does not appear. This excitatory effect of diphenylhydantoin to lower the CD_{50} of pentylenetetrazol is probably due to blockade of presynaptic inhibition, as shown by its enhancement of picrotoxin seizures. After 14 days of age, diphenylhydantoin raises the CD_{50} of pentylenetetrazol, an effect that decreases with age. When tested against strychnine [24], diphenylhydantoin increases the CD_{50} after day 14, as it does for pentylenetetrazol, and this effect also decreases with age until day 36, at which time the CD_{50} of strychnine is not affected by the anticonvulsant drug.

Conclusions on Effects of Diphenylhydantoin on the Developing CNS. It has been shown that the most prominent feature of the mechanism of action of diphenylhydantoin at the cellular level may be the ability of this drug to stabilize excitable membranes against a variety of agents and conditions which ordinarily lead to hyperexcitability [25]. Moreover, the ultimate basis of membrane threshold-stabilizing action of the drug may be stimulation of the metabolic sodium *pump,* although other mechanisms are conceivable.

In the developing animal, the neuronal, glial, and interstitial compartments and electrolyte distribution in these compartments reach adult patterns around 3 weeks of age and coincide with the age period at which predominance of the net anticonvulsant effect of diphenylhydantoin becomes apparent. The immaturity, therefore, of neuronal-interstitial-glial interrelationship may be an important contributing factor in the excitatory action of diphenylhydantoin during early CNS development.

GENERAL CONCLUSION

Evidence is presented that some excitatory systems are mature at birth and that inhibitory systems develop rapidly during the first three weeks after birth. During early development, therefore, the nervous system represents a physiological model *focus* deprived of inhibition and vulnerable to a variety of stimuli. With such a model, mechanisms of seizure activity can be explored further, and the actions of anticonvulsant drugs can be more precisely localized.

REFERENCES

1. Casper, R., Vernadakis, A., and Timiras, P. S. Influence of estradiol and cortisol on lipids and cerebrosides in the developing brain and spinal cord of the rat. *Brain Res.* 5:524, 1967.
2. Crain, S., and Peterson, E. R. Onset and development of functional interneuronal connections in explants of rat spinal cord-ganglia during maturation in culture. *Brain Res.* 6:750, 1967.
3. Esplin, D. W. Spinal cord convulsions. *Arch. Neurol.* (Chicago) 1:485, 1959.
4. Geel, S., and Timiras, P. S. The influence of neonatal hypothyroidism and thyroxine on the ribonucleic acid and deoxyribonucleic acid concentrations of rat cerebral cortex. *Brain Res.* 4:135, 1967.
5. Geel, S., Valcana, T., and Timiras, P. S. Effect of neonatal hypothyroidism and of thyroxine on L-[14C] leucine incorporation in protein *in vivo* and the relationship to ionic levels in the developing brain of the rat. *Brain Res.* 4:143, 1967.
6. Geel, S., and Timiras, P. S. Influence of neonatal hypothyroidism and of thyroxine on the acetylcholinesterase and cholinesterase activities in the developing central nervous system of the rat. *Endocrinology* 80:1069, 1967.
7. Hatotani, N., and Timiras, P. S. Influence of thyroid function on the postnatal development of the transcallosal response in the rat. *Neuroendocrinology* 2:147, 1967.
8. Lewin, J., and Esplin, D. W. Analysis of the spinal excitatory action of pentylenetetrazol. *J. Pharmacol. Exp. Ther.* 132:245, 1961.
9. Maletta, G. J., Vernadakis, A., and Timiras, P. S. Pre- and postnatal development of the spinal cord: Increased acetylcholinesterase activity. *Proc. Soc. Exp. Biol. Med.* 121:1210, 1966.
10. Maletta, G. J., Vernadakis, A., and Timiras, P. S. Acetylcholinesterase activity and protein content of brain and spinal cord in developing rats after prenatal X-radiation. *J. Neurochem.* 14:647, 1967.
11. Millichap, J. G. Seizure patterns in young animals. Significance of brain carbonic anhydrase, II. *Proc. Soc. Exp. Biol. Med.* 97:606, 1958.
12. Penfield, W., and Jasper, H. *Epilepsy and the Functional Anatomy of the Human Brain*. Boston: Little, Brown, 1954.
13. Pylkkö, O. O., and Woodbury, D. M. The effect of maturation on chemically-induced seizures in rats. *J. Pharmacol. Exp. Ther.* 131:185, 1961.
14. Timiras, P. S., Vernadakis, A., and Sherwood, N. Development and Plasticity of the Nervous System. In Assali, N. S. (Ed.), *Biology of Gestation*. New York: Academic, 1968, Vol. 2, Chap. 5.
15. Vernadakis, A. Spinal cord convulsions in developing rats. *Science* 137:532, 1962.
16. Vernadakis, A., and Burkhalter, A. Convulsive responses in developing chickens. *Proc. Soc. Exp. Biol. Med.* 119:512, 1965.
17. Vernadakis, A., and Timiras, P. S. Regulation of brain and spinal cord excitability by cortisol and estradiol in developing rats. *Proc. Second Int. Congr. on Hormonal Steroids*. Excerpta Med. 1966, No. 132, p. 908.
18. Vernadakis, A., and Timiras, P. S. Interrelation between convulsant drugs and X-radiation on the central nervous system. *Arch. Int. Pharmacodyn.* 170:146, 1967.
19. Vernadakis, A., and Woodbury, D. M. Electrolyte and amino acid changes in rat brain during maturation. *Amer. J. Physiol.* 203:748, 1962.
20. Vernadakis, A., and Woodbury, D. M. Effect of Subacute Administration of Diphenylhydantoin on Electroshock Threshold in Developing Rats. In Himwich, H. E., and Himwich, W. A. (Eds.), *The Developing Brain. Progress in Brain Research*. Amsterdam: Elsevier, 9:174, 1964.
21. Vernadakis, A., and Woodbury, D. M. Effects of cortisol and diphenylhydantoin

(Dilantin) on spinal cord convulsions in developing rats. *J. Pharmacol. Exp. Ther.* 144:316, 1964.

22. Vernadakis, A., and Woodbury, D. M. Effects of diphenylhydantoin on electroshock seizure thresholds in developing rats. *J. Pharmacol. Exp. Ther.* 148:144, 1965.

23. Vernadakis, A., and Woodbury, D. M. Cellular and extracellular spaces in developing rat brain. Radioactive uptake studies with chloride and inulin. *Arch. Neurol.* (Chicago) 12:284, 1965.

24. Vernadakis, A., and Woodbury, D. M. The developing animal as a model. *Epilepsia* (Amst.) 1969, in press.

25. Woodbury, D. M., and Esplin, D. W. Neuropharmacology and neurochemistry of anticonvulsant drugs. *Res. Publ. Ass. Res. Nerv. Ment. Dis.* 27:1, 1959.

20

Sensory Precipitation and Reflex Mechanisms[*]

REGINALD G. BICKFORD AND DONALD W. KLASS

SEIZURES that can be initiated by definable conditions of external or internal environment have assumed a prominent role in the study of epileptic mechanisms, whether observed in the patient, the experimental animal, or in the computer model of an unstable system. The purpose of these investigations has varied, but there have been certain principal motivations:

(1) The controllable nature of the seizure lends itself to experimental analysis since it can be produced repeatedly and can be measured with greater convenience and accuracy than more random types of events.

(2) Study of the initiation parameters may provide important insights into the seizure mechanism and at the same time reveal location and connections of central integrative systems.

(3) The large amplitude synchronized potentials often associated with epileptic phenomena lend themselves to simple and accurate electrographic analysis. Thus their clear definition avoids the necessity of signal extraction techniques such as averaging and thus retains the information value of individual events, which would seem to be the most important variants of neuronal function.

(4) The reactive nature of stimulus-induced seizures allows measurements of excitability of central mechanisms and their periodic changes with time (and with drugs) so that informed models incorporating cyclical changes in seizure threshold can be constructed.

(5) Their study has yielded significant diagnostic information in elucidation of obscure symptomology and furthermore may indicate novel forms of treatment (such as protective glasses and deconditioning).

(6) Finally there has been a growing conviction that in spite of relatively infrequent occurrence of these seizures, they might reveal mechanisms operative in the more commonly encountered *spontaneous* seizures. The latter may represent only a variety of the former in which external input factors are less powerful than the cyclical changes in internal excitability.

Boundaries of Discussion and Relevant Terminology

The title of this discussion, "Sensory Precipitation and Reflex Mechanisms," appears deceptively simple but in fact refers to a rather complex field with uncertain boundaries in which present terminology is often demonstrably inadequate. Patients are encountered in whom seizures can be reliably initiated by establishment of definable preconditions, which contrast with a large group whose seizures appear sporadically and without recognizable initiating factors. Understanding of causation in the first group is incomplete, and in some instances operational descriptions "of what has to be done" replace a clear definition

[*] Supported by PHS Research Grants NB02056 and NB07066 from National Institute of Neurological Diseases and Stroke.

of a causal stimulus. For example, in the primary type of reading epilepsy [11], a stimulus cannot be defined but it is known that an attack can be reliably precipitated by a period of reading. On the other hand, even noninitiable epilepsies are not entirely capricious since they may occur with greater probability at certain times when related to occurrences such as diurnal and menstrual cycles. A spectrum of causality ranges from clearly defined deterministic mechanisms at one end of the scale to probability effects or no definable causal relation at the other. This also suggests the need to regard epilepsy as a multivariant system with a number of external and internal factors which may be operative in a particular case. This orientation, which derives some stimulus from the general field of systems analysis, requires definition of minimal components necessary to describe behavior of the system.

A number of different descriptive terms have been applied to seizures that can be initiated by an appropriate input, which include such terms as *reflex, triggered, stimulus-sensitive, evoked,* and *precipitated.* Finding satisfactory terminology poses real problems since it is clear that varied mechanisms are operative in the initiation of seizures. At one end of the spectrum, a brief flash of light may initiate a petit mal seizure (Fig. 20-1) whereas half an hour of continuous reading may be necessary to precipitate the myoclonus of reading epilepsy and a further period to initiate grand mal seizure. A further difficulty is the number of instances where the precise initiating stimulus is not understood (for example, in reading epilepsy).

The term *reflex* has been employed in so many different contexts that it no longer has a precise meaning as a descriptor and its use in reference to seizure-induction is being discouraged. The term *stimulus-sensitive epilepsy* is legitimate for only those types in which a stimulus can be identified; it does not seem appropriate in the case of calculation epilepsies and perhaps those related to emotional factors. The term *trigger* has often been used to designate seizures that can be initiated by a clearly defined input. By convention, trigger is employed to designate the activation of a relatively large response (bomb explosion) by a small one whose energy and directional properties do not enter to an appreciable degree into the final process. While the neurophysiologic situations discussed here meet this criterion to a varying extent, its use can be supported when a relatively short-lived stimulus overcomes a threshold and activates more massive discharge differing in content and organization from the stimulus.

It should be noted that these studies fre-

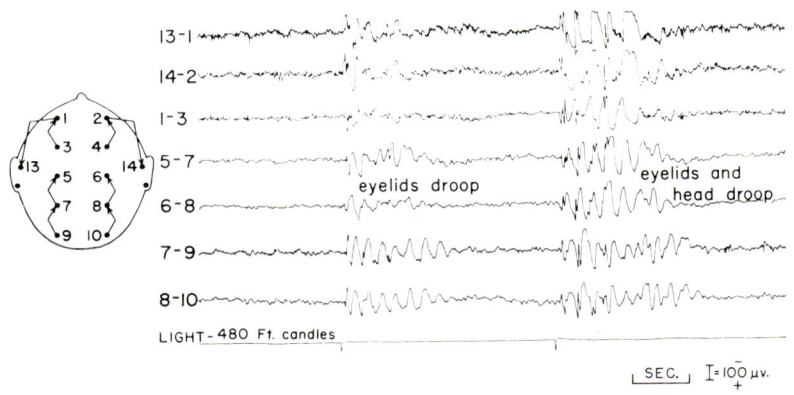

Fig. 20-1. Spike and wave discharges with associated seizure produced by a single light stimulus. Patient had petit mal attacks and mental retardation. Some attacks were induced by hand waving. Note widespread atypical spike-wave discharges produced by single light flash. There are differences in response to first flash (shorter and less spike component) in the EEG discharge and absence of head droop.

quently involve investigation of abortive mechanisms falling short of production of a seizure but often producing a characteristic electrographic signal. Here there is no completion of a reflex arc, and the effect can be more appropriately regarded as response of a convulsive type. Since they illuminate the general problem of seizure initiation, those seizures related to hyperventilation and to chemical stimulation should be included although they are not conventionally considered in the categories of trigger or reflex.

It has been clinically convenient to classify certain seizures by initiation mechanisms such as audiogenic and photogenic, but such classification does little justice to the complexity of epileptic processes, which have been shown to involve tightly interacting events of input, central, and output levels. In considering initiation mechanisms operative in precipitated seizures, it will be necessary to spend time with central processing and have some concern with output mechanisms; the latter are importantly operative in the feedback loop characteristic of self-induced seizures.

INDUCTION MECHANISMS IN EPILEPTIC PATIENTS

The data presented are studies by the authors on a population of approximately 40,000 patients referred from various sections of the Mayo Clinic for recordings in the EEG laboratory during the last 22 years. During this time many of the patients were studied repeatedly over periods of many years. Conventional recordings and those made by implanted depth leads have been used where the latter appeared to be therapeutically justified. Cinematographic recordings of the EEG alongside the patient were used to study induced seizures and more recently parallel techniques employing video tape. Computer studies were made using special purpose summating devices or the general purpose CDC 3200 time-share system with peripheral consoles incorporating a variety of EEG and field display options.

These data have been supplemented by extensive studies reported in the literature, summarized in a number of reviews [1, 22, 23, 36, 37, 41, 54, 61, 67, 68, 69]. (These should be referred to.)

PHOTOEPILEPSY. All authorities agree that seizures related to stimulation of the visual system are by far the most frequently induced attacks, accounting for about 2–4 percent of all epileptic patients in Mayo experience. It is not obvious why this should be so but perhaps relates to the fact that, in the normal subject, responses to photic stimulation occur more widely in the brain than those to any other sense modality; this is the only afferent system that can be effectively driven by outside stimuli at a cortical level.

Fluctuation of light stimulus appears necessary to induce an epileptic attack, although a single pulse of light may be effective as seen in Fig. 20-1. Any claims of observing seizure induction by continuous light can probably be discounted as due to interruptions of the beam by rapid flutter of eyelids, often seen in these cases (and at times a mechanism for self-induction). In general, photic stimuli are effective in proportion to their intensity, degree of modulation, frequency (the optimal usually considered as between about 10 and 15 cycles per second), and to the degree the visual field is filled. Monocular stimulation is of reduced effectiveness compared with binocular. Seizures are apparently more easily induced with eyes closed as compared with eyes open, a phenomenon partly due to *diffuser effect;* in addition, a factor of lower convulsive threshold is produced by reduction in visual pattern input.

Many claims in the literature for differential effects in spectral sensitivity have been made, mainly incriminating the red end of the spectrum as being more epileptogenic. In many instances there have not been adequate controls for changes in intensity when different colors are compared, bearing in mind the complex spectral emission of most light sources, problems of optimal filtering, and differential color sensitivity of the eye itself. In spite of these difficulties, in occasional cases there appears to be genuine red sensitivity, which can be largely eliminated by use of minus red glasses (Fig. 20-2), which have bluish color

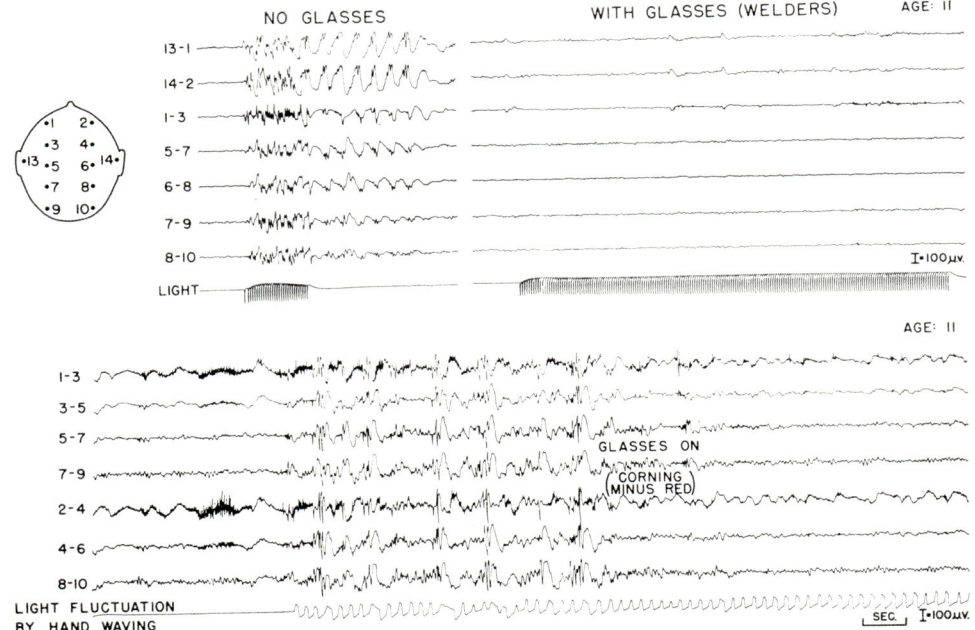

Fig. 20-2. Photoepilepsy with protection of welder's glasses (above). Self-induced attack with protection by red excluded lens (below). A photocell attached to face documents movements of hand; an approximate 5 per sec light fluctuation is produced. Note momentary arrest of hand movement following larger spike-wave complexes. (From Bickford [9].)

and do not reduce overall transmission markedly [16, 42].

Existence of epileptic sensitivity to more physiologic types of visual stimulation, as by pattern, and first described in 1954 [7, 9, 12, 49], is of considerable interest. These cases form a subgroup of photoepileptics with an incidence of about 5 percent. Twenty such cases have been investigated and some may show remarkable sensitivity to the directional orientation of visual pattern; for instance, the patient illustrated in Fig. 20-3 produced almost continuous spike-wave discharge when he viewed vertical patterns, an effect which disappeared at about 30 degrees, becoming entirely absent with horizontal patterns. Such effects are reminiscent of directionally sensitive unit discharges in cortex of cats described by Hubel and Weisel [44].

The hypothesis that could be considered is if pattern-sensitive patients exhibit a facilitation of the normal lambda mechanism, which is an evoked response known to be related in the normal subject to scanning of visual patterns. However, evidence is against such relationship since (1) patterns effective in triggering spike-wave discharges in the pattern-sensitive are usually geometric in type and different from the half-tone pattern stimuli shown to be optimal for producing lambda waves [60]; (2) in some pattern-sensitive patients, normal lambda response can be distinguished; and (3) lambda response is localized to the occipital-parietal region whereas spike-wave response of light sensitivity is widespread and often maximal in the frontal regions (Fig. 20-4). In some but not all pattern-sensitive cases, movement of the pattern may increase its effectiveness markedly (Fig. 20-4).

Although such cases are exceedingly rare, there appear to be occasional pattern sensitivities in which a specific object is involved such as the "safety pin case" of Mitchell et al. [56] and the observation of a child who precipitated massive spasm seizures in viewing his left hand [51]. Falconer et al. believe that conditioning influences were involved in the particular re-

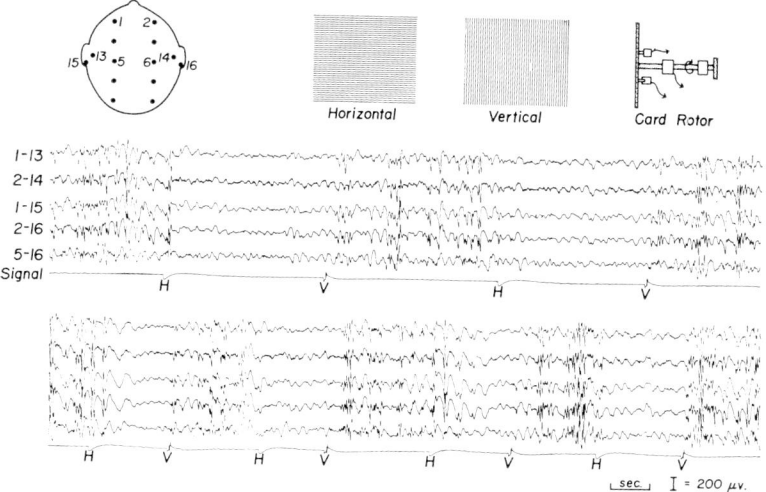

Fig. 20-3. Effect of pattern line direction in pattern-sensitive epileptic patient; child (age 8) had absence attacks on looking at geometric patterns. Signal documents direction of pattern lines as rapidly switched from horizontal (H) to vertical (V). Note sensitivity to vertical direction pattern.

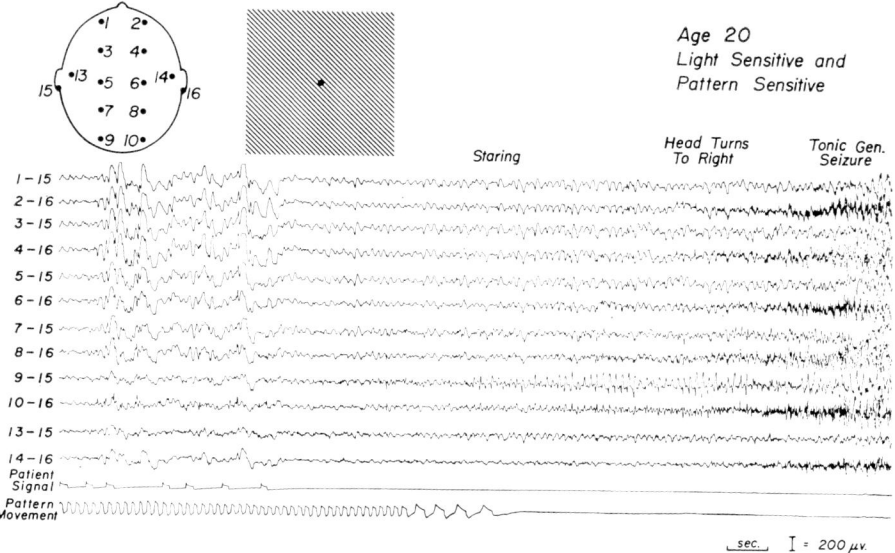

Fig. 20-4. Petit mal and generalized seizure (with some focal onset) produced by gazing at pattern which is moved sideways with frequency shown in bottom channel recorded by photocell. Patient (age 20) had infrequent seizures of petit mal type, was photic and pattern sensitive. Channel 15 is signal operated by patient, which he was told to press rapidly. Note that initially a generalized multiple spike-wave attack is induced with some motor arrest as indicated by patient's signal. Following this, there is the period of gradual buildup of theta frequency together with more focal spiking from left occipital (9–15), which eventually became a generalized tonic and clonic seizure. Transition here is from petit mal to automatismlike seizure via some focal occipital components into generalized seizure with ipsilateral head turning. Patient never had grand mal seizure before this maneuver.

sponse. These situations certainly seem to involve more complex mechanisms than those operative in visual-pattern epilepsy or in lambda response. In fact, they may be more directly related to the phenomenon of *semantic information* thought by Grey Walter to be involved in genesis of the contingent negative variation.

ELECTROGRAPHIC DISCHARGES EVOKED BY LIGHT STIMULATION. Photic stimulus has a tendency to activate diffuse spike-wave discharge and its many variants. Rather rarely does light activate or drive a spike focus confined to the occipital-parietal regions. Occasionally the spike-wave discharge builds up by recruitment from occipital regions. A photic stimulus activating a temporal lobe spike or changing its firing rate has not been observed.

Usually (but not always) associated with diffuse, paroxysmal spike-wave discharge set up by photic stimulus, there is evidence of a petit mal attack, although the degree of induced unresponsiveness may vary considerably from one induced episode to another in the same patient.

In line with the absence of photic effects on a temporal lobe spike, it is also very rare for a photic stimulus to induce a temporal-lobe type of seizure. However, these may be noted occasionally as a result of migration into the temporal lobe of a discharge originating elsewhere [31]. Grand mal seizures are very rarely induced directly by photic stimulus but usually may follow a period of induction of petit mal attacks (Fig. 20-4) or focal seizures.

The frequent characteristic of photic stimulation is completion of the response arc with the appearance of some kind of brief motor response usually termed myoclonus. In fact, a jerking response to light flashes in the facial muscles can be detected in a considerable number of the normal population and has been designated photomyoclonus [6, 8]. More recently, responses of about the same latency, but subliminal for movement and widespread in their distribution to the head and limb musculature, have been delineated by Bickford et al. [13, 14] using computer averaging techniques. They have been termed *microre-*

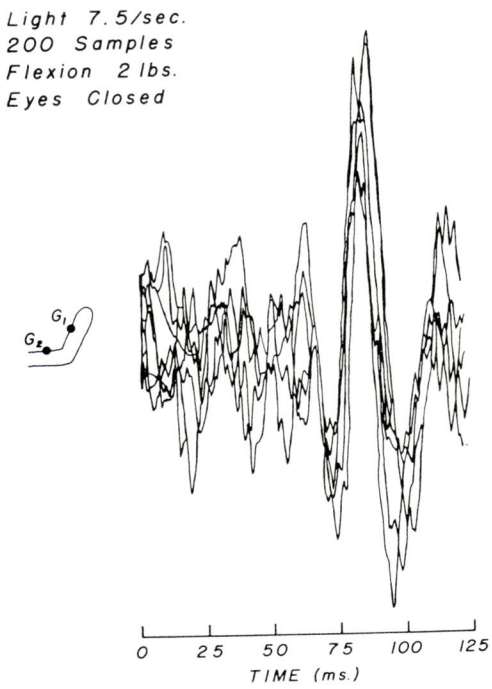

FIG. 20-5. Photomotor microreflex recorded in arm in normal subject. Electrodes placed on left arm and forearm shown in diagram; arm is supporting a two-pound weight. Light flashes of 7.5 per sec (intensity, 75,000 foot-candles), and there are five superimposed summations. Note clearly defined response commencing at about 55 msec with negative peak at 75 msec and large positive peak at 85 msec.

flexes (Fig. 20-5). There is no doubt that microreflexes are normal phenomena though they occur to different extents in members of the normal population. Photomyoclonus also occurs extensively in the normal population and in nonepileptic conditions, although observers have differed in their views on its relation to epilepsy [53].

On the other hand, a group of stimulus-sensitive myoclonus syndromes have clear organic pathology, are often related to diffuse degenerative disease [24, 70, 71]. Production of myoclonus in such a case is shown in Fig. 20-6. Note two important features of this mechanism: the latency is longer than that of the photomotor microreflex, which, when recorded in the arm or leg, is 50 or 75 msec respectively; there is considerable variability in latency from one

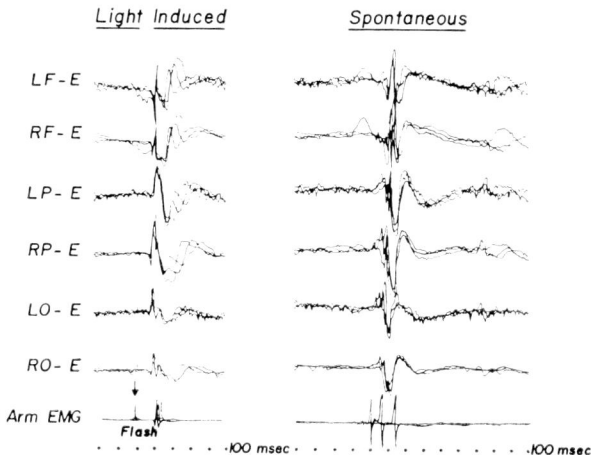

Fig. 20-6. Variability of myoclonus latency in patient with probable Jacob Creutzfeldt's disease (age 56, coma with stimulus-sensitive myoclonus). Light-induced myoclonus shown on left in which is superimposition of three cortical EEG traces and three EMG responses from right arm. Notice range in latency of about 100–140 msec. On right side, three spontaneous discharges superimposed on basis of frontal tracing; note wide range in myoclonus latency. In some instances, jerk appears to precede cortical event.

response to another suggesting that more complex pathways are operative as compared with normal photomotor response. This kind of myoclonic response seems to appear in a variety of degenerative conditions and is often associated with sensitivity to other sensory stimuli. This seems to be a condition of diffuse facilitation as indicated by ability to trigger responses from an implanted electrode at both cortical and subcortical levels.

The diagram in Fig. 20-7 summarizes these rather complex findings in the patient group, comparing them with a large variety of responses to light encountered in the normal population. Relatively few of the abnormal responses can be accounted for on the basis of exaggeration of a normal mechanism (columns 1–10) although Broughton [17] has shown that some cases of photic sensitivity have latencies that would be appropriate for facilitated photomotor (microreflex) response.

CENTRAL MECHANISMS IN PHOTOEPILEPSY. In producing a seizure response, the input volley resulting from stimulation of external receptors must reach the internal processors; the result of this interaction determines whether or not a seizure is initiated. That these internal processors have important bearing on the outcome is evidenced in Fig. 20-8. In this experiment, a patient sensitive to rhythmic photic stimulation signaled by production of spike-wave discharges was subjected to a long series of identical stimulus trains over a period of many minutes. During this period her eyes were closed, and every effort was made to maintain experimental conditions constant. It will be seen, however, that response obtained to the standard train of 10 stimuli is remarkably variable, at times resulting in no detectable change, at others in a self-sustained 10 sec spike-wave discharge; intermediately there were discharges of shorter duration. When the length of spike-wave discharge was plotted over the time period, cyclical changes were quite evident, but there was no very constant period. Evidence of cyclic variability in responsiveness of central mechanisms is crucial in the interpretation of both induced attacks and its implication for initiation mechanisms in epilepsy of an apparently untriggered variety; this evidence also leads directly to consideration of feasible models of the epileptic seizure process.

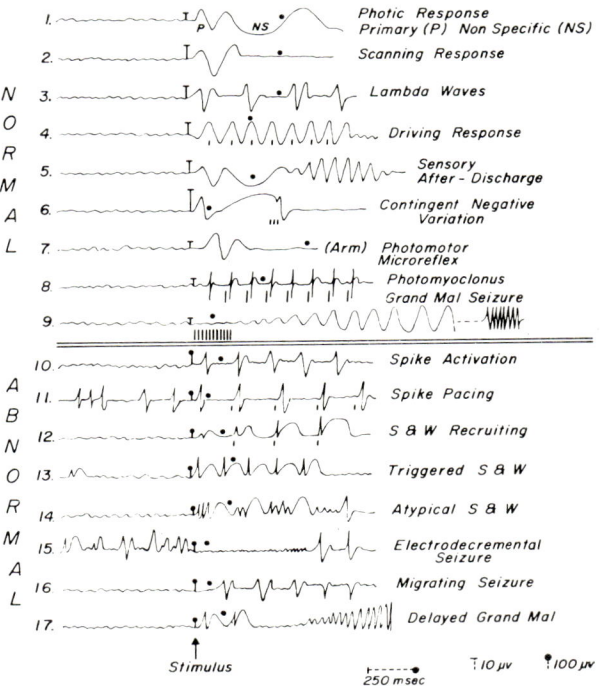

Fig. 20-7. Comparison of normal and epileptic responses to photic stimulus (diagram). Comparison of normal evoked responses to light above including grand mal seizure, which occurs in small percentage of normal subjects. Lower 8 traces illustrate varied mechanisms by which light induces change in epileptic patients. Since responses are viewed on various time scales, the 250-msec marker is shown above each tracing, and amplitude calibration is shown as stimulus artifact for each trace.

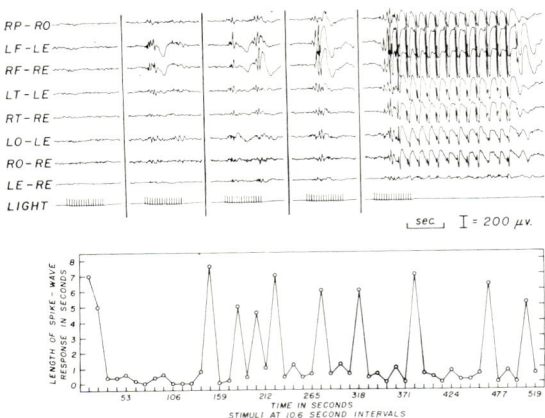

Fig. 20-8. Periodic variation in response to light. Identical and electronically timed stimulus trains applied to a photosensitive patient over period of 520 sec. Range of response to standard stimulus shown in section above, and graph below plots spike-wave response duration against time.

PHOTOEPILEPTIC SEIZURE MODELS. With the qualitative data concerning initiable seizures borne in mind, an attempt may be made to isolate the important components of a seizure system and consider interrelations required by the data. At first we will be concerned with relatively simple deterministic models with direct and feedback loops, remembering that in later models some probabilistic elements will have to be introduced. The model naturally falls into three compartments: input, brain or central processor, and output (Fig. 20-9).

Let us first consider how this model might operate in the common variety of photic epilepsy such as that illustrated in Fig. 20-1. Since a single pulse of light is effective here, it finds the visual system unprepared and makes its way through branch 1 on its way to occipital cortex but also affects pathway 2 (at a presently unknown anatomic site but possibly arising from the lateral geniculate) to activate the epileptogenic lesion 3. Whether a threshold of activation of this lesion can be reached will depend on a number of influences which are shown playing on system 3, namely, the level of brain excitability (which is pictured as undergoing periodic change), cyclic changes in the epileptic lesion itself that are known to occur (as evidenced by variations in spike discharge frequency), factors of CO_2 level, and the like. When the lesion fires, it shows tendency to produce a petit mal attack. The PM component has a threshold which determines whether the discharge will in fact activate seizure mechanisms to produce overt evidence of the petit mal attack.

If we now consider a repetitive series of stimuli, there is a possibility that feedback control loop 9 will start to influence the outcome since it will produce some closure of iris and possibly some inhibitory effect at the retinal level. The other feedback mechanism represented by pathway 8 is that which operates in the self-induced epilepsies [9, 49, 58, 63] (Fig. 20-2), shown here as originating in the voluntary motor center (6), where compulsive acts are presumably initiated, resulting in waving of the hand or clonus of the eyelids, which produces an interruption of light input. This may feed a new stimulus through the system resulting in myoclonus, which in itself will produce jerkiness of hand movements and eyelids so that additional stimuli are generated and a complete positive feedback system is initiated. Grand mal attacks are rarely induced by photic stimulation unless they are secondary to petit mal as shown by the loop between petit mal and grand mal. Occasionally, however, grand mal attacks result, such as those associated with drug action and withdrawal.

QUANTITATIVE MODELS (PHOTOEPILEPSY). To illustrate the systems approach, consider how the photoepilepsy model would function if we proceed to the next stage of assigning values and mathematical relations to the components illustrated. A simple

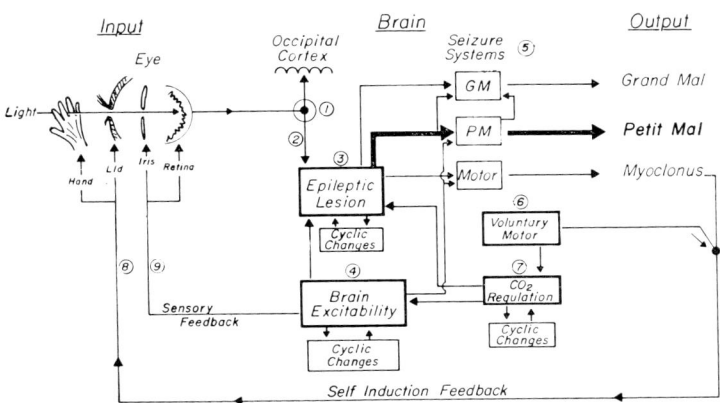

FIG. 20-9. Component model of photic epilepsy (see text).

deterministic model might operate in the manner illustrated in Fig. 20-10, which model assigns numeric values to fluctuations that the two main variables (brain lesion and excitability) undergo as the periodic function with time. Light stimulus is also given a numeric value that might be regarded as dependent on intensity. When light is repeated as in flicker, its value increases with each flash thus representing facilitatory effects. When addition of the three variables exceeds the threshold (40 in the diagram), it is assumed that the spike-wave mechanism is activated for a time that depends on the amount by which the sum exceeds the threshold. In the top part of the diagram, the resulting spike-wave episode is drawn. In the left half of the model, data are regarded as deterministic, but in the last section random functions are employed for all variables so that the model becomes stochastic.

Some examples may now be considered. At *A* a relatively low intensity flash fails to reach threshold because of relatively low values of both brain and lesion excitability. On the other hand, the same stimulus repeated in *B* exceeds the threshold and gives a short burst of spike-wave because it occurred at almost peak values of both the brain variables. The third stimulus (*C*) of the same intensity fails to initiate discharge because of low value of lesion excitability although we are here almost at the peak of the brain excitability cycle. The longest spike-wave episode is produced in *D* by a higher intensity flash associated with peak value of brain excitability and fairly high value of lesion excitability. In *E* we note the effect of repetitive flicker stimulation, which gives rise to increasing values of the stimulus until, in combination with the other two variables, it produces a short spike-wave discharge. The model also predicts at *F* what is commonly noted in these cases, that is, occasional occurrence of a spontaneous burst of spike and wave. In the model these occur because when there is coincidence of peak values in both brain excitability and lesion excitability, the threshold for discharge is exceeded. Finally, in *G*, when both brain variables are given probability values ranging about a mean and the same distribution applies also to flash intensity, there are possibilities of seizure induction, but these will now have a probability distribution rather than the certainty associated with a deterministic model.

Sound-Induced Seizures

Auditory stimulation is a relatively ineffective trigger for epileptic seizures in man. This perhaps relates to the difficulty

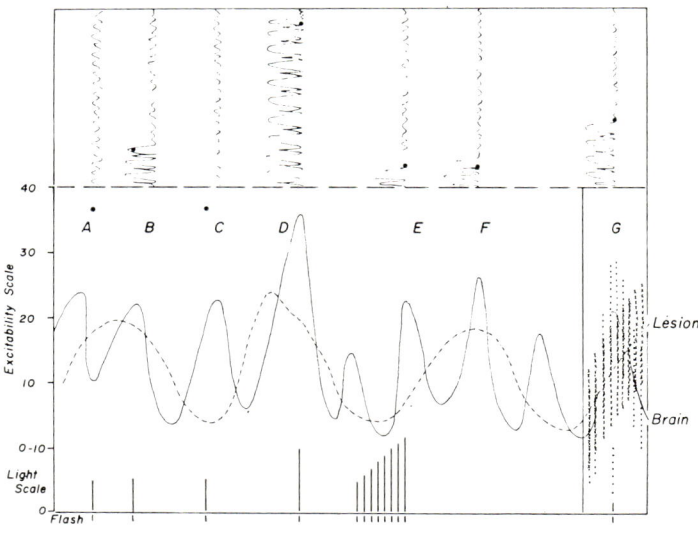

Fig. 20-10. Quantitative model of photoepilepsy (see text).

of recording evoked responses from the primary auditory cortex in man. Such responses have been recorded occasionally from depth electrodes and in the operating room [18]. Very rarely has it been possible to trigger epileptic spikes in the temporal lobe by auditory (click) stimuli. The recording of *driving* responses to rhythmic auditory stimuli in man has been claimed by some workers but in view of more recent work on sound-evoked microreflexes, the possibility that these rhythms arose from muscle still has to be considered.

An extremely rare type of seizure is that produced by music [21], and these cases are usually characterized by a highly specific stimulus, only certain forms of music being effective in any particular case. The necessary buildup time to induce this type of seizure is often long and may take many minutes. The syndrome is unusual among sensory-precipitated epilepsies insofar as the attack induced among the reported cases has commonly been a temporal lobe type of seizure. Little is known concerning the mechanism of this seizure induction although some attempts have been made at therapy by deconditioning procedures [32].

Probably the most frequent kind of seizure induced by sound (but still rare) is that induced by startle [2], sound being one of the most effective stimuli. An example is shown in Fig. 20-11. Notice here a switch from the widely synchronized sharp wave

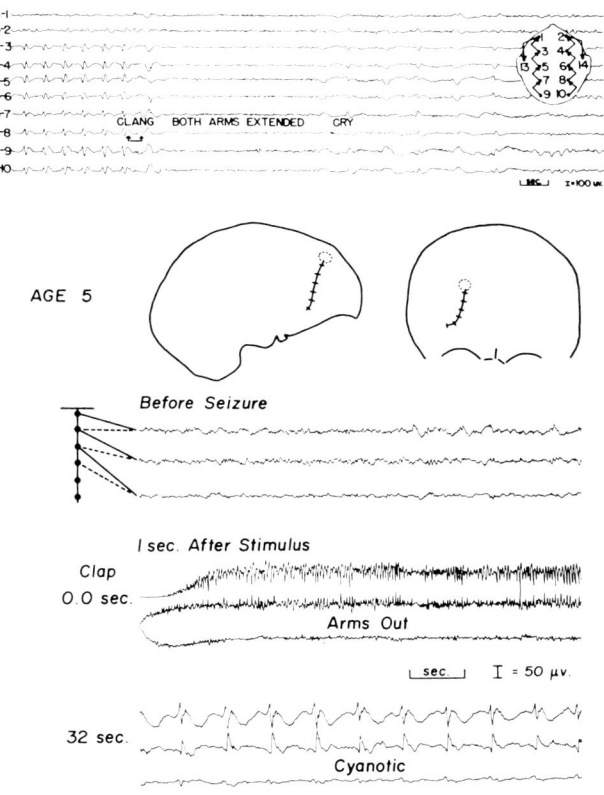

Fig. 20-11. Seizure induced by startling sound. Note widely synchronized sharp waves in recording before loud clang produced by metal sheets (upper traces), which caused sudden extension of arms and legs with tonic posture followed by cyanosis and crying. During seizure there is marked electrical decrement in presence of low voltage, fast activity seizure discharge recorded in depth electrodes (lower traces). On this occasion, EEG is less synchronized before induction of seizure by means of a clap. This resulted in widespread high voltage fast activity present in several depths of cortex (actually quite widespread as shown in other depth electrodes not illustrated in this diagram). Following fast activity, there is repetitive sharp-wave discharge.

pattern of the abnormal resting recording to an entirely different type of low voltage, fast discharge during the seizure. The latter could be distinguished only with difficulty in the conventional scalp recording but in depth it appeared as widespread, fast discharge of 15–30 cycles per second.

MODEL OF STARTLE EPILEPSY. Although we have little understanding of the startle mechanism, the probable components can at least be defined into a deterministic model similar to that for photoepilepsy seizures. The suggested model is shown in Fig. 20-12.

It should be noted that this is another situation where an epileptic condition seems to be grafted on to normal brain mechanisms represented by the startle system. The component labeled *epileptic lesion* is the only one not present in the normal brain. The concept in generation of startle is that input to the brain is continuously processed and cross-correlated with memory store, close coherence indicating that nothing unusual is being received. When the two are not coherent, however, the system is activated and an unusual event is defined and registered in the *novelty assessment* component. The signal is then passed on to the system that has the function of assessing its threat to integrity of the organism. Thus all high-energy, short-duration stimuli are likely to possess a high positive value. If this value is sufficiently positive, the startle system is activated; it must be borne in mind that the threshold of the startle system comes under several regulatory influences. Thus the *intellectual* center provides a general background tone of fear or confidence and the *brain excitability* center feeds in such influences as alertness or drowsiness to influence the startle threshold. When the startle threshold is activated as a result of these inputs, it will produce the well-known motor reaction. Additionally, in the case of the epileptic, an appropriate stimulus will be transmitted to the *epileptic lesion*. This component has cyclic inputs and is affected by brain excitability. Thus if a sufficiently large stimulus arises from the startle center at an appropriate phase in the excitability cycle, the lesion is activated and produces a petit mal or grand mal seizure, dependent on its predominant connections in the particular patient under consideration. It is, of course, characteristic of startle reactions that they can be influenced by both previous experience, which in this model is handled by the memory store, or by communicated information in the form of a message which plays on both the memory store and threat assessment, dependent on the nature of input from this source.

Somesthetic Induced Seizures. In rare instances, somesthetic stimuli, such as touch, will induce spike discharge or occasionally focal seizure in the appropriate cortical area [33]. On further investigation some of these cases turn out to be examples of startle effects which disappear if a patient is

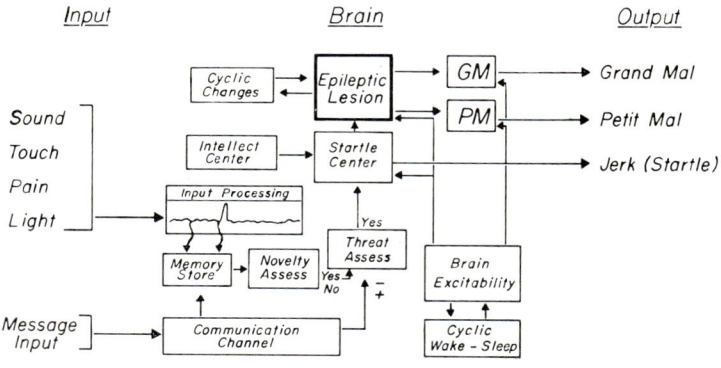

FIG. 20-12. Component model of startle epilepsy (see text).

expecting the stimulus. In the remaining cases, however, a touch (usually to a specific part of the cutaneous surface) will induce an attack. Goldie and Green [38] have described a case in which hypnotic suggestion of cutaneous stroking or thinking about this procedure would in itself initiate spike discharges. Unlike most other induction types, the somesthetic group have very frequently been associated with cortical lesions, and there are several instances in which excision of the epileptogenic focus has caused disappearance of the seizure syndrome.

Proprioceptive Induction. A classic study of proprioceptive triggering of myoclonic seizures by Dawson [25, 26] has established many of the physiologic properties of this syndrome, documenting its considerable dependence on spinal mechanisms. Unlike the somesthetic group, proprioceptive triggers commonly seem to activate seizure mechanism characterized by bilateral symmetric myoclonus, and the syndrome is frequently seen in degenerative conditions and in familial myoclonus epilepsy.

Reading Epilepsy. This condition, first described by Bickford [9, 11], is not so rare as some authorities have supposed; it is clear that many cases are misdiagnosed or never seek medical assistance. It has been divided into two groups: the primary group, a very specific syndrome in which seizures take the form of jaw myoclonus with electrographic accompaniment related to reading and often ending in a generalized seizure if reading continues; in the secondary group, reading is a nonspecific stimulus shared by many other stimuli such as may exist in pattern-sensitive patients or in calculation epilepsy. The group of primary reading epilepsy patients represents one of the most highly specific forms of epilepsy that has been observed. While in suitable patients the attack can be very reliably induced by reading (the material is usually not pertinent, and nonsense reading may be effective), the nature of the initiating stimulus has so far evaded definition. It seems likely that input from eye muscle proprioceptors [62] and from the jaw and laryngeal muscles combine with visual input so that we are probably dealing with a multisensory trigger.

Miscellaneous Varieties. In a considerable number of isolated cases, investigators have claimed induction through stimuli carried by vestibular [3], visceral [36], and olfactory [28] channels but, apart from the nature of the trigger, these cases do not seem to differ essentially from others in the sensory precipitation group.

Internal Epileptic Triggers. Some epileptic patients exhibit a situation in which an internal trigger in the form of an epileptic spike may excite the brain into epileptic oscillation. This syndrome has usually been called *secondary bilateral synchrony*. Thus there exists a complex situation in which one epileptic component interacts with a second. The mechanism by which spike discharge can initiate diffuse spike-wave reaction has been simulated in this patient by single pulse depth stimulation (Fig. 20-13). As the voltage of local stimulus is increased, there is gradual recruiting, first locally and finally triggering of generalized discharge. It was found that single pulse initiation of the spike-wave discharge could be accomplished over wide areas of the cortex and subcortex. Initiation of these spike-wave discharges from a single pulse stimulus is reminiscent of that illustrated in Fig. 20-1 from a single photic stimulus.

Emotional and Intellectual Induction. There has long been anecdotal evidence that the patient's emotional state affects and sometimes initiates a seizure. On the other hand, it has been hard to document this finding because it is difficult to control hyperventilation and afferent inflow influences, which might well account for triggering in some instances. However, a case has been reported [39] in which grand mal seizure was induced by an emotionally challenging conversation (with sexual connotations). Hyperventilation effects were carefully controlled, and yet there is clear evidence that seizure was induced in a patient who had not previously suffered from epileptic seizures. The fact that depth recording was available in this case also rules out artifact and recording uncertainties that usually accompany an emotional

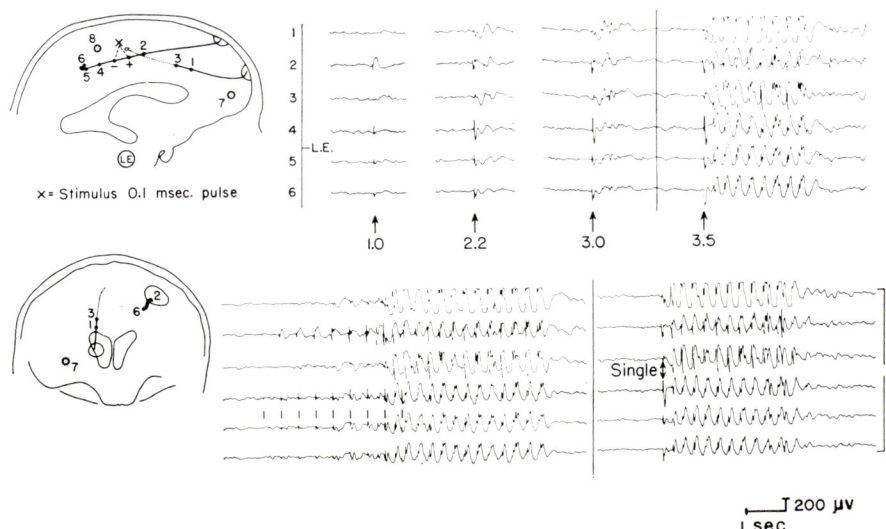

FIG. 20-13. Gradual recruiting of spike-wave episode following single-pulse depth stimulation. Notice gradual increase of first and local discharge, later more generalized as stimulus voltage is increased from 1–3.5 in upper part of diagram. At 3.5, self-sustained spike-wave discharge is induced with clinical evidence of petit mal attack. Similar series of events can be seen with repetitive stimulation as shown in lower part of diagram.

experience when conventional scalp recording is employed. Thus there seems to be valid evidence that emotional factors influence seizure states, although the precise degree for which these factors, rather than others secondary to them, influence the EEG is often difficult to assess.

In rare instances it is found that intellectual tasks such as recall and calculation will reliably precipitate seizure, such as the case illustrated in Fig. 20-14 and one recorded by Ingvar [47]. Both these cases involve unilateral myoclonus and are associated with multiple spike-wave discharges in the EEG. It is difficult to rule out some unrecognized, proprioceptive inflow as the trigger in these instances, since it is known that a number of *expressive phenomena* (eyelid flutter, frowning, and the like) are often associated with the act of calculation or recall. However, evidence suggests that internal triggering was in fact operative.

It might be expected that varied syndromes represented by sensory-precipitated epilepsy could be modified by conditioning procedures. On the whole, however, this has proved a disappointing endeavor in both the human and animal, although evidence can undoubtedly be found where conditioning has modified the effective trigger mechanism. Forster reported limited success in using such techniques in treatment of stimulus-sensitive epileptics [32], and Efron [28] has modified the effective stimulus by conditioning.

Chemical Induction. One of the most effective methods of triggering epileptic seizures is via the mechanism of lowering blood CO_2 associated with hyperventilation. There is a tendency here to petit mal seizures although temporal lobe seizures can occasionally be activated. The exact mechanism of chemical triggering is still not clearly understood, there probably being a combination of vascular effects leading to anoxia in addition to lowering of CO_2 and other ionic changes associated with it. Perhaps from the point of view of trigger epilepsies, the most important implication of the hyperventilation-induced seizure is that it can easily be associated with other induction types (emotional), thus rendering clear delineation of the causal stimulus difficult. Synergy between hyperventilation and photic stimulation can be easily demonstrated and supports

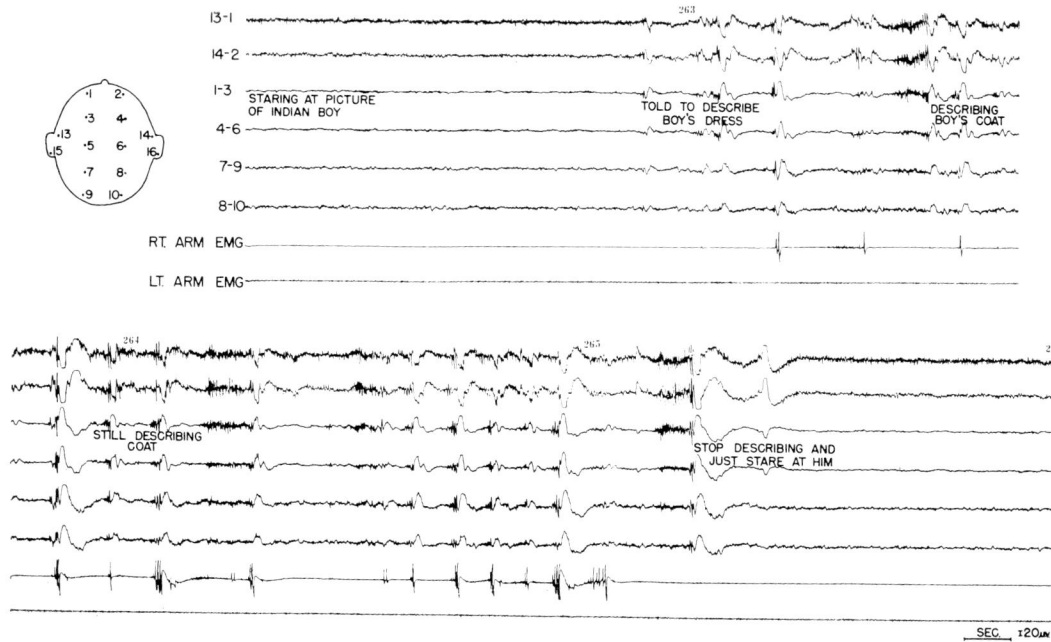

FIG. 20-14. Induction of multiple spike-wave discharges associated with right arm myoclonus in a patient in whom recall or calculation induced an attack. Resting record was normal except when patient was instructed to recall or calculate. Discharges occurred only when mental manipulation was in progress.

the concept of a multivariate system. This combination was included in the model (Fig. 20-9).

Convulsant Drug Induction. Comparative studies of seizures induced in the normal subject by drugs and electrical stimulation [19] indicate that at least a grand mal seizure may, from an electrographic and behavioral standpoint, involve rather identical induction mechanisms under influence of these rather differing triggers. These effects also provide evidence for existence of built-in seizure mechanisms in the normal subject.

Electrical Stimulation Induction. Triggering of seizures by electrical stimulation, particularly in observations made possible by intracerebral electrodes, has provided important information on the state of cerebral excitability and its periodic changes. This avoids complications and uncertainties of estimates dependent on external sensory stimulation. Varied and periodic response to a standard intracerebral stimulus can often be seen in terms of the afterdischarge produced. It is likely that such cyclical changes are paramount in determining onset of seizures both in triggered and spontaneous variety as indicated in our discussions of epilepsy models.

BIOLOGIC AND COMPUTER MODELS OF TRIGGER EPILEPSY

Natural Models. All neuronal systems are subject to oscillation. If electrical or chemical (convulsant) stimuli of sufficient strength are applied, seizures can be produced in all higher animals and man.

Turning now to less artificial and more physiologic stimuli, it has been known for many years that special genetic varieties of rodents (mouse, rat, rabbit) can be triggered into a seizure (usually associated with running and then a generalized convulsion) by a variety of auditory stimuli [4, 30, 55]. While a seemingly disproportionate amount of research has been done on these seizures, as yet there are few clearly defined data on the origin of the seizure, its electrographic components, or its relationship to human

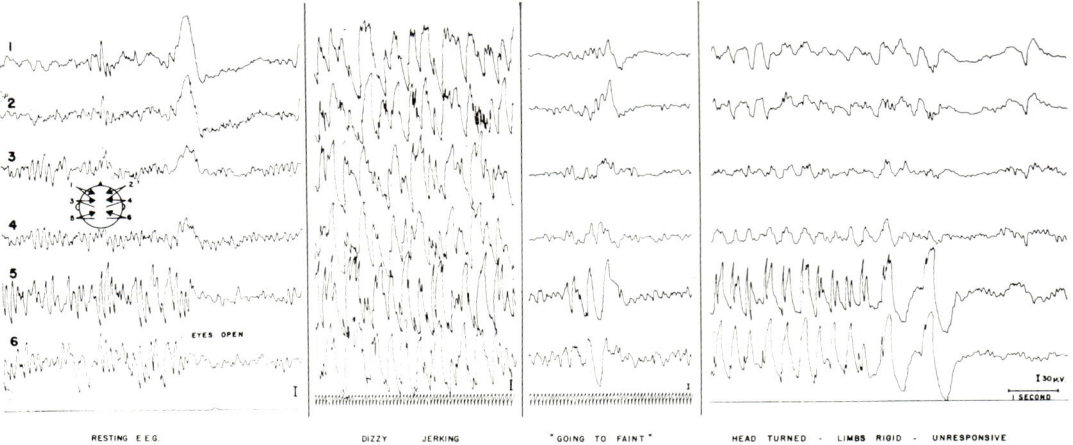

Fig. 20-15. Seizure induced by light stimulation in normal subject (18-year-old nurse). Stimulus generated by three-quarter blackened rotating disc in front of R2 floodlight. There is induction of diffuse high-voltage 3–6 per sec activity associated with dizziness and some generalized jerking; a few seconds later, discharge was more localized to occipital-parietal regions bilaterally. At this time there was head turning with limbs rigid and unresponsiveness.

epilepsy. Indeed there seems to be no direct human equivalent of the audiogenic seizure, which therefore reduces its interest from our standpoint. However, there have been extensive studies of intrinsic periodicity in this animal model.

The human provides his own model of photogenic epilepsy since it has been shown [5] that seizures can be induced in a small percentage (probably fewer than 2 percent) of the normal human population when subjected to flicker stimulation (Fig. 20-15). Usually the seizure induced has been of the grand mal type with atypical electrographic onset, but there have not been extensive studies of these seizures because of medical and ethical problems involved in induction of seizures in a normal subject.

An animal model of photogenic epilepsy was discovered in the baboon by Naquet, Killam, and collaborators [50, 57]. This model is of considerable interest since it seems to show both photomyoclonic and photoconvulsive effects and in this may indeed be very parallel to some phenomena that occur in the normal human. However, there seem to be differences from the human in the optimal flash rate for seizure induction.

Experimental Models

Electrographic Effects. After recognition of waveforms characteristic of epilepsy (such as spike and spike-wave) from the study of human material, there has been considerable research in animal preparations which can simulate this form of discharge. Extensive research indicated that a large variety of chemical substances applied to the cortex will produce periodic spike discharges. If these are located within the primary auditory or visual areas, these spikes can often be triggered or driven by photic or acoustic stimuli thereby simulating a rather uncommon variety of electrographic seizure discharge in the human EEG. In some of these cases, more rapid rates of stimulation will drive individual spike discharges into repetitive and self-sustained discharge. As Clementi [20] showed originally in the behaviorally alert animal, strychninization of the visual cortex results in a reflex myoclonus affecting muscles around the eyes. While this effect has some superficial resemblance to human photomyoclonus, its mechanism is almost certainly different.

In view of the usual association of photo-epilepsy in the human with widespread spike-wave discharge, many investigators have attempted to model this mechanism. Thus, Guerrero-Figueroa [40] has shown that injection of convulsant material into the brain stem in young kittens will produce an acceptable facsimile of widespread spike-wave discharge, and this can be triggered by photic stimulation. A different approach has been used by Stevens [65, 66] and by Hubel and Nauta [45], who combined epileptogenic lesions of visual cortex with brain stem lesions; this procedure provided animals showing excellent simulation of spike and wave and photosensitivity in addition to induced seizures. This work has drawn attention to possible need for two lesions, cortical and brain stem, for simulation of photoepilepsy.

Induction of Seizures. It is generally true in most higher animals and with many convulsive drugs (such as pentylenetetrazol, strychnine, picrotoxin, and others) that continuous administration of the drug, associated with periodic photic stimulation, eventually reaches a stage where the photic stimuli will trigger a seizure, usually the generalized motor type and often preceded by myoclonus. The level at which photically induced seizure can be initiated is usually lower as far as drug concentration is concerned than that of the spontaneous seizure that will ultimately occur with increasing dosage. These effects, however, are not of any great interest from the human standpoint, since this kind of situation is only encountered in the photo-pentylenetetrazol test [34] and is not a good model of naturally occurring photoepilepsy.

The classic work on simulation of spike-wave discharge associated with evidence of unresponsiveness in the animal remains that of Hunter and Jasper [46], who stimulated the diffuse thalamic system nuclei from implanted leads in the unrestrained animal. They obtained good reproduction of spike and wave with a stimulus frequency of about 3 per sec. These authors obtained arrest, stimulus-related myoclonus and some self-sustained discharge; all of these features tended to relate the phenomenon closely to that of petit mal.

However, further experience gained with animal preparations makes it now appear that arrest reaction may not be so specific a simulation as was first believed, since it can be obtained from many other regions of midbrain and brain stem. When photic stimulation is combined with administration of convulsant drugs such as pentylenetetrazol [35], an interesting preparation results in which it can be demonstrated that forward cortical spread occurs from the visual area, eventually involving the motor regions (*irradiation*). Again, relevance of this mechanism to the human disease may be questioned since no such spread or irradiation has been easily demonstrable in patients with photoepilepsy although this may be seen in rare cases.

Observation that spike-wave discharges associated with petit mal in the human can be initiated by single-pulse stimulation from a wide variety of cortical and subcortical areas [10] is of interest, since it indicates existence of a diffusely facilitated system, triggerable from many areas, and suggests perhaps that this is a model for trigger epilepsies in the human. An example is shown in Fig. 20-13.

Myoclonus Models. Many convulsant drugs given in increasing dosage to animals will set up a condition of myoclonus. In most instances, in a period before an overt seizure occurs the preparation is sensitive to sensory stimuli, each of which may cause generalized jerking. These mechanisms have been investigated extensively.

The myoclonus associated with administration of chloralose is one of the most interesting and appears to reproduce in many details the stimulus-sensitive myoclonus, which has already been noted as occurring in human degenerative conditions. In view of recent work on microreflexes, it is interesting to speculate whether the myoclonus response of the chloralose preparation evolved as an exaggeration of the normally present photomotor reflex pathways. The experiment is illustrated in Fig. 20-16. From this, it is clear that a later response occurs in the drug preparation involving more synapses or longer pathways, or both, and that the drug has a suppressive effect on the microreflex.

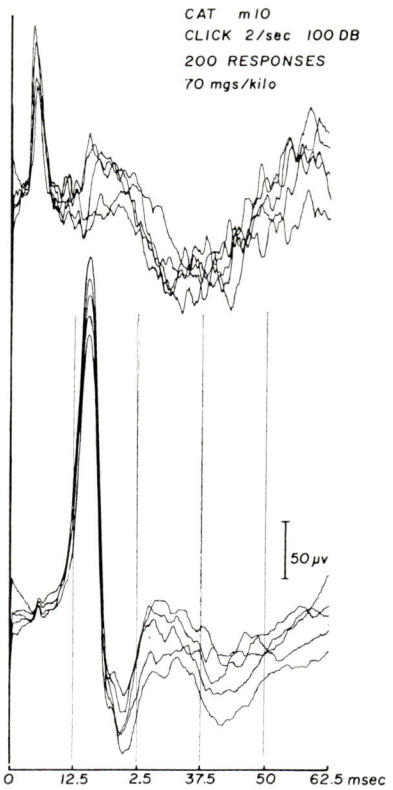

Fig. 20-16. Effect of chloralose on microreflex to click stimuli recorded in cat. Electrode bipolar in neck muscles (6 superimposed averages). Short duration latency microreflex to 100 db click stimuli in waking animal is shown in upper trace. Following intraperitoneal chloralose, 70 mg per kg, cat developed stimulus-sensitive myoclonus, and response in neck muscles is shown in lower trace. Note that main response associated with visible jerking is considerably longer with latency of about 11 msec whereas microreflex response with peak latency at about 6 msec is just visible but almost entirely suppressed. This is evidence that myoclonus does not occupy normal microreflex pathway.

Likewise, it has already been noted that in stimulus-sensitive myoclonus occurring in human patients with degenerative disease, the myoclonus is also of greater latency than the appropriate microreflex response. While the chloralose preparation seems an appropriate model for the human syndrome, particularly in view of the multisensory triggering which it exhibits, we have not observed variability in myoclonus latency which is often, but not invariably, encountered in the human disease.

It is known from the classical experiments of Clementi [20] that localized myoclonus of a stimulus-sensitive variety may occur from local strychninization of the cortex, although accurate latency data on the effects apparently are not available. In the human subject it is known that naturally occurring photomyoclonus can be markedly exaggerated by administration of pentylenetetrazol [6, 8]. Latency measures seem to indicate here that photomotor response to a single stimulus, the photomyoclonus obtained with repetitive stimuli, and possibly some forms of pathologic photomyoclonus all possess the same latency and presumably use the same pathways. This seems to be an example of invasion of a normal pathway by an epileptic process, a mechanism which is not observed very often in epileptic patient syndromes.

In a recent investigation [52], widely synchronized spikes or spike-wave complexes were consistently induced in EEGs of dogs rendered hyponatremic by selective hemodialysis. Intermittent photic stimulation effectively triggered discharges in most dogs exhibiting paroxysmal abnormalities; most of these animals also developed self-sustained electrographic seizure patterns. This animal model simulates the type of light sensitivity that can be acquired by biochemical alterations in patients with uremia and in uremic patients undergoing dialysis treatment. The model will also permit future investigations of the mechanism of light sensitivity in animals without local cerebral chemical or structural lesions.

Computer Models. Farley [29] was one of the first to set up a neuronal-network simulation model on a digital computer. He provided the neurons in this system with adjustable interneuron connections and threshold firing levels that could be changed within the model. He found that under certain conditions this neuronal model shows oscillatory behavior when it is fired from a localized stimulus. It is unfortunate that up to the present, this model cannot be made very realistic, since we do not possess required data on firing thresholds, connectivity, and the like, but as these data become available the model may have increasing relevance to epileptic problems.

DISCUSSION

The most obvious finding from these studies is the great number and variety of functional mechanisms that operate in trigger epilepsies. This raises a significant question as to whether there is an *epileptic disease* that has any uniformity of mechanism. Would it not be more in line with our findings to say that because of its high degree of connectivity and other interactive properties, neuronal tissue necessarily has a built-in mechanism for oscillation? This situation resembles that which occurs in complex servomechanisms in which unintended oscillation is the significant hazard faced by the designer. We know that the brain is particularly vulnerable because of evidence that its oscillatory properties can be manifest at any level of organization, ranging from single neurons through the nerve net of cortical-subcortical interrelations throughout the brain. Since self-perpetuated oscillation can occur at any of these levels, epilepsy syndromes are likely to be compounded from one or a combination of these processes. In this circumstance, well known by the systems engineer, it is very difficult to isolate causal mechanisms of the complete process even though contributing factors can be recognized at many levels by procedures which isolate part of the complete system.

In addition to complexities relevant to a multilevel, tightly linked, hierarchical system with potential for oscillation built in separately at all levels, experimental data indicate existence of many periodicities in oscillatory threshold among components of the system that generates the final oscillation. Finally, it is evident that most signals generated by these varied components are noisy and their random qualities can be handled only by appropriate statistical models.

With this potentially unstable neuronal network of the normal brain, it is evident that sensory inflow takes a significant share in shifting the balance in an oscillatory direction thereby producing the triggered seizure. However, seizures that result from these factors do not seem to differ significantly from those of patients with non-triggerable epilepsy, and some patients have both types of syndrome. For this reason, triggered seizures, which have great advantages for experimental investigation, provide a valid model of the more common spontaneous seizure, and the model presented for photoepilepsy (Fig. 20-10) functions for both types of seizure.

Complexity of processes involved in the induction of seizures has been amply illustrated by varied mechanisms presented by each patient. It is found that identical mechanisms are never encountered in two patients if the analysis is pressed to sufficient depth. Such variety can be appreciated by the fact that in one of the most elite subcategories of epilepsy, that of pattern precipitation, many variants of the initiation mechanism have been encountered. Thus, some patients are sensitive to direction of stripe, others not; and there are those who are markedly sensitive to movement of the pattern, yet others in whom this maneuver is entirely ineffective.

In epileptic conditions, complexity and variety of findings probably reflect the well-known redundancy in mechanisms that subserve the function of information transmission. The use of alternate pathways for producing the same final result is well illustrated in latency shifts that may be observed for myoclonus evoked by light in a number of degenerative syndromes, and in the experimental model when various ablations are made, as in the experiments of DeHaas et al. [27], on chemically induced myoclonus.

Finally, it may be suggested that if we accept a systems approach to epileptic mechanisms, the stimulus-sensitive variety will continue to provide the most appropriate material for further study. This will require application of *input forcing* techniques necessary for development of transfer functions within the various subsystems, which can then be used to build a mathematical model of the epileptic syndrome [15]. Such models would have to be custom built for each individual patient, but predictive properties could be expected which would be valuable to the patient in organizing his daily activities as well as for such factors as making appropriate adjustments in medication.

Little has been said concerning neuronal mechanisms underlying the triggering process [64] and the relative importance of excitatory and inhibitory mechanisms. Likewise, there has been little opportunity to discuss the diverse pathologic [70, 71] concomitants of stimulus-sensitive epilepsies and the important influence of genetic [43], metabolic [52], pharmacologic [48], and alertness factors [59]. Fortunately these topics will be discussed in other contributions.

REFERENCES

1. Ajmone-Marsan, C., and Ralston, B. L. *The Epileptic Seizure. Its Functional Morphology and Diagnostic Significance. A Clinical-Electrographic Analysis of Metrazol Induced Attacks.* Springfield, Ill.: Thomas, 1957.
2. Allen, J. Observations in cases of reflex epilepsy. *New Zeal. Med. J.* 44:135, 1945.
3. Behrman, S., and Wyke, B. Vestibulogenic seizures. *Brain* 81:529, 1958.
4. Bevan, W. Sound precipitated convulsions: 1947 to 1954. *Psychol. Bull.* 52:473, 1955.
5. Bickford, R. G. Electroencephalographic and clinical responses to light stimulation in normal subjects. *Electroenceph. Clin. Neurophysiol.* 1:126, 1949.
6. Bickford, R. G., Sem-Jacobsen, C. W., White, P. T., and Daly, D. Some observations on the mechanisms of photic and photo-metrazol activation. *Electroenceph. Clin. Neurophysiol.* 4:275, 1952.
7. Bickford, R. G., Daly, D., and Keith, H. Convulsive effects of light stimulation in children. *Amer. J. Dis. Child.* 86:170, 1953.
8. Bickford, R. G., White, P. T., Sem-Jacobsen, W., and Rodin, E. A. Components of the photomyoclonic response in man. *Fed. Proc.* 12:1, 1953.
9. Bickford, R. G. Sensory precipitation of seizures. *J. Mich. State Med. Soc.* 53:1018, 1954.
10. Bickford, R. G., Keith, H. M., and MacCarty, C. S. Symposium on electrical activity of subcortical centers: Some observations on the mechanism of petit mal. *Trans. Amer. Neurol. Ass.* 1955, p. 13.
11. Bickford, R. G., Whelan, J. L., Klass, D. W., and Corbin, K. B. Reading epilepsy. *Trans. Amer. Neurol. Ass.* 1956, p. 100.
12. Bickford, R. G., and Klass, D. W. Stimulus factors in the mechanism of TV induced seizures. *Trans. Amer. Neurol. Ass.* 87:176, 1962.
13. Bickford, R. G., Jacobson, J. L., and Cody, D. T. Nature of average evoked potentials to sound and other stimuli in man. *Ann. N.Y. Acad. Sci.* 112:204, 1964.
14. Bickford, R. G. Effect of facial expression on the averaged evoked response to light in man. *Electroenceph. Clin. Neurophysiol.* 23:88, 1967.
15. Blum, B., and Posener, L. N. A stochastic analysis of inter-ictal epileptiform activity. *Confin. Neurol.* 26:519, 1965.
16. Brausch, C., and Ferguson, J. Color as a factor in light sensitive epilepsy. *Neurology* (Minneap.) 2:154, 1965.
17. Broughton, R., Meier-Ewert, K., and Ebe, M. Evoked visual, somatosensory, myogenic, oculogenic and electroretinographic potentials of photosensitive epileptic patients and normal control subjects. *Electroenceph. Clin. Neurophysiol.* 23:492, 1967.
18. Chatrian, G. E., Petersen, M. C., and Lazarte, J. A. Responses to clicks from the human brain: Some depth electrographic observations. *Electroenceph. Clin. Neurophysiol.* 12:479, 1960.
19. Chatrian, G. E., and Petersen, M. C. The convulsive patterns provoked by Indoklon, Metrazol and electroshock. Some depth electrographic observations in human patients. *Electroenceph. Clin. Neurophysiol.* 12:715, 1960.
20. Clementi, A. Stricninizzazione della sfera corticale visiva ed epilessia sperimentale da stimuli luminosi. *Arch. Fisiol.* 27:356, 1929.
21. Critchley, M. Musicogenic epilepsy. *Brain* 60:13, 1937.
22. Critchley, M. Über reflex-epilepsie.

Schweiz. Arch. Neurol. Neurochir. Psychiat. 35:256, 1935.

23. Daube, J. Sensory precipitated seizures: A review. *J. Nerv. Ment. Dis.* 141:524, 1965.
24. Davison, S., and Watson, C. Hereditary light sensitive epilepsy. *Neurology* (Minneap.) 6:231, 1956.
25. Dawson, G. Investigations on a patient subject to myoclonic seizures after sensory stimulation. *J. Neurol. Neurosurg. Psychiat.* 10:141, 1947.
26. Dawson, G. The relation between the EEG and muscle action potentials in certain convulsive states. *J. Neurol. Neurosurg. Psychiat.* 9:5, 1946.
27. DeHaas, A. M. L., Lombroso, C., and Merlis, J. K. Participation of the cortex in experimental reflex myoclonus. *Electroenceph. Clin. Neurophysiol.* 5:177, 1953.
28. Efron, R. Conditioned inhibition of uncinate fits. *Brain* 80:251, 1957.
29. Farley, B. G. A neural network model and its possible relation to electrophysiology. *Proc. Fifth IBM Med. Sympos.* Endicott, N.Y. 1963, p. 391.
30. Finger, F. W. Convulsive behavior in the rat. *Psychol. Bull.* 44:201, 1947.
31. Fischer-Williams, M., Bickford, R. G., and Whisnant, J. P. Occipito-parieto-temporal seizure discharge with visual hallucinations and aphasia. *Epilepsia* (Amst.) 5:279, 1964.
32. Forster, F. M. Conditioning of cerebral dysrhythmia induced by pattern presentation and eye closure. *Cond. Ref.* 2:236, 1967.
33. Forster, F., Penfield, W., Jasper, H., and Madow, L. Focal epilepsy, sensory precipitation and evoked potentials. *Electroenceph. Clin. Neurophysiol.* 1:349, 1949.
34. Gastaut, H. Combined photic and Metrazol activation of the brain. *Electroenceph. Clin. Neurophysiol.* 2:249, 1950.
35. Gastaut, H., and Hunter, J. An experimental study of the mechanisms of photic activation in idiopathic epilepsy. *Electroenceph. Clin. Neurophysiol.* 2:263, 1950.
36. Gastaut, H., and Poirier, F. Experimental or "reflex" induction of seizures. Report of a case of abdominal (enteric) epilepsy. *Epilepsia* (Amst.) 5:256, 1964.
37. Gastaut, H., Regis, H., and Bostem, F. Attacks Provoked by Television and Their Mechanism. In Servit, Z., (Ed.), *Reflex Mechanisms in the Genesis of Epilepsy.* Amsterdam: Elsevier, 1963, p. 230.
38. Goldie, L., and Green, J. A study of the psychological factors in a case of sensory reflex epilepsy. *Brain* 82:505, 1959.
39. Groethuysen, U. C., Robinson, D. B., Haylett, C. H., Estes, H. R., and Johnson, A. M. Depth electrographic recording of a seizure during a structured interview. *Psychosom. Med.* 19:353, 1957.
40. Guerrero-Figueroa, R., Barros, A., Balbian Verster, F. de, and Heath, R. B. Experimental "petit mal" in kittens. *Arch. Neurol.* (Chicago) 9:297, 1963.
41. Henner, K. Reflex Epileptic Mechanisms. In Servit, Z., (Ed.), *Reflex Mechanisms in the Genesis of Epilepsy.* Amsterdam: Elsevier, 1963, p. 28.
42. Herberg, K. P., Duffy, F. M., and Lombroso, C. T. Visual evoked potentials to colored light in normal controls and light sensitive epileptics. *Electroenceph. Clin. Neurophysiol.* 24:284, 1968.
43. Herrlin, K. Epilepsy, light-sensitivity and left-handedness in a family with monozygotic triplets. *Pediatrics* 25:385, 1960.
44. Hubel, D. H., and Wiesel, T. N. Receptive fields of single neurones in the cat's striate cortex. *J. Physiol.* (London) 148:574, 1959.
45. Hubel, D. H., and Nauta, W. J. H. Electrocorticograms of cats with chronic lesions of rostral mesencephalic tegmentum. *Fed. Proc.* 19:287, 1960.
46. Hunter, J., and Jasper, H. Effects of thalamic stimulation in unanesthetized animals. *Electroenceph. Clin. Neurophysiol.* 1:305, 1949.
47. Ingvar, D. H., and Nyman, G. E. Epilepsia arithmetices. *Neurology* (Minneap.) 12:281, 1962.
48. Jasper, H., and Courtois, G. A practical method for uniform activation with intravenous metrazol. *Electroenceph. Clin. Neurophysiol.* 5:443, 1953.
49. Keith, H., Aldrich, R., Daly, D., Bickford, R., and Kennedy, R. Study of light induced epilepsy in children. *Amer. J. Dis. Child.* 83:408, 1952.
50. Killam, K. F., Killam, E. K., and Naquet, R. An animal model of light sensitive epilepsy. *Electroenceph. Clin. Neurophysiol.* 22:497, 1967.

51. Klass, D. W. and Daly, D. A. An unusual seizure induction mechanism (manugenic). *Electroenceph. Clin. Neurophysiol.* 12:756, 1960.

52. Klass, D. W., Wakim, K. G., and Johnson, W. J. Paroxysmal electroencephalographic abnormalities experimentally induced by electrolyte alterations. *Electroenceph. Clin. Neurophysiol.* In press.

53. Kooi, K., Thomas, M., Mortenson, F. Photoconvulsive and photomyoclonic responses in adults. *Neurology* (Minneap.) 10:1051, 1960.

54. Kreindler, A. *Experimental Epilepsy. Progress in Brain Research.* Amsterdam: Elsevier, 1965, Vol. 19.

55. Lindsley, D. B., Finger, F. W., and Henry, C. Some physiological aspects of audiogenic seizures in rats. *J. Neurophysiol.* 5:185, 1942.

56. Mitchell, W., Falconer, M., and Hill, D. Epilepsy with fetishism relieved by temporal lobectomy. *Lancet* 2:626, 1954.

57. Naquet, R., Balzano, E., and Poncet, M. The light sensitive epilepsy of *Papio papio*. Topographic study of corticosubcortical EEG paroxysmal activity. *Electroenceph. Clin. Neurophysiol.* 24:289, 1968.

58. Robertson, E. Photogenic epilepsy: Self-precipitated attacks. *Brain* 77:232, 1954.

59. Rodin, E., Daly, D., and Bickford, R. Effects of photic stimulation during sleep. *Neurology* (Minneap.) 5:149, 1955.

60. Scott, D. F., Groethuysen, U. C., and Bickford, R. G. Lambda responses in the human electroencephalogram. *Neurology* (Minneap.) 17:770, 1967.

61. Scollo-Lavizzari, G., and Hess, R. Sensory precipitation of epileptic seizures. *Epilepsia* (Amst.) 8:157, 1967.

62. Shanzer, S., April, R., and Atkin, A. Seizures induced by eye deviation. *Arch. Neurol.* (Chicago) 13:621, 1965.

63. Sherwood, S. Self induced epilepsy (collected cases). *Arch. Neurol.* (Chicago) 6:49, 1962.

64. Smith, T. G., Jr., and Purpura, D. P. Electrophysiological studies on epileptogenic lesion of cat cortex. *Electroenceph. Clin. Neurophysiol.* 12:59, 1960.

65. Stevens, J. R. Central and peripheral factors in epileptic discharge. *Arch. Neurol.* (Chicago) 7:330, 1962.

66. Stevens, J. R., Nakamura, Y., Milstein, V., Okuma, P., and Llinas, R. Central and peripheral factors in epileptic discharge. *Arch. Neurol.* (Chicago) 11:463, 1964.

67. Symonds, C. Excitation and inhibition in epilepsy. *Brain* 82:133, 1959.

68. Vizioli, R. The Problem of Human Reflex Epilepsy. In Servit, Z., (Ed.), *Reflex Mechanisms in the Genesis of Epilepsy.* Amsterdam: Elsevier, 1963, p. 85.

69. Walter, V. J., and Walter, W. G. The central effects of rhythmic sensory stimulation. *Electroenceph. Clin. Neurophysiol.* 1:57, 1949.

70. Watson, C. W., and Denny-Brown, D. Myoclonus epilepsy as a symptom of diffuse neuronal disease. *Arch. Neurol. Psychiat.* 70:151, 1953.

71. Watson, C. W., and Denny-Brown, D. Studies of the mechanism of stimulus-sensitive myoclonus in man. *Electroenceph. Clin. Neurophysiol.* 7:341, 1955.

Discussion

PHOTOGENIC SEIZURES IN THE BABOON
ROBERT NAQUET

The review by Bickford and Klass [3] brings up problems so numerous that it is not possible to discuss it in its entirety. Only some forms of reflex epilepsy will be studied, but we are in agreement with the authors that the term *reflex* is not precise. Our discussion will be limited to *stimulus-sensitive* epilepsy since the triggering stimulus can be demonstrated. We speak of *audiogenic, audiosensitive, photogenic*, or *photosensitive* epilepsy, although in agreement with Bickford and Klass [3] that these terms are disputable; attention will be focused on the triggering stimulus. Three aspects will be discussed:

(1) Triggers in two types of reflex epilepsy (so-called audiogenic seizures in the rodent and photosensitive epilepsy in man) are apparently multisensorial, as observed by Bickford and Klass [3] in some forms of evoked seizures in man, particularly in reading epilepsy. Also described were microreflexes in the normal subject and their role in reflex epilepsy. The role of multisensory triggers will be analyzed further.

(2) Recent data will be given on photosensitive epilepsy of the baboon, *Papio papio*, that is also probably multisensorial. These findings may partly explain why intermittent light stimulation (ILS) can induce widespread EEG manifestations in man.

(3) Evoked potentials in the baboon were studied with computers and a temporospatial map technique. Afterdischarge followed the evoked potential, and we suggest its relationship to epilepsy, as do Bickford and Klass [3]. In normal man, however, this afterdischarge is mainly occipitoparietal whereas in the epileptic baboon it is maximal in the frontal region.

Multisensory Triggers of Seizures

Previous authors were reluctant to compare experimental reflex epilepsy in animals with reflex epilepsy in man. Experimental reflex epilepsy of Amantea [2] and Clementi [7] was focal whereas in man the most common variety of reflex epilepsy (the photosensitive) was considered *centrencephalic* epilepsy [50].

Reflex epilepsies in animals are not always clearly focal, as exemplified by audiogenic seizures of the mouse, white rat [5, 26, 45, 47, 48], and probably rabbit [18]. The Czechoslovakian school emphasized three requisite factors: stimulus, focus, and global susceptibility [46]. In more recent work [36, 37] cochlear lesions were described in those animals which were most audiosensitive, perhaps causing hyperexcitability of auditory pathways. Aside from an excess of afferents (with or without cochlear lesion), there may be abnormal sensitivity of the specific auditory cortex (or another part of the cortex) caused by lesion or disturbed function. Global lowering of the convulsant threshold varies from one animal to another.

Aside from auditory stimuli, experimental conditions may alter the attack: immobilization with curare or with simple restraint lowers the percentage of seizures; unilateral section of the vibrissae changes direction of the animal's running, which leads to seizure [40]. This suggests that triggering stimuli are not only auditory but may be associated with behavioral changes or with a new type of stimulation from the vibrissae or the proprioceptors, or both, as the animal runs. Thus it may be not only an audiosensitive seizure but a more complex reflex epilepsy in which other factors, mainly sensory, act in a feedback system.

Audiogenic epilepsy does not exist in man, and these experimental data can be used only with reservations in human epilepsy. Some forms of reflex epilepsy do, however, exist in man, the commonest being photosensitive epilepsy [4, 51].

Appropriate photic stimulation, in certain subjects, may cause paroxysmal spike-wave discharges which are predominantly rolandic and may be followed by an attack generalized from the start. These events have usually been considered of centrencephalic origin [15, 16, 38]. Photic stimulation can also cause ictal discharges confined to the occipital region. These may remain localized or spread forward, following the pattern for propagation of occipital seizures, in which case they are accompanied by motor symptoms [1]. In such cases, a focal reflex mechanism may be invoked [9, 16, 33].

Photic stimulation can trigger paroxysmal events, some of which are considered focal and others centrencephalic. However, it was pointed out [33] that in certain subjects one or another type of seizure might be triggered depending on circumstances: stimulation might provoke seizure beginning in the occipital cortex and spreading, or remaining localized, or a grand mal attack preceded by generalized spikes and waves. The latter type of seizure occurs when spikes and waves are accompanied by violent myoclonic jerks, which suggests that the starting point of the seizure (although reflex) might be rolandic and not occipital, due to afferents associated with each clonus. Epileptic discharges arising in the rolandic region may resemble a seizure generalized from the start, and their threshold is very low [11].

Photic stimulation can therefore trigger different types of seizure in man depending upon whether it provokes only visual afferents or visual plus somatosensory afferents. If audiosensitive epilepsy may be compared with photosensitive epilepsy, it should be noted that reflex epilepsy may be pure for one type of stimulation or more complex and multisensorial. Multiple afferents are not necessary in either audiosensitive or photosensitive epilepsy. In some animals, probably the most sensitive, one sensory modality may be sufficient and seizure may occur with the subject paralyzed or immobilized. In others, secondary somatosensory afferents are required, but triggering of these afferents occurs through different sensory pathways, according to the species.

If intrinsic factors [16] are added to the extrinsic, evaluation of the role of specific afferents in triggering reflex epilepsy becomes even more complex. Our understanding of mechanisms of human photosensitive epilepsy remains limited because (1) these subjects do not justify surgical treatment and are rarely investigated stereotaxically, and (2) convulsive drugs such as pentylenetetrazol [12, 14, 25, 35] are required to reproduce this condition in an animal. In this situation, conditions would be so changed that the reflex factor would lose its specificity.

Understanding of mechanisms of photosensitive epilepsy were at this stage at the time of laboratory studies made with Killam et al. [19] on reflex epilepsy in a Senegal baboon, the *Papio papio*. The results with this new *animal model* [22] are summarized here.

REFLEX EPILEPSY IN THE *Papio papio*

Photosensitivity is common in all *Papio papio*, but its frequency depends on the region of Senegal from which the animals come. We showed that 60 percent of the animals living in Casamance are photosensitive [23] irrespective of age, sex, and living conditions. In a region 800 km from Casamance, photosensitive animals are only 10 to 20 percent [42], which is similar to other races and species of primates (*Erythrocebus patas, Cercopithecus sabaeus* [23, 24, 41, 49], but a great deal higher than in normal man [3, 17] and the chimpanzee [34].

Photosensitivity is manifested by clinical and electrographic signs during ILS at frequencies close to 25 cycles per second [10, 22, 32, 39].

CLINICAL SIGNS DURING ILS. These may be of several types.

(1) At first, clonus of the eyelids appears as bilateral, rhythmic, rapid, small-amplitude jerks. Movements may stop abruptly as ILS is continued or they may gradually increase in amplitude and become part of a more widespread response which affects successively muscles of the face, the back of the

neck, and then the whole body. Polygraphic studies show that eye clonus generally precedes those of the face, nape, and neck musculature by a fraction of a second up to several seconds.

(2) Violent jerks of the whole body occur with contraction of facial muscles, sudden flexion of head onto chest, extension of both upper limbs, and flexion of both lower limbs. These jerks, either single or in series, are often preceded by clonic contractions of eyelids and face.

(3) Onset is with clonic jerks of eyelids followed by spasm of face which spreads to the neck and is interrupted suddenly by a clonic jerk. Tonic contraction then occurs again, the animal's jaw is open slightly, and fairly fast clonic jerks interrupt this tonic contraction. The tonic spasm may spread to the whole body and be followed by generalized clonic contractions. The animal cries out during some of them and is often incontinent of urine. Polygraphic studies showed that tonic contraction of nape musculature was always later than the first clonus of eyes and preceded contraction of shoulder and trunk musculature.

SELF-SUSTAINED CLINICAL SIGNS CONTINUING AFTER THE END OF ILS. These also may be of several types:

(1) After photic stimulation, a few clonic jerks of eyelids and face and sometimes even the body may persist for several seconds, gradually decreasing.

(2) Fairly violent clonic manifestations may occur for many seconds. Violent clonic jerks are usually generalized, bilateral, and synchronous, followed by a *confusional state* lasting several seconds.

(3) After the final generalized clonic jerk provoked by the last flash, the animal cries out and goes into a tonicoclonic seizure: during the tonic phase, eyes are open, pupils dilated; a rictus exposes the teeth, jaws are clenched or half open, head extended; arms are adducted against the thorax, forearms flexed on upper arms, wrists flexed on forearms; thighs are flexed on the pelvis, legs flexed, feet in dorsiflexion and toes plantar-flexed. The clonic phase starts with small range movements which affect first the muscles of the face, then the entire musculature, while a certain tonic component persists. Clonic jerks increase gradually, causing eye closure, opening or increased opening of jaws upward and forward, extension of upper limbs, and flexion of lower limbs. Frequency and range of the jerk then decreases. Saliva runs from angle of the mouth, and then suddenly all motor signs stop and the animal enters a postictal *confusional phase*.

ELECTROGRAPHIC SIGNS OCCURRING DURING ILS. Electrographic activity was recorded from the external surface of the hemispheres and from 186 points in the cortex and deep structures.

(1) On the surface of the hemispheres: occipital driving is soon followed by paroxysmal discharges on frontal and precentral regions, corresponding to Brodmann's areas 6 and 8 and particularly to the frontal oculomotor fields (Fig. D20-1). These may be of large amplitude from onset or increase gradually (Fig. D20-2). They consist of polyspikes at a frequency close to that of the ILS, or independent of it, or of polyspikes and waves at approximately 3 per sec. In all cases the discharges seem bilateral, synchronous, and symmetrical. Their synchrony, however, is only relative as was

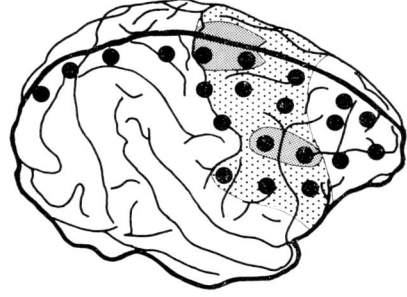

FIG. D20-1. Diagram of the spikes and waves repartition induced by ILS in a photosensitive *Papio papio* (P.P. 269). Large black dots correspond to real emplacement of electrodes in relation with explored convolutions in this chronic preparation. Dotted zones correspond to regions where spike discharges have been pointed out. Darkest zones correspond to regions where the spike discharges had their highest amplitudes.

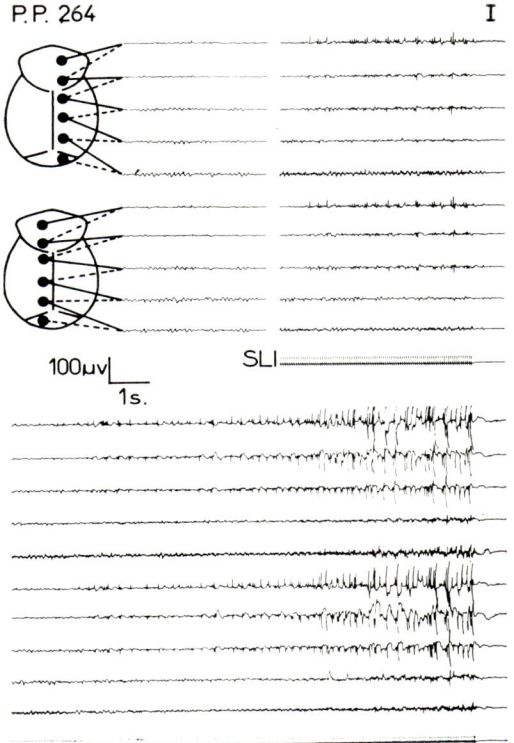

FIG. D20-2. Paroxysmal discharges induced by ILS in highly photosensitive *Papio papio* (P.P. 264). Above left: spontaneous pattern. Above right: under ILS at 25 per sec, manifestation of first paroxysmal discharges at low amplitude in frontal regions. Below: progressive increase of amplitude of paroxysmal discharges which ceases when ILS stops.

shown by Menini et al. [29] and Morrell et al. [31]. For a fairly long period, sometimes even throughout recording, paroxysmal activity remains localized while in the parieto-occipital cortex normal driving continues. Sometimes the discharges spread to the entire cortex. The occipital driving becomes interspersed and then replaced by polyspike and wave activity (at this stage, the paroxysmal activity consists more of polyspikes and waves than of polyspikes). These discharges may stop either spontaneously or with the ILS, but they may continue as self-sustained events.

(2) Frontal cortex and underlying white matter: paroxysmal activity during ILS from superficial part of frontal subcortex and cortex of medial surface of frontal lobe is similar to that from superficial frontal cortex. However, that recorded from medial frontal cortex occurs somewhat later.

(3) The deep structures: three types of activity were recorded during ILS and may occur in the same animal at different times. The more photosensitive the animals, the more complex are the types of activity.

Activity may continue unchanged during cortical spikes and waves. This occurs in the least photosensitive or in photosensitive animals with only small-amplitude frontal discharges not accompanied by myoclonus, and in the optic pathways. Here regular driving continues unchanged, and there are rarely spike and wave discharges, even when these are seen in other subcortical structures.

Paroxysmal discharges invade the deep structures when they increase on the cortex and when generalized myoclonus appears. Amount of invasion varies in the same animal from moment to moment and from one structure to another. Paroxysmal activity simultaneous with cortical discharges is much more common in the thalamus, internal capsule, pons, reticular formation, and certain hypothalamic structures than in the rhinencephalon.

The deep structures show characteristic changes. The following events may occur repetitively, especially in the most sensitive animals: spike and wave and polyspike and wave discharges are at first limited strictly to the frontal cortex. Suddenly frontal polyspikes and waves increase in amplitude. Certain deep structures are invaded by discharges similar to those on the cortex and by the slow wave component more than the polyspikes. Other structures (even the rhinencephalon) are invaded by rhythmic activity at a frequency near or identical to that of the photic stimulation. It appears as though two types of competing activity were simultaneous in the subcortical structures: driving at 25 per sec and spike and wave discharges related to those on the frontal cortex. Significance and mechanism of this global invasion of the brain by two types of rhythmic activity are complex and require further experimentation.

ELECTROGRAPHIC SIGNS OCCURRING AFTER ILS. In most cases, electrographic signs stop with the ILS, and the record returns to its prestimulation state. Sometimes, however, self-sustained electrographic activity occurs.

(1) When ILS ends, slow spikes or polyspikes and waves occur strictly frontal or in the frontocentral cortex and certain deep structures. These self-sustained activities differ in morphology from those recorded during ILS, probably because light afferents have stopped. This afterdischarge lasts 3–6 sec, stops abruptly, and there is no postictal flattening.

(2) Polyspike and wave discharges remain generalized in all recorded structures for many seconds, followed by generalized electrical silence.

(3) Photic stimulation is followed by electrical phenomena of a new type suggesting an ictal discharge (Fig. D20-3). This starts in the anterior and posterior frontal cortex and superficial part of the subcortex usually as fast, low-amplitude rhythmic activity followed by slow spike or high-amplitude rhythmic slow waves, gradually slowing. A few seconds later, activity of the deep structures becomes paroxysmal; evolution in various structures indicates that this is not direct invasion. Each structure seems to react characteristically to the propagation; the rhinencephalon is not usually involved. The parieto-occipital cortex is reached only secondarily, and ictal activity here is also characteristic at first.

During the following seconds, ictal discharge invades most of the cortex and subcortex except the rhinencephalon. At this stage, amplitude, frequency, and morphology of the rhythms vary greatly between structures. This is not a generalized bilateral, synchronous, and symmetrical discharge. Polyspikes and waves predominate in the cortex while slow, rhythmic waves predominate in the thalamus.

In the following seconds and minutes, the clonic phase occurs. Paroxysmal activity is progressively more rhythmic and of higher amplitude. Discharges in the cortex are rhythmic at 1–2 per sec, then 1 per sec, and finally 1 every 2 sec. These discharges are bilaterally generalized in the cortex

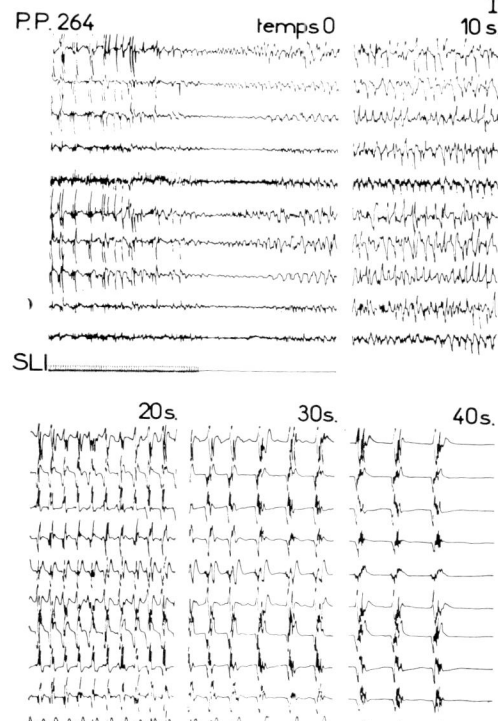

FIG. D20-3. Temporospatial evolution of self-sustained critical discharge in the same *Papio papio* (P.P. 264). A new ILS induces paroxysmal discharges in frontal regions even more ample than before. With cessation of ILS (*Temps 0* = time 0), critical discharge occurs in the two frontal regions, followed secondarily by seizure with different frequency depending on the territory. Seizure starts first in frontal region and propagates itself slowly in posterior region. Temporal evolution (here s. = seconds) of this critical discharge 10 sec, 20 sec, 30 sec, and 40 sec later. During this seizure, the animal has presented (from the clinical point of view) a tonicoclonic seizure.

(with synchrony between anterior and posterior regions) and also synchronous with most of the deep discharges, excluding the rhinencephalon. Morphologically, however, they are dissimilar: at the cortex, they are polyspikes and waves whereas in the deep structures, they are more likely spike-wave complexes. Spontaneous activity of the rhinencephalon is always changed at this time with either increase in amplitude or a few high voltage polyspike and wave discharges, or an ictal discharge develops independently in frequency and duration of the other discharge.

The final burst of polyspike and wave is followed by electrical silence in the neocortex and deep structures; silence may not develop in the rhinencephalon, or, if it does, it is shorter than elsewhere.

VARIATIONS IN ELECTRICAL SIGN. With curare, frontal paroxysmal discharges provoked by ILS are much diminished in the more photosensitive animals and disappear in the others. Rarely do self-sustained paroxysmal discharges occur after ILS; if they do, it is when curarization is becoming light. Other factors may affect intensity of the paroxysmal discharges. We have shown recently that paroxysmal discharges vary in frequency and extent with light intensity and are increased when the stroboscope is near the retinal field; mydriasis from homatropine facilitates them whereas miosis from pilocarpine reduces them [44]. Similar findings have been obtained with the *Galago senegalensis* [43].

EVOKED POTENTIALS IN THE *Papio papio*

This electroclinical study of paroxysms provoked by photic stimulation reveals two important facts: (1) Paroxysmal epileptic discharges caused by ILS always arise frontally, and visual and subcortical structures are only secondarily invaded. (2) When myoclonus, caused by ILS, is allowed to develop, paroxysmal discharges are favored; photosensitivity in *Papio papio* therefore may not be purely photosensitive reflex epilepsy but a more complex photosensitive and somatosensory association, the visual stimulus nevertheless being the major one.

We therefore studied responses evoked by different types of stimuli and compared visual responses from the most and the least photosensitive animals [8, 20, 21, 22, 27, 28, 30]. The evoked potential from the occipital cortex is remarkably similar to that of man [6, 13]. It shows several component waves: a low-amplitude positive wave at 25 msec, a very stable, high-amplitude negative wave at 40 msec followed by a series of later waves (III, IV, and V) lasting up to 150 msec. This response is sometimes followed by afterdischarge in the same territory, analogous to that seen in man [6]. It varies little from one animal to another, whether or not photosensitive.

When the excitability cycle of the occipital cortex is studied with flashes coupled at varied intervals, a refractory period of about 20 msec is noted after the first stimulus, followed by a facilitation phase from 120 to 200 percent; facilitation occurs from 40 to 200 msec after the stimulus.

With averaging, evoked responses can be obtained over most of the cortex, but these responses are smaller and far less stable. An important finding is late oscillation in the frontal region in the most photosensitive animals, and particularly in those self-sustained ictal discharges after ILS.

Studying the excitability cycle of the frontal cortex we note 500 to 700 percent facilitation, particularly for later components and for stimuli separated by 40–50 msec. Facilitation is maximal in the more photosensitive animals; it does not exceed 300 percent with mild or no photosensitivity. This facilitation phase appears as hypersynchronous, rhythmic oscillation of great amplitude, which may outlast stimulation by 700–800 msec.

We observed auditory and somatesthetic evoked responses on frontal cortex always as late responses.

A stable auditory evoked response can be averaged from the frontal cortex with a negative wave barely visible at 15 msec, followed by a positive wave at 35 msec, and finally a very large negative wave at 100 msec. Focus of this activity persists for about 500 msec.

The earliest evoked somatesthetic responses are in the postrolandic region contralateral to the stimulation. From 38 msec onward, however, a series of very high-amplitude oscillations appear in the frontal cortex and may last more than 500 msec. All components of this late response are also found with ipsilateral stimulation.

From these data, we propose that a convergence of afferents exists in frontal regions of the photosensitive *Papio papio*, involved in development of an attack. We emphasize the response evoked by coupled flashes 40 msec apart (corresponding to a frequency of 25 per sec) in areas 6 and 8 in the most photosensitive animals. However, more work is required to explain the mechanism that facilitates somatesthetic and light afferents in this region. Does their combination involve an excess of afferents locally, or is reactivity to normal afferents pathological in this territory? It is too early to say.

REFERENCES

1. Ajmone-Marsan, C., and Ralston, B. *The Epileptic Seizure. Its Functional Morphology and Diagnostic Significance. A Clinical Electrographic Analysis of Metrazol Induced Attacks.* Springfield, Ill.: Thomas, 1957, p. 251.
2. Amantea, G. Rapporto tra eccitamenti afferenti ed epilessia sperimentale. *Boll. Accad. Med. Roma* 46, 1920.
3. Bickford, R. G., and Klass, D. W. Sensory Precipitation and Reflex Mechanisms. In Jasper, H. H., Ward, A. A., Jr., and Pope, A. (Eds.), *Basic Mechanisms of the Epilepsies.* Boston: Little, Brown, 1969.
4. Bickford, R. G., Sem-Jacobsen, C. W., White, P. T., and Daly, D. Some observations on the mechanism of photic and photometrazol activation. *Electroenceph. Clin. Neurophysiol.* 4:275, 1952.
5. Busnel, R. G. *Psychophysiologie, neuropharmacologie et biochimie de la crise audiogène.* Paris: C.N.R.S. 1963, p. 531.
6. Ciganek, L. Potentiels corticaux chez l'Homme, évoqués par des stimuli photiques. *Rev. Neurol.* (Paris) 99:194, 1958.
7. Clementi, A. Striccnizzazione della sfera corticale visiva ed epilessia sperimentale da stimoli luminosi. *Arch. Fisiol.* 27:356, 1929.
8. Dimov, S., and Menini, C. Réponses corticales évoquées par la stimulation lumineuse chez le babouin. II. Étude de la réactivité corticale à l'aide de potentiels évoqués induits par des stimulations lumineuses multiples. To be published, 1969.
9. Fischer-Williams, M., Bickford, R. G., and Whisnant, J. P. Occipito-parieto-temporal seizure discharges with visual hallucinations and aphasia. *Epilepsia* (Amst.) 5:279, 1964.
10. Fischer-Williams, M., Poncet, M., Riche, D., and Naquet, R. Light-induced epilepsy in the baboon *Papio papio*: cortical and depth recordings. *Electroenceph. Clin. Neurophysiol.* 25:557, 1968.
11. French, J. E., Gernandt, B. E., and Livingston, R. B. Regional differences in seizure susceptibility in monkey cortex. *A.M.A. Arch. Neurol. Psychiat.* 75:260, 1956.
12. Gastaut, H. Combined photic and Metrazol activation of the brain. *Electroenceph. Clin. Neurophysiol.* 2:263, 1950.
13. Gastaut, H., Bostem, F., Waltregny, A., Poire, R., and Regis, H. Les activités cérébrales spontanées et évoquées, chez l'Homme. *Monographies de Physiologie causale.* Paris: Gauthier-Villars, 1967, Vol. VII.
14. Gastaut, H., and Hunter, J. An experimental study of the mechanism of photic activation in idiopathic epilepsy. *Electroenceph. Clin. Neurophysiol.* 2:263, 1950.
15. Gastaut, H., and Fischer-Williams, M. The Physiopathology of Epileptic Seizures. In Field, J. (Ed.), *Handbook of Physiology,* Baltimore: Williams and Wilkins, 1959, Sec. I, Vol. 1, pp. 329–363.
16. Gastaut, H., and Tassinari, A. Triggering mechanisms in epilepsy. The electroclinical point of view. *Epilepsia* (Amst.) 7:85, 1966.
17. Gastaut, H., Trevisan, C., and Naquet, R. Diagnostic value of electroencephalographic abnormalities provoked by intermittent photic stimulation. *Electroenceph. Clin. Neurophysiol.* 10:194, 1958.
18. Horak, F. Selection of strains of rabbits sensitive to an epileptogenic sound stimulus. *Physiol. Bohemoslov.* 14:495, 1965.
19. Killam, K. F., Killam, E. K., and Naquet, R. Mise en évidence chez certains singes d'un syndrome photomyoclonique. *C. R. Acad. Sci.* (Paris) 262:1010, 1966.
20. Killam, K. F., Killam, E. K., and Naquet,

R. Étude des réponses évoquées par la stimulation lumineuse intermittente chez des singes présentant des réponses paroxystiques à ce type de stimulation. *Rev. Neurol.* (Paris) 115:422, 1966.

21. Killam, K. F., Killam, E. K., and Naquet, R. Evoked potentials studies in response to light in the baboon (*Papio papio*). *Electroenceph. Clin. Neurophysiol.* Suppl. 26, 108, 1967.

22. Killam, K. F., Killam, E. K., and Naquet, R. An animal model of light sensitive epilepsy. *Electroenceph. Clin. Neurophysiol.* 22:497, 1967.

23. Killam, K. F., Naquet, R., and Bert, J. Paroxysmal responses to intermittent light stimulation in a population of baboons (*Papio papio*). *Epilepsia* (Amst.) 7:215, 1966.

24. Killam, E. K., Stark, L. G., and Killam, K. F. Photostimulation in three species of baboons. *Life Sci.* 6:1569, 1967.

25. Kreindler, A. *Experimental Epilepsy. Progress in Brain Research.* Amsterdam: Elsevier, 1965, Vol. 19.

26. Lehman, A. *Contribution à l'étude psychophysiologique et neuropharmacologique de l'épilepsie acoustique de la souris et du rat.* Thèse de Sciences, Paris, 1964.

27. Menini, C., Cacciuttolo, G., and Naquet, R. Étude morphologique et topographique des potentiels évoqués visuels d'un Cercopithecinae: le *Papio papio*. *Rev. Neurol.* 118:474, 1968.

28. Menini, C., and Dimov, S. Réponses corticales évoquées par la stimulation lumineuse chez le babouin. I. Étude des potentiels évoqués par des stimulations uniques. To be published, 1969.

29. Menini, C., Morrell, F., and Naquet, R. Enregistrements corticaux au moyen de microélectrodes chez le *Papio papio* photosensible. *J. Physiol.* (Paris) Suppl. 2, 60:698, 1968.

30. Menini, C., Vuillon-Cacciuttolo, G., and Lesèvre, N. Chronologie et topographie des réponses corticales évoquées par différents types de stimulations chez le *Papio papio*. *J. Physiol.* (Paris) Suppl. 1, 60:277, 1968.

31. Morrell, F., Naquet, R., and Menini, C. Microphysiology of cortical single neurons in *Papio papio*. Unpublished data, 1968.

32. Naquet, R., Balzano, E., and Poncet, M. The light sensitive epilepsy in *Papio papio*. Topographic study of cortico-subcortical EEG paroxysmal activity. *Electroenceph. Clin. Neurophysiol.* 24:289, 1968.

33. Naquet, R., Fegersten, L., and Bert, J. Seizure discharges localized to the posterior cerebral region in man, provoked by intermittent photic stimulation. *Electroenceph. Clin. Neurophysiol.* 12:305, 1960.

34. Naquet, R., Killam, K. F., and Rhodes, J. M. Flicker stimulation with chimpanzees. *Life Sci.* 6:1575, 1967.

35. Naquet, R., and Lanoir, J. Détermination de l'activité anti-épileptique expérimentale. Tests spéciaux. *The International Encyclopedia of Pharmacology and Therapeutics.* Oxford: Pergamon, to be published, 1969.

36. Niaussat, M. Caractère génétique de la dissociation entre le potentiel microphonique cochléaire et le potentiel d'action du nerf auditif de la souris audiogène. *C. R. Soc. Biol.* (Paris) 162:21, 1968.

37. Niaussat, M., and Legouix, J. P. Anomalies des réponses microphoniques cochléaires dans une lignée de souris présentant des crises convulsives au son. *C. R. Acad. Sci.* (Paris) 264:103, 1967.

38. Penfield, W., and Jasper, H. *Epilepsy and the Functional Anatomy of the Human Brain.* Boston: Little, Brown, 1954, p. 886.

39. Poncet, M. *L'épilepsie photosensible du singe Papio papio. Étude clinique et électrographique (structures corticales et profondes).* Thèse de Médecine, Marseille, 1968, p. 140.

40. Requin, J., and Paillard, J. Effects of Removing Vibrissae on Audiogenic Epilepsy in Mice. In Servit, Z. (Ed.), *Comparative and Cellular Pathophysiology of Epilepsy.* Proceedings of a Symposium held in Liblice near Prague. Prague: Czechoslovak Academy of Sciences and Excerpta Medica, 1966.

41. Rhodes, J. M. Personal communication.

42. Serbanescu, T., Bert, J., Guillon, R., and Naquet, R. Étude de la photosensibilité du *Papio papio* du Sénégal oriental. *J. Physiol.* (Paris) 60:399, 1968.

43. Serbanescu, T., Godet, R., Orsini, J. C., and Naquet, R. La stimulation lumineuse intermittente chez le *Galago sénégalensis*. *J. Physiol.* (Paris) 60:391, 1968.

44. Serbanescu, T., and Naquet, R. L'importance du degré d'illumination réti-

nienne dans le déclenchement des paroxysmes induits par la S.L.I. chez le *Papio papio* photosensible. To be published, 1969.

45. Servit, Z. Audiogenic epilepsy in rats as a model of reflex mechanisms in the pathogenesis of epileptic seizure. (An experimental approach to analysis of reflex arch topography). *J. Exp. Med. Sci.* (India) 3:37, 1959.

46. Servit, Z. The application of the reflex theory in the interpretation of the clinical picture, genesis and treatment of epilepsy. *Epilepsia* (Amst.) 3:209, 1962.

47. Servit, Z. Les mécanismes réflexes dans la pathologie des crises audiogènes. In *Psychophysiologie, neuropharmacologie et biochimie de la crise audiogène.* Paris: C.N.R.S., 1963.

48. Servit, Z. In Servit, Z., (Ed.), *Comparative and Cellular Pathophysiology of Epilepsy.* Proceedings of a Symposium held in Liblice near Prague. Prague: Czechoslovak Academy of Sciences and Excerpta Medica, 1966.

49. Stark, L. G., Joy, R. M., Hance, A. J., and Killam, K. F. Further studies of photic stimulation in subhuman primates. Unpublished data, 1968.

50. Vizioli, R. The problem of human reflex epilepsy and the possible role of masked epileptogenic factors. *Epilepsia* (Amst.) 3:293, 1962.

51. Walter, W. G., Walter, V. J., Gastaut, H., and Gastaut, Y. Une forme électroencéphalographique de l'épilepsie, l'épilepsie photogénique. *Rev. Neurol.* (Paris) 80: 613, 1948.

21
Synaptic Inhibition in Seizures*

W. ALDEN SPENCER AND ERIC R. KANDEL

THE ROLE of inhibition in the transformation of neural activity is being increasingly recognized in studies of the central nervous system. As long as studies of central synaptic action in the mammalian nervous system were limited to the spinal cord, neurons mediating inhibition were often thought to serve primarily as biochemical commutators designed to produce an inversion of the sign of postsynaptic response in a particular branch of an excitatory pathway [22, 24]. With the discovery that unusually large inhibitory potentials dominate the synaptic organization of more central regions of the brain [5, 6, 25, 34, 39, 47] and that neurons mediating inhibition can themselves be inhibited [25, 66], an increasingly important integrative role has been assigned to synaptic inhibition.

At least three roles can be demonstrated for inhibitory actions: *Surround inhibition* around a zone of excitation can serve to sharpen and limit excitatory actions; *reciprocal inhibition* can serve to suppress an antagonistic response; *feed-forward and recurrent inhibition* can serve to synchronize neurons. These actions can also generate patterns of neural activity (the sculpturing role of inhibition [25]) by superimposition of inhibition on an ongoing spontaneous firing pattern. The several inhibitory functions are not exclusive, and in any given neural transformation, several may coexist.

Given this rich repertoire of normal inhibitory functions, what role, if any, does inhibition serve in abnormal seizure activity? For example, does the normal functional effectiveness of inhibition explain why seizures usually do not occur, and can changes in the effectiveness of inhibitory actions lead to a seizure?

We shall examine these questions here by considering first several types of inhibition found in the nervous system and their integrative functions. To do this we shall draw largely on data obtained from studies of the mammalian cortex, but we shall also consider some examples from other preparations which have proven useful for studying the integrative function of inhibition. We will next review studies of seizure afterdischarge following tetanic stimulation of cortical pathways and interictal spikes and propagated discharges produced by epileptogenic agents such as penicillin and strychnine. Each of these techniques is useful for analyzing the various aspects of the seizure process and the results obtained with these two independent methods are consistent and complementary. Moreover, seizure has been studied in both archicortex and neocortex, and results from studies of both types of cortex are in substantial agreement. Consequently it is now possible to outline the basic features of alterations in cellular functions which occur during the seizure process, to specify the role of inhibition in seizure, and to formulate a number of specific hypotheses about the development, spread, and limitation of seizure in a population of neurons.

In four sections of this paper we will consider (1) mechanisms for generating in-

---

* Original research by the authors and their collaborators reported in this chapter supported by PHS Research Grant NB05980 from National Institute of Neurological Diseases and Stroke.

hibitory postsynaptic potentials, (2) integrative actions of inhibition and disinhibition, (3) occurrence and function of inhibition during seizure, and (4) the role of inhibition in the initiation and limitation of seizure activity.

Ionic Mechanisms of Inhibitory Postsynaptic Potentials

Inhibition can be mediated chemically or electrically [23, 28]. Only chemical inhibition will be considered since electrical inhibition appears to be rare and has not yet been encountered in mammals. Chemical inhibitory actions can be of two types: conductance IPSPs and electrogenic pump IPSPs.

CONDUCTANCE IPSPs. This is the common mode of chemical inhibition [22, 23]. The interaction between a chemical transmitter substance and a postsynaptic receptor causes an increased conductance to Cl^- or K^+ ions or both (Fig. 21-1A). These ions then move down their concentration gradients without requiring metabolic energy [5, 22, 23, 34]; this type of IPSP is a common feature of the organization of mammalian cortex [39, 47, 59, 61, 62]. The main features of the conductance IPSPs of cortical neurons are their large size and duration, and their effectiveness (Fig. 21-1B). This can best be illustrated by comparing the IPSP generated in pyramidal cells of the hippocampal archicortex by recurrent collateral pathways to the *direct* disynaptic IPSP generated in motoneurons by group 1a afferent fibers from antagonistic muscles (Fig. 21-1C).

ELECTROGENIC PUMP IPSP. This is a recently discovered and less common mode of chemical inhibition. It differs from the conductance IPSP by being directly dependent upon metabolism and not involving an increased conductance to ions (Fig. 21-2B, 2C; see also [45, 48]). This type of IPSP resembles the prolonged hyperpolarizing afterpotentials, due to activation of an electrogenic Na^+ pump, which follows the intense firing of certain neurons (Fig. 21-2$A1$, $A2$ and [15, 43, and 44]). In certain cells the chemical transmitter can also activate an electrogenic Na^+ pump which produces a flow of Na^+ against a concentration gradient from the inside of the cell to the outside, thereby generating a hyperpolarizing potential change. The active transport process involved in generating this IPSP (Fig. 21-2$B2$) appears to be a Na^+-K^+ activated ATPase identical to that which maintains the normal Na^+ and K^+ distribution across nerve cell membranes [58].

Electrogenic IPSPs have been encountered in the frog sympathetic ganglion [45] and in the *Aplysia* abdominal ganglion [48]. There is also some evidence that a similar, nonconductance IPSP may occur in the mammalian sympathetic ganglion [35]. The characteristic feature of the few electrogenic IPSPs that have so far been examined is their long duration (tens of seconds), compared to that of the conductance IPSP (Fig. 21-2$B1$), and their direct dependence on oxidative metabolism (Fig. 21-2$B2$).

The two types of chemical mechanisms for generating inhibitory synaptic potentials can be compared by means of a schematic diagram (Fig. 21-2C). The conductance IPSP mechanism can be depicted as a switch bringing a battery of about -65 mV and its low series resistance in parallel with the resting membrane. The electrogenic IPSP can be depicted as a switch bringing a constant current generator with its high internal impedance in parallel with the resting membrane potential.

The two types of synaptic channels for inhibition have very different properties. The synaptic current flowing in the conductance channel can be activated only by the appropriate chemical transmitter acting on the external surface of the membrane, not by voltage or ionic changes within the postsynaptic cell. By contrast, the pump channel triggered by the transmitter appears identical to that which contributes to the resting potential. This pump channel can be activated in two quite different ways: on the external surface of the membrane by the transmitter released by the presynaptic neuron and on the internal surface by an increase in intracellular Na^+

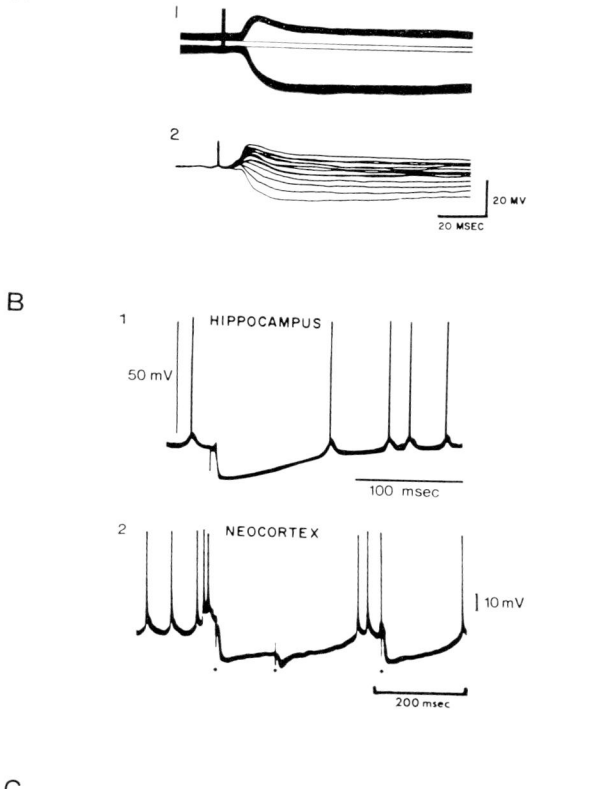

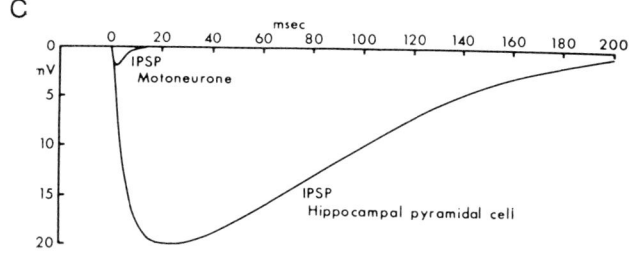

FIG. 21-1. Properties of conductance IPSPs in hippocampus and neocortex. (*A*) Inversion of hyperpolarizing to depolarizing IPSP in hippocampal pyramidal cell as a result of the diffusion of Cl^-. (1) The initial IPSP before inversion (lower trace) and the final PSP after inversion (upper trace). (2) Sequence of inversion with superimposed fine line tracings. (From Kandel, Spencer, and Brinley [34].)

(*B*) Comparison of prolonged IPSP in hippocampal (1) and neocortical (2) neurons. (1) Stimulus to fornix. (From Spencer and Kandel [59].) (2) Stimuli to unspecific thalamus (center median). The dots signal the stimulations. (From Lux and Klee [39].)

(*C*) Schematic comparisons of IPSPs in motoneuron and hippocampal pyramidal cell. Same voltage and time coordinates are used to illustrate an IPSP on a motoneuron following a single inhibitory volley in Group Ia afferent fibers and an IPSP in a hippocampal pyramidal cell in response to fornix stimulation. (From Hamlyn [31].)

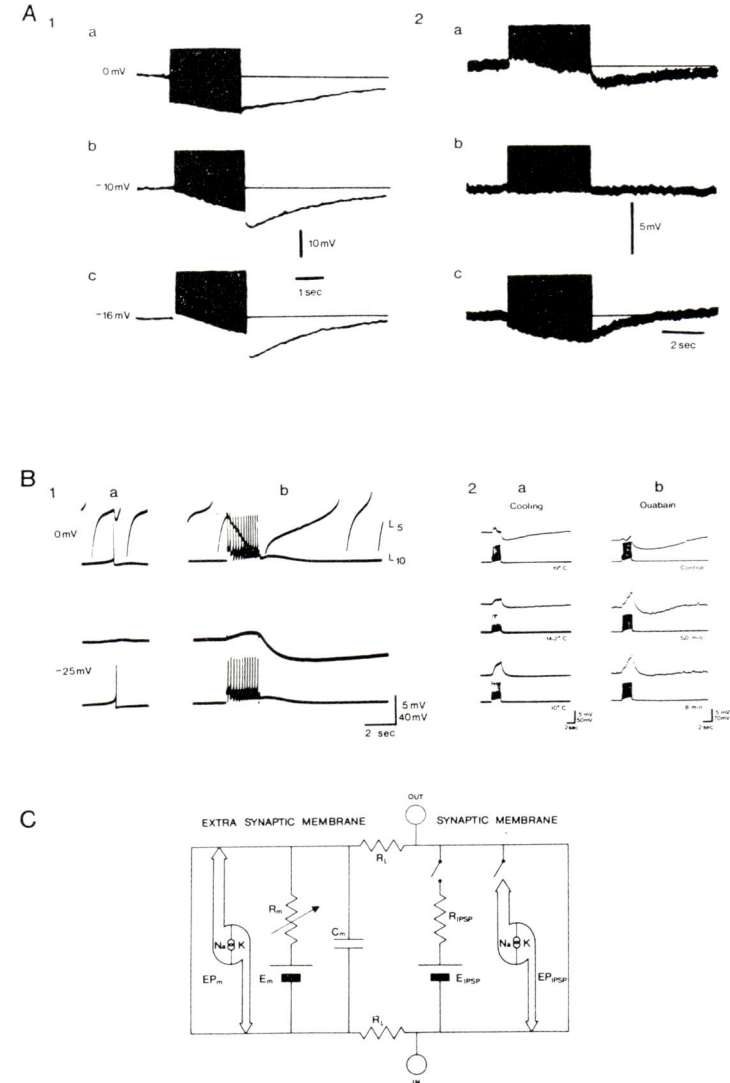

Fig. 21-2. Spike and synaptic activation of an electrogenic Na+ pump. (A) Spike activation of an electrogenic Na+ pump. (1) Effects of hyperpolarization on the afterpotentials in crayfish stretch-receptor neuron. Changes in membrane potential are indicated in left-hand column as millivolts of hyperpolarization, starting from 0 mV at the resting level of membrane potential. When the membrane is hyperpolarized, the brief hyperpolarizing afterpotential, due to an increased K+ conductance, is reversed. The posttetanic hyperpolarization, however, is not reversed but actually becomes larger. (2) Effect of 2,4 dinitrophenol, which blocks active transport, on the posttetanic hyperpolarization: (a) control in normal solution; (b) after application of DNP; (c) after return to normal solution. (Modified from Nakajima and Takahashi [43].)

(B) Synaptic activation of an electrogenic Na+ pump. (1) The effects of changing membrane potential on conductance and pump IPSPs in *Aplysia*. Interneuron mediating inhibition (bottom trace) and follower cell (top trace). (a) Single spike in the interneuron produced only an elementary (early) IPSP in the follower cell. This IPSP was nullified at an equilibrium potential of about −20 mV of hyperpolarization. (b) When the interneuron was depolarized so as to discharge a train of spikes, a second synaptic component became evident. At the resting level (0 mV hyperpolar-

concentration such as that produced by a long series of action potentials in the postsynaptic cell.

INTEGRATIVE ACTIONS OF INHIBITION

Some features of the integrative actions of inhibition can be particularly well demonstrated in preparations simpler than the mammalian cortex, such as the abdominal ganglion of the marine mollusc *Aplysia*. In this ganglion an identified interneuron mediating inhibition, and its follower cells, can be impaled under direct vision with both stimulating and recording microelectrodes [32]. The follower cells can be shown to have an endogenous rhythm due to a pacemaker property intrinsic to the neuron, which persists in the complete absence of synaptic input [2, 27, 63]. The monosynaptic IPSP produced by the interneuron is large and provides the main synaptic modulating drive for the endogenous rhythm of the follower cells. In this preparation several integrative functions of inhibition, including its sculpturing role, can be examined in some detail.

SERIES INHIBITORY CONNECTIONS: INHIBITION AND DISINHIBITION. We shall first consider a direct series inhibitory connection. In studies of *Aplysia* [32], the abrupt turning-on of activity in an interneuron mediating inhibition produces a slowing, and at higher frequencies, a complete suppression of the follower cell's endogenous rhythm. After some seconds, the follower cell's rhythm accommodates slightly to the inhibition and again fires, but at a much reduced rate (Fig. 21-3A1, A2). Turning the interneuron off results in disinhibition, an apparent excitation which results in the return to full activity of the follower neuron (Fig. 21-3A3).

Inhibition and disinhibition illustrated in Fig. 21-3A result from direct stimulation of a neuron-mediating inhibition. Similar modulation is produced in this interneuron by convergent inhibitory controls. Thus, neurons mediating inhibition can themselves be innervated by other neurons mediating inhibition, thereby forming a three-stage neuron chain connected by inhibitory synapses. Addition of a third element in the series-inhibitory chain has two obvious consequences. First, a *low* frequency burst of spikes in the higher order interneuron produces an inhibition of the lower order interneuron and a disinhibition of the

---

ization), this second component manifested itself only as a slowed return of the early IPSP and a delayed firing of the endogenously active follower cell. As the membrane potential was raised beyond the equilibrium potential of the early IPSP, the second component failed to invert and was clearly evident as a late hyperpolarization. (From Pinsker and Kandel [48].) (2) Effects of metabolic inhibitors on early conductance IPSP and late pump IPSP. Experimental set-up as in (1); interneuron (bottom trace); follower cell (top trace). (*a*) Reducing the temperature from 19° to 10°C produced a progressive and selective decrease in the late IPSP. The increase in the early IPSP is an unmasking of its true size following blockade of the late IPSP. (*b*) Ouabain (2×10^{-4}M), a specific inhibitor of the Na^+-K^+ activated ATPase, selectively decreased the late IPSP when added to the bathing solution. Because a component of the resting membrane potential is due to an electrogenic Na^+ pump, ouabain produced a depolarization in both the follower cell and the interneuron; only the change in follower cell was compensated for. As a result, increase in early IPSP represents in part a more effective train in L10 as well as an unmasking of the early IPSP. (From Pinsker and Kandel [48].)

(*C*) Schematic diagram depicting membrane components responsible for the resting potential (extrasynaptic membrane) and for early and late IPSPs (synaptic membrane). Generators for the resting membrane potential are depicted as consisting of two components: a conductance channel —a battery (E_m) in series with a variable, anomalously rectifying resistor (R_m)—in parallel with an electrogenic Na^+ pump (EP_m). Generators for the two PSPs are depicted as parallel with each other and operated by two independent switches (receptors). Early IPSP is generated by usual conductance increase to Cl^-, which results from throwing a switch connecting a battery (E_{IPSP}) and its series resistance (R_{IPSP}) into a parallel arrangement with generators of the resting membrane potential. Late IPSP is generated by an electrogenic pump (EP_{IPSP}), which acts as charge generator because it transports more Na^+ out than K^+ in. (From Pinsker and Kandel [48].)

follower neuron similar to that illustrated in Fig. 21-3A. Second, a *high* frequency burst of spikes in the higher order interneuron produces a large inhibition followed by rebound excitation in the lower order element and a disinhibition followed by inhibition in the follower neuron. This transformation is illustrated schematically in Fig. 21-3C.

An apparent excitation due to disinhibi-

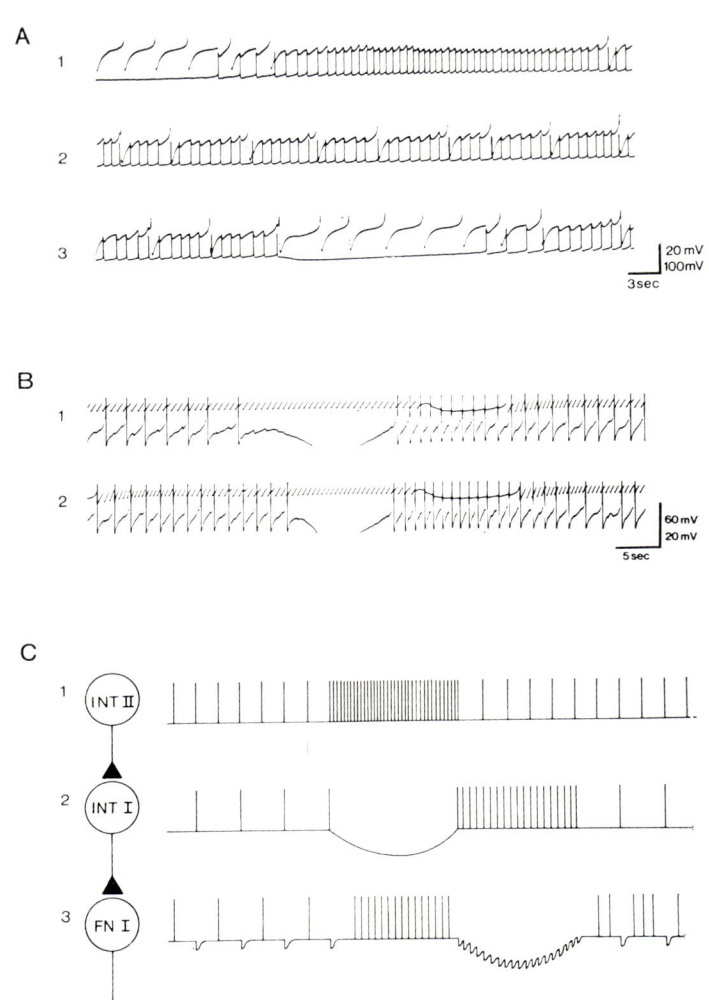

FIG. 21-3. Series inhibitory connections. (A) Modulation of regular firing rhythm of a follower neuron in *Aplysia* by a neuron mediating inhibition. The follower cell is in the upper tracing; the interneuron is in the lower tracing. (1) and (2) Onset of activity on the interneuron leads to sustained slowing of follower neuron. (3) Sudden turning off of interneuron leads to disinhibition of follower neuron and a return of its regular firing. (B) Disinhibition followed by delayed inhibitory action. Inhibition of interneuron mediating inhibition by prolonged and large IPSP is followed by rebound excitation in interneuron and disinhibition followed by delayed inhibition in follower neuron. (C) Schematic representation of the neural transformations occurring in (B) to illustrate how burst of spikes in higher order interneuron (Interneuron II) can lead to inhibition followed by rebound excitation in Interneuron I resulting in disinhibition followed by inhibition in the follower neuron (FN I). All data based upon the same interneuron and follower cells. (From Kandel et al. [32].)

tion, similar to that illustrated here, was first demonstrated in motoneurons [66]; also, it has been found in the cells of Deiter's nucleus and in the cells of other cerebellar nuclei [25]. Disinhibition may be important also in the development of certain types of seizure activity, as will be discussed subsequently.

PARALLEL INHIBITORY CONNECTIONS: SYNCHRONIZATION OF A FOLLOWER CELL POPULATION. An interneuron-mediating inhibition typically innervates many cells in parallel (Fig. 21-4A), and the inhibitory actions and subsequent rebound can serve to synchronize the firing pattern of the follower cell population. This type of inhibitory synchronization also occurs in the mammalian brain (Fig. 21-4B) and has been postulated to be responsible for the phasing of EEG waves in the hippocampus [59] and, more recently, in thalamocortical pathways as well [3, 4].

The synchronizing capabilities of a multibranched inhibitory interneuron (Fig. 21-4C) can be readily demonstrated in the abdominal ganglion of *Aplysia* [65].

MUTUALLY INHIBITORY CONNECTIONS AMONG NEURONS. It has been indicated previously that neurons mediating inhibition can make series connections. Here we consider, as a final case, the consequences of mutual inhibitory connections between two cells mediating inhibition, each of which makes parallel connections with a population of follower cells. As a result of such mutual inhibition between cells, activity can alternate between the two.

The following sequence of interactions can be demonstrated in *Aplysia* (Fig. 21-5 and [32]). A burst of spikes in one cell (Interneuron I) inhibits the other (Interneuron II). Inhibition of the second cell (Interneuron II) is followed by disinhibition and rebound excitation leading to inhibition of the first cell (Interneuron I). The inhibition of the first cell (Interneuron I) is followed by disinhibition and rebound excitation which again leads to inhibition of the second cell (Interneuron II). This mutual inhibition of the two interneurons, followed by disinhibition and rebound excitation in each, leads to an alternation of activity which can be sustained for several minutes (Fig. 21-5).

To summarize: series, parallel, and mutual inhibitory connections exist between cells in the CNS and can provide considerable flexibility in transforming neural information. In chains of endogenously active cells connected by only inhibitory connections, decrements and increments of inhibitory drive are comparable in importance and opposite in sign and provide as much flexibility in transforming neural activity as do independent excitatory and inhibitory drives. Indeed, cells that are interconnected by inhibitory synapses can maintain persistent alternation of activity in a closed two-neuron loop as a result of reciprocal phasing of inhibition and disinhibition.

Given the variety of integrative functions of different inhibitory actions, their role in seizure has been investigated in two standard types of acute experimental epilepsy. One of these is the sustained seizure which occurs as an afterdischarge following tetanic stimulation of the cortex or of pathways leading to it. The other is the spiking epileptic focus produced by the topical application of epileptogenic agents. We shall first consider seizure afterdischarge.

THE ROLE OF INHIBITION DURING SEIZURE AFTERDISCHARGE

Much of the recent progress in understanding cerebral physiology in general and seizure states in particular derives from advances in electroanatomy. As a result of these advances it is now possible to study selectively, and in some detail, several specific cortical inhibitory pathways [23, 24]. From studies of such pathways it is possible to ask the following questions: Does inhibition occur during a seizure? Does this inhibition involve an increased conductance to Cl^- or the activation of an electrogenic Na^+ pump? Does a decrease in inhibition (disinhibition) have a function in the onset of seizure? Does an increase in inhibition have a role in terminating the seizure?

The cortical inhibitory pathway which has been most thoroughly studied is the recurrent inhibitory pathway of the fornix

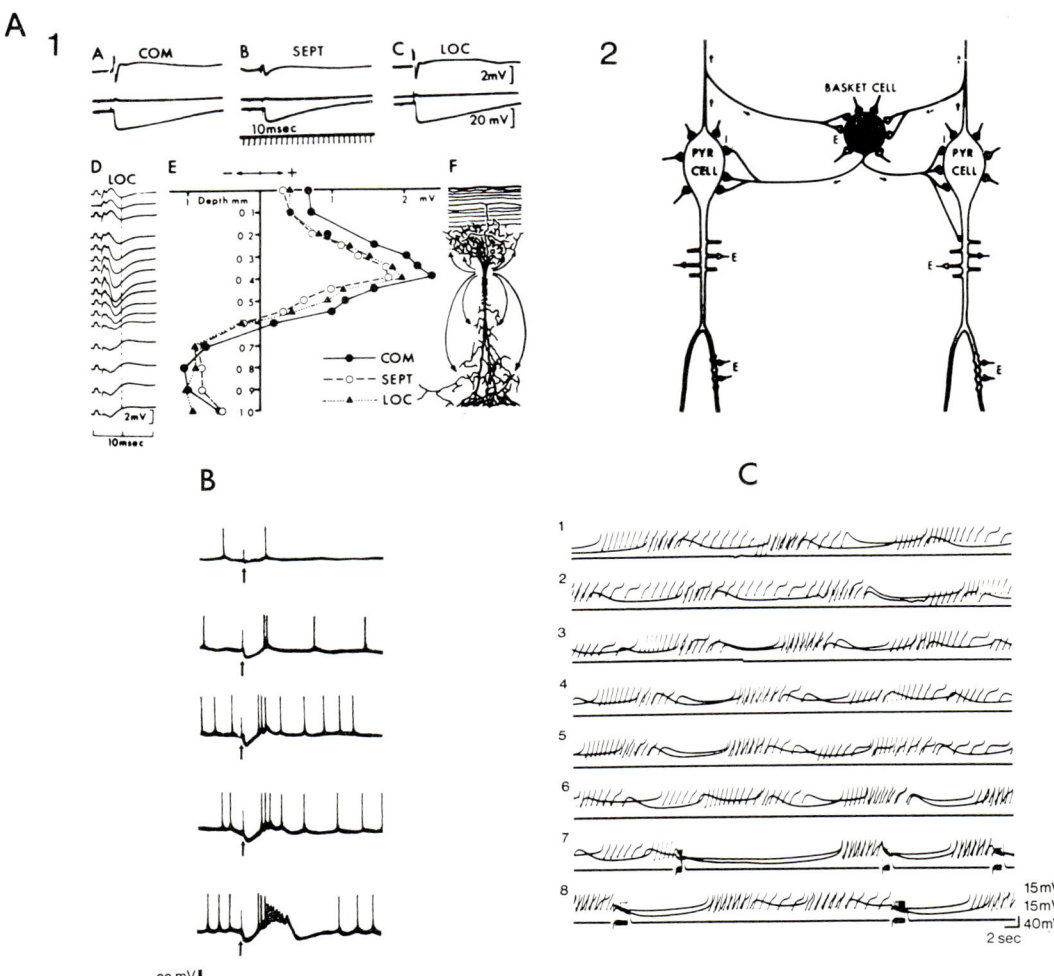

FIG. 21-4. Parallel inhibitory connections. (*A*1) Recurrent inhibitory connections in hippocampus. Intracellular and extracellular potentials generated by the recurrent inhibitory pathway in the hippocampus. (*A*1A) through (*A*1C) Surface responses, top lines; intracellular recordings, bottom line; and extracellular field potentials immediately outside cell, middle line; in response to commissural, septal, and local stimulation. (*A*1D) through (*A*1F) Extracellular records obtained at the indicated depths of the field CA3 in response to commissural septal and local stimulation. Responses (*A*1D) are shown in graphic presentation at (E) and are related to a diagram of a CA3 pyramidal cell (F). (From Andersen, Eccles, and Løyning [5].) (*A*2) Operational diagram of postulated recurrent inhibitory pathway involving basket cell with extensive terminals on pyramidal cell soma. (From Eccles [26].)

(*B*) Inhibition and rebound in a hippocampal pyramidal cell following stimulation of the deafferented fornix at progressively increasing stimulus intensities. Note progressive increase in inhibition and postinhibitory rebound as stimulus strength is increased, leading in last trace to recycling of inhibitory activity. (From Spencer and Kandel [59].)

(*C*) Synchronizing effects of interneuron mediating inhibition (bottom trace) on bursting rhythm of two different follower neurons (top two traces) in the abdominal ganglion of *Aplysia*. In (1) through (6), follower neurons are bursting spontaneously, and interneuron is silent. In (7) and (8), interneuron is activated and pulls follower cells into a synchronous beat. (From Waziri and Kandel [65].)

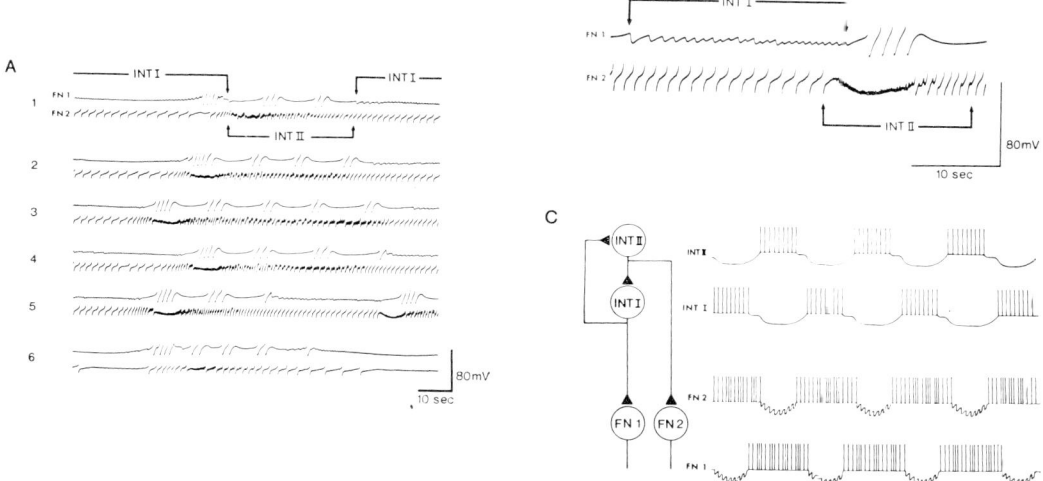

FIG. 21-5. Alternation of activity produced by two interneurons with mutually inhibitory connections. (A) Simultaneous recording, from follower neuron 1 (top trace) and follower neuron 2 (bottom trace) in the abdominal ganglion of *Aplysia*, showing alternating bursts of IPSPs. Bursts of IPSPs in FN 1 are due to a connection from Interneuron I, and bursts of IPSPs in FN 2 are attributable to a connection from Interneuron II. (1) through (5) Continuous records; (6) taken 22 min later. Alternating bursts continued without interruption for slightly more than 30 min. (B) Enlargement of segment of part (A) to show detail of alternating bursts of IPSPs. (C) Schematic representing alternating activity in closed neural chain (Interneuron I and Interneuron II connected by mutually inhibitory connections) and consequences of this alternating activity on two follower cells, FN 1 and FN 2. (From Kandel et al. [32].)

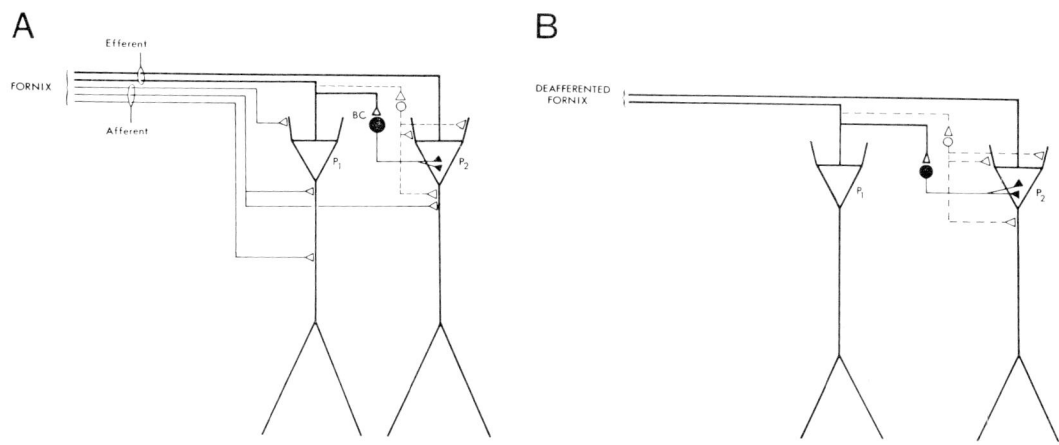

FIG. 21-6. Schematic of recurrent connections in normal fornix (A) and deafferented fornix (B). (A) Normal fornix contains afferent fibers which impinge on basal dendrites and shafts of apical dendrites of the hippocampal pyramidal cells. Collateral from P_1 axon shown synapsing with a basket cell (BC) which in turn synapses with soma of P_2. Basket cells and terminals drawn in black to represent presumed inhibitory role. Pathway (dashed lines) represents possibility that there may be recurrent excitatory pathways. (B) Fornix several weeks after operative section contains no afferent fibers. Recurrent systems are intact. Electrical stimulation of deafferented fornix can activate pyramidal cells only antidromically or through recurrent pathways.

fibers of the hippocampal pyramidal cells [5, 6, 14, 34, 38, 59]. The fornix, the outflow tract of the hippocampus, contains both afferent and efferent fibers; these can be functionally separated (as shown in Fig. 21-6) by deafferenting the fornix by chronic transection of the fornix so that the afferent fibers degenerate [34, 59].

The deafferented fornix is similar to a ventral root, it contains outgoing fibers only, and activation of this structure produces purely antidromic impulses in the hippocampal pyramidal cells. This permits selective activation of recurrent inhibitory pathways, as distinct from pathways subserving feed-forward inhibition. Fornix tetanization can be used to initiate hippocampal seizure, and pyramidal cell activity has been studied in both intact and deafferented fornix preparations. Hippocam-

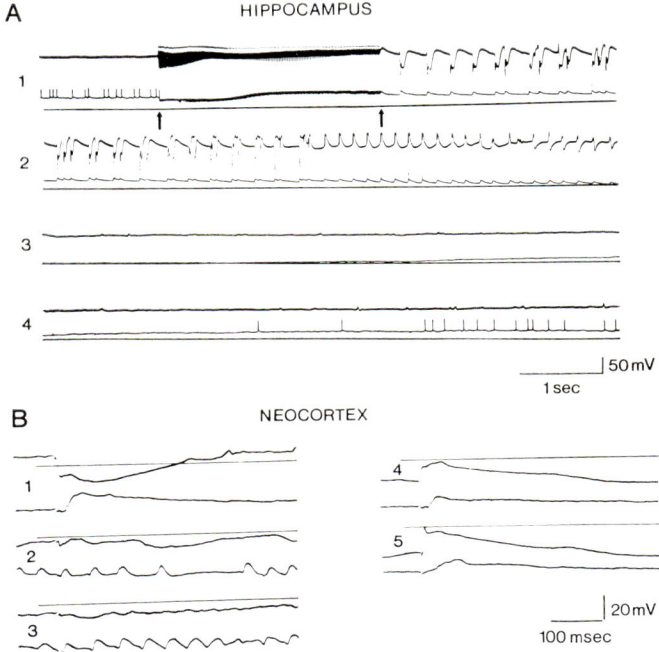

FIG. 21-7. Termination of excitatory seizure by hyperpolarization. (A) Hippocampal seizure in an intact fornix preparation. Upper line: surface recording; middle line: intracellular recording; lowest line: arbitrary baseline. Interval between arrows (in line 1) indicates a period of fornix tetanization. Note that seizure begins with sustained depolarization during tetanus, which persists and is associated with humplike depolarizing transients. During line 2, membrane undergoes hyperpolarization which becomes very large in line 3 and slowly declines in line 4. This hyperpolarization is much larger than sustained IPSP which developed during early phase of fornix tetanus in line 1. (From Kandel and Spencer [33].)

(B) Effect of very intense, sustained hyperpolarization in neocortical cell which developed spontaneously during tonic and clonic phases of seizure in penicillin-treated preparation, on IPSPs generated by stimulation of VL. Upper tracing: intracellular recording; middle: arbitrary reference line; lower: electrocorticogram. VL stimulation during interictal period (B1) is followed by large IPSP, probably mixed with EPSPs. During tonic seizure (B2) resting membrane displays steady 10 mV hyperpolarization. Brief hyperpolarizations of only 3–4 mV are triggered by VL stimulation. Later, during tonic seizure (B3), resting membrane potential hyperpolarized an additional 7–8 mV, and attains 17–18 mV more than at interictal level. At this level apparently no synaptic potentials follow VL stimulus. During the clonic phase (B4, 5), when resting membrane potential reached largest values of hyperpolarization (B5 is 34 mV), VL stimulus evokes depolarizing potential of approximately same time course as hyperpolarization seen in B1 (Ayala et al. [11].)

pal seizure can be produced with equal facility in both intact and deafferented preparations, but large differences exist between seizures generated in these two preparations; these can be shown to result from the different cortical circuits involved.

THE EXCITATORY SEIZURE OF THE INTACT FORNIX PREPARATION. Stimulation of the intact fornix activates excitatory afferents in addition to recurrent inhibitory pathways [34, 54, 59]. Stimulation of the intact fornix produces the characteristic features of hippocampal afterdischarge [33]. During seizure produced by tetanization of the intact fornix (Fig 21-7A), the membrane potential is markedly depolarized either during the initiating tetanus itself or shortly thereafter. This depolarizing shift is up to 30 or 40 mV in amplitude. Superimposed upon the crest of the steady membrane depolarization are large depolarizing oscillations, which sometimes, but not always, triggered abortive spikes; however, in all cases the oscillations and spikes differed from those encountered in normally firing cells.

The distinctive feature of seizures elicited in the intact preparation is the extraordinary depolarization and oscillation in membrane potential of the pyramidal cell. Patterns such as these have been noted in several different types of neocortical seizure [11, 37, 42, 56].

The nature of these peculiar oscillations is obscure, as is also the source of the underlying steady depolarization. It is clear, however, that the cell body is inactivated during these periods of excessive depolarization and that all-or-nothing somatic action potentials are not generated. This does not mean, of course, that the axon is not being fired; the first or second node may become the trigger zone under these circumstances. It is also of interest that reduced action potentials often arise directly out of the elevated base line, suggesting a remote site of impulse initiation (Fig. 21-8A). Full-blown spikes of this sort, but rising from a large resting potential, have been demonstrated by Purpura et al. [53] following tetanic stimulation of temporoammonic pathway (Fig. 21-8B).

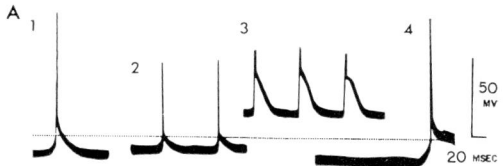

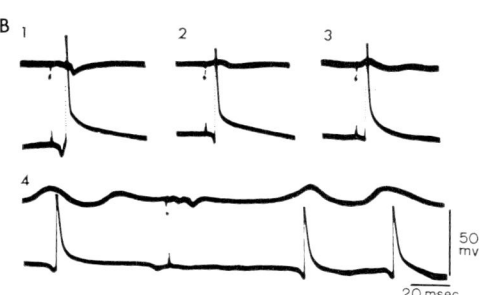

FIG. 21-8. Altered modes of impulse initiation in hippocampal pyramidal cells during seizure. (A) Instances (3) of small amplitude spikes arising out of baseline during steady depolarization associated with seizure initiated by tetanization of intact fornix (Kandel and Spencer [33].) (B) Spike potentials arising in different ways during and after repetitive subiculum stimulation. (1) Single shock subiculum stimulation elicits field response seen as negative deflection intracellularly. Rapid depolarizing prepotential is produced, which triggers spike discharge. Latter is succeeded by prolonged depolarizing afterpotential. (2) During repetitive stimulation, spikes (elicited on declining phases of depolarizing afterpotential of a preceding discharge) lack fast prepotential. (3) With continued stimulation, orthodromic spike without depolarizing prepotential indicates conduction into soma from dendritic sites. (4) *Spontaneous* discharges with negative deflections preceding spikes which lack depolarizing prepotentials. These discharges were initiated during seizure activity as noted in upper channel hippocampal surface records (Purpura et al. [53].)

Another feature of the fornix excitatory seizure is the extremely large inhibitory hyperpolarization associated with termination of the seizure (Fig. 21-7A). This, then, is the first suggestion that inhibition can have an important role in seizure states. To examine the functional role of inhibition further, we examined the deafferented fornix preparation, where the recurrent inhibitory system could be stimulated selectively.

INHIBITORY SEIZURE OF THE DEAFFERENTED FORNIX PREPARATION. Seizure discharge could be initiated in the deafferented fornix preparation by delivering a 5–10 sec tetanus to the fornix (Fig. 21-9). The distinctive feature of seizure in these preparations was the long period of time during which the soma membrane remained hyperpolarized and spike generation was inhibited. This ranged from 50 to 80 percent of the total seizure period [33]. This sustained hyperpolarization had characteristics of a conductance IPSP.

Although seizure onset was immediately evident in the surface record after cessation

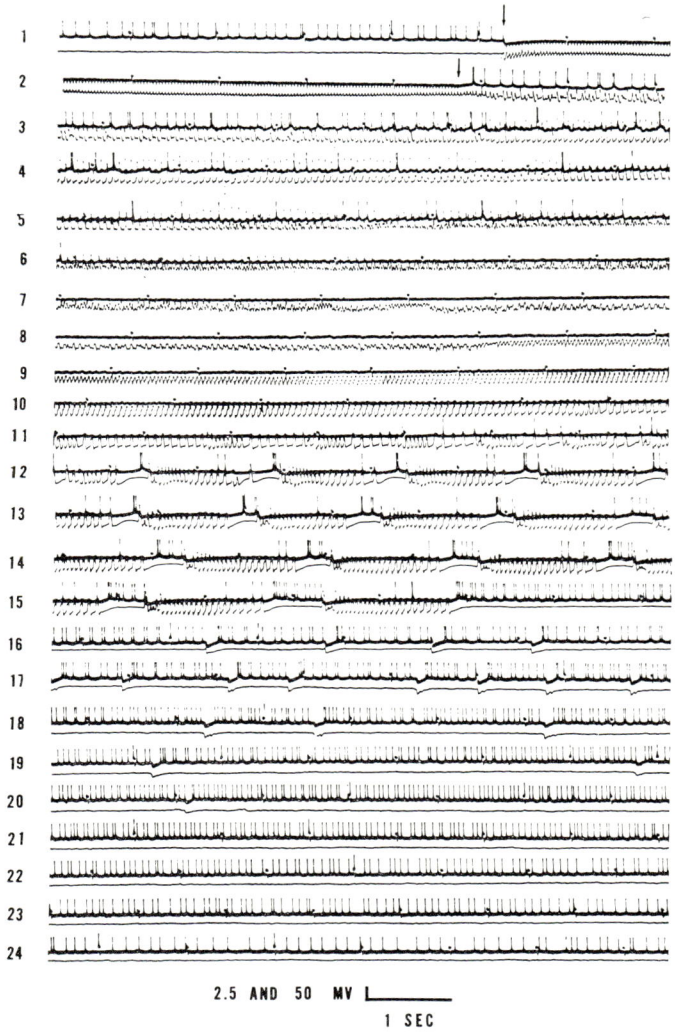

FIG. 21-9. Continuous record of seizure in deafferented fornix preparation. Top record from intracellular microelectrode. Bottom record from surface monitor. Arrows in lines 1 and 2 indicate onset and termination of the fornix tetanus. Voltage calibration refers to both surface (2.5 mV) and intracellular (50 mV) records. Intracellular record also has a constant-voltage (10 mV), 20-msec calibration pip that occurs 1 per sec. Note sustained inhibition in lines 6–11 and intermittent inhibition during clonic and later phase, lines 12–20. (From Kandel and Spencer [33].)

of the tetanus, the intracellular record did not at first show any significant changes from the control firing of the unit. There was characteristically a latency of several seconds, after the end of the tetanus, before the membrane potential first began to show evidence that it had become involved in the seizure process.

The persistent hyperpolarization which characterized these seizures was terminated by the appearance of the clonic phase (lines 11 and 12 of Fig. 21-9). During this phase, interruptions of the surface oscillations were accompanied by a burst of activity in the pyramidal cell. When the surface oscillations finally terminated, steady firing of the pyramidal cell returned. Occasionally the isoelectric surface tracing characteristic of this phase of the seizure showed interruptions by surface transients which were accompanied by corresponding transients in the intracellular tracing. Unitary firing often continued at a higher than control rate for as long as half a minute after cessation of all surface activity, as shown in Fig. 21-9.

Thus, in the CA2 and CA3 regions of the hippocampus, stimulation of the deafferented fornix leads to what is essentially an inhibitory seizure, presumably mediated by the recurrent inhibitory pathways. Not only are pyramidal cells strongly inhibited during the major portion of such seizures, but it seems likely that the bursts of pyramidal cell activity during the clonic phase and the increased firing at the end of the seizure represent disinhibition and rebound, similar to that considered earlier (compare with Fig. 21-3).

MECHANISMS OF SEIZURE IN DEAFFERENTED AND INTACT FORNIX PREPARATIONS. In comparing seizure in the deafferented and intact fornix preparations, the striking difference is that inhibition predominated in one situation and excitation in the other. Two points are relevant here: (1) the different types of neuronal behavior during seizure in the two preparations result not from a permanent change in the intrinsic properties of the cells but rather from a difference in the synaptic bombardment which initiates the seizure in each case, and (2) inhibitory mechanisms can be importantly involved in seizure activity.

The sustained hyperpolarization seen in the deafferented fornix seizures appears to be due to abnormal inhibitory synaptic bombardment on the pyramidal cells of CA2 and CA3 sampled by our recording microelectrodes. In support of this notion is the observation that these hyperpolarizations are chloride sensitive just as are the isolated recurrent IPSPs (Fig. 21-1). This line of reasoning would suggest that these cells serve as a follower region for a population of pacemaker neurons located in other parts of the hippocampus. On the other hand, if the abnormal depolarizations in the *intact* fornix preparations are accompanied by axon discharges, this behavior might be considered as characteristic of a population of hippocampal neurons acting as pacemaker neurons. *The finding that the cells in CA2 and CA3 act as follower neurons in the deafferented fornix preparation and as pacemaker neurons in the intact fornix preparation suggests that a group of cells can behave as either follower or pacemaker neurons depending upon the nature of the afferent synaptic drive converging upon them.*

In addition to these general findings, numerous studies have now examined some detailed factors related to the onset of seizure afterdischarge. For example, some degree of inhibitory decrement [56] may be a factor in the initiation of excitatory seizure. Consistent with this idea is the finding that, in the hippocampus, recurrent inhibitory action shows some decrement following repetitive stimulation. (See Fig. 5 in [59]; also [8].) An additional factor in the initiation of hippocampal seizure may be the tendency of excitatory synaptic actions to increase in amplitude with high frequency activation. (See Fig. 6 in [59], Fig. 6 in [33]; also [8].) The combination of IPSP decrement and EPSP frequency potentiation (with temporal summation) may explain the remarkable depolarizing onset of intact fornix seizures as shown in Fig. 21-7A [33].

Finally, the finding that there is good correlation between surface and intracellular recording suggests that many neurons are involved in synchronous inhibitory activity. The mechanism for this is obscure, but such synchrony could be provided by parallel pathways from common inhibitory interneurons with widespread connections, such as the basket cells. This synchronizing function of inhibition has been discussed previously (Fig. 21-4). Similarly alternating inhibitory interactions (Fig. 21-5) could account for reciprocal patterns in surface and intracellular records during seizure (Fig. 21-9).

COMPARISON OF INHIBITORY AND EXCITATORY ACTIONS IN NEOCORTICAL AND HIPPOCAMPAL AFTERDISCHARGE. The basic features noted in studies of hippocampal seizure have also been identified in seizures in the neocortex. As in the hippocampus, states of excessive depolarization have been found in neocortex [1, 11, 30, 37, 41, 42, 51, 56], as have pronounced inhibitory states [1, 11, 30, 41, 42, 50, 53, 56]. Thus, it may be hoped that continued study of hippocampal seizure may yield principles which are also applicable to neocortex. In turn, studies of neocortical seizure can clarify features of hippocampal seizure. An example of this interdigitation of findings is provided by the elegant experiments of Ayala et al. [11] on the later hyperpolarization which terminates seizure afterdischarge in the pyramidal cells of the motor neocortex (Fig. 21-7B). These extreme states of hyperpolarization produce an inversion of the thalamically evoked IPSPs (Fig. 21-7B) suggesting that the membrane has hyperpolarized beyond the equilibrium potential for the IPSP. Thus, the sustained hyperpolarization may involve a completely different mechanism from the conductance mechanism generating the phasic IPSPs. These facts suggest that the hyperpolarizing potential, which terminates seizure afterdischarge, may be generated by an electrogenic Na^+ pump. As a result of an excitatory seizure, neurons presumably take up a great deal of Na^+ and accumulate K^+ on their outside surfaces, thereby providing a powerful double stimulus for the action of an electrogenic Na^+ pump. Therefore, two mechanisms for producing inhibitory actions may become manifest during seizures: one, a Cl^- dependent IPSP; the other, a hyperpolarization due to the activity of an electrogenic Na^+ pump.

THE ROLE OF INHIBITION IN GENERATION OF INTERICTAL SPIKES

Studies of seizure afterdischarge illustrate the importance of inhibitory actions in seizure states for both the pacemaker population, where inhibition may terminate the seizure, and for certain follower populations, where inhibition may actually dominate the seizure state. But these studies fail to explain the topographical relationships which exist between pacemaker and follower cell populations. In contrast, studies of interictal spikes have proven very useful in this regard.

Interictal spikes [1, 10, 11, 18, 19, 20, 21, 41, 50, 51, 52] are abortive seizures, and the question naturally arises whether inhibitory mechanisms are important in preventing them from developing into full-blown seizures.

Regularly recurring and large *interictal spikes* can be produced experimentally by applying penicillin or strychnine in high concentration to the surface of the hippocampus or neocortex. After penicillin or strychnine application, a variety of stimuli can also trigger the all-or-nothing interictal discharges at short latencies, and the responses can thus be brought under experimental control. The interictal discharges do not usually progress spontaneously to full seizures unless elicited several times in quick succession. Intracellular recordings reveal a picture that is similar in both archicortex and neocortex. The key finding is that in each case there is a topographical distribution of inhibitory and excitatory actions so that the cellular pattern of response differs markedly in the center and in the periphery of the seizure focus. Cells in the center of the focus (Fig. 21-10) show large early depolarizing and late hyperpolarizing responses, whereas cells in the periphery (Fig. 21-11) show primarily large hyperpolarizing responses.

In the hippocampus [18, 19, 20], the triggered responses in the center of the focus provide an interesting contrast to those evoked by a similar stimulus in a normal

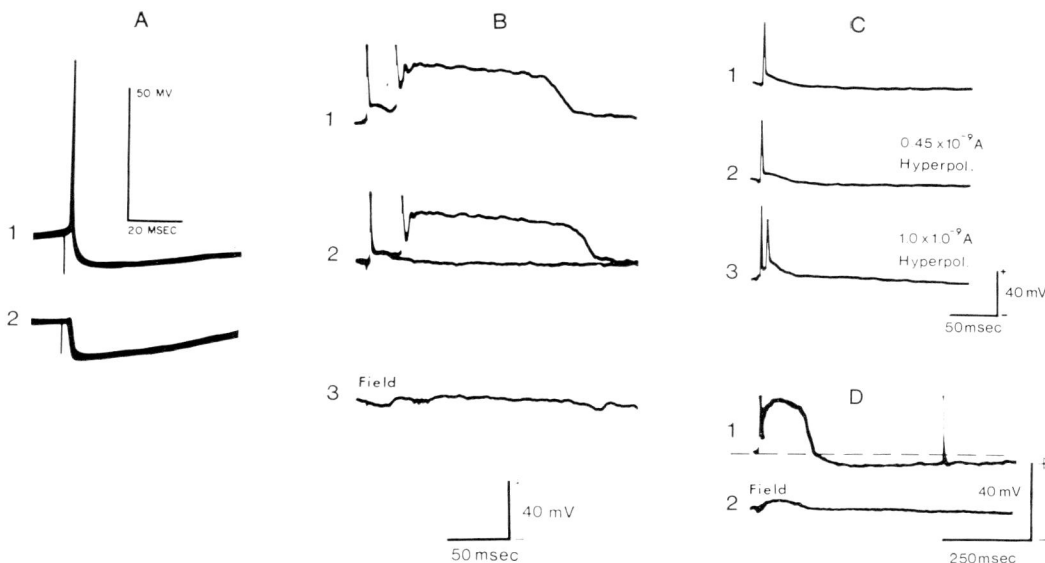

Fig. 21-10. Inhibitory actions, in normal and penicillin-treated preparations, in response to stimulation of fornix. (*A*) Normal preparation: fornix stimulus gives antidromic spike (1) and recurrent IPSP (1) and (2). (From Kandel, Spencer, and Brinley [34].) (*B*) through (*D*) Penicillin-treated preparation: fornix stimulus triggers all-or-nothing depolarizing wave (*B*1) and (*B*2) and reduced inhibition when stimulus is below triggering threshold (*B*2) and (*C*1, 3). Inhibition is not abolished, however, since it is often seen following depolarizing wave, shown in (*D*). Passage of hyperpolarizing current (*C*2) and (*C*3) disclosed brief early excitatory actions. (From Dichter [18].)

preparation (Fig. 21-10). When the fornix stimulus is subthreshold for triggering the interictal discharge, the antidromic spike is followed by a small depolarizing potential, and the usual IPSP is not seen. Even with stimuli which are suprathreshold for the interictal spikes, the recurrent IPSP, although present, is reduced in size suggesting that the epileptogenic agent may reduce recurrent inhibition. Although these agents may reduce inhibitory actions, they do not completely abolish them in the hippocampus [7]. In fact, both in neocortex and archicortex, the large interictal depolarizing potentials are often followed by long-lasting hyperpolarizations which can last up to several seconds (Figs. 21-10 and 21-13).

CELLULAR MECHANISMS OF DEPOLARIZING AND HYPERPOLARIZING POTENTIALS. Characteristic features of the interictal discharge are (1) a large depolarization in the center of the focus followed by a hyperpolariza-tion, and (2) a large hyperpolarization in the surround. What are these large depolarizing and hyperpolarizing potentials which occur during the paroxysmal penicillin and strychnine interictal discharge?

The depolarizing potential is not due to any gross abnormality in the impulse generating mechanism of the pyramidal cell [10, 11, 18, 19, 21]. The electrophysiological characteristics of the pyramidal cells seem normal, except that the amplitude of action potentials is often somewhat reduced, perhaps due to background depolarization. In order to differentiate between possible synaptic and ephaptic origins for the depolarizing potential, intracellular hyperpolarizing and depolarizing currents have been utilized in several different studies [1, 11, 18, 19, 20, 21, 41, 50, 51]. Figures 21-12 and 21-13 illustrate the results of these experiments for cells of both neocortex and archicortex. Hyperpolarizing the cells caused the depolarizing potential to increase whereas depolarizing the cells

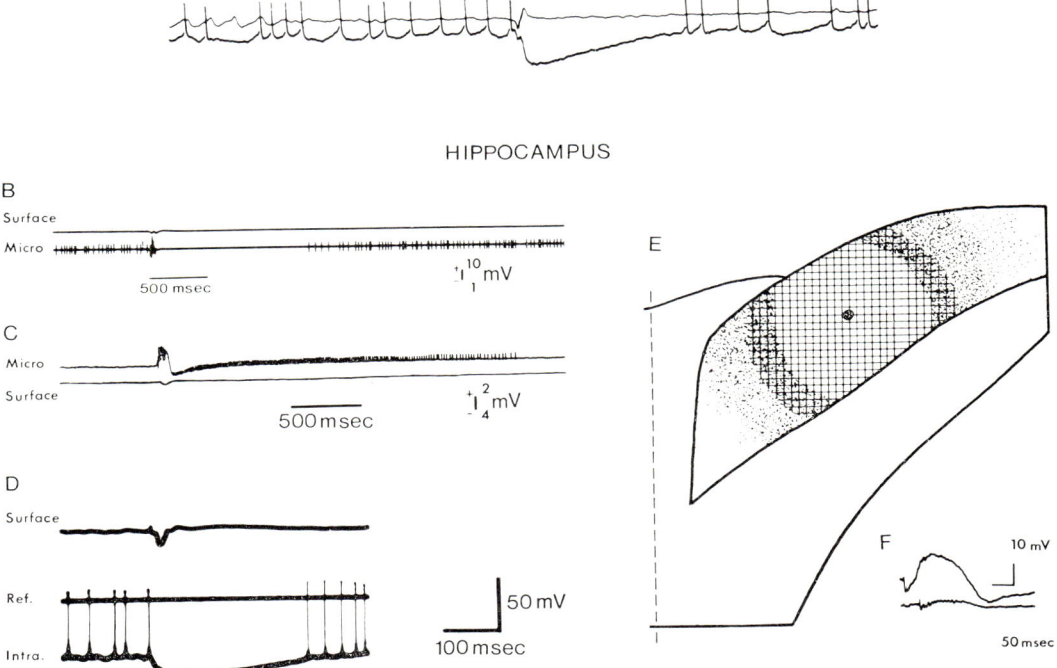

FIG. 21-11. Peripheral inhibition of interictal *spikes* in neocortex and hippocampus. (A) Surface (upper) and intracellular (lower) recordings at margin of focus showing large IPSP (From Prince and Wilder [52].) (B) Extracellular recordings from pyramidal cell in hippocampus at periphery of focus showing inhibitory pause in firing. (C) Extracellular recording from presumed inhibitory interneuron showing sustained, high frequency firing pattern which is inverse to that of pyramidal cells. (D) Intracellularly recorded inhibition from periphery of epileptic focus. (E) Schematic representation of epileptic focus showing central excitatory zone (cross bars), peripheral inhibitory areas (stippling), and mixed zone (region of overlap). (F) Intracellular recording (upper trace) with field (lower trace) taken from intermediate zone. Note hyperpolarizing, depolarizing, hyperpolarizing sequence. (From Dichter [18].)

caused the depolarizing potential to decrease. In some cells, Ayala et al. [11] have been able actually to invert depolarizing potential with large depolarizing current pulses (Fig. 21-13). The alterations in the amplitude of the depolarizing potential with changes in membrane potential indicate that the depolarizing potential has a specific equilibrium potential which lies close to the zero level of the resting potential. These findings suggest that the depolarizing potential is a greatly enlarged EPSP.

A similar analysis has been carried out on the late hyperpolarizing potentials that are seen both in the center of the focus and in the peripheral ring of cortex around the discharging center (Figs. 21-12 and 21-13). Such analyses have suggested that these hyperpolarizing components are IPSPs [11, 18, 20, 21, 50]. Of special interest is Prince's demonstration [50] that these can be inverted by Cl$^-$ injection. Some occult inhibition may exist during the depolarizing waves (see diagram of Fig. 21-12), but it seems unlikely that this can explain all the changes.

PATHWAYS MEDIATING DEPOLARIZING AND HYPERPOLARIZING POTENTIALS. What are the anatomical pathways mediating these postsynaptic potentials? Dichter and Spencer [18, 19, 20, 21] have analyzed these pathways in the hippocampus by examining the

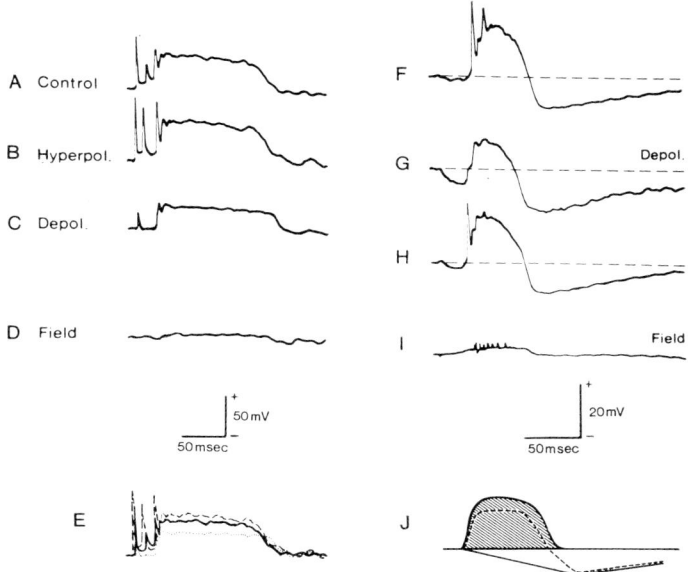

FIG. 21-12. Effects of polarizing currents on excitatory and inhibitory actions associated with interictal spikes in hippocampus. (A) and (B) Background hyperpolarizing current (0.67×10^{-9} amp) increases amplitude of the depolarizing wave. (C) Illustrates that background depolarizing current (0.71×10^{-9} amp) reduces its amplitude. (E) Superimposed tracings delineate these effects. (F) through (I) Effects of background depolarizing current (0.83×10^{-9} amp) on early and late inhibitory components (G). (J) Hypothesis according to which depolarizing contributions dominate early phase of response, inhibitory components the later phases. However, potential actually recorded in absence of polarizing current represents algebraic interaction of two types of conductance changes. (From Dichter [18].)

triggering of interictal spikes in both the intact and deafferented fornix preparation (Fig. 21-14). It was found that purely antidromic stimuli could trigger interictal penicillin discharges in the deafferented fornix preparation identical to those in the intact preparation [18, 19, 20, 21]. This finding strongly suggests that the large EPSP must reflect the activity of axon collaterals of pyramidal cells; in other words, the large EPSP is produced by a recurrent excitatory action and hence is a *giant recurrent* EPSP. The activity in a recurrent excitatory system could also account for the extreme synchrony among pyramidal cells during the interictal discharges because of the recruiting potentialities of such a pathway. Work in progress, by Lebovitz, Dichter, and Spencer [36], indicates that it is possible to demonstrate a rather weak recurrent excitation even when the hippocampus has not been treated with penicillin (Fig. 21-14).

The exact anatomical pathways mediating recurrent excitation have not been identified; nor has the exact mechanism by which penicillin or strychnine produces such gross enhancement in the effectiveness of these pathways been determined. However, in any positive feedback system such as this, alterations at *any one of a number of different sites* [12, 40] might all produce the same end result: a huge increase in recurrent EPSP amplitude. Thus, the presence of the giant recurrent EPSPs does not necessarily imply a specific synaptic action of these epileptogenic agents. Several possible sites for drug action are shown diagrammatically in Fig. 21-14. The reduction in recurrent IPSP amplitude induced by these agents (Fig. 21-6) might provide further support for positive feedback actions.

Studies with iontophoretic application of strychnine [12] have suggested a nonspecific direct excitatory action on neocortical deep pyramidal cells. Although several different

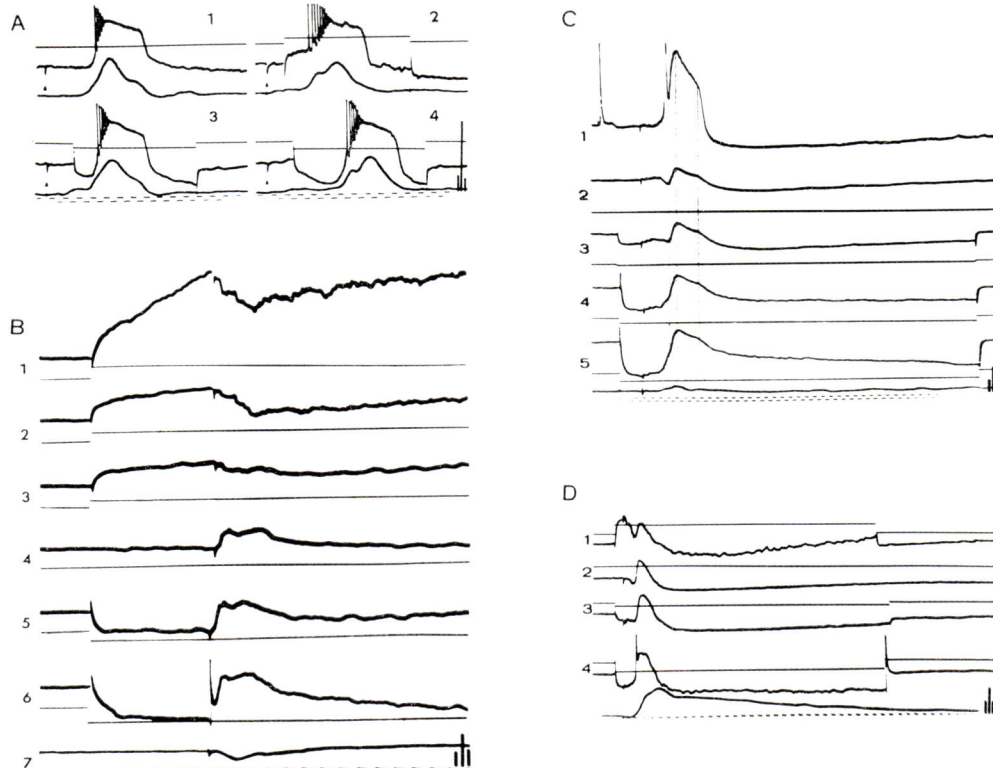

FIG. 21-13. Alterations in amplitude of depolarizing and hyperpolarizing phases of intracellularly recorded responses associated with interictal spikes in neocortical cells. (*A*) Amplitude of paroxysmal depolarizing shift increased by inward current (3) and (4) and decreased by outward current (2). (*B*) Outward currents capable of reversing the polarity of depolarizing shift (1) and (2), but only in deteriorated cells. Current injections did not affect latency of depolarizing waves. (*C*) Reversal of late hyperpolarization (4) and (5) by injection of hyperpolarizing current pulses. (*D*) Augmentation and diminution of both early and late hyperpolarizing phases by background membrane polarization. (From Ayala et al. [11].)

hypotheses have been advanced to explain strychnine IPSP reduction (or inversion) in neocortex [49, 57], it seems probable that these effects do not reflect a specific synaptic action, such as that on cord inhibition [7, 16], since they are seen only with topical application, which would involve very high and nonuniform drug concentrations [17]. Recent studies by Ayala on the crayfish stretch receptor [9] have demonstrated a low-level sustained depolarization upon application of penicillin, which is not associated with a conductance increase, suggesting that the penicillin has blocked an electrogenic Na^+ pump.

The late IPSP of the interictal discharge is also obtained by stimulating the deafferented fornix, indicating that it is probably generated by the normally powerful recurrent inhibitory system mentioned before; the depth analyses of the field potentials associated with the late IPSP, also the surround IPSPs, are consistent with this view since they show greatest amplitude in the cell body layer [5, 6, 18].

In summary, during the triggered interictal spike discharge, pyramidal cells in the center of both archicortical and neocortical foci show a large depolarizing potential often followed by a long-lasting hyperpolar-

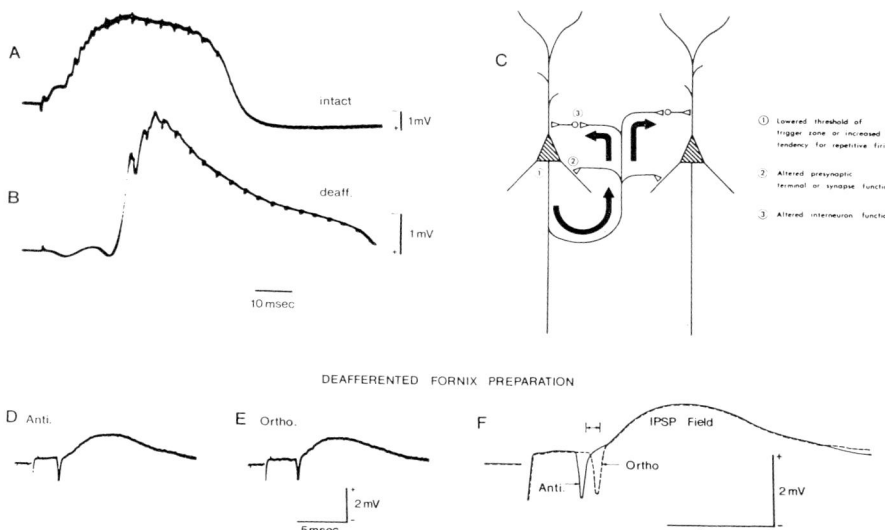

Fig. 21-14. Evidence that recurrent excitatory pathways exist in hippocampus and may play key role in generation of interictal spikes. (A) Surface recording of interictal spike triggered by stimulus to intact fornix.

(B) Surface recording of interictal spike triggered by stimulus to chronically deafferented fornix. These interictal spikes were identical to those triggered by stimuli to intact fornix, thus depolarizing potentials represent type of recurrent excitation. (From Dichter [18].)

(C) Diagram illustrating postulated positive feedback system formed by recurrent excitatory pathways, their recruiting and synchronizing potential, and way in which drug-induced changes at any one of a number of different sites might increase overall effectiveness of recurrent excitatory pathways.

(D) through (F) Evidence that recurrent excitatory pathways exist in non-penicillin-treated deafferented fornix preparation that has not been treated with penicillin. (D) and (E) show antidromic and orthodromic type responses to stimulation of deafferented fornix with strong and weak stimuli respectively. Stronger stimulus (D) activated the axon of unit yielding antidromic response which followed at frequencies in excess of 100 per sec and showed no latency jitter. This identifies this unit as a pyramidal cell. Weaker stimulus elicited unitary spikes at longer and variable latencies (E) which showed jitter and failed to follow at high frequencies. These *orthodromic* responses are believed to arise by action of recurrent pyramidal cell axon collaterals. In (F) are superimposed tracings of the two types of responses. Bidirectional arrow shows range of onset latencies for orthodromic (i.e., recurrent) unitary responses. This jitter is characteristic of transsynaptic modes of activation. (From Lebovitz, Dichter, and Spencer [36].)

ization. In the hippocampus, the potential sequence can be triggered by activating purely antidromic pathways, indicating that both the depolarizing and the hyperpolarizing components are mediated by recurrent collateral pathways. Both Ramón y Cajal [14] and Lorente de Nó [38] describe local direct collateral pathways to pyramidal cells, which may be those mediating the recurrent excitatory actions which we believe play a critical role in the development of the interictal spike.

MECHANISMS IN GENERATION OF INTERICTAL SPIKES: DUAL RECURRENT SYSTEM HYPOTHESIS. During the interictal spike, the central zone of excitation is surrounded by a peripheral zone of inhibition in both neocortex and archicortex (Fig. 21-11). In addition, in the hippocampus an intermediate zone containing a hyperpolarizing-depolarizing-hyperpolarizing sequence has been found (Fig. 21-11). The existence of these three zones led to the suggestion, by Dichter and Spencer [18–21], of a *dual recurrent*

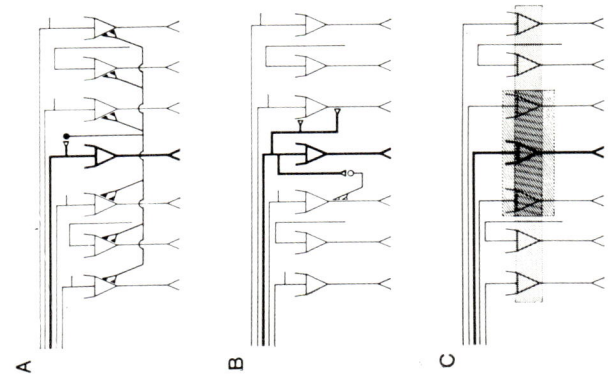

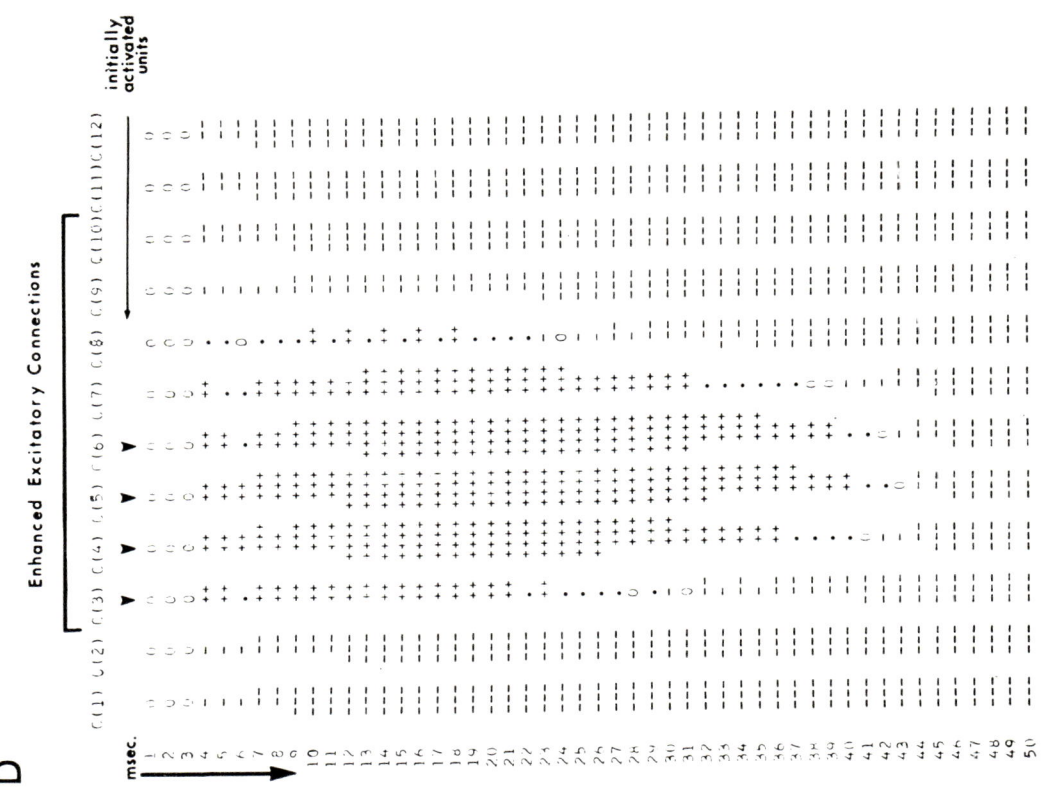

594

FIG. 21-15. Model of interictal spikes. (A) through (C) Schematic of the postulated lateral distribution patterns of recurrent inhibitory and recurrent excitatory synaptic connections. Such connections illustrated only for central cell (drawn with thicker outline) but would apply for all cells. (A) Recurrent inhibition with its wide lateral distribution, presumably mediated through basket cell connections. (B) Recurrent excitation with rather restricted distribution. Connections may be direct or indirect. (C) Superimposition of recurrent excitatory areas (stripes) and inhibitory areas (stippling). Exact lateral extent of each component is arbitrary, but pattern is not.

(D) Computer presentation on right shows *interictal discharge* pattern for 12 units (12 rows of symbols) with respect to time (vertical, downward axis). Each unit has equal recurrent inhibitory action on all other units, but diminishing recurrent excitatory action on 3 adjacent units in either direction. Cells (3), (4), (5), and (6) were initially activated (arrows) to trigger the discharge. (·) represents depolarization of the unit below threshold. (++) represents depolarization above threshold. (+++) and (++++) represent larger amounts of depolarization. Minus signs indicate inhibitory actions. Note the fluctuations in depolarization of cells (3) through (8) between 4 and 8 msec, relatively steady state between 9 and 18 msec, and peripheral to central encroachment of inhibition between 18 and 42 msec, at which point depolarization is finally terminated in all the cells. (From Dichter [18].).

system hypothesis for the origin and restriction of the interictal spike discharge. In some manner, which cannot as yet be precisely specified, penicillin and strychnine lead to an enhanced action of the recurrent excitatory system. The triggering fornix stimulus activates a small group of pyramidal cells. The enhanced effectiveness of the recurrent excitation, probably coupled with decreased recurrent inhibition, produces positive feedback within this population of cells, which recruits a large number of them into hypersynchronous activation resulting in the all-or-nothing discharge. Meanwhile, the pyramidal cells are slowly accumulating the longer lasting and more widespread recurrent inhibition which eventually terminates the depolarization. The widespread recurrent inhibition also establishes a ring of peripheral inhibition around the spiking focus, which serves to restrict the spatial spread of the discharge [18, 19]. This hypothesis embodies many of the feedback principles suggested by Gloor et al. [29] from extracellular field analyses of hippocampal seizure. The dual recurrent system hypothesis [18–21] has been specified by developing a computer model demonstrating many of the same features as the naturally occurring interictal spike discharge [Fig. 21-15]. Such computer models exhibit several parametric features of interictal spikes; for example, the discharges are nearly all-or-nothing spikes and show latency shifts with changes in the number of pyramidal cells activated to trigger them (Fig. 21-16).

RESTRICTION AND PROPAGATION OF THE INTERICTAL SPIKE: TRANSITION TO SEIZURE. The importance of inhibition in restricting the interictal spike to an isolated discharge can also be seen during the transition of the spiking focus into seizure. If the interictal spikes are triggered at intervals of one every one or two seconds, a repetitive afterdischarge develops in the surface spike. With repeated triggering, the afterdischarge grows, and a seizure finally develops as an uncontrolled extension of the discharge. This has been demonstrated in both neocortex and archicortex [1, 11, 18, 42, 55].

During the transition to seizure, the normal EPSP–IPSP sequence in pyramidal cells usually undergoes the following changes: First the late IPSP disappears, and then small afterdepolarizations occur which are synchronous with the surface spike afterdischarges. Matsumoto and Ajmone-Marsan [1, 41, 42] were the first to describe this transitional pattern in their studies of neocortical cells (Fig. 21-17). In the hippocampus, Dichter and Spencer [18, 21] have occasionally recorded extracellularly from cells which discharge long trains of action potentials during and after the isolated interictal discharge (Fig. 21-18); these are postulated to be inhibitory interneurons, perhaps the basket cells. Prince and Wilder [52] previously noted similar cells in neocortex. These cells are also believed to be the inhibitory interneurons responsible for the prolonged period of pyramidal cell inhibition after the paroxysmal interictal discharges. As seizure develops in the hippocampus following repeated fornix stimulation, there is a progressively longer delay in the onset of the *interneuron* discharge (Fig. 21-18). Once the discharge pattern does get under way, the interneuron fires for approximately the same time that it would when only the interictal spike is generated. Eventually the interneuron ceases to respond as the system approaches the seizure state.

These preliminary data suggest that during the transitions from isolated interictal spiking to the development of the full-blown seizure afterdischarge there is an accompanying blockade within the recurrent inhibitory pathway. We would suggest that for some reason the interneurons in the recurrent inhibitory pathways no longer respond to the interictal discharges; perhaps they have become inactivated by an excessive depolarizing action. Whatever the mechanism, a blockade within the inhibitory pathway could explain some of the existing data on the transition from interictal spiking to full seizure.

We have therefore examined the transition from interictal to full seizure in our computer model, using a reduced intensity of the recurrent inhibition. With this modification the model does show a sustained

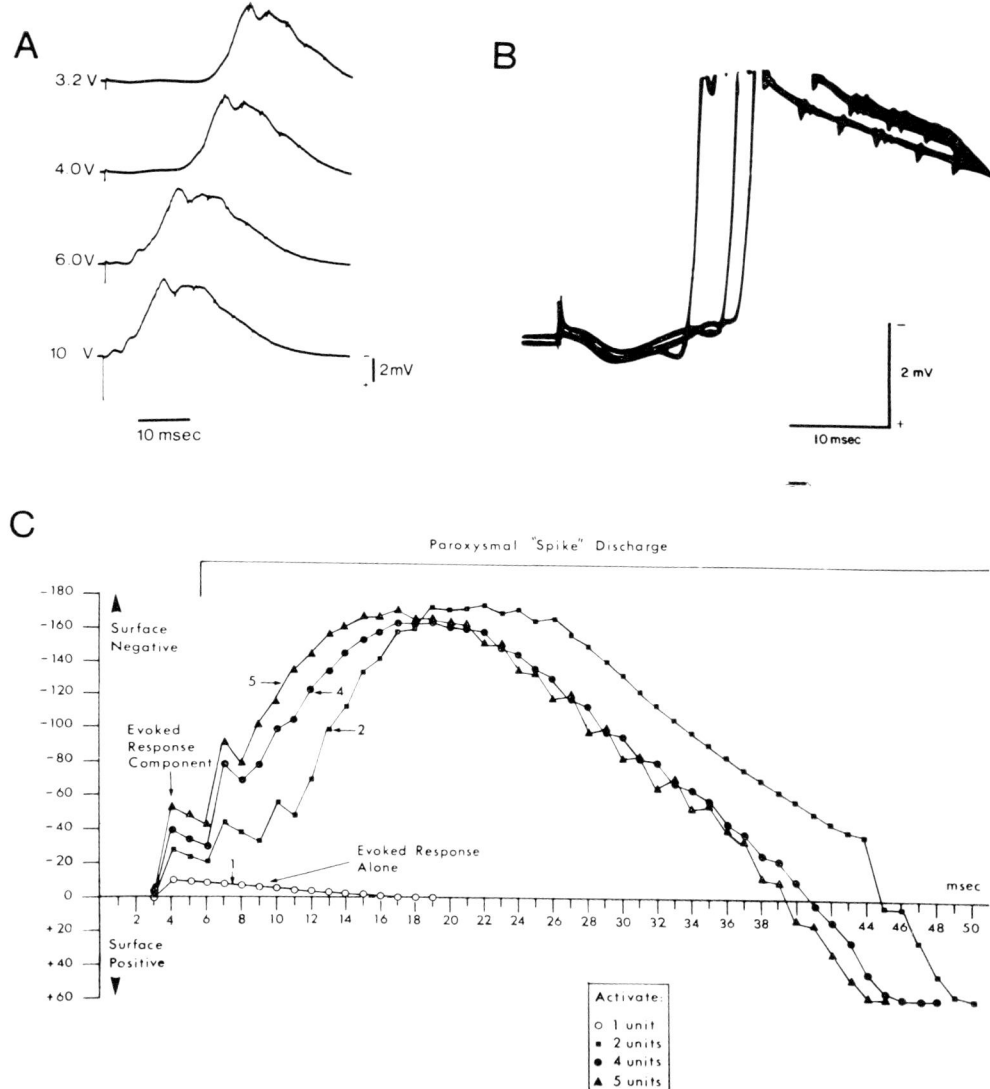

Fig. 21-16. Parametric features common to hippocampal penicillin interictal spike surface recordings and computer model. (A) Graded stimuli to fornix elicit all-or-nothing *spike*, recorded from hippocampal surface, at progressively shorter latencies. Note graded evoked response at foot of spike. (B) Constant triggering stimuli trigger interictal *spikes* (surface recording) at variable latency. (C) Computer model. Graph of the sum of the PSPs of 4 cells in array, used as approximation for *surface gross recording*, against time, in millisecond units for 4 different initial activating conditions. (○) Response to activating one cell in array. (■) Response to activating two cells in array. (●) Response to activating four cells in array. (▲) Response to activating five cells in array. Note graded *evoked response* component of each curve at arrow, and all-or-nothing *paroxysmal "spike" discharges* which occur in response to 2 or more stimuli with shifting peak latency. These curves are considered analogous to the change in latency with changes in stimulus strength for eliciting all-or-nothing penicillin discharge. Amplitude units are arbitrary. (From Dichter [18].)

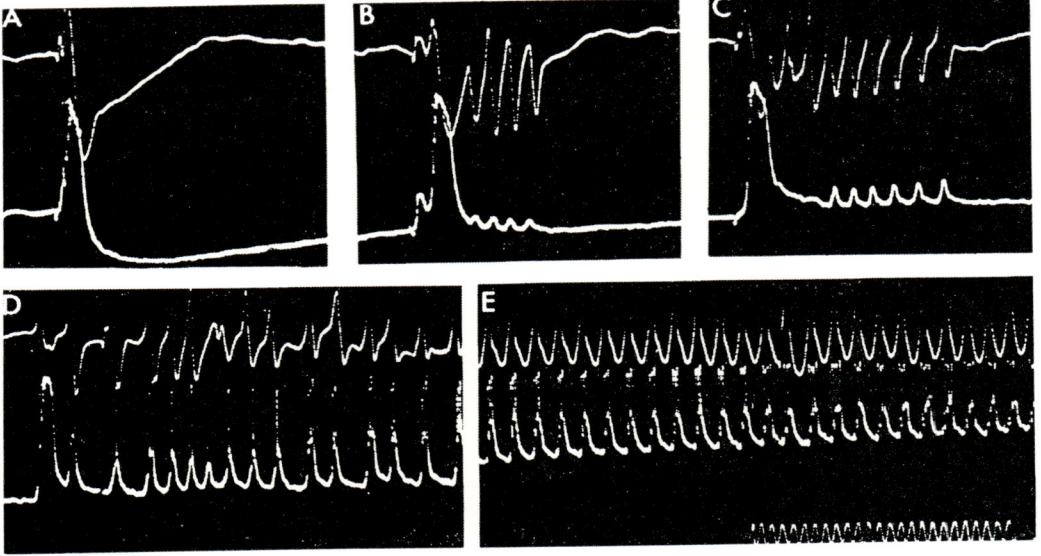

Fig. 21-17. Epileptogenic focus (penicillin) induced in cortex of posterior sigmoid gyrus. Intracellular recording. In each record upper channel is from a gross surface electrode, lower one from micropipette. Five records (A) through (E) are from same experiments and follow each other at variable intervals. Note how hyperpolarizing shift, present in (A) is substituted by depolarization of progressively longer duration (B, C) until an ictal episode develops (D, E). In (A) through (C) paroxysmal discharges are *triggered* by stimulus applied to contralateral homologous region. Calibrations: 1 mV and 10 mV respectively for surface and intracellular tracings; 50 cycles per sec. (From Ajmone-Marsan [1].)

state of depolarization developing in the cells in the center part of the focus. As with interictal spikes, the seizure model shows sustained peripheral inhibition.

These data indicate that alterations in the recurrent collateral systems of the hippocampus may be responsible for both the origin and restriction of the interictal penicillin spike discharge and for the escape from such restriction when a seizure develops. A corollary to this idea is that only structures that have well-developed, recurrent excitatory and inhibitory systems are capable of developing the highly synchronous activity characteristic of cortical epilepsy. Perhaps the inability of a structure such as the cerebellum to develop interictal spikes when strychnine is applied locally (Fig. 21-19), despite the fact that Purkinje cells are directly excited [13], can be due to the lack of recurrent excitatory connections in this structure [25].

DISCUSSION

The characteristic feature of integrative action of the central nervous system is a balanced interaction of synaptic excitation and inhibition. This balance appears to exist at all levels of the neuraxis, and, indeed, synaptic inhibition has been found to coexist with synaptic excitation in most regions examined. The effects of this balance are likely to be particularly critical in the cerebral cortex where prolonged inhibitory postsynaptic potentials dominate the synaptic organization.

Perhaps the simplest way to summarize the data reviewed on the role of inhibition in cortical epilepsy is to state that during the seizure state the balanced interaction between inhibition and excitation is radically altered for a short period so that in certain regions excitation dominates over inhibition, whereas in others inhibition dominates

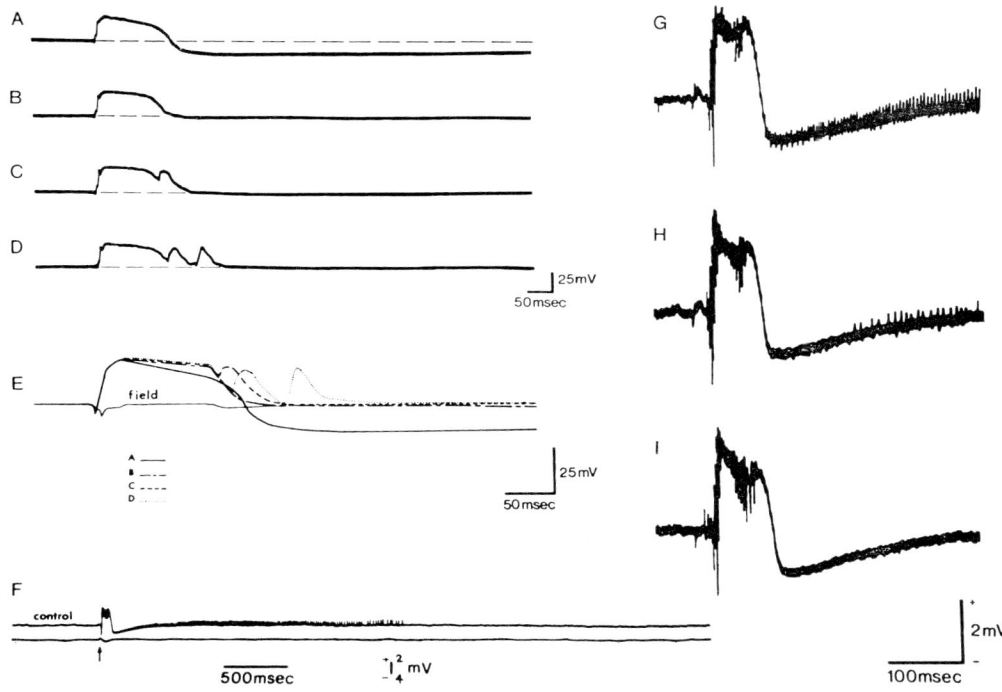

FIG. 21-18. Transition from interictal spiking to seizure in hippocampus. (A) through (E) Recordings of slow potentials (PSPs) associated with transition to seizure in hippocampal pyramidal cell, spike generator inactivated. (A) through (D) Intracellular recordings (dc) of successive triggered interictal spikes. (A) Normal depolarizing-hyperpolarizing sequence (with the dashed line indicating baseline). (B) Depolarizing potential after dropout of late hyperpolarization. (C) and (D) Single and double late depolarizing potentials which would be associated with surface afterdischarge. (E) Four traces are superimposed, extracellular field added. (F) Full duration of postulated inhibitory interneuron response to isolated fornix triggering stimulus. (G) Early phase of same response at high gain. (H) and (I) Progressive dropout of interneuron firing upon repeated stimulation. Note delayed onset of interneuron firing in (H) and the absence of firing in (I). Large spikes during discharge itself probably originate from pyramidal cells. It is suggested that failure of inhibitory interneuron action may be partly responsible for dropping out of pyramidal cell inhibition and prolongation of pyramidal cell depolarization. (From Dichter [18].)

over excitation. This is evident both in hippocampal afterdischarge and in focal interictal spikes, where regions of excessive excitation are surrounded by regions of excessive inhibition. Stated another way, in both types of experimental epilepsy a common topographical picture of synaptic imbalance occurs whereby an excitatory pacemaker region is surrounded by a powerful ring of inhibition.

How does this spatial separation of excitatory and inhibitory functions come about? And what are its consequences for the genesis of seizure?

Perhaps the main reason for the development of a spatial separation of inhibitory and excitatory zones lies in the nature of the operational wiring diagrams of the cerebral cortex. Characteristically, the neurons of both neocortex and archicortex give rise to recurrent collateral systems capable of exerting feedback control. In hippocampus these are of two types: a powerful inhibitory system which appears to have a widespread distribution and a weaker, shorter duration excitatory system, which appears to have a very limited distribution. The chapters by Szentágothai

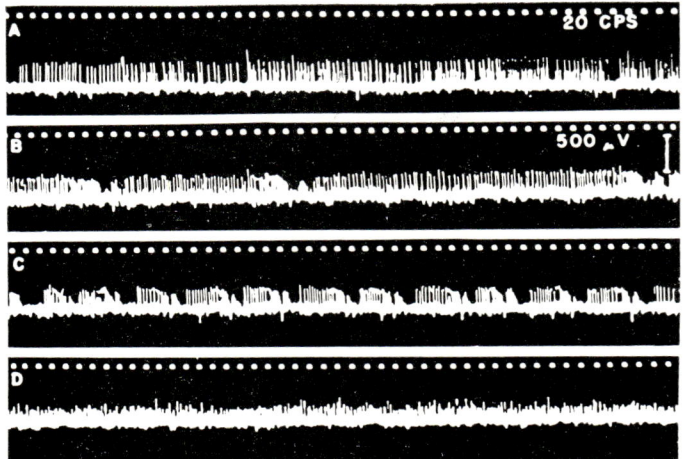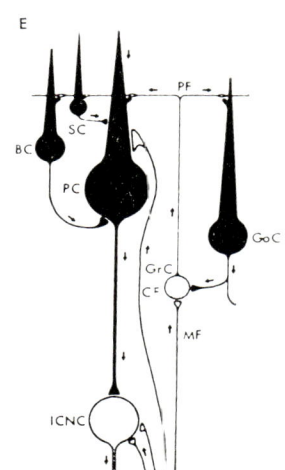

FIG. 21-19. Excitatory effects of strychnine on cells of cerebellar cortex not accompanied by surface spikes, presumably because neuronal circuitry fails to provide essential features for postulated positive and negative feedback actions. (A) through (D) Avalanching outbursts in cerebellar cortex following local strychninization. Decerebrate cat. Glass micropipette in right lobulus paramedianus. (A) Normal multiunit discharge which had been in progress for 7 min. (B) Nine minutes after application of 3 percent strychnine locally near tip of electrode. Note long outbursts with terminal increase in frequency. (C) One minute after (B). Convulsive outbursts are shorter and more frequent, with higher initial frequency. (D) Strychnine removed and area washed with saline solution 14 min after application. Record taken 1 hr after application of strychnine. Convulsive outbursts have disappeared. Time and sensitivity constant throughout as indicated. (From Brookhart, Moruzzi, and Snider [13].)

(E) Diagram of most significant neuronal connections in cerebellum. Open cells are excitatory, filled cells inhibitory. PC = Purkinje cell; BC = basket cell; SC = stellate cell; GoC = Golgi cell; GrC = granule cell; CF = climbing fiber; MF = mossy fiber; PF = parallel fiber; ICNC = intracerebellar nuclei cell. Note circuit lacks recurrent excitatory actions, which are postulated to be necessary for synchronized reactions. Also, although there are recurrent Purkinje cell inhibitory connections which are not shown, these are relatively weak. (From Eccles [24].)

[64] and Oshima [46] in this volume contain suggestions that similar arrangements may obtain in the neocortex. We would suggest that the primary trigger in the seizure process in both hippocampal afterdischarge and focal spiking produces an increased activity in the recurrent facilitatory system giving rise locally to the characteristic regenerative pacemaker activity. The regenerative activity of the pacemaker region in turn activates the widespread recurrent inhibitory system with the result that the pacemaker region will be spatially surrounded by a region dominated by synaptic inhibition. The nature of the cortical neuronal circuitry is such that increased activity in the recurrent facilitatory system will produce not only regenerative activity in that system but also increased activity in the recurrent inhibitory system.

This schema is probably highly simplified, but it is useful for explaining a number of the electrophysiological features of the seizure state. First, this view suggests that the fundamental defect in the seizure state probably reflects less an abnormality of the neuron than it reflects an abnormal utilization of the circuitry to which cortical neurons belong. Seizure is therefore ultimately a manifestation of a system defect although the initial trigger may be an abnormality in a number of cells. Once triggered, any cell seems capable of being drawn into either the excitatory-pacemaker or the inhibitory-follower region. Second, the interactions of excitatory and inhibitory zones may explain certain temporal and spatial features of the seizure. For example, the existence of a zone of inhibition around the pacemaker focus is important for limiting the *spatial spread* as well as the duration of the seizure. Indeed there is the suggestion from preliminary data that as long as the inhibitory surround can be effectively maintained, seizure spread will be limited both in space and time. The breakdown of the surround, by disinhibition due to inactivation of the interneuron mediating inhibition, seems to lead to propagated and more prolonged seizure activity. As in the normal functioning of cortex, the multiple integrative capabilities of inhibition clearly appear to be important in the restriction and genesis of seizure activity.

REFERENCES

1. Ajmone-Marsan, C. Micro-Structural Mechanisms of Seizure Susceptibility. In Servit, Z. (Ed.), *Comparative and Cellular Pathophysiology of Epilepsy*. Prague: Czechoslovak Academy of Sciences and Excerpta Medica, 1966.
2. Alving, B. O. Spontaneous activity in isolated somata of *Aplysia* pacemaker neurons. *J. Gen. Physiol.* 51:29, 1968.
3. Andersen, P., and Andersson, S. *Physiological Basis of the Alpha Rhythm*. New York: Appleton-Century-Crofts, 1968.
4. Andersen, P., and Eccles, J. C. Inhibitory phasing of neuronal discharge. *Nature* (London) 196:645, 1962.
5. Andersen, P., Eccles, J. C., and Løyning, Y. Location of postsynaptic inhibitory synapses on hippocampal pyramids. *J. Neurophysiol.* 27:592, 1964.
6. Andersen, P., Eccles, J. C., and Løyning, Y. Pathway of postsynaptic inhibition in the hippocampus. *J. Neurophysiol.* 27:608, 1964.
7. Andersen, P., Eccles, J. C., Løyning, Y., and Voorhoeve, P. E. Strychnine resistant inhibition in the brain. *Nature* (London) 200:843, 1963.
8. Andersen, P., and Lømo, T. Counteraction of Powerful Recurrent Inhibition in Hippocampal Pyramidal Cells by Frequency Potentiation of Excitatory Synapses. In Von Euler, C., Skoglund, S., and Soderberg, U. (Eds.), *Structure and Function of Inhibitory Neuronal Mechanisms*. Oxford: Pergamon, 1968, p. 335.
9. Ayala, G. F. Unpublished data, 1968.
10. Ayala, G. F., Matsumoto, H., and Gumnit, R. J. Betz cell spike generating mechanisms during experimental focal seizures. *Neurology* (Minneap.) 17:282, 1967.
11. Ayala, G. F., Matsumoto, H., and Gumnit, R. J. Unpublished data, 1968.
12. Biscoe, T. J., and Curtis, D. R. Strychnine and cortical inhibition. *Nature* (London) 214:914, 1967.
13. Brookhart, J. M., Moruzzi, G., and Snider, R. S. Spike discharges of single units in the cerebellar cortex. *J. Neurophysiol.* 13:465, 1950.
14. Cajal, S. R. *Histologie du système nerveux de l'Homme et des vertébrés*. Paris: A. Maloine, 1911. Vol. II.
15. Connelly, C. M. Recovery processes and metabolism of nerve. *Rev. Mod. Phys.* 31:475, 1959.
16. Curtis, D. R. Pharmacological investigations upon inhibition of spinal neurons. *J. Physiol.* (London) 145:175, 1959.
17. Curtis, D. R. Pharmacology and Neurochemistry of Mammalian Central Inhibitory Processes. In Von Euler, C., Skoglund, S., and Soderberg, U. (Eds.), *Structure and Function of Inhibitory Neuronal Mechanisms*. Oxford: Pergamon, 1968, p. 429.
18. Dichter, M. *Experimental Penicillin Epilepsy in the Cat Hippocampus*. Ph. D. Thesis. New York University Medical School, 1963.
19. Dichter, M., and Spencer, W. A. Origin and inhibitory restriction of hippocampal epileptic spikes. *Physiologist* 10:166, 1967.
20. Dichter, M., and Spencer, W. A. An analysis of focal epilepsy induced by penicillin. *Fed. Proc.* 27:387, 1968.
21. Dichter, M., and Spencer, W. A. Hippocampal penicillin spike discharge: Epileptic neuron or epileptic aggregate. *Neurology* (Minneap.) 18:282, 1968.
22. Eccles, J. C. *The Physiology of Nerve Cells*. Baltimore: Johns Hopkins Press, 1957.
23. Eccles, J. C. *The Physiology of Synapses*. Berlin: Springer, 1964.

24. Eccles, J. C. Postsynaptic Inhibition in the Nervous System. In Quarton, G., Melnechuck, T., and Schmidt, F. O. (Eds.), *The Neurosciences*, New York: Rockefeller University Press, 1967, p. 408.

25. Eccles, J., Ito, M., and Szentágothai, J. *The Cerebellum as a Neuronal Machine*. New York: Springer, 1967.

26. Eccles, J. C. Inhibition in thalamic and cortical neurones and its role in phasing neuronal discharges. *Epilepsia* (Amst.) 6:89, 1968.

27. Frazier, W. T., Kandel, E. R., Kupfermann, I., Waziri, R., and Coggeshall, R. E. Morphological and functional properties of identified cells in *Aplysia californica*. *J. Neurophysiol*. 30:1288, 1967.

28. Furukawa, T., and Furshpan, E. J. Two inhibitory mechanisms in Mauthner neurons of goldfish. *J. Neurophysiol*. 26:140, 1963.

29. Gloor, P., Sperti, L., and Vera, C. L. A consideration of feedback mechanisms in the genesis and maintenance of hippocampal seizure activity. *Epilepsia* (Amst.) 5:213, 1964.

30. Goldensohn, E. S., and Purpura, D. P. Intracellular potentials of cortical neurones during focal epileptogenic discharges. *Science* 139:840, 1963.

31. Hamlyn, L. H. An electron microscopic study of pyramidal neurons in the Ammon's horn of the rabbit. *J. Anat*. 97:189, 1963.

32. Kandel, E. R., Frazier, W. T., and Wachtel, H. Organization of inhibition in the abdominal ganglion of *Aplysia*. I. The role of inhibition and disinhibition in transforming neural activity. *J. Neurophysiol*. 1969, in press.

33. Kandel, E. R., and Spencer, W. A. Excitation and inhibition of single pyramidal cells during hippocampal seizure. *Exp. Neurol*. 4:162, 1961.

34. Kandel, E. R., Spencer, W. A., and Brinley, F. J. Electrophysiology of hippocampal neurons. I. Sequential invasion and synaptic organization. *J. Neurophysiol*. 24:225, 1961.

35. Kobayashi, H., and Libet, B. Generation of slow potentials without increase in ionic conductance. *Proc. Nat. Acad. Sci. U.S.A*. 60:1304, 1968.

36. Lebovitz, R., Dichter, M., and Spencer, W. A. Recurrent excitation in hippocampus. *Fed. Proc*. 28:455, 1969.

37. Li, C.-L. Functional properties of cortical neurones with particular reference to strychninization. *Electroenceph. Clin. Neurophysiol*. 7:475, 1955.

38. Lorente de Nó, R. Studies on the structure of the cerebral cortex. II. Continuation of the study on the ammonic system. *J. Psychol. Neurol*. (Lpz.) 46:113, 1934.

39. Lux, H. D., and Klee, M. R. Intracelluläre Untersuchungen über den Einfluss hemmender Potentiale im mortorischen Cortex. I. Die Wirkung elektrischer Reizung unspecifischer Thalamuskerne. *Arch. Psychiat. Nervenkr*. 203:648, 1963.

40. Maruhashi, J., Otani, T., and Yamada, M. On the effects of strychnine upon the myelinated nerve fibers of toads. *Jap. J. Physiol*. 6:174, 1956.

41. Matsumoto, H., and Ajmone-Marsan, C. Cortical cellular phenomena in experimental epilepsy: Interictal manifestations. *Exp. Neurol*. 9:286, 1964.

42. Matsumoto, H., and Ajmone-Marsan, C. Cortical cellular phenomena in experimental epilepsy: Ictal manifestations. *Exp. Neurol*. 9:305, 1964.

43. Nakajima, S., and Takahashi, K. Post-tetanic hyperpolarization and electrogenic Na^+ pump in stretch receptor neurone of crayfish. *J. Physiol*. (London) 187:105, 1966.

44. Nicholls, J. G., and Baylor, D. A. Long lasting hyperpolarization after activity of neurons in leech central nervous system. *Science* 162:279, 1968.

45. Nishi, S., and Koketsu, K. Origin of ganglionic inhibitory postsynaptic potential. *Life Sci*. 6:2049, 1967.

46. Oshima, T. Studies of Pyramidal Tract Cells. In Jasper, H. H., Ward, A. A., Jr., and Pope, A. (Eds.), *Basic Mechanisms of the Epilepsies*. Boston: Little, Brown, 1969.

47. Phillips, C. G. Actions of antidromic pyramidal volleys on single Betz cells in the cat. *Quart. J. Exp. Physiol*. 44:1, 1959.

48. Pinsker, H., and Kandel, E. R. Synaptic activation of an electrogenic sodium pump. *Science* 163:931, 1969.

49. Pollen, D., and Ajmone-Marsan, C. Cortical inhibitory postsynaptic potentials and strychninization. *J. Neurophysiol*. 28:342, 1965.

50. Prince, D. Inhibition in "epileptic" neurons. *Exp. Neurol*. 21:307, 1968.

51. Prince, D. The depolarization shift in "epileptic" neurons. *Exp. Neurol.* 21:467, 1968.
52. Prince, D., and Wilder, B. J. Control mechanisms in cortical epileptogenic foci. *Arch. Neurol.* (Chicago) 16:194, 1967.
53. Purpura, D., McMurtry, J., Leonard, C., and Malliani, A. Evidence for dendritic origin of spikes without depolarizing prepotentials in hippocampal neurons during and after seizure. *J. Neurophysiol.* 29:954, 1966.
54. Raisman, G., Cowan, W. M., and Powell, T. P. S. The extrinsic afferent, commissural and association fibers of the hippocampus. *Brain* 88:963, 1965.
55. Ralston, B. L. The mechanism of transition of interictal spiking foci into ictal seizure discharges. *Electroenceph. Clin. Neurophysiol.* 10:217, 1958.

Ramón y Cajal, see Cajal.

56. Sawa, M., Maruyama, N., and Kaji, S. Intracellular potential during electrically induced seizures. *Electroenceph. Clin. Neurophysiol.* 15:209, 1963.
57. Sawa, M., Maruyama, N., Kaji, S., and Nakamura, K. Action of strychnine to cortical neurons. *Jap. J. Physiol.* 16:126, 1966.
58. Skou, J. C. Enzymatic basis for active transport of Na+ and K+ across cell membrane. *Physiol. Rev.* 45:596, 1965.
59. Spencer, W. A., and Kandel, E. R. Hippocampal neuron responses to selective activation of recurrent collaterals of hippocampofugal axons. *Exp. Neurol.* 4:149, 1961.
60. Spencer, W. A., and Kandel, E. R. Electrophysiology of hippocampal neurons. III. Firing level and time constant. *J. Neurophysiol.* 24:260, 1961.
61. Stefanis, C., and Jasper, H. Intracellular microelectrode studies of antidromic responses in cortical pyramidal tract neurons. *J. Neurophysiol.* 27:828, 1964.
62. Stefanis, C., and Jasper, H. Recurrent collateral inhibition in pyramidal tract neurons. *J. Neurophysiol.* 27:855, 1964.
63. Strumwasser, F. The Demonstration and Manipulation of Circadian Rhythm in a Single Neuron. In Aschoff, J. (Ed.), *Circadian Clocks*. Amsterdam: North Holland Publishing Co., 1965, p. 442.
64. Szentágothai, J. Architecture of the Cerebral Cortex. In Jasper, H. H., Ward, A. A., Jr., and Pope, A. (Eds.), *Basic Mechanisms of the Epilepsies*. Boston: Little, Brown, 1969.
65. Waziri, R., and Kandel, E. R. Organization of inhibition in the abdominal ganglion of *Aplysia*. II. Two interneurons mediating inhibition. *J. Neurophysiol.* 1969, in press.
66. Wilson, V. J., and Burgess, P. R. Disinhibition in the cat spinal cord. *J. Neurophysiol.* 25:392, 1962.

Discussion

ORGANIZATION AND FREQUENCY DEPENDENCE OF HIPPOCAMPAL INHIBITION

P. ANDERSEN AND T. LØMO

Experiments performed by our group on organization of the hippocampal neurons fully support the interpretation of Spencer and Kandel in the first part of this chapter that inhibition plays an important role in the sculpturing of epileptic activity.

In all areas of the hippocampus, it is quite evident that an afferent volley initially excites a relatively small number of cells. Subsequently, surrounding cells will be inhibited over recurrent pathways in the hippocampus proper as well as in the dentate fascia [1, 7, 12].

Some recent data on the organization of the hippocampal cortex may be relevant in this connection. As far as we know, the main afferent supply of the hippocampus derives from the entorhinal area [3, 9, 10]. The fibers from this area constitute the perforant path, which enters the hippocampal formation in the way illustrated in Fig. D21-1B, and run parallel and deep to the angular bundle. After a shorter or longer course in the subicular area, fibers turn to travel across the hippocampal fissure and end in the molecular layer of the dentate fascia (Fig. D21-1B) very nearly parallel to the midline in the dorsal part of the hippocampal formation (Fig. D21-1C). The next neuron in the chain, the dentate granule cell, sends its axon through the hilus toward the CA3 area. Again, these fibers are arranged strictly parallel to each other, so that a small group of granule cells activates a similarly small region of the CA3. The direction of the mossy fibers is in exactly the same plane as that of the incoming perforant path fibers. The CA3 neurons send their axons into the fimbria. From each axon, one large myelinated collateral curves back, reenters the hippocampal formation, and travels in a caudal direction in the deeper part of the CA1 to activate a remote part of the apical dendrites. These so-called Schaffer collaterals course in the same plane as that of the perforant path and mossy fibers. Therefore, the three-neuron chain in the hippocampal formation, consisting of the perforant path, mossy fibers and Schaffer collaterals are contained within a slice-shaped block of tissue. In Fig. D21-1B, one such segment or *slice* can be seen. In addition, the CA3 and CA1 axons destined for the fimbria or the alveus, respectively, travel in the same plane.

At each relay of the hippocampal formation, cells are profoundly inhibited following initial excitation. In the dentate granule cells, this inhibition lasts up to 100 msec, whereas the duration of the inhibition in CA3 and CA1 is 200–300 msec. The degree of inhibition produced by a conditioning stimulus, delivered at various distances from the beam, is found to be maximal on either side of the excited strip (Fig. D21-1C). The excited beam produced by the perforant path volley is hatched; black zones on each side of the excited beam indicate areas of inhibition. Similar arrangements were found for the mossy-fiber excitation of the CA3 area as well as for the Schaffer collateral excitation of the CA1 area.

Thus, in all three parts of the three-membered neuronal loop, there is a central beam of excited cells bordered on each side by a zone of inhibited cells.

With the use of deafferented hippocampal preparations, Spencer and Kandel [12] showed that inhibition in the CA3 hippocampal pyramids was of the recurrent type. Similarly, Andersen et al. [1] suggested that the powerful inhibition of the dentate granule cells also was of a recurrent nature. Recently, Lømo [7] has provided new evi-

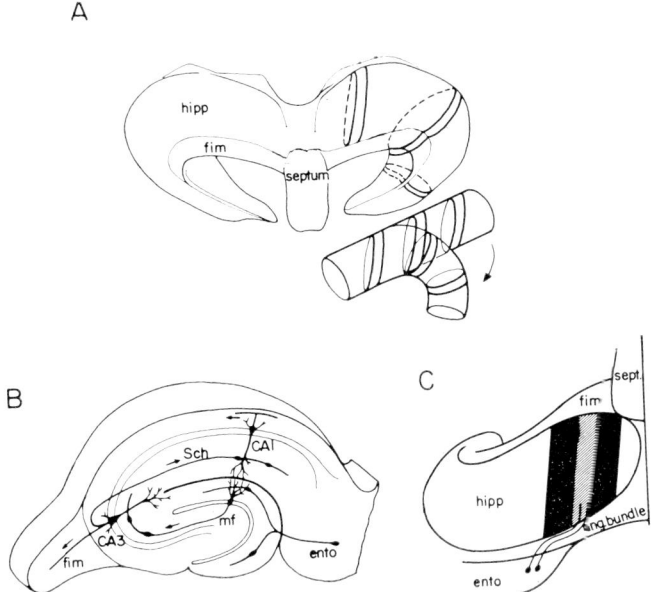

Fig. D21-1. Schematic drawing of hippocampal formation in rabbit. (A) Hippocampal formation viewed from above; heavy lines indicate *slices* (see text). Inset shows relative position of slices in a curved and straight tissue cylinder. (B) Diagram of tissue slice with four-neuronal chain, arranged in the plane of the slice. (C) Diagram of hippocampal formation viewed from above with an excited beam of cells (hatched), bordered on each side by a strip of inhibited neurons (black).

dence which strongly supports this notion. In this region the population spike in response to a perforant path volley is composed of a large number of granule cell discharges. When this test response was preceded by a conditioning stimulus given through the same electrode at certain intervals, there was marked increase of the test-population spike. This effect has a dual explanation: it is partly due to increased release of transmitter and partly to activation of a facilitatory pathway operated through excitatory interneurons [6, 8]. It is similar to the scheme suggested for the hippocampus proper by Spencer and Kandel in this chapter. However, as soon as the strength of the conditioning stimulus increased above the threshold for eliciting a spike, there was a dramatic decrease of the population spike; this reduction is exactly paralleled by growth of the conditioning spike. In other words, as soon as the granule cells discharge, they elicit the inhibitory effect through the recurrent inhibitory path.

Similar arrangements were found for the mossy-fiber activation of CA3 cells and for Schaffer collateral excitation of CA1 pyramids.

Another important organizational feature is the synapse type: the fibers have a large number of *en passage* boutons along their entire length. Therefore, excitation takes the form of a narrow strip bordered on each side by a longitudinal trough of inhibition. In the present context, hippocampal seizure activity will, therefore, confine itself to a striplike area. Recurrent inhibition restricts the spread of excitation laterally and medially as pointed out by Spencer and Kandel.

FREQUENCY POTENTIATION OF EXCITATORY SYNAPSES

A remarkable phenomenon in the hippocampal cortex is the ability of tetanic stimulation to increase the excitatory post-synaptic potentials (EPSP). In the train, subsequent stimuli produce successively augmenting EPSPs that summate and cause a large depolarization of the cells. This phenomenon has been called *frequency potentiation* [2]; typically, the response to tetanic stimulation starts with hyperpolarization lasting a few seconds (Fig. D21-2), which is due, no doubt, to summation of recurrent inhibitory potentials. The hyperpolarization is terminated by a prolonged phase of depolarization, which is associated with a successive increase in size and duration of the EPSP. Eventually, these get so large that they completely counteract the recurrent IPSPs. Summation of the EPSPs causes the large depolarization which leads to repeated discharges followed by depolarization block.

It appears likely that the process of frequency potentiation is instrumental in the buildup of intense depolarization of hippocampal cells which leads to the tonic phase of a seizure [5]. This may explain why the deafferented fornix preparation behaves so differently from the intact fornix preparation. In the deafferented preparation, frequency potentiation presumably is weak due to the fact that the fibers which normally conduct orthodromic impulses to the hippocampal neurons have degenerated.

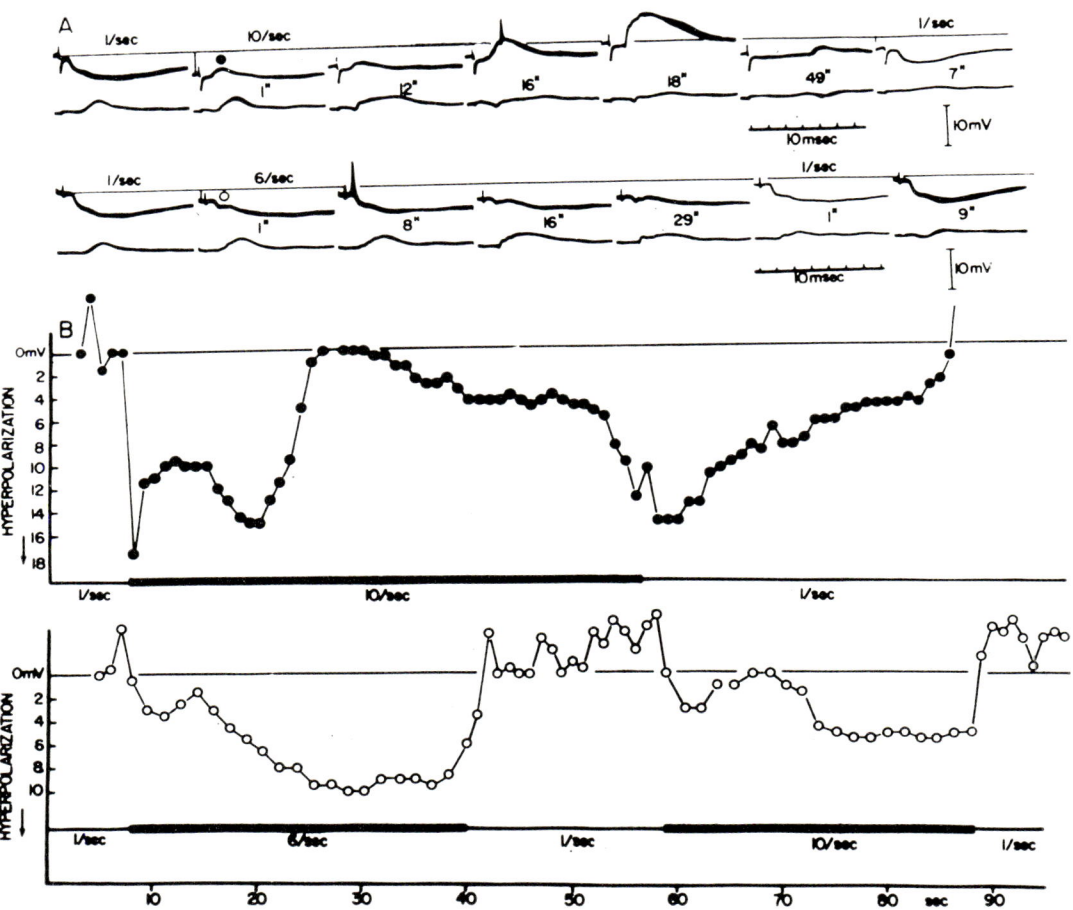

Fig. D21-2. Frequency potentiation of CA3 pyramidal cells. (*A*) Sample records taken from a CA3 pyramidal cell in response to 1 and 10 per sec stimulation of the commissural pathway. Numbers between records indicate time after onset of tetanic stimulation. Upper line: intracellular record; lower line: surface record. (*B*) Membrane potential changes caused by a long-lasting tetanic stimulation of 10 per sec. Lower half gives effect of 6 per sec and 10 per sec tetani.

In short, it is possible that the powerful increase of synaptic transmission, which is a notable feature of the hippocampal neuronal systems, may be important in the buildup of seizure activity. This represents an alternative to the hypothesis that depolarization is due to lack of inhibition. Unfortunately, no technique is available to determine whether profound depolarization in response to tetanic stimulation is due to active increase of synaptic excitation or due to lack of inhibition.

FREQUENCY SENSITIVITY OF RECURRENT INHIBITION

The experiment illustrated in Fig. D21-3 is pertinent to the discussion of whether recurrent inhibition breaks down with high frequency stimulation. In this particular experiment, frequency potentiation of excitatory synapses was very slow and of relatively small amplitude. Normally, frequency potentiation starts after 2–4 sec and usually overwhelms the recurrent inhibitory period, as shown in Fig. D21-2. However, the sweep is very slow in Fig. D21-3 so that recurrent IPSPs occur as vertical, downward deflections. The membrane potential of this CA3 pyramidal cell was around -60 mV. Fimbrial stimulation elicited an ordinary recurrent IPSP which brought the membrane potential to approximately -80 mV. At 5-per-sec stimulation, the IPSPs that were produced occurred with normal amplitude. At 50-per-sec stimulation for 8 sec (A), the IPSP summed with a virtual clamping of the membrane potential at about -80 mV. After the first 4 sec, however, there was a slight decline of the membrane potential. Following this tetanic period, the first single-volley recurrent IPSP increased the membrane potential to -78 mV only; and the duration of this IPSP was markedly prolonged. The second and third IPSPs had normal shape and peak potential level, but full restitution was not obtained until after about 10 sec. Between (A) and (B), there were four 8-sec periods with tetanic stimulation at 50 per sec. The fifth period was longer than the other periods, lasting for about 12 sec.

During the tetanic stimulation, there was clearly decline of the membrane potential, perhaps due to reduced release of inhibitory transmitter. This conclusion was drawn because the first three IPSPs after the tetanic period elicited by a low stimulus rate were less effective than the control record. A relatively good restitution was obtained after about 10 sec, but full restitution of the recurrent inhibitory process was not obtained until after about one minute.

These experiments suggest a possibility of reducing the efficacy of recurrent inhibition by longstanding tetanic stimulation. However, the stimulation must last for several tens of seconds to produce a marked deficit of recurrent inhibition. From such evidence it appears likely that the frequency potentiation process is more important for development of seizures than for withdrawal or depression of the inhibitory system. However, since the inhibition is shown to be frequency sensitive, this last possibility

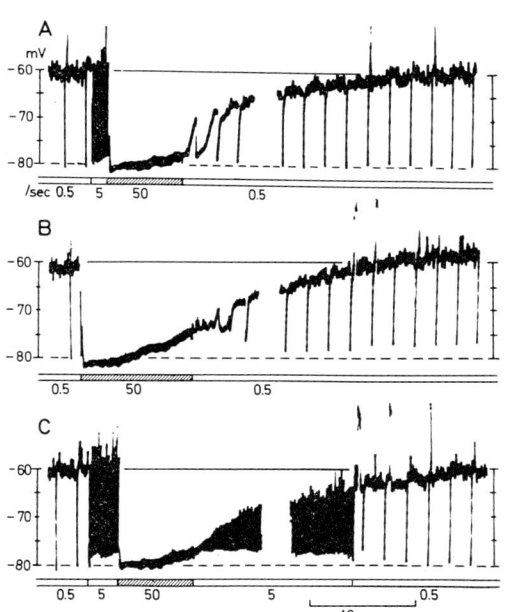

FIG. D21-3. Frequency sensitivity of recurrent inhibition. Intracellular records from a CA3 pyramidal cell in response to fimbrial stimulation at rates indicated by figures below each record. Note slow reduction of hyperpolarization during high frequency tetanus and relatively fast recovery. Between (A) and (B), three similar tetanic periods were given. (C) Followed 1 min after (B).

may also play a certain role in development of seizure activity.

REGIONAL VARIABILITY IN SEIZURE SUSCEPTIBILITY

A remarkable feature of the hippocampal formation is the ease with which seizure discharges can be produced [4], a phenomenon which has been repeatedly confirmed by a number of investigators. Although seizures are easily produced in CA1 and CA3 regions, containing mostly pyramidal cells, it has been impossible to ascribe any seizure activity to granule cells of the dentate fascia. So far, no adequate explanation can be offered for this striking discrepancy; both granule cells and hippocampal pyramidal cells are subject to effective excitatory synaptic activation. Furthermore, in both areas there are powerful recurrent inhibitory mechanisms. A possible explanation of the different seizure tendencies, although tentative, might be sought in the smaller relative increase in the granule cell compound discharge as compared with pyramidal cell discharge during frequency potentiation conditions.

In the dentate fascia, granule cells are relatively easily excited by an afferent perforant path volley from the entorhinal area. Although frequency potentiation of granule cell discharges is easily produced, the relative increase is less than the potentiation of pyramidal cells. In the anesthetized preparation, a single volley usually produces a relatively small number of discharged pyramidal cells. However, with frequency potentiation, the number of cells increases by a factor of several hundred. Thus, the more effective frequency potentiation in hippocampal pyramidal cells may perhaps be responsible for the seizure tendency in this region. Admittedly, there are a number of alternative explanations for this difference, such as a greater number of synapses and a larger tendency to recurrent facilitatory systems among pyramidal cells.

CONCLUSION

The process of frequency potentiation of excitatory synapses is offered as an alternative hypothesis for the initiation of seizure activity. This may occur in addition to the postulated depression of the inhibitory mechanism. Frequency potentiation increases the ability of an afferent path to excite the neurons and may thereby overcome the powerful recurrent inhibition which is found in all parts of the hippocampal system; the inhibition affects mainly the cells on each side of an excited beam. In the dorsal part of the hippocampus, this excited beam is found in a slice of hippocampal tissue, oriented nearly parallel to the midline. In more lateral positions, the slices are oriented homologously, but with increased tilting corresponding to the curvature of the hippocampal formation. This arrangement may account for the initial tendency to suppress the spreading of a seizure. However, due to profound depolarization, even this powerful inhibition is overridden by the excitatory process, and the seizure activity may then spread to the rest of the hippocampal formation as well as to the other side.

REFERENCES

1. Andersen, P., Holmqvist, B., and Voorhoeve, P. E. Entorhinal activation of dentate granule cells. *Acta Physiol. Scand.* 66:448, 1966.
2. Andersen, P., and Lømo, T. Control of Hippocampal Output by Afferent Volley Frequency. In Adey, W. R., and Tokizane, T. (Eds.), *Structure and Function of the Limbic System. Progress in Brain Research.* Amsterdam: Elsevier, 1967, vol. 27.
3. Blackstad, T. W. On the termination of some afferents to the hippocampus and fascia dentata. *Acta Anat.* (Basel) 35:202, 1958.
4. Jung, R. Der Elektrokrampf in corticalen und subcorticalen Hirngebieten. Demonstration und Diskussion des zentralen Krampfmechanismus. *Ber. Ges. Physiol.* 139:211, 1950.
5. Kandel, E. R., and Spencer, W. A. Excitation and inhibition of single pyramidal cells during hippocampal seizure. *Exp. Neurol.* 4:162, 1961.
6. Lømo, T. Potentiation of monosynaptic

EPSPs in cortical cells by single and repetitive volleys. *J. Physiol.* (London) 194:84, 1968.
7. Lømo, T. Recurrent inhibition of dentate granule cells. 1968, unpublished data.
8. Lømo, T. Mechanisms of late facilitation of dentate granule cells. 1968, unpublished data.
9. Lorente de Nó, R. Studies on the structure of the cerebral cortex. II. Continuation of the study of the ammonic system. *J. Psychol. Neurol.* 46:113, 1934.
10. Ramón y Cajal, S. *Histologie du système nerveux de l'Homme et des vertébrés.* Paris: Maloine, 1911, vol. 2.
12. Spencer, W. A., and Kandel, E. R. Hippocampal neuron responses to selective activation of recurrent collaterals of hippocampofugal axons. *Exp. Neurol.* 4:149, 1961.

22
Neurochemical Mechanisms

DONALD B. TOWER

EPILEPSY is symptomatic of a great variety of derangements of, or interferences with, neuronal function, so that the number of possible mechanisms could be potentially very large. However, the recordable characteristics of neurons during spontaneous or induced paroxysmal discharges are much less diverse; in fact, they tend to be very similar or almost stereotyped for many different agents or conditions. Hence it may be reasonable to suppose that there is a final common mechanism or set of mechanisms responsible for epileptogenicity. If it is not yet possible to specify the nature of such a set of mechanisms, certain models can be utilized to define many of the characteristics of these mechanisms and to indicate appropriate directions for future investigations.

Before considering such models in some detail, it is important to discuss briefly some of the problems which the neurochemist faces in studies on epilepsy. Ideally one should study human material but there are serious limitations to this approach. Availability of suitable patients and cooperation of a neurosurgeon oriented to epilepsy are essential. There are procedures (such as isotope tracer studies) which are difficult or impossible to carry out on human subjects. Experimental and sampling procedures must always be subordinated to the welfare of the patient and the demands of good surgical practice. Thus, a biopsy of human brain tissue may, of necessity, be a rather lengthy affair involving a considerable interval of circulatory arrest that could significantly alter or obscure metabolic or compositional characteristics of the sample. The majority of epileptic patients who are currently candidates for surgery do not usually present simple or easily defined epileptogenic foci. And since the patients are epileptic, it is questionable whether one can obtain from them at surgery truly normal samples to serve as controls for the presumed epileptogenic samples.

The alternative use of experimental animal preparations poses equally serious problems. With few exceptions the brains are very small for many of the requisite biochemical techniques. Induced focal epileptogenic lesions are likewise small and difficult to study. There are few problems with regard to availability of normal control samples of tissue but the experimental counterparts of clinical epilepsy are few indeed. Such preparations as penicillin focus, alumina cream focus, and freezing lesion may be relatively similar to clinical foci, but the simpler and more widely utilized techniques, such as electroshock, pentylenetetrazol, strychnine and the like, are hardly comparable. Given a sufficient and appropriate stimulus, any normal neuron will discharge paroxysmally. However, when the stimulus is withdrawn or dissipated, such cells revert to normal with no apparent trace of the episode imprinted for later analytical evaluation and no residual tendency for subsequent spontaneous paroxysmal firing.

Any models which might be proposed should have similar or closely analogous counterparts in man, preferably in the setting of clinical epilepsy. And these models or the mechanisms which are suggested by them should accommodate in a reasonable fashion other well-established aspects of human epilepsy. The latter include such facets as the numerous and diverse precipitating factors (hyperventilation, photic stimulation, sleep, water intoxication, alcohol ingestion, and induction of or withdrawal from narcosis) as well as the actions of anticonvulsant drugs. In many clinical cases there are demonstrable pathological lesions present. Some of them are associated with seizures in a causal relationship. Others are either incidental or are themselves the consequences of seizure activity. Clearly, seizures can and do occur in the absence of any visibly demonstrable lesion, so that a basic premise for subsequent discussions is that many or most cases of epilepsy involve a biochemical lesion as the underlying or final common mechanism. The models or analogies presented here will indicate those types of biochemical lesions which are likely candidates in this context [192].

SELECTED MODEL MECHANISMS

1. Anticholinesterases and the Role of Acetylcholine

The first model to be considered is perhaps the most clear-cut and thoroughly documented. By now it is well established that at or near neuromuscular junctions and many central synapses there is a system for the synthesis (choline acetylase, hemicholiniums), storage (synaptic vesicles), release (stimulation, botulin toxin), reception (atropine, curare), and inactivation (acetylcholinesterase, organophosphates) of acetylcholine. Furthermore it is generally accepted that acetylcholine functions as a physiological transmitter initiating excitation in the postsynaptic effector unit served by the exciting neuron [39, 85].

When acetylcholine is liberated onto the receptive surface of the postsynaptic membrane, it produces prompt depolarization of some 6–30 mV, recordable as an excitatory postsynaptic potential (EPSP). If the EPSP is of sufficient magnitude, alterations in membrane conductance for sodium and potassium occur, which in turn initiate and propagate an action potential along the conducting membrane of the postsynaptic effector cell. It has been estimated that 10^5 or 10^6 moles of sodium and potassium ions move across the membrane per mole of acetylcholine released [39]. The process is normally self-limiting as the liberated acetylcholine is removed by means of hydrolytic inactivation by acetylcholinesterase and to a small extent by diffusion.

In the presence of a potent cholinesterase inhibitor, such as diisopropylfluorophosphate (DFP) or tetraethylpyrophosphate (TEPP), the accumulation of unhydrolyzed acetylcholine and the concomitant development of seizures can be clearly demonstrated, as in the studies reported by Stone [180]. He employed morphinized dogs, prepared to counteract systemic effects of the inhibitor with atropine (0.075 mg per kg) and artificial respiration. A dose of 2 mg per kg body weight of TEPP was administered intravenously. Within 5–10 min characteristic epileptiform activity appeared in the EEG (Fig. 22-1) associated with frank convulsions and markedly elevated levels of acetylcholine in brain samples (Table 22-1) biopsied after freezing the cerebral cortex

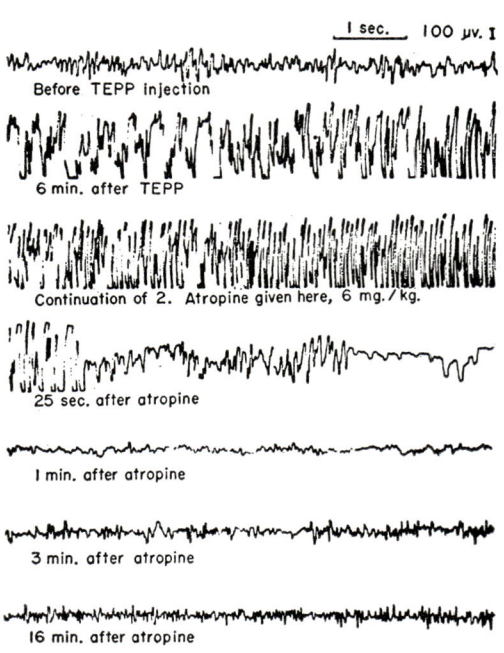

Fig. 22-1. Epileptiform activity in the EEG of a dog after intravenous administration of 2 mg per kg of TEPP, and its suppression by intravenous administration of atropine. (Reproduced from Fig. 7, Stone [180], by permission of the author and the publishers of *Amer. J. Phys. Med.*)

TABLE 22-1. Effects of TEPP on Various Constituents of Dog Cerebral Cortex

Constituents	Controls $n=11$	After TEPP[a] $n=5$	After Atropine[b] $n=2$
Acetylcholine micromoles/kg	6.8 (± 1.1)	9.95 (± 1.35)	24.4; 28.6
Lactic acid micromoles/g	1.1	4.9	4.0
Creatine P micromoles/g	2.3	2.0	1.8
Inorganic P micromoles/g	3.0	3.4	3.0
Acid-labile P micromoles/g	5.9	5.3	5.3

[a] Within 2–15 min after TEPP, 2 mg per kg intravenously, with epileptiform activity present in the EEG and seizures observed.
[b] After seizures were abolished by atropine sulfate, 6 mg per kg intravenously, 13–21 min before biopsy.
Data taken from Stone [180].

in situ with liquid air. At this time there was no activity of acetylcholinesterase measurable in the cerebral tissues of these dogs. The epileptiform activity in the EEG and the accompanying clinical convulsions could be abolished by large doses (6 mg per kg intravenously) of atropine (Fig. 22-1), despite persistence of elevated levels of acetylcholine in the brain (Table 22-1), these observations clearly indicating that the cerebral, cholinergic postsynaptic receptor sites could be protected by atropine from the excessive amounts of acetylcholine impinging upon them.

Similarly Baker and Benedict [15] have shown that microinjections of DFP (30 µg) directly into the hippocampus of the cat would elicit within 7 min paroxysmal discharges which persisted uninterruptedly for several hours. As the effect wore off, injections of normally ineffective doses of acetylcholine (1–5 µg) would reactivate or potentiate the discharges. These effects could be antagonized by intrahippocampal scopolamine (30 µg) within about 20 min after injection and dramatically reversed by injections of 50 µg of the cholinesterase reactivator, pyridine-2-aldoxime methiodide (P-2-AM), within 10 min. These effects of acetylcholine and of P-2-AM were restricted to experiments involving DFP and could not be demonstrated with discharges induced by other classes of convulsants.

The inhibitors of acetylcholinesterase employed in the foregoing experiments belong to the class of organophosphorus nerve gases and insecticides which inactivate the enzyme temporarily or permanently. It is of interest that TEPP was synthesized by Philippe de Clermont in 1854 [45] ten years before Jobst and Hesse [95] isolated physostigmine from the Calabar bean. Yet the toxicity of TEPP was not discovered until the work of Lange and Schrader in the 1930s [88, 89], whereas the Calabar bean was well known as the "ordeal" poison used by West African natives and many of its pharmacological properties had been demonstrated prior to the identification of its principal active ingredient as physostigmine [107].

On the basis of extensive studies by Wilson and his colleagues, it is now known that the hydrolysis of acetylcholine by acetylcholinesterase involves an acetylation of the enzyme, as the choline moiety is released, followed by rapid reaction with water to release the acetate moiety and regenerate the enzyme [213]; the action of the organophosphorus inhibitors is to phosphorylate the enzyme, forming a bonding which is only slowly or not at all susceptible to hydrolysis with water [130] and yielding an inactive enzyme. Although subsequent studies have indicated that such anticholinesterases as DFP also react with a number of other esterases and proteases and that in each case the phosphorylation appears to involve a serine residue in the region of the active site of the enzyme protein [46], the toxicity of the organophosphorus compounds in vivo seems to be clearly restricted to their effects upon cholinesterases [77].

With the growth since World War II of the industrial manufacture and agricultural use of the organophosphorus compounds, many thousands of cases of poisoning and hundreds of deaths from these agents have been reported [1, 77, 78, 131]. Grob et al. [78] have provided details on 40 cases of accidental poisoning with parathion involving 6 deaths. Of the 8 patients who went into coma, 6 exhibited concomitant convulsions. Determinations of the levels of cholinesterase activity in samples from two of the fatalities showed plasma levels at 0–5 percent of normal, erythrocyte levels at 11–22 percent of normal, and cerebral cortex levels at 22–31 percent of normal. The studies by Wilson on the mechanisms of hydrolysis and of inhibition led him to trials of hydroxylamine and related oximes, which proved to be highly effective in reactivating the inhibited enzyme by virtue of the ability of the oxime to displace and combine with the phosphoryl group [214]. The most useful reactivator has proved to be P-2-AM (pyridine-2-aldoxime methiodide) available for human therapy as pralidoxime chloride [107, 212]. Following its introduction there have been numerous reports of its efficacy in reversing the signs and symptoms of toxicity in clinical cases of organophosphorus poisonings [78, 131] in conjunction with supportive therapy with atropine [74] and other appropriate measures [77].

This first model of epileptogenicity implies that derangements of normal functioning of the acetylcholine transmitter system could be a factor in the final common mechanism of epileptogenicity. It is now quite clear that not all central synapses are cholinergic and that not all convulsant agents operate by means of derangements of cholinergic systems [15, 180]. However, there is evidence to indicate a normally close association between levels of cerebral activity and levels of cerebral acetylcholine [42, 118] as well as circumstantial evidence suggesting the possibility of alterations in the acetylcholine system in clinical epilepsy [143, 196, 197].

In confirmation of the earlier experiments of MacIntosh and Oborin [118], Celesia and Jasper [42] demonstrated a significant correlation between the level of cerebral activity in cats (under local anesthesia and immobilization with gallamine triethiodide) and the release of acetylcholine into a perfusion chamber fitted over the surface of the cerebral cortex. At rest in the waking state, there was a release of 2–4 ng (mμg or 10^{-9} gm) of acetylcholine per cm^2 of cortex per minute into the collection chamber. In light sleep the rate decreased to about 2 ng per min and under deep barbiturate anesthesia to less than 1 ng per min; whereas seizures induced by pentylenetetrazol were associated with a twofold to fourfold increase in the rate of release of acetylcholine. Thus, it is not surprising that acetylcholine is readily detectable in many samples of cerebrospinal fluid from patients with epilepsy but is seldom demonstrable in CSF samples from nonepileptic controls [197].

Samples of cerebral cortex from experimentally induced epileptogenic foci in monkeys [143] and from foci identified at craniotomy on epileptic patients [196] exhibit significant elevations of cholinesterase activity compared to appropriate control samples. In addition, the latter samples, upon incubation, may fail to synthesize the "bound" or storage form of acetylcholine at the normal rate [196], although the validity of this observation remains somewhat in doubt at present [139, 192]. It is difficult to judge whether such metabolic abnormalities relate to the cause of the epileptogenicity or merely reflect the consequences thereof. Nevertheless the circumstantial evidence is sufficient to warrant serious consideration of the factors implicit in this first model mechanism.

2. Vitamin B_6 Dependency and the Role of γ-Aminobutyric Acid

In 1934 György [81] demonstrated a growth factor in the vitamin B complex which he named vitamin B_6 and which over the next decade was identified as a pyridine derivative [83, 112] that could exist in the several forms of pyridoxine, pyridoxal, and pyridoxamine [173, 176] and when phosphorylated as pyridoxal-5'-phosphate or PLP [79], functioned as coenzyme for the enzymatic decarboxylation or transamination of amino acids [68, 114, 159]. In 1949 Roberts and Frankel [151] found in chromatographed extracts of fresh brain tissue an unknown ninhydrin-positive substance which was identified during the following year as γ-aminobutyric acid [13, 152, 199] and shown to be restricted in distribution in animal tissues to brain and spinal cord [5, 17, 148, 151]. The presence of γ-aminobutyric acid in bacteria [5, 67] and in plant tissues [5, 185] had already been established.

This unique tissue distribution reflected distribution of the synthesizing enzyme, glutamic decarboxylase, which was found to be limited to central nervous tissues [7, 17, 153, 154]. The brain enzyme resembled plant and bacterial glutamic decarboxylases in requiring for its optimal activity pyridoxal-5′-phosphate as coenzyme [154, 156]. The complete system for synthesis and metabolism of γ-aminobutyric acid in brain was subsequently demonstrated in detail, comprising, in addition to glutamic decarboxylase, the transaminase converting γ-aminobutyric acid to succinic semialdehyde [26, 150, 158] and the aldehyde dehydrogenase completing its conversion to succinate [9]. It was immediately recognized that this pathway for synthesis and metabolism of γ-aminobutyric acid provided an alternative or shunt to the classical Krebs cycle steps from α-ketoglutarate to succinate in the oxidation of intermediary metabolites in brain [5, 9, 26, 150]. Evidence that this shunt could indeed function was provided by the studies of Tsukada et al. [198] and McKhann and co-workers [119, 121, 122].

Three independent sets of clinical observations in the period 1953–1954 set the stage for convergence of the foregoing metabolic data onto problems of epilepsy and thereby provide a second model mechanism. After identification of the chemical nature of vitamin B_6, reports rapidly accumulated indicating that severe dietary deficiency of vitamin B_6 was associated in a variety of avian and mammalian species with convulsions which promptly responded without exception to supplements of pyridoxine [187]. Evidence for inclusion of man in the foregoing generalization was first provided by Snyderman et al. [177], who observed convulsions responsive to pyridoxine in a human infant 76 days after institution of a B_6-deficient diet. Dramatic confirmation of the human nutritional requirement for vitamin B_6 was provided by the "epidemic" of some 300 convulsing infants reported in 1954 following a change in the processing of a liquid infant formula that inadvertently destroyed its B_6 content [2, 24, 48, 49, 126, 128]. Coursin [48, 49] studied a number of these infants in detail and demonstrated termination of seizures and normalization of EEGs within minutes after the intravenous administration of pyridoxine hydrochloride—a rapidity of response clearly indicative of a neurochemical lesion. At this same time Hunt et al. [90] reported the first case of pyridoxine or vitamin B_6 dependency: a human infant who developed in the immediate neonatal period seizures unresponsive to the usual anticonvulsants but completely controlled by a daily maintenance dose of 10 mg or more of pyridoxine. At age 6 years [178], the effects of withdrawal of vitamin B_6 therapy were still readily demonstrable; EEG abnormalities and clinical seizures appeared within 72 hr after withdrawal and were dramatically reversed within 2 min by an intravenous dose of 15 mg of pyridoxine-HCl (Fig. 22-2). This youngster continues to be severely retarded mentally and at last report at age 12 years was still dependent upon daily vitamin B_6 supplementation for control of seizures [51].

Reports of other cases of vitamin B_6 dependency have followed (Table 22-2). In the original report by Hunt et al. [90] there was a history of two previous siblings, one normal, the other dying with intractable convulsions in the immediate neonatal period. This indication that vitamin B_6 dependency might be a familial syndrome has received strong support from several subsequent reports of documented occurrence of the disorder in more than one sibling of the same family [125, 201], as well as strong circumstantial evidence from a number of other reports (Table 22-2). Thus this relatively rare clinical syndrome provides a model mechanism for epilepsy that appears to involve a readily reversible neurochemical lesion which is genetically determined.

Like many genetically determined disorders, there may be several variants of the vitamin B_6 dependency syndrome. Scriver has proposed that the apparently familial "deficiency syndrome" in which there is a lesser daily requirement for vitamin B_6 supplementation but widespread evidence of

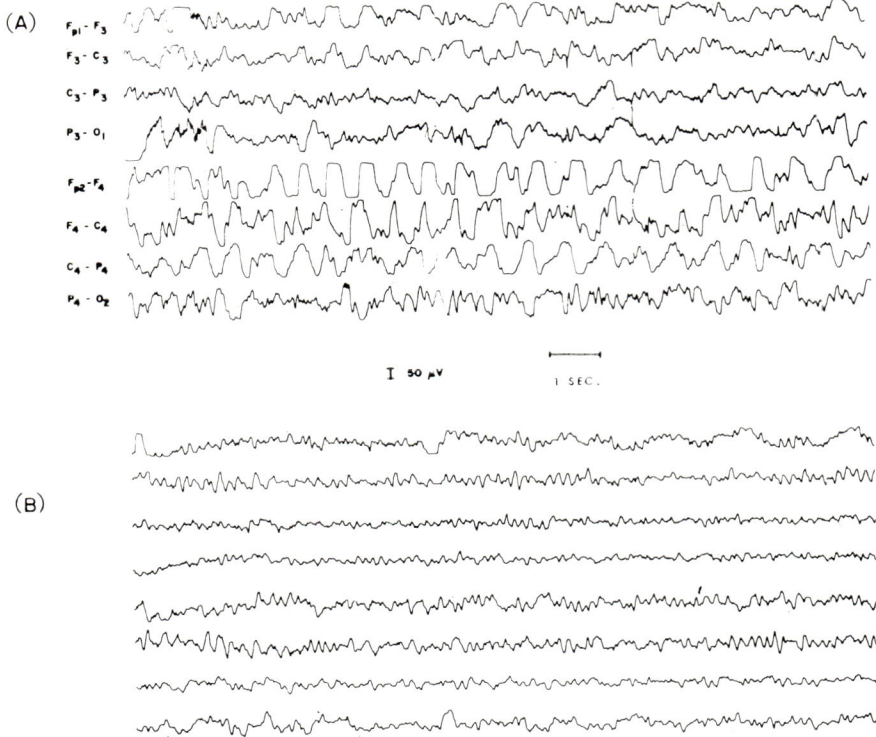

Fig. 22-2. EEG records taken from a 6-year-old child with vitamin B_6 dependency. *Upper record* illustrates epileptiform activity present 72 hr after withdrawal of maintenance dose of pyridoxine. *Lower record* shows the normalization achieved within 2 min after the intravenous administration of 15 mg of pyridoxine [178].

malfunction of vitamin B_6-dependent systems (tryptophan metabolism, cystathionine metabolism, hematopoiesis, and seizures) may be related to "vitamin B_6 dependency with seizures" as a more general disorder of vitamin B_6 utilization or metabolism or both [165, 167].

Subsequent studies correlating γ-aminobutyric acid metabolism and the functional roles of the B_6 vitamers have elucidated the details of the model. A number of antagonists of the B_6 vitamers, such as deoxypyridoxine and methoxypyridoxine [14, 69, 146], and compounds, principally of the hydrazide group, which chemically inactivate the coenzyme pyridoxal-5′-phosphate (PLP) as a hydrazone complex [14], can elicit in both experimental animals and man seizures which are exquisitely amenable to therapy with vitamin B_6 or γ-aminobutyric acid or both [14, 69, 105, 187, 192]. When the intake of B_6 vitamers is prevented by deficient diets there is considerable variation in vulnerability of the bodily enzymes requiring PLP as coenzyme [187], but one of the enzymes most sensitive to B_6-deficiency is glutamic decarboxylase [17, 156, 187] which in animals is uniquely localized to the central nervous system. This same enzyme is also especially sensitive to the effects of neurotoxic hydrazides [17, 103, 104, 153, 154].

Baxter and Roberts [17] have adduced evidence that the relative affinities of the PLP coenzyme for mouse brain apoenzymes is in the ratio of 1:10 for glutamic decarboxylase versus γ-aminobutyrate transaminase, so that dissociation of the coenzyme from the decarboxylase apoenzyme would occur very much more readily. After seizures have been induced by hydrazides, Bain and Williams [14] found that brain

TABLE 22-2. Reported Cases of Vitamin B_6 Dependency[a]

Case No.	Reported by	Ref. No.	Onset of Seizures at Age	Age B_6 Begun	With-drawal Test	Maint. on B_6	Re-tarded[b]	Affected[c] / Total Siblings
1	Hunt et al., 1954	90	3 hr	1 mo	+	+	+	2/3
2	Bessey et al., 1957; Adam and Hansen, 1958	25 3	58 hr	5 da	+	+	0	1/2
3	Marie et al., 1959, 1961	124	5 da	2 mo	+	+	+	2/3
4		125	5 da	5 da	+	+	0	
5	Scriver, 1960	164	7 da	10 da	+	+	0	2/3
6	Nordio et al., 1961, 1962	134	8 da	1 mo	+	+	0	2/2
7	Garty et al., 1962	70	Birth	11 da	+	+	?	3/10
8	Waldinger and Berg, 1963	201	3 hr	22 da	+	+	+	3/4
9		201	3 hr	1 da	+	+	0	
10	Zunin and Vallarino, 1963	220	< 20 da	5 mo	+	+	?	2/2
11	French et al., 1965	64	28 hr	5 mo	+	+	+	1/?
12	Robins, 1966	157	Birth	1 mo	+	+	0	2/2
13	Bejšovec et al., 1967	21	In utero	Birth	+	+	0	3/3
14	Gentz et al., 1967	71	21 da	3 mo	+	+	?	1/6[d]
Total	[12 families]							24/41

[a] Only those cases were included which satisfied the following criteria: (1) onset of generalized seizures at or shortly after birth; (2) refractoriness of seizures to usual types of anticonvulsant therapy; (3) immediate response to oral or parenteral vitamin B_6; (4) intolerance to withdrawal of vitamin B_6; hence requirement for permanent maintenance dose (usually about 10 mg orally per day); and (5) no evidence of dietary B_6 deficiency, i.e., negative tryptophan load tests, etc. On this basis, one case of Bessey et al. [25] and cases reported by Denève and Jongbloet [58], Scriver and Hutchinson [167], Scriver and Cullen [166], Christiaens et al. [44], and Schmidt [160] were excluded. A report by Rezzonico and Funes [147] was unavailable for evaluation. The tabulation is not necessarily complete since exhaustive search of the world literature has not been undertaken.

[b] Conclusions regarding presence or absence of mental retardation must be cautious since some of the evaluations were reported at ages too early for reliable assessment. In addition, it seems evident that some variation in severity of the syndrome may be present (as judged from the time of onset of seizures) so that any potential association between time of initiating vitamin B_6 therapy and presence or absence of subsequent mental retardation would be difficult to establish.

[c] The total number listed as *affected* includes siblings, other than the 14 documented cases, in which circumstantial evidence from the history was sufficient to warrant a strong suspicion that such siblings were also vitamin B_6 dependent.

[d] Two siblings were known to have epilepsy but of a type responsive to usual anticonvulsants and unresponsive to vitamin B_6.

levels of pyridoxal-5′-phosphate were approximately 25 percent of normal control levels, and Killam [103, 104] demonstrated that the effects of the hydrazides were limited to inhibition (at about 50 percent of normal) of cerebral glutamic decarboxylase together with reduction (by about 50 percent) of brain levels of γ-aminobutyric acid. The administration of vitamin B_6 intravenously or of γ-aminobutyric acid locally to the brain (topical or intraventricular) resulted in prompt abolition of the seizure activity and reversion of the EEG to normal [105].

Thus, there was increasing evidence favoring the view that interference with the production and/or the maintenance of γ-aminobutyric acid in the central nervous system would result in seizures. If this were so and if the γ-aminobutyric acid shunt functioned significantly in substrate oxidations in brain, depression of the latter ought to be demonstrable when cerebral glutamic decarboxylase was inhibited either by vitamin B_6 deficiency or by hydrazides. Studies by McKhann et al. [119, 120] provided support for this view by showing that in kittens fed a vitamin B_6-deficient diet to the point of convulsions, the oxygen consumption of incubated slices of cerebral cortex was 80–85 percent of pair-fed controls, but could be increased to control values by addition of pyridoxal-5′-phosphate; comparable depressions of oxygen consumption were exhibited by incubated slices of cerebral cortex from mice convulsing after administration of thiosemicarbazide or L-2,4-diaminobutyric acid. These studies indicated that as much as 20–40 percent of the substrate metabolized by neural cells in the stage between α-ketoglutarate and succinate might be metabolized via the γ-aminobutyric acid shunt pathway [119, 122], although other more recent work suggests that for some species at least the contribution of the shunt pathway may be considerably less [16].

It is of considerable interest in this regard that when the original case of vitamin B_6 dependency reported by Hunt et al. [90] was restudied at age 6 years by Sokoloff et al. [178], measurements of cerebral oxygen consumption while the patient was convulsing in the depleted state (Fig. 22-2) gave a value significantly lower than that measured immediately following repletion with 15 mg of pyridoxine-HCl intravenously. The respective values (in micromoles of O_2 per 100 gm of brain per min) were 147 (depleted) and 197 (after repletion) compared to mean values of 211 for epileptic children interictally and of 201 for mentally retarded children [192]. Furthermore, when Marie et al. [125] studied one of their vitamin B_6-dependent patients during the depleted state, they were able on two occasions to stop the seizures and obtain normalization of the EEG by intravenous administration of 2 gm of γ-aminobutyric acid (Fig. 22-3).

None of these observations can be considered more than circumstantial evidence, and much of the data is susceptible to alternative interpretations. But there are additional findings from other types of seizure preparations and clinical epilepsy which also tend to implicate the γ-aminobutyrate system. When slices of cerebral cortex taken from animals with seizures induced by a variety of agents (methionine sulfoximine, 3,3-methylethylglutarimide (bemegride), thiosemicarbazide) are incubated under optimal conditions in vitro, the levels of glutamic acid after incubation for one hour are only about 50 percent (or less) of levels in normal control slices [190,

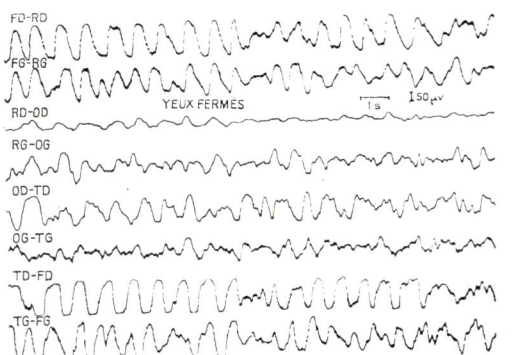 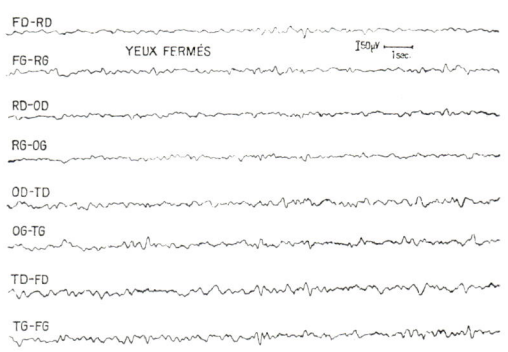

FIG. 22-3. EEG records taken from an 11-month-old child with vitamin B_6 dependency. *Left record* illustrates epileptiform activity present 6 days after withdrawal of maintenance dose of pyridoxine. *Right record* shows the normalization achieved within 25 min after intravenous administration of 2 gm of γ-aminobutyric acid. (Reproduced from Figs. 2a and b of Marie et al. [125] by permission of the authors and of the publishers of *Rev. Neurol.*)

192]. Incubated slices from human cerebral cortex are comparable, the control values being 10.0 (±0.95) micromoles of glutamic acid per gram fresh weight compared to 5.15 (±0.95) for samples from epileptogenic foci [190]. Analogous findings have been reported by Berl et al. [22], who produced cortical foci by ethyl chloride spray; coincident with the onset of spiking in the focus, the level of glutamic acid in the focus was found to have decreased about 46 percent from pre-ictal and control samples but no changes in levels of γ-aminobutyrate were detected. These investigators suggested that depletion of glutamate might reflect attempts to maintain γ-aminobutyrate levels and they demonstrated the efficacy of intravenous glutamate or γ-aminobutyrate in suppression of these focal epileptic discharges. Neither glutamic acid or γ-aminobutyric acid penetrate the central nervous system compartment readily in normal subjects [163, 200] but when the blood-brain barrier systems are impaired, as in the experiments of Berl et al. [22], delivery to the brain can be achieved. Whether this situation obtains in other cases where γ-aminobutyrate has proved efficacious remains to be established, but the reports by Hawkins and Sarett [84] for animals convulsed with 3,3-methylethylglutarimide or pentylenetetrazol and by Tower [191] for some patients with clinical epilepsy (Fig. 22-4) clearly demonstrate the anticonvulsant efficacy of γ-aminobutyric acid in these specific instances.

On the basis of some of the foregoing observations, attempts have been made to alter pharmacologically the levels of γ-aminobutyric acid in brain. By the use of the carbonyl reagents, hydroxylamine and amino-oxyacetic acid, which differentially inhibit the γ-aminobutyrate transaminase, it is possible to produce significant and long-lasting increases in the levels of γ-aminobutyric acid in many brain areas [18, 202]. While these effects are associated with anticonvulsant effects under some conditions [40, 63, 149], the situation is not that simple, since thiosemicarbazide will still induce seizures in the presence of hydroxylamine-induced elevations of brain γ-aminobutyrate [155]; L-2,4-diaminobutyric acid produces seizures and markedly elevated

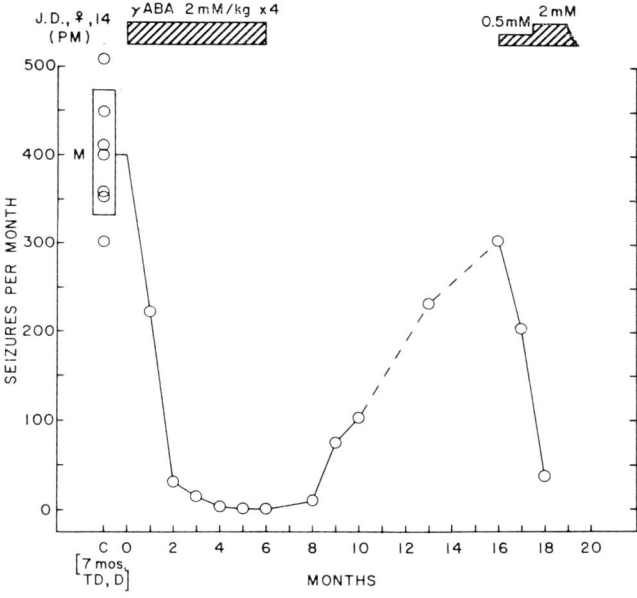

FIG. 22-4. Monthly seizure record of a 14-year-old patient with petit mal. During 7-month control period on trimethadione and diphenylhydantoin therapy, seizures averaged 402 (±68) per month. Effect of oral doses of γ-aminobutyric acid (2 mM per kg four times daily) is shown [191].

brain γ-aminobutyrate levels [119]; and both hydroxylamine and amino oxyacetic acid can themselves produce seizures [127, 202]. One conclusion that has been suggested for these rather confusing observations is that the important factor may not be the brain level per se of γ-aminobutyric acid, but the maintenance of metabolism through the γ-aminobutyric acid-shunt pathway [119, 183].

Finally, account must be taken of the recently established role for γ-aminobutyric acid as a mediator of inhibitory transmission at various invertebrate and mammalian synapses. Initial studies of the topical or local effects of γ-aminobutyric acid on neural systems were suggestive of a role as an inhibitory transmitter [91, 111] or at least as a modulator of neuronal activity [20, 55, 56, 62], but almost a decade passed before definitive evidence to support these views was obtained. It was soon noted that in the crayfish stretch-receptor preparation or at the lobster neuromuscular synapse, γ-aminobutyric acid clearly mimicked the effect of stimulation of the inhibitory nerve [110]. In the latter system Kravitz and Potter [108] found a distribution of γ-aminobutyric acid content in the ratio for inhibitory versus excitatory axons of 100:1, and Otsuka et al. [137] demonstrated that only the inhibitory nerves released γ-aminobutyric acid on stimulation, the amount per stimulus being 1 to 4×10^{-14} moles. Shortly after these observations, Krnjević and Schwartz [109] and Obata [136] provided evidence that the effects of γ-aminobutyric acid applied iontophoretically to neurons of sensorimotor cortex or Deiter's nucleus, respectively, of the cat duplicated those of central postsynaptic inhibition, including hyperpolarization of the cells. In addition, recent observations have suggested a correlation between the level of cerebral activity and release of amino acids into a perfusion chamber fitted over the surface of the cerebral cortex. These observations were analogous to those on acetylcholine by Celesia and Jasper [42] cited above. Jasper et al. [93] showed that during "arousal," the release of γ-aminobutyrate averaged about 12 ng per cm^2 of cortex per min compared to a rate of release of about 33 ng per min during sleep. There were reciprocal changes in release of glutamic acid but no effects on glutamine or aspartic acid. Altogether the foregoing data argue strongly for identification of γ-aminobutyric acid as a physiological transmitter initiating inhibition in the postsynaptic effector unit served by the inhibiting neuron. As such, it might be considered a natural anticonvulsant [192].

This discussion has dealt at some length with the question of why the syndrome of vitamin B_6 dependency and other related conditions are associated with seizure states or epilepsy. The nature of the neurochemical lesion itself also deserves consideration in order to appreciate the full dimensions of this model mechanism for epilepsy. Several investigators [51, 82, 165] have discussed many of the possible alternatives, which may be summarized thus:

POSSIBLE MECHANISMS FOR REDUCTION OF THE EFFECTIVE PYRIDOXAL-5'-PHOSPHATE POOL SIZE

Factors of Supply

A. Primary intake inadequate (*dietary deficiency*)
B. Faulty delivery
   1. Defective intestinal absorption
   2. Defective cellular penetration
C. Excessive excretion
   1. Lowered renal threshold
   2. Increased oxidation to 4-pyridoxic acid

Factors of Metabolism

A. Increased demand (*pregnancy, fever, aging*)
B. Impaired phosphorylation
   1. Defective pyridoxal kinase (*genetic*)
   2. Inhibition of pyridoxal kinase (*pyridoxal hydrazones*)
   3. Faulty energy generation (*lack of ATP*)
C. Chemical inactivation (*hydrazides*) or competition of antimetabolites

Factors Associated with the Apoenzyme

A. Absence of apoenzyme (*genetic deletion*)
B. Altered affinity of apoenzyme for coenzyme
C. Impaired complexing of holoenzyme with substrate

Some may be eliminated at once. There is no evidence that the primary dietary intake is generally inadequate, since a cardinal feature of vitamin B_6 dependency is the absence of the usual features of B_6 deficiency such as positive tryptophan load tests, cystathioninuria, or anemia. Similarly faulty delivery or impaired phosphorylation may be ruled out since the response to oral or parenteral administration of pyridoxine is dramatically prompt, indicating rapid absorption and cellular penetration and functionally effective conversion to the coenzyme form.

Details of the metabolism and coenzyme functions of the B_6 vitamers have been reviewed by Snell [174, 175]. Among the important contributions by Snell and co-workers is the demonstration that the hydrazones of pyridoxal formed from various hydrazides and carbonyl reagents are potent inhibitors of pyridoxal kinase [115, 116], acting at concentrations a thousand-fold less than the concentrations necessary to inhibit such enzymes as glutamic decarboxylase. As Snell [174] has pointed out, reduced activity of pyridoxal kinase, either genetically determined or chemically induced, would drastically curtail the supply of pyridoxal-5′-phosphate despite adequate dietary intake of B_6 vitamers; simply increasing the intake would be of little value in alleviating the situation. If the usual types of increased demand are eliminated and if chemical inactivation can be considered unlikely, the possibilities are narrowed to excessive excretion or to abnormalities directly related to the specific apoenzyme (presumably glutamic decarboxylase) of brain.

On the basis of various metabolic studies in rats by Johansson et al. [96] and in human subjects by Coursin [50] and by Baysal et al. [19] after dietary depletion of vitamin B_6, it is evident that dietary deficiency is associated with a rapid decrease in urinary output of B_6 vitamers and their principal oxidation product, 4-pyridoxic acid, as well as marked reduction of circulating amounts and tissue stores of B_6 vitamers (Table 22-3). Analyses of the contents of B_6 vitamers in specific tissues are consonant with these conclusions [14, 184]. After administration orally or parenterally to rats (Table 22-3) or to man (Table 22-4), tritium-labeled pyridoxine distributes to two gross "compartments," one (A) comprising 5–10 percent of the total body B_6 with a rapid turnover (half-life less than one day) and the other (B) representing the body storage or tissue pool with a turnover at the slow rate of about 1–4 percent of the total body store per day. Dietary deficiency does not alter these turnover rates significantly. In a study of the original case of vitamin B_6 dependency [90], Coursin [50] reported normal blood levels but markedly increased urinary excretion of B_6 vitamers with less than the normal percentage as urinary 4-pyridoxic acid.

In his original report on another case of vitamin B_6 dependency, Scriver [164] also suggested, on the basis of the 4-pyridoxic acid excretion pattern, that excessive renal clearance of B_6 vitamers appeared to be the responsible factor. However, Scriver and Cullen [166] were subsequently unable to demonstrate an abnormality in 4-pyridoxic acid or B_6 vitamer excretion patterns in this same case or in several others. Similarly, Johansson et al. [97] and Gentz et al. [71], utilizing tritium-labeled pyridoxine (Table 22-4), found that the rate of elimination of B_6 vitamers from the body reser-

TABLE 22-3. Metabolism of ^{3}H-Labeled Pyridoxine by Normal and Vitamin B_6-Deficient Rats

Distribution	Pool Sizes (micromoles)		Turnover Rate ($T\frac{1}{2}$)	
	Normal	Deficient	Normal	Deficient
Storage compartment (B)	11–32	2.3–4.7	71 days	110 days
↕ Daily transfer	0.4–0.8	0.18	(1%/day)	(0.5–1%/day)
"Circulating" compartment (A)	0.3–5	0.12–0.27	13 hr	21 hr
↓				
Daily urine output	0.15–0.47	0.02–0.035		
(% as 4-pyridoxic acid)	(30%)	(10–20%)		

Data taken from Johansson et al. [96].

TABLE 22-4. Metabolism of ^{3}H-Labeled Pyridoxine by Normal Human Subjects and a B_6-Dependent Patient

Distribution	Pool Sizes (micromoles)		Turnover Rate ($T\frac{1}{2}$)	
	Normal[a]	B_6-dependent[b]	Normal	B_6-dependent
Storage compartment (B)	215–800	2860	18–38 days	21 days
⇅ Daily transfer	58.5–130	160	(2–3%/day)	(3%/day)
"Circulating" compartment (A)	17–83	219	15–17.5 hr	16 hr
↓				
Daily urine output	10–21	237		
(% as 4-pyridoxic acid)	(20–40%)	(21%)		
	(33–55%)[c]			

[a] Vitamin B_6 intake in the range of 10–12 micromoles per day. Note that daily urinary excretion usually approximates daily dietary intake.

[b] Studies on a 3-month-old patient were made during maintenance on 40–80 mg (237–475 micromoles) of pyridoxine per day over several months.

[c] Percentage of urinary excretion as 4-pyridoxic acid for normal subjects given daily pyridoxine supplementation of 20–200 mg.

^{3}H-labeled pyridoxine, 50 μg of specific activity 1 μc per μg, was administered intravenously to each subject. Data taken from Johansson et al. [97] and Gentz et al. [71].

voirs of normal human subjects was 2–3 percent per day and that the rate for their vitamin B_6-dependent patient was 3 percent. The turnover rates for the two compartments in this patient were in the normal range and the urinary pyridoxic acid excretion was, if anything, slightly subnormal. These authors concluded that the mechanism of dependency is not an inability to retain B_6 vitamers in the body but could be a consequence of structural abnormalities of one or more apoenzymes resulting in increasing requirements for the coenzyme pyridoxal-5′-phosphate [71]. A precedent for this situation has been reported by Frimpter [65] who found in cases of cystathioninuria no evidence for B_6 deficiency or lack of cystathionase apoenzyme despite correction of the metabolic abnormalities by extra vitamin B_6; however, investigation of the liver enzyme (on biopsy) indicated an impaired ability of the apoenzyme to bind the pyridoxal-5′-phosphate coenzyme.

It must be emphasized that vitamin B_6 dependency is a very rare condition (Table 22-2) and that the vast majority of cases of clinical epilepsy fail to respond at all to massive doses of B_6 vitamers [51, 187]. Coursin [51], Scriver [165], and others have called attention to various small groups of patients not characteristic examples of the dependency syndrome but with increased daily requirements for vitamin B_6, usually accompanied by signs of deficiency (abnormal tryptophan load tests, anemia, and cystathioninuria). Some cases exhibit seizures and in a number of cases there appears to be a familial incidence. These groups may well represent other variants or extensions of the dependency syndrome, as Scriver [165] has suggested. For this reason he has proposed that the classic cases of vitamin B_6 dependency be termed dependency "with convulsions."

Despite the fact that vitamin B_6 dependency is almost a clinical curiosity, it does provide a model for epileptogenicity which emphasizes several factors that may prove to be highly relevant to the final common mechanisms of epileptogenicity. The importance of vitamin B_6 nutrition and function to neuronal function and in particular to the metabolism of cerebral amino acids, notably γ-aminobutyric acid, points to the strategic situation of this set of systems in the metabolic and functional economy of the neuron. The seizures resulting from dysfunctions of these systems may reflect the impairment of energy generation (if γ-aminobutyrate oxidation is critical) or interference with inhibitory processes (if the transmitter role of γ-aminobutyrate is paramount) or both. Further studies of this type of model are likely to prove extremely fruitful.

3. Hypoxia and the Role of Cellular Energy Metabolism

The third model of epileptogenicity has been known for at least three centuries and is deceptively simple. The prototype is provided by a series of experiments reported by Robert Boyle [35] in 1660. Together with Robert Hooke, Boyle had modified the vacuum pump of Otto Gericke so that he could observe the effects of "exsuction of the air" by his "pneumatical engine" upon such living creatures as a "large Flesh-fly," an "Humble Bee," several snails, a "white Butter-fly," an eel, a lark, a hen sparrow, a number of mice, and a cat [35, 36]. His experimental arrangement is illustrated in Fig. 22-5.

Upon "exsuction of the air," Boyle observed that the insects simply expired but that the birds and mammals exhibited convulsions before they died. He describes the experiment on the lark as follows.

The Vessel being hastily, but carefully clos'd, the Pump was diligently ply'd, and the Bird for a while appear'd lively enough; but upon greater Exsuction of the Air, she began manifestly to droop and appear sick, and very soon after was taken with as violent and irregular Convulsions, as are wont to be observ'd in Poultry, when their heads are wrung off: For the Bird threw herself over and over two or three times, and dyed with her Breast upward, and her Head downwards, and her Neck awry. And though upon the appearing of these convulsions, we turn'd the Stopcock, and let in the Air upon her, yet it came too late; where upon, casting our eyes upon one of those accurate Dyals that go with a *Pendulum,* and were of late ingeniously invented by the Noble and Learned *Hugenius,* we found that the whole Tragedy had been concluded within ten Minutes of an hour, part of which time had been imploy'd in cementing the Cover to the Receiver [35, p. 328].

The description is classic for avian seizures. Similar observations were reported for mice subjected to the same procedure. On the basis of these and numerous control experiments and autopsies, Boyle commented:

. . . there appear'd not much cause to doubt, but that the death of the fore-mention'd Animals proceeded rather from want of Air . . . [35, p. 332].

These Experiments seem'd the more strange, in regard, that during a great part of those few minutes, the Engine could but considerably rarefie the Air (and that too, but by degrees) and at the end of them there remain'd in the Receiver no inconsiderable quantity . . . [35, p. 331].

And then Boyle concluded with the following challenge:

. . . that in almost all the destructive Experiments made in our Engine, the Animals appear'd to die with violently Convulsive Motions: From which, whether Physicians can gather any thing towards the Discovery of the Nature of Convulsive Distempers I leave them to consider [35, p. 332].

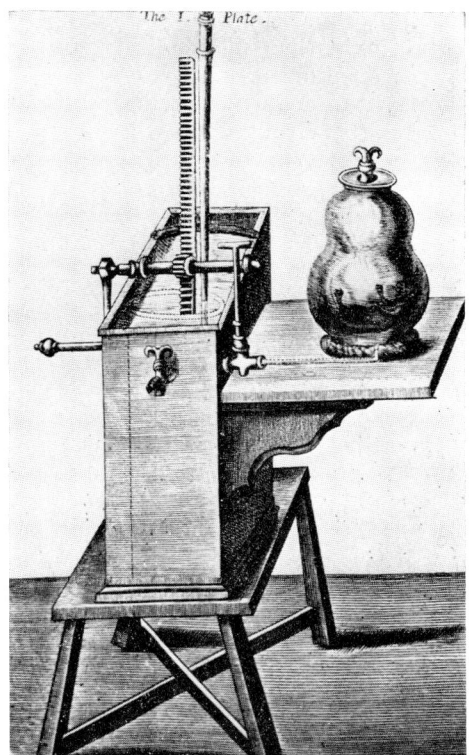

FIG. 22-5. Engraving of Boyle's drawing of his "pneumatical engine," showing a cat having a typical generalized seizure in the evacuated bell jar [36, 192].

Today we know a great deal more about the metabolic circumstances associated with hypoxia or other interferences with supplies of energy-yielding substrates to the central nervous system, but the exact link between failure of energy supplies and the development of seizures is still elusive.

It is firmly established that for normal functioning, the central nervous system is dependent upon continuing delivery via the cerebral circulation of adequate supplies of oxygen and glucose, the latter serving essentially as the sole substrate for cerebral oxidative metabolism. Thus it is not surprising that although the human brain comprises only a small proportion of the total body mass (6 percent in a 6-year-old child and 2 percent in the adult), it commands at rest a significant proportion of the total cardiac output and total bodily oxygen consumption (in the child, 40–50 percent of each; in the adult, 20 percent of each), as well as the major share (65 percent in the adult) of total bodily glucose utilization [192]. When the delivery of supplies is compromised, the consequences are promptly manifest as cerebral dysfunction. The clinical situations of circulatory insufficiency or arrest (stroke, Adams-Stokes syndrome), of hypoxia (such as from high altitude), and of hypoglycemia (functioning pancreatic islet-cell adenoma) are familiar examples of conditions in which convulsions often occur. Experimental interference with glucose utilization by 2-deoxy-D-glucose [188], with oxidative steps in the Krebs cycle by fluorocitrate [140, 141] or by hyperbaric oxygen [129, 215–217], or possibly by ammonia [23, 123, 132, 133], and with the energy-yielding "transducers" of the electron transport system by cyanide [4, 101, 204] are all frequently associated with convulsions.

Yet the search for evidence of specific derangements at some stage in cerebral oxidative metabolism in clinical epilepsy has been rather fruitless, with the possible exception of the γ-aminobutyrate shunt pathway already discussed. Many changes are known to occur coincident with or after the onset of seizures: notably marked increases of cerebral blood flow, cerebral oxygen, and glucose consumption; production by brain of lactic acid; and depletion of tissue levels of oxygen, glucose, and energy-rich phosphates [192]. Despite the increased rates of supply, the demands for energy-rich phosphates appear to outstrip the rate of metabolic generation and thus deplete the brain reserves. However, a series of recent studies by Plum and associates [142, 144] indicates that if the considerable metabolic demands of convulsing skeletal muscles are eliminated (by gallamine triethiodide immobilization), the brain can instantaneously adjust its vascular bed and the systemic blood pressure to meet its metabolic demands, so that during seizures cerebral blood flow and cerebral oxygen supply exceed oxidative demands and only minimal or no output of lactate from brain occurs. As Elliott [61] has concluded, none of the observations indicates that there is necessarily any derangement of, or interference with, the energy-producing potentialities of cerebral tissue that might be involved in initiating seizures. In fact energy production from cerebral oxidative metabolism must be maintained above some critical level to sustain seizure activity. Cerebral anoxemia induced either from circulatory arrest or anoxia promptly arrests on-going seizure activity and produces flattening of the EEG, with rapid reversion to the previous seizure state when the anoxemia is relieved [52, 80, 92].

Even if the hypoxia model is imperfect in the sense that it is not possible to identify specific neurochemical abnormalities, it may still serve to allow us to "gather [some] thing towards the Discovery of the Nature of Convulsive Distempers. . . ." As this author has pointed out in a previous publication [192], a great variety of factors or agents can cause seizures and by their very variety seem to contradict any idea of a unitary mechanism or set of mechanisms; yet the majority of these factors or agents can be interrelated by the fact that they are directly or indirectly implicated in interference with some stage of cerebral oxidative metabolism. The clue would seem to lie in identifying the cerebral system or systems that are critically dependent upon cerebral oxidative metabolism.

McIlwain [117] has emphasized that the metabolic requirements of neural cells for cell maintenance and basal functioning involve only a fraction (certainly less than half) of the total energy which the cells are capable of generating under optimal conditions in vivo. The balance of energy available is presumably channeled primarily into the cation transport systems which provide the basis for differential distribution of sodium and potassium across neural membranes and for consequent excitability of and conduction by these membranes. It has been estimated that 25–50 percent of the energy derived from cerebral respiratory metabolism may be devoted to the fueling of cation transport [99, 102, 117, 205, 206]. Certainly one of the most dramatic consequences of subjecting neural tissue to anoxia or deprivation of glucose is rapid and complete depletion of intracellular potassium and its replacement by sodium chloride, with concomitant edema and depolarization of the cells [34, 188]. And, in fact, both Keynes [102] and Whittam [205, 206] have proposed that the active (energy-dependent) transport of cations in brain serves as a pacemaker of cerebral respiratory metabolism.

4. Ouabain and the Role of Cerebral Electrolyte Metabolism

The fourth and final model of epileptogenicity is particularly relevant to the immediately preceding discussion. Of the four models it is the newest, probably the least understood, and very possibly the most significant. It had been recognized for some years that the differential distribution of monovalent cations across cell membranes, specifically the apparent exclusion of sodium ion from various cells, could be explained if the sodium ions were extruded from the cells as fast as they entered by some active process [57] linked to cellular respiratory metabolism [179]. But it was not until about a decade ago that some understanding of the mechanisms for accomplishing active, energy-linked transport of cations began to emerge.

The occurrence and characteristics of the Mg-dependent, Na-K-activated adenosine triphosphatase (Na-K-ATPase) in the membrane of crab nerve and of human erythrocytes led Skou [169, 170], Post et al. [145], and Dunham and Glynn [60] to suggest that the activity of this enzyme was intimately associated with, if not an integral part of, the active transport system for sodium and potassium. Numerous subsequent reports have indicated: parallel asymmetries of the enzyme and the transport system [60, 87, 207]; correlations in a variety of tissues, including brain and nerve, of enzyme activity with cation fluxes [31]; parallelism of inhibitory effects of ouabain on both systems [32, 145, 170, 171, 205]; and characteristic association of the enzyme system with membrane-rich, subcellular fractions, especially from neural tissues [11, 32, 54, 59, 162, 169, 170, 209]. In addition, as already mentioned, Whittam and colleagues have suggested a close correlation of the activities of the cation transport system and its associated ATPase with cellular respiratory metabolism [205, 206], such that 30–50 percent of cellular energy generation is controlled by the rate of cation transport, mediated via the cellular level of ADP, which in turn is governed by the activity of the Na-K-ATPase [29, 208, 209, 211].

The effects of ouabain on sodium and potassium transport by neural tissues and preparations in vitro is well documented [34, 94, 161, 182, 205, 206, 219]. At concentrations of $10^{-5}M$ or greater, there is essentially total inhibition of the active transport of sodium and potassium, so that such ouabain-inhibited samples of neural tissue show an electrolyte composition close to that of the surrounding extracellular fluid. As an example, slices of cat cerebral cortex incubated under optimal conditions in vitro were found to have concentrations in microequivalents per milliliter of K, Na, and Cl in the non-inulin (intracellular) spaces of the slices of 119, 29.5, and 37, respectively; replicate slices incubated with $10^{-5}M$ ouabain exhibited concentrations of 38.5, 83.5, and 88.5, respectively, compared in each case to incubation media containing K 29.5, Na 122, Cl 122 [34]. On the basis of such experiments the concentration of ouabain producing in cerebral cortex 50 percent inhibition of potassium maintenance and sodium extrusion has been estimated to be 5 to 8 × $10^{-7}M$ [34

206], a value almost identical with that reported for half-maximal inhibition of brain and cortical Na-K-ATPase [11, 32, 171, 206]. It was this sort of correlation together with effects of ouabain on oxygen consumption and parallel results with sodium-free (choline) media that led to the proposals by Whittam and colleagues formulated in the preceding paragraph.

More recent studies have concentrated on elucidating the mechanism of action of the Na-K-ATPase (cf. reviews by Skou [172], Albers [6], and Albers and Siegel [10]), including the interactions of ouabain with the enzyme [8, 73]. Earlier studies had indicated that the action of ouabain is limited to the extracellular aspect of cell membranes [41, 60] and that direct exposure of mitochondria to ouabain fails to affect their respiratory metabolism or ion transport systems [30, 181]. Thus Caldwell and Keynes [41] reported that exposure of the intracellular or axoplasmic surface of the squid axon to $10^{-3}M$ ouabain had no effect on outward transport of sodium, whereas such transport was markedly inhibited by external application of $10^{-5}M$ ouabain.

On the basis of studies on purified preparations of Na-K-ATPase isolated from neural tissues (which are the richest source of the enzyme [32, 33]), Albers et al. [8] have proposed that a phosphorylated enzyme mediates the vectorial work of transport by virtue of allosteric transitions. They have shown that several compounds, such as N-ethyl maleimide, BAL-arsenite, and oligomycin act on the enzyme to activate a Na-dependent ATP-ADP exchange, increasing the sensitivity of the system to sodium ions, abolishing its response to potassium ions, and inhibiting ATP hydrolysis without interfering with the capacity of the enzyme to be phosphorylated by ATP. The authors suggested that these effects indicate stabilization of the *cis* forms of the enzyme by such inhibitions. By contrast, inhibition by cardiac glycosides such as ouabain is not accompanied by such effects. It was originally postulated that ouabain combined with the phosphorylated enzyme to inhibit the K-dependent dephosphorylation. Now Albers et al. [8] have found that as a consequence of the essentially irreversible combination of ouabain with Na-K-ATPase, the enzyme rapidly incorporates orthophosphate whereas only ATP is effective for phosphorylation of the native enzyme. These investigators have concluded that in addition to the effect of ouabain in abolishing the effect of potassium ions on dephosphorylation of the enzyme, ouabain must reduce the free energy difference between the phosphorylated and nonphosphorylated forms of the enzyme, that is, the free energy change must be attributed to the conformational potential of the system such that the combination of ouabain with the enzyme in the Na-ATPase form may remove a constraint on the structure of the enzyme which is normally a consequence of phosphorylation.

If effects on enzyme preparations may be translated into effects on the transport systems in neuronal membranes, the actions of ouabain at the external surface of the membranes would be in the nature of conformational changes of the membrane. One consequence might be a labilization of the membrane by the "mobilization" of calcium ions therein since calcium has generally been considered to be a stabilizer of excitable membranes [168, 186]. Such a mobilizing action of ouabain has been clearly shown for cardiac muscle [72, 75, 76, 100, 106], and the recent studies of Fujisawa et al. [66] and of this author [194] indicate that ouabain may have similar effects on neural membranes.

This author [194] found that incubation of slices of cerebral cortex with inhibitory concentrations of ouabain resulted in significantly elevated tissue levels of calcium ions, the increase being almost entirely accounted for in the mitochondrial fraction isolated from such tissue samples. Since mitochondria from various tissues including brain were known to accumulate calcium as insoluble Ca-phosphates [37, 43, 203], the foregoing observations seem to provide the explanation for the fact that ouabain-inhibited slices of cerebral cortex incubated in calcium-containing media respire initially at significantly higher-than-normal rates (presumably as a consequence of mitochondrial uptake of calcium and the concomitant uncoupling effect on respira-

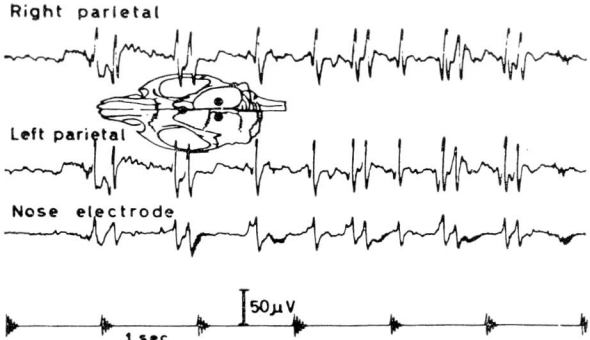

FIG. 22-6. EEG recorded by implanted skull electrodes and a nasal lead from a rat 2 hr after intracranial injection of 0.4 to 0.8 μmole of ouabain. Record is interictal, illustrating continuous bursts of high voltage spikes at 1–2 sec. (Reproduced from Fig. 1 of Bignami and Palladini [27] by permission of the authors and of the publishers of *Nature* [London].)

tion), whereas respiration of such slices incubated in calcium-free media is significantly inhibited [34, 94, 161, 182, 194, 205, 206, 210]. Whether such effects of ouabain are directly related to its obvious interaction with the membrane-bound Na-K-ATPase or whether its "mobilization" of membrane-bound calcium represents a separate effect remains to be elucidated.

Against the foregoing extensive and complex background provided by studies on the effects of ouabain on neural electrolyte metabolism in vitro, the very recent observations in vivo, which provide the fourth model for epileptogenicity, become considerably more meaningful. Within the last 2 to 3 years the first reports of the effects of ouabain on the central nervous system in vivo have appeared [12, 27, 53, 98]. Since ouabain does not penetrate the central nervous system compartment from the general circulation, all these observations were obtained using ventriculocisternal perfusion or intracerebral injection.

Exhibition of ouabain directly to the central nervous system is followed by severe, often fatal, convulsions (Fig. 22-6)* [27, 53,

* After completion of this paper, a more detailed report has come to my attention on the clinical and EEG manifestations following intracerebral injection of 10^{-5} to 10^{-4} M (approximate brain concentrations) ouabain in rats and guinea pigs [Maccagnani, F., Bignami, A., and Palladini, G. *Rev. Neurol.* 115:211, 1966].

98], associated with significant loss of brain-tissue potassium [12, 53, 98] and characteristic neuropathology [27, 28]. With regard to the last aspect, Birks [28] has published a very relevant correlation of morphological and biochemical parameters. He examined by electron microscopy sections of cat superior cervical ganglia fixed after perfusion with cat plasma with or without digoxin (a cardiac glycoside with properties very similar to those of ouabain). In the ganglia perfused with digoxin there was extensive edema of neuronal cytoplasm, of rough endoplasmic reticulum, and of dendrites and axon terminals plus severe changes of the neuronal mitochondria, characterized by a shrunken, dense appearance. No abnormalities were observed for Schwann cells in the same ganglia. Most of these alterations (except those of mitochondria) could be prevented by perfusion of the ganglia with digoxin in a chloride-free (sulfated) plasma, and all abnormalities could be prevented by perfusing with digoxin in a low sodium (sucrose-containing) plasma. Thus it would seem that the effects on cellular morphology were a reflection of the disturbances in electrolyte metabolism induced by the cardiac glycoside.

Clearly the finding that perfusion or injection of the brain with ouabain causes depletion of tissue potassium is to be expected if ouabain inhibits sodium and potassium transport in brain in vivo, as it does in vitro. The concomitant convulsions strongly implicate such interference with cation transport as the epileptogenic factor, since failure of mechanisms normally responsible for maintaining intraneuronal potassium and extruding sodium and the consequent leakage of potassium are associated with depolarization, membrane instability, and repetitive paroxysmal discharges.

Evidence from patients with epilepsy or animals with induced seizures in support of the foregoing implication is scanty and still highly circumstantial. Pappius and Elliott [138] were unable to demonstrate any significant differences of sodium or potassium content between samples of human cerebral cortex taken from epileptogenic foci and those from normal controls. Analyses of biopsies taken after the onset of experimentally induced seizures in animals indicate a shift of electrolytes characterized by decreased intracellular potassium and increased intracellular sodium [38, 47, 218]. In one such group of experiments in which the seizures were induced by withdrawal of anesthetizing doses of carbon dioxide (inhalation of 50 percent CO_2), Woodbury et al. [218] observed a shift in the ratio of $[Na]_o/[Na]_i$ from a control value of 10.5 to an ictal value of 6.8 and they reported that this shift appeared to precede the onset of detectable seizure activity.

A preliminary study of the electrolyte metabolism in incubated slices of human cerebral cortex [192, 193], suggests that the ability of slices from epileptogenic foci to reaccumulate lost potassium is impaired (Table 22-5). Total ATPase activity in comparable samples did not differ from normal [138] but more specific examination of Na-K-ATPase, as in recent experimental studies [113], might be more revealing. The crucial experiments designed to evaluate fluxes of sodium and potassium between extracellular and intracellular compartments of human samples taken from epileptogenic foci remain to be done. Nevertheless these fragmentary data and the ouabain model emphasize the relevance of factors in cerebral electrolyte metabolism to mechanisms of epileptogenicity.

CONCLUDING DISCUSSION

The four models presented here with the intent of focusing on the factors in or characteristics of a final common mechanism or set of mechanisms responsible for epileptogenicity have many aspects in common. Figure 22-7 represents an attempt to interrelate these models at what seems to be the focal point for the final common mechanisms, the excitable membrane of the neuron [192]. Models 1 and 2 provide evidence for a role of excitatory (acetylcholine) and inhibitory (γ-aminobutyric acid) transmitters. Increased amounts of the former (as found in organophosphorus toxicity) or decreased amounts of the latter (as found in vitamin B_6 deficiency or hydrazide toxicity) impinging upon the synaptic area would favor lowered thresholds to excitation and spontaneous firing. Model 3 and perhaps also to some extent Model 2 emphasize the

TABLE 22-5. Potassium Levels in Incubated Slices of Human Cerebral Cortex

	"Normal" Samples (4)		Epileptogenic Samples (4)	
	Slice Swelling %	K+ Content μeq/gm	Slice Swelling %	K+ Content μeq/gm
Initial slices	27.5 (±5.2)	72.2 (±3.8)	24.2 (±2.9)	72.3 (±6.1)
Incubated 1 hr	37.6 (±5.5)	100.2 (±9.4)	38.1 (±4.7)	80.6 (±2.5)
Δ swelling	+10.1		+13.9	
Δ K+		+28.0		+8.3

Slices (av. 250 mg) were incubated aerobically at 37°C in bicarbonate-saline-glucose medium containing 27 mM K+. Initial slices were immersed in the medium during gassing and equilibration (20 min) and were removed for analysis at the start of incubation. Swelling or imbibition of fluid (weight gain of slices) is expressed as percentage of the initial fresh weight of tissue. Potassium was determined by emission flame photometry and is expressed as content per gram of initial fresh weight of tissue. Values tabulated represent means (± S.D.) for the number of experiments indicated at the top of each column [193].

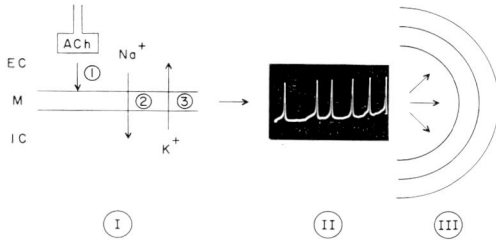

FIG. 22-7. Diagrammatic summary of probable final primary events in development of seizure activity at cellular level. (I) At the excitable membrane (M) oscillations of membrane potential and lowered threshold to excitation may result from (1) increased amounts of excitatory transmitter or decreased amounts of inhibitory transmitter; (2) by failure of energy supplies for or (3) interference directly with the active transport of Na and K between extracellular (EC) and intracellular (IC) compartments. (II) As a result, spontaneous repetitive spike discharges are generated. (III) If such activity becomes sufficiently intense and prolonged, spread to adjacent and distant normal neurons may ensue and lead to development of a full-blown seizure [192].

underlying importance of cerebral oxidative metabolism to fuel the critical processes involved in maintenance of membrane stability. Foremost among the latter is the system pinpointed by Model 4 which maintains intracellular potassium and extrudes excess sodium so that the potential energy in the form of ionic gradients is available to support the controlled responses to incoming impulses. As Models 3 and 4 indicate, any specific (ouabain) or general (hypoxia) interference with the operation or fueling of the cation pump mechanisms results in leakage of sodium and potassium down their concentration gradients, and depolarization of the membrane so that it becomes unstable and may fire spontaneously. As a consequence of any one or several of these factors, spontaneous repetitive spike discharges are generated which, if of sufficient intensity and duration, will spread to adjacent and distant normal neurons to develop into a full-blown seizure (Fig. 22-7).

By localizing the final common set of mechanisms responsible for epileptogenicity at the excitable membrane of the neuron, it is possible to accommodate numerous other aspects of epilepsy, such as the efficacy of anticonvulsant drugs and the effects of induction of and withdrawal from narcosis, both of which are involved in direct physicochemical interactions with membrane components. Other factors like hyperventilation, water intoxication, photic stimulation, or sleep activation may each be thought of as impinging directly on the membrane or on one of its key component systems. At this writing it cannot be said with certainty which aspect or aspects of the excitable membrane are deranged and hence responsible in the majority of cases of human epilepsy. But it seems likely that the example provided by Model 4 will prove to be a leading candidate, if the data in Table 22-6 can be substantiated by more precise evaluations.

This foregoing hardly constitutes an original suggestion since some 250 years ago Johann Thomas Hensing, one of the first pioneers in brain chemistry [189, 195], wrote very succinctly:

The immediate proximal cause of Epilepsy is the disorderly, rapid and most violent influx of spirits from the substance of the cerebral marrow into the nerves and by them into the muscles; this acknowledges another cause, irritation of the membranes and substance of the brain and nerves, which, passing by various means in the brain itself and the origin of the nerves, takes firm root there, or, harassing the processes in more remote parts of the nerves, draws these impetuous spirits from the brain into the muscles themselves . . . [86, p. 42].

Perhaps as a result of the kinds of data discussed above, our knowledge of the nature of these harassments and irritations is more extensive and precise but we still need those additional details which will, in Hensing's words, make possible that:

. . . specific and appropriate means of restoring the temperament of the spirits and rectifying their movements should be rationally determined [86, p. 43].

REFERENCES

1. Abrams, H. K., Hamblin, D. O., and Marchand, J. F. Pharmacology and toxicology of certain organic phosphorus insecticides: Clinical experience. *J.A.M.A.* 144:107, 1950.

2. Adam, D. J. D., Bessey, O. A., Bussey, D. R., and Hansen, A. E. Vitamin B_6 requirement in relation to convulsive seizures in infants. *Amer. J. Dis. Child.* 88:623, 1954.

3. Adam, D. J. D., and Hansen, A. E. Vitamin B_6 in relation to convulsions in infants. *Indian J. Pediat.* 25:210, 1958.

4. Albaum, H. G., Tepperman, J., and Bodansky, O. The *in vivo* inactivation by cyanide of brain cytochrome oxidase and its effect on glycolysis and on the high energy phosphorus compounds in brain. *J. Biol. Chem.* 164:45, 1946.

5. Albers, R. W. The Distribution of Gamma-Aminobutyrate and Related Enzyme Systems. In Roberts, E. (Ed.), *Inhibition in the Nervous System and Gamma-Aminobutyric Acid.* New York: Pergamon, 1960, p. 196.

6. Albers, R. W. Biochemical aspects of active transport. *Ann. Rev. Biochem.* 36:727, 1967.

7. Albers, R. W., and Brady, R. O. The distribution of glutamic decarboxylase in the nervous system of the rhesus monkey. *J. Biol. Chem.* 234:926, 1959.

8. Albers, R. W., Koval, G. J., and Siegel, G. J. Studies on the interaction of ouabain and other cardioactive steroids with sodium-potassium-activated adenosine triphosphatase. *Molec. Pharmacol.* 4:324, 1968.

9. Albers, R. W., and Salvador, R. A. Succinic semialdehyde oxidation by a soluble dehydrogenase from brain. *Science* 128:359, 1958.

10. Albers, R. W., and Siegel, G. J. Nucleoside Triphosphate Phosphohydrolases. In Lajtha, A. (Ed.), *Handbook of Neurochemistry.* New York: Plenum, 1969, vol. IV.

11. Aldridge, W. N. Adenosine triphosphatase in the microsomal fraction from rat brain. *Biochem. J.* 83:527, 1962.

12. Ames, A., III, Higashi, K., and Nesbett, F. B. Effects of Pco_2, acetazolamide and ouabain on volume and composition of choroid plexus fluid. *J. Physiol.* (London) 181:516, 1965.

13. Awapara, J., Landua, A. J., Fuerst, R., and Seale, B. Free γ-aminobutyric acid in brain. *J. Biol. Chem.* 187:35, 1950.

14. Bain, J. A., and Williams, H. L. Concentrations of B_6 Vitamers in Tissues and Tissue Fluids. In Roberts, E. (Ed.), *Inhibition in the Nervous System and Gamma-Aminobutyric Acid.* New York: Pergamon, 1960, p. 275.

15. Baker, W. W., and Benedict, F. Analysis of local discharges induced by intrahippocampal microinjection of carbachol or diisopropylfluorophosphate (DFP). *Int. J. Neuropharmacol.* 7:135, 1968.

16. Baláz̆s, R., Biesold, D., and Magyar, K. Some properties of rat brain mitochondrial preparations: Respiratory control. *J. Neurochem.* 10:685, 1963.

17. Baxter, C. F., and Roberts, E. Gamma-Aminobutyric Acid and Cerebral Metabolism. In Brady, R. O., and Tower, D. B. (Eds.), *The Neurochemistry of Nucleotides and Amino Acids.* New York: Wiley, 1960, p. 127.

18. Baxter, C. F., and Roberts, E. Elevation of γ-aminobutyric acid in brain: Selective inhibition of γ-aminobutyric-α-ketoglutaric acid transaminase. *J. Biol. Chem.* 236:3287, 1961.

19. Baysal, A., Johnson, B. A., and Linkswiler, H. Vitamin B_6 depletion in man: Blood vitamin B_6, plasma pyridoxal-phosphate, serum cholesterol, serum transaminases and urinary vitamin B_6 and 4-pyridoxic acid. *J. Nutr.* 89:19, 1966.

20. Bazemore, A. W., Elliott, K. A. C., and Florey, E. Isolation of factor I. *J. Neurochem.* 1:334, 1957.

21. Bejs̆ovec, M., Kulenda, Z., and Ponc̆a, E. Familial intrauterine convulsions in pyridoxine dependency. *Arch. Dis. Child.* 42:201, 1967.

22. Berl, S., Purpura, D. P., Gonzalez-Monteagudo, O., and Waelsch, H. Effects of Injected Amino Acids on Metabolic Changes Occurring in Epileptogenic and Non-Epileptogenic Lesions of the Cerebral Cortex. In Roberts, E. (Ed.), *Inhibition in the Nervous System and Gamma-Aminobutyric Acid.* New York: Pergamon, 1960, p. 445.

23. Berl, S., Takagaki, G., Clarke, D. D., and Waelsch, H. Carbon dioxide fixation in the brain. *J. Biol. Chem.* 237:2570, 1962.
24. Bessey, O. A., Adam, D. J. D., Bussey, D. R., and Hansen, A. E. Vitamin B_6 requirements in infants. *Fed. Proc.* 13:451, 1954.
25. Bessey, O. A., Adam, D. J. D., and Hansen, A. E. Intake of vitamin B_6 and infantile convulsions: A first approximation of the requirements of pyridoxine in infants. *Pediatrics* 20:33, 1957.
26. Bessman, S. P., Rossen, J., and Layne, E. C. γ-aminobutyric acid–glutamic acid transamination in brain. *J. Biol. Chem.* 201:385, 1953.
27. Bignami, A., and Palladini, G. Experimentally produced cerebral status spongiosus and continuous pseudorhythmic electroencephalographic discharges with a membrane-ATPase inhibitor in the rat. *Nature* (London) 209:413, 1966.
28. Birks, R. I. The effects of a cardiac glycoside on subcellular structures within nerve cells and their processes in sympathetic ganglia and skeletal muscle. *Canad. J. Biochem. Physiol.* 40:303, 1962.
29. Blond, D. M., and Whittam, R. Effects of Na and K on oxidative phosphorylation in relation to respiratory control by a cell-membrane ATPase. *Biochem. Biophys. Res. Commun.* 17:120, 1964.
30. Blond, D. M., and Whittam, R. The regulation of kidney respiration by sodium and potassium ions. *Biochem. J.* 92:158, 1964.
31. Bonting, S. L., and Caravaggio, L. L. Studies on sodium-potassium-activated adenosinetriphosphatase. V. Correlation of enzyme activity with cation flux in six tissues. *Arch. Biochem.* 101:37, 1963.
32. Bonting, S. L., Caravaggio, L. L., and Hawkins, N. M. Studies on sodium-potassium-activated adenosinetriphosphatase. IV. Correlation with cation transport sensitive to cardiac glycosides. *Arch. Biochem.* 98:413, 1962.
33. Bonting, S. L., Simon, K. A., and Hawkins, N. M. Studies on sodium-potassium-activated adenosinetriphosphatase. I. Quantitative distribution in several tissues of the cat. *Arch. Biochem.* 95:416, 1961.
34. Bourke, R. S., and Tower, D. B. Fluid compartmentation and electrolytes of cat cerebral cortex *in vitro*. II. Sodium, potassium and chloride of mature cerebral cortex. *J. Neurochem.* 13:1099, 1966.
35. Boyle, R. *New Experiments Physico-Mechanicall, Touching the Spring of Air, and its Effects.* Oxford: H. Hall, 1660.
36. Boyle, R. *A Continuation of New Experiments Physico-Mechanicall, Touching the Spring and Weight of Air, and their Effects.* Oxford: H. Hall, 1669.
37. Brierly, G. P. Ion Accumulation in Heart Mitochondria. In Chance, B., (Ed.), *Energy-Linked Functions of Mitochondria.* New York: Academic, 1963, p. 237.
38. Brodie, D. A., and Woodbury, D. M. Acid-base changes in brain and blood of rats exposed to high concentrations of carbon dioxide. *Amer. J. Physiol.* 192:91, 1958.
39. Burgen, A. S. V., and MacIntosh, F. C. The Physiological Significance of Acetylcholine. In Elliott, K. A. C., Page, I. H., and Quastel, J. H., (Eds.), *Neurochemistry* (1st ed.). Springfield, Ill.: Thomas, 1955, p. 311.
40. Busnel, R. G., and Lehmann, A. Démonstration expérimentale du rôle du GABA dans l'épilepsie acoustique de la souris. *Abstr. II Internat. Pharmacol. Mtg.* (Prague) [*Biochem. Pharmacol.* 12:Suppl.]: 98, 1963.
41. Caldwell, P. C., and Keynes, R. D. The effect of ouabain on efflux of sodium from a giant squid axon. *J. Physiol.* (London) 148:8P, 1959.
42. Celesia, G. C., and Jasper, H. H. Acetylcholine released from cerebral cortex in relation to state of activation. *Neurology* (Minneap.) 16:1053, 1966.
43. Chance, B. Calcium-Stimulated Respiration in Mitochondria. In Chance, B., (Ed.), *Energy-Linked Functions of Mitochondria.* New York: Academic, 1963, p. 253.
44. Christiaens, L., Briet, B., and Dehaene, P. Un cas familial de convulsions pyridoxino-sensibles. *Pédiatrie* 17:162, 1962.
45. Clermont, P. de. Note sur la préparation de quelques éthers. *C. R. Acad. Sci.* (Paris) 39:338, 1854.
46. Cohen, J. A., and Oosterbaan, R. A. The Active Site of Acetylcholinesterase and Related Esterases and Its Reactivity Towards Substrates and Inhibitors. In Koelle, G. B., (Ed.), *Handbuch der experimentellen Pharmakologie, Supplement 15: Cholinesterases and Anticholinesterase*

47. Colfer, H. F., and Essex, H. E. Distribution of total electrolyte, potassium and sodium in cerebral cortex in relation to experimental convulsions. *Amer. J. Physiol.* 150:27, 1947.
48. Coursin, D. B. Convulsive seizures in infants with pyridoxine-deficient diet. *J.A.M.A.* 154:406, 1954.
49. Coursin, D. B. Vitamin B_6 deficiency in infants: A follow-up study. *Amer. J. Dis. Child.* 90:344, 1955.
50. Coursin, D. B. Seizures in Vitamin B_6 Deficiency. In Roberts, E., (Ed.), *Inhibition in the Nervous System and Gamma-Aminobutyric Acid*. New York: Pergamon, 1960, p. 294.
51. Coursin, D. B. Vitamin B_6 metabolism in infants and children. *Vitamins Hormones* (N.Y.) 22:755, 1964.
52. Crossland, J. The significance of brain acetylcholine. *J. Ment. Sci.* 99:247, 1953.
53. Cserr, H. Potassium exchange between cerebrospinal fluid, plasma and brain. *Amer. J. Physiol.* 209:1219, 1965.
54. Cummins, J., and Hydén, H. Adenosine triphosphate and adenosine triphosphatases in neurons, glia and neuronal membranes of the vestibular nucleus. *Biochim. Biophys. Acta* 60:271, 1962.
55. Curtis, D. R., Phillis, J. W., and Watkins, J. C. The depression of spinal neurones by γ-amino-n-butyric acid and β-alanine. *J. Physiol.* (London) 146:185, 1959.
56. Curtis, D. R., and Watkins, J. C. The pharmacology of amino acids related to gamma-aminobutyric acid. *Pharmacol. Rev.* 17:347, 1965.
57. Dean, R. B. Theories of electrolyte equilibrium in muscle. *Biol. Sympos.* 3:331, 1941.
58. Denève, V., and Jongbloet, P. Convulsies in de neonatale periode beïnvloedbaar door pyridoxine. *Maandschr. Kindergeneesk.* 29:177, 1961.
59. Deuel, D. H., and McIlwain, H. Activation and inhibition of adenosine triphosphatases of subcellular particles from the brain. *J. Neurochem.* 8:246, 1961.
60. Dunham, E. T., and Glynn, I. M. Adenosine triphosphatase activity and the active movements of alkali metal ions. *J. Physiol.* (London) 156:274, 1961.
61. Elliott, K. A. C. Chemical Studies in Relation to Convulsive Conditions. In Elliott, K. A. C., Page, I. H., and Quastel, J. H., (Eds.), *Neurochemistry* (1st ed.). Springfield, Ill.: Thomas, 1955, p. 677.
62. Elliott, K. A. C., and Jasper, H. H. Gamma-aminobutyric acid. *Physiol. Rev.* 30:383, 1959.
63. Essig, C. F. Anticonvulsant effect of amino-oxyacetic acid during barbiturate withdrawal in the dog. *Int. J. Neuropharmacol.* 2:199, 1963.
64. French, J. H., Grueter, B. B., Druckman, R., and O'Brien, D. Pyridoxine and infantile myoclonic seizures, *Neurology* (Minneap.) 15:101, 1965.
65. Frimpter, G. W. Cystathioninuria: Nature of the defect. *Science* 149:1095, 1965.
66. Fujisawa, H., Kajikawa, K., Ohi, Y., Hashimoto, Y., and Yoshida, H. Movement of radioactive calcium in brain slices and influences on it of protoveratrine, ouabain, potassium chloride and cocaine. *Jap. J. Pharmacol.* 15:327, 1965.
67. Gale, E. F. The bacterial amino acid decarboxylases. *Advances Enzym.* 6:1, 1946.
68. Gale, E. F., and Epps, H. M. R. Studies on bacterial amino-acid decarboxylases. I. l(+)-lysine decarboxylase. *Biochem. J.* 38:232, 1944.
69. Gammon, G. D., Gumnit, R., Kamrin, R. P., and Kamrin, A. The Effect of Convulsant Doses of Analeptic Agents upon the Concentration of Amino Acids in Brain Tissue. In Roberts, E., (Ed.), *Inhibition in the Nervous System and Gamma-Aminobutyric Acid*. New York: Pergamon, 1960, p. 328.
70. Garty, R., Yonis, Z., Braham, J., and Steinitz, K. Pyridoxine-dependent convulsions in an infant. *Arch. Dis. Child.* 37:21, 1962.
71. Gentz, J., Hamfelt, A., Johansson, S., Lindstedt, S., Perrson, B., and Zetterström, R. Vitamin B_6 metabolism in pyridoxine dependency with seizures. *Acta Paediat. Scand.* 56:17, 1967.
72. Gersmeyer, G., and Holland, W. C. Influence of ouabain on contractile force, resting tension, Ca^{++} entry and tissue Ca content in rat atria. *Circ. Res.* 12:620, 1963.
73. Glynn, I. M. The action of cardiac glycosides on ion movements. *Pharmacol. Rev.* 16:381, 1964.
74. Gordon, A. S., and Frye, C. W. Large doses of atropine: Low toxicity and effec-

tiveness in anticholinesterase intoxication. *J.A.M.A.* 159:1181, 1955.

75. Govier, W. C., and Holland, W. C. Effects of ouabain on tissue calcium and calcium exchange in pacemaker of turtle heart. *Amer. J. Physiol.* 207:195, 1964.

76. Govier, W. C., and Holland, W. C. The relationship between atrial contractions and the effect of ouabain on contractile strength and calcium exchange in rabbit atria. *J. Pharmacol. Exp. Ther.* 148:284, 1965.

77. Grob, D. Anticholinesterase Intoxication in Man and Its Treatment. In Koelle, G. B., (Ed.), *Handbuch der experimentellen Pharmakologie, Supplement 15: Cholinesterases and Anticholinesterase Agents.* Berlin: Springer, 1963, p. 989.

78. Grob, D., Garlick, W. L., and Harvey, A. M. The toxic effects in man of the anticholinesterase insecticide Parathion (*p*-nitrophenyl diethyl thionophosphate). *Bull. Hopkins Hosp.* 87:106, 1950.

79. Gunsalus, I. C., Bellamy, W. D., and Umbreit, W. W. A phosphorylated derivative of pyridoxal as the coenzyme of tyrosine decarboxylase. *J. Biol. Chem.* 155:685, 1944.

80. Gurdjian, E. S., Webster, J. E., and Stone, W. E. Cerebral metabolism in metrazol convulsions in the dog. *Res. Publ. Ass. Res. Nerv. Ment. Dis.* 26:184, 1947.

81. György, P. Vitamin B_6 and the pellagra-like dermatitis in rats. *Nature* (London) 133:498, 1934.

82. Hagberg, B., Hamfelt, A., and Hansson, O. Tryptophan load tests and pyridoxal-5-phosphate levels in epileptic children. II. Cryptogenic epilepsy. *Acta Paediat. Scand.* 55:371, 1966.

83. Harris, S. A., and Folkers, K. Synthesis of vitamin B_6. *J. Amer. Chem. Soc.* 61:1245, 1939.

84. Hawkins, J. E., and Sarett, L. H. On the efficacy of asparagine, glutamine, γ-aminobutyric acid and 2-pyrrolidinone in preventing chemically induced seizures in mice. *Clin. Chim. Acta* 2:481, 1957.

85. Hebb, C. O., and Krnjević, K. The Physiological Significance of Acetylcholine. In Elliott, K. A. C., Page, I. H., and Quastel, J. H., (Eds.), *Neurochemistry* (2d ed.). Springfield, Ill.: Thomas, 1962, p. 452.

86. Hensing, J. T. *Dissertatio inauguralis chymico-medica de Vitriolo.* Giessen: Vulpius, 1710.

87. Hoffman, J. F. Cation transport and structure of the red-cell plasma membrane. *Circulation* 26:1201, 1962.

88. Holmstedt, B. Pharmacology of organophosphorus cholinesterase inhibitors. *Pharmacol. Rev.* 11:567, 1959.

89. Holmstedt, B. Structure-Activity Relationships of the Organophosphorus Anticholinesterase Agents. In Koelle, G. B., (Ed.), *Handbuch der experimentellen Pharmakologie, Supplement 15: Cholinesterases and Anticholinesterase Agents.* Berlin: Springer, 1963, p. 428.

90. Hunt, A. D., Stokes, J., McCrory, W. W., and Stroud, H. H. Pyridoxine dependency: Report of a case of intractable convulsions in an infant controlled by pyridoxine. *Pediatrics* 13:140, 1954.

91. Iwama, K., and Jasper, H. H. The action of gamma aminobutyric acid upon cortical electrical activity in the cat. *J. Physiol.* (London) 138:365, 1957.

92. Jasper, H., and Erickson, T. C. Cerebral blood flow and pH in excessive cortical discharges induced by metrazol and electrical stimulation. *J. Neurophysiol.* 4:333, 1941.

93. Jasper, H. H., Khan, R. T., and Elliott, K. A. C. Amino acids released from the cerebral cortex in relation to its state of activation. *Science* 147:1448, 1965.

94. Joanny, P., and Corriol, J. Influence de l'ouabaïne sur les mouvements ioniques, la respiration et le glycolyse aérobie du cortex cérébrale isolé de mammifère. *Arch. Sci. Physiol.* (Paris) 18:325, 1964.

95. Jobst, J., and Hesse, O. Ueber die Bohne von Calabar. *Ann. d. Chem. u. Pharm.* 129:115, 1864.

96. Johansson, S., Lindstedt, S., and Register, U. Metabolism of labelled pyridoxine in the rat. *Amer. J. Physiol.* 210:1086, 1966.

97. Johansson, S., Lindstedt, S., Register, U., and Wadström, L. Studies on the metabolism of labelled pyridoxine in man. *Amer. J. Clin. Nutr.* 18:185, 1966.

98. Katzman, R., Graziani, L., Kaplan, R., and Escriva, A. Exchange of cerebrospinal fluid potassium with blood and brain. *Arch. Neurol.* (Chicago) 13:513, 1965.

99. Keesey, J. C., and Wallgren, H. Movements of radioactive sodium in cerebral-cortex slices in response to electrical stimulation. *Biochem. J.* 95:301, 1965.

100. Keeton, W. F., and Briggs, A. H. In vivo effects of ouabain on calcium metabolism in rabbit hearts and plasma. *Proc. Soc. Exp. Biol. Med.* 118:1127, 1965.

101. Keilin, D., and Slater, E. C. Cytochrome. *Brit. Med. Bull.* 9:89, 1953.

102. Keynes, R. D. Electrolytes and Nerve Activity. In Richter, D., (Ed.), *Metabolism of the Nervous System.* New York: Pergamon, 1957, p. 159.

103. Killam, K. F. Convulsant hydrazides. II. Comparison of electrical changes and enzyme inhibition induced by the administration of thiosemicarbazide. *J. Pharmacol. Exp. Ther.* 119:263, 1957.

104. Killam, K. F., and Bain, J. A. Convulsant hydrazides. I. *In vitro* and *in vivo* inhibition by convulsant hydrazides of enzymes catalyzed by vitamin B_6. *J. Pharmacol. Exp. Ther.* 119:255, 1957.

105. Killam, K. F., Dasgupta, S. R., and Killam, E. K. Studies of the Action of Convulsant Hydrazides as Vitamin B_6 Antagonists in the Central Nervous System. In Roberts, E., (Ed.), *Inhibition in the Nervous System and Gamma-Aminobutyric Acid.* New York: Pergamon, 1960, p. 302.

106. Klaus, W., Kuschinsky, G., and Lüllmann, H. Über den Zusammenhang zwischen positiv inotroper Wirkung von Digitoxigenin, Kaliumflux und intracellularen Ionenkonzentrationen im Herzmuskel. *Arch. exp. Path. u. Pharmakol.* 242:480, 1962.

107. Koelle, G. B. Anticholinesterase Agents. In Goodman, L. S., and Gilman, A., (Eds.), *The Pharmacological Basis of Therapeutics* (3d ed.). New York: Macmillan, 1965, p. 441.

108. Kravitz, E. A., and Potter, D. D. A further study of the distribution of γ-aminobutyric acid between excitatory and inhibitory axons of the lobster. *J. Neurochem.* 12:323, 1965.

109. Krnjević, K., and Schwartz, S. Is γ-aminobutyric acid an inhibitory transmitter? *Nature* (London) 211:1372, 1966.

110. Kuffler, S. W. Excitation and Inhibition in Single Nerve Cells. *Harvey Lect.* 1958–59, 1960, p. 176.

111. Kuffler, S. W., and Edwards, C. Mechanism of gamma-aminobutyric acid (GABA) action and its relation to synaptic inhibition. *J. Neurophysiol.* 21:589, 1958.

112. Kuhn, R., Westphal, K., Wendt, G., and Westphal, O. Synthese des Adermins. *Naturwissenschaften* 27:469, 1939.

113. Lewin, E., and McCrimmon, A. ATPase activity in discharging cortical lesions induced by freezing. *Arch. Neurol.* (Chicago) 16:321, 1967.

114. Lichstein, H. C., Gunsalus, I. C., and Umbreit, W. W. Function of the vitamin B_6 group: Pyridoxal phosphate (codecarboxylase) in transamination. *J. Biol. Chem.* 161:311, 1945.

115. McCormick, D. B., Guirard, B. M., and Snell, E. E. Comparative inhibition of pyridoxal kinase and glutamic decarboxylase by carbonyl reagents. *Proc. Soc. Exp. Biol. Med.* 104:554, 1960.

116. McCormick, D. B., and Snell, E. E. Pyridoxal phosphokinase. II. Effects of inhibitors. *J. Biol. Chem.* 236:2085, 1961.

117. McIlwain, H. Electrical influences and speed of chemical change in the brain *Physiol. Rev.* 36:355, 1956.

118. MacIntosh, F. C., and Oborin, P. E. Release of Acetylcholine from Intact Cerebral Cortex. *Abstr. Commun. XIX Internat. Physiol. Congr. (Montreal, 1953),* 1953, p. 580.

119. McKhann, G. M., Albers, R. W., Sokoloff, L., Mickelsen, O., and Tower, D. B. The Quantitative Significance of the Gamma-Aminobutyric Acid Pathway in Cerebral Oxidative Metabolism. In Roberts, E., (Ed.), *Inhibition in the Nervous System and Gamma-Aminobutyric Acid.* New York: Pergamon, 1960, p. 169.

120. McKhann, G. M., Mickelsen, O., and Tower, D. B. Oxidative metabolism of incubated cerebral cortex slices from pyridoxine-deficient kittens. *Amer. J. Physiol.* 200:34, 1961.

121. McKhann, G. M., and Tower, D. B. Gamma-aminobutyric acid: A substrate for oxidative metabolism of cerebral cortex. *Amer. J. Physiol.* 196:36, 1959.

122. McKhann, G. M., and Tower, D. B. The regulation of γ-aminobutyric acid metabolism in cerebral cortex mitochondria. *J. Neurochem.* 7:26, 1961.

123. McKhann, G. M., and Tower, D. B. Ammonia toxicity and cerebral oxidative metabolism. *Amer. J. Physiol.* 200:420, 1961.

124. Marie, J., Hennequet, A., Lyon, G., Debris, P., and LeBalle, J.-C. Les crises convulsives pyridoxino-sensibles du nou-

veau-né et du nourisson. *Sem. Hôp.* (Paris) 35:(197) 1411, 1959.

125. Marie, J., Hennequet, A., Lyon, G., Debris, P., and LeBalle, J.-C. Le pyridoxino-dépendance, maladie métabolique s'exprimant par des crises convulsives pyridoxino-sensibles (première observation familiale). *Rev. Neurol.* 105:406, 1961.

126. May, C. D. Vitamin B_6 in human nutrition: A critique and an object lesson. *Pediatrics* 14:269, 1954.

127. Maynert, E. W., and Kaji, M. K. On the relationship of brain γ-aminobutyric acid to convulsions. *J. Pharmacol. Exp. Ther.* 137:114, 1962.

128. Molony, C. J., and Parmalee, A. H. Convulsions in young infants as a result of pyridoxine (vitamin B_6) deficiency. *J.A.M.A.* 154:405, 1954.

129. Myles, W. S., and Wood, J. D. The effect of hyperbaric oxygen on the GABA shunt pathway in brain homogenates. *Canad. J. Physiol. Pharmacol.* 46:669, 1968.

130. Nachmansohn, D., and Wilson, I. B. The enzymic hydrolysis and synthesis of acetylcholine. *Advances Enzym.* 12:259, 1951.

131. Namba, T., and Hiraki, K. PAM (pyridine-2-aldoxime methiodide) therapy for alkylphosphate poisoning. *J.A.M.A.* 166:1834, 1958.

132. Naruse, H., Cheng, S.-C., and Waelsch, H. CO_2 fixation in the nervous system. IV. CO_2 fixation and citrate metabolism in lobster nerve. *Exp. Brain Res.* 1:284, 1966.

133. Naruse, H., Cheng, S.-C., and Waelsch, H. CO_2 fixation in the nervous system. V. CO_2 fixation and citrate metabolism in rabbit nerve. *Exp. Brain Res.* 1:291, 1966.

134. Nordio, S., Segni, G., and Gandulla, E. Convulsioni piridossini-dipendenti: primo contributo della letteratura italiana. *Minerva Pediat.* 13:925, 1961.

135. Nordio, S., Segni, G., Romano, C., and Bianchi, M. L. G. Seltene Krankheiten, die einer Behandlung mit Pyridoxin zugänglich sind. *Mschr. Kinderheilk.* 110:116, 1962.

136. Obata, K. Pharmacological Study on Postsynaptic Inhibition of Deiter's Neurones. *Abstr. Commun. XXIII Internat. Congr. Physiol. Sci. (Tokyo, 1965)*, 1965, p. 406.

137. Otsuka, M., Iversen, L. L., Hall, Z. W., and Kravitz, E. A. Release of gamma-aminobutyric acid from inhibitory nerves of lobster. *Proc. Nat. Acad. Sci. USA* 56:1110, 1966.

138. Pappius, H., and Elliott, K. A. C. Adenosine triphosphatase, electrolytes, and oxygen uptake rates of human normal and epileptogenic cerebral cortex. *Canad. J. Biochem. Physiol.* 32:484, 1954.

139. Pappius, H. M., and Elliott, K. A. C. Acetylcholine metabolism in normal and epileptogenic brain tissue: Failure to repeat previous findings. *J. Applied Physiol.* 12:319, 1958.

140. Peters, R. A. Mechanism of the toxicity of the active constituent of *Dichapetalum cymosum* and related compounds. *Advances Enzym.* 18:113, 1957.

141. Peters, R. A., and Wakelin, R. W. The synthesis of fluorocitric acid and its inhibition in acetate. *Biochem. J.* 67:280, 1957.

142. Plum, F., Posner, J. B., and Troy, B. Cerebral metabolic and circulatory responses to induced convulsions in animals. *Arch. Neurol.* (Chicago) 18:1, 1968.

143. Pope, A., Morris, A. A., Jasper, H., Elliott, K. A. C., and Penfield, W. Histochemical and action potential studies on epileptogenic areas of cerebral cortex in man and the monkey. *Res. Publ. Ass. Res. Nerv. Ment. Dis.* 26:218, 1947.

144. Posner, J., and Plum, F. Cerebral metabolism during electrically-induced seizures in man. *Trans. Amer. Neurol. Ass.* 93:84, 1968.

145. Post, R. L., Merritt, C. R., Kinsolving, C. R., and Albright, C. D. Membrane adenosine triphosphatase as a participant in the active transport of sodium and potassium in the human erythrocyte. *J. Biol. Chem.* 235:1796, 1960.

146. Purpura, D. P., Berl, S., Gonzalez-Monteagudo, O., and Wyatt, A. Brain Amino Acid Changes during Methoxypyridoxine-Induced Seizures (Cat). In Roberts, E., (Ed.), *Inhibition in the Nervous System and Gamma-Aminobutyric Acid*. New York: Pergamon, 1960, p. 331.

147. Rezzonico, C. A., and Funes, H. R. Convulsiones sensibles a la administración de piridoxina. *Arch. Argent. Pediat.* 57:9, 1962. Cited by French et al. [64].

148. Roberts, E. Formation and Utilization of γ-Aminobutyric Acid in Brain. In Korey, S. R., and Nurnberger, J. I., (Eds.), *Progress in Neurobiology I. Neurochemistry*. New York: Hoeber, 1956, p. 11.

149. Roberts, E., Baxter, C. F., and Eidelberg, E. Some Aspects of Cerebral Metabolism and Physiology of γ-Aminobutyric Acid. In Tower, D. B., and Schadé, J. P., (Eds.), *Structure and Function of the Cerebral Cortex.* Amsterdam: Elsevier, 1960, p. 392.

150. Roberts, E., and Bregoff, H. M. Transamination of γ-aminobutyric acid and β-alanine in brain and liver. *J. Biol. Chem.* 201:393, 1953.

151. Roberts, E., and Frankel, S. Free amino acids in normal and neoplastic tissues of mice studied by paper chromatography. *Cancer Res.* 9:645, 1949.

152. Roberts, E., and Frankel, S. γ-aminobutyric acid in brain: Its formation from glutamic acid. *J. Biol. Chem.* 187:55, 1950.

153. Roberts, E., and Frankel, S. Glutamic decarboxylase in brain. *J. Biol. Chem.* 188:789, 1951.

154. Roberts, E., and Frankel, S. Further studies of glutamic acid decarboxylase in brain. *J. Biol. Chem.* 190:505, 1951.

155. Roberts, E., Wein, J., and Simonsen, D. G. γ-Aminobutyric acid (γ ABA), vitamin B_6, and neuronal function—a speculative synthesis. *Vitamins Hormones* (N.Y.) 22:503, 1964.

156. Roberts, E., Younger, F., and Frankel, S. Influence of dietary pyridoxine on glutamic decarboxylase activity of brain. *J. Biol. Chem.* 191:277, 1951.

157. Robins, M. M. Pyridoxine dependency convulsions in a newborn. *J.A.M.A.* 195:491, 1966.

158. Salvador, R. A., and Albers, R. W. The distribution of glutamic-γ-aminobutyric transaminase in the nervous system of the rhesus monkey. *J. Biol. Chem.* 234:922, 1959.

159. Schlenk, F., and Snell, E. E. Vitamin B_6 and transamination. *J. Biol. Chem.* 157:425, 1945.

160. Schmidt, E. Zum Krankheitsbild der Vitamin-B_6-(Pyridoxin)-Abhängigkeit beim Neugeborenen. *Z. Kinderheilk.* 89:211, 1964.

161. Schwartz, A. The effect of ouabain on potassium content, phosphoprotein metabolism and oxygen consumption of guinea pig cerebral tissue. *Biochem. Pharmacol.* 11:389, 1962.

162. Schwartz, A., Bachelard, H. S., and McIlwain, H. The sodium-stimulated adenosine-triphosphatase activity and other properties of cerebral microsomal fractions and subfractions. *Biochem. J.* 84:626, 1962.

163. Schwerin, P., Bessman, S. P., and Waelsch, H. Uptake of glutamic acid and glutamine by brain and other tissues of rat and mouse. *J. Biol. Chem.* 184:37, 1950.

164. Scriver, C. R. Vitamin B_6 dependency and infantile convulsions. *Pediatrics* 26:62, 1960.

165. Scriver, C. R. Vitamin B_6 deficiency and dependency in man. *Amer. J. Dis. Child.* 113:109, 1967.

166. Scriver, C. R., and Cullen, A. M. Urinary vitamin B_6 and 4-pyridoxic acid in health and in vitamin B_6 dependency. *Pediatrics* 36:14, 1965.

167. Scriver, C. R., and Hutchinson, J. H. The vitamin B_6 deficiency syndrome in human infancy: Biochemical and clinical observations. *Pediatrics* 32:161, 1963.

168. Shanes, A. M. Electrochemical aspects of physiological and pharmacological action in excitable cells. *Pharmacol. Rev.* 10:59, 1958.

169. Skou, J. C. The influence of some cations on an adenosine triphosphatase from peripheral nerves. *Biochim. Biophys. Acta* 23:394, 1957.

170. Skou, J. C. Further investigations on a Mg^{++} and Na^+-activated adenosinetriphosphatase, possibly related to the active, linked transport of Na^+ and K^+ across the nerve membrane. *Biochim. Biophys. Acta* 42:6, 1960.

171. Skou, J. C. Preparation from mammalian brain and kidney of the enzyme system involved in active transport of Na^+ and K^+. *Biochim. Biophys. Acta* 58:314, 1962.

172. Skou, J. C. Enzymatic basis for active transport of Na^+ and K^+ across cell membrane. *Physiol. Rev.* 45:596, 1965.

173. Snell, E. E. The vitamin B_6 group. I. Formation of additional members from pyridoxine and evidence concerning their structure. *J. Amer. Chem. Soc.* 66:2082, 1944.

174. Snell, E. E. Summary of session I and some notes on the metabolism of vitamin B_6. *Vitamins Hormones* (N.Y.) 22:485, 1964.

175. Snell, E. E., Fasella, P. M., Braunstein, A. E., and Rossi-Fanelli, A., (Eds.), *Chemical and Biological Aspects of Pyridoxal Catalysis.* New York: Pergamon, 1963.

176. Snell, E. E., Guirard, B. M., and Williams, R. J. Occurrence in natural products of a physiologically active metabolite of pyridoxine. *J. Biol. Chem.* 143:519, 1942.
177. Snyderman, S. E., Holt, L. E., Jr., Carretero, R., and Jacobs, K. Pyridoxine deficiency in the human infant. *J. Clin. Nutr.* 1:200, 1953.
178. Sokoloff, L., Lassen, N. A., McKhann, G. M., Tower, D. B., and Albers, W. Effects of pyridoxine withdrawal on cerebral circulation and metabolism in a pyridoxine-dependent child. *Nature* (London) 173:751, 1959.
179. Stiehler, R. D., and Flexner, L. B. A mechanism of secretion of the choroid plexus: The conversion of oxidation-reduction energy into work. *J. Biol. Chem.* 126:603, 1938.
180. Stone, W. E. The role of acetylcholine in brain metabolism and function. *Amer. J. Phys. Med.* 36:222, 1957.
181. Swanson, P. D. Effects of ouabain on acid-soluble phosphates and electrolytes of isolated cerebral tissues in presence and absence of calcium. *J. Neurochem.* 15:57, 1968.
182. Swanson, P. D., and McIlwain, H. Inhibition of the sodium-ion-stimulated adenosine triphosphatase after treatment of isolated guinea pig cerebral cortex with ouabain and other agents. *J. Neurochem.* 12:877, 1965.
183. Tapia, R., Pasantes, H., Pérez de la Mora, M., Ortega, B. B., and Massieu, G. H. Free amino acids and glutamate decarboxylase activity in brain of mice during drug-induced convulsions. *Biochem. Pharmacol.* 16:483, 1967.
184. Thiele, V. F., and Brin, M. Chromatographic separation and microbiologic assay of vitamin B_6 in tissues from normal and vitamin B_6 depleted rats. *J. Nutr.* 90:347, 1966.
185. Thompson, J. F., Pollard, J. K., and Steward, F. C. Investigation of nitrogen compounds and nitrogen metabolism in plants. III. γ-Aminobutyric acid in plants, with special reference to the potato tuber and a new procedure for isolating amino acids other than α-amino acids. *Plant Physiol.* 28:401, 1953.
186. Tobias, J. M. A chemically specified molecular mechanism underlying excitation in nerve: A hypothesis. *Nature* (London) 203:13, 1964.
187. Tower, D. B. Neurochemical aspects of pyridoxine metabolism and function. *Amer. J. Clin. Nutr.* 4:329, 1956.
188. Tower, D. B. The effects of 2-deoxy-D-glucose on metabolism of slices of cerebral cortex incubated *in vitro*. *J. Neurochem.* 3:185, 1958.
189. Tower, D. B. Origins and development of neurochemistry. *Neurology* (Minneap.) 8 (suppl. 1):3, 1958.
190. Tower, D. B. Glutamic Acid Metabolism in the Mammalian Central Nervous System. In Brücke, F., (Ed.), *Biochemistry of the Central Nervous System* (Vol. 3, Proc. IV Internat. Biochem. Congr., Vienna). London: Pergamon, 1959, p. 213.
191. Tower, D. B. The Administration of Gamma-Aminobutyric Acid to Man: Systemic Effects and Anticonvulsant Action. In Roberts, E., (Ed.), *Inhibition in the Nervous System and Gamma-Aminobutyric Acid*. New York: Pergamon, 1960, p. 562.
192. Tower, D. B. *Neurochemistry of Epilepsy*. Springfield, Ill.: Thomas, 1960.
193. Tower, D. B. Problems associated with studies of electrolyte metabolism in normal and epileptogenic cerebral cortex. *Epilepsia* ser. 3, (Amst.) 6:183, 1965.
194. Tower, D. B. Ouabain and the distribution of calcium and magnesium in cerebral tissues *in vitro*. *Exp. Brain Res.* 6:273, 1968.
195. Tower, D. B. [Biography of] Johann Thomas Hensing. In Haymaker, W. (Ed.), *Founders of Neurology* (2d ed.). In press.
196. Tower, D. B., and Elliott, K. A. C. Activity of acetylcholine system in human epileptogenic focus. *J. Applied Physiol.* 4:669, 1952.
197. Tower, D. B., and McEachern, D. Acetylcholine and neuronal activity. II. Acetylcholine and cholinesterase activity in the cerebrospinal fluids of patients with epilepsy. *Canad. J. Res., E.* 27:120, 1949.
198. Tsukada, Y., Nagata, Y., and Takagaki, G. Metabolism of γ-aminobutyric acid in brain slices. *Proc. Jap. Acad.* 33:510, 1957.
199. Udenfriend, S. Identification of γ-aminobutyric acid in brain by the isotope derivative method. *J. Biol. Chem.* 187:65, 1950.
200. Van Gelder, N. M., and Elliott, K. A. C. Disposition of γ-aminobutyric acid ad-

ministered to animals. *J. Neurochem.* 3:139, 1958.

201. Waldinger, C., and Berg, R. B. Signs of pyridoxine dependency manifest at birth in siblings. *Pediatrics* 32:161, 1963.

202. Wallach, D. P. Studies on the GABA pathway. I. The inhibition of γ-aminobutyric acid-α-ketoglutaric acid transaminase in vitro and in vivo by U-7524 (amino-oxyacetic acid). *Biochem. Pharmacol.* 5:323, 1960.

203. Weinbach, E. C., and Brand, T. v. The isolation and composition of dense granules from Ca^{++} loaded mitochondria. *Biochem. Biophys. Res. Commun.* 19:133, 1965.

204. Wheatley, M. D., Lipton, B., and Ward, A. A., Jr. Repeated cyanide convulsions without central nervous pathology. *J. Neuropath. Exp. Neurol.* 6:408, 1947.

205. Whittam, R. Active cation transport as a pace-maker of respiration. *Nature* (London) 191:603, 1961.

206. Whittam, R. The dependence of the respiration of brain cortex on active cation transport. *Biochem. J.* 82:205, 1962.

207. Whittam, R. The asymmetrical stimulation of a membrane adenosine triphosphatase in relation to active cation transport. *Biochem. J.* 84:110, 1962.

208. Whittam, R., Agar, M. E., and Wiley, J. S. Control of lactate production by membrane adenosine triphosphatase activity in human erythrocytes. *Nature* (London) 202:1111, 1964.

209. Whittam, R., and Blond, D. M. Respiratory control by an adenosine triphosphatase involved in active transport in brain cortex. *Biochem. J.* 92:147, 1964.

210. Whittam, R., Blond, D. M., and Ruscak, M. The influence of ions on the metabolism of brain-cortex slices. *Biochem. J.* 96:47P, 1965.

211. Whittam, R., Wheeler, K. P., and Blake, A. Oligomycin and active transport reactions in cell membranes. *Nature* (London) 203:720, 1964.

212. Wilson, I. B. Molecular complementarity and antidotes for alkylphosphate poisoning. *Fed. Proc.* 18:752, 1959.

213. Wilson, I. B., Bergmann, F., and Nachmansohn, D. Acetylcholinesterase. X. Mechanism of the catalysis of acylation reactions. *J. Biol. Chem.* 186:683, 1950.

214. Wilson, I. B., and Meislich, E. K. Reactivation of acetylcholinesterase inhibited by alkylphosphates. *J. Amer. Chem. Soc.* 75:4628, 1953.

215. Wood, J. D., Stacey, N. E., and Watson, W. J. Pulmonary and central nervous system damage in rats exposed to hyperbaric oxygen and protection therefrom by gamma-aminobutyric acid. *Canad. J. Physiol. Pharmacol.* 43:405, 1965.

216. Wood, J. D., and Watson, W. J. The effect of intraperitoneal injections of hyperosmotic solutions on convulsions induced by drugs and hyperbaric oxygen. *Canad. J. Physiol. Pharmacol.* 46:649, 1968.

217. Wood, J. D., Watson, W. J., and Clydesdale, F. M. Gamma-aminobutyric acid and oxygen poisoning. *J. Neurochem.* 10:625, 1963.

218. Woodbury, D. M., Rollins, L. T., Gardner, M. D., Hirschi, W. L., Hogan, J. R., Rallison, M. L., Tanner, G. S., and Brodie, D. A. Effects of carbon dioxide on brain excitability and electrolytes. *Amer. J. Physiol.* 192:79, 1958.

219. Yoshida, H., Nukada, T., and Fujisawa, H. Effect of ouabain on ion transport and metabolic turnover of phospholipid of brain slices. *Biochim. Biophys. Acta* 48:614, 1961.

220. Zunin, C., and Vallarino, G. Le crisi convulsive sensibili alla piridossina. *Minerva Pediat.* 15:975, 1963.

Discussion

CEREBRAL BLOOD FLOW AND ENERGY METABOLISM
LOUIS SOKOLOFF

Cells and tissues are, generally speaking, energy transducers that liberate chemical energy by the metabolism of foodstuffs and then either store it again as chemical energy in newly synthesized constituent molecules or, as is more often the case, convert it into mechanical or physicochemical work. Thus, cardiac and skeletal muscles perform obvious mechanical work, the former in the ejection and propulsion of blood against a pressure head and a variety of hydrodynamic resistances, and the latter in the support and translation of body masses. Glands synthesize and secrete complex molecules, and the kidneys reabsorb water and solutes against osmotic and concentration gradients. The work of the brain is more difficult to define. Presumably, it is represented in electrical activity, and chemical energy provided by cerebral metabolism is utilized mainly for the establishment, maintenance, and restoration of membrane potentials essential for neuronal excitability.

In organs which perform mechanical and physical work, increased functional activity is generally associated with increased metabolic rate. This relationship was first clearly enunciated as a basic physiological principle in 1914 by Joseph Barcroft [1], who stated, "There is no instance in which it can be proved that an organ increases its activity, under physiological conditions, without also increasing its demand for oxygen." Experience since that time has amply supported the validity of this principle. Only in the case of the brain has there been difficulty in clearly establishing this relationship. In nervous tissues outside the central nervous system, recorded electrical activity is quantitatively related to the degree of metabolic activity; for example, in such structures as the sympathetic ganglia or postganglionic axons, increased electrical activity produced by preganglionic electrical stimulation is definitely associated with an increased consumption of oxygen [2, 7, 17–19]. In the brain, however, the overall electrical activity recorded in the electroencephalogram represents the summated activity of heterogeneous units and cannot readily be interpreted quantitatively in terms of overall functional activity. Correlation of single unit electrical and metabolic activities would be desirable but is technically very difficult.

In the absence of a definitive measure of the work of the brain, convulsive seizures have been generally considered to represent states of enhanced cerebral functional activity. Although many types of seizures are manifested by increased activity of the recorder pens of the electroencephalograph or motor activity of innervated skeletal muscle, the association between convulsions and increased cerebral *work* is based more on impression than decisive deductive logic. Nevertheless, studies of various types of seizures have demonstrated that most of them are characterized by increases in cerebral metabolic rate. It should be noted, however, that most of these studies were carried out in convulsive states experimentally induced by drugs or electroshock, and there is no assurance that such experimental states accurately reflect the situation in spontaneous epileptiform convulsions in man.

BLOOD VESSELS OF THE EPILEPTIC BRAIN

The normal regulation of the cerebral circulation is accomplished chiefly by chemical mechanisms mediated mainly by the tonic cerebral vasodilator action of carbon dioxide [29, 31]. Operation of the regulating mechanisms is very much like that of a servomechanism designed to maintain the carbon dioxide tension and, to a lesser extent, the oxygen tension of the cerebral tissues at a constant level [29]. Since CO_2 production in the brain is determined by the cerebral metabolic rate, the blood flow under ordinary circumstances is adjusted to the metabolic needs of the brain tissue. Inferences concerning cerebral metabolic rate can, therefore, often be drawn from observations of the blood flow, and early studies of convulsive states were limited to blood flow because of lack of suitable methods for measuring cerebral metabolic rate. These studies uniformly provided, at least, qualitative evidence of cerebral vasodilatation and increased blood flow during seizures. Gibbs, Lennox, and associates, for example, obtained evidence by means of thermocouple techniques that cerebral blood flow was increased during experimental convulsions in animals [8] and spontaneous epileptic seizures in man [9]. Similar observations were made by Penfield and his associates [23, 24], who also noted in animals that the increase in blood flow was localized to the portion of *motor* cortex involved in the seizure and extended into other areas of both hemispheres only when the convulsion became generalized. The change in blood flow never preceded but lagged behind the onset of the electroencephalographic and muscular manifestations of the seizure by a few seconds and disappeared again soon after the convulsion was terminated.

Direct visualization of the pial vessels in man during spontaneous or induced convulsions has led to similar conclusions [23]. Cerebral vascular pulsation ceases after onset of the seizure and returns only after its termination. Cessation of vascular pulsation is consistent with vasodilatation. The postconvulsive state is marked by a reactive hyperemia in the epileptogenic focus, surrounded by areas of pallor or cerebral vasoconstriction. Reactive hyperemia suggests, of course, a preceding relative vascular insufficiency.

None of these studies provided any support for the once popular hypothesis that cerebral ischemia precedes and initiates convulsions. Cerebral anemia can, of course, lead to seizures, but it is apparently not a necessary antecedent in their pathogenesis. On the contrary, a cerebral vasodilatation, probably secondary to increased metabolic demand, follows the onset of the convulsive state.

CEREBRAL BLOOD FLOW AND METABOLIC RATE IN DRUG-INDUCED CONVULSIONS

The first direct evidence of increased cerebral oxygen consumption during convulsions was acquired by Davies and Rémond [3], who placed an oxygen electrode on the surface of the suprasylvian gyrus of the cat and observed an accelerated decline in oxygen tension during seizures induced by pentylenetetrazol. Since the increased oxygen consumption either coincided with or followed onset of the seizure, it was concluded that increased oxygen consumption was the consequence of increased neuronal functional activity occurring in the convulsive state. Similar results have been obtained in the perfused cat brain [6].

The degree of change of cerebral blood flow and metabolic rate during drug-induced convulsions was quantified by Schmidt, Kety, and Pennes [28] in the rhesus monkey. Their data are summarized in Table D22-1. Both cerebral blood flow and oxygen consumption were approximately doubled during the convulsion. Similar changes in blood flow have been observed in drug-induced seizures in human epileptic patients [34]. Following the convulsion and in association with a profound depression of consciousness, there was a marked reduction in cerebral metabolic rate, far below even the level of the resting

TABLE D22-1. Effects of Pentylenetetrazol Convulsions on Cerebral Blood Flow and Metabolism in the Monkey[a]

State of Animal	Cerebral Blood Flow[b]	Cerebral O_2 Consumption[b]
Control natural respiration	29.2	2.30
Pentylenetetrazol convulsion	59.8	4.13
Postconvulsive, 15 min	20.6	0.85

[a] Data taken from Schmidt et al. [28].
[b] Milliliters per 100 gm per min.

state. Cerebral blood flow was only moderately reduced below the control level, suggesting that some consequence of the preceding convulsion was maintaining blood flow above and beyond the metabolic needs of the brain. The nature and possible causes of the postictal depression will be discussed below. Increased cerebral blood flow was, at least in part, unquestionably the result of increases in CO_2 production and oxygen utilization in the cerebral tissues and the role of such changes in the regulation of cerebral blood flow [29, 31]. Plum and his associates [25] have recently suggested that blood pressure increases may also be contributory.

Postconvulsive Depression

The immediate postconvulsive period is characterized by depression of neuronal activity, coma, and paralysis. It is also associated with a constriction of the cerebral vessels [23], depression of cerebral blood flow [13, 28], and marked reduction in cerebral metabolic rate [13, 28]. The postconvulsive depression has generally been attributed to a failure of the cerebral blood flow to increase sufficiently to meet the enormously augmented metabolic needs of the brain during the seizure. Relative cerebral vascular insufficiency is presumed to lead to depletion of substrate stores, anoxia, and accumulation of acidic metabolic products in the cerebral tissues, which must be relieved during the postconvulsive period before normal cerebral function can resume. The oxygen tension of the cerebral cortex has, indeed, been found to fall during drug-induced convulsions [3, 4, 21], and there are some data suggesting that the tissue anoxia may be responsible for spontaneous termination of the seizure as well as for postconvulsive depression. For example, Meyer and Portnoy [21] have reported that pentylenetetrazol-induced convulsions terminate when the cortical pO_2 falls below a certain level and resume only when it has returned to the normal level. The breathing of high oxygen mixtures has also been reported to prolong the duration of seizures and shorten the interval between successive seizures [27]. There is also some evidence to suggest the development of cerebral tissue acidosis during the seizure. Jasper and Erickson [11] observed a fall in pH in the cerebral cortex of the cat during seizures induced by pentylenetetrazol or electroshock, and Meyer and Gotoh [22] have reported an excellent correlation between the fall in pH of the cerebral venous blood and postconvulsive depression of neuronal activity following epileptic seizures in man.

Plum and his associates [25] have recently questioned whether cerebral circulation is in fact incapable of adjusting adequately to increased metabolic demands of the brain during convulsions. They observed that in dogs, which were artificially ventilated with oxygen and paralyzed with neuromuscular blocking agents, induced convulsions caused a tremendous increase in cerebral blood flow which was more than adequate to prevent development of cerebral anoxia and acidosis. A marked hypertensive response contributed to the unusually large rise in cerebral blood flow; when the increase in blood pressure was prevented by ganglionic blockade, the rise in cerebral blood flow was more usual, and only then did evidence of cerebral anoxia and acidosis during the convulsion appear. The seizures terminated spontaneously whether or not anoxia occurred, but no information regarding postconvulsive depression was reported. However, inasmuch as artificial ventilation with oxygen and muscular paralysis are hardly conditions which normally obtain, there is some question as to the relevance of these studies to clinical epilepsy. They do serve the useful purpose of challenging the popular concept of the mechanism of postconvulsive depression. The metabolic deprivation hypothesis has certainly not been proved, and it may be fruitful to entertain alternative hypotheses. Other neuronal mechanisms may be considered, for example, spreading cortical depression like that produced by application of K^+ extracellularly in the cerebral cortex.

Interseizure Period

Chronic convulsive disorders do not appear to have any permanent effects on cerebral circulation and metabolism. Cerebral blood flow and oxygen consumption in human adult epileptic patients are normal during the interseizure period [10]. These functions also remain normal after a protracted series of seizures associated with electroconvulsive therapy [35]. Kennedy et al. [12] have reported a slight reduction in cerebral blood flow, but no significant change in cerebral metabolic rate, in epileptic children during the interseizure period. The types of epileptic seizures represented in the children's series were broader in scope than those of the adults studied by Grant et al. [10]; some were undoubtedly sequelae of perinatal accidents, and it is likely that disturbances in cerebral blood flow were not so much the consequence of convulsive disorders as an independent manifestation of the effects of perinatal trauma. There is no convincing evidence that convulsive episodes leave any residual effects on the cerebral circulation and energy metabolism beyond the immediate postconvulsive period.

Intermediary Energy Metabolism During Convulsions

Direct measurement of the levels in the cerebral tissues of intermediates and energy-rich products of energy-yielding metabolic pathways has provided additional evidence of increased energy metabolism in convulsive seizures [15, 33]. Convulsions induced by drugs or electroshock rapidly deplete the substrate and high energy reserves in the brain. Glycolysis is increased as evidenced by reduction in glycogen and glucose contents and accumulation of lactic acid [15, 16, 33]. The latter may be largely responsible for the fall in cerebral cortical pH which has been reported to occur during seizures [11]. High energy phosphates are more rapidly utilized than they can be resynthesized, and creatine phosphate and ATP levels decline and ADP and inorganic phosphate contents increase [5, 15]. The elegant studies of King et al. [15] have demonstrated that these changes develop within seconds following onset of convulsions and occur even when gross manifestations of seizure are suppressed by depressant drugs. They also demonstrated that energy utilization during convulsions exceeds energy replenishment; energy reserves in the cerebral tissues were markedly reduced despite increased glucose uptake and metabolism to lactic acid and beyond. These changes occurred too early and were of too great a magnitude to be accounted for by the apnea and anoxia which frequently accompany convulsions. The energy deficit in the cerebral tissues during convulsions is clearly the result of increased utilization.

CONVULSIONS ASSOCIATED WITH
PYRIDOXINE DEFICIENCY

In most of the studies demonstrating increased cerebral metabolic rates in convulsive states, seizures were induced by electroshock or analeptic drugs. Increased energy utilization is not, however, an essential component of the convulsive process. Indeed, convulsions may be induced by impairment of the energy generating system, caused, for example, by deficiency of oxygen or oxidizable substrate. Anoxia, fluoroacetate poisoning, and hypoglycemia all produce seizures without increasing cerebral metabolic rate. Hypoglycemic convulsions are, in fact, associated with slower than normal rates of cerebral oxygen and glucose consumption [13] and with no apparent depletion of high energy phosphate stores [15].

Our laboratory has had the rare opportunity to study cerebral circulation and metabolism in man during seizures associated with pyridoxine insufficiency [32]. The results indicate that at least as regards cerebral energy metabolism, this type of convulsive disorder resembles the substrate-deficiency type. The patient was a 6-year-old girl who, since birth, suffered from seizures which did not respond to the usual anticonvulsant drugs but only to pyridoxine administration. From 2 years of age she had been maintained free of convulsions by means of pyridoxine supplementation of the normal diet. At the time of the study, she exhibited no gross abnormalities other than severe mental retardation. Seizure activity, manifested both in motor activity and the electroencephalogram, could be induced in this patient by withholding pyridoxine supplementation for 72 hours

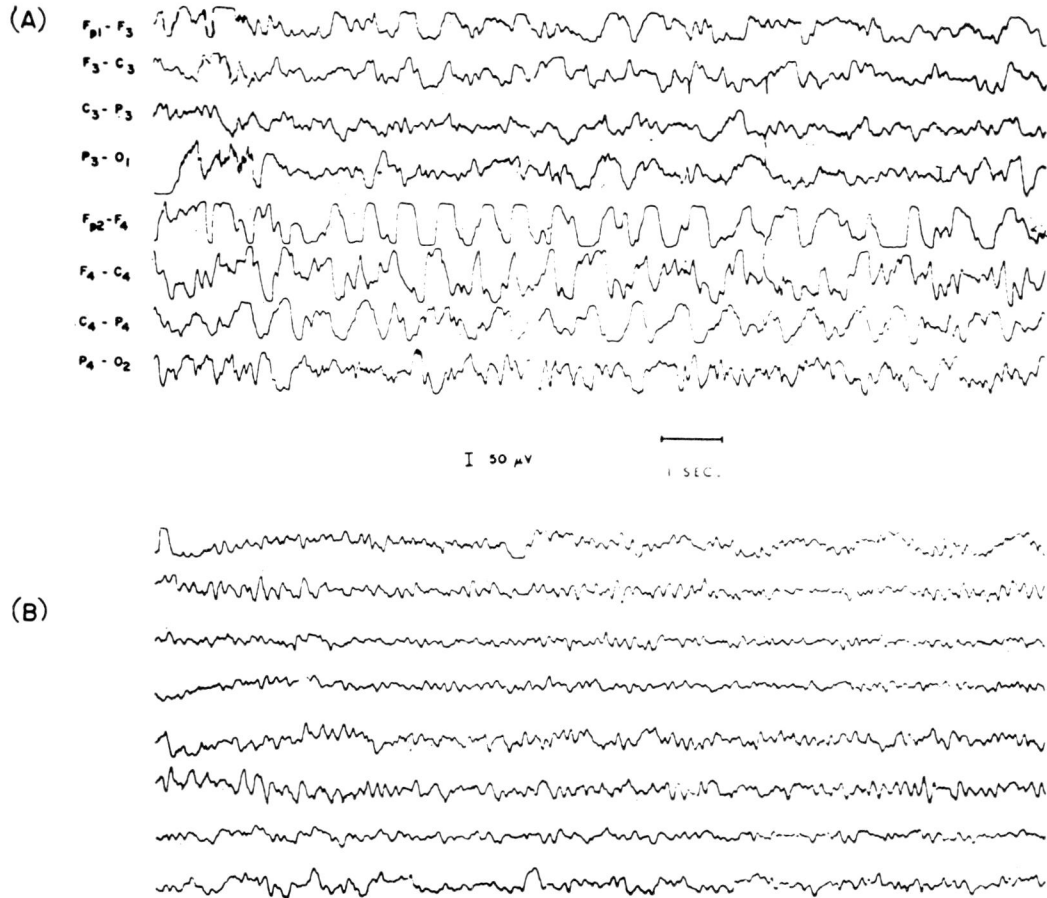

FIG. D22-1. Electroencephalographic tracings of pyridoxine-dependent child: (A) 72 hr after withdrawal of pyridoxine maintenance dose; (B) 2 min after intravenous administration of 15 mg of pyridoxine to terminate the seizure observed in (A).

and completely terminated within 2 minutes by an intravenous injection of pyridoxine (Fig. D22-1). Cerebral circulation and metabolic studies were performed in the midst of a seizure and immediately after its termination.

Cerebral oxygen consumption, blood flow, arteriovenous oxygen difference, and respiratory quotient (R.Q.) were all markedly reduced below the normal level during the seizure and were increased toward normal following cessation of the seizure activity (Table D22-2). Cerebral R.Q., in fact, completely returned to its normal level of approximately unity [30]; cerebral oxygen consumption and blood flow, although increased following the convulsion, did not entirely achieve normality but were no lower than the levels observed in mentally retarded children of the same age [30]. The reduction of cerebral energy metabolism during the seizure clearly indicates that convulsions of pyridoxine deficiency are more like those induced by substrate insufficiency than by electroshock or analeptic drugs. The low cerebral R.Q. during the seizure also suggests that the brain, which normally utilizes carbohydrate almost exclusively as the ultimate substrate for its oxidations [30], may have been diverted, perhaps, by lack of an essential substrate, to oxidation of other substances.

TABLE D22-2. Effects of Convulsions Due to Pyridoxine Deficiency on Cerebral Blood Flow and Metabolism in a Pyridoxine-Dependent Child[a]

Function	During Seizure	Following Termination of Seizure
Cerebral blood flow (ml/100 gm/min)	63	70
Cerebral O_2 consumption (ml/100 gm/min)	3.3	4.4
Cerebral arteriovenous oxygen difference (vol%)	5.26	6.23
Cerebral respiratory quotient (R.Q.)	0.85	0.96

[a] Data from Sokoloff et al. [31]. Conditions of the study are described in the legend to Fig. D22-1.

The convulsive disorder in this pyridoxine-dependent child is probably very similar to those induced experimentally by convulsant hydrazides or pyridoxine antagonists, inasmuch as all probably result from a deficiency of pyridoxal phosphate in the tissues. This coenzyme functions in various transamination and amino acid decarboxylations, including the decarboxylation of glutamate to γ-aminobutyric acid (GABA). Pyridoxal phosphate deficiency or antagonism leads to a decline in GABA levels in the tissues of the brain [14]. It has been suggested that the ketoglutarate-glutamate-GABA-succinic-semialdehyde-succinate pathway may constitute a shunt around the ketoglutarate-succinyl-CoA-succinate steps in the Krebs cycle within the brain [26].

McKhann et al. [20] have obtained evidence that as much as 40–50 percent of the flux from ketoglutarate to succinate may proceed via this shunt. Pyridoxine deficiency may slow the shunt pathway, since most of its steps involve pyridoxal phosphate-dependent enzymes, and thereby reduce the cerebral metabolic rate during the seizure. It would seem then that GABA, in addition to its role as a neurohumoral mediator of inhibitory function, may also serve as a vital metabolic intermediate in energy-yielding processes in the central nervous system.

Conclusions

Convulsions are associated with profound changes in the circulation and metabolism of the brain. There is no evidence that cerebral ischemia ordinarily initiates the convulsion; the changes in blood flow and oxygen consumption generally follow onset of the seizure. Cerebral blood flow and metabolic rate are increased in most types of convulsions, for example, those caused by analeptic drugs, electroshock, and perhaps also idiopathic epilepsy, and are reduced in the immediate postconvulsive period. On the other hand, seizures may also be caused by substrate deficiencies, such as hypoglycemia, and in these cases energy metabolism is depressed. Pyridoxine deficiency leads to a substrate-deficiency type of convulsion with reductions in cerebral blood flow and oxygen consumption. Since seizures can occur in the presence of either an increased or decreased metabolic rate, it is doubtful that changes in energy metabolism are fundamental to the mechanism of seizures. It seems rather that they reflect ancillary events.

REFERENCES

1. Barcroft, J. *The Respiratory Function of the Blood.* New York: Macmillan, 1914.
2. Bronk, D. W., Larrabee, M. G., and Davies, P. W. The rate of oxygen consumption in localized regions of the nervous system: In presynaptic endings and in cell bodies. *Fed. Proc.* 5:11, 1946.
3. Davies, P. W., and Rémond, A. Oxygen consumption of the cerebral cortex of the cat during metrazol convulsions. *Res. Publ. Ass. Res. Nerv. Ment. Dis.* 26:205, 1946.
4. Davis, E. W., McCulloch, W. S., and Roseman, E. Rapid changes in the oxygen tension of cerebral cortex during induced convulsions. *Amer. J. Psychiat.* 100:825, 1944.
5. Dawson, R. M. C., and Richter, D. Effect

of stimulation on the phosphate esters of the brain. *Amer. J. Physiol.* 160:203, 1950.
6. Geiger, A., and Magnes, J. The isolation of the cerebral circulation and the perfusion of the brain in the living cat. *Amer. J. Physiol.* 149:517, 1947.
7. Gerard, R. W. Nerve metabolism. *Physiol. Rev.* 12:469, 1932.
8. Gibbs, F. Cerebral blood flow preceding and accompanying experimental convulsions. *Arch. Neurol. Psychiat.* 30:1003, 1933.
9. Gibbs, F., Lennox, W., and Gibbs, E. Cerebral blood flow preceding and accompanying epileptic seizures in man. *Arch. Neurol. Psychiat.* 32:257, 1934.
10. Grant, F. C., Spitz, E. B., Shenkin, H. A., Schmidt, C. F., and Kety, S. S. The cerebral blood flow and metabolism in idiopathic epilepsy. *Trans. Amer. Neurol. Ass.* 72:82, 1947.
11. Jasper, H., and Erickson, T. C. Cerebral blood flow and pH in excessive cortical discharge induced by metrazol and electrical stimulation. *J. Neurophysiol.* 4:333, 1941.
12. Kennedy, C., Anderson, W., and Sokoloff, L. Cerebral blood flow in epileptic children during the interseizure period. *Neurology* (Minneap.) 8:100, 1958, suppl. 1.
13. Kety, S. S., Woodford, R. B., Harmel, M. H., Freyhan, F. A., Appel, K. E., and Schmidt, C. F. Cerebral blood flow and metabolism in schizophrenia. The effects of barbiturate seminarcosis, insulin coma, and electroshock. *Amer. J. Psychiat.* 104:765, 1948.
14. Killam, K. F., and Bain, J. A. Convulsant hydrazides. I. In vitro and in vivo inhibition by convulsant hydrazides of enzymes catalysed by vitamin B_6. *J. Pharmacol. Exp. Ther.* 119:255, 1957.
15. King, L. J., Lowry, O. H., Passoneau, J. V., and Venson, V. Effects of convulsants on energy reserves in the cerebral cortex. *J. Neurochem.* 14:599, 1967.
16. Klein, J. R., and Olsen, N. S. Effect of convulsive activity upon the concentration of brain glucose, glycogen, lactate, and phosphate. *J. Biol. Chem.* 167:747, 1947.
17. Larrabee, M. G. Effects of Anesthetics on Oxygen Consumption and Synaptic Transmission in Sympathetic Ganglia. *The Biology of Mental Health and Disease*. New York: Hoeber, 1952.
18. Larrabee, M. G., and Bronk, D. W. Metabolic requirements of sympathetic neurons. *Sympos. Quant. Biol.* 17:245, 1952.
19. Larrabee, M. G., Ramos, J. G. and Bülbring, E. Effects of anesthetics on oxygen consumption and on synaptic transmission in sympathetic ganglia. *J. Cell Comp. Physiol.* 40:461, 1952.
20. McKhann, G. M., Albers, R. W., Sokoloff, L., Mickelson, O., and Tower, D. B. The Quantitative Significance of the Gamma-Aminobutyric Acid Pathway in Cerebral Oxidative Metabolism. In Roberts, E. (Ed.), *Inhibition in the Nervous System and γ-Aminobutyric Acid*. Oxford: Pergamon, 1960.
21. Meyer, J. A., and Portnoy, H. D. Postepileptic paralysis. *Brain* 82:163, 1959.
22. Meyer, J. A., and Gotoh, F. Cerebral metabolism during epileptic seizures in man. *Trans. Amer. Neurol. Ass.* 90:23, 1967.
23. Penfield, W. The circulation of the epileptic brain. *Res. Publ. Ass. Res. Nerv. Ment. Dis.* 28:605, 1938.
24. Penfield, W., von Santha, K., and Cipriani, A. Cerebral blood flow during induced epileptiform seizures in animals and man. *J. Neurophysiol.* 2:257, 1939.
25. Plum, F., Posner, J. B., and Troy, B. Cerebral metabolic and circulatory responses to induced convulsions in animals. *Arch. Neurol.* (Chicago) 18:1, 1968.
26. Roberts, E. Formation and Utilization of γ-Aminobutyric Acid in Brain. In Korey, S. R., and Nurnberger, J. I. (Eds.), *Progress in Neurobiology. I. Neurochemistry*. New York: Hoeber, 1957.
27. Ruf, H. Experiments on the prolongation of induced epileptiform convulsions in the cat. *J. Ment. Sci.* 98:454, 1952.
28. Schmidt, C. F., Kety, S. S., and Pennes, H. H. Gaseous metabolism of the brain of the monkey. *Amer. J. Physiol.* 143:33, 1945.
29. Sokoloff, L. The action of drugs on the cerebral circulation. *Pharmacol. Rev.* 11:1, 1959.
30. Sokoloff, L. Metabolism of the Central Nervous System In Vivo. In Field, J., Magoun, H. W., and Hall, V. E. (Eds.), *Handbook of Physiology—Neurophysiology*. Washington, D.C.: American Physiological Society, 1960, vol. III.

31. Sokoloff, L., and Kety, S. S. Regulation of cerebral circulation. *Physiol. Rev.* 40: 38, 1960.
32. Sokoloff, L., Lassen, N. A., McKhann, G. M., Tower, D. B., and Albers, R. W. Effects of pyridoxine withdrawal on cerebral circulation and metabolism in a pyridoxine-dependent child. *Nature* (London) 183:751, 1959.
33. Stone, W. E., Webster, J. E., and Gurdjian, E. S. Chemical changes in the cerebral cortex associated with convulsive activity. *J. Neurophysiol.* 8:233, 1945.
34. White, P. T., Grant, P., Mosier, J., and Craig, A. Changes in cerebral dynamics associated with seizures. *Neurology* (Minneap.) 11:354, 1961.
35. Wilson, W. P., Schieve, J. F., and Scheinberg, P. Effect of series of electric shock treatments on cerebral blood flow and metabolism. *Arch. Neurol. Psychiat.* 68: 651, 1952.

23

Mechanisms of Action of Anticonvulsants*

DIXON M. WOODBURY†

DESPITE AN ABUNDANCE of knowledge in clinical and experimental epilepsy and on the drugs effective in the treatment of this disease, a full understanding of the metabolism and mechanisms of action of anticonvulsant agents is still lacking. Although much information has accumulated on physiological and biochemical effects of anticonvulsants, the ultimate basic effect, defined as the *action,* has not been elucidated. Even a simple ionic molecule such as bromide, the anticonvulsant property of which has been known for over 100 years, has not yielded its secrets to the neurophysiologists or the biochemists. However, recent evidence has pushed back the frontier considerably, which will be discussed.

In this chapter, the metabolism of selected anticonvulsants will not be discussed except as it contributes knowledge to the elucidation of their mechanisms of action. Emphasis instead will be limited to the neurophysiological and biochemical effects of these agents that yield insight into the mechanisms by which they act. A host of anticonvulsants has been tested in the laboratory against experimental seizures, and, subsequently, many were found useful in the therapy of epilepsy in man. However, only a few have been subjected to sufficiently intensive experimental and clinical study to allow intelligent conclusions or speculations about their actions. Consequently, only certain drugs, as prototypes, will be discussed in this chapter.

Since the anticonvulsant agent, diphenylhydantoin (DPH), has been studied most intensively by others and by this author, the discussion will be centered largely around it. However, trimethadione and bromide appear to have mechanisms distinct from that of DPH and from each other. Therefore, they will also be considered in some detail. Although a large literature is available on phenobarbital, its effects appear to be a combination of the effects of one or more of the drugs mentioned above. Consequently, it will be considered only as it contributes knowledge to a specific mechanism being discussed.

Several reviews have discussed the mechanisms of action of anticonvulsants as well as their pharmacology [16, 72, 111, 112, 135]. The structures of the prototype drugs to be discussed are shown in Fig. 23-1.

These drugs will be considered in the order listed, and the approach will be directed toward the prototype drugs. Space limitations preclude a discussion of the anticonvulsant mechanism of action of the carbonic anhydrase inhibitors (such as acetazolamide). A review by Woodbury and Karler [137] includes a discussion of their mechanism of action and that of carbon dioxide.

DIPHENYLHYDANTOIN

EXCITABLE TISSUES
Effects on the Nervous System

The effects of DPH on different levels of the neuraxis in adult as well as in maturing

---

* Original investigations reported herein supported by PHS Program–Project Grant 5–P01–NB04553 from National Institute of Neurological Diseases and Stroke and by Department of Pharmacology, University of Leiden, Leiden, Netherlands, during the tenure of the author's stay there as the Boerhaave Professor.

† Recipient of a PHS Research Career Program Award 5–K6–NB18838 from National Institute of Neurological Diseases and Stroke.

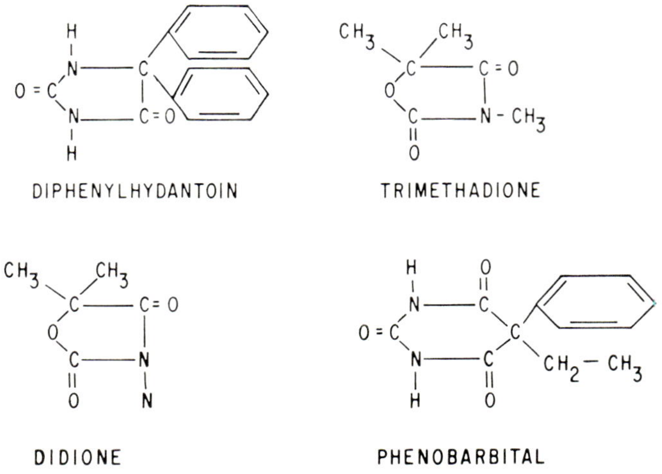

FIG. 23-1. Structures of prototype drugs discussed.

animals will be considered first. Its effects on experimentally induced seizures (electrical and chemical), already extensively documented, will be mentioned only briefly here [16, 72, 111, 112, 135]. The introduction of DPH thirty years ago by Merritt and Putnam [69] was a signal advance in antiepileptic therapy, demonstrating the feasibility of anticonvulsant testing in laboratory animals and that a drug need not be a sedative to be an effective antiepileptic agent. Since that time, the drug has been studied intensively in the laboratory because it provides a valuable laboratory tool for elucidation of the neurophysiological and neurochemical basis of seizures.

Mature Nervous System. One of the most easily demonstrated properties of DPH in adult animals of all species is its ability to limit the development of maximal seizure activity and, probably related to this, its ability to reduce spread of the seizure process from an active focus. Both these features are undoubtedly related to clinical usefulness of the drug in the treatment of grand mal epilepsy and of various lesser convulsive disorders other than the petit mal group. Since this chapter is concerned with the mechanisms by which anticonvulsants act, the question involved is how DPH acts neurophysiologically and neurochemically to limit development and reduce spread of the seizure process.

It is necessary, first, to consider briefly the possible mechanisms by which the anticonvulsant group of drugs might act [16, 72, 111, 112, 135]. The more plausible mechanism will then be discussed for each drug considered. General types of effects might include: (1) effects on nonneural systems to prevent changes which might precipitate or facilitate seizure activity; (2) effects confined to the pathologically altered neurons of the seizure focus to prevent their excessive discharge; and (3) effects on normal neurons to prevent their detonation by the seizure focus. It is likely that the last-named effect applies to most of the antiepileptic drugs presently available. This is particularly evident in that all produce one or more CNS side effects not related to obtundation of the seizure process (such as sedation, analgesia, and excitation).

Unlike phenobarbital, DPH, in *single acute* doses in adult animals of various laboratory species, does not elevate the threshold for seizures induced by 60-cycle alternating current (ac) stimulation of the brain or by injection of such convulsant drugs as strychnine, picrotoxin, or pentylenetetrazol. In fact, it may potentiate a subconvulsant dose of pentylenetetrazol and enhance seizures induced by inhalation of 30 percent CO_2, by withdrawal from 50 percent CO_2, and by high doses of salicylate [137, 139]. (The explanation of these effects is discussed in the next section dealing with the influence of DPH on CNS in the developing animal.) However, DPH does elevate (but not nearly as much as do phenobarbital and trimethadione) electroshock seizure threshold induced by low frequency (lf, 6 per second) stimulation of the brain (see [135] for summary); it also elevates toward normal the ac seizure threshold abnormally lowered by acute hyponatremia or by administration of cortisone or thyroxine [36, 108, 136]. Thus, the drug restores excitability to normal when it has been abnormally increased.

The ability of DPH to elevate the lf but not the ac electroshock seizure threshold appears to be related to the mechanism of these two types of seizures. Most anticonvulsants are more effective in elevating the lf than the ac threshold. The greater sensitivity of the former is probably due to the lf stimulus exciting the collection of neurons (conveniently called the oscillator) involved in producing sustained clonic discharge, the endpoint of this seizure test, with maximum efficiency. Discharge elicited by the 60-cycle ac threshold method is more intense and spreads over a wider area. Spread to other areas undoubtedly involves subcortical excitatory pathways that enhance the discharge to cortex, making it more difficult for DPH to elevate the ac threshold than is the case with the lf threshold. The inability of DPH to raise the ac threshold and its limited ability to elevate the lf threshold as compared with other drugs, such as phenobarbital and trimethadione, are probably related to the fact that this anticonvulsant, in addition to suppressing excitatory systems, can also block inhibitory systems to a certain extent (to be discussed below). This explains at least some of the excitatory effects of DPH. Such excitatory effects would probably counteract the threshold-elevating influence of the drug on the lf threshold (where little spread is involved) and would prevent its threshold-raising effects on the ac threshold (where a great deal of spread from subcortical pathways is involved).

With electrical and chemical stimuli substantially above threshold, a tonic-clonic seizure replaces the purely clonic minimal seizure. This convulsion has a characteristic stereotyped pattern consisting of tonic flexion, tonic extension, and clonus [114]. A distinctive qualitative difference between this maximal seizure and a threshold convulsion concerns the extent of spread of seizure discharge, which in the maximal seizure involves the entire cerebrospinal axis. The *pattern* of the convulsion is therefore independent of the seizure threshold and of factors which alter seizure threshold per se. Conceivably, drugs may alter pattern and duration of the maximal seizure by affecting the degree of spread of discharge throughout the brain, as well as by the two mechanisms concerned in elevation of seizure threshold: increasing the threshold of neurons to excitation or decreasing the ease with which neurons discharge repetitively once they are activated.

Probably the most significant effect of DPH is its ability to modify the pattern of maximal (tonic-clonic) electroshock seizures elicited in animals by supramaximal current; the characteristic tonic phase can be abolished completely by the drug; the resultant purely clonic seizure may be exaggerated and prolonged, but the EEG during such modified seizures shows reduction both in voltage and frequency of convulsive discharges [4, 114]. DPH produces similar alterations in the character of convulsions in psychiatric patients undergoing electroconvulsive therapy [113]. The ability to abolish the tonic phase of maximal seizures is not limited to electroshock seizures, since it can be demonstrated in animals with maximal seizures induced by picrotoxin or pentylenetetrazol. However, DPH does not abolish the tonic seizure induced by strychnine in experimental animals. This lack of effect is not unexpected since strychnine (and its close congener, brucine) is unique among the convulsant agents in that it acts by blockade of postsynaptic inhibition [25], and (as will be discussed) most of the effects of DPH in the brain of the adult animal appear to be related to presynaptic events rather than to effects on the postsynaptic membrane.

The effect of DPH to abolish the tonic phase of the maximal seizure is also not limited to the cerebrum. It can be demonstrated in laboratory animals decerebrated at the midcollicular level and exhibiting maximal seizures induced by electrical stimulation, pentylenetetrazol, or picrotoxin. Furthermore, experiments carried out in our laboratory by Esplin and colleagues [30, 31] demonstrated that massive stimulation of the spinal cord results in a sequence of motor events identical to those observed in an intact animal during maximal electroshock seizure. Thus the initial latent phase, the brief tonic flexion, and the abrupt change from flexion to extension are responses of the spinal cord stimulated maximally. DPH blocks the tonic phase of maximal seizure in the spinal animal, but a higher dose is required than that to abolish the tonic phase in the intact animal.

The effects of DPH at various levels of the CNS have been studied in more detail and reveal certain differences that are relevant to its mechanism of action. The threshold for afterdischarge obtained by electrical stimulation of cerebral cortex and thalamus is slightly elevated by DPH but it is less effective than trimethadione in raising the threshold of the thalamus; however, the latter does not affect the threshold of the cortex [101]. Thus, there is a distinct difference between the two drugs in this respect. Also, DPH decreases duration of afterdischarge response and reduces its amplitude in cortex, thalamus, and hippocampus, whereas trimethadione reduces duration only in the thalamus. The small but definite increase in 1f electroshock seizure threshold induced by DPH, which probably represents mainly cortical discharge, is consonant with the increase in cerebral-cortical threshold observed by Schallek and Kuehn [101]. It is evident, therefore, that DPH is effective in reducing spread of seizure discharge in all areas but has only a selective effect on seizure threshold, namely, elevation of the cortical threshold. Other data also demonstrate the ability of DPH in various species to elevate the seizure threshold of the cortex [3, 20, 44, 106, 118] and to reduce duration and amplitude of the seizure discharge, that is, to prevent seizure spread [106, 118]. It also elevates the threshold of hippocampus, amygdala, and anterior dorsal nucleus of the thalamus [3, 20]. However, unlike phenobarbital, it does not affect the threshold of the reticular activating system nor prevent activation of the cortex, either in the normal EEG or when the reticular activating system is stimulated electrically [94]. Furthermore, Blum [9] found no influence of anticonvulsant doses of DPH on sensory relay paths to the pyramidal tract, but did find that such doses depressed the motor cortical and thalamic pathways to the pyramidal tract. Indirect pathways involving more synapses were depressed more readily, again an indication of effectiveness of the drug in blocking spread of discharge.

The threshold for stimulation of the diencephalon was found to be elevated by DPH, according to Gangloff and Monnier [44]. However, Morrell et al. [75] found no influence of DPH on the diencephalon nor did they find an effect of the drug, in contrast to phenobarbital and trimethadione, on discharge induced by pentylenetetrazol activation of chronic experimental foci in visual cortex of rabbit. Also, it did not prevent projection of the focus to the diencephalon, but was definitely superior to phenobarbital in blocking cortical spread of seizure activity from the focus; trimethadione was inactive in this respect. Thus, the predominant effect of DPH in these experiments was its antispreading effect on maximal seizure patterns and on seizure discharges elicited by other means. Morrell et al. [75] consider this effect to be of particular significance in its clinical action. This correlates with observations in patients that DPH therapy can induce complete remission of grand mal or certain types of partial seizures, but does not completely abolish sensory aura or other prodromal signs; there also remains a localized focus of seizure activity in the EEG.

DPH has, in addition, been tested for its effects on peripheral nerve. For example, various isolated nerve preparations normally respond to supramaximal rapid stimuli with prolonged increase in excitability, also by repetitive firing to a single shock (see [110] for review). These responses are abolished by prior exposure of the nerve preparation to DPH, either in vitro or in nerves tested in situ in animals treated with an anticonvulsant dose of the drug [74]. It also stabilizes nerve fibers from various species against hyperexcitability caused by low calcium or a combination of low calcium and magnesium [61, 95, 110]. It should be emphasized that this anticonvulsant exerts its stabilizing influence on hyperexcitable nerves without impairing the ability of the nerve fiber to carry impulses even at high frequency, nor does it elevate threshold or otherwise alter normal excitation and response properties of neurons. DPH thus has a stabilizing effect on all neural membranes, probably on all excitable and even nonexcitable membranes, but does not appear to interfere with normal function of excitable cells, except in near toxic doses.

Since the predominant effects of DPH are inhibition of spread of seizure activity to involve the entire brain and thereby prevention of seizures, and causing stabilization of excitable membranes, it is pertinent to discuss the effects of this drug on neurons or neuronal patterns that might explain its action. One of the most significant findings concerning DPH which helps to elucidate the mechanism involved in its action is its ability to reduce posttetanic potentiation (PTP) of synaptic transmission within the spinal cord, as well as in the stellate ganglion of the cat, as described by Esplin [28]. The marked effect of the drug on PTP correlates well with its ability to modify the pattern of maximal seizures. Arguments concerning the role of PTP in spread of seizure discharge presented in detail by Esplin [28] will be outlined only briefly here.

PTP is a general synaptic property and appears to be a normal consequence of synaptic excitation. It is an enhancement of synaptic transmission following rapid, repetitive presynaptic stimulation. While PTP is most easily demonstrated following tetanic stimulation, it is apparent that the tendency toward increased transmission potentiality is also present during tetanization, although it is then intermingled with refractoriness and subnormality. Considered in this light, PTP appears to be concerned in all functions of the nervous system characterized by repetitive activity. The process of potentiation acts to oppose neuronal subnormality; but, more significantly with regard to epilepsy, PTP allows the zone of postsynaptic discharge to include neurons not ordinarily concerned in a specific pathway. A clear example of this may be seen in the spinal cord. During PTP it is possible for afferents from one muscle to discharge the motoneurons of another muscle through the monosynaptic pathway. Thus, synaptic connections which normally exert only facilitatory influences actually become excitatory as a result of PTP. It is likely that the intense activity of a seizure focus [76, 83, 96, 125] in the brain leads to potentiation sufficient to produce activity in pathways not ordinarily excited by neurons at the site of the focus. Discharges by these new excitatory connections would then produce potentiation in their axon terminals; the result of this cumulative process would be rapid and progressive detonation of virtually all neurons of the brain. Ward and Schmidt [125], for example, by means of ultramicroelectrodes have measured activity from single cells in seizure foci of patients with epilepsy. In contrast to normal areas, the foci often showed cells with intermittent bursts of high frequency spikes up to 800 per sec and occasionally prolonged high frequency trains of impulses. These high frequency discharges probably cause PTP which is, therefore, a vital link in explaining the observation that seizure discharges travel through cerebral pathways not active under normal conditions. Since DPH exerts its principal effect on the progressive spread of seizure discharge in the brain, the effect of this agent to inhibit PTP is in harmony with the anticonvulsant properties of the drug.

The experiments of Raines and Standaert [88, 89] provide further evidence for an effect of DPH on posttetanic phenomena. In the cat soleus neuromuscular junction they showed that this drug suppresses generation of posttetanic repetitive afterdischarges in the motor nerve [88]. In addition, in anticonvulsant doses, it abolishes posttetanic hyperpolarization originating in the central terminals of dorsal root fibers of spinal cats [89]. Also, Franz and Esplin [42] have demonstrated that DPH prevents the posttetanic enhancement of negative afterpotentials in mammalian C fibers.

The basic mechanism of posttetanic hyperpolarization has not been completely elucidated, but present evidence indicates that this hyperpolarization is dependent upon transport of ions across the membrane during the recovery process (see, for example, [19, 87]). The hyperpolarization is due to summation of positive afterpotentials following tetanic stimulation. DPH thus prevents hyperpolarization by preventing summation of the positive afterpotentials. The possible manner in which this is accomplished will be discussed in a later section.

Posttetanic hyperpolarization is a fundamental neuronal property and appears to be the basic phenomenon that leads to augmentation of the terminal action potential and, hence, activation of a larger proportion of the postsynaptic motor pool which leads to PTP. In the soleus motor nerve, hyperpolarization of terminals probably leads to prolongation of negative afterpotential and formation of a generator potential which reexcites the axon to repetitive discharge. DPH, by suppressing posttetanic hyperpolarization of presynaptic terminals, thereby prevents PTP and posttetanic repetitive discharge which are related to seizure discharge as described above.

Immature Nervous System. The effects of anticonvulsant agents on the immature CNS in developing animals have had little study. Another article in this volume, by Vernadakis and Woodbury (Chap. 19), discusses this aspect; only the results contributing to the mechanism of action of DPH will be considered here.

In developing mice, DPH administered acutely does not significantly influence the lf electroshock seizure threshold prior to 17 days of age but markedly increases the threshold in the older age groups studied [123]. Lack of effect of this drug on the lf threshold in mice prior to 17 days of age is due to this threshold being already very high; the neuronal system on which this threshold depends is not mature, therefore cannot be further elevated by DPH.

In rats up to about 16 days of age, DPH increases the 60 cycle per sec ac seizure threshold but does not change it thereafter [123]; this effect is greatest at 13 days. However, when the drug is given chronically to developing rats from the eighth to the eleventh day after birth, the ac electroshock threshold is lowered [121]. Lack of effect of DPH in rats older than 16 days of age and excitatory effects when the drug is given chronically to developing rats are probably due to the depressant effect of the drug on a central inhibitory system which is developing during this age period. This conclusion is reinforced by experiments in which the effects of DPH on chemically induced seizures in maturing rats have been determined [124]. DPH lowers the median effective dose (CD_{50}) for picrotoxin at all age periods. Hence, it appears to act like picrotoxin in that it blocks presynaptic inhibition, which appears to be the predominant effect of this convulsant agent (see [32] for summary).

When tested against seizures induced by pentylenetetrazol, a drug that produces seizures by activation of excitatory pathways that are unopposed by inhibition [63], DPH has a biphasic effect. Prior to 14 days it lowers the CD_{50} of pentylenetetrazol, and the peak in the CD_{50} that occurs at 12 days of age in the rats given only pentylenetetrazol does not appear. This excitatory effect of DPH to lower the CD_{50} of pentylenetetrazol is probably due to its blockade of presynaptic inhibition as indicated from its enhancement of picrotoxin seizures. Also, in rats between 8 and 12 days of age, DPH lowers the CD_{50} of strychnine, a drug that acts by selectively blocking postsynaptic inhibition. This effect also could be due to its blocking effect on presynaptic inhibition. Thus, in young animals DPH produces excitatory effects as assessed by the responses to all three seizure-inducing agents and by its ability to lower the electroshock seizure threshold on chronic administration. Its basic excitatory effect, which persists in the adult animal, appears to be blockade of presynaptic inhibition, and this would explain its lack of effect on electroshock seizure threshold, as described above, and its excitatory effects in high doses.

In rats after 14 days of age, DPH raises the threshold for pentylenetetrazol-induced seizures, an effect which decreases with age. When tested against strychnine seizures, DPH increases the threshold for the convulsant after the fourteenth postnatal day, as it does for pentylenetetrazol, and this effect also decreases with age until the thirty-sixth day, at which time the threshold for strychnine is not altered by the anticonvulsant. Correspondence between the effects of DPH on strychnine and pentylenetetrazol seizures after the fourteenth day suggests that the decrease in excitation is due to enhancement of postsynaptic inhibition by the drug. In 4-day-old animals DPH elevates the threshold for strychnine. This is presumably due to enhancement of postsynaptic inhibition in the spinal cord, which is mature in this age period [119]. It is clearly evident from these studies that the net effect of DPH depends on the particular system (excitatory or inhibitory) that predominates in the CNS at the age period tested. When these stages have been defined, the developing animal is useful for describing selective mechanisms of action of anticonvulsant agents.

In contrast to its effects on the thresholds for minimal seizures, DPH markedly raises the threshold for evoking the tonic-flexor component of maximal electroshock seizures at all age periods [123]. Flexor-extensor spinal cord convulsions can be elicited by electrical stimulation of the cord in 1-day-old rats [119]. The flexion-extension frequency curve obtained in 12-day-old rats is similar to the response observed in adult rats, which indicates that the spinal cord convulsive pattern has developed by the twelfth day. When administered acutely to rats who are 4, 8, and 12 days old, DPH significantly reduces the duration of tonic hindlimb extension of spinal cord convulsions [122]. It is evident, therefore, that at all age periods and at all levels of the cerebrospinal axis, DPH has a remarkable ability to modify the pattern of maximal seizures by preventing spread of seizure activity, presumably by its effects on PTP.

In summarizing the effects of DPH in developing animals, the evidence strongly suggests that during early postnatal development, the drug exerts net excitatory effects on the CNS by blocking presynaptic, inhibitory systems which predominate at this time. At later stages of development and in adulthood, this excitatory effect of DPH is counteracted by slight activation of postsynaptic inhibitory systems that have developed during this time and by marked depression of spread of seizure discharges as a result of its effects on PTP. Hence, the net anticonvulsant effect of the drug becomes predominant in rats only after 3 weeks of age. The biochemical mechanisms involved in these neurophysiological effects of DPH are discussed below.

Effects on Cardiac Muscle and Vascular Smooth Muscle

DPH exerts a marked effect on the excitable tissues of the heart and vascular system (see [67] for review), as is the case for CNS. Although it is more effective when the system is hyperexcitable, this anticonvulsant exerts an effect on normal tissue. In 1941, soon after its introduction as an anticonvulsant, Baudouin and Hazard [6] noted in intact dogs a diminution in myocardial contractile force and arterial pressure following intravenous administration of 5 mg per kg. Since that time, numerous observations (to be summarized here) have established the effects of DPH on the cardiovascular system and its place in therapy.

Contractility. A direct myocardial depressant effect (negative inotropic effect) of DPH has been demonstrated in various species of animals both in vivo [6, 50, 70, 71, 97] and in vitro [68]. For example, Mixter et al. [71] found that the most pronounced cardiovascular effect of DPH, in intact dogs and in dogs whose cardiopulmonary and systemic circulations were separated from each other, is direct myocardial depression of contractility. In addition, they found a reflex cardiac depression when the peripheral vasculature was exposed to the drug. The effect was abolished by denervation, an indication of the reflex nature of the effect. This could, however, be due to release of acetylcholine by DPH from the vagus nerve endings to the heart. Indeed, small doses of DPH have been shown to produce vagal stimulation which results in atrioventricular block [17].

The effects of atropine on the reflex myocardial depression produced by DPH and stimulatory effects of the anticonvulsant on the vagus should be investigated. Stimulation of the vagus causes release of acetylcholine which produces a negative inotropic effect on the heart and causes atrioventricular block. Further evidence for a stimulatory effect of DPH on nerve endings to release acetylcholine is derived from studies on isolated ileum of the rat, as discussed below; this effect is blocked by atropine. Ventricular function curves in dogs have demonstrated a negative inotropic effect of DPH on the heart [70]; repeated injection of the drug produces a cumulative negative inotropic effect. However, Helfant et al. [54] and Lüllman and Weber [64] found that DPH could block the arrhythmias produced by digitalis without blocking its positive inotropic effects. This should be tested in the isolated perfused heart. In isolated beating heart cells in tissue culture, DPH decreases the number of cells beating (automaticity) and antagonizes the digitalis-induced increase in automaticity [68]. Also, in a Langendorff preparation of a rat heart, DPH produces marked decrease in myocardial contraction, an effect which is antagonized by ouabain; DPH also antagonizes the increased force of contraction (positive inotropic effect) induced by ouabain [138]. The nature of the DPH-ouabain antagonism is discussed below.

Automaticity, Excitability, Conduction Velocity, and Refractory Period. In chick embryo heart cells, dissociated by trypsin and then grown in tissue culture, spontaneous beating occurs in most cells. Addition of DPH (50 μg per ml) to such cells caused reduction in the total percentage of cells beating [68]. Digoxin effectively antagonizes the depressant effect of DPH on the automaticity of these beating cells. DPH also depresses ventricular automaticity in vivo in the normal heart and suppresses the enhanced automaticity which leads to arrhythmias induced by digitalis [53]. Thus, automaticity of the heart is reduced by DPH. The antiarrhythmic effect of DPH (see below) may be due, at least in part, to depression of automaticity.

A prolongation of atrioventricular conduction time by DPH was noted by Scherf and by Sasyniuk and Dresel [100, 102]. The latter also noted marked influence of the drug to increase the atrioventricular nodal conduction delay of an extrasystole. In contrast, enhanced atrioventricular conduction by DPH in the normal heart [8, 53, 94] and antagonism by it of the action of digitalis on the atrioventricular node [53] have been reported. Higher doses lead to idioventricular rhythms, severe bradycardia, and eventual cardiac arrest. Dreifus et al. [22] have shown that this drug diminishes conduction time between myocardial fibers. Thus, in addition to its effects of decreasing the force of myocardial contraction, DPH causes myocardial depression (decreased excitability).

Blood Pressure, Cardiac Output, Coronary Circulation, and Peripheral Circulation. Rapid intravenous injection of DPH generally results in a decreased blood pressure. This is due, at least in part, to the negative inotropic effect of the drug and, more importantly, initially to its direct vasodilating effect on vascular smooth muscle [6, 50, 71, 97]. Cardiac output may initially increase but later it is decreased due to myocardial depression. Dilatation of vascular smooth muscle produced by the drug also occurs in coronary vessels and results in increased coronary blood flow [50], but this is variable and difficult to assess [97]. In man, however, contrary to the effects noted in animals, doses of DPH effective in preventing cardiac arrhythmias (in patients undergoing routine cardiac catheterization) had no hemodynamic effects [18]. Thus, there was no change in cardiac output, peripheral resistance, pulmonary pressures, or electrocardiogram (EKG); higher doses, however, do cause some changes in these parameters. Thus, the excitable tissues of the heart and vascular smooth muscle, as for the brain, are depressed by DPH.

Electrical Activity of the Heart. The observations of Harris and Kokernot in 1950 [51] that DPH was effective in abolishing ventricular tachycardia produced in anesthetized dogs by acute ligation of a branch of the left coronary artery engendered much interest. This drug held interest not only as a therapeutic agent for treatment of various types of cardiac arrhythmias, but also for its heuristic value in studying the mechanism of its suppressant effect on excitable tissues. The antiarrhythmic effect of the drug has been demonstrated for arrhythmias that occur in acutely induced myocardial infarction in animals and in naturally occurring disease in man [5, 143], for various other cardiac arrhythmias [7, 103], and for digitalis-induced arrhythmias in animals and man [7, 17, 52, 53, 54, 62, 77, 144]. Chronic treatment prevents recurrence of the arrhythmias [7, 54]. Atrial flutter and fibrillation induced by local application of aconitine and delphinine to the atria are prevented by low doses of DPH [102].

Thus, the drug appears to prevent arrhythmias by blocking the spread of excessive electrical activity originating at the focus, an action similar to its blockade of spread of seizure activity from a focus in the brain. Changes in the EKG are produced by DPH, and typical changes in the EKG induced by overdosage with ouabain are antagonized by the drug [22, 38, 64, 102, 126]. By itself, the drug causes prolongation of atrioventricular conduction (increased PR interval), although enhancement of such conduction has been reported by others [53]; widening of QRS in high doses leading to cardiac standstill; decreased T-wave; and increased QT interval. In guinea pigs given ouabain [126] or digoxin [64], DPH increases the LD_{50} of these digitalis glycosides (decreases mortality); it also counteracts the resultant EKG changes, due, in this case at least in part, to K accumulation in plasma as a result of the inhibition of the Na pump in cells induced by ouabain, and prevents to a large extent the resulting loss of K and gain of Na in heart cells [126].

One of the most striking illustrations of the antagonistic effects of DPH and ouabain was observed by J. W. Woodbury [141]. The effects of these two drugs on the intracellular action potential measured by ultramicroelectrodes in frog heart muscle were tested. Digitalis markedly shortened duration of the action potential, whereas DPH prolonged it. The shortened potential produced by digitalis could be prevented by simultaneous exposure to DPH. This effect of DPH to prolong the action potential has been interpreted by J. W. Woodbury to be a result of the stimulatory effect of this anticonvulsant agent on the Na pump, as previously proposed by D. M. Woodbury for the brain [131]. This seems reasonable, since it antagonizes ouabain which inhibits the Na pump. Similar antagonistic effects of DPH on ouabain-induced changes in the intracellular action potential have been noted by Lüllman and Weber [64].

It is clear from these studies that most of the effects of digitalis on the heart can be antagonized by DPH and vice versa. These two drugs, therefore, appear to be rather selective antagonists. The antagonism applies not only to their effects on the heart, but also to their effects on the brain (see above), on the thyroid gland [133], and on the gastrointestinal tract as discussed below. Possible mechanisms of this antagonism and their relation to the Na pump and to the mechanism of action of DPH are discussed below.

Effects on Skeletal Muscle

Although DPH depresses myocardial and vascular smooth muscle and the contraction of gastrointestinal smooth muscle, as discussed below, its effects on the contraction of skeletal muscle have been studied little. In cat soleus muscle, DPH modifies the tetanic contraction and often increases twitch tension by a direct effect on muscle [88]. Preliminary data [138] obtained from a rat phrenic nerve-diaphragm preparation in vitro suggest that DPH, after initial stimulation, blocks the effects of direct lf electrical stimulation of the muscle, without altering the response to indirect stimulation through the phrenic nerve. This suggests, as will be shown below for smooth muscle, that the drug inhibits either excitation-contraction coupling or the contractile process. It also blocks the contraction of frog rectus abdominus muscle induced by acetylcholine and potassium [115]. Further work is obviously needed.

Effects on Smooth Muscle

The contraction in response to various agents and the spontaneous activity of gastrointestinal smooth muscle are markedly diminished by DPH in anticonvulsant doses [23, 43, 45, 92]. In isolated rabbit intestine, DPH reduces tone, amplitude, and rate of contraction in doses as low as 5 μg per ml (2×10^{-5}M); doses of 80 μg per ml (3×10^{-4}M) completely abolish the contractions. This effect is rapidly reversible when the drug is washed out [23]. These observations were extended by van Rees et al. [92] to the isolated ileum of the rat. DPH in doses as low as 0.1 μg per ml causes an initial stimulation of gut contraction and the effect is blocked by atropine. This indicates that DPH might cause release of acetylcholine from parasympathetic nerve endings in the wall of isolated ileum. On the other hand, in higher doses, this drug, as depicted in the dose effect curves of Fig. 23-2, progressively inhibits contraction of the ileum produced by acetylcholine, an effect previously noted by Gayet-Hallion [45]. Analysis of these results from the dose-effect curves and by Lineweaver-Burke plots shows that this effect is mainly of the noncompetitive type of inhibition (that is, decreased maximal effect with only a slight change in Km). However, part of the effect appears to be competitive to acetylcholine (increased Km) and this is further demonstrated by the fact that DPH enhances the competitive effect of atropine on acetylcholine-induced contractions of the gut. That the noncompetitive inhibition of the response to acetylcholine, which is the majority of the effect, is due to an action on excitation-contraction coupling or the contractile process is indicated by experiments with $BaCl_2$.

Barium has a direct stimulatory effect on the contraction of smooth muscle. The marked increase in contraction induced by barium ion is blocked noncompetitively by DPH [43, 92]. The doses are in the same range as those that inhibit acetylcholine-

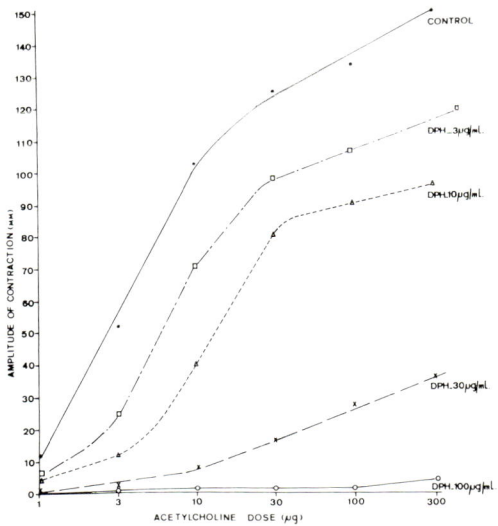

FIG. 23-2. Effect of diphenylhydantoin (DPH) at various dose levels on contraction of isolated ileum of rat exposed to various concentrations of acetylcholine. Temperature, 37°C. Ileum bathed in Tyrode's solution. Ordinate is amplitude of contraction of ileum in millimeters and abscissa is dose in micrograms of acetylcholine added to the bath. Graph plotted from unpublished data of van Rees et al. [92]. See text for discussion.

induced contractions. Doses of 30–100 μg per ml completely abolish barium-induced contractions of the muscle. This is the same dosage range found by Druckman and Moore [23] to abolish spontaneous contractions, as described above. DPH also blocks the contractions of smooth muscle induced by the convulsants pentylenetetrazol and nikethamide [43].

It appears that this anticonvulsant can cause acetylcholine release from the parasympathetic nerve endings in the intestinal tract as well as in the heart (see above). The stimulation of contraction of intestinal smooth muscle induced by DPH as a result of acetylcholine release is evident only at low doses of the drug. At higher doses, acetylcholine release is probably still present, but manifestation of the effect in the smooth muscle is absent because these high doses directly inhibit the influence of the released acetylcholine on the muscle. Whether acetylcholine release in response to the drug also occurs in the brain and could account for central excitatory effects is discussed in a later section.

The inhibitory influence of DPH, not only on spontaneous contractions of the gut but also on contractions induced by acetylcholine and barium, suggests that it affects the excitable membrane of the muscle and excitation-contraction coupling, or the contractile process itself. In intestinal smooth muscle, acetylcholine increases membrane permeability to Na, K, and Cl which leads to depolarization and contraction. That portion of the effect of DPH which cannot be attributed to blocking of the barium effect antagonizes acetylcholine and enhances the atropine blockade of the acetylcholine response. At least part of the action of DPH appears to be due to competition with acetylcholine for the receptor site on the muscle; it thereby prevents this mediator from acting to increase permeability. It could, however, antagonize the increased permeability induced by acetylcholine in some other manner. Further studies are necessary in order to learn the mechanism of this effect. It is not known how barium acts to stimulate contraction of the muscle. It might act, as does calcium, by enhancing excitation-contraction coupling or by affecting ATPase activity and thereby stimulating the contractile process. However, elucidation of the mechanism of DPH antagonism of the barium-induced contraction should provide further information on the mechanism of action not only of barium but also of the anticonvulsant. DPH counteracts the ouabain-induced contraction of rat ileum smooth muscle, also the ouabain-induced blockade of acetylcholine contractions; yet given alone, DPH by itself blocks the same process, as has been recently described [92]. Whether ouabain antagonizes barium-induced contraction of the ileum and whether this effect is prevented by DPH are questions now being studied in the Department of Pharmacology at the University of Leiden, where this work on the smooth muscle effects of DPH is being conducted.

DPH antagonism of the ouabain effect on acetylcholine-induced contractions of the gut again suggests that at least part of the action of DPH is stimulation of the Na pump (as in heart and brain), or at least antagonism of the ouabain-induced inhibition of the pump; other actions are possible, however. Further evidence for this will be discussed below.

DPH in small doses (6 µg per ml) inhibits contractions and decreases tonus of the isolated, nonpregnant rabbit uterus, also decreases tonus in the uterus of the rabbit and cat in vivo [21, 45].

It is apparent from all the studies reviewed here that this drug has a general effect to depress contractility of smooth muscle. It does, however, increase contractions in low doses by causing acetylcholine release from nerve endings in the wall of the muscle.

Effects on Biochemical Processes
Effects on Electrolyte and Acid-Base Metabolism

Throughout this presentation, allusion has been made to the effects of DPH on electrolyte metabolism and ionic fluxes. It is now germane to document these effects.

The first indication that DPH affected electrolyte metabolism was the observations of Woodbury [131] that 40 mg per kg of the drug given every 6 hours in a series of 4 doses produced marked decrease in total Na content and Na space of cerebral cortex in rats, with no significant change in total K concentration. Calculation of intracellular Na concentration from the Cl space in cerebral cortex indicated that DPH decreases Na concentration in the cell but does not alter intracellular K concentration. It is obvious now that Cl is present not only in the extracellular space of brain but also in neuronal and glial cells; hence, measurement of extracellular space by this means is inaccurate, and the calculated intracellular Na is lower than the real value. Also, location of the cellular Na is not known because of its presence in both glial and neuronal cells. However, despite these reservations about the absolute value of cell Na concentration and uncertainty of its exact distribution, since the Cl space was not significantly changed by DPH treatment, decrease in nonchloride-space Na induced by the drug is real. If the data are recalculated on the basis of an inulin space of 14 percent, the correct extracellular space of cerebral cortex of the rat [142], there is a decrease in the noninulin-space Na concentration induced by the drug. Location of this decrease in Na concentration, whether glial or neuronal or both, has not been assessed as yet.

DPH also decreases Na space and intracellular Na concentration in the cerebral cortex of rats made hyponatremic by intraperitoneal injection of isosmotic glucose solution; in such animals without the drug, Na space and intracellular Na concentration are increased above normal. Furthermore, decrease in brain K concentration that results from hyponatremia is nearly prevented by the drug. In addition, DPH reduces the rise in cerebral cortical non-chloride-space Na that follows maximal electroshock seizures [131]. Thus, Na concentration in the brain is reduced by this anticonvulsant both in normal animals and in animals made hyperexcitable either by hyponatremia or by electrically induced seizures.

Accompanying the decrease in non-chloride-space Na concentration induced by DPH, there is an increase in the rate of turnover of radiosodium in the cerebral cortex. The most logical interpretation of these data is that DPH causes increased movement of Na out of the nonchloride space of cerebral cortex and lowers its concentration there; that is, it increases active Na transport in the cerebral cortex. The calculated concentration of K in brain cells after DPH treatment does not change, except after its reduction in the animals made hyperexcitable by intraperitoneal administration of glucose solution. However, K is high in both neuronal and glial cells and, in order to determine its concentration in each cell type, the proportion of neurons to glia and the concentration of K in at least one of these cells must be known. If glial cells serve as a sink for K during nervous activity, as has been postulated, then stimulation of the brain sufficient to cause a seizure would shift K from neurons to glia without changing total K content in brain, since extracellular K concentration is low. Therefore, it is possible that DPH increases K concentration in neurons and decreases it in glial cells without changing total K concentration of the brain. In order to measure such a change, compartmentalization of K by means of kinetic analysis of radioactive K-uptake curves is necessary. Since, in brain cells, the active extrusion of Na is generally coupled to inward transport of K, DPH probably also increases intracellular K concentration.

Other data have since corroborated the above observations of a stimulatory effect of DPH on the Na pump not only in brain but also in other tissues. In synaptosomes isolated from rat cerebral cortex, Festoff and Appel [35] found that DPH, in low doses, stimulates Na-K-ATPase activity maximally when the ratio of Na to K was 50:1, but inhibited activity of this enzyme when the Na to K ratio was 5:1 or less. A close link has been established between Na-K-ATPase activity and cation transport in many tissues including brain [24, 130]. Since this enzyme is present in synaptic endings which have the ability to transport Na and K actively in a coupled system, enhancement of activity of this enzyme by DPH when the Na to K ratio is high probably has direct pertinence to its anticonvulsant effects. This is, in particular, the case since Escueta and Appel [27] have demonstrated that DPH stimulates K accumulation in incubated synaptosomes of the cortex. During seizures, neuronal concentration of Na is increased and that of K decreased. In red blood cells, activity of Na-K-ATPase is determined by Na concentration internal to the membrane and K concentration external to the membrane. Therefore, increased Na and decreased K concentrations in neurons induced by seizures increase the Na to K ratio, a situation which in vitro at least is favorable for stimulation of Na-K-ATPase activity by DPH. Enhanced active transport of Na out of the cell and K into the cell would stabilize the membrane in the nerve endings (synaptosomes) and prevent further seizure activity. Blockade of PTP by DPH could be a result of stabilization of the membrane by enhanced active transport of Na and K; this would prevent hyperpolarization from summation of the positive afterpotentials at the nerve endings and thereby reduce PTP.

Rawson and Pincus [90] have shown that DPH causes inhibition of Na-K-ATPase activity in microsomal fractions of rat and guinea pig brain and in whole homogenates of human brain when the Na to K ratio is low. Thus, under normal conditions of the brain, the enzyme may be inhibited by DPH and this may account for the initial excitatory effects of the drug in the adult. Evidence for this viewpoint is strengthened by observations cited above that in neonatal rats up to 12 days of age, DPH decreases threshold to seizures induced by electroshock, strychnine, picrotoxin, and pentylenetetrazol. In such animals, where the Na and K concentrations in cells can be measured because glial cells are few in number, the blood-brain barrier is not well developed, and the extracellular space can be determined [34]; DPH, in the same doses that increase excitability, increases intracellular Na and decreases intracellular K concentration [134]. In these young animals, K concentration in cerebrospinal fluid (CSF), and presumably in the interstitial space of the brain, is higher than in adult animals because the transport system for its exit from the brain is not well developed. The ratio of Na to K is thus lower, and this would favor inhibition of the enzyme by DPH. These data provide strong evidence for a role of the enzyme in the active transport of Na and K.

Further evidence is derived from the effects of DPH on tissues other than brain. In cardiac muscle, the drug slightly decreases intracellular Na concentration but does not affect intracellular K concentration; the turnover of radiosodium is slightly increased [131]. DPH prolongs duration of the action potential of frog ventricle fibers, when given alone or given to counteract the shortened duration caused by ouabain; this effect has been interpreted to be due to an enhancing action of the drug on active Na transport [141]. In K-free perfusion medium the action-potential duration was prolonged at least fivefold by DPH as compared with twofold in normal Ringer's solution. The effect occurred within 20 min after exposure to the drug. Decreased K permeability or increased Na permeability or both, of the membrane during the plateau phase of the action potential could also produce the observed effects. This is, however, unlikely since DPH antagonizes the shortened duration induced by ouabain, a glycoside that blocks the pump and which has not been shown to affect permeability. Data to be presented at this point also suggest an effect of DPH on Na transport in the heart. Enhancement by the drug of the effect of low K on the action potential is of interest because of the observations of Festoff and Appel [35] that a high Na to K ratio favors activation of Na-K-ATPase by DPH. This provides further evidence for an enhancement of active transport in the heart by this drug.

Helfant et al. [52] have demonstrated that decrease in arterial-coronary sinus K difference induced by toxic doses of digitalis is prevented by DPH and, at the same time, arrhythmias induced by digitalis are abolished. The increased rate of loss of radioactive rubidium induced by toxic doses of digitalis in isolated guinea pig atrial tissue is also prevented by DPH [144]. Thus, increased K and Rb loss from the heart induced by digitalis is prevented by this anticonvulsant. Decreased loss of K and Rb as a result of DPH could be due to decreased permeability of the cardiac muscle cell membrane or to stimulation of the active Na-K coupled transport system of the cell. Since K and Rb loss caused by digitalis is due to inhibition of the Na-K pump and since DPH antagonizes both the positive inotropic and electrophysiological effects of digitalis, it is likely that the anticonvulsant acts on the heart through enhancement of Na transport, as it does on the brain. Further evidence for this is provided by the studies of Watson and Woodbury [126], who demonstrated that increase in Na concentration and decrease in K concentration induced by toxic doses of ouabain in guinea pig hearts in vivo are prevented by DPH, and arrhythmias produced by ouabain were also prevented. The evidence, therefore, strongly favors a stimulatory effect of DPH on the Na-K active transport system in the heart. The effect is more prominent when the pump is compromised by digitalis, and this may provide the ionic explanation for marked ability of DPH to restore excitability to normal when it is abnormally increased and the lesser effect of the drug on normal cardiac tissue. Influence of DPH on cardiac muscle Na-K-ATPase activity in media containing various Na to K ratios should be assessed in the presence and absence of digitalis.

In isolated peripheral nerve, Pincus and colleagues [84] found that DPH decreased the concentration of intracellular Na. Also, the radioactive sodium experiments reported by Woodbury [131] for frog sciatic nerve in vitro indicated that this anticonvulsant increased the efflux of Na from such nerves made hyperexcitable by immersion in isotonic phosphate solution. These data are consistent with its effects on brain to decrease Na concentration in cells and increase radiosodium turnover as a result of enhanced active transport of Na.

Figure 23-3 shows that DPH increases the rate of absorption of a NaCl solution from ligated sections of the jejunum [92]. Under normal conditions Na is absorbed against a concentration and electrical gradient. Such absorption involves active transport of Na from the luminal fluid into the blood across the epithelial cells of the mucosa. DPH increases the Na concentration difference across the mucosal cells and enhances the rate of absorption of Na, Cl, and water (Fig. 23-3). It increases also the concentration difference of K in the other direction, that is, between blood and luminal fluid. Furthermore, Na concentration in the intestinal wall is decreased, and K concentration is increased by the drug during the period of its enhancement of NaCl absorption. It is therefore evident that in the intestine DPH stimulates active transport of Na across the mucosal epithelium. Since ouabain blocks absorption of NaCl via inhibition of the Na pump, enhancement of absorption of DPH is probably due to stimulation of the pump. Experiments to test the effects of DPH on the ouabain-induced blockade of absorption and on intestinal Na-K-ATPase activity are now in progress. The ratio of Na to K exposed to the Na transport system across the mucosal epithelium (luminal Na, extracellular K if the Na pump is on the membrane toward the serosal side of the cell) is in the range (50:1) that Festoff and Appel [35]

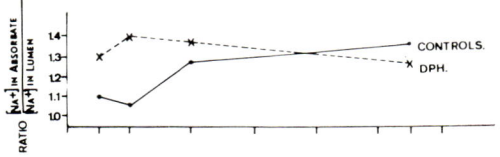

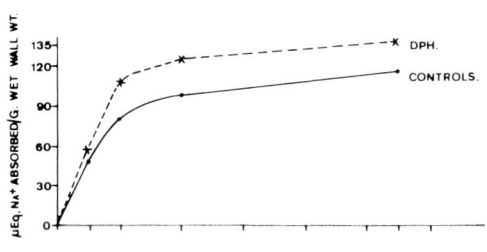

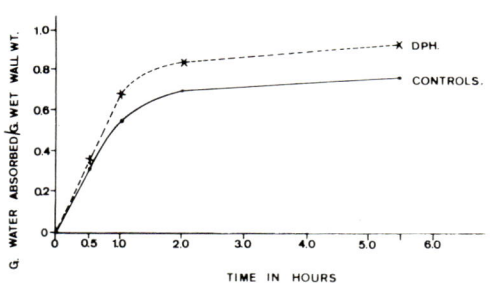

FIG. 23-3. Effect of DPH (100 μg per ml, 4×10^{-4}M) on transfer of Na and water across mucosa of jejunal sections of rat intestine. Ordinate in lower graph is grams of water absorbed per gram wet weight of intestinal wall; in middle graph it is μEq Na absorbed per gram wet weight of intestinal wall; and in upper graph it is ratio of Na concentration in absorbate fluid to that in luminal water in control and DPH-treated rats. Abscissa is time in hours after injection of 0.5 ml of 0.9 percent NaCl solution into each of ligated gut sections in which absorption was tested. At all time periods tested, concentration of Na in absorbate fluid was higher than its concentration in luminal water; ratio between the two was greater in the DPH-treated group than in the controls except at 5.5 hours [92]. See text for further explanation.

found was most favorable for stimulation of activity of Na-K-ATPase activity by DPH.

Earlier studies by Woodbury [134] showed that the same doses of this anticonvulsant that were effective in decreasing Na concentration in brain and heart also decreased total Na concentration in the gastrointestinal tract plus its contents. In addition, he noted that the drug decreased concentration of Na in skin and liver and markedly increased K concentration in liver.

Absorption of Na across renal tubules in dog kidney is increased by DPH, an effect attributed by Koch et al. [59] to enhancement of active Na transport. Preliminary data from our laboratory [55] suggest that the active process that transports Na across epithelial cells of the choroid plexus is enhanced by DPH. However, flux-rate studies with radioactive Na and determination of the effect of ouabain on the process are necessary before final conclusions are warranted. If this proves to be the case, it could also explain the observations of Aird and Strait [1] that DPH decreases uptake of convulsive doses of cocaine into brain and CSF, which these authors interpreted as due to DPH-induced decrease in permeability of the blood-brain barrier to cocaine. Enhanced transport and secretion of CSF caused by DPH would accelerate loss of the cocaine via the CSF and arachnoid villi pathway as the result of the well-known sink effect of the CSF. Further experiments are obviously necessary in this area.

DPH does not produce any acid-base alterations in brain or blood of rats given anticonvulsant doses of the drug [135]. It also does not affect carbonic anhydrase activity [73].

Effects on Energy, Carbohydrate, Protein, Lipid, and Nucleic Acid Metabolism

Since DPH stimulates transport of Na across cell membranes, a process that requires energy and also in many tissues appears to increase growth of epithelial and parenchymatous cells and of connective tissue elements, it is pertinent to summarize the effects of this drug on various metabolic processes in order to elucidate, if possible, their biochemical bases.

Energy and Carbohydrate Metabolism. DPH is not a general depressant of the nervous system. Hence, unlike large doses of phenobarbital and trimethadione, it does not depress the respiration of cerebral tissue. In patients with epilepsy during the interseizure period, brain respiration is not affected by either DPH or phenobarbital in anticonvulsant doses [58]. In vitro, respiration of isolated cerebral tissues in media containing a variety of oxidizable substrates (pyruvate, lactate, or glucose) is unaffected by $10^{-4}M$ to $10^{-3}M$ (25 to 250 μg per ml) DPH or trimethadione; also unaffected is the metabolism of glutamic acid by brain slices [48]. Respiration of brain slices stimulated by 2,4-dinitrophenol, by 50 mM KCl, and by guanidines is also unaltered by DPH or trimethadione. However, in media containing glucose, pyruvate, or lactate, increases in respiration and anaerobic glycolysis induced in brain slices by electric stimulation with alternating currents of 500 or 2000 cycles per sec are selectively inhibited by $10^{-4}M$ to $4 \times 10^{-4}M$ DPH and by $10^{-3}M$ trimethadione, whereas increased respiratory and anaerobic glycolytic responses to currents of 50 cycles per sec or to brief condensor pulses of 100 per sec are not affected by the two drugs. Decreased creatine phosphate and increased inorganic phosphate levels that result from high frequency stimulation are not, however, affected by the anticonvulsants; nonselective depressants antagonize the increase in respiration brought about by all frequencies examined [40, 48]. DPH thus blocks the effects of high frequency stimulation on the energy metabolism of brain slices, but not those of low frequency stimulation. This probably has some pertinence to the effects of the drug to block PTP and posttetanic hyperpolarization, processes which are undoubtedly involved in the genesis of epileptic discharges (see above) and during which excessive oxygen consumption occurs during the hyperpolarization stage following the tetanus (see [86]).

Effects of DPH on energy and carbohydrate metabolism in brain, other than those mentioned above, have been studied little. It has been observed that xylose transport in brain slices is a carrier-mediated process, susceptible to the effects of anticonvulsants [46]. DPH decreases rate of transport and intracellular concentration of xylose when the incubating medium contains a low concentration of xylose, but it is without effect when the xylose concentration is high. Phenobarbital and didione, however, accelerate transport of xylose when its concentration in the medium is low and decrease it when its concentration is high. The mechanism of these effects of DPH, phenobarbital, and didione on xylose transport and its relation to their anticonvulsant effects, are not clear at the present time.

Acute single doses of DPH increase the concentration of glycogen in brain, liver, and skeletal muscle of intact rats, but the effect is absent in adrenalectomized or hypophysectomized animals. Thus, on acute administration, the increase is due to release of glucocorticoids [130, 140]. However, more prolonged administration decreases glycogen in liver but increases it in brain at a time when initial adrenocortical stimulation has disappeared; the decrease in liver glycogen is associated with an increase in blood sugar. Enhanced glycogenesis in brain would thus appear to be due initially to adrenocortical stimulation by DPH and subsequently to a direct effect of the drug. Such a direct effect on brain glycogen is also consonant with observations of Broddle and Nelson [11] that DPH in very high single doses (200 mg per kg) increases the levels of glucose (eightfold) and glycogen (twofold) in the brain of mice 15 hr after administration. They also noted that lactate levels were decreased (by 40 percent) and that phosphocreatine concentrations were increased at 7 and 15 hr after giving the drug, but that ATP levels were unchanged. The brain to serum glucose ratio is increased by the drug, a possible indication that the carrier-mediated transport of glucose into the brain, unlike that of xylose, is increased. However, these two effects, increased glucose and glycogen concentration in brain, could be due to stimulation of the adrenal cortex produced by acute single doses of the drug.

In anticonvulsant, nontoxic doses (20 mg per kg), DPH did not change the above-named metabolite levels in brain. The same authors noted that the rate of change of these metabolites after decapitation, a measure of metabolic rate, was modified by DPH at the high-dose level. A 40 percent reduction in high-energy phosphate utilization and a 60 percent reduction in glucose utilization were noted in the treated animals, but glycogen levels did not change. Since the animals exhibited lethargy, after initial hyperexcitability, beginning an hour after treatment with this large dose, it is difficult to assess whether the increased levels of high-energy phosphate in the brain and their decreased utilization after decapitation are a direct effect of the drug or of the decrease in excitability noted at the time of the measurements. Since no effects were noted with anticonvulsant doses, it is difficult to relate the observed alterations to its anticonvulsant actions.

Greengard and McIlwain [48] observed no change in inorganic phosphate or creatine phosphate content of unstimulated or stimulated isolated cerebral cortical slices after either DPH or trimethadione treatment. Nor did Fingl et al. [37] find an effect of DPH on the rate of incorporation of radiophosphate into the acid-soluble fraction of frog sciatic nerve rendered hyperexcitable by immersion in high phosphate concentrations, although the drug inhibited the rate of incorporation of radiophosphate into the phospholipid fraction.

In summarizing the effects of DPH on energy and carbohydrate metabolism, we note that the drug appears to inhibit oxygen uptake when the brain is subjected to high frequency stimulation, and to increase the glycogen content of cells by an as yet unknown direct action as well as by an indirect effect through adrenocortical stimulation. Other effects are noted only in high doses, hence their relevance to the anticonvulsant effect cannot be assessed.

Amino Acid, Protein, Lipid, and Nucleic Acid Metabolism. The effects of DPH on amino acid metabolism in brain in vivo have been described by Vernadakis and Woodbury ([120], see also [135]). The most prominent effect is decrease in glutamic acid and increase in glutamine concentrations in the brain; the ratio between the two concentrations is markedly decreased. These changes occur in intact rats, adrenalectomized rats, and adrenalectomized rats given a maintenance dose of adrenal-cortical extract, hence are independent of the adrenal cortex. Gamma-aminobutyric acid (GABA) concentration in brain is also increased by the drug, but the change is much greater in adrenalectomized than in intact animals; the electroshock seizure threshold is also higher in adrenalectomized rats. Thus, the adrenocortical steroids released as a result of DPH treatment antagonize direct effects of the anticonvulsant to elevate GABA concentration in brain, also its ability to elevate seizure threshold (see subsequent discussion).

These metabolic effects of DPH on glutamic acid, glutamine, and GABA metabolism in brain can be explained by the following hypothesis. Since conversion of glutamic acid to glutamine is an energy-dependent process that requires ATP, enhancement of this conversion by DPH suggests that this drug makes more energy available for the occurrence of such a reaction. This is also consonant with its enhancement of transport of electrolytes as presented above, another energy-dependent process. It would appear from these observations that the availability of high-energy phosphates is increased by the drug, but further work is required to prove this effect. In addition to enhancement of glutamine and GABA production from glutamic acid, DPH promotes conversion of glutamic acid to Krebs cycle intermediates via formation of α-ketoglutarate and possibly enhances protein synthesis. Enhanced protein synthesis is also suggested by some of the reported effects of the drug on gingival tissue, skin, and liver and by some observations to be discussed later for brain. The enhanced glycogen synthesis in the brain induced by DPH could result from increased utilization of glutamic acid via the Krebs cycle, an effect that would be enhanced by its concurrent effect to stimulate adrenocortical secretion. Since alternative explanations for these effects of DPH on amino acid metabolism are possible, further work is indicated.

It has been suggested (see [135]) that inasmuch as changes in amino acids induced by DPH seem to be specifically related to changes in the glutamic acid and glutamine system, and since an inverse correlation has been shown between the ratio of brain extracellular to intracellular Na concentration and the ratio of glutamic acid to glutamine concentrations in brain, the active transport of Na may be closely coupled to this system. The role of the glutamic acid and glutamine system in Na-K transport has not been demonstrated. But in view of the fact that these amino acids and GABA may serve as an alternative pathway for aerobic metabolism by the brain, it is possible that enhancement of the Na-K pump by DPH is evoked by its activation of this alternative pathway via glutamic acid and the resultant increase in rate of production of high-energy phosphates. This enhanced production of high-energy phosphate would be accompanied by such factors as increased utilization by the Na pumping process and enhanced glycogen and protein synthesis. Hence, turnover of high-energy phosphates would increase but their total concentrations would not necessarily change.

It is clear that turnover studies with radioactive metabolites and phosphate are necessary in order to establish whether this drug acts to mobilize high-energy compounds and, if so, whether it does this by action on glutamic acid metabolism. McIlwain and colleagues [48], however, found no influence of DPH on the metabolism of glutamic acid in brain slices in vitro, as noted above. The increase in brain phosphocreatine levels by toxic doses of DPH, described above [11], could be due to increased production of this high-energy compound coupled with decreased utilization due to the marked depressant effect of large doses. Amino acid levels should be measured under the same conditions, but the observations are in line with the hypothesis just discussed.

That protein synthesis is increased by DPH appears likely from observations already discussed. Chronic administration of the drug enhanced regeneration of liver parenchymal tissue following partial hepatectomy, fibroblastic activity, growth of gingival and connective tissue, and wound healing in skin. Biochemical studies indicate that in skin and gingivae, which have been studied most extensively, there is increased synthesis of various soluble and insoluble collagens, as measured by increased tissue content of hydroxyproline, mucopolysaccharides (increased hexosamine content), and glycoproteins, and by enhanced incorporation of hydroxyproline into collagen. However, Forscher et al. [41] noted that in mucosal tissue from the soft palate, in which an inflammatory response had been induced, DPH did not change the tissue content of tyrosine, proline, hydroxyproline, hexosamine, RNA, DNA, and inorganic or residue phosphate, but that it decreased the acid-soluble fraction of phosphate; this fraction contains the high-energy phosphate compounds. In gingival tissues from very young rats, cats, and dogs after prolonged administration of DPH and a close congener, 3-carbethoxy-5,5-diphenyl-hydantoin, in doses of 50 mg per kg (rats) twice weekly for 5 weeks or 100 mg per kg for 14 to 16 months (cats and dogs), no hyperplasia of the gingivae was noted [79]; in the skin, levels of insoluble hydroxyproline were decreased, but no effects were noted for total soluble and insoluble fractions of hexosamine; histological studies were not made, however, to determine if increased amounts of collagen were present. A marked decrease in dermal total lipids, cholesterol, triglycerides, and phospholipids was noted in the treated groups as well as inhibition of incorporation of acetate-1-^{14}C into dermal total lipids, monoglycerides, diglycerides, triglycerides, cholesterol, and phospholipids. These effects of DPH on lipids were previously noted by Houck and colleagues [14, 15] who found that treatment of rats with a fairly large dose (100 mg per kg) for 10–12 days decreased concentration of neutral glycerides (particularly diglycerides), total lipids, and phospholipids in skin and decreased concentration of neutral glycerides in both aorta and liver. They also noted that in skin, in which histological examination showed that chronic DPH treatment increased collagenization and keratinization, the amounts of soluble and insoluble collagens were increased, as measured by hydroxyproline and hexosamine contents.

It is clear that most of the experimental evidence indicates protein synthesis in skin and gingivae as measured by collagen production is increased by DPH and that this is accomplished at the expense of fat, which presumably supplies the energy for the synthetic process. Decreased incorporation of acetate-^{14}C into lipids of skin would suggest that the drug decreased synthesis rather than increasing utilization of lipids. This is in agreement with the observation that incorporation of radiophosphate into the phospholipid fraction of frog sciatic nerve exposed to normal Ringer's solution or made hyperexcitable by immersion in isotonic phosphate solution is decreased by DPH [37].

The evidence in liver, skin, and gingival tissue indicates that chronic administration of DPH increases protein synthesis. The pertinent question, then, is whether this phenomenon is related to the anticonvulsant effect of the drug. Also: what is the mechanism of the drug-induced increase in protein synthesis?

Studies by Kemp and Woodbury [56, 57] utilizing ^{14}C-DPH and ^{14}C-orotic acid have helped to answer these questions, at least in part. It was observed by Noach et al. [81] in rats, by Firemark et al. [39] in cats, and by Nakamura et al. [80] in cats and dogs that, if the ratio of total brain DPH concentration to total plasma concentration is calculated, the value is greater than 1.0 and may be as high as 10. This ratio is even higher if calculated on the basis of the unbound drug concentration in plasma (approximately 20 percent of total plasma drug concentration). Firemark et al. [39] speculated that the drug was bound to protein constituents of brain.

The nature of binding of 4-^{14}C-DPH to subcellular fractions of brain and its subcellular distribution were studied in rats by Kemp and Woodbury [56]. It is shown in Fig. 23-4 that DPH is found in all subcellular fractions, but a definite sequence of its movements is noted. The ordinate is the percent of total radioactivity in cerebral cortex in each fraction tested and the abscissa is the time in hours after injection of

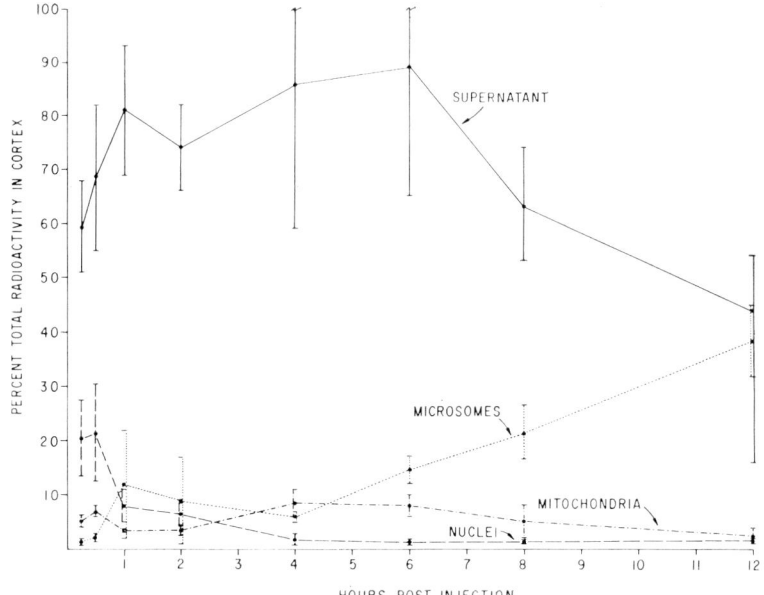

Fig. 23-4. Subcellular distribution of ^{14}C-DPH in cerebral cortex of rats as a function of time. Ordinate is ratio in percent of concentration of ^{14}C-DPH in subcellular fractions to concentration of the drug in the whole homogenate from which fractions were taken. Abscissa is time in hours after injection of the radioactive drug. Each point on the curve is the mean value of three observations. Vertical-bracketed lines represent standard error of the mean. See text for explanation. (From Kemp and Woodbury [56].)

the 4-^{14}C-DPH. DPH enters very rapidly and just as rapidly leaves the nuclei of the brain cells; the amount remaining at the end of 12 hr is practically zero. Activity in the supernatant fraction reaches a peak at 4–6 hr and then falls off with time. Activity in the microsomes, however, is low at first but increases markedly with time; at 12 hours it is considerably higher than in any other fraction except the supernatant. If concentration of the drug per unit wet weight is calculated, concentration in microsomes at 12 hr is higher than in all the other fractions. Thus, these data demonstrate the remarkable affinity of the microsomal fraction for DPH. At 30 min, 20 percent of the activity is in the nuclei, about 70 percent in the supernatant fraction, 8 percent in the mitochondria, and only 2 percent in microsomes. In contrast, at 12 hr, nuclei contain only 2 percent of the activity, supernatant 44 percent, and mitochondria 8 percent, but microsomes contain 38 percent of total radioactivity in the homogenate of cortex. At 24 hr (not shown in Fig. 23-4) most of the remaining drug in the brain is in the microsomal fraction. This finding accounts for the marked accumulation of DPH in the brain, as described above.

The nature of the drug accumulated in the microsomes was investigated by chromatographic procedures. The drug in the microsomes remained at the origin of the chromatogram, associated with the proteins, and had high affinity for them, but could be released by alkaline hydrolysis to give free, unchanged DPH. The drug in the nuclei at the early period was also found to be tightly bound to the protein of this fraction; but, as in microsomes, free DPH could be released by alkaline hydrolysis. It appears, therefore, that this drug enters the nucleus, is bound to some substance there, probably protein or nucleoprotein, then leaves the nucleus in this form and is transfered to the endoplasmic reticulum (microsomal fraction) in the same form, where it accumulates. Since accumulation in nuclei and microsomes can be blocked by actinomycin and that in the microsomes by puromycin, and since DPH enhances incorporation of orotic acid into nucleic acids of the nuclei and inhibits its incorporation into microsomes [57], it is speculated that this drug is incorporated into messenger RNA and may thereby affect protein synthesis by the ribosomal system. Incorporation of DPH into RNA could occur since there is similarity of structure between orotic acid and the hydantoin ring. Also, in the bacterium, *Zymobacterium oroticum,* orotic acid can be converted to 5-carboxymethyl hydantoin. That the bound form of the drug, the nature of which requires further elucidation, is involved in its anticonvulsant actions is indicated by the fact that nearly all the drug in the brain is in the microsomes as the bound form, at a time after single injection when the anticonvulsant effect is still present.

These data suggest an effect of DPH on nucleic acid metabolism. Since this anticonvulsant enhances active Na transport, probably increases availability of high-energy phosphates, and enhances protein synthesis, its effects are similar to those of aldosterone as described by Edelman and colleagues [26]. (See also review by Sharp and Leaf [104].) Aldosterone enhances active Na transport probably by increasing the synthesis of protein enzymes concerned with energy metabolism for the transport process. This effect is exerted through an action on nucleic acid metabolism, it is thought, since aldosterone is localized in the nuclei of cells, as is DPH. The steroid enhances radioactive uridine incorporation into RNA, as DPH does the incorporation of orotic acid, and its stimulation of Na transport is blocked by actinomycin, which inhibits synthesis of messenger RNA; by puromycin, which inhibits ribosomal assembly of protein; and by other inhibitors of the RNA protein-synthesizing system. The effects of these agents on DPH-induced enhancement of Na transport have not yet been tested. These data strongly suggest an effect of this drug on nucleic acid metabolism. Studies are in progress in our laboratory further to characterize this effect.

An influence of DPH, phenobarbital, and primidone on nucleic acid (or at least on one-carbon) metabolism is suggested by the observation that folic acid treatment of epileptic patients with folic acid deficiency induced by these anticonvulsants partially reverses the antiepileptic effect of these drugs (increased the number of seizures), yet improved the mental state resulting from the folic acid deficiency [93]. This would suggest that the deficiency, or at least the interference with the metabolism of folic acid, was involved in the anticonvulsant effects of these drugs. However, part of the deficiency, in the case of DPH at least, is a result of interference with intestinal absorption of folate polyglutamates. This intriguing possible relation between therapeutic effectiveness of the drugs and folic acid deficiency induced by them should be examined further.

Effects on Neurotransmitters

Since the most striking effect of DPH is to delimit the spread of seizure activity, a process that involves synaptic transmission, it seems reasonable that part of its action is due to an effect on the release, synthesis, storage, or metabolism of neurotransmitters. Very little work has been done on this aspect of the effects of DPH. The various putative transmitters in the CNS are reviewed by Curtis in this volume (Chap. 5) and will not be discussed here. The discussion will consider the effects only of DPH on the known peripheral neurotransmitters and those thought to be transmitters in the CNS.

Acetylcholine. Studies on isolated ileum of rat (discussed above) indicate that DPH in low doses stimulates release of acetylcholine from the parasympathetic nerve endings in the wall of the ileum and also from the intramural ganglia. The released acetylcholine stimulates contraction of the ileum. Evidence for these effects is provided by the fact that contraction of the ileum induced by DPH is blocked by atropine and partially by hexamethonium, a ganglionic blocking agent. Physostigmine enhances the effect of DPH. Stimulation of vagal nerve endings in the heart is also produced by DPH; the effect is blocked by atropine. That stimulation of acetylcholine release by DPH may also occur in the brain was shown by McLennan and Elliott [66], who observed that production of free acetylcholine by brain slices is stimulated by low concentrations of phenobarbital and DPH and depressed by high concentrations. Acetylcholine is probably an excitatory transmitter in the brain; hence the initial enhanced release of acetylcholine with low doses of anticonvulsant could account for at least some of its excitatory effects, and subsequent depression of its release with higher doses or chronic administration could be the reason for at least part of its subsequent anticonvulsant effects.

Although Tower [117] noted a biochemical lesion in human epileptogenic cerebral cortex characterized by failure in production of bound acetylcholine and that phenobarbital and DPH, but not trimethadione, counteracted this defect, Pappius and Elliott [82] could not repeat these results. This aspect is, therefore, as yet unresolved. However, it seems probable (from the above-mentioned observations) that DPH stimulates release of acetylcholine from the brain, as it does in peripheral parasympathetic nerve endings and probably in certain autonomic ganglia, and it is likely that some of its excitatory effects may be due to this action.

Biogenic Amines. DPH has been shown to elevate the concentration of 5-hydroxytryptamine (5HT) in the brain [10]. This substance has been implicated as a CNS transmitter (see Chap. 5 by Curtis in this volume). Other experiments [2], however, have demonstrated that other agents which elevate 5HT levels in the brain have no anticonvulsant action, also that the time course of change in 5HT levels induced by DPH does not correspond with the time course of its anticonvulsant effects [2]. That there is no correlation between anticonvulsant activity and 5HT levels in brain was thus concluded. It is possible that increased availability of energy resulting from DPH might increase synthesis of 5HT, a possibility that is readily testable. The drug might also alter the metabolism of 5HT in brain.

Original observations of Chen et al. [13] were subsequently confirmed by others [98, 99], that reserpine and certain other biogenic amine-depleting agents and α-adrenergic blocking agents antagonize the inhibiting effect of DPH on the tonic phase of the maximal electroshock seizure in mice. These findings suggest a role of biogenic amines in the anticonvulsant effect of this drug. However, since not all depleting agents and only phenoxybenzamine of the α-adrenergic blocking group antagonize the effect of DPH on maximal seizures, the effect has been attributed not to biogenic amine depletion but to other, as yet unknown, actions of reserpine and related depleting agents [98, 99].

Evidence indicates that an effect of DPH on biogenic amines is not a major mechanism of its anticonvulsant action.

Amino Acids. The effects of DPH on GABA, glutamic acid, and glutamine metabolism in the brain are discussed above under *Amino Acid, Protein, Lipid, and Nucleic Acid Metabolism.* This drug increases GABA and decreases glutamic acid levels in cerebral cortex of the rat. Various studies have shown that GABA might well be an inhibitory transmitter in the cerebral cortex and that glutamic acid has excitatory properties and is probably an excitatory transmitter in the spinal cord (see Chap. 5, by Curtis). Thus, both increase in GABA and decrease in glutamic acid induced by this drug are changes that would inhibit transmission across synapses and prevent spread of seizure discharges. A highly significant correlation between electroshock seizure threshold and GABA concentration in cerebral cortex has been reported [135]. It is possible, therefore, that DPH-induced changes in GABA and glutamic acid may play a role in mediating its anticonvulsant effect. Effects of the drug on glycine, thought to be the inhibitory mediator in the spinal cord, have not been assessed; but in view of the fact that DPH has some effect on postsynaptic inhibition, even though small, its effect on this amino acid should be evaluated. It is evident from this brief summary that much more work is necessary to elucidate the effects of DPH on CNS transmitters.

SUMMARY

DPH influences most of the body tissues tested, which indicates a general effect on a basic cellular process. Evidence suggests that it plays a role in increasing the availability of high-energy phosphates for enhancement of active Na transport and synthesis of new protein. This, it is postulated, occurs as a result of an action on nucleic acids, which are involved in the regulation of protein synthesis.

The most impressive effects of DPH are on excitable tissues, where it stabilizes membranes, at least in part, by enhancing active Na transport, particularly when they are hyperexcitable. The anticonvulsant effect is accomplished largely by inhibition of spread of excessive discharges as a result of blocking posttetanic potentiation, an action that accounts for its therapeutic effectiveness in grand mal epilepsy. The ability of the drug to stabilize excitable membranes also accounts for its antiarrhythmic effect and its depression of smooth muscle. Under conditions where active transport of Na may be compromised, DPH is particularly effective in enhancing activity of the Na pump and thereby restoring function to normal.

Excitatory effects of DPH are seen in the CNS. Excitation may be due in part to stimulation of acetylcholine release in the brain, similar to its release of acetylcholine from parasympathetic nerve endings in the wall of gastrointestinal smooth muscle and in the heart.

TRIMETHADIONE AND DIDIONE (DIMETHADIONE, DMO)

Much less is known about the neurophysiological and biochemical properties of trimethadione and its N-demethylated product in the body, 5,5-dimethyl-2,4-oxazolidinedione (didione), than is known about DPH. Consequently, the approach to these drugs will be to describe how they differ from DPH in therapeutic usefulness and in their mechanism of action.

EFFECTS ON THE NERVOUS SYSTEM

The discovery of trimethadione provided the first indication that drugs could be developed which were selective for different kinds of epilepsy, in this case, petit mal. It was synthesized and first reported to have analgesic properties by Spielman (see [16]), and subsequently shown by Everett and Richards [33] to raise the threshold for both chemically and electrically induced seizures. These studies were extended by Goodman and colleagues (see [112] for review) with a battery of assay methods. They concluded that the outstanding property of trimethadione was its protective effect against pentylenetetrazol-induced seizures, in which property it differs markedly from DPH. It is far inferior to DPH in its ability to modify maximal electroshock seizure pattern. In laboratory animals given nondepressant doses, trimethadione prevents all evidence of central excitation, including EEG signs, from pentylenetetrazol. Conversely, central depression produced by large doses of the drug can be antagonized by pentylenetetrazol. Thus there is a mutual antagonism between the two. Didione is like trimethadione in all respects, but is generally less potent as well as less toxic [128].

More detailed studies on the effectiveness of trimethadione in elevating thresholds in selective areas of the brain have shown that it differs in many respects from DPH. Schallek and Kuehn [101] found that trimethadione was capable of considerably raising the threshold for seizure discharge by repetitive stimulation of the central lateral nucleus of the thalamus of the cat, in doses lower than those required for other areas; DPH did not affect this region of the thalamus. Morrell and co-workers [75] noted that trimethadione depressed the projection of seizure activity from cortical foci to thalamus while leaving cortical spread relatively unaffected, quite a different effect on seizure spread from that of DPH. Trimethadione also elevates cortical seizure threshold [20]; however, the thalamus appears to be particularly sensitive to the drug.

On the spinal cord, trimethadione selectively depresses polysynaptic transmission in acute spinal cats without affecting monosynaptic transmission, an effect different from that of CO_2 and acetazolamide (see [111]); it also reverses effects of pentylenetetrazol on the spinal cord. In spinal cord stimulation experiments by Esplin and Freston [30], trimethadione modified the induced spinal convulsions by markedly diminishing duration of poststimulation discharge, but did not block initiation of these discharges. The effects of trimethadione on spinal cord synaptic transmission have also been studied ([29], see also [135]). This drug, more effective in elevating electrical seizure threshold than is DPH, markedly decreases spinal cord transmission during repetitive stimulation; however, it does not alter the ability to transmit single impulses. This effect to reduce transmission during repetitive stimulation is also observed in the stellate ganglion, which responds to anticonvulsant drugs qualitatively, similarly to the spinal cord. However, trimethadione does not affect PTP in the spinal cord or stellate ganglion. These effects correlate with anticonvulsant actions of the drug, since it would be expected that an agent which reduces transmission during repetitive stimulation would decrease the tendency to self-sustained discharges in a given neuronal system. This property probably underlies its ability to raise electrical seizure threshold. Its ability to raise pentylenetetrazol seizure threshold may, however, be due to the additional factor of direct antagonism of this convulsant agent.

It is clear, therefore, that trimethadione does not act to intensify presynaptic inhibition nor to alter postsynaptic inhibition, since it does not inhibit strychnine-induced seizures. In addition, it does not raise the resting threshold for synaptic excitation. Trimethadione does, however, intensify posttransmission depression and is competitive with pentylenetetrazol, an agent which is thought to stimulate excitatory synapses. Thus trimethadione probably acts in a manner opposite to that of pentylenetetrazol on excitatory synapses. Its main action is then to block transmission of repetitive impulses without impairing transmission of single impulses. The nature of postactivity depression and its intensification by trimethadione are not known and require much further investigation. It is of interest, however, that pentylenetetrazol has been reported as stimulating contractions of isolated ileal preparations from the guinea pig, an effect that is blocked by atropine [43]. This is probably due to the pentylenetetrazol-induced release of acetylcholine from the parasympathetic nerves in the wall of the intestine.

If the effect of pentylenetetrazol to release acetylcholine from nerve endings also occurs in the nervous system and if acetylcholine is a neurotransmitter at central excitatory synapses, this could explain the facilitatory effect of pentylenetetrazol on excitatory synapses. Trimethadione could act by preventing the pentylenetetrazol-induced release of acetylcholine without affecting its normal rate of release from nerve endings. It is of interest that in this connection pentylenetetrazol has been found to increase the synthesis of acetylcholine as measured by an increase in choline acetylase activity, a very slight decrease in cholinesterase activity, and an increase in the sensitivity of the frog rectus abdominus muscle to acetylcholine and K-induced contractions [115]. Trimethadione does not affect any of these systems, which indicates that it does not affect normal transmission, but it has not been tested against the enhanced effects produced by pentylenetetrazol. If it is found to block these enhanced effects produced by the convulsant in a competitive manner, the action of trimethadione would be partly explained. The effects of trimethadione against pentylenetetrazol on the above-mentioned systems should be tested.

Unlike DPH, trimethadione in concentrations up to 10 mM per liter has no effect on normal properties of peripheral nerves or on the excitatory effects induced by excessive stimulation or calcium deficit (see [110]).

Since the thalamocortical system appears to be particularly important in the genesis of petit mal epilepsy, the selective sensitivity of the thalamus to trimethadione probably accounts for its therapeutic effectiveness in this disease.

In the chronic treatment of petit mal

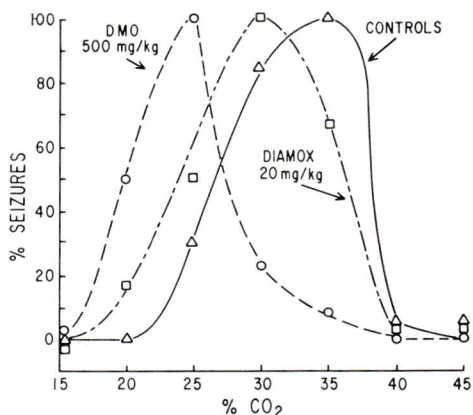

FIG. 23-5. Effect of didione and acetazolamide on seizures induced in rats by exposure to various concentrations of CO_2. Ordinate is percent of animals exhibiting seizures and abscissa is percent CO_2 to which animals were exposed. See text for explanation. (From Withrow et al. [128]. Used by permission of *Journal of Pharmacology and Experimental Therapeutics*.)

epilepsies with trimethadione, part of its anticonvulsant effects are due to accumulation of its metabolite didione. This N-demethylated derivative is very slowly excreted in the urine, hence accumulation in the body fluids occurs. It has been demonstrated that didione has the same anticonvulsant spectrum as its parent compound, but it is less potent [128].

One of the effects of both trimethadione and didione is the protective ability against seizures induced in rats by 30 percent CO_2 and the seizures resulting from withdrawal from 50 percent CO_2 (CO_2 withdrawal seizures) [128, 139]. DPH, except in very high doses, enhances such seizures, but acetazolamide prevents them [128, 139]. The effect of didione to prevent CO_2-induced seizures is similar to that of acetazolamide, which suggests that at least some of their actions may be similar (see Fig. 23-5).

EFFECTS ON BIOCHEMICAL PROCESSES

Very few biochemical effects of trimethadione and didione have been examined. Some of the described effects, however, provide additional evidence for their mechanism of action.

Effects on Electrolyte and Acid-Base Metabolism

The effects of trimethadione and didione on electrolytes and acid-base metabolism of the brain have been studied little. Chronic administration of trimethadione to rats for 25 days produces no striking changes in electrolyte concentrations of plasma, muscle, or brain, nor does it alter the marked changes in electrolytes in these tissues produced by chronic treatment with deoxycorticosterone acetate (DCA) when given in combination with DCA; however, it antagonizes the elevation of threshold to electrically induced seizures produced by DCA, after an initial potentiation of the effect of the DCA on threshold [129]. These results suggest that the anticonvulsant effect of trimethadione is not related to electrolyte changes in the brain, but do not rule out an effect of trimethadione on acid-base balance. The effects of didione on electrolyte have not been assessed.

The acid-base effect of trimethadione and didione, however, are of interest. The anticonvulsant effect of didione requires relatively large doses of the drug, both in experimental animals and in man. In rats, the median effective doses for protection against maximal electroshock seizures and for raising electroshock seizure threshold are around 600–700 mg per kg body weight or 4–5 mM per kg. The pKa of this compound is 6.1 so that at the pH of plasma (7.4) it exists predominantly in the anionic form. In experimental animals given unneutralized didione, an extracellular metabolic acidosis results which is characterized by decrease in pH and bicarbonate and increase in the nonlabile didione anion [127]. This also occurs in patients on chronic trimethadione medication, since its N-demethylated product, didione, accumulates in the blood. Thus this drug, like acetazolamide, results in an extracellular acidosis, but the mechanism of its production is different from that of acetazolamide.

As a result of this acidosis, more of the didione enters the brain because the proportion of nonionized to ionized didione is increased by the lowered pH and presumably only the nonionized form can cross the membrane and enter the brain cell. In the brain cells, the nonionized form dissociates according to the pH of the cell into ionized and nonionized forms. The amount in the brain appears to be directly proportional to plasma pH, which in turn is dependent on the amount of drug given. High levels of didione anion necessary to produce an anticonvulsant effect result in an increase in the nonlabile anion in brain cells; this could result in marked changes in acid-base metabolism of the cell and disruption of metabolic processes. If the total CO_2 content of the brain is measured after administration of didione, alone and in combination with acetazolamide, it is found to be increased by didione alone, acetazolamide alone, and to a greater extent by the combination of the two. Thus effects of didione on the brain are similar to those of acetazolamide. This is also the case for the effects of didione on CO_2-induced seizures, as shown in Fig. 23-5. The increase in total brain CO_2 after administration of didione, acetazolamide, and the combination of the two is accompanied by marked increase in concentration of didione in the brain. Extracellular pCO_2 is lower than normal since there is a metabolic acidosis. Consequently, increased total CO_2 in brain is not due to inhibition of red-blood-cell carbonic anhydrase or respiratory depression since, in both conditions, plasma pCO_2 should increase.

These data, considered in connection with the similarity in effect of didione and acetazolamide against CO_2-induced seizures and CO_2-withdrawal seizures, suggest that at least part of the action of didione as an anticonvulsant is like that of acetazolamide, that is, to cause accumulation of CO_2 in brain cells [127]. Whether didione acts like acetazolamide to inhibit brain carbonic anhydrase, which appears unlikely, thereby to increase brain CO_2, or whether the CO_2 accumulation in brain cells is a result of high concentration of nonlabile didione anion which causes disruption of brain cell metabolism with respect to H^+ ion transport, CO_2 production, oxygen consumption, and decarboxylation reactions awaits further biochemical studies. It is possible that pH alterations in brain cells induced by didione, the nature of which is now being analyzed in our laboratory, change the activity of key pH-dependent enzymes in the brain and thereby alter brain metabolism. It is apparent, however, that the anticonvulsant activity of didione (and perhaps trimethadione) is intimately related to an effect on acid-base metabolism in brain cells.

Effects of trimethadione and didione on transport processes have been described and must be considered in relation to the anticonvulsant effects of these drugs. The rate of cellular transport of xylose into brain slices in vitro is accelerated by didione when xylose concentration in the medium is low, decreased by the drug when concentration is high [46]. This effect is opposite to that of DPH. The mechanism of the effect and its relation to the anticonvulsant effect of the drug await further experimentation. In CSF, the experiments of Reed et al. [91] indicate that didione anion is transported out of the CSF into blood. If this is substantiated, it may be that the transport involves the same system which moves many other organic anions (such as probenecid, penicillin, and PAH) against an electrochemical gradient from CSF to blood. If this is the case, large doses of didione necessary for anticonvulsant effects may saturate this carrier-mediated process and inhibit its transport out of CSF. This would increase levels of didione in CSF and also in the brain, since CSF is in intimate relation to the extracellular fluid of the brain. The resulting increased drug anion in the brain would cause the acid-base effects noted above. The nature of this transport process and effects of anticonvulsant doses of didione on it are now being studied in our laboratory. The similarity of this postulated process to the known effects of bromide is striking (see below).

Effects on Energy, Carbohydrate, Protein, Lipid, and Nucleic Acid Metabolism

The effects of trimethadione on the respiration of brain in vitro have been studied by a number of investigators [40, 48, 107, 109]. High concentrations of trimethadione (35 mM) slightly inhibit oxygen uptake of motor cortex removed from dogs, but do not significantly affect oxygen consumption of the sensory cortex [107]. A slight depressant effect on mouse brain has also been noted [109]. The lack of effect of trimethadione in anticonvulsant doses on oxygen consumption of brain tissues is consistent with observation that, in vitro, low concentrations do not affect the activity of cytochrome oxidase [116]. Depression by large doses is not unexpected since such doses have sedative effects when administered in vivo. In contrast, increases in respiration and anaerobic glycolysis induced in brain slices by electrical stimulation with high frequency currents are inhibited by trimethadione, as by DPH, but responses at low frequency currents are not affected. This is consonant with its effects to block repetitive but not single impulses [40, 48].

Effects of trimethadione and didione on other biochemical processes have not been assessed. Consequently, the metabolic basis, other than accumulation of CO_2 as just described, of the acid-base changes produced by didione administration has not been elucidated. Obviously further work is necessary. However, trimethadione does not affect the activity of carbonic anhydrase and hence it does not act by this means to inhibit seizures [73]; but this conclusion has not been established for didione.

Effects on Neurotransmitters

The effects of these two anticonvulsants on the possible neurotransmitters discussed above in connection with DPH have been studied little. Trimethadione has been reported to have no effect on activity of choline acetylase obtained from frog brain or on the activity of cholinesterase obtained from frog brain and human serum, in drug concentrations that ranged from 10^{-6}M to 10^{-2}M [115]. Effects on the biogenic amines and amino acid transmitters have not been described.

BROMIDE AND OTHER MONOVALENT ANIONS

Bromide is the oldest of the antiepileptics, but is largely outmoded because of its toxicity and sedative properties. Chemically it is the simplest of all the anticonvulsant agents, yet very little is known about its mechanism of action. However, newer knowledge on the transport of cations and anions across cell membranes and effects of bromide and other monovalent anions thereon has given some clues to possible mechanisms of the anticonvulsant activity of this drug. In addition, studies of the movement of bromide and related anions into and out of the brain and CSF have increased our understanding of the role of CSF as the environment of brain and in the regulation of anion entry into and exit from the brain. It is, therefore, pertinent to review these data which are probably related to the mechanism of the anticonvulsant effect of bromide. It is also germane to discuss together the effects of bromide on the nervous system and on biochemical processes.

Bromide is effective as an anticonvulsant only in doses that produce some sedation; at higher dose levels, psychoses, neurological disturbances, and dermatitis occur [112]. In experimental animals, bromide antagonizes the effects of pentylenetetrazol and some other convulsants and antagonizes direct stimulation of the motor cortex. It raises electroshock seizure threshold of animals and abolishes the tonic extensor component of maximal seizure in animals and man in doses that cause neurological signs. Elevation of electroshock seizure threshold by the drug is long lasting; the peak time of effect of a single dose is 4–24 hr, and the effect persists for 96 hr [12]. Relatively high doses are required to produce its effects: the ED_{50} for modifying the pattern of maximal electroshock seizures in rats is 26 mEq per kg body weight; for elevating seizure threshold by 20 percent, 18 mEq per kg; for antagonizing pentylenetetrazol-induced seizures, 8.7 mEq per kg; and the toxic dose (TD_{50}) is 20.6 mEq per kg [49]. Thus bromide is more effective against pentylenetetrazol than against electrically induced seizures. However, it is clinically useful in grand mal, only slightly effective against psychomotor types of seizures, and reported to exacerbate petit mal attacks. Efficacy of the drug against the various above-mentioned laboratory tests, used to assess its anticonvulsant spectrum, correlates linearly with the plasma bromide level [49]; correlation with brain or CSF levels of bromide has not been made.

Other monovalent anions, especially nitrate [60], and to a lesser extent iodide [134], have anticonvulsant effects as assessed by the maximal electroshock seizure test. In contrast, the monovalent anions thiocyanate [134] and perchlorate [134], which, like nitrate and bromide, are actively transported across the choroid plexus (see below), have excitatory and in higher doses convulsant effects on the CNS. Seizures produced by these anions closely resemble those produced by strychnine [134]. In subconvulsant doses both perchlorate and thiocyanate markedly shorten the duration of the flexor and lengthen duration of the extensor phase of maximal seizure; seizures are precipitated, as is the case with strychnine, by sensory stimulation.

Some effects of bromide and nitrate on the neuromuscular junction are pertinent to a discussion of the mechanism of action of these anions. Recordings of intracellular potentials from the end-plate region of frog sartorius muscle in Ringer's solution containing either chloride, bromide, or nitrate were made by Muchnik and Gage [78]. When sodium bromide was substituted for sodium chloride and the potassium concentration was 10 mEq per liter, frequency and amplitude of miniature end-plate potentials increased. No alteration in membrane potential of the muscle was observed when bromide replaced chloride. Also, sodium bromide in concentrations as low as 20 mEq per liter, which are in the anticonvulsant range, decreased the quantal content of an average end-plate potential when the muscle was in high magnesium–low calcium solution, an effect that was reversible when chloride was returned to the medium. Nitrate anion also reduced quantal content and hyperpolarized the muscle slightly, an indication that muscle is more permeable to nitrate ion than to chloride ion.

These effects of bromide and nitrate ions to increase frequency of miniature end-plate potentials and reduce quantal content of an average end-plate potential are similar to the effects of presynaptic membrane depolarization. Reduction of chloride concentration per se is not the cause of the bromide or the nitrate effect since such a reduction does not cause increase in miniature end-plate potentials; this indicates that the presynaptic membrane is not significantly depolarized. Muchnik and Gage [78] therefore postulated that the sedative, and presumably anticonvulsant effects of these anions are related to a pharmacological *presynaptic inhibition* in the CNS, brought about by adsorption of ions to the outer surface of the presynaptic membrane. This would result in change in the electric field across the membrane in such a way that efficacy of synaptic transmission is reduced. However, other possibilities are equally likely.

In the sympathetic chain of the lumbar region of the frog, synaptic transmission was measured by an electrode inserted into a postganglionic ramus or from individual cells by means of an intracellular electrode. When chloride was replaced by bromide in this system, synaptic transmission through the ganglia was not impaired [47]. The procedure changed neither the amount of transmitter released nor the number of quanta released per stimulus. But in these experiments, quantal release was measured in solutions containing physiological concentrations of calcium and magnesium, hence the experimental conditions were different from those utilized by Muchnik and Gage; also a different synaptic system was used. Thus the reported differences in effect of bromide on transmission across synapses remain unresolved.

The experiments of Pollay [85] on bromide and of Woodbury [132, 134] on perchlorate cast additional light on the mechanism of action of these anions and support the concept of Muchnik and Gage that bromide and nitrate act by influencing synaptic processes. These investigators measured the movement of bromide, an anticonvulsant, and perchlorate, a convulsant, simultaneously from the plasma into the brain and CSF; in the case of bromide, its movements out of CSF into brain and plasma and into CSF and brain during ventriculocisternal perfusion with an artificial CSF were also measured.

Previous studies have demonstrated that

secretion of CSF is an active process involving transport of Na and probably Cl across the choroid plexus. The flow of CSF in ventricular and subarachnoid cavities from the choroid plexus to the arachnoid villi provides a continuous drainage route for substances that enter the brain via its capillaries and subsequently leave by entrance into the CSF. Substances entering the CSF from the brain can exit by way of the arachnoid villi; in addition to this route of exit, substances such as monovalent anions (Br, I, SCN, and ClO_4) and some weak electrolytes leave the CSF and enter the blood by active transport across the ependymal cells of the choroid plexus. For example, if active transport of monovalent anions across the choroid plexus is blocked by inhibitors of this system (large loads of these same monovalent anions), their concentration in CSF is increased; since CSF is in intimate contact with the interstitial fluid of the brain, there is a concomitant rise in the brain concentration of these anions. The magnitude of such increases is directly proportional to the dose of anion used until a maximal effect is reached. It is thus clear that the concentration of these anions in brain can be markedly affected by changing their concentration in CSF, either by affecting CSF secretion rate or by altering their transport out of the CSF if such outward transport is present. This is the case for the monovalent anions, which may be either convulsant (SCN^-, ClO_4^-) or anticonvulsant (Br, I, NO_3). However, the final effect of the anion, that is, whether it produces or prevents seizures, depends on its direct effect on brain cells.

Distribution of these anions in brain when their active transport out of CSF has been blocked by a large load of the requisite anion is different for bromide and chloride than for the convulsant agents, perchlorate and thiocyanate. In the case of bromide, concentration in brain is increased to a greater extent than in CSF whereas the reverse is true for perchlorate and thiocyanate. Calculations of the concentration of bromide and perchlorate in the brain cells from the CSF and the extracellular space data indicate that bromide loads increase brain cell bromide concentration relative to the CSF whereas perchlorate loads decrease brain cell perchlorate and increase brain cell chloride concentrations relative to the CSF.

Pollay [85] has provided evidence that there is active transport of bromide into the brain cells and that this transport is blocked by large loads of bromide. In the case of perchlorate, large loads of the anion decrease brain cell levels of the ion but result in an increase in brain cell chloride concentration. If the ratio between cellular and extracellular concentrations of perchlorate and chloride is calculated and compared with the ratio for passive distribution according to the resting potential, it appears that both the ions are probably actively transported into brain cells; the same conclusion applies to bromide. However, when large loads of the anions are given, the transport process of these anions is blocked, and concentration ratios across the cells for all three ions approach each other at the passive distribution ratio. However, the calculated equilibrium potential for perchlorate ($E_{ClO_4^-}$) is considerably lower than E_{Cl^-}, which is slightly less than E_{Br^-} in the nonloaded control animals. In the animals loaded with perchlorate, $E_{ClO_4^-}$ increases as compared with the control whereas E_{Cl^-} decreases; in the brain cells of bromide-loaded rats, E_{Br^-} decreases as compared with its control. It appears from these data that the monovalent anions are transported actively into brain cells, that perchlorate ion has a greater affinity for the carrier than does chloride ion, and that in large doses perchlorate also reduces permeability of the brain cells to chloride. The result of a large load would therefore be replacement of chloride in the cell with perchlorate at a higher concentration. The net effect would be depolarization sufficient to cause convulsions. If this occurred at synapses where the inhibitory mediator acts, the result would be an effect on chloride permeability opposite to that of the inhibitory mediator, presumably glycine in the spinal cord and GABA in the cortex. This would produce a seizure like that produced by strychnine; both perchlorate and thiocyanate do produce such a seizure.

Bromide and chloride compete for the carrier that transports these anions into the brain cell. Since bromide has a lower affinity for the carrier, this would reduce chloride entry and drive the potential toward the resting potential; the net effect would be hyperpolarization. The data could also be explained by a greater permeability of the cells to bromide than to chloride, as is true for nitrate. This also would cause hyperpolarization of inhibitory postsynaptic potentials and would explain the anticonvulsant effects of bromide and nitrate.

Much further work is obviously necessary to test this hypothesis, but the results so far suggest an action of bromide and other monovalent anions on the transport of anions into brain cells. The opposite effects of bromide and nitrate on one hand and perchlorate and thiocyanate on the other can be rationally explained on this basis.

PHENOBARBITAL

The effects of phenobarbital and the other barbiturates on the CNS and on biochemical processes have been so extensively studied that a separate review would be necessary to do them justice. However, the mechanism of the fairly selective anticonvulsant effect of phenobarbital and a few related barbiturates (mephobarbital, metharbital) has still not been elucidated. Anticonvulsant barbiturates exhibit anticonvulsant effects only in doses that usually cause some sedation. The anticonvulsant effects of phenobarbital (elevation of the seizure thresholds for 60-cycle and 1f electroshock and for pentylenetetrazol, abolition of the tonic extensor component of the maximal seizure, prevention of repetitive firing in peripheral nerves stimulated by supramaximal currents or produced by immersion in low calcium solutions, clinical effectiveness mainly in grand mal and focal seizures of the tonic or clonic type and in status epilepticus and withdrawal types of seizures) are multiple and rather nonselective as compared with the rather *pure* effects possessed by DPH, trimethadione, and acetazolamide. This indicates multiple actions of the drugs to cause such changes as inhibition of PTP, reduction of transmission during repetitive discharge, depression of certain pathways in which the safety factor for transmission is low, as well as others. These processes and the effects of phenobarbital thereon must be studied further to define the multiple effects of this drug and elucidate its actions.

The effects of phenobarbital on various areas of the nervous system have been discussed above in comparison with DPH and trimethadione. In general, it elevates the threshold for electrical or chemical stimulation in all areas studied. Thus no real selectivity is noted. This is compatible with a general sedative effect on the CNS; however, some selectivity as compared to the nonanticonvulsant barbiturates is present.

The biochemical effects of phenobarbital are even more complex. Effects such as inhibition of oxidative metabolism, actions on acetylcholine metabolism, alterations of transport of sugars, uncoupling of oxidative phosphorylation, inhibition of enzymes, and effects on nucleic acids have been described, but none of these has as yet clearly defined the actions of the drug. The results are encouraging, however, and much progress has been made. Further work is obviously necessary.

SUMMARY

It is evident from the results summarized in this chapter that much progress has been made in elucidating the neurophysiological and biochemical bases for anticonvulsant drug action. However, it is also evident that much more research must be done before the anticonvulsant actions can be defined precisely. An attempt has been made to describe the problems that need to be solved, and possible lines of approach for solving these problems have been indicated. A two-pronged assault on the action of these drugs by use of biophysical and biochemical techniques, which are now delineating the nature of cell membranes, transport processes, and cell metabolism, is necessary before the mechanisms of their actions will be elucidated. Our knowledge so far has clarified mainly the effects, not the basic actions, of these drugs.

REFERENCES

1. Aird, R. B., and Strait, L. Mode of action of sodium diphenylhydantoinate (Dilantin) in epilepsy. *J. Pharmacol. Exp. Ther.* 103:136, 1951.
2. Anderson, E. G., Markowitz, S. D., and Bonnycastle, D. D. Brain 5-hydroxytryptamine and anticonvulsant activity. *J. Pharmacol. Exp. Ther.* 136:179, 1962.
3. Aston, R., and Domino, E. F. Differential effects of phenobarbital, pentobarbital and diphenylhydantoin on motor cortical and reticular thresholds in the rhesus monkey. *Psychopharmacologia* 2:304, 1961.
4. Barany, E. H., and Stein-Jensen, E. The mode of action of anticonvulsant drugs on electrically induced convulsions in the rabbit. *Arch. Int. Pharmacodyn.* 73:1, 1946.
5. Bashour, F. A., Jones, R. E., and Edmondson, R. Ventricular tachycardia in acute myocardial infarction. Preliminary report on the prophylactic use of Dilantin. *Clin. Res.* 13:399, 1965.
6. Baudouin, A., and Hazard, R. Action cardiovasculaire dépressive exercée par la diphénylhydantoine et son dérivé sodique par injection intraveineuse. *Bull. Acad. Nat. Med.* (Paris) 125:39, 1941.
7. Bernstein, H., Gold, H., Lang, T. W., Pappelbaum, S., Bazika, V., and Corday, E. Sodium diphenylhydantoin in the treatment of recurrent cardiac arrhythmias. *J.A.M.A.* 191:695, 1965.
8. Bigger, J. T., Jr., Harris, P. D., and Weinberg, D. I. Effects of diphenylhydantoin on cardiac conduction and repolarization. *Amer. J. Cardiol.* 19:119, 1967.
9. Blum, B. A differential action of diphenylhydantoin on the motor cortex of the cat. *Arch. Int. Pharmacodyn.* 149:45, 1964.
10. Bonnycastle, D. D., Giarman, N. J., and Paasonen, M. K. Anticonvulsant compounds and 5-hydroxytryptamine in rat brain. *Brit. J. Pharmacol.* 12:228, 1957.
11. Broddle, W., and Nelson, S. R. The effect of diphenylhydantoin on energy levels in brain. *Fed. Proc.* 27:751, 1968.
12. Chakravarty, N. L., and Woodbury, D. M. Unpublished data, 1968.
13. Chen, G., Ensor, C. R., and Bohner, B. A facilitation action of reserpine on the central nervous system. *Proc. Soc. Exp. Biol. Med.* 86:507, 1954.
14. Chung, A. C., Duren, B. Y., and Houck, J. C. Effect of diphenylhydantoin administration upon concentration of liver and aortic lipids. *Proc. Soc. Exp. Biol. Med.* 110:788, 1962.
15. Chung, A. C., and Houck, J. C. Connective tissue. VI. Dermal lipid response to diphenylhydantoin. *Proc. Soc. Exp. Biol. Med.* 109:454, 1962.
16. Close, W. J., and Spielman, M. A. Anticonvulsant Drugs. In Hartung, W. H. (Ed.), *Medicinal Chemistry*. New York: Wiley, 1961, vol. V, chap. 1.
17. Conn, R. D. Diphenylhydantoin sodium in cardiac arrhythmias. *New Eng. J. Med.* 272:277, 1965.
18. Conn, R. D., Kennedy, J. W., and Blackman, J. R. Hemodynamic effects of diphenylhydantoin. *Amer. Heart J.* 73:500, 1967.
19. Coombs, J. S., Eccles, J. C., and Fatt, P. The electrical properties of the motoneuron membrane. *J. Physiol.* (London) 130:291, 1955.
20. Delgado, J. M. R., and Mihailović, L. Use of intracerebral electrodes to evaluate drugs that act on the central nervous system. *Ann. N.Y. Acad. Sci.* 64:644, 1956.
21. Drake, M. E., Haury, V. G., and Gruber, C. M. The actions of sodium diphenylhydantoinate (Dilantin) on the excised and intact uterus. *Arch. Int. Pharmacodyn.* 63:288, 1939.
22. Dreifus, L. S., Robbins, M. D., and Watanabe, Y. Newer agents in the treatment of cardiac arrhythmias. *Med. Clin. North Amer.* 48:371, 1964.
23. Druckman, R., and Moore, F. J. Effects of sodium diphenylhydantoinate upon isolated small intestine of the rabbit. *Proc. Soc. Exp. Biol. Med.* 90:173, 1955.

24. Dunham, E. T., and Glynn, I. M. ATPase activity and the active movements of alkali metal ions. *J. Physiol.* (London) 156:274, 1961.
25. Eccles, J. C. *The Physiology of Synapses.* New York: Academic, 1964.
26. Edelman, I. S., Bogoroch, R., and Porter, G. A. On the mechanism of action of aldosterone on sodium transport: the role of protein synthesis. *Proc. Nat. Acad. Sci. U.S.A.* 50:1169, 1963.
27. Escueta, A. V., and Appel, S. H. Personal communication, 1968.
28. Esplin, D. W. Effects of diphenylhydantoin on synaptic transmission in cat spinal cord and stellate ganglion. *J. Pharmacol. Exp. Ther.* 120:301, 1957.
29. Esplin, D. W., and Curto, E. M. Effects of trimethadione on synaptic transmission in the spinal cord; antagonism between trimethadione and pentylenetetrazol. *J. Pharmacol. Exp. Ther.* 121:457, 1957.
30. Esplin, D. W., and Freston, J. W. Physiological and pharmacological analysis of spinal cord convulsions. *J. Pharmacol. Exp. Ther.* 130:68, 1960.
31. Esplin, D. W., and Laffan, R. J. Determinants of flexor and extensor components of maximal seizures in cats. *Arch. Int. Pharmacodyn.* 113:189, 1957.
32. Esplin, D. W., and Zablocka, B. Central Nervous System Stimulants. In Goodman, L. S., and Gilman, A. (Eds.), *Pharmacological Basis of Therapeutics* (3d ed.). New York: Macmillan, 1965, chap. 18.
33. Everett, G. M., and Richards, R. K. Comparative anticonvulsive action of 3,5,5-trimethyloxazolidine-2,4-dione (Tridione), dilantin and phenobarbital. *J. Pharmacol. Exp. Ther.* 81:402, 1944.
34. Ferguson, R. K., and Woodbury, D. M. Penetration of ^{14}C-inulin and ^{14}C-sucrose into brain, cerebrospinal fluid, and skeletal muscle of developing rats. *Exp. Brain Res.* 7:181, 1969.
35. Festoff, B. W., and Appel, S. H. Effect of diphenylhydantoin on synaptosome sodium-potassium-ATPase. *J. Clin. Invest.* 47:2752, 1968.
36. Fingl, E., Olsen, L. J., Harding, B. W., Cockett, A. T., and Goodman, L. S. Effects of chronic anticonvulsant administration upon cortisone-induced brain hyperexcitability. *J. Pharmacol. Exp. Ther.* 105:37, 1952.
37. Fingl, E., Woodbury, D. M., Ward, J. R., Toman, J. E. P. Effect of diphenylhydantoin, temperature, and phosphate concentration on P^{32} uptake by frog sciatic nerve. *Fed. Proc.* 9:172, 1950.
38. Finkleman, I., and Arieff, A. J. Untoward effects of phenytoin sodium in epilepsy. *J.A.M.A.* 118:1209, 1942.
39. Firemark, H., Barlow, C. F., and Roth, L. J. The entry, accumulation and binding of diphenylhydantoin-2-C^{14} in brain. Studies on adult, immature and hypercapnic cats. *Int. J. Neuropharmacol.* 2:25, 1963.
40. Forda, O., and McIlwain, H. Anticonvulsants and electrically stimulated metabolism of separated mammalian cerebral cortex. *Brit. J. Pharmacol.* 8:225, 1953.
41. Forscher, B. F., and Cecil, H. C. Biochemical studies on acute inflammation. II. The effect of Dilantin. *J. Dent. Res.* 36:927, 1957.
42. Franz, D. N., and Esplin, D. W. Prevention by diphenylhydantoin of posttetanic enhancement of action potentials in nonmyelinated nerve fibers. *Pharmacologist* 7:174, 1965.
43. Frommel, Ed., Radouco, C., Gold, Ph., Burgermeister-Guex, G., and Ducommum, M. De l'action périphérique des anticonvulsivants (phénobarbital, phényléthylacétylurée ou S46, diphénylhydantoine). *Schweiz. Med. Wschr.* 83:681, 1953.
44. Gangloff, H., and Monnier, M. The action of anticonvulsant drugs tested by electrical stimulation of the rabbit cortex, diencephalon and rhinencephalon in the unanesthetized rabbit. *Electroenceph. Clin. Neurophysiol.* 9:43, 1957.
45. Gayet-Hallion, Th. Action de certains anticonvulsivants sur le muscle lisse. *C. R. Soc. Biol.* (Paris) 138:332, 1944.
46. Gilbert, J. C., Ortiz, W. R., and Millichap, J. G. Effects of anticonvulsant drugs on the permeability of brain cells to sugars. *Proc. Inst. Med. Chicago* 25:258, 1965.
47. Ginsborg, B. L. Effect of bromide ions on junctional transmission. *Nature* (London) 218:363, 1968.
48. Greengard, O., and McIlwain, H. Anticonvulsants and the metabolism of separated mammalian cerebral tissues. *Biochem. J.* 61:61, 1955.
49. Grewal, M. S., Swinyard, E. A., Jensen, H.

V., and Goodman, L. S. Correlation between anticonvulsant activity and plasma concentration of bromide. *J. Pharmacol. Exp. Ther.* 112:109, 1954.

50. Gupta, D. N., Unal, M. O., Bashour, F. A., and Webb, W. R. Effects of diphenylhydantoin (Dilantin) on pheripheral and coronary circulation and myocardial contractility in the experimental animal. *Dis. Chest* 51:248, 1967.

51. Harris, A. S., and Kokernot, R. H. Effects of diphenylhydantoin sodium (Dilantin sodium) and phenobarbital sodium upon ectopic ventricular tachycardia in acute myocardial infarction. *Amer. J. Physiol.* 163:505, 1950.

52. Helfant, R. H., Ricciutti, M. A., Scherlag, B. J., and Damato, A. N. Effect of diphenylhydantoin sodium (Dilantin) on myocardial A-V potassium difference. *Amer. J. Physiol.* 214:880, 1968.

53. Helfant, R. H., Scherlag, B. J., and Damato, A. N. The electrophysiological properties of diphenylhydantoin sodium as compared to procaine amide in the normal and digitalis-intoxicated heart. *Circulation* 36:108, 1967.

54. Helfant, R. H., Scherlag, B. J., and Damato, A. N. Protection from digitalis toxicity with the prophylactic use of diphenylhydantoin sodium: an arrhythmic-inotropic dissociation. *Circulation* 36:119, 1967.

55. Kemp, J. W., and Woodbury, D. M. The influence of diphenylhydantoin on cerebrospinal fluid electrolytes. *Pharmacologist* 8:199, 1966.

56. Kemp, J. W., and Woodbury, D. M. Subcellular distribution of 4-C^{14}-diphenylhydantoin in rat brain. Submitted for publication, 1968.

57. Kemp, J. W., and Woodbury, D. M. Unpublished data, 1968.

58. Kennedy, C., Anderson, W. B., and Sokoloff, L. Cerebral blood flow in epileptic children during the interseizure period. *Neurology* (Minneap.) Suppl. 1, 8:100, 1958.

59. Koch, A., Higgins, R., Sande, M., Tierney, J., and Tulin, R. Enhancement of renal Na+ transport by dilantin. *Physiologist* 5:168, 1962.

60. Koch, A., and Woodbury, D. M. Effects of carbonic anhydrase inhibition on brain excitability. *J. Pharmacol. Exp. Ther.* 122:335, 1958.

61. Korey, S. R. Effect of dilantin and mesantoin on the giant axon of the squid. *Proc. Soc. Exp. Biol. Med.* 76:297, 1951.

62. Leonard, W. A. The use of diphenylhydantoin (Dilantin) sodium in the treatment of ventricular tachycardia. *Arch. Intern. Med.* 101:714, 1958.

63. Lewin, J., and Esplin, D. W. Analysis of the spinal excitatory action of pentylenetetrazol. *J. Pharmacol. Exp. Ther.* 132:245, 1961.

64. Lüllman, H., and Weber, R. Inhibition of cardiac glycoside-induced arrhythmia by phenytoin. *Arch. Exp. Path. Pharm.* 259:182, 1968.

65. Martin, W. R., Vernier, V. G., and Unna, K. R. Effects of Dilantin and phenobarbital on the response of the cortex to stimulation of the activating center. *J. Pharmacol. Exp. Ther.* 110:35, 1954.

66. McLennan, H., and Elliott, K. A. C. Effect of convulsant and narcotic drugs on acetylcholine synthesis. *J. Pharmacol. Exp. Ther.* 103:35, 1951.

67. Mercer, E. N., and Osborne, J. A. The current status of diphenylhydantoin in heart disease. *Ann. Intern. Med.* 67:1084, 1967.

68. Mercer, E. N., Ziegler, W. G., Wickland, G. F., and Dower, G. E. The effect of diphenylhydantoin upon beating of heart cells grown in vitro. *J. Pharmacol. Exp. Ther.* 155:267, 1967.

69. Merritt, H. H., and Putnam, T. J. A new series of anticonvulsant drugs tested by experiments on animals. *Arch. Neurol. Psychiat.* 39:1003, 1938.

70. Mierzwiak, D. S., Mitchell, J. H., and Shapiro, W. Effect of diphenylhydantoin (Dilantin) on left ventricular function in dogs. *Clin. Res.* 14:42, 1966.

71. Mixter, C. G., Moran, J. M., and Austen, W. G. Cardiac and peripheral vascular effects of diphenylhydantoin sodium. *Amer. J. Cardiol.* 17:332, 1966.

72. Millichap, J. G. Anticonvulsant Drugs. In Root, W. S., and Hofman, F. G. (Eds.), *Physiological Pharmacology*. New York: Academic, 1965, vol. 2.

73. Millichap, J. G., Woodbury, D. M., and Goodman, L. S. Mechanism of the anticonvulsant action of acetazolamide, a carbonic anhydrase inhibitor. *J. Pharmacol. Exp. Ther.* 115:251, 1955.

74. Morrell, F., Bradley, W., and Ptashne, M.

Effect of diphenylhydantoin on peripheral nerve. *Neurology* (Minneap.) 8:140, 1958.

75. Morrell, F., Bradley, W., and Ptashne, M. Effect of drugs on discharge characteristics of chronic epileptogenic lesions. *Neurology* (Minneap.) 9:492, 1959.

76. Moruzzi, G. General mechanisms of seizure discharges. *Electroenceph. Clin. Neurophysiol.* 4:221, 1955, suppl.

77. Mosey, L., and Tyler, M. D. The effect of diphenylhydantoin sodium (Dilantin), procaine hydrochloride, procaine amide hydrochloride and quinidine hydrochloride upon ouabain-induced ventricular tachycardia in unanesthetized dogs. *Circulation* 10:65, 1954.

78. Muchnik, S., and Gage, P. W. Effect of bromide ions on junctional transmission. *Nature* (London) 217:373, 1968.

79. Nakamura, K., and Masuda, Y. Effects of 5,5-diphenylhydantoin and 3-ethoxycarbonyl-5,5-diphenylhydantoin (P-6127) on the dermal and gingival tissues of experimental animals. *Arch. Int. Pharmacodyn.* 162:255, 1966.

80. Nakamura, K., Masuda, Y., Nakatsuji, K., and Hiroka, T. Comparative studies on the distribution and metabolic fate of diphenylhydantoin and 3-ethoxycarbonyl-diphenylhydantoin (P–6127) after chronic administration to dogs and cats. *Naunyn Schmiedeberg. Arch. Pharm. Exp. Path.* 254:406, 1966.

81. Noach, E. L., Woodbury, D. M., and Goodman, L. S. Studies on the absorption, distribution, fate and excretion of 4-C^{14}-labeled diphenylhydantoin. *J. Pharmacol. Exp. Ther.* 122:301, 1958.

82. Pappius, H. M., and Elliott, K. A. C. Acetylcholine metabolism in normal and epileptogenic brain tissue; failure to repeat previous findings. *J. Appl. Physiol.* 12:319, 1958.

83. Penfield, W., and Jasper, H. *Epilepsy and the Functional Anatomy of the Human Brain.* Boston: Little, Brown, 1954.

84. Pincus, J. H. Presented at meeting of American Academy of Neurology, April 1968.

85. Pollay, M. The processes affecting the distribution of bromide in blood, brain, and cerebrospinal fluid. *Exp. Neurol.* 17: 74, 1968.

86. Rang, H. P., and Ritchie, J. M. The dependence on external cations of the oxygen consumption of mammalian non-myelinated fibres at rest and during activity. *J. Physiol.* (London) 196:163, 1968.

87. Rang, H. P., and Ritchie, J. M. On the electrogenic sodium pump in mammalian non-myelinated nerve fibres and its activation by various external cations. *J. Physiol.* (London) 196:183, 1968.

88. Raines, A., and Standaert, F. G. Pre- and post-junctional effects of diphenylhydantoin at the cat soleus neuromuscular junction. *J. Pharmacol. Exp. Ther.* 153: 361, 1966.

89. Raines, A., and Standaert, F. G. An effect of diphenylhydantoin on posttetanic hyperpolarization of intramedullary nerve terminals. *J. Pharmacol. Exp. Ther.* 156: 591, 1967.

90. Rawson, M. D., and Pincus, J. H. The effect of diphenylhydantoin on sodium, potassium, magnesium-activated adenosine triphosphatase in microsomal fractions of rat and guinea pig brain and on whole homogenates of human brain. *Biochem. Pharmacol.* 17:573, 1968.

91. Reed, D. J., Withrow, C. D., and Woodbury, D. M. Electrolyte and acid-base parameters of rat cerebrospinal fluid. *Exp. Brain Res.* 3:212, 1967.

92. Rees, H. van, Woodbury, D. M., and Noach, E. L. Unpublished data, 1968.

93. Reynolds, E. H. Effects of folic acid on the mental state and fit-frequency of drug-treated epileptic patients. *Lancet* 1:1086, 1967.

94. Rosati, R. A., Alexander, J. A., Schaals, S. F., and Wallace, A. G. Influence of diphenylhydantoin on electrophysiological properties of the canine heart. *Circ. Res.* 21:757, 1967.

95. Rosenberg, P., and Bartels, E. Drug effects on the spontaneous electrical activity of the squid giant axon. *J. Pharmacol. Exp. Ther.* 155:532, 1967.

96. Rosenblueth, A. and Cannon, W. B. Cortical responses to electric stimulation. *Amer. J. Physiol.* 135:690, 1942.

97. Rowe, G. G., McKenna, D. H., Sialer, S., and Corliss, R. J. Systemic and coronary hemodynamic effects of diphenylhydantoin. *Amer. J. Med. Sci.* 254:534, 1967.

98. Rudzik, A. D., and Mennear, J. H. The mechanism of action of anticonvulsants. I. Diphenylhydantoin. *Life Sci.* 4:2373, 1965.

99. Rudzik, A. D., and Mennear, J. H.

Antagonism of anticonvulsants by adrenergic blocking agents. *Proc. Soc. Exp. Biol. Med.* 122:278, 1966.

100. Sasyniuk, B., and Dresel, P. E. The effect of diphenylhydantoin on conduction in isolated, blood-perfused dog hearts. *J. Pharmacol. Exp. Ther.* 161:191, 1968.

101. Schallek, W., and Kuehn, A. Effects of trimethadione, diphenylhydantoin, and chlordiazepoxide on after-discharges in brain of cat. *Proc. Soc. Exp. Biol. Med.* 112:813, 1963.

102. Scherf, D. Changes in the electrocardiogram after intravenous administration of phenytoin sodium (Dilantin) in the acute experiment. *Bull. N.Y. Med. Coll.* 6:82, 1943.

103. Scherf, D., Blumenfeld, S., Taner, D., and Yildiz, M. The effects of diphenylhydantoin (Dilantin) on atrial flutter and fibrillation provoked by focal application of aconitine or delphinine. *Amer. Heart J.* 60:936, 1960.

104. Sharp, G. W. G., and Leaf, A. Mechanism of action of aldosterone. *Physiol. Rev.* 46:593, 1966.

105. Skou, J. C. Enzymatic aspects of active linked transport of Na^+ and K^+ through the cell membrane. *Progr. Biophys.* 14:133, 1964.

106. Strobos, R. R. J., and Spudis, E. V. Effect of anticonvulsant drugs on cortical and subcortical seizure discharges in cats. *Arch. Neurol.* (Chicago) 2:399, 1960.

107. Struck, H. C., Stumpff, D. L., and Caffrey, R. J. Effect of tridione (3,5,5-trimethyl oxazolidine-2,4-dione) on the oxygen uptake of motor and sensory cortex of dog brain. *Fed. Proc.* 9:123, 1950.

108. Swinyard, E. A., Toman, J. E. P., and Goodman, L. S. The effect of cellular hydration on experimental electroshock convulsions. *J. Neurophysiol.* 9:47, 1946.

109. Taylor, J. D., Richards, R. K., and Everett, G. M. Effect of tridione (3,5,5-trimethyl-2,4-oxazolidinedione) on the oxygen uptake of mouse brain. *J. Pharmacol. Exp. Ther.* 98:392, 1950.

110. Toman, J. E. P. Neuropharmacology of peripheral nerve. *Pharmacol. Rev.* 4:168, 1952.

111. Toman, J. E. P. Drugs Effective in Convulsive Disorders. In Goodman, L. S., and Gilman, A. (Eds.), *Pharmacological Basis of Therapeutics* (3d ed.). New York: Macmillan, 1965, chap. 13.

112. Toman, J. E. P., and Goodman, L. S. Anticonvulsants. *Physiol. Rev.* 28:409, 1948.

113. Toman, J. E. P., Loewe, S., and Goodman, L. S. Physiology and therapy of convulsive disorders. I. Effect of anticonvulsant drugs on electroshock seizures in man. *Arch. Neurol. Psychiat.* 58:312, 1947.

114. Toman, J. E. P., Swinyard, E. A., and Goodman, L. S. Properties of maximal seizures and their alterations by anticonvulsant drugs and other agents. *J. Neurophysiol.* 9:231, 1946.

115. Torda, C., and Wolff, H. G. Effect of convulsant and anticonvulsant agents on acetylcholine metabolism (activity of choline acetylase, cholinesterase) and on sensitivity to acetylcholine of effector organs. *Amer. J. Physiol.* 151:345, 1947.

116. Torda, C., and Wolff, H. G. Effect of convulsant and anticonvulsant agents on the activity of cytochrome oxidase. *Proc. Soc. Exp. Biol. Med.* 74:744, 1950.

117. Tower, D. B. Nature and extent of the biochemical lesion in human epileptogenic cerebral cortex: an approach to its control in vitro and in vivo. *Neurology* (Minneap.) 5:113, 1955.

118. Vastola, E. F., and Rosen, A. Suppression by anticonvulsants of focal electrical seizures in the neocortex. *Electroenceph. Clin. Neurophysiol.* 12:327, 1960.

119. Vernadakis, A. Spinal cord convulsions in developing rats. *Science* 137:532, 1962.

120. Vernadakis, A., and Woodbury, D. M. Effects of Diphenylhydantoin and Adrenocortical Steroids on Free Glutamic Acid, Glutamine, and Gamma-Aminobutyric Acid Concentrations of Rat Cerebral Cortex. In Roberts, E. (Ed.), *Inhibition in the Nervous System and Gamma-Aminobutyric Acid.* New York: Macmillan (Pergamon), 1960.

121. Vernadakis, A., and Woodbury, D. M. Effect of acute and subacute administration of diphenylhydantoin on electroshock threshold in developing rats. In Himwich, H. E., and Himwich, W. A. (Eds.), *The Developing Brain. Progress in Brain Research.* Amsterdam: Elsevier, 1964, vol. 9.

122. Vernadakis, A., and Woodbury, D. M. Effects of cortisol and diphenylhydantoin on spinal cord convulsions in developing rats. *J. Pharmacol. Exp. Ther.* 144:316, 1964.

123. Vernadakis, A., and Woodbury, D. M. Effects of diphenylhydantoin on electroshock seizure thresholds in developing rats. *J. Pharmacol. Exp. Ther.* 148:144, 1965.

124. Vernadakis, A., and Woodbury, D. M. The developing animal as a model. *Epilepsia* (Amst.) 1968, in press.

125. Ward, A. A., Jr., and Schmidt, R. P. Some properties of single epileptic neurones. *Arch. Neurol.* (Chicago) 5:308, 1961.

126. Watson, E. L., and Woodbury, D. M. Unpublished data, 1968.

127. Withrow, C. D., Barton, L. J., and Woodbury, D. M. Acid-base effects of 5,5-dimethyl-2,4-oxazolidinedione (DMO) in rat muscle and brain. Manuscript in preparation, 1968.

128. Withrow, C. D., Stout, R. J., Barton, L. J., Beacham, W. S., and Woodbury, D. M. Anticonvulsant effects of 5,5-dimethyl-2,4-oxazolidinedione (DMO). *J. Pharmacol. Exp. Ther.* 161:335, 1968.

129. Woodbury, D. M. Effect of anticonvulsants alone and in combination with desoxycorticosterone on electroshock seizure threshold. *J. Pharmacol. Exp. Ther.* 103:366, 1951.

130. Woodbury, D. M. Effects of hormones on brain excitability and electrolytes. *Recent Progr. Hormone Res.* 10:65, 1954.

131. Woodbury, D. M. Effect of diphenylhydantoin on electrolytes and radiosodium turnover in brain and other tissues of normal, hyponatremic and postictal rats. *J. Pharmacol. Exp. Ther.* 115:74, 1955.

132. Woodbury, D. M. Distribution of nonelectrolytes and electrolytes in the brain as affected by alterations in cerebrospinal fluid secretion. *Progr. Brain. Res.* 29:297, 1968.

133. Woodbury, D. M. Role of pharmacological factors in the evaluation of anticonvulsant drugs. *Epilepsia* (Amst.) 1969, in press.

134. Woodbury, D. M. Unpublished data, 1968.

135. Woodbury, D. M., and Esplin, D. W. Neuropharmacology and neurochemistry of anticonvulsant drugs. *Proc. Ass. Res. Nerv. Ment. Dis.* 37:24, 1959.

136. Woodbury, D. M., Hurley, R. E., Lewis, N. G., McArthur, M. W., Copeland, W. W., Kirschvink, J. F., and Goodman, L. S. Effect of thyroxin, thyroidectomy and 6-n-propyl-2-thiouracil on brain function. *J. Pharmacol. Exp. Ther.* 106:331, 1952.

137. Woodbury, D. M., and Karler, R. Role of carbon dioxide in the nervous system. *Anesthesiology* 21:686, 1960.

138. Woodbury, D. M., Rees, H. van, and Noach, E. L. Unpublished data, 1968.

139. Woodbury, D. M., Rollins, L. T., Gardner, M. D., Hirschi, W. C., Hogan, J. R., Rallison, M. L., Tanner, G. S., and Brodie, D. A. Effects of carbon dioxide on brain excitability and electrolytes. *Amer. J. Physiol.* 192:79, 1958.

140. Woodbury, D. M., Timiras, P. S., and Vernadakis, A. Influence of adrenocortical steroids on brain function and metabolism. In Hoagland, H. (Ed.), *Hormones, Brain Function and Behavior.* New York: Academic, 1957.

141. Woodbury, J. W. Interrelationships between ion transport mechanisms and excitatory events. *Fed. Proc.* 22:31, 1963.

142. Woodward, D. L., Reed, D. J., and Woodbury, D. M. The extracellular space of rat cerebral cortex. *Amer. J. Physiol.* 212:367, 1967.

143. Zeft, H. J., Whalen, R. E., Ratliff, N. B., Jr., Davenport, R. D., Jr., and McIntosh, H. D. Diphenylhydantoin therapy in experimental myocardial infarction. *J. Pharmacol. Exp. Ther.* 162:80, 1968.

144. Zwieten, P. A. van. The influence of cardiac glycosides on membrane permeability in guinea-pig atrial tissue, determined by means of ^{86}Rb. *J. Pharm. Pharmacol.* 20:731, 1968.

Discussion

FURTHER OBSERVATIONS ON DIPHENYLHYDANTOIN*

JAMES E. P. TOMAN

Anticonvulsant Actions at Various CNS Levels

That diphenylhydantoin has effects upon every kind of excitable tissue, well documented by Woodbury's review, certainly suggests the possibility that the drug exerts manifold effects through possibly one, but at most a few, mechanisms common to cell membranes.

Role of Posttetanic Potentiation. If we confine our attention to nerve cells, central or peripheral, it is evident that basic membrane action becomes manifest as a stabilization of the cell against various but not all forms of induced hyperexcitability and hyperresponsiveness. In particular, as demonstrated by Esplin [2], at the simplest levels of synaptic transmission in both spinal cord and in autonomic ganglia, the physiologic phenomenon, posttetanic potentiation (PTP), can be selectively suppressed by diphenylhydantoin without noteworthy impairment of other parameters of excitation or response. In addition, the drug has the well-known property of preventing the tonic phase of seizures induced by electroshock or by some (but not all) convulsant drugs. Thus, there is reason to believe that the tonic phase of such seizures required the development of PTP and, conversely, that certain other types of seizure manifestations do not require the development of PTP. It seemed of interest to explore seizure activity at various levels of the nervous system, even in a pseudomodel preparation, in order to distinguish between diphenylhydantoin-sensitive and insensitive forms of seizure activity.

Cortical Focal Seizures. A standard preparation used for many years in drug studies is the restrained, unanesthetized rabbit with sets of epidural needles implanted on each side in the sensorimotor cortex [19]. Stimulation is bipolar (2 mm), and recordings can be taken monopolarly from 2 mm away on the ipsilateral side, also from the contralateral electrodes. Ordinarily this system is used with slowly repeated stimuli to study the complex, nonconvulsive evoked EEG response, which includes some initial fast events, a so-called *dendritic* potential, a negative *slow hump* potential with peak at about 200 msec, and some 10-per-sec *spindle* activity corresponding to the 14 per sec sleep spindles in man (obtainable here by stimulation even in an awake animal). Spread of this nonconvulsive evoked response to the contralateral side is opposed by alerting stimuli or by neutral stimuli previously paired with painful stimulation. Spread to the opposite side is actually favored by sedatives including sedative anticonvulsants, but is also promoted by both pentylenetetrazol, a threshold decreaser, and by procaine, a threshold increaser for local response. Among the anticonvulsants, trimethadione is a more effective threshold raiser than the barbiturates, but is also less effective in enhancing the spindle portion of response. Diphenylhydantoin has relatively little effect on any component of the response and no consistent action on threshold or spread.

In contrast to the foregoing evoked potential, which can be elicited for hours at one-second intervals with no apparent local fatigue or any notable disturbance of the animal's spontaneous behavior, a focal seizure response can be set up by moderate increase in voltage and frequency of stimu-

---

* Supported in part by PHS Grant 5–RO1–MH5503–06 from National Institute of Mental Health.

lation (6-per-sec stimulation was usually used). During stimulation the evoked response undergoes marked changes in all of its components, the slow hump, in particular, being converted to a briefer and larger 50-msec spike of changing and bizarre form similar to the spontaneous-seizure repetitive spike, which continues as an afterdischarge for 20 sec or so following cessation of stimulation. It is followed in turn by a period of postictal depression characterized by increased threshold and altered form of the nonconvulsive test response. The ipsilateral focal seizure is accompanied by behavioral changes, ranging from mere cessation of spontaneous movement to tonic adversive seizures, facial movements, squealing, and other types of submaximal seizure responses. Associated seizure discharges of repetitive spike type usually remain confined to the stimulated side, but each such spike elicits a relatively normal-appearing nonconvulsive evoked response on the contralateral side. The contralateral response shows no evidence of postictal fatigue, therefore appears to be projected evoked activity, rather than true spread of convulsive activity.

The threshold for ipsilateral focal-seizure response can be markedly raised by trimethadione and also by carbon dioxide inhalation. In contrast, diphenylhydantoin has small and variable effect on threshold; the afterdischarges actually become considerably longer in duration and more stable in repetition rate. It also fails to abolish high frequency, small spikes of A fiber type associated with the seizure discharge.

According to these criteria, diphenylhydantoin would scarcely be considered an anticonvulsant. However, when stimulus conditions were modified to permit more generalized seizures to develop from focal stimulation (higher frequency and a wider electrode separation were usually necessary), then the ability of the drug to limit the extent and severity of the seizure became evident.

The results are comparable with those previously found in various laboratory species when gross corneal electrodes were used for stimulation [11]. Diphenylhydantoin had little effect on the threshold or form of the limited seizure obtained at threshold voltage with high frequency stimulation, or with 6 per sec stimulation and supramaximal voltage. In fact such seizures were longer on the average in the drug-treated animals. However, the same dosage level was effective in preventing tonic seizure activity in response to typical, high frequency EST stimulation with voltages exceeding threshold by a factor of 10. In contrast, while trimethadione raised the threshold for the EST seizures, it did not prevent emergence of a tonic phase when shock voltage was increased. This difference between trimethadione and diphenylhydantoin has been demonstrated in humans undergoing electroshock therapy [14].

Assuming that the most relevant action of diphenylhydantoin is reduction or abolition of PTP, the foregoing experiments would indicate that PTP is not essential for induction of focal-seizure circuits involving high frequency burst activity as in the rabbit ipsilateral-evoked discharges, nor for the induction of presumed limited seizure pathways obtained by gross stimulation at low frequency in various species. Conversely, it could be held that PTP is essential for progressive involvement of additional brain areas in seizure activity, as in the development of maximal tonic seizures. The next step in this discussion will be to examine some aspects of the pharmacology of tonic convulsions.

Seizure Patterns after Brain Stem Transection. In a few rabbits and an extensive series of mice, the effect of progressive transection of brain was studied in relation to type of seizure evocable by electroshock and seizure modification by drugs [12]. The usual succession of tonic flexor, tonic extensor, clonic, and abrupt change to postictal activity was still seen, even with sections intruding upon the upper mesencephalon. But below this level, the evoked seizures were of tonic extensor type and tended to fade away smoothly, as in some spasms of decerebrate rigidity, rather than abruptly, as in convulsions with cerebrum intact. As long as the full tonic-clonic seizures were obtainable, their tonic phases could be abolished by diphenylhydantoin, leaving clonic activity intact and even prolonged. However, the decerebrate type of tonic spasm was not abolished by diphenylhydantoin, in contrast to typical central-depressant barbiturates and anticonvulsants.

Thus, not tonic spasms as such, but a more involved aspect of the organization of seizures, resulting in severe but abruptly terminating tonic activity, appears to require development of PTP and to be abolishable by diphenylhydantoin. The best interpretation, we feel, is that the upper brain stem contains feedback circuits normally involved in various roles in reflex postural adjustments, but is capable of being brought into concurrent, maximal, positive feedback activity by forced development of PTP. This results in maximal facilitation of tonic medullary mechanisms, the more caudal and stronger extensor system eventually predominating in most mammalian species. Inhibitory mechanisms are also activated and help to bring tonic facilitation to an abrupt conclusion at some critical level of PTP fatigue. Below this level of PTP, or when PTP has been sufficiently reduced by drug action, interplay between hyperactive positive and negative feedback circuits results in interrupted spasms of clonic activity until further fatigue lowers feedback gain below a critical value for self-sustained activity. Incidentally, the general tendency for seizures of clonic type to become more prolonged after administration of diphenylhydantoin would seem to indicate the normal role of PTP in inhibitory as well as in excitatory systems. In contrast, the lower brain stem is relatively lacking in local, negative feedback pathways; the clonic mechanism is therefore absent, and the resultant cascade type of tonic spasm thus diminishes with fatigue, rather than being abruptly overwhelmed by inhibition.

Decerebration experiments should not be interpreted as showing that maximal seizures in the intact brain originate and are confined to the upper brain stem, or that this is the sole site of diphenylhydantoin action in changing seizure pattern. What is demonstrated is that a relatively small amount of brain tissue superimposed on medullary and spinal mechanisms is sufficient for these phenomena.

Strychnine Seizures. In maximal seizures induced either by pentylenetetrazol (a presumed excitatory facilitator), or by picrotoxin (a presumed blocker of presynaptic inhibition), the tonic phase of seizure can be prevented by diphenylhydantoin without reduction in clonic activity or increase in threshold. With strychnine (a presumed blocker of postsynaptic inhibition), the story is somewhat different. When high doses are used, or after repeated seizures, attacks become purely tonic with smooth termination; under these circumstances diphenylhydantoin cannot prevent spasms or convert them to sustained clonus. With subconvulsive strychnine dosage and use of electroshock to initiate seizure, the role of inhibition can be evaluated. The latency to onset of tonic-extensor phase (which is interpreted as due to activation of inhibitory systems) is reduced and finally abolished by increasing strychnine dosage. Concomitantly the terminal clonus and abruptness of seizure-phase change is eradicated, and diphenylhydantoin becomes incapable of restoring the clonus or abolishing the tonic phase. These experiments are roughly comparable with the decerebrate observations. Both illustrate the principle that it is not upon tonic mechanisms as such, but rather upon facilitation of such mechanisms by driving systems made hyperactive by PTP, that diphenylhydantoin exerts its curious qualitative action in favoring clonic discharges.

ACTIONS ON PERIPHERAL NERVE

Our observations on seizurelike behavior evoked in peripheral nerve and its modification by anticonvulsant drugs were recently reviewed [15]. Omitting a detailed recapitulation here, it is sufficient to say that certain phenomena of hyperexcitability and hyperresponsiveness can be evoked in typical vertebrate myelinated nerve by means of excessive repetitive electrical stimulation, through decalcifying agents such as phosphate ion and by various other procedures (but not, incidentally, by typical convulsant drugs). Induced hyperactivity can be prevented by diphenylhydantoin in relatively physiologic concentrations, as well as by other drugs capable of abolishing the tonic phase of maximal seizures induced by supramaximal electroshock stimulation in intact animals. But this would not be the case with other types of anticonvulsants such as trimethadione, or with typical barbiturates such as pentobarbital.

A contrasting type of phenomenon is repetitive firing induced in earthworm giant fibers with high calcium concentration; this hyperactivity is more readily abolished with trimethadione than with other types of anticonvulsants [15, 16]. Earthworm fibers are, however, also susceptible to diphenylhydantoin blockade of hyperexcitability induced by excessive stimulation. Thus, both types of anticonvulsant action can be shown in a simple axonal preparation and are not confined to some special mechanism of synaptic transmission.

A pseudomodel of the seizure process can be made by feeding back the amplified action potential to the stimulating electrodes [17]. This has been done principally with frog sciatic nerve, but also with rabbit vagus nerve and other preparations. The resultant feedback discharge shows such seizure-like features as threshold, recruitment, and abrupt termination. Furthermore, if a low level of background stimulation is maintained, the *tonic* seizure is followed by repeated *clonic* spasms, before onset of *postictal depression*. In the case of rabbit vagus feedback preparation, records are remarkably like those of electrically induced focal-cortical seizures in the same rabbit, in spike form and frequency, recruitment, and total duration.

With regard to drug alteration of behavior in this nerve system, diphenylhydantoin does not raise the threshold for initiation of seizure. It does, however, prevent development of hyperexcitability due to repetitive activity, the nerve equivalent of PTP; therefore there is less recruitment and lower peak voltage of synchronized, repetitive-action potential spikes. The stabilized discharge tends to persist longer, however. When clonus is made possible by means of background stimulation, it tends to be of higher frequency than in the control, something we have also noted in animal experiment clonic seizures. However, when feedback gain is increased to the point where behavior of the preparation is essentially all or none, and therefore PTP can play no additional role, the difference between control and drug-treated preparations largely disappears.

ACTIONS ON OTHER THAN CONVULSIVE PHENOMENA

Because of current interest in our laboratories, brief mention will be made of some studies on systems unrelated to the seizure paradigm, particularly those with diphenylhydantoin. Although relating more to other possible uses of this drug or to its side effects, some light may also be cast on possible alternative modes of anticonvulsant action, or perhaps may expand the definition of anticonvulsant to types of phenomena not properly described as seizures, which are nevertheless related to common features of instability of excitable membranes.

ACTIONS ON THE HEART. Little can be added to Woodbury's review of the cardiac actions of diphenylhydantoin. Ludmer [9] has been studying the actions of a number of drugs on the transmembranal action potential of isolated frog ventricle. He has noted, with regard to diphenylhydantoin, that drug prolongation of the plateau phase is less marked in calcium-free Ringer's solution, that there is essentially no effect on the initial rate of rise and peak potential commonly attributed to sodium influx followed by inactivation. This again raises the question of whether the drug exerts its effects only through the sodium mechanism, or whether calcium is also involved, in view of the role of calcium in maintenance of the plateau phase. In the stimulus-driven preparation, diphenylhydantoin protects against the occurrence of premature beats. Here, again, some questions need to be resolved concerning the role of a calcium prepotential in initiation of spontaneous beats and the action of diphenylhydantoin thereupon.

ACTIONS ON HUMAN BEHAVIOR. Many anticonvulsants have sedative and hypnotic properties which set an upper limit to effective dosage. That central depression is not essential to the anticonvulsant effect is illustrated by the common practice of adding an amphetamine or other analeptic drug; antiepileptic activity may sometimes be enhanced [7]. This common central depression is not notably different from that of barbiturates and minor tranquilizers in general. However, some drugs present additional features. Thus phenacemide has been implicated in occasional cases of psychotic manifestations despite suppression of psychomotor seizures for which the drug was prescribed [3]; the mechanism is unclear.

Recently there has been some renewal of interest in possible psychological effects of diphenylhydantoin in nonepileptic patients. It should be recalled that in the early days of clinical trial of this drug, considerable attention was given to its use in a variety of cases of paroxysmal minor disturbances in motor, sensory, autonomic, and psychic function, sometimes classed together as epileptic equivalents, although not always verified by the finding of relevant EEG abnormalities [3].

A number of relatively new reports on diphenylhydantoin treatment of nonepileptic behavior disturbances have been brought together in a symposium [18], but have been criticized in turn because of popularization in the lay press [8]. These reports, although covering several rather different types of patient population, have a feature in common in that patients with impulsive or compulsive characteristics of behavior and mentation showed most subjective benefit. This led the present author to speculate that there may be an unrecognized class of behavioral disturbances, characterized physiologically by excessive posttetanic potentiation (PTP), since this is the most obvious neurophysiological parameter suppressible by the drug [13]. Although the reasoning is circular, implying a pathophysiologic diagnosis based on the positive effects of a medication, it is no more so than a post hoc diagnosis of epileptic diathesis based on the same result in the absence of EEG or other confirmation. The same question is raised concerning the occasional benefit of diphenylhydantoin, as well as of amphetaminic analeptics, in hyperkinetic children without demonstrable neurological findings or EEG evidence of convulsive disorder [10].

Considering the selective actions on animal conditioned-behavior mentioned in this discussion, it seemed worthwhile to study diphenylhydantoin in a group of aged, institutionalized patients by means of a substantial battery of psychological tests. In this double-blind study, Gordon and Tobin [6] found no overall, significant, objective changes in the total population. However, they were able to identify a subset of patients by psychological criteria who were likely, at a significant level of expectation, to report subjective benefit in coping with memory problems and similar disabilities.

Thus, while it is evident that diphenylhydantoin is relatively lacking in universal and dramatic effects on personality or behavior comparable even to those of the common barbiturates, there remains a residue of nonepileptic patients with minor disturbances amenable to management by this drug. The problem is worth exploration with other anticonvulsants and with a search for possible relevant EEG correlates.

ACTIONS ON ANIMAL BEHAVIOR. Gordon et al. [4, 5, 6] have reported effects of diphenylhydantoin on conditioned behavior in the rat, in comparison with effects of other drugs. Gordon studied a conditioned avoidance reaction in rats of various ages, with and without sodium depletion brought about by the administration of intraperitoneal glucose solution. Diphenylhydantoin had no noteworthy action on the performance of young rats, but partly restored toward normal the impaired performance of aged rats. In young rats whose performance had been impaired by sodium depletion, diphenylhydantoin could restore conditioned avoidance behavior toward normal. From the experiments of Doty and Gordon, it is evident that this drug is by no means a universal *memory-enhancer*, but rather that it is selective in its actions. Indeed, Bogdanove [1] noted that in a conditioned water-reward leverpress system there may be deterioration of performance in young animals: pentobarbital, in contrast, produces some enhancement of leverpress activity in the lower part of the dosage range and up to the level of motor impairment. All the above studies with diphenylhydantoin used dosage levels below that causing motor impairment. The curious selective profile of this drug on conditioned behavior merits further study.

ACTIONS ON POLYNUCLEOTIDE SYSTEMS. Gordon and his group [5] are devoting considerable effort to the study of biochemical effects of anticonvulsants and other drugs on aspects of polynucleotide chemistry in brain and in other tissues as well, in addition to in vitro systems. One phenomenon under study has been the apparent ability of diphenylhydantoin to enhance the activity of DNAase. This effect seems to depend upon the presence of an unknown inhibitor substance present in some but not all preparations of DNAase; the action of diphenylhydantoin therefore seems to be disinhibition of the enzyme rather than direct enhancement. Some in vivo actions of diphenylhydantoin include: alterations in composition and content of DNA; shifts in molecular-size profile of brain in RNA; changes in profile of uptake of amino acids in protein synthesis. Since diphenylhydantoin effects are seen in other tissues in addition to brain, they may have some relevance to the variety of somatic side effects known to occur with this drug.

CONCLUSION

The foregoing discussion has been limited primarily to some notes on a variety of effects of diphenylhydantoin, the most thoroughly investigated of the anticonvulsant drugs. Are all these effects attributable to a single mechanism of action at the molecular level? A fair case could be made, for example, for its role in stabilizing and enhancing the sodium pump, particularly if attention is confined to central neurons and convulsive behavior. The antiPTP effect can also be demonstrated in nerve in such a manner as to suggest a possible interaction with calcium-binding properties of the membrane. This suspicion is increased when turning to the action of diphenylhydantoin on the heart.

The behavorial effects of diphenylhydantoin, although minor, bring attention to the important actions of this drug on polynucleotide biochemistry, but this information cannot yet be related to the above-mentioned ionic mechanisms. The eclectic conclusion would probably be that diphenylhydantoin, and by inference some other drugs of the same anticonvulsant class, have more than one mode of action at the molecular level and that more than one such mode contributes to anticonvulsant properties. But the possibility of a single basic mechanism yet unrecognized will undoubtedly continue to foster fundamental research in this field, to which Woodbury has so prodigiously contributed.

REFERENCES

1. Bogdanove, L. Unpublished data, 1968.
2. Esplin, D. W. Effects of diphenylhydantoin on synaptic transmission in cat spinal cord and stellate ganglion. *J. Pharmacol. Exp. Ther.* 120:301, 1957.
3. Gibbs, F. A., and Stamps, F. W. *Epilepsy Handbook.* Springfield, Ill.: Thomas, 1958.
4. Gordon, P. Diphenylhydantoin and procainamide: normalization of suboptimal learning behavior. *Recent Advances Biol. Psychiat.* 10:121, 1968.
5. Gordon, P., Callahan, O., and Doty, B. Diphenylhydantoin effects on nucleic acid biochemistry, learning and neoplasm. *Pharmacologist* 10:169, 1968.
6. Gordon, P., Tobin, S. S., Doty, B., and Nash, M. Drug effects on behavior of aged animals and man: diphenylhydantoin and procainamide. *J. Geront.* 23:434, 1968.
7. Lennox, W. G., and Lennox, M. A. *Epilepsy and Related Disorders.* Boston: Little, Brown, 1960.
8. Livingston, S. Diphenylhydantoin in emotional disorders. *J.A.M.A.* 204:549, 1968.

9. Ludmer, R. I., and Toman, J. E. Some drug effects on cardiac transmembranal potentials. *Fed. Proc.* 24:303, 1968.
10. Pieper, W., and Abrams, N. Unpublished data, 1968.
11. Toman, J. E. P. Neuropharmacological considerations in psychical seizures. *Neurology* (Minneap.) 1:444, 1951.
12. Toman, J. E. P. Mechanisms of Action of Convulsant and Anticonvulsant Drugs. *Proc. XII Internat. Physiol. Congr.* (Sympos.) 1959, pp. 158–162.
13. Toman, J. E. P. Neuropharmacology of diphenylhydantoin. *Int. J. Neuropsychiat.* 3:s57–s62, 1967, suppl. 2.
14. Toman, J. E. P., Loewe, S., and Goodman, L. S. Studies on the physiology and therapy of convulsive disorders. I. The effect of anticonvulsant drugs on electroshock seizures in man. *Arch. Neurol. Psychiat.* 58:312, 1947.
15. Toman, J. E. P., and Sabelli, H. C. Comparative neuronal mechanisms. *Epilepsia* (Amst.), 1969, in press.
16. Toman, J. E. P., and Sabelli, H. C. Neuropharmacology of earthworm giant fibers. *Int. J. Neuropharmacol.* 1969, in press.
17. Toman, J. E. P., and Toman, M. E. Seizures in a peripheral nerve model with feedback. *Fed. Proc.* 11:162, 1952.
18. Turner, W. J. (Ed.) Symposium: Diphenylhydantoin—its usefulness in disorders of a nonepileptic nature. *Int. J. Neuropsychiat.* 1967, vol. 3, suppl. 2.
19. Vazquez, A. J., Sabelli, H. C., Ludmer, R. I., and Toman, J. E. P. Pharmacological analysis of evoked potentials in rabbit cortex. *Recent Advances Biol. Psychiat.* 8:51, 1966.

24

Genetics of Seizure Susceptibility*

GUY M. McKHANN† AND ERIC M. SHOOTER

OTHER AUTHORS contributing to this volume have focused attention on the relationships between seizures and abnormalities of the neuron and of neuronal membranes. It seems appropriate to include within the scope of this presentation not only a discussion of the genetics of seizure disorders of the human, but also a review of basic genetic mechanisms as they may apply to neuronal structure and function. This presentation will be in three parts: mechanisms of gene action; altered gene function in relationship to seizure disorders; and, finally, in the Discussion, Metrakos will review data relating to genetics of human seizure disorders.

Mechanism of Gene Action

The ultimate products of gene action are proteins. Details of how the linear coding of information in the genome DNA is transformed into the three-dimensional structure of proteins have been firmly established in bacterial systems (Fig. 24-1) [49]. Genetic information from the continuous series of base triplets in one strand of DNA is transcribed by the enzyme RNA polymerase into single-stranded molecules of messenger RNA. The latter attach via their 5'-termini to the ribosomes. In turn, the triplet codons of messenger RNA are recognized sequentially by the triplet anticodons of transfer RNA species to each of which is attached a particular amino acid [32].

Translation of the messenger RNA begins at the 5'-terminus, which corresponds to the amino terminal end of the polypeptide chain, and proceeds three bases or one amino acid at a time to the 3'-terminus of the messenger RNA or the carboxyterminal end of the polypeptide chain. The completed polypeptide chain folds spontaneously into a unique three-dimensional structure whose conformation is determined by the interactions between the amino acid residues of the chain [12]. Thus, genetic information encoded in DNA dictates not only the amino acid sequence, but also final structural relationships of the protein molecule. In so doing, it generates a structure endowed with its own specific biological property.

The principle of self-organization applies also to larger aggregates. If the folded polypeptide chain is one subunit of a multisubunit protein, then the initial folding also generates the binding sites on the subunit, which allow it to combine spontaneously with other subunits in the assembly [14, 17]. Even assemblies containing heterologous subunits can arise by the same mechanism. For example, the RNA-containing viruses, such as tobacco mosaic virus, are spontaneously generated from mixtures of their protein subunits and the appropriate long RNA strand [13]. At even higher levels of complexity, there is evidence that at least some part of membrane structures are self-

---

* These studies supported by the Joseph P. Kennedy, Jr., Foundation, the John A. Hartford Foundation, PHS Research Grants NB05300 and NB04270 from National Institute of Neurological Diseases and Stroke and PHS Research Grant HD02147 and PHS Training Grant HD00049 from National Institute of Child Health and Human Development.

† Joseph P. Kennedy, Jr., Foundation Senior Research Scholar and John and Mary R. Markle Scholar in Academic Medicine.

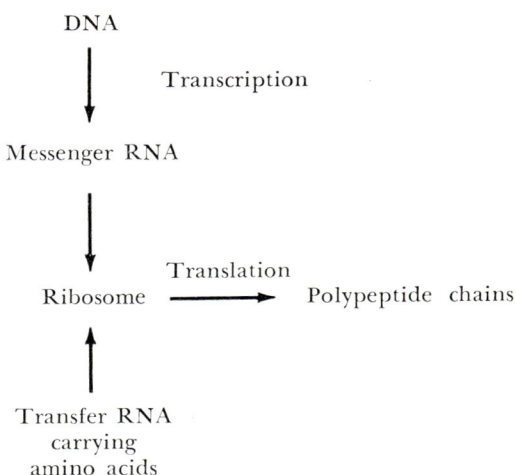

Fig. 24-1. Transformation of DNA into three-dimensional structure of proteins.

assembling, although the assembly of the complete membrane may require a primer [44]. Information in the triplet code of the genome is therefore sufficient for specification of synthesis of all biological macromolecules and of many more complex supramacromolecular assemblies. Within this body of information are also the elements which regulate cellular activity via induction or repression of enzyme synthesis [40] and the allosteric control of enzymatic activity [28].

The principle of self-assembly stops short at the organelle level since organelles apparently require some preexisting structure to make growth and replication possible [24]. It has recently been established, for example, that mitochondria have their own unique DNA [31] which is passed on, by division of mitochondria, to all daughter cells, which are therefore responsible for mitochondrial replication [22, 23]. Mitochondria participate actively in protein synthesis by mechanisms not entirely similar to those of ribosomal protein synthesis, and they appear to be important elements in the determination of cytoplasmic inheritance and thus of differentiation [20].

The same basic mechanisms of gene action apply to mammalian systems and, as far as is known from data currently available, operate also in nervous system cells [7, 8, 50]. Much of the structure and activity of the neuronal and glial elements is thus determined by the nuclear DNA, but a significant part may well be controlled at the level of mitochondria [8]. Also, there is recent evidence for protein synthesis in axons [11] and in isolated nerve-ending particles [2]. It should be emphasized that the significance of these possible alternate control sites in the nervous system remains to be explored, but the possibility exists that some proteins required for normal neuronal functioning may be synthesized at local sites within the neuron.

The consequences of mutations in the genome or of errors in transcription or translation have, again, been well documented in bacterial systems. Examples of altered physiological function in man arising from single base changes in the genome are also known and will be discussed shortly. In general, however, it should be clear from the preceding discussion that the ultimate physiological outcome of a mutation may be expressed at one or more levels. If the primary gene product is, like hemoglobin, a protein with a major and readily observable function, then it is possible to relate changes in function directly to changes in protein structure. On the other hand, the altered gene product may be an enzyme involved in the synthesis of an essential membrane component. Lack of this component, or its overproduction, or simply some subtle change in its structure may produce diverse effects on membrane function and in turn apparently unrelated disease processes. The latter may even be such as to not immediately implicate abnormal membrane structure or function.

MODEL SYSTEMS

There are a number of diseases of genetic origin in which the development or function of the nervous system is altered. However, despite the fact that enzymatic defect is recognizable in these conditions and that altered metabolism can be detected, little is known about the mechanisms underlying the altered neural function. For example, although the defect in phenylalanine hydroxylase is well documented in phenylketonuria and the accumulation of products of phenylalanine easily demonstrated, the mechanism for production of seizures and of mental deficiency is not known [27]. In a disorder of lipid metabolism, metachromatic leukodystrophy, there is accumulation of large amounts of a normal lipid component of the myelin sheath, sulfatide, secondary to the functional absence of a catabolic enzyme [1, 26, 30]. Here again, even though the metabolic error is known, the mechanism is not known by which accumulation of sulfatide results in mental deterioration, altered motor function, and eventually seizures. However, in this instance, it is possible to speculate about altered membrane functions in association with altered membrane composition [35].

The clearest example in man of the relation between altered gene product and altered function comes from the study of the hemoglobinopathies. In order to be effective in oxygen transport, hemoglobin must be able to combine with oxygen in the lungs and be able to deliver oxygen to tissues for diffusion to intracellular sites. Normal human hemoglobin has these properties. Of the large number of genetic abnormalities of human hemoglobin which have been discovered, a few have been found to have altered oxygen-binding properties. An example of this form of hemoglobinopathy is provided by hemoglobin Yakima [18, 33].

Hemoglobinopathy and Hemoglobin Yakima. Hemoglobin Yakima differs from normal hemoglobin only in the substitution of a histidine residue for the usual aspartic acid residue at one position, β99, in the β chain. This site is in the plane of contact between the β and the α chains and the amino acid substitution apparently so alters the interaction between the two chains that hemoglobin Yakima has a higher affinity for oxygen than does normal hemoglobin. Thus, the physiological defect is a difficulty in delivery of oxygen at the level of tissues. The body compensates for this difficulty by increasing the synthesis of hemoglobin. Thus, the heterozygote may be asymptomatic except for erythrocytosis.

Homozygote persons are not found and the homozygote condition is presumably lethal. Another physiological effect of this increased oxygen binding occurs in pregnant mothers who are heterozygotes. In this situation, the mother's blood will probably have at least as high an affinity, if not higher, for oxygen than that of the fetus. Since hemoglobin Yakima is a β-chain variant, very little of the abnormal hemoglobin will be present in fetal red cells. The latter will have their usual content of normal fetal hemoglobin in which fetal γ chains substitute for the adult β chains. Thus, there may well be lower transplacental oxygen flow in the fetus, and the fetuses rarely survive.

There are at least two other hemoglobinopathies in which the physiological defect is an increased binding of oxygen, and familial erythrocytosis occurs. In one of these, hemoglobin Kempsey [37], there is a substitution in the same place in the β chain as in hemoglobin Yakima. However, in this instance, it is a substitution of an asparagine for an aspartic acid residue. In a third instance, hemoglobin Chesapeake [9], the amino acid substitution, leucine for arginine, is in the α rather than β chain. The position of the substitution, however, is still in the contact region between unlike chains. Thus, three different genetically determined abnormalities in hemoglobin structure resulting in changes in the interaction between the subunits give rise to essentially the same physiological defect, that is, an increased binding of oxygen.

Relation of Genetic Defects to Abnormal Neural Function. This model of abnormal hemoglobins may have particular relevance to discussion of the relationship of genetic defects to abnormal neural function. Analysis of this model suggests that a defect in a gene product can result not only in an absence of a physiological function, but also in variation in a physiological function, that a number of different genetic abnormalities resulting in different gene products may all result in a similar alteration of physiological function, and that abnormality may often be detected by the secondary response of the host, for example, an erythrocytosis in the examples given above. It would also be expected that clinical manifestations of this disease would be altered by changes in environmental conditions; for the hemoglobin model this could be high altitude or, as has been mentioned, the effects of the physiological defect on oxygen transport to the fetus.

Is it possible to analyze disorders of neural function in the same fashion that disorders of hemoglobin function have been detailed? The answer to this question depends partly on the ability to isolate and characterize the primary gene products in the nervous system, the neural proteins, and also partly on identification of the function of these proteins. Steps have been taken in both directions.

Before proceeding to a discussion of proteins in the central nervous system, it should be pointed out that proteins as structural components of membranes are constituents of complex macromolecules consisting not only of proteins, but also lipids, and possibly mucopolysaccharides. Genetically determined defects in membrane structure and function could be related to disorders of synthesis or maintenance of these other components of membranes as well as proteins.

PROTEINS OF THE NERVOUS SYSTEM

A number of investigations have concentrated on the isolation and characterization of proteins unique to the nervous system. An excellent example is the group of acidic proteins, of which the S-100 protein is one, which Moore has shown to exist only in nervous system cells, and they are apparently of neuroglial origin [29]. They are sufficiently well characterized so that it would now be possible to look for conditions where one or more of these proteins is missing, or altered, and thus gain some insight into their structure-function relationships. In principle, this could also be done for many of the water-soluble proteins from nervous tissue since resolution of even these complex mixtures by current chromatographic, electrophoretic, and sedimentation techniques is possible.

Water-soluble proteins do not, however, constitute the main fraction of neural proteins. In the nervous system tissues, membranes are a major structural component and a substantial portion of the enzyme complement of neuronal and glial cells are firmly bound to, or incorporated within these membranes. In addition, there are the usual structural proteins of the membranes. Together, these water-insoluble membrane enzymes and proteins amount to at least two-thirds of the total protein of nervous tissue.

The search for abnormal neural proteins associated with abnormal function of the nervous system is, therefore, closely allied to the development of techniques for solubilization and fractionation of water-insoluble membrane proteins. Based on earlier reports of the effect of nonionic [6] and ionic detergents [5], a method has been developed for the virtually quantitative solubilization of membrane proteins of mouse brain [16] in two major fractions. After efficient removal of the soluble cytoplasmic proteins which surround and are contained within the organelles of the cells, optimum concentrations of the nonionic detergent, alkyl aryl polyether alcohol (Triton X-100) solubilize an additional 35 percent of the total brain protein. This pool of detergent-soluble protein cannot be increased by subsequent extraction of the remaining organelles with additional volumes of higher concentrations of the detergent. The remaining protein is, however, soluble in the ionic detergent, sodium lauryl sulfate. Each type of detergent thus solubilizes a finite pool of membrane proteins suggesting that the differential solubility properties may also correspond to different morphological localization.

Of equal importance was the finding that the membrane proteins solubilized in sodium lauryl sulfate could be separated by electrophoresis in polyacrylamide gels containing this detergent. Moreover, the nonionic detergent in the detergent-solubilized pool could be displaced by addition of sodium lauryl sulfate and the protein in this pool thereby also separated by electrophoresis. The extent of the separation of proteins in the two pools is illustrated in Fig. 24-2A, where it can be seen that they contain essentially two different groups of proteins.

It is apparent that the two detergents selectively disaggregate the membranes of nervous tissue as they do membranes from

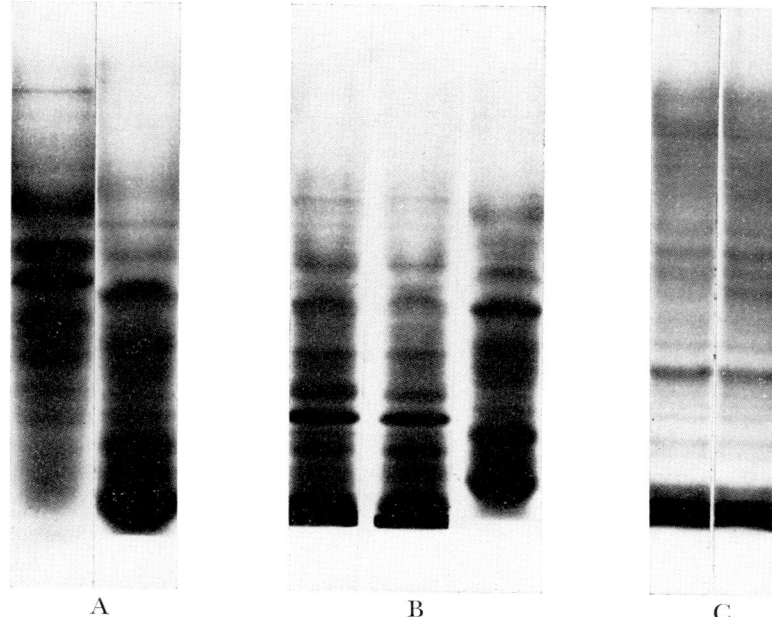

FIG. 24-2. Electrophoretic analysis of some membrane proteins from brain. (A) Analysis of protein solubilized by 1 percent alkyl aryl polyether alcohol (Triton X-100), left, and subsequently by 0.1 percent sodium lauryl sulfate, right, from a lysed subcellular fraction of whole adult mouse brain. (B) Analysis of protein solubilized by 0.1 percent sodium lauryl sulfate from brains of mice 17 and 20 days after fertilization, left and center respectively, and of an adult mouse, right. (C) Analysis of protein solubilized by 0.1 percent sodium lauryl sulfate from brains of C57/B6, left, and AKR, right, strains of mice of comparable age. Electrophoretic analyses carried out in porosity gradient polyacrylamide gels at pH 9.6 incorporating 0.025 percent sodium lauryl sulfate in (A) and (B) and 0.1 percent sodium lauryl sulfate in (C).

other tissues. These methods of extraction and separation have been applied to the subcellular organelles derived from whole brain, myelin, nuclei, mitochondria, synaptosomes, and ribosomes and each organelle gives a characteristic pattern [48]. The search for abnormal brain proteins (or for proteins from more closely defined regions of the nervous system) in disease conditions can thus be extended to membrane proteins at the level of the whole tissue or of the functional organelles. A necessary precaution is to compare proteins from brain or organelles at similar stages of development, since protein type and distribution vary with age, as is indicated in Fig. 24-2B for whole-brain membrane protein of prenatal and adult mice. Examples of the occurrence of variants of membrane proteins can be found in inbred strains of mice. The two strains C57/B1 and AKR are from quite different origins. On the basis of the above criteria, no differences were detected in the water-soluble or detergent-soluble protein groups. However, one major difference was noted in the group soluble in sodium lauryl sulfate (Fig. 24-2C): one main protein band in C57/B1 was replaced by another protein band of somewhat higher mobility in AKR. This type of analysis should now be extended to certain of the neurological mutant strains of mice to inquire whether other genetic variants of nervous system protein appear in these conditions.

ENZYMATIC DEFECTS RESULTING IN ABNORMAL NEURAL FUNCTION

Proteins, as mentioned previously, have not only a structural role but also a functional role: either as structural components of membranes or as enzymes. In a number of genetically determined diseases, the defect is in enzymatic function. In most instances, these "inborn errors of metabolism" have been recognized and studied on the basis of their disturbed metabolism, either in terms of accumulation of specific substances or by direct demonstration of altered metabolism. In only a few instances has the altered metabolism been correlated with alterations in structure of the enzyme protein. The central nervous system is affected in a number of these metabolic errors. In most instances, effect on the nervous system is secondary to effects of an enzymatic defect in liver or a generalized defect in metabolism. For example, the seizures and mental retardation in one form of glycogen storage disease are secondary to a defect in glucose 6-phosphatase in liver, and the resulting deficiency of free blood sugar. In other instances, accumulation of substances resulting from a defect in metabolism, such as galactose in galactosemia or phenylalanine in phenylketonuria, may have direct damaging effects on the metabolism of the developing nervous system.

Gangliosides. Of greater pertinence to the present discussion are metabolic defects in which enzymatic functions present in brain are altered. In a group of progressive, degenerative diseases of the nervous system in children, the neuronal storage diseases, particular neuronal compounds accumulate to great excess. Clinical features are progressive dementia, intractable seizures, and eventual death. The metabolic defect in all of these conditions has not been determined. In some, however, the condition has been quite well defined. The best examples are those diseases in which there is the abnormal accumulation of gangliosides, a group of complex glycosphingolipids containing N-acetylneuraminic acid (NANA). In the central nervous system, gangliosides are located primarily within neurons, are probably associated with synaptic membranes [10, 19]. Their normal physiological role is not clear. In certain neuronal storage diseases, particular gangliosides accumulate within neurons to great excess.

In Tay-Sachs disease, a particular ganglioside accumulates, GM_2, in the terminology of Svennerholm [43] (Fig. 24-3). This accumulation is presumably secondary to the absence of a lipid hexosaminase, which would normally split off the terminal N-acetylhexosamine [42]. The genetics of this condition have been well studied; the frequency of the heterozygous state in Jewish persons is one in 30–40 [47]. The inheritance of Tay-Sachs disease is as an autosomal recessive with complete penetrance. Despite the extent of our knowledge of the chemical pathology and biochemistry of this disease, the mechanism by which the ganglioside accumulation alters neuronal function is not known. Perhaps before we can attain such knowledge we will have to wait for further information about the normal role of gangliosides in neural function. Of interest in relation to study of the effects of ganglioside accumulation on neural function is the maintenance of isolated involved neurons in tissue culture. These cells (Fig. 24-4) were obtained from the cortex of a patient with Tay-Sachs disease and isolated by the technique of Varon and Raiborn [45]. The involved cells could be maintained for 8–10 days, during which time material continued to accumulate [25].

Another form of ganglioside-storage disease is marked by accumulation of a different ganglioside than the one which accumulates in Tay-Sachs disease. This molecule, GM_1, accumulates because a β-galactosidase, which should split off the terminal galactose, is missing [34] (Fig. 24-5).

In this disease, there is the accumulation of material within other organs, such as liver and spleen. However, material in the somatic organs is not ganglioside, but a form of mucopolysaccharide, probably

$$(GM_2) \quad \begin{array}{c} \text{Fatty Acid} \\ | \\ \text{Sphingosine-Glucose-Galactose-N-Acetylgalactosamine} \\ | \\ \text{NANA} \end{array}$$

FIG. 24-3. The ganglioside GM_2 that accumulates in Tay-Sachs disease.

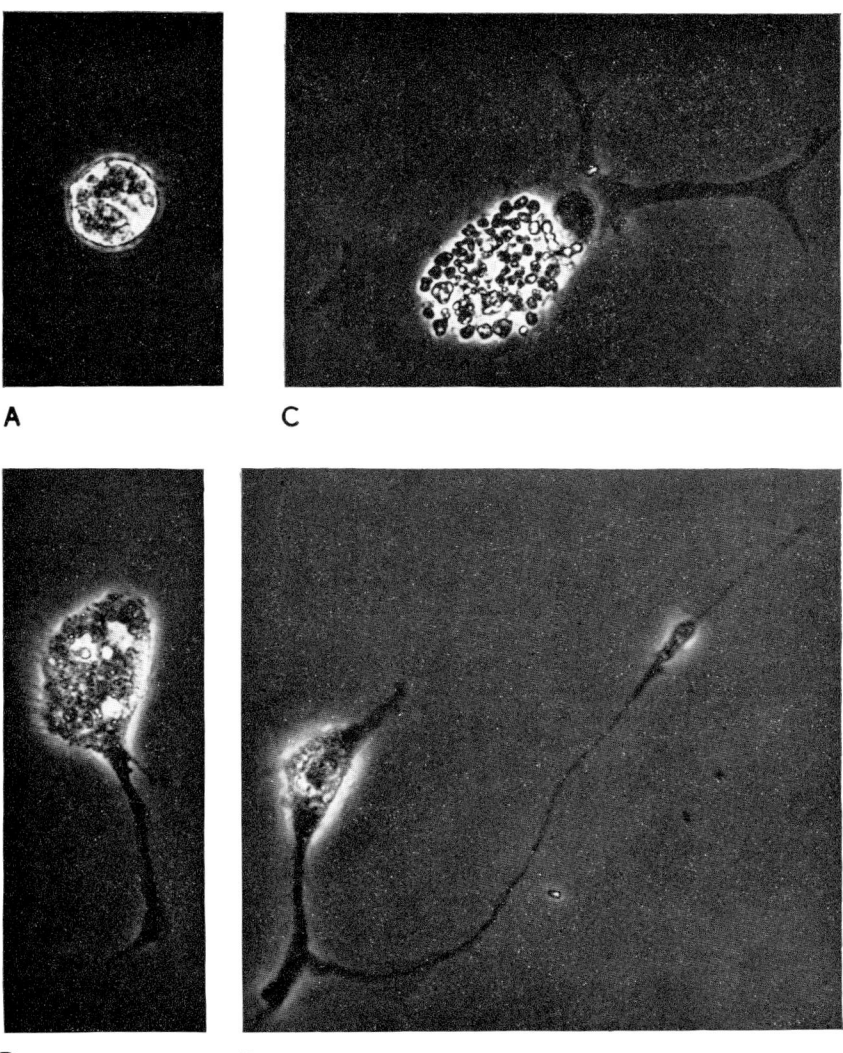

Fig. 24-4. Isolated cells from cerebral biopsy of patient with Tay-Sachs disease, maintained in tissue culture. (A) An involved cell after dissociation and before culture. The cell processes have been sheared off by the dissociation procedure. (B) The appearance after 24 hours in culture. (C) The appearance after 144 hours in culture. (D) The appearance of another cell after 144 hours in culture. The highly refractile material is positive for PAS and Oil-Red-O and easily extractable with lipid solvents.

keratin-sulfate [41]. This mucopolysaccharide accumulation in peripheral organs may be secondary to a defect in the same enzyme, β-galactosidase. Presumably, in liver, the normal substrate for this enzyme is mucopolysaccharide and in brain, ganglioside. The findings in generalized gangliosidosis are of particular importance to clinical investigators, who have tried to draw conclusions about the possible chemical pathology of the nervous system on the basis of study of somatic organs.

Lipid Components of Membranes. Despite the fact that the accumulating products may differ, the enzymatic defect in brain and other organs may be similar. Brady and colleagues have taken advantage of this fact for demonstration of the enzy-

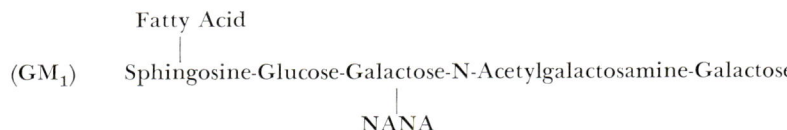

Fig. 24-5. The GM_1 ganglioside that accumulates in brain in generalized gangliosidosis.

matic defect in a group of diseases involving defects in metabolism of membranous lipids, the sphingolipidoses, using leukocytes as the source of enzyme [3]. An example of the use of this readily available tissue for demonstration of an enzymatic defect involving a lipid component of membranes is in the studies by Percy and Brady, who found the following values for arylsulfatase A activity in leukocytes of patients with metachromatic leukodystrophy (MLD) and controls (adapted from Percy and Brady [36]):

Controls (16 patients) 100.9 ± 6.5 units
MLD (6 patients) 11.7 ± 2.4 units

This reaction is the release of sulfate from p-nitrocatechol sulfate. The units refer to the amount of p-nitrocatechol sulfate released per hour per milligram of protein from leukocytes. The markedly decreased enzymatic activity in the MLD patients results in failure of catabolism of sulfatides and subsequent accumulation of these sulfolipids [26]. The affected patients had barely detectable activity of arylsulfatase in their leukocytes. So far, enzymatic assays of leukocytes have not been sensitive enough to detect the heterozygote.

There are two extensions of these studies of isolated, involved cells which may have significance in regard to human disease. Preliminary evidence from Brady's laboratory and from others indicates that the enzymatic defect is present in human amniotic cells [4]. Use of this source of tissue may provide not only early detection of affected fetuses, but also a cell line, containing the metabolic defect, which can be propagated.

A second extension of these studies relates to the varying clinical forms of the sphingolipidoses. For example, Gaucher's disease, a disease involving the accumulation of glucocerebroside, has various forms varying in age of onset, rate of progression, and distribution of involvement. Studies of leukocytes in the various forms of Gaucher's disease suggest that the later life forms may be related to partial genetic defects, with residual enzymatic activity present [3]. In this kind of model, the appearance of clinical symptoms may be associated with the gradual accumulation of a material or the sudden overwhelming of deficient enzymatic systems by increased demands.

There are enzymes which are located primarily within neurons, such as glutamic decarboxylase. Other authors in this volume have outlined the possible role of amino acids as transmitters, glutamic acid being excitatory and γ-aminobutyric acid and glycine being inhibitory. It is apparent that alterations in metabolism of these compounds could have profound effects on neural function.

Trophic Factors. Finally, to complete the spectrum of enzymatic defects in relation to the nervous system, trophic factors which affect development must be considered. The best studied of these is nerve growth factor (NGF), a protein required for the normal growth of autonomic and peripheral sensory neurons [21]. The protein-subunit structure of one form of NGF has been recently elucidated [46]. Of the three different types of subunits found in this protein, only one, the β subunits, elicits biological response. The second type, the γ subunits comprising three major components, has enzymatic activity against argininyl esters or amides [15]. The remaining γ subunits comprise a family of closely related acidic proteins. It is not known how many genetic loci control the synthesis of these multiple subunits and thus of NGF itself, but it is clear that genetically determined deficits could arise in the synthesis of one or more subunits which might then result in altered sympathetic or sensory neuronal development.

In the central nervous system, there are a number of parameters of neuronal growth and development which might be under the control of similar trophic factors, such as neuronal migration or cell-to-cell recognition. The possibility that these aspects of neuronal development are under genetic control is raised by the studies by Sidman of the *reeler* mouse [39]. In this inherited developmental disease, the mutant neurons are abnormally positioned and poorly interconnected in regions of brain, such as cerebellum, cerebral isocortex, and hippocampal formation, where synaptic specificity is thought to be acquired by cell-to-cell recognition during neuroblast migration. Thus, a consideration of genetically determined seizure disorders in the human must include cases with seizures associated with defects of cortical layering and neuronal migration. Unfortunately, most such children die without adequate pathological study; genetic data for comparison of human developmental disorders with those in experimental animals are not available.

So far we have discussed the genetic control of protein synthesis and the role of proteins as structural components or as enzymes. However, it should be emphasized that the regulation of cellular and metabolic activity includes not only the synthesis of protein, but also their subsequent removal. Knowledge about this removal process is fragmentary at best. However, studies from a number of laboratories, recently reviewed by Schimke [38], indicate that protein turnover and its regulation can be important in determining the levels and response of specific proteins to hormonal, pharmacologic, and nutritional variables.

As Schimke emphasizes, the turnover of protein is an active process and in itself may be under genetic control. For example, the level of the enzyme catalase in a number of mouse strains is regulated by the rate of turnover of this enzyme. This turnover is regulated by genetically distinct locus in which rapid turnover is dominant. Thus, there must be included in the interpretation of the genetic control of protein synthesis not only the control of amino acid sequence and ultimate structure, but also the rate of metabolism of particular proteins. In addition, clearly extragenetic factors can enhance or retard membranous protein or enzyme inactivation or degradation. As Schimke concluded, "The best model to observe dynamics of independent synthesis and turnover of membrane proteins would appear to be that of a mosaic of proteins which are synthesized and are degraded at different rates in response to different physiologic stimulae" [38].

CONCLUSION

In this chapter, an outline of the genetic control of protein synthesis has been presented. We have tried to point out that proteins have a number of potential roles in the nervous system and that defects in their synthesis, function, or turnover could result in abnormal neural functioning. In addition, it is worth emphasizing that the observed clinical phenomenon may be difficult to relate to a single enzymatic function or a single abnormal protein. Further, extragenetic effects may influence the genetic expression of the organism and such factors as degree of development, body temperature, hormonal state, and rates of neuronal activity may all influence the metabolism or function of neural proteins.

On a note of optimism, it should be pointed out that techniques are available for isolation and characterization of proteins and protein-containing complexes from whole brain, regions of brain, isolated neurons, and specific neural membranes. What remains to be done is to apply these techniques to the study of genetically determined seizures.

REFERENCES

1. Austin, J., Armstrong, D., and Shearer, L. Metachromatic form of diffuse cerebral sclerosis. *Arch. Neurol.* (Chicago) 13:593, 1965.
2. Austin, L. J. Unpublished data, 1968.
3. Brady, R. O. Enzymatic abnormalities in diseases of sphingolipid metabolism. *Clin. Chem.* 14:565, 1967.

4. Brady, R. O. Unpublished data, 1968.
5. Brunngraber, E. G., and Abood, L. T. Mitochondrial glycolysis of rat brain and its relationship to the remainder of cellular glycolysis. *J. Biol. Chem.* 235:1847, 1960.
6. Brunngraber, E. G., and Aguilar, L. Fractionation of brain macromolecules. I. Chromatography on hydroxylapatite of enzymes solubilized by Triton X-100 from the rat brain mitochondrial fraction. *J. Neurochem.* 9:451, 1962.
7. Campagnoni, A. T., and Mahler, H. R. Isolation and properties of polyribosomes from cerebral cortex. *Biochemistry* 6:956, 1967.
8. Campbell, M. K., Mahler, H. R., Moore, W. J., and Tewari, S. Protein synthesis systems from rat brain. *Biochemistry* 5:1174, 1966.
9. Charache, S., Weatherall, D. J., and Clegg, J. B. Polycythemia associated with a hemoglobinopathy. *J. Clin. Invest.* 45:813, 1966.
10. Derry, D. M., and Wolfe, L. S. Gangliosides in isolated neurons and glial cells. *Science* 158:1450, 1967.
11. Edström, A. Inhibition of protein synthesis in Mauthner nerve fiber components by actinomycin-D. *J. Neurochem.* 14:239, 1967.
12. Epstein, C. J., Goldberger, R. F., and Anfinsen, C. B. The genetic control of tertiary protein structure: Studies with model systems. *Sympos. Quant. Biol.* 28:439, 1963.
13. Fraenkel-Conrad, H., and Williams, R. C. Reconstitution of active tobacco mosaic virus from its inactive protein and nucleic acid components. *Proc. Nat. Acad. Sci. U.S.A.* 41:695, 1955.
14. Gerhart, J. C., and Schachman, H. K. Distinct subunits for the regulation and catalytic activity of aspartate transcarbamylase. *Biochemistry* 4:1054, 1965.
15. Greene, L. A., Shooter, E. M., and Varon, S. Enzymatic activities of mouse nerve growth factor and its subunits. *Proc. Nat. Acad. Sci. U.S.A.* 60:1383, 1968.
16. Grossfeld, R. M., and Shooter, E. M. Unpublished data, 1968.
17. Huehns, E. R., and Shooter, E. M. The reaction of hemoglobin α-A with hemoglobin H. *Nature* (London) 193:1083, 1962.
18. Jones, R. T., Osgood, E. E., Brimhall, B., and Koler, R. D. Hemoglobin Yakima. I. Clinical and biochemical studies. *J. Clin. Invest.* 46:1840, 1967.
19. Lapetina, E. G., Soto, E. F., and De Robertis, E. Gangliosides and acetylcholinesterase in isolated membranes of rat brain cortex. *Biochim. Biophys. Acta* 135:33, 1967.
20. Lehninger, A. L. Cell Organelles: The Mitochondria. In Quarton, G. C. (Ed.), *The Neurosciences.* New York: Rockefeller Univ. Press, 1967.
21. Levi-Montalcini, R., and Angeletti, P. U. Nerve growth factor. *Physiol. Rev.* 48:534, 1968.
22. Luck, D. J. L. Formation of mitochondria in *neurospora crassa*. A quantitative radioautographic study. *J. Cell. Biol.* 16:483, 1963.
23. Luck, D. J. L. Formation of mitochondria in *neurospora crassa*. A study based on mitochondrial density changes. *J. Cell. Biol.* 24:461, 1965.
24. Lukins, H. B., Tham, S. H., Wallace, P. G., and Linnane, A. W. Correlation of membrane bound succinate dehydrogenase with the occurrence of mitochondrial profiles in *succharomyces cerevisiae*. *Biochem. Biophys. Res. Commun.* 23:363, 1966.
25. McKhann, G. M., Ho, W., Raiborn, C., and Varon, S. Isolation of neurons from normal and abnormal human cerebral cortex. *Arch. Neurol.* (Chicago) 20:542, 1969.
26. Mehl, E., and Jatzkewitz, H. Evidence for the genetic block in metachromatic leucodystrophy. *Biochem. Biophys. Res. Commun.* 19:407, 1965.
27. Menkes, J. H. The pathogenesis of mental retardation in phenylketonuria and other inborn errors of amino acid metabolism. *Pediatrics* 39:297, 1967.
28. Monod, J., Changeux, J. P., and Jacob, F. Allosteric proteins and cellular control systems. *J. Molec. Biol.* 6:306, 1963.
29. Moore, B. W., Perez, V. J., and Gehring, M. Assay and regional distribution of a soluble protein characteristic of the nervous system. *J. Neurochem.* 15:265, 1968.
30. Moser, H. W., Moser, A. B., and McKhann, G. M. The dynamics of a lipidosis. *Arch. Neurol.* (Chicago) 17:494, 1967.

31. Nass, M. M. K. The circularity of mitochondrial DNA. *Proc. Nat. Acad. Sci. U.S.A.* 56:1215, 1966.
32. Nirenberg, M., Caskey, T., Manhall, R., Brunacombe, R., Kellogg, D., Doctor, B., Hatfield, D., Levin, J., Rottman, F., Pestka, S., Wilcox, M., and Anderson, F. The RNA code and protein synthesis. *Sympos. Quant. Biol.* 31:11, 1966.
33. Novy, M. J., Edwards, M. J., and Metcalfe, J. Hemoglobin Yakima. II. High blood oxygen affinity associated with compensatory erythrocytosis and normal hemodynamics. *J. Clin. Invest.* 46:1848, 1967.
34. O'Brien, J. S. Personal communication.
35. O'Brien, J. S., and Sampson, E. L. Myelin membrane: A molecular abnormality. *Science* 150:1613, 1965.
36. Percy, A. K., and Brady, R. O. Metachromatic leucodystrophy: Diagnosis with samples of venous blood. *Science* 161:594, 1968.
37. Reed, C. S., Hampson, R., Gordon, S., Jones, R. T., Novy, M. J., Brimhall, B., Edwards, M. J., and Koler, R. D. Unpublished data, 1968.
38. Schimke, R. T., Ganschow, R., Doyle, D., and Arias, I. M. Regulation of protein turnover in mammalian tissues. *Fed. Proc.* 37:1223, 1968.
39. Sidman, R. L. Cell Proliferation and Migration in the Developing Brain. In McKhann, G. M. and Yaffee, S. J. (Eds.), *Drugs and Poisons in Relation to the Developing Nervous System*. Bethesda: U.S. Department of Health, Education and Welfare, Pub. No. 1791, 1968.
40. Stent, G. S. Induction and Repression of Enzyme Synthesis. In Quarton, G. C. (Ed.), *The Neurosciences*. New York: Rockefeller Univ. Press, 1967.
41. Suzuki, K. Cerebral G_{M1}-Gangliosidosis: Chemical pathology of visceral organs. *Science* 159:1471, 1968.
42. Svennerholm, L. S. Personal communication, 1968.
43. Svennerholm, L. S. The gangliosides. *J. Lipid Res.* 5:145, 1964.
44. Thompson, T. E. The Properties of Biomolecular Phospholipid Membranes. In Locke, M. (Ed.), *Cellular Membranes in Development*. New York: Academic, 1964.
45. Varon, S., and Raiborn, C. Unpublished data, 1968.
46. Varon, S., Nomura, J., and Shooter, E. M. Reversible dissociation of the mouse nerve growth factor protein into different subunits. *Biochemistry* 7:1296, 1968.
47. Volk, B., Schneck, L., Saifer, A., and Aronson, S. W. *Tay-Sachs Disease*. New York: Grune & Stratton, 1964.
48. Waehneldt, T., and Shooter, E. M. Unpublished data, 1969.
49. Watson, J. D. *Molecular Biology of the Gene*. New York: W. A. Benjamin, 1965.
50. Zomzely, C. E., Roberts, S., Gruber, C. P., and Brown, D. M. Cerebral protein synthesis. *J. Biol. Chem.* 243:5396, 1968.

Discussion

GENETIC STUDIES IN CLINICAL EPILEPSY*

JULIUS D. METRAKOS AND KATHERINE METRAKOS

We live because we have enzymes. Everything we do—walking, thinking, reading these lines—is done with some enzymatic process.—ERNEST BOREK

In their assessment of modern molecular biology as it applies to the epilepsies, McKhann and Shooter pointed out that enzymes are proteins which have been coded and synthesized by genes. By this token, Ernest Borek could have said, "We live because we have genes."

In the study of disease at the molecular and developmental levels, any lines of demarcation that may have existed previously all but disappear between heredity and environment as etiological factors. If genes are involved in everything we do and if heredity and environment interact and cannot be clearly separated, it is not surprising that genes have been implicated in the most frequently occurring of constitutional diseases, including heart disease, cancer, diabetes, and the epilepsies.

From the geneticist's point of view, it is not presumptuous to state that the most basic of the mechanisms of the epilepsies is the minute gamete and the genes which it carries from one generation to the next. There will be no attempt made here to outline basic principles of genetics and various modes of inheritance; these may be found in any standard textbook of human genetics such as *Genetics in Medicine* by Thompson and Thompson [26]. Instead, the discussion will be limited to: (1) certain basic concepts and *mechanisms* of which the genetic epileptologist must be aware in his search for genetic factors in the epilepsies and (2) that which the committee for this volume referred to as an original contribution expected of each discussant. Hopefully, these two additions will serve suitably as adjuncts to the contributions of McKhann and Shooter, to help underscore the basic biochemical genetics concepts presented.

SEARCH FOR GENETIC FACTORS IN THE EPILEPSIES

The genetic epileptologist, in his search for genetic factors in the epilepsies, may think and proceed along certain avenues.

Clinical and Genetic Heterogeneity

First of all, it must be appreciated that the epilepsies constitute a highly heterogeneous group of diseases, that the heterogeneity is not only clinical but also genetic. Genetic heterogeneity refers to different genetic situations, both at the chromosomal and genic levels, which may be capable of producing similar clinical pictures (phenotypes) as far as seizure patterns are concerned. For example, we know of a chromosomal disease, the D1 trisomy, where part of the syndrome is minor motor seizures and where the EEG frequently shows atypical spike-wave complexes [25]. Many hereditary diseases also affect the brain whose genes produce seizures as part of their pleiotropic effect. Examples of these are autosomal dominant tuberose sclerosis, autosomal recessive galactosemia, and sex-linked recessive hydrocephalus. Many other examples may be found in Pratt's *The Genetics of Neurological Disorders* [20] and in McKusick's *Mendelian Inheritance in Man* [12]. Of primary interest here is whether part of this genetic heterogeneity is due to specific *epilepsy per se* genes, capable

---

* This review article based on investigations supported by PHS Research Grant NB00706-14 from National Institute of Neurological Diseases and Stroke.

of producing epilepsy alone with no other obvious clinical symptomatology.

Familial and Genetic Epilepsy

When a well-defined clinical form of epilepsy is distinguished, the first question to investigate is whether it is familial. Familial means simply whether near relatives of an affected individual are similarly affected more often than near relatives of a comparable unaffected individual. This step is not as simple as it sounds since numerous biases may creep in and distort the answer. The first problem is to set criteria for *affected* and *unaffected*. If the genes involved result in variable severity (expressivity), then it is essential to decide at which point of severity and at which level of examination a near relative will be considered as affected similarly to the patient (proband). Is one convulsion sufficient? Are borderlands of epilepsy to be included? Is an epileptiform EEG without clinical seizures sufficient? Does a specific aminoaciduria with no other signs or symptoms indicate the presence of a single dose of a recessive pathological gene (heterozygous carrier)?

These and other biases have caused and continue to cause considerable confusion in the literature. A more detailed account of some of these has been given elsewhere [14]. However, when these biases are minimized and investigation is properly controlled, it is generally found that the prevalence of individuals with a history of seizures or cerebral dysrhythmias or both, is higher among near relatives of epileptics than among near relatives of nonepileptics.

Since familial predisposition does not necessarily mean that the condition is genetic, other investigations are needed to establish that genes are indeed involved. Pedigree, twin, and sibling studies have supported the conclusion that resistance or susceptibility to epilepsy in general is under genetic control. Unfortunately, at the present time our knowledge concerning these genes is very limited. For example, we know little if anything about such matters as the following.

Mode of Inheritance. Although the mode of inheritance is known for many rare cerebral diseases where epilepsy is part of the syndrome, for the commoner forms of epilepsy, the inheritance pattern remains unclear and seemingly complex. If these forms of epilepsy are due to interaction of two or more genes, which is the case with common diseases, the answer would be very difficult to obtain. Even if it is due to a single pathological gene, the answer may be complicated by phenomena of variability of expression and age of onset and lack of penetrance. The fact that in *centrencephalic* epilepsy there is an optimum age at which the *centrencephalic EEG trait* can be demonstrated (that is, an aspect of lack of penetrance) made it difficult for a long time to realize that the major gene in this form of epilepsy is an irregular, autosomal, dominant gene [16]. How many modifying genes may be involved still remains unclear.

Gene Frequency and Mutation Rate. When a gene has been identified and its mode of inheritance is known, several other questions concerning it are then raised. What is the relative frequency of the pathological allele to its normal allele? The answer to this question will provide an estimate of the number of affected individuals and of the number of carriers for any particular recessive form of epilepsy. In this context, the rate at which the normal allele mutates to its pathological form and selective factors becomes important. Except for very few hereditary cerebral diseases mentioned above, nothing is known about gene frequency and mutation rate of epilepsy genes.

Phenocopy. When an environmental factor produces a clinical picture closely resembling that produced by a gene, the affected individual is referred to as a phenocopy. In the epilepsies, of course, it is important to establish whether environment or heredity is the primary etiological factor. Both type of treatment and what is said in genetic counseling would depend on this distinction. It is of interest to note here that whether a phenocopy results from an environmental agent (for example, trauma or febrile disease) may well depend on threshold genes controlling resistance or susceptibility of the individual. This is another example of the futile attempt to separate environmental and genetic factors.

Linkage and Association. If a gene exists, it must occupy a locus on a particular chromosome. Genes whose loci are on the same chromosome show linkage relationships with one another. At the moment we know of no such linkages between epilepsy genes and marker genes, for example, blood groups. It is important to differentiate between linkage and association. For example, if migraine headache, criminality, suicide, and psychosis are more apt to appear among family members of epileptics than in the general population, this would be a mere association, and no genetic linkage should be implied. (Incidentally, such an association between the conditions mentioned and epilepsy has not, in the opinion of the authors, been established.)

Mode of Gene Action. In recent years, biochemical genetics has become the most fundamental and most important aspect of genetics, that branch of genetics which deals with how genic DNA produces its ultimate effect. This topic, amply reviewed by McKhann and Shooter, will not be expanded other than to point out that in the epilepsies, seizure as an end product of a gene is undoubtedly very far removed, by many steps, from the primary product of the gene. As suggested by McKhann and Shooter, it may well be that the end product of the gene is formation of an abnormal protein and the seizure is a far-removed neurophysiological consequence. Wide as this gap may be, it is of utmost importance that it be bridged and that intermediate steps become known. It is a sad commentary that although more is known about the genetics of the erythrocyte than about any other differentiated cell of the human body, the reverse is probably true about the neuron. The task of isolating and characterizing proteins specific to the nervous system is just beginning.

Gene Regulation. For the sake of simplicity, discussion so far has been in terms of single epilepsy genes of different categories. However, when it is recalled that no gene acts solely by itself but is dependent upon the whole genotype, probably some 10,000 gene pairs, it is unnecessary to mention that biochemical products of each gene interact, directly or indirectly, with biochemical products of all other genes of the individual. Modern gene concepts state that all major genes have not only pleiotropic effects but that their action is delicately balanced by a number of controlling genes. Some of the controlling genes act as inducers, while others act as inhibitors. Several adjacent genes concerned with the same synthetic process, with a *switch* gene at one end, and a regulator gene elsewhere, are in a state of dynamic equilibrium—the *operon*. Whether epilepsy operons exist, or whether operons exist at all in man, has not been established; but it is clear that with common diseases of man, such as epilepsy, in addition to major genes there are a number of modifying genes resulting in multifactorial inheritance or (if a threshold is involved) quasi-continuous variation. Thus, although a single major gene may be responsible for the *centrencephalic EEG trait*, a number of other genes may be controlling such factors as its variability in age of onset, sex distribution, and severity into typical and atypical.

Balanced Polymorphism

When the genetic structure of a population is such that several forms of a gene (alleles) are maintained in various but specific frequencies, such a population is referred to as exhibiting balanced polymorphism. Of such a polymorphic population for a particular type of genetic epilepsy, several questions could be asked. Why is the disease so common? What is the relative fertility of affected and unaffected individuals? What are natural and artificial selection pressures? Do genetic carriers show hybrid vigor? Are there any racial or ethnic differences? At the moment there are no answers to any of these questions.

Animal Studies

In a review of comparative genetics in mammals, Nachtsheim [18] lists 40 hereditary diseases of mammals of which counterparts are also found in man. Epilepsy is one of these diseases. Sidman et al. [24] have cataloged no less than 90 neurological mutants in inbred strains of mice. At least 15 of these exhibit epileptic seizures. What a wealth of material is here for the clinical epileptologist to pursue parallel animal studies!

The complexity of the genetic mechanism has been demonstrated in the case of audiogenic seizures in mice. It has been found that not only is susceptibility to audiogenic seizures hereditary but also the ability to recover [5]. Furthermore, genes responsible for susceptibility and for recovery segregate independently from one another. More recently Meier [13], Rauch [21], and others [9, 23] have shown association between phenylalanine metabolism and susceptibility to audiogenic seizures in mice. Finding an inhibitor of phenylalanine hydroxylase in *dilute* mice (that is, the susceptible strain) suggests that seizures may result from accumulation of phenylalanine metabolites which have been shown to inhibit decarboxylases. In particular, 5-hydroxytryptophan decarboxylase is inhibited [28]. This enzyme, it will be recalled, is responsible for synthesis of serotonin, the substance which is selectively concentrated in certain brain regions, for example, limbic system. Inasmuch as phenylketonuria and seizures are also found together in man, parallel studies between man and other mammals become essential and should prove most productive.

Therapy and Pharmacogenetics

The present treatment of epilepsy has been described as the *brute force* approach (surgery) and the *trial-and-error* approach (anticonvulsant therapy). These two approaches will undoubtedly continue to serve the epileptic well for many years to come. However, if certain forms of epilepsy can be traced to genes, then an understanding of their biosynthetic pathways becomes essential for a more scientific program of therapy. Just as genetic blocks (absent enzymes) at specific points in the biosynthetic pathways have been identified in phenylketonuria and galactosemia, so too, in genetic forms of epilepsy, it should be possible to identify enzymatic accumulations or deficiencies. If intermediate substances are accumulating, an understanding of their biochemical nature and position in the biosynthetic pathway would make their removal possible. If the deficiency is due to an absent enzyme, then at least theoretically, substitution is possible. Recently Hagberg [8] reported on a group of epileptic children with disturbed tryptophan metabolism who were treated with vitamin B_6.

The term pharmacogenetics, first used by Vogel in 1959 [27], denotes genetic variation of response to drugs. Pharmacogenetics, therefore, is a special aspect of therapy. Genetically determined variations of response to several drugs are now known [6]. For example, it has been well established that the rate of isoniazid metabolism in man is controlled by an autosomal pair of genes. Similar studies have been conducted with such drugs as the muscle relaxant, suxamethonium, with sensitivity to primaquine, and with psychotherapeutic drugs such as the phenothiazines. In all these studies, evidence for genetically determined variations has been found. References to these and other studies may be found in Kalow's *Pharmacogenetics. Heredity and the Response to Drugs* [11], where three of the nine chapters are devoted to heritable factors recognized in man through the use of drugs.

It is conceivable and highly likely that response to some anticonvulsant drugs may be under the control of genes. Such a finding would answer the present puzzling question of why, in two seemingly identical clinical cases of epilepsy, one responds well to a given anticonvulsant to which the other remains resistant.

Genetic Counseling

An ultimate objective in any genetic investigation of man is the transfer and application of genetic knowledge to genetic counseling situations. If I marry, what is the risk that my children will be epileptic as I am? I have an epileptic child, what is the risk that my next child will also be epileptic? The answers to these questions have been discussed elsewhere [17] in connection with *centrencephalic* epilepsy.

If accurate, empirical-risk figures exist, then genetic counseling can be given with confidence. However, it is unlikely that reliable, empirical-risk figures for different classes of relatives can be determined without knowledge and appreciation of the questions considered under the above five headings.

ORIGINAL CONTRIBUTION TO MONOGRAPH

Investigations conducted in the last 15 years have added substantially to the conclusion that hereditary factors are implicated in the etiology of the epilepsies. The results of pedigree, electroencephalographic, twin, animal, and biochemical studies by many investigators have compounded the evidence. Thus the problem is no longer whether or not genes are important in the epilepsies, but rather (1) to identify which genes are acting in which of the epilepsies, and (2) to determine which of these genes may be common to more than one type of epilepsy. Because of its significance, only the second question will be considered here, by reviewing briefly four different but related studies. For simplicity, in all four studies, observations will be confined mainly to siblings of four different types of *epileptic* probands. Although significant differences have been demonstrated between brothers and sisters in one of these studies, for the purpose of this discussion this separation will not be made.

Spike-Wave Epilepsy
(383 Siblings)

Evidence has been presented elsewhere [15, 16] supporting the hypothesis that the EEG showing a relatively good background pattern but with interspersed paroxysmal, bilaterally synchronous bursts of 2.5–3.5 cycles per second (cps) spike-wave complexes is inherited as an autosomal dominant trait, that additional factors, environmental and genetic, interact to precipitate the clinical seizures.

In trying to keep up with recommended changes in terminology, we have, unfortunately, referred to this type of epilepsy in the past as both *centrencephalic* and *epilepsy of subcortical origin*. This means being guilty of contributing to confusion which exists presently regarding the neurophysiological significance of generalized, bilaterally synchronous spike-wave discharges.

For clarification, before proceeding further, an individual is said to have *the spike-wave EEG trait*, if (1) at any time his electroencephalogram shows bursts of paroxysmal, bilaterally synchronous spike-wave complexes occurring rhythmically at a frequency of 2.5–3.5 cps; (2) his record shows a relatively good background pattern and no localizing features; and (3) the trait is obtained spontaneously in the resting record and/or during hyperventilation, and/or during photic stimulation. (Intermittent photic stimulation is carried out with eyes closed at frequencies of 3, 15, 18 alpha, 20 and 25 flickers per second for 6–8 seconds; and at intensity, full, 16.) In other words, several levels of penetrance are considered when deciding whether or not the trait is present. An individual with the trait may or may not have a history of clinical seizures. It should also be pointed out that an individual may exhibit the trait with activation only in one record and spontaneously in the resting record at another time. Thus, approximately 85 percent of probands who usually have several EEGs show the trait in the resting record, approximately 10 percent show the trait with hyperventilation, and 5 percent with photic stimulation. On the other hand, with siblings who usually have only one EEG, only approximately 60 percent show the trait in the resting record; the remainder show the trait either with hyperventilation (35 percent) or with photic stimulation (5 percent).

The studies to be reported here simply attempt to estimate prevalence of the spike-wave EEG trait in siblings of different groups of epileptic probands. Whether this type of EEG originates from only subcortical or only cortical or from both mechanisms is beyond our competence to decide; the polemics are accordingly left to those better fortified to reach a conclusion. Whether or not the EEGs are *over-read* so that prevalence of positive EEGs is higher than it should be is of importance and of concern. However, if this type of subjective error is of the same order of magnitude and in the same direction in the control EEGs of siblings of nonepileptic probands, then our concern is lessened. Since EEGs are read without prior knowledge of which group they belong to, dangers of this type of bias are minimized.

In the study referred to [15, 16], approximately 37 percent of the siblings of probands with spike-wave epilepsy have the spike-wave EEG trait, compared with 5 percent of comparable controls (Fig. D24-1). For other types of cerebral dysrhythmia, there is no essential difference between the experimental and control groups.

It is clear from the distribution curve that age has an important bearing on whether the EEG trait will be present in the siblings (Fig. D24-2). The trait is not fully developed at birth, but its prevalence rises rapidly, so that in the age group of 5–15 years more than 40 percent of the siblings show the trait. For older age groups, the trait tends to disappear and by 40 years of age it is very seldom present, as evidenced by low prevalence in the parents. This higher prevalence of paroxysmal, bilaterally synchronous spike-wave discharges has been found in siblings of at least three other groups of probands with clinical seizures.

Febrile Convulsions (147 Siblings)

By observing certain strict criteria, Escala, one of our colleagues, obtained EEGs of siblings of children who developed brief, generalized convulsions in association with fever for the first time between the ages of 6 months and 5 years.

Prevalence of EEG abnormalities among the siblings is significantly higher than among siblings of comparable control probands (Fig. D24-3). It is of interest that approximately 21 percent of siblings of the experimental group had the spike-wave EEG trait.

Probands with Focal EEG (127 Siblings)

Changing concepts regarding focal epilepsy prompted a study to test the hypothesis that a familial *convulsive tendency*, as expressed in the EEG, may be an underlying factor in this form of symptomatic epilepsy. In order to avoid subjective interpretations, probands were chosen on the

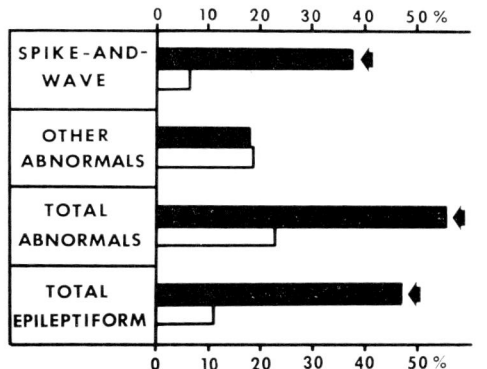

FIG. D24-1. EEG abnormalities in siblings of probands with spike-wave epilepsy. (Arrows = $p = 0.02$.)

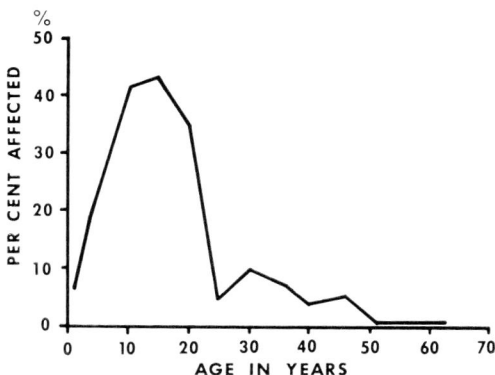

FIG. D24-2. Influence of age on spike-wave EEG trait. (Up to about age 20 years, distribution is based mainly on siblings; after that, based mainly on parents. However, both classes of relatives have a coefficient of relationship of $r = 0.5$.)

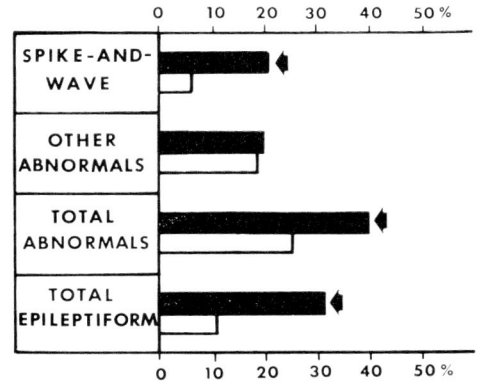

FIG. D24-3. EEG abnormalities in siblings of probands with febrile convulsions.

basis of the single objective criterion of having a focal EEG abnormality; however, surgical intervention was not indicated in any of the probands chosen.

Prevalence of abnormal EEGs among siblings of the focal group is significantly higher than among siblings of a control group (Fig. D24-4). More specifically, prevalence of individuals with the spike-wave EEG trait is significantly higher in the experimental than in the control group. Prevalence of cerebral dysrhythmias among siblings of probands with a focal EEG abnormality is approximately the same as that reported above for siblings of probands with spike-wave epilepsy; however, distribution of types of abnormalities is different.

Probands Treated Surgically for Focal Epilepsy (63 Siblings)

Presently, Eva Andermann, another of our colleagues, is studying families of epileptics who have been operated on for focal epilepsy at The Montreal Neurological Institute. To date only 48 families have been studied and EEGs have been taken on only 63 siblings; however, it is already apparent that on the whole, prevalence of EEG abnormalities among the siblings, parents, and offspring of epileptic probands is significantly higher than among the same class of relatives of the control group (Fig. D24-5).

When siblings are considered separately (Fig. D24-6), it is found that only approxi-

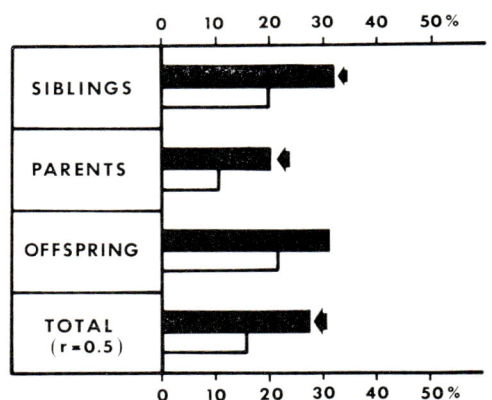

Fig. D24-5. EEG abnormalities in siblings, parents, and offspring of probands operated on for focal epilepsy.

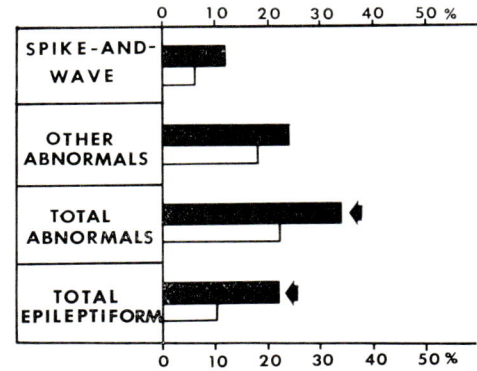

Fig. D24-6. EEG abnormalities in siblings of probands operated on for focal epilepsy.

mately 10 percent have the spike-wave EEG trait. This prevalence is far smaller than for the other three studies; with the small numbers involved, it is not significantly different from that found in controls. However, an explanation that accounts for most of this difference is that the mean age of siblings of this group is much higher (22 yr) than that of the other three groups (6–8 yr). This point has been discussed in more detail elsewhere [2].

The four studies are summarized on the basis of percentage of siblings showing the spike-wave EEG trait (Fig. D24-7). In each of these studies, whenever higher prevalence of epileptiform EEG abnormalities is found in siblings of epileptic groups than in siblings of control groups,

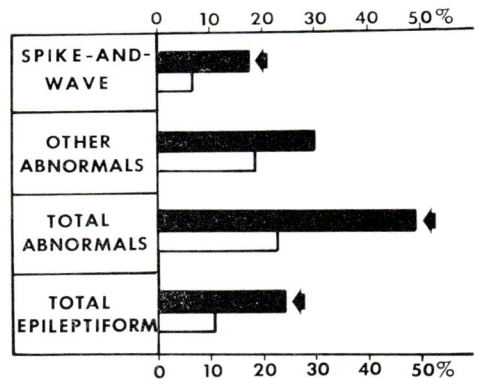

Fig. D24-4. EEG abnormalities in siblings of probands with focal EEG change irrespective of any other findings.

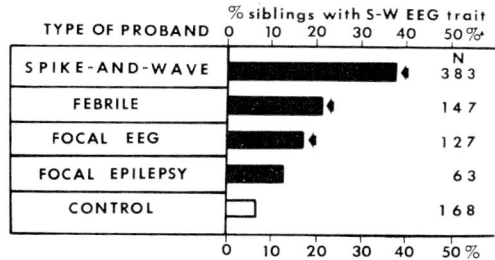

FIG. D24-7. Spike-wave EEG trait in siblings of 4 different types of probands with seizures compared with siblings of nonepileptic probands.

most of the elevation appears to be due to higher prevalence of individuals with the spike-wave EEG trait.

This observation suggests that perhaps several of the *epilepsies,* including febrile convulsions, have at least one genetic factor in common which may well be the autosomal dominant gene responsible for the spike-wave EEG trait. Whether or not the EEG trait is due to an autosomal dominant gene or to quasi-continuous variation would not alter the empirical risk figure reported. On the basis of the former hypothesis, frequency of this major pathological gene is high, $p = 0.02$, so that it is carried by approximately 4 percent of a randomly mating population. Its presence may be demonstrated in the resting record or elicited with hyperventilation or intermittent photic stimulation. But whether or not it can be demonstrated depends in great part on the age of the individual at the time the EEG is taken. Thus, in the population as a whole, when all age groups are included, the spike-wave EEG trait may not be demonstrable in more than one percent of those tested.

Many investigators representing different disciplines have suggested, in the last few years, the need for a complete reevaluation of our concepts of epilepsy. In the words of Niedermeyer [19], "Decades of heated discussions have taught us that no straight line can be drawn between the focal, presumably acquired type and the generalized, presumably predispositional type of convulsive disorder." Ajmone-Marsan [1] and Gloor [7] have expressed this same view in different ways. Rodin [22], Bray [3, 4], Hughes [10], and several others have produced data, in the last two years, in support of genetic factors in the so-called *focal* epilepsies.

Gloor [7], in a most recent provocative review of pathophysiological bases of generalized bilaterally synchronous spike-wave discharge, proposes that this type of generalized seizure is the result of an abnormal interaction of both cortical and subcortical grey matter; for this reason he suggests using the term "generalized cortico-reticular epilepsies" when describing epilepsies characterized by this specific type of electroencephalogram. (For the moment, we shall resist the temptation to adopt the new terminology.)

SUMMARY

In terms of recent developments in molecular biology and particularly in biochemical genetics, the clinical seizure observed in an epileptic is very far removed from the primary product of any gene which may be involved. In the strictest sense, clinical seizure has no ordinal position in a biosynthetic pathway, not even as an end product. This also applies to cerebral dysrhythmias recorded in the electroencephalogram. Important as electroencephalography is in studying convulsive disorders, it has no role in the biochemical identification of disease. It would be as if an electrocardiogram were taken in order to ascertain the blood group of the patient. However, both clinical seizure and cerebral dysrhythmia may well be the neurophysiological consequence of a genetically controlled biosynthetic pathway. In this context, it would have to be admitted that knowledge of genetic factors in the epilepsies is still negligible.

Such knowledge may remain negligible, it is feared, unless the neurophysiologist, the neurobiochemist, the neuropharmacologist, the neurobiophysicist—in short, the contributors to and readers of this volume—aid the geneticist and enter the exciting and rewarding field of biochemical genetics referred to by McKhann, Shooter, and Tower. Because this era is one of molecular biology, there is little if any doubt that the breakthrough in epilepsy, when it comes, will be in the discipline of biochemical genetics. It is surmised that the answer will probably be, to our surprise and delight, a relatively simple one.

REFERENCES

1. Ajmone-Marsan, C. Changing concepts in focal epilepsy. Clinical-EEG considerations. *Epilepsia* (Amst.) 2:217, 1961.
2. Andermann, E., and Metrakos, J. D. EEG studies of relatives of probands with focal epilepsy who have been treated surgically. *Abstracts of the American Epilepsy Society*. New York. 1968.
3. Bray, P. F., and Wiser, W. C. Evidence for a genetic etiology of temporal-central abnormalities in focal epilepsy. *New Eng. J. Med.* 271:926, 1964.
4. Bray, P. F., and Wiser, W. C. Hereditary characteristics of familial temporal-central focal epilepsy. *Pediatrics* 36:207, 1965.
5. Coleman, D. L. Phenylalanine-hydroxylase activity in dilute and non-dilute strains in mice. *Arch. Biochem.* 91:300, 1960.
6. Evans, D. A. P. Pharmacogenetics. *Amer. J. Med.* 34:639, 1963.
7. Gloor, P. Generalized cortico-reticular epilepsies. *Epilepsia* (Amst.) 9:249, 1968.
8. Hagberg, B., Hamfelt, A., and Hansson, O. Epileptic children with disturbed tryptophan metabolism treated with vitamin B_6. *Lancet* 1:145, 1964.
9. Huff, S. D., and Fuller, J. L. Audiogenic seizures, the dilute locus, and phenylalanine hydroxylase in DBA/1 mice. *Science* 144:304, 1964.
10. Hughes, J. R. EEG epileptiform abnormalities at different ages. *Epilepsia* (Amst.) 8:93, 1967.
11. Kalow, W. *Pharmacogenetics. Heredity and the Response to Drugs*. Philadelphia: Saunders, 1962.
12. McKusick, V. A. *Mendelian Inheritance in Man*. Baltimore: Johns Hopkins Press, 1967.
13. Meier, H. Phenylketonuria and susceptibility to audiogenic seizures in mice. *Roscoe B. Jackson Memorial Laboratory, Supply Bulletin* no. 351, 1964, p. 1.
14. Metrakos, J. D., and Metrakos, K. Genetics of convulsive disorders. I. Introduction, problems, methods and base-lines. *Neurology* (Minneap.) 10:228, 1960.
15. Metrakos, J. D. Heredity as an Etiological Factor in Convulsive Disorders. In Fields, W. S., and Desmond, M. M. (Eds.), *Disorders of the Developing Nervous System*. Springfield, Ill.: Thomas, 1961.
16. Metrakos, K., and Metrakos, J. D. Genetics of convulsive disorders. II. Genetic and electroencephalographic studies in centrencephalic epilepsy. *Neurology* (Minneap.) 11:474, 1961.
17. Metrakos, J. D., and Metrakos, K. Childhood epilepsy of subcortical ("centrencephalic") origin. *Clin. Pediat.* (Phila.) 3:625, 1966.
18. Nachtsheim, J. Problems of comparative genetics in mammals. *Proc. X Int. Congr. Genet.* 1:187, 1958.
19. Niedermeyer, E. Considerations of the centrencephalic (generalized) type of epilepsy. *Delaware Med. J.* 38:341, 1966.
20. Pratt, R. T. C. *The Genetics of Neurological Disorders*. London: Oxford University Press, 1967.
21. Rauch, H., and Yost, M. Phenylalanine metabolism in dilute-lethal mice. *Genetics* 48:1487, 1963.
22. Rodin, E., and Gonzales, S. Hereditary components in epileptic patients. *J.A.M.A.* 198:221, 1966.
23. Schlesinger, K., Elston, R. C., and Boggan, W. The genetics of sound induced seizure in inbred mice. *Genetics* 54:95, 1966.
24. Sidman, R. L., Green, M. C., and Appel, S. H. *Catalog of the Neurological Mutants of the Mouse*. Cambridge: Harvard University Press, 1965.
25. Smith, D. W., Patau, K., Therman, E., Inhorn, S. L., and DeMars, R. I. The D_1 trisomy syndrome. *J. Pediat.* 62:326, 1963.
26. Thompson, J. S., and Thompson, M. W. *Genetics in Medicine*. Philadelphia: Saunders, 1966.
27. Vogel, F. Moderne Probleme der Humangenetik. *Ergebn. Inn. Med. Kinderheilk* 12:52, 1959.
28. Woolley, D. W., and van der Hoeven, T. Prevention of a mental defect of phenylketonuria with serotonin congeners such as melatonin or hydroxytryptophan. *Science* 144:1593, 1964.

25

Systemic Electrolyte and Neuroendocrine Mechanisms*

J. GORDON MILLICHAP

SEIZURES are a frequent and well-known complication of systemic electrolyte and endocrine disorders but the possible significance of electrolyte and endocrine imbalance in the mechanism of the epilepsies is undetermined. Data have been obtained from clinical observations in both nonepileptic and epileptic patients and from laboratory studies in animals with experimentally induced seizures. The evidence concerning the relationship of systemic electrolytes and endocrines to epilepsy may be subdivided and reviewed as follows:

(1) abnormalities of serum electrolytes and endocrine function complicated by a lowered seizure threshold in nonepileptic patients and in experimental animals;

(2) electrolyte metabolism and endocrine function in epileptic patients;

(3) changes in electrolyte and endocrine balance induced by anticonvulsant therapy and their relation to control of epilepsy.

SYSTEMIC ELECTROLYTE MECHANISMS

Electrolyte Disorders that Predispose to Seizures

Sodium, calcium, and magnesium levels in the serum have been closely correlated with seizure thresholds in both clinical and laboratory studies. Depletion of these electrolytes deranges the balance of extracellular and intracellular cations essential to neuronal stability and may predispose to seizures in nonepileptic as well as epileptic patients [40]. The causes of electrolyte disorders are usually systemic in nature but disturbances of central nervous system regulatory mechanisms may also be invoked. Evidence for a central control of electrolyte metabolism is based principally on disturbances in sodium balance associated with brain pathology and reference to calcium deficiency related to cerebral disease is less frequently documented. The mechanism of seizures in these cases may involve both the primary central disease and the secondary systemic electrolyte imbalance.

Hyponatremia and Seizures. In laboratory studies [19, 74], hypoelectrolytemia and water intoxication produced by the intraperitoneal injection of 5.5 percent glucose solution are associated with a lowered threshold to seizures, experimentally induced by electroshock, chemoshock, and fever [38, 41, 58, 59]. Clinically, hyponatremia and disturbance in the balance of cerebral electrolytes may be caused by the following conditions: (1) sodium depletion as a result of diarrhea or prolonged fever and excessive sweating; (2) low intake of sodium due to inadequate diet or hypotonic parenteral fluid therapy; (3) water intoxication due to excessive thirst or the administration of tap water enemas; and (4) an expansion of the plasma volume and reduction in the extracellular sodium caused by fever [41], acute extracerebral or

---

* Original investigations supported by PHS Research Grant NB05161–05 from the National Institute of Neurological Diseases and Stroke, and by the Epilepsy Foundation of America.

intracerebral infections, or both, and the administration of morphine and ether [40]. In cases of hyponatremia associated with acute bacterial meningitis and encephalitis [48], reduction in extracellular sodium represents a primary water retention due to stimulation of the supraoptic nuclei of the hypothalamus and an excessive release of antidiuretic hormones. A similar mechanism may explain the complication of water intoxication following administration of ether or morphine.

Hypernatremia and Seizures. Cerebral lesions that may be complicated by hypernatremia and seizures usually involve the frontal lobes and the hypothalamus. Primary systemic causes include: (1) diarrhea with dehydration and sodium retention; (2) reduced intake of water or excessive ingestion of salt; (3) the feeding of a high solute skimmed-milk formula; and (4) an impairment of renal function. In infants with hypertonic dehydration the occurrence of seizures may be explained by a subdural hygroma or subdural hemorrhages [34] caused by rupture of veins which bridge the enlarged gap between the superior sagittal sinus and the superficial cerebral veins. Contributory factors in the causation of seizures are hypocalcemia, a concomitant electrolyte abnormality, and an alteration in the permeability of the nerve-cell membrane, disturbing normal balance of intracellular and extracellular concentrations of sodium. Occurrence of seizures during correction of hypertonic dehydration is related more closely to the rate of administration of the fluid and electrolytes than the type of parenteral fluid employed [10, 15].

Hypocalcemia and Seizures. Normal amounts of ionized calcium in the serum are needed for the selective permeability of cell membranes to sodium and potassium, and hypocalcemia is associated with an instability of cell membranes and signs of neuromuscular irritability. Convulsions may be associated with a reduction of the diffusible ionized calcium in the following conditions: (1) neonatal tetany; (2) cryptogenic or traumatic hypoparathyroidism; (3) pseudohypoparathyroidism; (4) rickets; (5) steatorrhea; (6) during treatment of acidosis and dehydration; (7) treatment of hypertonic dehydration; and (8) chronic renal insufficiency. A primary neurogenic lesion is suspected if an immediate anticonvulsant response to intravenous calcium is absent or equivocal. Cerebral pathology reported in association with hypocalcemia and seizures includes injury from anoxia or hemorrhage at birth and intracranial tumor [39], findings suggestive of a central regulatory mechanism for calcium metabolism.

Magnesium Depletion and Seizures. Seizures may occur as a complication of magnesium depletion in such disorders as malnutrition, particularly in alcoholics; severe diarrhea and vomiting; renal insufficiency; hyperparathyroidism, especially following parathyroidectomy; hyperthyroidism; hepatic insufficiency; acute pancreatitis; and vitamin D intoxication. The understanding of the symptoms and signs of magnesium disorders is incompletely defined because magnesium is largely an intracellular ion and serum levels may be misleading. Other electrolyte disorders occur together with magnesium deficiency and may account for some of the symptomatology [49, 85].

Electrolyte Metabolism in Epileptic Patients

Fluctuations in the urinary excretion of electrolytes have been correlated with changes in frequency of seizures in children and adults with centrencephalic epilepsy. Schneider [51] found in patients with petit mal that phases of electroclinical exacerbation coincided with marked decrease in urinary sodium whereas periods of remission were associated with an increase in sodium and water excretion. Changes in urinary excretion occurred when clinical improvement was spontaneous or induced by effective antiepileptic medications of the oxazolidinedione class, alone or combined with corticotropin (ACTH). Clinical improvements which coincided with sodium diuresis appeared to be antagonized by increases in potassium excretion, and an exacerbation of seizures, usually associated with sodium retention, was modified by concomitant retention of potassium. Calcium excretion paralleled that of sodium whereas magnesium excretion was unrelated to excretion of sodium, potassium, or calcium, or to the occurrence of seizures. Treatment with corticotropin controlled the petit mal and was associated with initial retention of potassium and intermittent increases in calcium excretion followed by a sodium diuresis.

Millichap and Jones [43] studied the balance of electrolytes during 6-day periods in four children with petit mal (Figs. 25-1, 25-2). The regular diet was of known composition, the patient was weighed in the morning and evening of each day, and urine output and fluid intake were measured daily. Specimens of blood obtained on two days in each balance period and 24-hr specimens of urine and stool were analyzed for sodium, potassium, calcium, magnesium, and phosphorus. Electroencephalograms were recorded on the third or fourth day of each balance period. During control periods when antiepileptic treatment was withheld, occurrence of petit mal and prolongation of spike-wave discharges in the electroencephalograms were unassociated with any constant and specific electrolyte balance. Retention of sodium previously postulated as a prerequisite for seizure exacerbation in untreated patients was not confirmed, and the possible significance of systemic electrolyte imbalance in the mechanism of epilepsy was studied further by observations of the effects of anticonvulsant treatments [43].

Etiologic Significance of Electrolyte Imbalance in Epilepsy

A positive balance of electrolytes observed in some patients with petit mal was converted to a negative balance during treatment and successful control of seizures with the ketogenic diet and acetazolamide (Fig. 25-1) [44]. However, the positive balance of sodium was accentuated by treatment with other anticonvulsant therapies that included trimethadione, methsuximide, mephobarbital, and corticotropin (Fig. 25-2) [43]. Control of petit mal seizures was obtained in response to all therapies and showed no constant correlation with the balance of electrolytes (Table 25-1). The possible importance of a systemic electrolyte imbalance in the etiology of petit

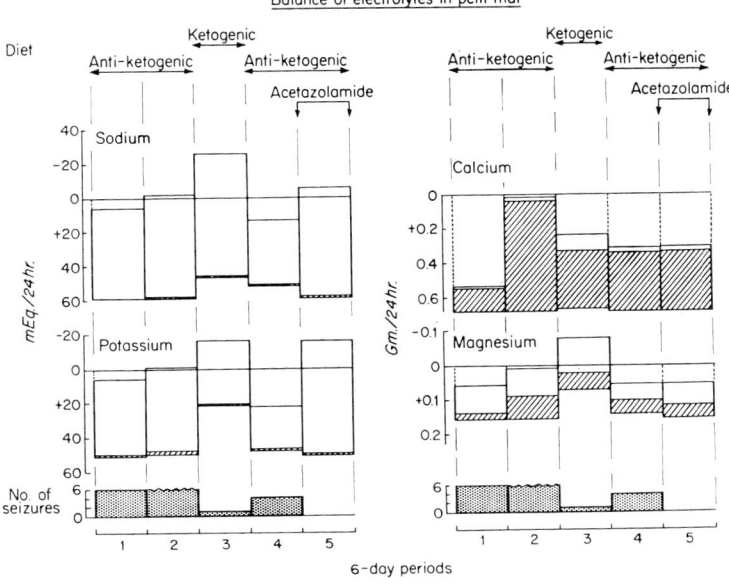

FIG. 25-1. Balance of electrolytes in girl aged 14 years with petit mal, and effects of ketogenic diet and acetazolamide. Columns below baseline: intake of electrolytes; shaded columns: fecal excretion; unshaded columns: urinary excretion of electrolytes. (From Millichap, J. G., Jones, J. D., and Rudis, B. P. [44].)

712 SYSTEMIC ELECTROLYTE AND NEUROENDOCRINE MECHANISMS

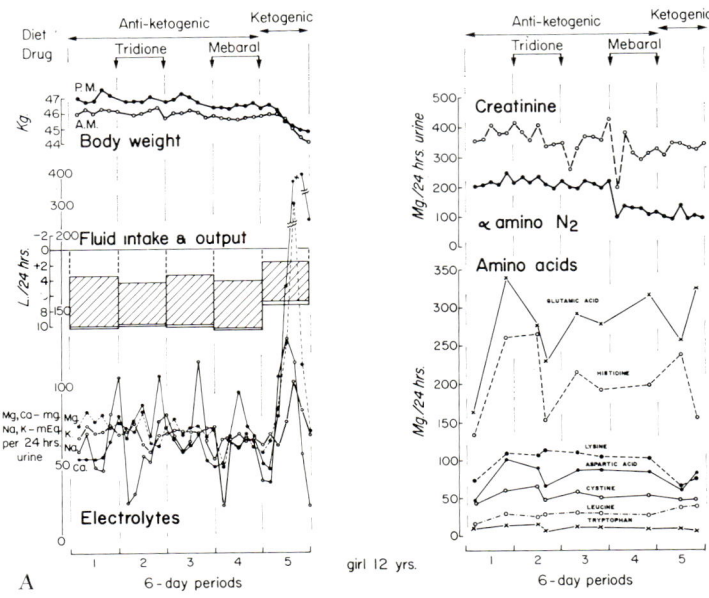

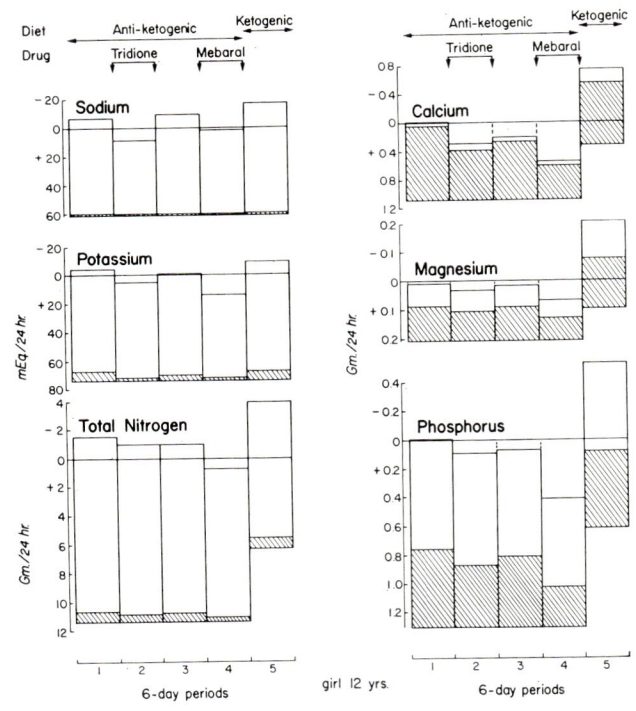

Fig. 25-2. Effects of trimethadione and mephobarbital compared with ketogenic diet on (*A*) urinary excretion of electrolytes and amino acids and (*B*) balance of electrolytes, in a girl aged 12 years with petit mal. (From Millichap, J. G., and Jones, J. D. [43].)

TABLE 25-1. Directional Changes in Acid-Base, Electrolyte and Nitrogen Balance in Children with Petit Mal Controlled by Diet and Drugs[a]

	Ketogenic Diet	Diamox	ACTH	Celontin	Tridione	Mebaral
Urine						
Volume	D[a]	I[a]	D[a]	—	D	—
Sodium	I	I	D	D	D	D
Potassium	I	I	D	D	D	D
Calcium	I	I	—	—	—	—
Magnesium	I	—	D	—	—	D
Phosphorus	I	I	D	—	—	D
Total nitrogen	—	—	I	D	—	D
α Amino N_2	D	—	I	D	—	D
Free amino acids	—	—	I	D	D	—
Blood						
pH	D	D	I	I	I	I
pCO_2	D	D	I	D	I	D
Base	D	D	I	I	I	—
Balance						
Sodium	D	D	I	I	I	I
Potassium	D	D	I	I	I	I
Calcium	D	—	D	I	I	I
Magnesium	D	—	I	I	I	I
Phosphorus	D	—	I	—	I	I
Nitrogen	D	—	I	I	I	I

[a] D, decrease; I, increase; —, no change. (From Millichap, J. G., and Jones, J. D. [43].)

mal was minimized by the results of these investigations, although observations in larger numbers of patients and controls would be required for a satisfactory statistical analysis of the findings. It was suggested that systemic metabolic defects other than electrolyte imbalance or primary neurogenic lesions should be considered as more likely factors in the etiology and mechanism of petit mal epilepsy.

SYSTEMIC ACID-BASE MECHANISMS

Acid-Base Changes and Seizures

Whereas alterations of blood pH and pCO_2 have been found to affect responses of the cerebral cortex to direct electrical and chemical stimulation, acute changes in the blood acid-base balance have only minimal effects on the threshold and pattern of experimental seizures and excitability of the brain as a whole [40, 84]. For example, a moderate to severe metabolic acidosis or alkalosis in rabbits produced no significant effect on the electroencephalogram at rest or after treatment with subconvulsive doses of pentylenetetrazol. The threshold for seizures induced by electroshock or injection of convulsant drugs in rats was not affected by mild acidemia produced either by injection of ammonium chloride or inhalation of carbon dioxide, nor by severe respiratory acidemia. A severe metabolic acidosis produced by maximal oral tolerated doses of ammonium chloride modified the maximal electroshock seizure pattern in only 16 percent of mice tested [40]. Furthermore, the anticonvulsant activity of acetazolamide was independent of the metabolic acidosis which results from inhibition of carbonic anhydrase in the kidney [37, 45].

In more recent studies in rats and mice [79], however, Woodbury and co-workers (1958) [80] and Woodbury and Karler (1960) [78] have shown that inhalation of increasing concentrations of carbon dioxide produces a progressive increase in the electroconvulsive threshold up to a peak with

12–15 percent carbon dioxide, after which the seizure threshold falls and seizures may be precipitated by inhalation of 30 percent carbon dioxide [8, 27]. The inhibition of carbonic anhydrase activity by acetazolamide that results in an increased concentration of carbon dioxide in the brain has been shown to prevent electroshock seizures in animals in a manner similar to the inhalation of carbon dioxide. Evidence derived from studies of the mechanism of anticonvulsant action of acetazolamide [45] indicates that changes in the excitability of cerebral neuronal systems are not affected by alterations in arterial pH per se, but only by blood pH changes that are associated with a variation in arterial and brain pCO_2 [84].

Acid-Base Changes in Epileptic Patients

Lennox and co-workers [31] showed that low CO_2 concentrations in the blood of patients with petit mal tended to precipitate seizures and abnormally high CO_2 levels had an anticonvulsant effect. In periods of spontaneous exacerbation of seizures, the CO_2 content of the arterial blood was usually lower than in periods of spontaneous remission [22]. In contrast to these observations, Millichap and associates [43, 44] found in four patients with petit mal that the blood pCO_2 was elevated when seizures were untreated (Fig. 25-3). It was suggested that the respiratory acidosis might possibly represent an autogenous attempt at an antiepileptic mechanism. Another report [69] of an epileptic patient with chronic hypoventilation tended to corroborate this observation, but subsequent studies in our clinic showed that a respiratory acidosis in patients with petit mal was not an invariable finding.

Significance of Acid-Base Changes in Epilepsy

Petit mal seizures were controlled with a number of antiepileptic therapies but the response showed no constant correlation with the acid-base metabolism (Table 25-1). The ketogenic diet and acetazolamide caused reductions in the blood pH, pCO_2 and standard bicarbonate (Fig. 25-3), whereas treatment with trimethadione and corticotropin was associated with increases in the pH and pCO_2. The control of petit mal seizures by the ketogenic diet was not antagonized by administration of bicarbonate and correction of metabolic acidosis. The antiepileptic effect was independent of

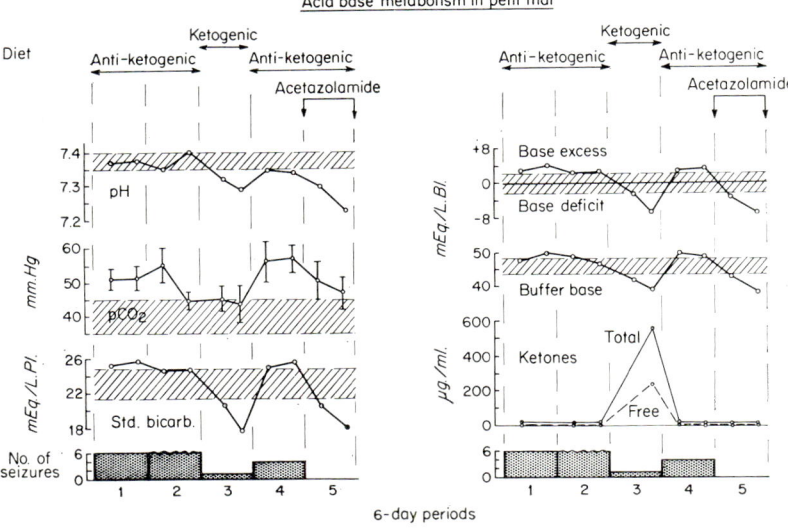

Fig. 25-3. Acid-base metabolism in petit mal, before and during treatment with ketogenic diet and acetazolamide. (From Millichap, J. G., Jones, J. D., and Rudis, B. P. [44].)

either a respiratory or metabolic acidosis and was correlated most closely with a negative balance of sodium and potassium. Effects of the diet on the systemic electrolyte and acid-base balance of patients with petit mal were almost identical to those of acetazolamide. Lack of a constant correlation between acid-base balance and petit mal seizures in this study was in agreement with the opinion of MacQuarrie and Keith [35] who postulated that a change in the acid-base balance in certain cases of epilepsy was probably not the factor of chief importance in the mechanism of the seizures.

AMINO ACID MECHANISMS

Amino Acid Disorders Complicated by Seizures

An elevation of certain amino acids in the serum occurs in primary aminoacidopathies and some of these diseases are complicated by seizures. A primary aminoaciduria represents a specific defect in an enzymatic step in the metabolic pathway of one or more amino acids, as in phenylketonuria and maple-syrup urine disease; alternatively the defect is found in a protein mediator which is necessary for transport of certain amino acids into or out of cells, as in Hartnup disease. In the primary aminoacidurias the enzymatic defect leads to accumulation of one or more amino acids in blood and tissues and aminoaciduria occurs because of increased glomerular filtration. Renal aminoaciduria, in contrast to the primary variety of these disorders, is due to defective renal tubular reabsorption of one or more amino acids, the blood concentration of the amino acids being normal or low [17].

Phenylketonuria and maple-syrup urine disease are the primary overflow aminoacidurias most likely to be associated with seizures. Phenylketonuria is characterized by an increased level of phenylalanine in the serum and a deficiency of phenylalanine hydroxylase in the liver. In maple-syrup urine disease, valine, leucine, isoleucine, and alloisoleucine are present in increased amounts in the blood, and the enzyme deficiency involves the branched chain keto acid decarboxylase in the leukocytes. In both of these conditions the administration of a diet low in the particular amino acid involved may result in a change in seizure frequency and may prevent development of mental retardation and other neurologic abnormalities. Other less well-known primary overflow aminoacidurias associated with seizures include the following: hyperlysinemia, ornithinemia, carnosinuria, hyperbeta-alaninemia, and hyperprolinemia, types I and II. Renal aminoacidurias complicated by seizures include methionine malabsorption syndrome (Oast House urine disease) and severe prolinuria (Joseph's syndrome). The relation of the increased susceptibility to seizures to the hyperaminoacidemia in the primary aminoacidopathies is not definitely determined.

Amino Acid Metabolism in Epileptic Patients

An abnormal aminoaciduria and aminoacidemia have been reported in patients with cryptogenic seizures and particularly in children with petit mal [42]. Choremis and co-workers [12] found hyperaminoaciduria in 13 of 16 patients with grand mal but the authors considered the abnormalities to be secondary and related to the severity of convulsions, having no etiologic significance. In a later publication from the same laboratory [13] an abnormal aminoaciduria discovered in 9 of 11 patients with infantile myoclonic spasms and hypsarrhythmia showed no correlation with the incidence of seizures.

In a preliminary communication in 1962, Millichap and Ulrich [42] reported a significant increase in the urinary excretion of isoleucine, leucine, cystine, histidine, tryptophan, aspartic acid, glutamic acid, and lysine in 10 children with petit mal epilepsy (Fig. 25-4). The hyperaminoaciduria was not associated with obvious renal disease or with transient renal tubular dysfunction secondary to grand mal seizures and could not readily be explained as a side effect of anticonvulsant drugs. In a further study of 40 patients with petit mal, Millichap and his associates [46] confirmed

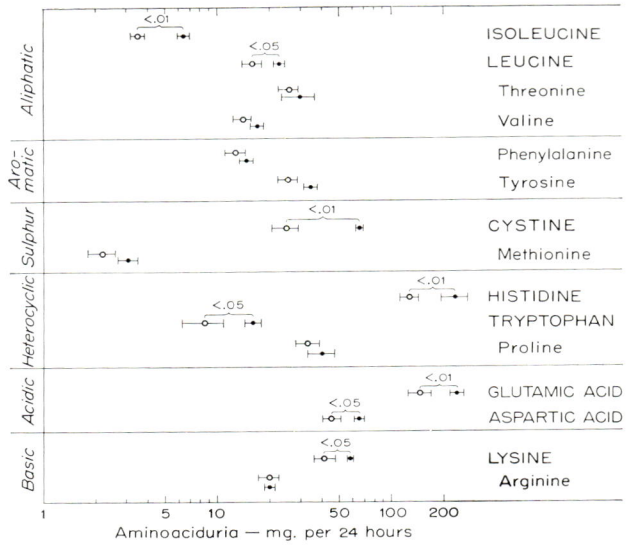

Fig. 25-4. Abnormal aminoaciduria in petit mal epilepsy. (From Millichap, J. G., and Ulrich, J. A. [42].)

the hyperaminoaciduria in association with idiopathic epilepsy and found that the pattern of the abnormality was more extensive, with significant increases demonstrated in the excretion of 13 of 15 amino acids estimated. In 1963, Gordon and Wilson [25] reported an excess of cystine, glutamic acid, or taurine in the urine of 47 of 63 patients with epilepsy of unclassified type, and the abnormalities could not be explained by the occurrence of convulsions or by the administration of anticonvulsant drugs. More recently, in 1965, Stemmerman [55] reported transient increases in cystinuria in several patients with petit mal and consistently abnormal aminoacidurias in 5 of 16 young retarded children with minor motor seizures and generalized multiple spike and slow-wave discharges in the electroencephalogram. The occurrence of hyperaminoaciduria in a significant number of patients with idiopathic epilepsy and particularly petit mal seems to be established, but the nature of these metabolic disorders and their relation to the seizure mechanism are incompletely determined. The occurrence of relatively high levels of amino acids in the serum suggests a prerenal disorder of amino acid metabolism, although the number of patients studied was limited.

Etiologic Significance of Amino Acid Disorders in Epilepsy

The possible significance of abnormalities of amino acid metabolism in the etiology of certain epilepsies has been investigated by observations of the effects of anticonvulsant drugs. Treatment of petit mal with trimethadione, an anticonvulsant that occasionally may cause nephrosis, did not exacerbate the abnormal aminoaciduria, and a drug-induced defect in the renal tubular reabsorption of amino acids was excluded. Indeed, the urinary excretion of amino acids in patients who received trimethadione, phenobarbital, or mephobarbital was normal or at least lower than in untreated patients, and the values for leucine, proline, and valine were significantly reduced.

The ketogenic diet and acetazolamide also modified the excretion of amino acids and alpha-amino nitrogen. The abnormally high urinary excretion of histidine, phenylalanine, tryptophan, tyrosine, and alpha-amino nitrogen was significantly decreased by the diet to levels that approximated or were below normal, whereas that of leucine was significantly increased. Acetazolamide tended to correct the hyperaminoaciduria, but the changes were not statistically significant. In four patients treated with the ketogenic diet, the mean levels of histidine and leucine in the serum were modified in the same directions as the urinary excretion of these amino acids; the level of serum histidine was decreased, whereas serum leucine was increased significantly. Similar changes in serum amino acids were obtained in a 14-year-old boy treated with acetazolamide; the level of the serum histidine and lysine fell from 3.4 and 6.6 mg per 100 ml to 2.0 and 3.1 mg per 100 ml, respectively, and the level of serum leucine was increased from 4.4 to 6.6 mg per 100 ml. Values in control healthy children were not available for comparison, but the levels of serum amino acids for adults obtained in this same laboratory were: histidine, 2.3 ± 0.19; lysine, 3.3 ± 0.35; and leucine, 2.4 ± 0.22—expressed as the mean and standard deviation of the mean in mg per 100 ml of serum.

The relation of the hyperaminoaciduria to the etiology and mechanism of petit mal is unclear. The diet and drug-induced modifications of the urinary excretion and serum levels of amino acids were accompanied by a remission of seizures, suggesting a correlation between the hyperaminoaciduria and epilepsy. However, the increase in concentrations of leucine induced by the diet and the lack of a specific pattern of aminoaciduria are difficult to reconcile with this explanation. The possibility of systemic metabolic defects other than those determined in these studies or of hyperaminoaciduria secondary to dysfunction of the central nervous system should be considered further.

NEUROENDOCRINE MECHANISMS

A close relationship between the nervous and endocrine systems is well documented, the secretion of hormones being subject to neural control and, at the same time, influencing the activity of the nervous tissues [11]. Some endocrine secretions are concerned with metabolic processes affecting the brain as well as the body as a whole and the hormones of the thyroid gland, the gonads, and the adrenal cortex play a particularly significant and frequently specific role in regulating the growth and activity of the brain. The frequency of alpha rhythm of the electroencephalogram is related to metabolic rate; it is increased by administration of thyroxine and reduced in hypothyroid states. Hormones have been studied in relation to the changes they induce in the excitability of nervous tissue and susceptibility to seizures.

Pituitary-Adrenal Imbalance and Seizures

A reciprocal relationship between blood levels of adrenal corticoids and adrenocorticotrophic hormone (ACTH) secretion has been demonstrated, and high levels of adrenocortical hormones act directly upon anterior pituitary cells and upon the hypothalamus to inhibit release of ACTH and formation of a corticotrophin releasing factor. Feedback action of target hormones involving an increase or decrease in the formation of corticotrophin may explain in part the variable convulsant or anticonvulsant effects reported in patients treated with corticotrophin (ACTH) or cortisone.

An anticonvulsant action of ACTH was first reported in 1950 by Klein and Livingston [29], who observed a temporary beneficial response in 6 epileptic children. In 1958, Sorel and Dusaucy-Bauloye [53] gave ACTH to infants with myoclonic spasms, a form of epilepsy refractory to conventional therapies, and a dramatic improvement was noted in 6 of 7 patients. Subsequently, the anticonvulsant efficacy of ACTH was confirmed in larger groups of patients with myoclonic seizures [40, 54] and in children with petit mal [47], but the mechanism of its action was undetermined. It was equally effective in patients with cryptogenic seizures and in those with a history of acquired brain lesions and the response appeared to be unrelated to the etiology of the seizures. In one controlled trial the effect appeared to be independent of the release of hydrocortisone from the adrenal cortex; 6 of 10 patients treated with ACTH were benefited, whereas cortisone had no effect. In some reports, however, cortisone and prednisone have been advocated in the treatment of myoclonic spasms and an effect of ACTH mediated through the adrenals seems possible.

That the control of petit mal and myoclonic seizures by ACTH cannot be correlated with changes induced in electrolyte metabolism is suggested by the results of recent balance studies in children. The effects obtained were similar to those expected in hypercorticism and the opposite of those induced by anticonvulsants such as acetazolamide and the ketogenic diet.

In animal studies, Woodbury [73] has reported that ACTH increased the threshold to electroshock seizures in adult rats. Torda and Wolff [64] found that the effects of ACTH on the electrical activity of the brain of rats and on the sensitivity to pentylenetetrazol varied with the duration of treatment and the amount administered. Single injections or injections repeated from two to four times resulted in paroxysmal bursts of high voltage waves and occasional spiking and a reduction in the threshold to pentylenetetrazol-induced seizure discharges in the electroencephalogram. Repeated administration of ACTH for three or four days decreased the sensitivity to pentylenetetrazol. The authors suggested that ACTH modifies the activity of the brain by at least two mechanisms. A shift in the electrolytes was postulated to explain the decrease in electrical activity following prolonged administration of large concentrations and a mechanism independent of the effect on the adrenal cortex was considered necessary for the induction of hyperexcitability by single injections of ACTH.

A study in our own laboratory showed that ACTH caused a significant reduction in the threshold to minimal clonic electroshock seizures in young rats, and this effect was noted in both intact and adrenalectomized animals. The effect was therefore independent of the action of ACTH on the adrenal glands. The variability of the effect of ACTH on seizure thresholds observed in both laboratory and clinical studies is not easily explained by the available data. The importance of age is indicated by the superior anticonvulsant effects in young infants and children compared with older children and adolescents.

A relation between the adrenal glands and convulsions [23] was postulated by Fischer [see 73]. He noted that susceptibility to convulsions in rabbits decreased with a decrease in adrenal substance and susceptibility increased with hyperfunction of the adrenal glands. His work led to clinical trial of partial adrenalectomy for seizures refractory to medications but the results were equivocal. McQuarrie and his colleagues [see 40] and later Aird and Gordan [1] showed that deoxycorticosterone acetate had some anticonvulsant activity in patients with epilepsy. Woodbury [71, 72, 73, 76] and Timiras [63] have examined the effects of hormones on brain excitability of rats in an extensive series of experiments. They found that adrenocortical insufficiency increased brain excitability and decreased the electroshock seizure threshold. Hypophysectomy caused an initial increase and later a decrease in brain excitability. Diphenylhydantoin stimulated the pituitary-adrenal system and its anticonvulsant effect was antagonized by the release of adrenocortical steroids; an elevation of the electroshock threshold to minimal clonic seizures in response to diphenylhydantoin was obtained only in adrenalectomized animals. Woodbury and his colleagues [81] concluded that the adrenal cortex has a regulatory effect on central nervous system function and acts to restore brain excitability to normal.

The mechanism of the effects of adrenal pituitary hormones on brain excitability may be related to electrolyte changes; deoxycorticosterone [66, 75], hypophysectomy, and adrenalectomy caused changes in concentrations and the balance of electrolytes in the plasma and brain, whereas cortisone [67] and related C-11-oxysteroids altered brain excitability without effect on electrolyte metabolism. In our own laboratory [68] the changes in electrolyte balance observed after ACTH therapy in adrenalectomized animals were those previously correlated with a reduction in seizure threshold. An increase in the intracellular concentration of sodium in the brain was the only change in electrolytes common to both adrenalectomized and intact animals treated with ACTH. Animals with the highest intracellular sodium concentration had the lowest threshold to electroshock seizures. A direct effect of ACTH on neuronal cell membranes or on inhibitory seizure mechanisms might explain the anticonvulsant response obtained in infants with myoclonic epilepsy.

Thyroid Imbalance and Seizures

Timiras and her colleagues have shown in rats that thyroxine and triiodothyridine increased brain excitability [60, 61]. The authors suggested that the effects of thyroid hormones are mediated by a dual mechanism: direct stimulation of the central nervous system and indirect stimulation which results from an increased secretion of 11-oxysteroids from the adrenal cortex. Woodbury [77] found in the rat that the threshold and duration of seizures were increased by thyroidectomy and reduced by giving thyroid hormone. The alterations in brain excitability could be correlated with changes in brain electrolytes.

In clinical studies concerning the relationship of thyroid function to the central nervous system, the electroencephalogram has been examined in patients with myxedema. Abnormalities of the electroencephalogram consist mainly of a reduction of rate of alpha activity and in general amplitude of the recording. Among 56 cases of adult myxedema with neurological complications, 10 presented with epilepsy or syncope and 6 with coma or stupor. The clinical patterns of epilepsy were grand mal, confusional states, drop seizures, and attacks difficult to differentiate from syncope. Cerebral ischemia was thought to underlie many of the attacks resembling syncope. Epilepsy was most likely to appear in myxedema coma, but there was no simple relationship with the degree of hypothyroidism or with the electroencephalographic abnormalities. The seizures responded fairly well to thyroid treatment.

Parathyroid Deficiency and Seizures

The occurrence of seizures has been reported in patients with idiopathic, postoperative, and pseudohypoparathyroidism [4, 9, 20, 26, 52, 57, 70]. At least two-thirds of all reported cases of idiopathic hypoparathyroidism and pseudohypoparathyroidism are complicated by epileptic seizures of various patterns, including grand mal as well as minor or partial seizures. In many cases the characteristic features of the grand mal convulsion, such as aura, tongue biting, loss of consciousness, and tonic-clonic movements, may be absent and the seizure is manifested by psychomotor disturbances or athetoticlike spasms of extremity and trunk muscles. The response of seizures in hypoparathyroidism to anticonvulsant medication such as diphenylhydantoin and phenobarbital is erratic, varying from fair to poor control.

In most patients with hypoparathyroidism and seizures, the electroencephalogram is abnormal [24], showing paroxysmal sharp waves, spike discharges, and atypical slow spike-wave complexes. The spike discharges and spike-wave complexes are more common in children with this disorder than in adults. Occasionally, focal or unilateral abnormalities are present. Electroencephalographic abnormalities are increased during hyperventilation and a low threshold to photic pentylenetetrazol activation has been described.

The mechanism of production of the seizures and the electroencephalographic abnormalities in hypoparathyroidism is not clearly determined. Hypocalcemia and possibly an increased cerebral hydration are invoked, but an intravenous infusion of calcium often does not correct the electroencephalographic abnormality. Furthermore, many patients with severe hypocalcemia and tetany do not have seizures or an abnormal electroencephalogram. These conflicting findings have been related to lags or other variations in calcium ion transport between the blood and cerebral neurons. In some instances the hypocalcemia may act as a precipitating mechanism in an individual predisposed to seizures.

Insulin Excess, Hypoglycemia, and Seizures

Gibbs and his associates [see 43] reported that the 3-per-sec spike-wave discharge in the electroencephalogram of patients with petit mal was exacerbated by hypoglycemia, and Gellhorn [21] found that fasting increased the severity of seizures induced by electroshock in rats. The tendency for insulin excess and hypoglycemia to promote convulsions is well documented [28, 62], but a close correlation between the degree of hypoglycemia and the incidence of seizures has not been established in clinical studies. Indeed, in some patients both the hypoglycemia and seizures may be caused by a primary lesion in the central nervous system that results in failure of a blood glucose regulatory mechanism. Etheridge and Millichap [18] found evidence of brain lesions preceding the onset of symptoms in 10 of 20 children with cryptogenic hypoglycemia, and Broberger and Zetterstrom [7] and Van Wyk [65] have emphasized the frequent history of obstetric complications or perinatal difficulties in children who develop hypoglycemic episodes in late infancy or childhood.

Etheridge has reviewed the relationship of hypoglycemia and central nervous system function. The neurologic symptoms resulting from abnormal cerebral metabolism secondary to hypoglycemia may depend on the rate of fall of blood sugar, duration and severity of low levels of blood sugar, age at which the hypoglycemia occurs, and existence of previous or concurrent damage to the central nervous system [6]. Damage to the hypothalamic control of the sympathetic system may result in failure of compensatory hyperadrenalism secondary to insulin-induced hypoglycemia. In some patients the abnormal adrenal medullary function and seizures may be manifestations of primary central nervous system disease.

Hyperglycemic Effect of Seizures. Hyperglycemia following convulsive seizures has been noted clinically and in laboratory studies. The elevation of blood sugar in rabbits with electroshock convulsions was related directly to strength of the current stimulus and severity of the seizure. Phenobarbital prevented the convulsion and blood sugar elevation after electroshock, whereas the administration of diphenylhydantoin was accompanied by significant increase in blood sugar despite the absence of convulsive response [5] (Fig. 25-5). It was concluded that the blood sugar elevation that follows an electroshock stimulus is unrelated to convulsive movements per se and may be explained by central nervous excitation and stimulation of the sympathetico-adrenal system. The hyperglycemic effect of diphenylhydantoin first described as a result of these laboratory investigations [5] has been confirmed in patients with epilepsy.

Sex Hormones and Seizures

Estrogens, progesterone, and androgens may modify brain excitability and the periodic fluctuations in the secretion of these hormones may account in part for the remissions and exacerbations of epileptic seizures.

Animal Studies. The effects of female sex hormones on electroshock convulsions in the rat have been studied by Timiras and Woolley [82, 83]. Administration of estradiol to intact mature males and to ovariectomized immature and mature females markedly lowered seizure thresholds. Similar effects of estradiol were observed in hypophysectomized rats, demonstrating that

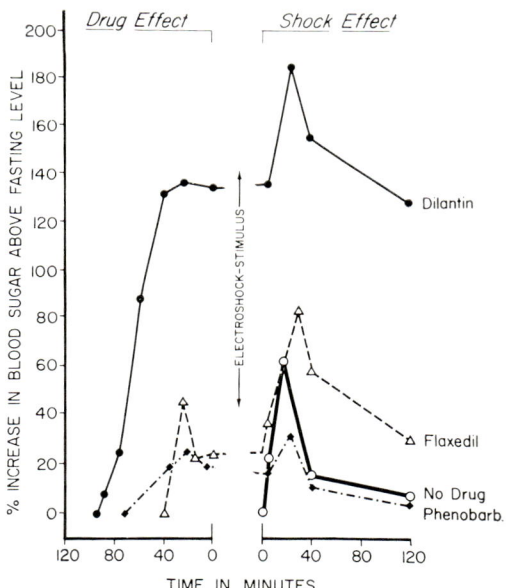

Fig. 25-5. Hyperglycemic effects of electroshock convulsions and diphenylhydantoin in rabbits. (From Belton, N. R., Etheridge, J. E., Jr., and Millichap, J. G. [5].)

the convulsant action of the hormone was not mediated through the pituitary trophic hormones. Estradiol appeared to have a more marked central excitatory action than progesterone, testosterone, or methyl androstenediol. In addition, progesterone exhibited both an anticonvulsant and a convulsant action in female rats, the effect depending on duration of treatment. It was concluded that sex steroids are capable of altering the seizure threshold and brain excitability and thus play a basic role in aspects of central nervous system physiology [36] other than those exclusively concerned with sexual functions. An epileptogenic effect of estrogens was confirmed by Logothetis and associates [33], who studied the results of local application of conjugated estrogenic substances to experimentally induced cortical lesions in rabbits.

Stitt and Kinnard [56] confirmed the effect of progestins and estrogens on the threshold of electrically induced seizure patterns in rats and cats, and these authors employed deoxycorticosterone-trimethylacetate to induce water retention resembling a premenstrual state in women. The expected fall in the seizure threshold as a result of water retention was not observed and a direct suppressant effect of desoxycorticosterone on cortical excitability was postulated.

Sex Hormones in Epileptic Patients. Logothetis and associates [33] examined the effects of injection of conjugated estrogenic substances in 16 patients with epilepsy. They observed activation of electroencephalographic abnormalities in 11 of 16 patients examined, and a clinical seizure was induced in one patient. An exacerbation of epilepsy may occur immediately before or at the time of menstruation, but a relationship between the rhythmic occurrence of seizures and menstruation is inconstant. However, Laidlaw [30] found unequivocal evidence of catamenial epilepsy in a 25-year study of 33,000 seizures in 50 epileptic women.

Most investigators have maintained that seizures are exacerbated shortly before or during menstruation in about 50 percent of epileptic women, and a worsening of attacks is noted at the menarche. The menopause seems to have a significant depressant effect on the incidence of seizures and ovariectomy has been reported to relieve human epilepsy and to elevate the seizure threshold in animals.

Mechanism of Catamenial Epilepsy. In addition to the controversy regarding the relationship between seizures and menstruation there is also considerable difference of opinion regarding the pathogenesis of catamenial exacerbation of seizures. Factors considered in etiology include estrogenic excess, water retention, progesterone withdrawal, and psychic disturbances. Logothetis and co-workers [33] found that 64 percent of patients had onset of seizures at about the time of the menarche and spells tended to cluster during and immediately before menstruation. A single patient in the group had serial electroencephalograms recorded at different phases of the menstrual cycle. A moderate dysrhythmia occurred at the luteal phase and was exaggerated on the first and third days of menstruation, at which time slow paroxysmal waves appeared in both hemispheres. The record was less abnormal one day after the cessation of the menses. Similar aggravation of preexisting convulsive discharges at the menstrual period was noted by Lin and associates [32], and Dusser De Barenne and Gibbs [16] found a significant change in the electroencephalograms at the onset of menses in normal females. The authors concluded that catamenial exacerbation of seizures in epileptic patients must be related to the increased estrogenic activity during the immediate premenstrual period.

Ansell and Clarke [3] studied the role of water retention in the catamenial exacerbation of epilepsy, and found that a disturbance of water storage in the body was not primarily responsible for seizures. In seven epileptic patients the total body water estimated by the antipyrine method was normal and patients with and those without a menstrual aggravation of seizures showed no differences. Estimations repeated in five of the patients after their seizures had been satisfactorily controlled with acetazolamide or diphenylhydantoin were unchanged, and control of epileptic seizures was independent of an alteration in body water.

Reynolds [50], in more recent investigations using isotope methods, found that whereas the total body water remains constant, the distribution of extracellular and intracellular water may be altered significantly in epileptic patients.

In Laidlaw's study [30] of the relationship of seizures to menstruation in 50 epileptic patients, a reduction of seizures occurred during the luteal phase and an irregular increase immediately before, during, and after menstruation. The midluteal reduction but not the menstrual increase of seizures was greater during regular menstruation. It was concluded that catamenial epilepsy may be due to an anticonvulsant action of progesterone with an exacerbation of seizures when its secretion stops. In this analysis no attempt was made to correlate a rhythm of seizures with an assumed rhythm of the menstrual cycle. Since it is known that in the nonpregnant woman progesterone is produced only during the luteal phase and only during ovular cycles, the catamenial pattern and accentuation of this pattern during phases of regular menstruation could be explained if it were assumed that progesterone exerted a slight but significant anticonvulsant action. The exacerbation of seizures would then be the result of cessation of progesterone secretion and comparable to the effect of withdrawal of anticonvulsant drugs. Costa and Bonnycastle [14], investigating the ability of various steroids to protect dogs from agene-induced convulsions, found that progesterone not only had a considerable anticonvulsant action but also was the most effective of the steroids tested. In contrast to these investigations demonstrating a relationship between menstruation and seizures, Almquist [2] has shown that the rhythm of epileptic attacks occurs as frequently in male as in female patients and is not confined to the reproductive age, a history of rhythmicity occurring in infancy and childhood as well as in adults. It seems probable, therefore, that the periodicity of attacks may be determined also by a basic rhythmicity of certain biological constants independent of the sex hormones.

Summary

Systemic electrolyte disorders, particularly hyponatremia, hypernatremia, hypocalcemia, and magnesium deficiency, may be associated with an increased susceptibility to seizures, but abnormalities of electrolyte and acid-base metabolism show no constant correlation with the exacerbation or remission of seizures in patients with epilepsy. The effect of systemic electrolyte imbalance on seizure thresholds appears to have no significant relation to the basic etiology and mechanism of epilepsy.

Hyperaminoaciduria has been demonstrated and confirmed in a significant number of patients with petit mal and other idiopathic epilepsies. The abnormal aminoaciduria was possibly related to a prerenal defect of amino acid metabolism in some patients and was modified by anticonvulsant therapies.

Effects of pituitary-adrenal hormones, thyroid disorders, parathyroid deficiency, insulin excess, and sex hormones on seizure susceptibility have been reviewed and the pathogenesis of catamenial epilepsy discussed. The influence of hormones on seizures and brain excitability may be correlated with changes in electrolyte and water balance, but a direct depressant or excitant effect on neuronal cell membranes and inhibitory or facilitatory cerebral mechanisms must also be postulated.

References

1. Aird, R. B., and Gordan, G. S. Anticonvulsive properties of desoxycorticosterone. *J.A.M.A.* 145:715, 1951.
2. Almquist, R. The rhythm of epileptic attacks and its relationship to the menstrual cycle. *Acta Psychiat. Scand.* 1955, suppl. 105.
3. Ansell, B., and Clarke, E. Epilepsy and menstruation. The role of water retention. *Lancet* 271:1232, 1956.

4. Bartter, F. C. The parathyroid gland and its relationship to disease of the nervous system. *Res. Publ. Ass. Res. Nerv. Ment. Dis.* 32:1, 1953.

5. Belton, N. R., Etheridge, J. E., Jr., and Millichap, J. G. Effects of convulsions and anticonvulsants on blood sugar in rabbits. *Epilepsia* (Amst.) 6:243, 1965.

6. Blattner, R. J. Central nervous system damage and hypoglycemia. *J. Pediat.* 72:904, 1968.

7. Broberger, O., and Zetterstrom, R. Hypoglycemia with an inability to increase the epinephrine secretion in insulin-induced hypoglycemia. *J. Pediat.* 59:215, 1961.

8. Brodie, D. A., and Woodbury, D. M. Acid-base changes in brain and blood of rats exposed to high concentrations of carbon dioxide. *Amer. J. Physiol.* 192:91, 1958.

9. Bronsky, D., Kushner, D. S., Dubin, A., and Snapper, I. Idiopathic hypoparathyroidism and pseudohypoparathyroidism; case reports and review of the literature. *Medicine* (Balt.) 37:317, 1958.

10. Bruck, E., Abal, G., and Aceto, T., Jr. Therapy of infants with hypertonic dehydration due to diarrhea. *Amer. J. Dis. Child.* 115:281, 1968.

11. Campbell, H. J., and Eayrs, J. T. Influence of hormones on the central nervous system. *Brit. Med. Bull.* 2:81, 1965.

12. Choremis, C., Kyriakides, V., and Karponzas, J. Aminoaciduria in epilepsy. *J. Pediat.* 55:593, 1959.

13. Choremis, C., Kyriakides, V., and Basti-Maounis, V. Aminoaciduria in infantile spasms with hypsarrhythmia. *Excerpta Medica Int. Congr. Ser.* 37:159, 1961.

14. Costa, P. J., and Bonnycastle, D. D. Steroids and convulsions in dogs. *Arch. Int. Pharmacodyn.* 91:330, 1952.

15. Dodge, P. R., Sotos, J. F., Gamstorp, I., DeVivo, D., Levy, M., and Rabe, T. Neurophysiologic disturbances in hypertonic dehydration. *Trans. Amer. Neurol. Ass.* 87:33, 1962.

16. Dusser De Barenne, D., and Gibbs, F. A. Variations in the EEG during the menstrual cycle. *Amer. J. Obstet. Gynec.* 44:687, 1942.

17. Efron, M. L., and Ampola, M. G. The Aminoacidurias. In Millichap, J. G. (Ed.), *Pediatric Neurology. Pediat. Clin. N. Amer.* 14:881, 1967.

18. Etheridge, J. E., Jr., and Millichap, J. G. Hypoglycemia and seizures in childhood. *Neurology* (Minneap.) 14:397, 1964.

19. Faris, A. A., and Poser, C. M. Experimental production of focal neurologic deficit by systemic hyponatremia. *Neurology* (Minneap.) 14:206, 1964.

20. Frame, B., and Carter, S. Pseudohypoparathyroidism. Clinical picture and relation to convulsive seizures. *Neurology* (Minneap.) 5:297, 1955.

21. Gellhorn, E. *Physiological Foundations of Neurology and Psychiatry*. Minneapolis: University of Minnesota Press, 1953.

22. Gibbs, E. L., Lennox, W. G., and Gibbs, F. A. Variations in the carbon dioxide content of the blood in epilepsy. *Arch. Neurol. Psychiat.* 43:223, 1940.

23. Glaser, G. H. On the relationship between adrenal cortical activity and the convulsive state. *Epilepsia* (Amst.) 2:7, 1953.

24. Glaser, G. H., and Levy, L. L. Seizures and idiopathic hypoparathyroidism. A clinical EEG study. *Epilepsia* (Amst.) 1:454, 1960.

25. Gordon, N., and Wilson, V. K. Abnormal amino-acid excretion in cerebral disease. *Develop. Med. Child. Neurol.* 5:586, 1963.

26. Grant, D. K. Papilloedema and fits in hypoparathyroidism. *Quart. J. Med.* 22:243, 1953.

27. Holmberg, G. The effect of carbon dioxide on convulsions induced by electric shock treatment. *Acta Psychiat. Neurol. Scand.* 29:99, 1954.

28. Holmberg, G. The effect of different blood-sugar concentrations on convulsions induced by electric shock treatment. *Acta Psychiat. Neurol. Scand.* 29:89, 1954.

29. Klein, R., and Livingston, S. The effects of adrenocorticotropic hormone in epilepsy. *J. Pediat.* 37:733, 1950.

30. Laidlaw, J. Catamenial epilepsy. *Lancet* 271:235, 1956.

31. Lennox, W. G., Gibbs, F. A., and Gibbs, E. L. Effect on the electroencephalogram of drugs and conditions which influence seizures. *Arch. Neurol. Psychiat.* 36:1236, 1936.

32. Lin, T.-Y., Greenblatt, M., and Solomon,

H. C. A polygraphic study of one case of petit mal epilepsy. Effects of medication and menstruation. *Electroenceph. Clin. Neurophysiol.* 4:351, 1952.

33. Logothetis, J., Harner, R., Morrell, F., and Torres, F. The role of estrogens in catamenial exacerbation of epilepsy. *Neurology* (Minneap.) 9:352, 1959.

34. Luttrell, C. N., Finberg, L., and Drawdy, L. P. Hemorrhagic encephalopathy induced by hypernatremia. II. (Experimental observations on hyperosmolarity in cats.) *Arch. Neurol.* (Chicago) 1:153, 1959.

35. McQuarrie, I., and Keith, H. M. Experimental study of the acid-base equilibrium in children with idiopathic epilepsy. *Amer. J. Dis. Child.* 37:261, 1929.

36. Michael, R. P. Oestrogens in the central nervous system. *Brit. Med. Bull.* 2:87, 1965.

37. Millichap, J. G. Anticonvulsant action of Diamox in children. *Neurology* (Minneap.) 6:552, 1956.

38. Millichap, J. G. Studies in febrile seizures. II. Febrile seizures and the balance of water and electrolytes. *Neurology* (Minneap.) 10:312, 1960.

39. Millichap, J. G. Unpublished observations, 1962.

40. Millichap, J. G. Anticonvulsant Drugs. In Root, W. S., and Hofmann, F. A. (Eds.), *Physiological Pharmacology*. New York: Academic, 1965, vol. 2.

41. Millichap, J. G. *Febrile Convulsions*. New York: Macmillan, 1968.

42. Millichap, J. G., and Ulrich, J. A. Abnormal urinary excretion of amino acids in children with petit mal epilepsy. Preliminary communication. *Mayo Clin. Proc.* 37:307, 1962.

43. Millichap, J. G., and Jones, J. D. Acid-base, electrolyte, and amino-acid metabolism in children with petit mal. Etiologic significance and modification by anticonvulsant drugs and the ketogenic diet. *Epilepsia* (Amst.) 5:239, 1964.

44. Millichap, J. G., Jones, J. D., and Rudis, B. P. Mechanism of anticonvulsant action of ketogenic diet. *Amer. J. Dis. Child.* 107:593, 1964.

45. Millichap, J. G., Woodbury, D. M., and Goodman, L. S. Mechanism of the anticonvulsant action of acetazolamide, a carbonic anhydrase inhibitor. *J. Pharmacol. Exp. Ther.* 115:251, 1955.

46. Millichap, J. G., Jones, J. D., and Etheridge, J. E., Jr. The abnormal aminoaciduria in petit mal epilepsy. *Neurology* (Minneap.) 16:569, 1966.

47. Miribel, J., and Poirier, F. Effects of ACTH and adrenocortical hormones in juvenile epilepsy. *Epilepsia* (Amst.) 2:345, 1961.

48. Nyhan, W. L., and Cooke, R. E. Symptomatic hyponatremia in acute infections of the central nervous system. *Pediatrics* 18:604, 1956.

49. Paunier, L., Radde, I. C., Kooh, S. W., Conen, P. E., and Fraser, D. Primary hypomagnesemia with secondary hypocalcemia in an infant. *Pediatrics* 41:385, 1968.

50. Reyolds, E. H. Personal communication, 1968.

51. Schneider, J. Urinary excretion of electrolytes in centrencephalic epileptics. *Epilepsia* (Amst.) 2:358, 1961.

52. Simpson, J. A. The neurological manifestations of idiopathic hypoparathyroidism. *Brain* 75:76, 1952.

53. Sorel, L., and Dusaucy-Bauloye, A. A propos de 21 cas d'hypsarythmia de Gibbs. Treatment spectaculaire par l'ACTH. *Rev. Neurol.* (Paris) 99:136, 1958.

54. Stamps, F. W., Gibbs, F. A., and Gibbs, E. L. Treatment of hypsarhythmia with ACTH. *J.A.M.A.* 171:408, 1959.

55. Stemmerman, M. G. Metabolic errors and seizures. *Epilepsia* (Amst.) 6:16, 1965.

56. Stitt, S. L., and Kinnard, W. J. The effect of certain progestins and estrogens on the threshold of electrically induced seizure patterns. *Neurology* (Minneap.) 18:213, 1968.

57. Sugar, O. Central neurological complications of hypoparathyroidism. *A.M.A. Arch. Neurol. Psychiat.* 70:86, 1953.

58. Swinyard, E. A. Effect of extracellular electrolyte depletion on brain electrolyte pattern and electroshock seizure threshold. *Amer. J. Physiol.* 156:163, 1949.

59. Swinyard, E. A., Toman, J. E. P., and Goodman, L. S. The effect of cellular hydration on experimental electroshock convulsions. *J. Neurophysiol.* 9:47, 1946.

60. Timiras, P. S., Woodbury, D. M., and Agarwal, S. L. Effect of thyroxine and triiodothyronine on brain function and electrolyte distribution in intact and adrenalectomized rats. *J. Pharmacol. Exp. Ther.* 115:154, 1955.

61. Timiras, P. S., and Woodbury, D. M. Effect of thyroid activity on brain function and brain electrolyte distribution in rats. *Endocrinology* 58:181, 1956.

62. Timiras, P. S., Woodbury, D. M., and Baker, D. H. Effect of hydrocortisone acetate, desoxycorticosterone acetate, insulin, glucagon and dextrose, alone or in combination, on experimental convulsions and carbohydrate metabolism. *Arch. Int. Pharmacodyn.* 105:450, 1956.

63. Timiras, P. S., Woodbury, D. M., and Goodman, L. S. Effect of adrenalectomy, hydrocortisone acetate and desoxycorticosterone acetate on brain excitability and electrolyte distribution in mice. *J. Pharmacol. Exp. Ther.* 112:80, 1954.

64. Torda, C., and Wolff, H. G. Effects of various concentrations of adrenocorticotrophic hormone on electrical activity of brain and on sensitivity to convulsion-inducing agents. *Amer. J. Physiol.* 168:406, 1952.

65. Van Wyk, J. J. Unpublished observations. (Quoted in Etheridge, J. E., Jr., *Pediat. Clin. N. Amer.* 14:865, 1967.)

66. Vernadakis, A., and Woodbury, D. M. Effect of cortisol and deoxycorticosterone (DCA) on electroshock seizure patterns in developing rats. *Fed. Proc.* 19:153, 1960.

67. Vernadakis, A., and Woodbury, D. M. Effect of cortisol on the electroshock seizure thresholds in developing rats. *J. Pharmacol. Exp. Ther.* 139:110, 1963.

68. Wasserman, M. J., Belton, N. R., and Millichap, J. G. Effect of corticotropin (ACTH) on experimental seizures. Adrenal independence and relation to intracellular brain sodium. *Neurology* (Minneap.) 15:1136, 1965.

69. Wells, C. A. Chronic hypoventilation in an epileptic patient. *Neurology* (Minneap.) 6:744, 1956.

70. Willison, R. G., and Whitty, C. W. M. Parathyroid deficiency presenting as epilepsy. *Brit. Med. J.* 1:802, 1957.

71. Woodbury, D. M. Extrarenal effects of desoxycorticosterone, adrenocortical extract and adrenocorticotrophic hormone on plasma and tissue electrolytes in fed and fasted rats. *Amer. J. Physiol.* 174:1, 1953.

72. Woodbury, D. M. Effect of adrenocortical steroids and adrenocorticotrophic hormone on electroshock seizure threshold. *J. Pharmacol. Exp. Ther.* 105:27, 1952.

73. Woodbury, D. M. Effect of hormones on brain excitability and electrolytes. In *Recent Progress in Hormone Research, The Proceedings of the Laurentian Hormone Conference.* New York: Academic, 1954, vol. X.

74. Woodbury, D. M. Effect of acute hyponatremia on distribution of water and electrolytes in various tissues of the rat. *Amer. J. Physiol.* 185:281, 1956.

75. Woodbury, D. M., and Davenport, V. D. Brain and plasma cations and experimental seizures in normal and desoxycorticosterone-treated rats. *Amer. J. Physiol.* 157:234, 1949.

76. Woodbury, D. M., Emmett, J. W., Hinckley, G. V., Jackson, N. R., Newton, J. D., Bateman, J. H., Goodman, L. S., and Sayers, G. Antagonism of adrenocortical extract and cortisone to desoxycorticosterone: Brain excitability in adrenalectomized rats. *Proc. Soc. Exp. Biol. Med.* 76:65, 1951.

77. Woodbury, D. M., Hurley, R. E., Lewis, N. G., McArthur, M. W., Copeland, W. W., Kirschvink, J. F., and Goodman, L. S. Effect of thyroxin, thyroidectomy and 6-N-propyl-2-thiouracil on brain function. *J. Pharmacol. Exp. Ther.* 106:331, 1952.

78. Woodbury, D. M., and Karler, R. The role of carbon dioxide in the nervous system. *Anesthesiology* 21:686, 1960.

79. Woodbury, D. M., Rollins, L. T., Henrie, J. R., Jones, J. C., and Sato, T. Effects of carbon dioxide and oxygen on properties of experimental seizures in mice. *Amer. J. Physiol.* 184:202, 1956.

80. Woodbury, D. M., Rollins, L. T., Gardner, M. D., Hirschi, W. L., Hogan, J. R., Rallison, M. L., Tanner, G. S., and Brodie, D. A. Effects of carbon dioxide on brain excitability and electrolytes. *Amer. J. Physiol.* 192:79, 1958.

81. Woodbury, D. M., Timiras, P. S., and Vernadakis, A. Influence of Adrenocorti-

cal Steroids on Brain Function and Metabolism. In *Hormones, Brain Function, and Behavior*. New York: Academic, 1957.

82. Woolley, D. E., Timiras, P. S., and Woodbury, D. M. Some effects of sex steroids on brain excitability and metabolism. *Proc. West. Pharmacol. Soc.* 3:11, 1960.

83. Woolley, D. E., and Timiras, P. S. The gonad-brain relationship: Effects of female sex hormones on electroshock convulsions in the rat. *Endocrinology* 70:196, 1962.

84. Wyke, B. *Brain Function and Metabolic Disorders*. London: Butterworth, 1963.

85. Zimmet, P., Breidahl, H. D., and Nayler, W. G. Plasma ionized calcium in hypomagnesaemia. *Brit. Med. J.* 1:622, 1968.

Discussion

ROLE OF HORMONES IN DEVELOPMENT OF SEIZURES*

PAOLA S. TIMIRAS

Millichap has considered some of the important relationships that exist between electrolyte balance and endocrine function in the occurrence of epilepsy. Attention will be focused here on the developmental aspects of seizure activity and an examination of the regulatory role of hormones.

Morphological, biochemical, and functional studies of the central nervous system (CNS) in many mammals, including man, indicate that CNS development is characterized by periods of accelerated growth during which both internal and external stimuli exert profound effects. Studies in the developing rat brain have demonstrated that the response of the CNS to hormones varies with respect to the maturational timetable of a specific brain area, presence of the blood-CNS barrier, affinity of a discrete area for a particular hormone, and level of the hormone present in the circulation, all of these factors being integrally related [19, 20, 27].

Recent work from our laboratories and others has shown that postnatal development of generalized and localized seizure activity can be influenced by administration of a specific hormone at a critical stage of CNS maturation. Mechanisms underlying these hormonal effects have been studied both in vivo and in vitro in terms of ionic, lipid, and protein metabolism, and increasingly appear to involve the direct action of hormones on neural cells at identifiable periods of CNS growth.

DEVELOPMENT OF GENERALIZED SEIZURE ACTIVITY

The development of electroconvulsive responses, routinely used as an index of functional maturation of neural units involved in seizure activity, was followed in rats from birth until adulthood. It is known that the brain of the rat at birth is relatively immature and undergoes rapid development in the first three postnatal weeks. Maximal electroshock stimulation during this period produces a sequence of characteristic seizure patterns—hyperkinesia, clonus, tonic flexion, tonic extension—the full tonic-clonic seizure typical of adult animals occurring at 21 days, coincident with the end of the period of accelerated growth [13, 28]. Similarly, seizure threshold undergoes characteristic changes with age, from high values at birth to a minimum at approximately 2 weeks of age when it begins to increase progressively to adult values [28, 29].

Experiments were conducted to assess the effects of several steroid hormones—cortisol, deoxycorticosterone, estradiol, and testosterone—on the development of seizure activity in rats. Cortisol was found to accelerate the appearance of seizure activity when administered between the eighth and sixteenth postnatal days [27, 28]. Before or after this time period, it is without any significant effect on seizure patterns. Estradiol, on the other hand, induces precocious seizure activity when administered prior to the eighth postnatal day [12, 13]. Beyond that time, its influence is not significant. These findings suggest not only the existence of hormonal-age specificity, but also that the systems affected by cortisol develop later than those influenced by estradiol. Further evidence of hormonal specificity is demonstrated in the case of deoxycorticosterone which induces

---

* This research supported in part by PHS Research Grant GM-09267 from National Institute of General Medical Sciences, and Grant AT(11-1)-34 Project 82 from U.S. Atomic Energy Commission.

no alterations in seizure responses during development [27].

The physiological role of estradiol in influencing brain excitability is supported by the finding that both male and female animals show the same intensity of seizure activity until the age of sexual maturation, when the female shows increased convulsibility [34, 35]. In addition, seizure activity varies throughout the estrous cycle, being lowest during diestrus and highest during estrus when the level of circulating estrogens is also highest [32]. These observations coincide with those discussed by Millichap regarding the relationship between seizures and menstruation in humans. Seizure activity in rats has also been found to fluctuate according to the time of day. The circadian rhythm of convulsibility has been suggested to be related to alterations in the levels of adrenocortical hormones [32].

Another aspect of the influence of hormones on the development of seizure activity has emerged from experiments using testosterone. In the adult rat, testosterone is capable of both convulsant and anticonvulsant action, depending on the age of the animal, the dose used, and the type of seizure pattern under study [31]. During development, testosterone is believed to be the hormone that triggers the differentiation of the hypothalamus leading to the male pattern of gonadotropin secretion [10]. When administered to newborn rats, testosterone does not affect seizure responses. Yet lack of physiological levels of the hormone, as in rats that have been castrated neonatally, results in delayed appearance of the maximal seizure pattern [14]. From these studies, it appears that certain hormones may influence CNS development by a "permissive" rather than a regulatory action [27].

The effects of hormones on seizure activity may also differ according to the reciprocal stage of development of CNS excitatory and inhibitory systems [20]. During the early postnatal period, the subcortical centers are predominant, and seizure responses at this time may result either from stimulation of subcortical areas or indirectly from impaired inhibitory activity from the less mature cortical centers. For example, seizure threshold in neonatally thyroidectomized animals is markedly lower 2 weeks after birth than in controls but gradually increases as the higher CNS centers mature [22]. In contrast, as pointed out by Millichap, the adult hypothyroid animal shows decreased brain excitability—an effect which is reversed in hyperthyroidism. The differential effects of thyroid hormones on seizure activity in the young and in the adult correlate with those observed in brain electrolytes with age [21, 23, 24].

Spinal reflex systems are known to play an important role in integrating maximal seizure discharge into motor patterns; consequently, the effects of cortisol, estradiol, and testosterone on spinal cord convulsions, elicited by direct electrical stimulation of the spinal cord, were studied in developing rats. Administration of these hormones was found to intensify spinal cord convulsions, suggesting that increased spinal reflex activity may contribute to the enhancement of electroshock responses [27].

Development of Localized Seizure Activity

Studies in awake, unrestrained rats chronically implanted with electrodes have demonstrated that hormones are also capable of influencing localized seizure activity. For example, changes in seizure threshold were observed in discrete structures of the limbic system during the estrous cycle, after ovariectomy, and following administration of estrogen or progesterone [17]. Seizure threshold in the dorsal hippocampus and the medial part of the amygdala was significantly decreased during proestrus and estrus, whereas that of the lateral part of the amygdala was significantly increased during the same period and decreased during diestrus (Fig. D25-1). Ovariectomy of young adult rats eliminated the cyclic aspects of activity in the limbic system, but a dampened cyclicity was restored by a single injection of estradiol (Fig. D25-2). The same dose of estrogen was somewhat less effective in older ovariectomized rats and failed to establish cyclicity in rats that had been ovariectomized at birth (Fig. D25-3). Progesterone in relatively high doses affected seizure threshold only slightly and,

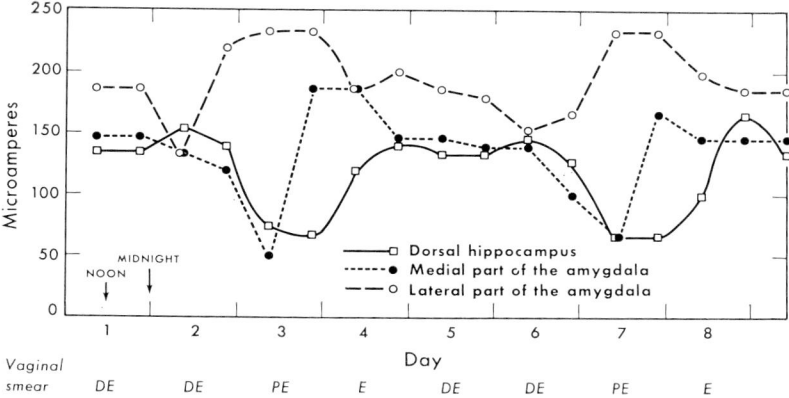

FIG. D25-1. Comparison of localized seizure threshold curves of 3 structures of limbic system during 2 estrous cycles. Data on hippocampus and lateral part of amygdala from one rat; data for medial part of amygdala from another rat. DE, diestrous day; E, estrous day; PE, proestrous day.

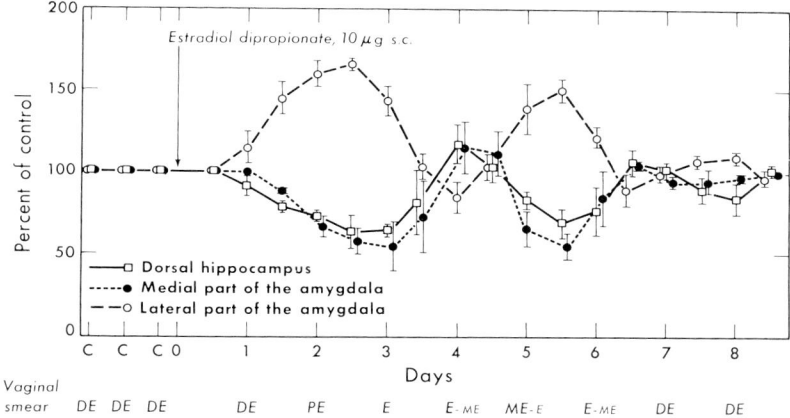

FIG. D25-2. Effect of 10 μg of estradiol dipropionate on localized seizure thresholds in limbic areas of ovariectomized rats. (Values are expressed with mean and standard errors as a percentage of control values.) E-ME: Nearly all the animals show cornified vaginal smears, but some animals show metestrous smears. ME-E represents the reverse situation. (In time legend, C indicates control. Other abbreviations are the same as in Fig. D25-1.)

generally, its effects were opposite to those of estradiol. These data indicate that estrogen plays a role not only in the regulation of seizure activity of the hippocampus and the amygdala in the adult animal, but also on its development.

Such observations as those just cited have led to investigation of the development of seizure activity in specific CNS areas from birth to sexual maturity in the rat. In order to assure accurate placement of electrodes in developing CNS structures, a stereotaxic atlas of the developing rat brain was prepared [16]. Experiments were designed to explore the development of seizure activity in the dorsal hippocampus and the medial part of the amygdala in intact female rats, rats ovariectomized at birth, and rats in which precocious puberty was induced by injection of gonadotropin [18]. The results show significant change in seizure activity with age in both structures; in the amygdala, seizure threshold dropped sharply around 30 days of age, a few days

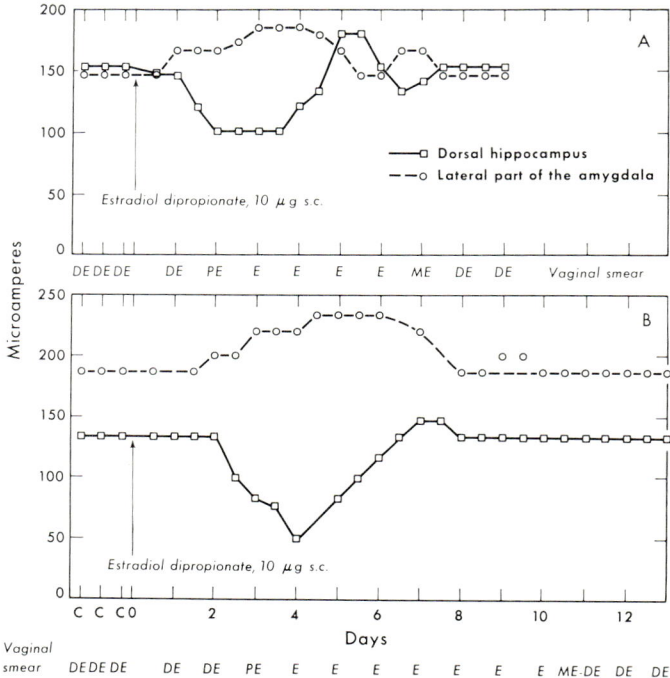

Fig. D25-3. (A) Effect of 10 μg of estradiol dipropionate on localized seizure thresholds in rats of advanced age ovariectomized in adulthood. (B) Effect of 10 μg of estradiol dipropionate on localized seizure thresholds in adult rats ovariectomized at birth.

before the onset of puberty (as evidenced by vaginal and ovarian signs), whereas no such changes occurred in the ovariectomized animals. When puberty was accelerated by administration of gonadotropin, amygdaloid threshold similarly dropped preceding the onset of sexual function (Fig. D25-4).

From these findings several important physiological conclusions can be drawn: The development of seizure activity in the limbic system and especially in the amygdala is influenced by gonadal hormones. Indeed, it may be postulated that estrogens have an *organizing* action in the amygdala comparable to that of androgens in the hypothalamus; that is, these hormones are indispensable to normal functional differentiation at a specific neonatal age. It can also be inferred from these studies that maturation of specific CNS structures and their changing sensitivity to gonadal hormones may be key factors in the onset of puberty. Finally, it is possible that transitory hormonal disturbances at critical periods during CNS maturation may produce permanent neurogenic alterations implicated in the etiology of epilepsy.

DEVELOPMENT OF ASSOCIATIVE ACTIVITY

In view of the reverberative nature of seizure activity, it is important to study the possible hormonal effects on maturation of the *association* systems in the brain. Although little research has yet been conducted in this area, the available data suggest that some of these systems may be influenced by hormonal changes. For example, the development of evoked transcallosal response is retarded in hypothyroid rats and generally accelerated in hyperthyroid rats [11]. The retarded maturation of this response may be related to delayed myelination and hypoplasia of the cortical neuropil consequent to thyroid deficiency; the precocious maturation attendant to hyperthyroidism, conversely, may result from its effect in accelerating myelination.

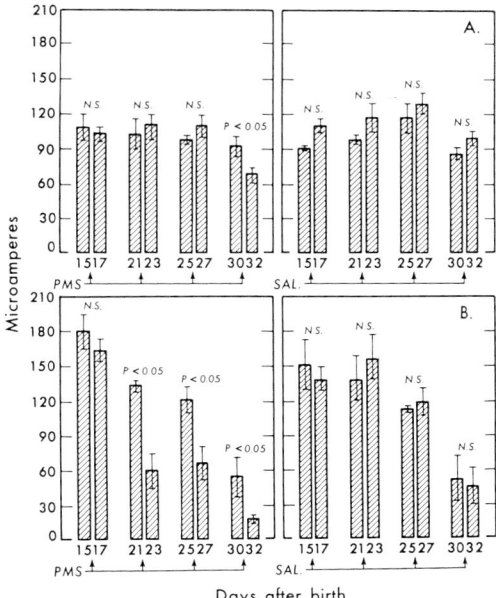

Fig. D25-4. Localized seizure thresholds (mean ± standard error) in (A) hippocampus, and (B) amygdala before and after 30 IU (0.6 cc) pregnant mare serum (PMS) injection and 0.66 cc of saline (SAL) injection at ages 15, 21, 25, 30 days. Each group consisted of 5 rats; p values (based on t test) are given where threshold levels before and after injection are significant; N.S. = not statistically significant.

In contrast to thyroid hormones, estradiol has less effect on the development of evoked transcallosal response or evoked responses of other systems, again illustrating hormonal and structural specificity [2].

CNS BIOCHEMICAL DEVELOPMENT RELATED TO SEIZURE ACTIVITY AND ENDOCRINE FUNCTION

As stated by Millichap, both systemic and neurogenic alterations in metabolism have been considered as causative or contributory factors in the occurrence of seizures. In some cases, metabolic changes have been induced for therapeutic purposes. Whether specific metabolic alterations are related to certain types of epilepsy, or, more generally, whether seizures can be explained in terms of CNS biochemical changes, remains to be conclusively demonstrated. On the other hand, it is well known that hormones profoundly influence metabolic patterns of muscle, liver, and kidney, and evidence has been accumulating in the last few years to show that their effects on metabolism extend also to the brain.

Although it has not yet been clarified which hormones are most critical in regulating CNS metabolism, or the precise cellular and molecular mechanism(s) underlying their effects, important correlations are being made between the effects of hormones on the biochemical development of the brain and the development of seizure patterns. Such investigations are both theoretically and practically significant in understanding the pathogenesis of epilepsy and planning effective therapy. The experiments summarized here represent only a few of those currently conducted in this relatively new but promising area of study.

IONIC METABOLISM. Thyroid hormones significantly influence ionic metabolism in developing animals, as in the adult. Recent studies have investigated the role of thyroid hormones on Na^+-K^+-activated ATPase, an enzyme associated with the active transport of Na and K, and on the distribution of Na, K, Cl, and Mg in cerebral cortex and cerebellum of the developing rat [23, 24]. The Na^+-K^+-activated ATPase, known to be highly localized in the synaptosomal fraction of the brain, exhibits rapid increase during the period of morphological and functional growth of the brain similar to that of cholinesterases [15]. Neonatal hypothyroidism significantly depresses the specific activity of Na^+-K^+-activated ATPase (but not that of Mg^{++} ATPase) in both brain areas studied (Fig. D25-5). Inasmuch as the decrease was observed in enzymes extracted from total homogenate of these tissues as well as in heavy microsomal fraction, this change may be related to a reduced synthesis of the enzyme and/or its properties of association to the cellular membranes [23]. The alteration in enzymatic activity is accompanied by marked increase in cerebral and cerebellar Na and Cl content and decrease in K content, changes which can be interpreted as reflective of intracellular change resulting from a depressed Na-K pump. In addition to the

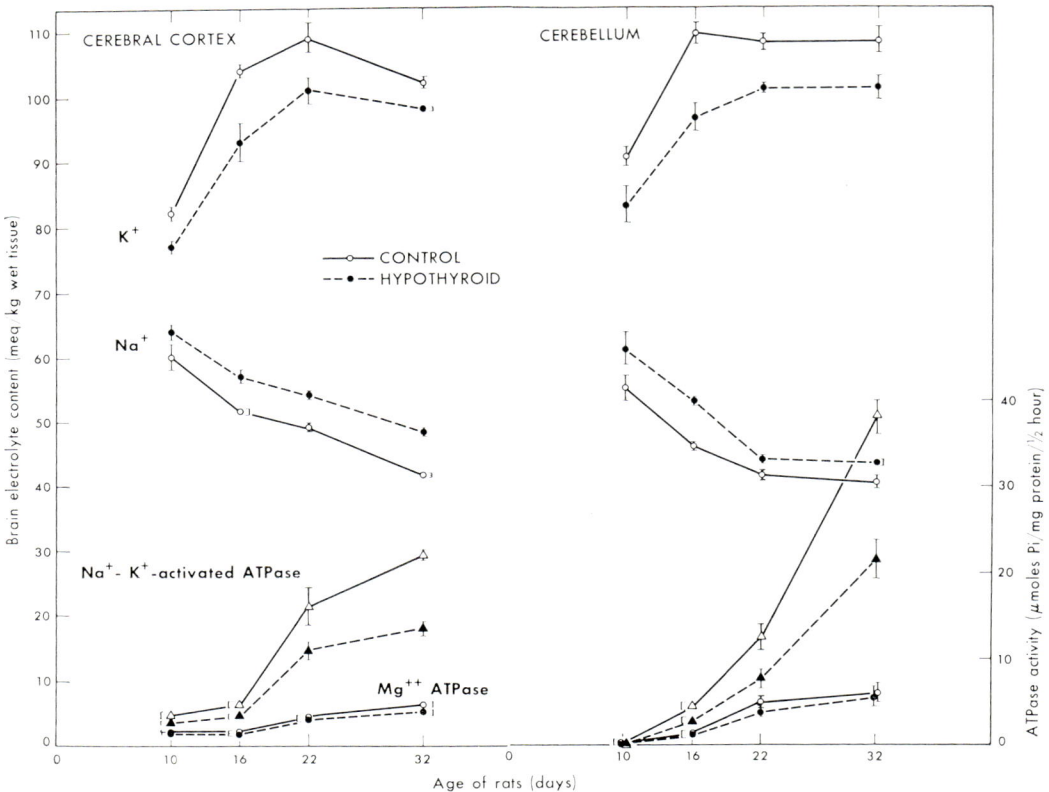

Fig. D25-5. Effects of neonatal hypothyroidism on Na+ and K+ contents, Mg++ ATPase, and Na+-K+-activated ATPase activity in the cerebral cortex and cerebellum of the rat during development. For ATPase activity, each point represents mean ± standard error of duplicate determinations from 16 enzyme preparations, and, for Na+ and K+ contents, each point represents mean ± standard error of 8 or more samples.

Na and K changes, neonatal hypothyroidism leads to a decrease in Mg ions in the brain as well as in plasma. The altered Mg metabolism in the developing hypothyroid rat may influence brain excitability, particularly with reference to seizure responses, as indicated by Millichap. These studies reveal again a differential effect between the adult and immature brain. The Na content is decreased in the hypothyroid adult rat whereas it is increased in the developing animal. These differences are also reflected in seizure activity of the hypothyroid animal, which is decreased in the adult and increased in the young. When thyroid hormone was restored from an early age, the biochemical alterations described above were not observed.

It is conceivable that the effects of thyroid hormones on ionic metabolism may underlie many of the physiological deviations attendant to hypothyroidism, including altered seizure susceptibility. In view of the characteristic sensitivity of the brain-synthesizing system to ionic environment, it is also possible that ionic changes induced by thyroid hormone deficiency may be related to the concomitant alterations in protein biosynthesis [7, 8].

Other hormones are probably involved in regulation of electrolyte metabolism in the immature brain but their effects have not yet been extensively studied. Experiments designed to assess the effects of estradiol and cortisol on ionic content in the developing rat brain have demonstrated an age-specific response that may be related to the stage of development of the specific brain area studied [25, 33]. The data presented in Table D25-1 illustrate the effects of estradiol on Cl concentration in the developing and mature rat brain. The increase observed in Cl content may reflect changes in glial cell distribution inasmuch as these cells are believed to be high in Cl concentration. Since glial cells are thought to modify neuronal activity, such changes in these cells may, in turn, contribute to changes in brain excitability.

LIPID METABOLISM. Although the role of hormones on lipid metabolism has been little studied as yet, it has been reported that when estradiol or cortisol is administered to developing rats [1, 3] or chicks [9], myelination is accelerated. This effect has been observed both biochemically and histologically. Myelination increases conduction velocity, thus facilitating the generation of reverberating circuits. It would seem justified to associate the early appearance of seizure response induced by these hormones, at least in part, to accelerated myelination.

Proceeding on this hypothesis, it is possible to relate the age-specific effects of hormones on discrete brain structures to the stage of development of lipid metabolism in these areas. For example, tritiated estradiol administered to infant and adult rats shows differences in its distribution with the age of the animal [30]. The immature brain, low in lipids, appears to be less able to concentrate estradiol than the adult brain, as shown by the lower plasma-tissue ratio observed in the pituitary, hypothalamus, and cerebral cortex of these animals. In the mature brain, the relatively higher uptake of tritiated estradiol by the brain stem than by the other areas studied may be explained by the high lipid levels of this area in the adult animal.

It should be emphasized that many factors may be implicated in the differential sensitivity of the brain to hormones with age. Numerous studies have shown that the blood-CNS barrier to many substances, including hormones, develops with age. Glial cells play an important role in the development of the blood-CNS barrier and are also affected by hormones [25, 27, 33].

PROTEIN METABOLISM. Despite striking advances in our knowledge of the regulatory role of hormones in the protein synthetic activity of target cells, a recent review on the role of hormones in cerebral protein metabolism discloses that little information is available on this aspect of CNS-endocrine relationships [7]. Yet in terms of structure and function, the requirement for protein is perhaps more important in the brain than in any other organ. Most of the investigations thus far conducted in this area have been concerned with thyroid hormones, probably because of their well-known actions on development and function

TABLE D25-1. Effect of Estradiol Treatment on Chloride Concentrations (mEq per kg Wet Tissue) in Various Brain Areas of Adult and Developing Rats

Experimental Groups	Adult Rats[a]			Developing Rats[b]	
	Cerebral Cortex	Brain Stem	Cerebellum	Cerebellum	Spinal Cord
Oil vehicle (controls)	31.40 ± 0.32	34.71 ± 0.51	30.65 ± 0.48	26.89 ± 0.38	32.10 ± 0.56
Estradiol dipropionate	33.14 ± 0.55 ($p < 0.01$)[c]	36.57 ± 0.66 ($p < 0.01$)	31.91 ± 0.68	29.26 ± 0.65 ($p < 0.01$)	33.75 ± 0.75

[a] 500 μg of estradiol per 100 gm body weight was injected daily to male adult rats for 20 days.
[b] 100 μg of estradiol per 100 gm body weight was injected daily to developing male and female rats from the 6th to the 10th day after birth; animals were sacrificed at 12 days of age.
[c] Values are means ±S.E.; figures in parentheses are p values (t test) representing significant differences between control and estradiol-injected groups.

of the CNS in young and adult animals, including man.

Recent studies have demonstrated that neonatal hypothyroidism depresses whereas hormone therapy stimulates protein synthesis in the immature brain, as measured by the incorporation of labeled leucine into cerebral cortical protein [8]. Further studies on the mode of action of thyroid hormones in the developing brain have shown that neonatal hypothyroidism produces a significant decrease in nuclear and cytoplasmatic RNA content of the cerebral cortex [5, 6]. The changes observed in RNA content are accompanied by significant increase in DNA content, probably reflecting the increase in packing density of cerebral cortical cells and corresponding decrease in dendritic branching that has been described by several investigators. Even though the net RNA content of cerebral cortical fractions is reduced in thyroid-deficient rats, the rate of protein synthesis as measured by incorporation of labeled orotic acid into RNA, appears to be unaltered. It would seem that thyroid hormones control the rate of utilization or breakdown of RNA species [6].

Information on the effects of other hormones on protein metabolism in the brain is fragmentary and largely based on indirect evidence. Some observations in rats seem to indicate that growth hormone administered prenatally increases DNA content in the brain and induces neuronal hyperplasia. Other studies, however, do not seem to support this view; for example, growth hormone does not restore to normal the altered nucleic acid metabolism characteristic of hypothyroidism [6].

Hormonal effects on protein metabolism are also evidenced by changes in enzymatic activity during development. A clear illustration of the dependency of enzymatic activity on thyroid hormones during critical periods of CNS development is represented by the significant decrease that occurs in acetylcholinesterase and cholinesterase activities following hypothyroidism and by its return to normal following replacement therapy [4]. Inasmuch as acetylcholinesterase has been implicated in synaptic transmission in the CNS, it may be expected that alterations in the activity of this enzyme would be reflected in changes in seizure responses. Indeed, tissue culture studies have demonstrated that cortisol and estrogen exert a direct effect on acetylcholinesterase activity in the spinal cord and cerebellum and, further, that this effect varies depending on the stage of maturation of these structures at the time the hormone is added to the medium [26].

Concluding Remarks

The foregoing discussion briefly covers our own research on the regulatory role of hormones on the development of seizure activity and suggests the complexity of interrelating factors involved in this area of inquiry. Our findings thus far, while fragmentary and scattered, indicate clear avenues for further investigation. It is possible that no one theory will emerge to cover seizure phenomena in young and adult or in the brain as a whole, and indeed, the evidence increasingly indicates that a multiplicity of interdependent actions underlies seizure responses. Our continued study and collaborative efforts will yield the answers to the questions that remain.

REFERENCES

1. Casper, R., Vernadakis, A., and Timiras, P. S. Influence of estradiol and cortisol on lipids and cerebrosides in the developing brain and spinal cord of the rat. *Brain Res.* 5:524, 1967.

2. Curry, J. J., III. *Evoked Responses in Some Specific Brain Systems during Development after Neonatal Administration of Estradiol.* (Ph.D. thesis) Berkeley: University of California, 1968.

3. Curry, J. J., III, and Heim, L. M. Brain myelination after neonatal administration of oestradiol. *Nature* (London) 209:915, 1966.

4. Geel, S. E., and Timiras, P. S. Influence of neonatal hypothyroidism and of thyroxine on the acetylcholinesterase and cholinesterase activities in the developing central nervous system of the rat. *Endocrinology* 80:1069, 1967.

5. Geel, S. E., and Timiras, P. S. The influence of neonatal hypothyroidism and of thyroxine on the ribonucleic acid and deoxyribonucleic acid concentrations of rat cerebral cortex. *Brain Res.* 4:135, 1967.

6. Geel, S. E., and Timiras, P. S. The role of thyroid and growth hormones on RNA synthesis in the developing brain. Presented at the Conference on Hormones in Development, Nottingham, England, 1969, in press.

7. Geel, S. E., and Timiras, P. S. The Role of Hormones in Cerebral Protein Metabolism. In Lajtha, A. (Ed.), *Protein Metabolism of the Nervous System.* New York: Plenum Press, 1969, in press.

8. Geel, S. E., Valcana, T., and Timiras, P. S. Effect of neonatal hypothyroidism and of thyroxine on L-[^{14}C] leucine incorporation in protein in vivo and the relationship to ionic levels in the developing brain of the rat. *Brain Res.* 4:143, 1967.

9. Granich, M., and Timiras, P. S. Mechanism of action of cortisol in maturation of brain lipid patterns in embryonal and young chicks. Presented at the Conference on Hormones in Development, Nottingham, England, 1969, in press.

10. Harris, G. W. Sex hormones, brain development and brain function. *Endocrinology* 75:627, 1964.

11. Hatotani, N., and Timiras, P. S. Influence of thyroid function on the postnatal development of the transcallosal response in the rat. *Neuroendocrinology* 2:147, 1967.

12. Heim, L. M. Effect of estradiol on brain maturation: Dose and time response relationships. *Endocrinology* 78:1130, 1966.

13. Heim, L. M., and Timiras, P. S. Gonad-brain relationship: Precocious brain maturation after estradiol in rats. *Endocrinology* 72:598, 1963.

14. Irvine, G., Ransom, T. W., Westbrook, W. H., and Timiras, P. S. A Regulatory Role of Testosterone in the Development of the Central Nervous System and Sexual Behavior of the Rat. In *Abstracts of Papers Presented at the Second International Congress on Hormonal Steroids.* Amsterdam: Excerpta Medica, 366:211, 1966.

15. Maletta, G. J., Vernadakis, A., and Timiras, P. S. Acetylcholinesterase activity and protein content of brain and spinal cord in developing rats after prenatal X-irradiation. *J. Neurochem.* 14:647, 1967.

16. Sherwood, N. M., and Timiras, P. S. *Stereotaxic Atlas of the Developing Rat Brain.* Berkeley: Univ. California Press, 1969.

17. Terasawa, E., and Timiras, P. S. Electrical activity during the estrous cycle of the rat: Cyclic changes in limbic structures. *Endocrinology* 83:207, 1968.

18. Terasawa, E., and Timiras, P. S. Electrophysiological study of the limbic system in the rat at onset of puberty. *Amer. J. Physiol.* 215:1462, 1968.

19. Timiras, P. S., and Vernadakis, A. Brain Plasticity: Hormones and Stress. In Jasmin, G. (Ed.), *Endocrine Aspects of Disease Processes.* St. Louis: Warren H. Green, Inc., 1968.

20. Timiras, P. S., Vernadakis, A., and Sherwood, N. Development and Plasticity of the Nervous System. In Assali, N. S. (Ed.), *Biology of Gestation.* New York: Academic, 1968, vol. II.

21. Timiras, P. S., and Woodbury, D. M. Effect of thyroid activity on brain function and brain electrolyte distribution in rats. *Endocrinology* 58:181, 1956.

22. Valcana, T., Meisami, E., and Timiras, P. S. Effect of neonatal hypothyroidism on the development of electroshock seizure threshold in rats. In preparation.

23. Valcana, T., and Timiras, P. S. Effect of thyroid hormones on ionic metabolism of the developing rat brain. Presented at the Conference on Hormones in Development, Nottingham, England, 1969, in press.

24. Valcana, T., and Timiras, P. S. Effect of hypothyroidism on ionic metabolism and Na+-K+-activated ATPase in the developing rat brain. *J. Neurochem.* 1969, in press.

25. Valcana, T., Vernadakis, A., and Timiras, P. S. Influence of estradiol and cortisol on electrolytes in the central nervous system of developing rats. *Neuroendocrinology* 2:326, 1967.

26. Vernadakis, A., and Timiras, P. S. Effects of estradiol and cortisol on neural tissue in culture. *Experientia* 23:467, 1967.

27. Vernadakis, A., and Timiras, P. S. Regulation of Brain and Spinal Cord Excitability by Cortisol and Estradiol in

Developing Rats. In Martini, L., and Motta, F. F. M. (Eds.), *Proceedings of the Second International Congress on Hormonal Steroids*. Amsterdam: Excerpta Medica, 1967, pp. 908–912.

28. Vernadakis, A., and Woodbury, D. M. Effect of cortisol on the electroshock seizure thresholds in developing rats. *J. Pharmacol. Exp. Ther.* 139:110, 1963.

29. Vernadakis, A., and Woodbury, D. M. Effects of diphenylhydantoin on electroshock seizure thresholds in developing rats. *J. Pharmacol. Exp. Ther.* 148:144, 1965.

30. Woolley, D. E., Holinka, C. F., and Timiras, P. S. Changes in ^{3}H-estradiol distribution with development in the rat. *Endocrinology* 84:157, 1969.

31. Woolley, D. E., and Timiras, P. S. Gonad-brain relationship: Effects of castration and testosterone on electroshock convulsions in male rats. *Endocrinology* 71:609, 1962.

32. Woolley, D. E., and Timiras, P. S. Estrous and circadian periodicity and electroshock convulsions in rats. *Amer. J. Physiol.* 202:379, 1962.

33. Woolley, D. E., and Timiras, P. S. Water and electrolyte alterations in plasma, brain and liver of rats after castration and sex hormone administration. *Acta Endocr.* (Kobenhavn) 46:12, 1964.

34. Woolley, D. E., Timiras, P. S., Rosenzweig, M. R., Krech, D., and Bennett, E. L. Sex and strain differences in electroshock convulsions of the rat. *Nature* (London) 190:515, 1961.

35. Woolley, D. E., Timiras, P. S., Rosenzweig, M. R., Krech, D., and Bennett, E. L. Strain differences in seizure responses and brain cholinesterase activity in rats. *Proc. Soc. Exp. Biol. Med.* 112:781, 1963.

26
Neuroglial-Neuronal Interactions

RICHARD K. ORKAND

THE CELLS that make up the central nervous system (CNS), neurons and neuroglia, are usually separated by narrow intercellular clefts 200–300 Å wide [15]. At certain regions the structure of apposed cells is modified to form a specialized contact; for example, a chemical synapse [29]. At this type of synapse the neurons are still separate; the synaptic cleft is continuous with and about as wide as the intercellular clefts found elsewhere. In a few special situations the intercellular cleft separating the membrane outer leaflets of two neurons appears to be only 20–30 Å wide, forming a *gap junction*. Under certain conditions, lanthanum hydroxide and peroxidase can be shown to penetrate the intercellular cleft system, synaptic cleft, and gap junctions, whereas a larger molecule, ferritin, cannot penetrate the gap junction [4]. The remarkable coincidence in occurrence of gap junctions and electrical synaptic transmission makes it likely that these structures have relatively low electrical resistance and provide for electrical continuity between neurons [2, 12].

To a large extent neurons are apposed to glial cells rather than to other neurons. Glial cells can be clearly differentiated from neurons by a number of light and electron microscopic histological criteria [30, 37]. One type of glial cell, the oligodendrocyte, enwraps the axons of some neurons forming a myelin sheath which increases the velocity of the propagated action potential [31]. Functions of the great number of other glial cells, the astroglia, are still largely speculative [20]. One type of specialized contact occurs frequently between glial cells, the *gap junction*.

Specialized structural contacts have not been found between astroglia and neurons. Thus, the usual means of intercellular communication, chemical synapses, or direct electrical connections are apparently not available for the transfer of information between neurons and glia.

Diffusion through Intercellular Clefts

In early anatomic studies [14], glial cells were found to be interposed between capillaries and neurons, which gave rise to speculation that substances moving between blood and neurons were transported through glial cells. An alternate hypothesis is that exchange takes place by diffusion through the system of narrow intercellular clefts. Present evidence indicates many substances can diffuse through the intercellular clefts; a clear demonstration of transport through glia is still lacking [20].

Electron microscopic studies have shown that relatively large electron-dense molecules, such as ferritin, move through the intercellular clefts [3]. Physiological studies indicate that substances such as sodium and sucrose also diffuse through the clefts rather than through the glial cytoplasm. If the physiological solution which surrounds either the leech CNS or the *Necturus* optic nerve is exchanged for a solution where sodium is replaced by sucrose, the action potentials in the neurons are rapidly blocked [21, 27]. During this exchange the glial membrane potential remains essentially constant, suggesting that the ionic content of glia is affected very little. The rate of exchange is slowed only slightly by cooling to 1–4°C; it is unlikely that active processes, pinocytosis, or transport play an important role. The time course of exchange is in quantitative agreement with that expected from calculations of diffusion of molecules, such as sodium and sucrose through 150 Å channels. Thus, the extracellular cleft system permits the diffusion of ions and small molecules throughout the nervous system.

Blood-Brain Barrier

The conglomeration of neurons and glia floats in a modified ultrafiltrate of blood plasma, the cerebrospinal fluid (CSF), secreted primarily by the choroid plexus and circulated through and around the CNS through a series of ventricles and canals. In addition, the nervous system is penetrated by a rich network of capillaries. This raises the question of whether the immediate environment of the neurons is constituted by the CSF or by the blood. Before discussing the physiological experiments relevant to this question, the histology of the structures involved will be considered.

In most body tissues the cells are surrounded by fluid in equilibrium with blood plasma. The capillaries are permeable to small molecules. As a result, changes in composition of the blood produce rapid changes in the fluid surrounding the cells. To a large extent, changes in the composition of the plasma do not produce comparable changes in the composition of CSF. In fact, under equilibrium conditions there are important differences in the concentrations of ions between CSF and blood plasma [9]. Large molecules injected into the blood get into the environment of most body cells but not into the neurons and glia of the CNS. These observations have led to the conclusion that there is a barrier between blood and CSF. Recent anatomical studies provide a structural basis for a barrier preventing the penetration of large molecules into the central nervous system [33].

One hypothesis for the structural basis of the blood-brain barrier was that the astroglial end-feet surrounding blood vessels prevented the movement of substances out of the capillary. This hypothesis is apparently incorrect. The astroglia are occasionally closely apposed, forming gap junctions. However, these are merely spots of attachment and can be circumvented by large molecules which reach the extravascular space. It now appears that the endothelial cells which line the capillaries form the only continuous barrier between the blood plasma and the extracellular clefts of the nervous system [33].

Endothelial cells in central nervous system capillaries differ from those found elsewhere in that at points of apposition, the outer leaflets of the unit membranes are fused, forming a *tight* junction; in other capillary beds, endothelial cells are separated by 200–300 Å gaps. The *tight* junctions between CNS endothelial cells are discontinuous but overlapping and form a barrier to proteins and colloids [4].

In the region of the choroid plexus, large molecules pass through the fenestrated capillaries but cannot enter the CSF because of tight junctions between the choroid epithelial cells. In special regions, such as the median eminence and area postrema, large molecules pass through fenestrated capillaries but cannot enter the ventricular system because of tight junctions between ependymal cells in these regions. Elsewhere, ependymal cells joined by gap junctions permit passage of large molecules from the ventricles to the vicinity of the neurons and glia [4].

Figure 26-1 illustrates some of the relations between cells in the nervous system outlined above.

FLUID ENVIRONMENT OF NEURONS AND GLIA

The ionic composition of blood plasma and CSF differ. Does the immediate environment of the neurons and glia resemble the composition of the blood, the ventricular CSF, or is it some compromise between the two? In this connection, it should be noted that CNS capillaries penetrate within about 100 μ of all neurons and glia, whereas the ventricular fluid is frequently much more distant. It has not been possible to sample directly the fluid in contact with the neurons and glia for chemical analysis. It has been possible, however, to utilize physiological responses of the cells to bio-

NEUROGLIAL-NEURONAL INTERACTIONS 739

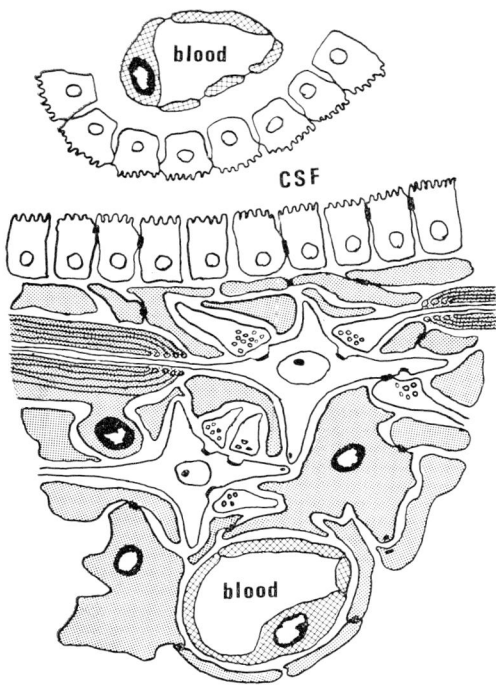

FIG. 26-1. Some cellular relations in the vertebrate nervous system. Top: Blood capillary perfusing choroid epithelium. Endothelial cells lining capillary have fenestrated walls which permit passage of large molecules. Below capillary are choroid epithelial cells. These cells secrete the CSF, are joined by tight junctions which form a continuous barrier. Below CSF are ependymal cells, joined only by spots of attachments, *gap junctions,* allowing diffusion from CSF to intercellular clefts. Below ependymal cells are glial cells (shaded areas), which are occasionally joined by spotlike gap junctions. Two types of neuronal contacts are shown. Chemical synapses with presynaptic terminals containing synaptic vesicles and separated from postsynaptic cell by synaptic cleft and combination electrical-chemical synapse where part of presynaptic terminal forms a gap junction with postsynaptic neuron. Two axons are covered with myelin sheaths formed by oligodendroglia. Brain capillary, bottom, is surrounded by astroglial end-feet, occasionally joined by gap junctions, permitting diffusion from extravascular space to intercellular clefts. Endothelial cells of capillary are joined by tight junctions and form a continuous barrier between blood plasma and intercellular cleft system. Basement lamina surrounding capillaries not shown. (Based primarily on [4].)

assay fluid in the intercellular clefts. One test utilized the sensitivity of activity in respiratory neurons to changes in pH [10].

Variations in the pH, pCO_2, and HCO_3^- in blood and CSF were produced by chronic administration to goats of either NH_4Cl or $NaHCO_3$. In these experiments, the plasma HCO_3^- varied from 10–45 mM; the CSF HCO_3^- varied only between 15–25 mM, providing evidence not only for differences between CSF and plasma composition but also for a homeostatic process tending to keep the composition of the CSF constant. Changes in alveolar ventilation when alveolar pCO_2 was varied were measured. The results were clear: the activity of the respiratory neurons could not easily be related to blood pH or pCO_2, but was rather a single exponential function of the pH of the CSF. These results were entirely consistent with the view that the $[H^+]$ around the respiratory neurons is similar to that in CSF rather than in plasma.

Cohen, Gerschenfeld, and Kuffler [7] used the glial membrane potential in the optic nerve of *Necturus* as an indicator of $[K^+]$ in the intercellular clefts. The plasma $[K^+]$ was increased from 2–9 mM by maintaining the animals in potassium-rich water. Under these conditions the CSF $[K^+]$ increased from 2 mM to only 4 mM. Figure 26-2A shows that the relation between membrane potential and log CSF $[K^+]$ had a slope of 58 mV, the same as found in vitro (see below). By contrast, the relation between glial membrane potential and blood $[K^+]$ (Fig. 26-2B) had a slope of only 22 mV. The membrane potential of skeletal muscle fibers changed as expected from changes in blood potassium. It was concluded that potassium concentration of the fluid immediately surrounding the glial cells was more than 90 percent determined by the $[K^+]$ of the CSF.

These experiments demonstrate that the composition of the fluid surrounding neurons and glia under steady-state conditions resembles the CSF rather than the blood.

Changes in blood composition can rapidly affect neuronal activity, and it is known that substances such as CO_2, glucose, and K^+ exchange rapidly between blood and CSF [9]. Thus, although there is a

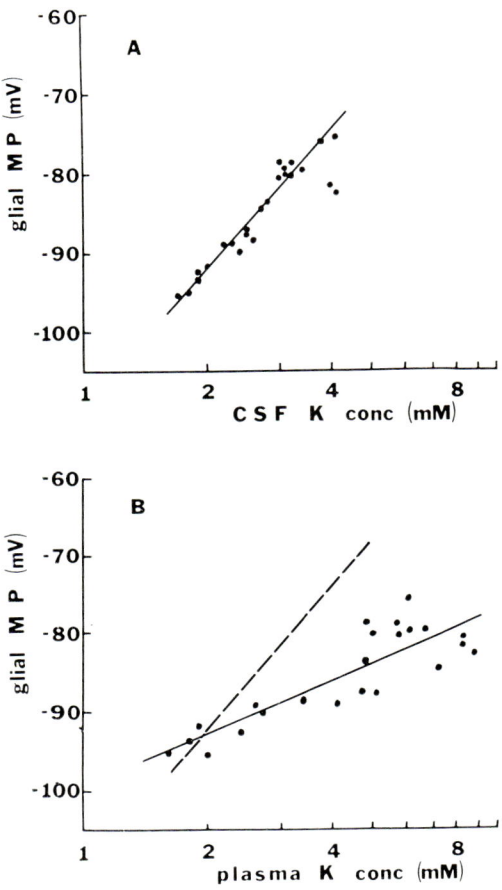

Fig. 26-2. Relation between glial membrane potential and potassium concentration (log scale) in CSF (*A*) and in plasma (*B*). (*A*) Solid line drawn with slope of 59 mV, according to the Nernst equation. (*B*) Solid line calculated to fit points (slope of 22 mV) and is significantly different from dashed line with slope of 59 mV. (From [7].)

structural *barrier* to large molecules, small molecules can penetrate the CNS but their concentrations surrounding neurons and glia are controlled presumably by active processes. The study of these processes has been impeded by thinking of the environment of neurons and glia as being surrounded by a mysterious barrier. The actual situation is probably related to that found in the kidney, with the sequence of events somewhat reversed. The last step in the process, reabsorption of the CSF, appears to involve passive filtration from the subarachnoid space through the arachnoid villi into venous sinuses. The initial step, production of CSF, involves active transport and other regulatory processes requiring metabolic energy. To attribute these complex processes to a *barrier* is analogous to explaining the difference in concentration of glucose in blood and urine to a blood-urine barrier.

Regulation of Cerebrospinal Fluid

Under steady-state conditions the composition of the CSF remains remarkably constant despite wide fluctuations in plasma composition. This is of physiological importance in that neuronal function is critically dependent upon the ionic environment. For example, Leusen [23] found that perfusion of cerebral ventricles of anesthetized dogs with varying concentrations of Ca^{++}, Mg^{++}, and K^+ produced dramatic changes in the function of the vasomotor system. The CSF concentrations of K^+, Ca^{++}, Mg^{++}, and HCO_3^- are so well controlled that their levels in CSF appear to be remarkably independent of their levels in plasma [9, 10, 31].

The complexity of the processes involved can be appreciated by considering the relation of CSF $[K^+]$ to plasma $[K^+]$ in patients with hypokalemia and hyperkalemia [8]. In the former, CSF $[K^+]$ is greater than plasma and in the latter, less. These results suggest an ability of the CSF regulating mechanisms to actively transport ions in both directions. Some, but not all, of the regulation is accomplished by the choroid plexus [1], which can secrete a fluid of low $[K^+]$ while being perfused with a solution of high $[K^+]$. Pappenheimer [30] suggests that $[HCO_3^-]$ in CSF is maintained by a system located in the vicinity of capillaries. CNS capillary endothelial cells form a continuous barrier [32], and it is conceivable that pumping activity in these cells participates in the regulation. The ependymal cells and glial cells might also play some role [18]; at present there is no direct evidence to support this view.

PHYSIOLOGICAL PROPERTIES OF GLIAL CELLS

The physiological properties of glial cells have been the subject of recent reviews [19, 20] and will be summarized briefly here. First, glial cells have high resting potentials of about 90 mV, which is 20 mV greater than that of neurons. The magnitude of the resting potential depends on the [K+] of the extracellular fluid, the same as in neurons and muscle fibers. In Fig. 26-3 the relation between membrane potential and external [K+] is shown for both glial cells in the isolated optic nerve of *Necturus* [21] and isolated myelinated frog axons [16]. It can be seen that at approximately normal values of [K+], 2–3 mEq per liter, the glial membrane potential is not only higher than that of the axons but also more sensitive to variations in [K+]$_o$. In fact, for [K+]$_o$ greater than about 1.5 mEq per liter, the glial cell membrane behaves as an accurate potassium electrode. The slope of the K+ membrane potential relation is predicted by the Nernst equation,

$$E = \frac{RT}{zF} \ln \frac{[K^+]_o}{[K^+]_i}$$

and at 25°C is 59 mV for a tenfold change in [K+]$_o$. The lesser slope for nerve at near normal [K+] suggests that the resting axon is more permeable to Na+ than is the glial cell.

The deviation from linearity of the glial membrane potential vs log [K+] relation at low [K+]$_o$ may reflect a small resting permeability of the glial cell to Na+ or other ions. Alternatively, the [K+] surrounding the glial cell may be greater than that applied to the preparation. At low [K+]$_o$, potassium would leak out of the neurons or glia or both and accumulate in the intercellular clefts [11]. The above calculation of glial membrane potential at varying [K+]$_o$ assumes that [K+]$_i$ is constant. Good agreement between prediction and observation suggests that (1) the glial cells under these conditions do not modify [K+] in the clefts, and (2) the [K+]$_i$ remains constant despite variations in [K+]$_o$. However, because [K+]$_i$ is large, the results are not sufficiently precise to rule out the possibility that changes in [K+]$_i$ of a few percentages occur when [K+]$_o$ is altered.

It follows from the above considerations that when [K+]$_o$ = [K+]$_i$, the membrane potential of both nerve and glial cell should be abolished. Therefore, in these experiments, [K+]$_i$ in both axon and glia can be estimated to be approximately 100 mEq per liter.

When the membrane potential of the neuron is decreased by 10–20 mV, the cell gives rise to an all-or-none propagated action potential. By contrast, the membranes of glial cells do not respond with an electrical response if the membrane potential is either increased or decreased up to 100 mV by current passed through an intracellular microelectrode; the glial membrane behaves as a passive electrical circuit of a resistor and capacitor in parallel (cf. [36]). Difficulties in determining the membrane areas of neuroglia have so far precluded determination of the specific membrane resistance and capacitance.

Except in those few cases in which electrical synaptic transmission has been found to occur [2, 12], neurons are electrically isolated from one another. However, glial cells

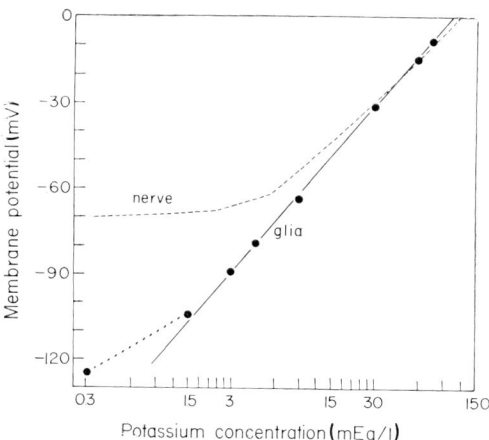

FIG. 26-3. Relation between membrane potential and external potassium concentration (log scale) for nerve and glia. Solid line has slope of 59 mV, according to the Nernst equation. Points are membrane potentials from glial cells in *Necturus* optic nerve [20]. Dashed line is relation found for frog myelinated nerve fibers [16].

are attached by specialized gap junctions which apparently provide a low-resistance pathway permitting ionic currents to flow between the cells. Thus, the glial cells form an electrical syncytium [21]. The function of these pathways between glial cells is not known. It appears that neurons and glia are electrically isolated from each other. That is, an action potential in an axon does not, by itself, produce a detectable potential change across the glial membrane. Transmembrane currents are shunted by the low-resistance intercellular cleft system [22].

Effect of Nerve Activity on Neuroglia

A hypothesis for coordination of neuronal and glial function implies a mechanism whereby neuronal activity signals the gial cell. It has been found that impulses in unmyelinated axons produce a depolarization of slow time course in the surrounding glia [28]. Figure 26-4A shows that following the passage of a single, synchronous nerve-volley in the optic nerve of *Necturus*, the glial cell slowly depolarizes. In Fig. 26-4B it can be seen that this depolarization disappears with a time course of seconds. If a series of shocks is delivered to the nerve, there is summation of the glial depolarizations. The magnitude of glial depolarization, it has been found, depends on the number of active axons and on the frequency of their discharge. Subsequent analysis revealed that glial depolarization is produced in a manner analogous to the negative afterpotential in axons [11, 28]. Potassium is liberated from the active axons and accumulates in the intercellular clefts between glial cells and neurons. As a result, the glial cell becomes depolarized. A similar effect of neuronal activity on *idle* cells in the mammalian cortex has been demonstrated [17].

With prolonged, repetitive neuronal discharge, the accumulation of potassium and concomitant glial depolarization can be surprisingly large. In the experiment illustrated in Fig. 26-5, the axons were stimulated at 10 per sec for 27 sec. The glial cell was depolarized by 48 mV, indicating that the [K+] in the clefts increased from 3 to 20 mEq per liter. It is known that synchronously stimulated, unmyelinated axons cannot follow frequencies much greater than 10 per sec [25]. At these high frequencies, conduction is apparently blocked in small-diameter axons by the dual effect of an increase in external potassium and increase in internal sodium. As indicated above, the linear relation between glial membrane potential and log $[K^+]_o$ suggests that when the whole nerve is exposed to varying concentrations of potassium, the

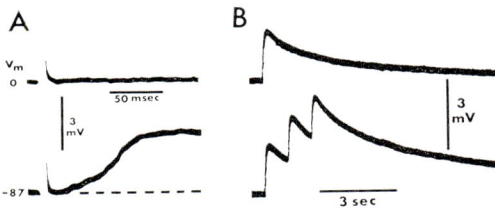

Fig. 26-4. Depolarization of glial cell produced by nerve impulses in *Necturus* optic nerve. (*A*) Top record: Microelectrode within optic nerve was "extracellular," $V_m = 0$, and nerve was stimulated by maximal electrical stimulus (shock artifact recorded, nerve action current not measurable). Bottom record: Electrode slightly advanced and glial membrane potential of −87 mV recorded. Same electrical stimulus produced a glial depolarization of 3.1 mV, which reached a peak in about 75 msec. (*B*) Top: Record of change in glial membrane potential following nerve stimulation shown on a much slower time scale. Bottom: Stimulus is repeated 3 times at 1-sec intervals, and there is summation of glial depolarizations [27].

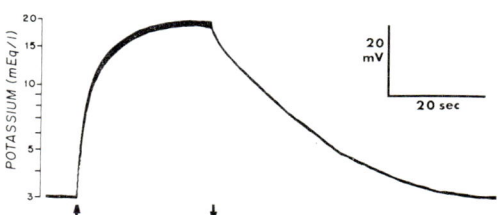

Fig. 26-5. Record of change in glial membrane potential with maximal stimulation of axons in *Necturus* optic nerve at 10 per sec for 27 sec. Resting potential was 86 mV. Arrows show duration of stimulation. On left is scale indicating concentration of external potassium which would produce equivalent depolarization. (Modified from [27].)

glial cells do not modify the potassium in intercellular clefts and the internal potassium remains constant.

These results do not rule out the possibility that glial cells play a role in equalizing the concentration of K+ in various portions of the intercellular cleft system when neuronal activity is not artificially synchronized. In fact, current through the glial syncytium will tend to equalize the potassium concentration throughout the cleft system. The actual mechanism of this *spatial buffering* can be simple. Depolarization of a portion of the glial syncytium apposed to active axons is probably produced by a small inward movement of potassium. As a result there will be a potential gradient between the depolarized part of the syncytium and a part where the membrane potential is normal. The current flow will cause potassium to leave the glial cells in regions not apposed to active axons. If the glial cell is primarily permeable to potassium, the net effect will be to move K+ from a region of high K+ to one of low K+. As long as a potential gradient remains between different portions of the syncytium, the current will continue to flow. When potassium distribution is uniform throughout the clefts, the glial membrane potential will be equal everywhere and there will be no further current flow.

This process does not necessarily involve active transport or a change in ionic concentrations of the glial cells. If, in addition, the glial cell $[K^+]_i$ increases by some active process, the concentration of potassium in the cleft would be further reduced. An increase in $[K^+]_i$ in the glia of only a few millimoles would produce a large decrease in the potassium concentration of the clefts because the volume of the glial cells is roughly ten times that of the cleft system [21]. The usefulness of such a process in neuronal recovery can be questioned, however, because neurons probably pump out sodium more rapidly in the presence of an increase in $[K^+]_o$. Specific details concerning the rate and magnitude of the redistribution and regulation of $[K^+]_o$ can be worked out only after the specific membrane permeabilities and physiological properties of the glial cells and the geometrical relations of the glial syncytium are better known.

In the above discussion it was postulated that the glial cell acts as a barrier to the diffusion of K+ away from active axons. Recently, Nicholls and Baylor [26] obtained direct evidence of this in studies of leech ganglia. They compared the accumulation of K+, produced by repetitive nerve activity, outside neurons surrounded by glia and in those where the glial cell was cut away. In the latter case the accumulation of K+ around the neuron was markedly reduced.

The question of whether glial cells modify the ionic environment of less active neurons has been subjected to a direct test in the isolated leech central nervous system [27]. The activity of neurons was recorded in one neuron when the glial covering was intact and in a second neuron after surgical disruption left the surface of a considerable part of the neuron naked to the bathing solution. External sodium and potassium concentrations were varied, and it was found that the resting and action potentials of the two neurons changed in similar fashion. As expected, changes in the naked neuron were produced more rapidly due to removal of diffusion barriers. These results indicate that at equilibrium both neurons were surrounded by the same fluid, and it can be concluded that (1) glia do not modify the sodium and potassium concentrations surrounding resting neurons, and (2) glial covering is not necessary for the signaling activity of neurons. Additional evidence that glial cells are not necessary for the signaling activity of neurons comes from studies of neocortex of newborn kittens. In these preparations the neurons are active prior to development of the glial elements [35].

Consequences of Potassium Accumulation

It can be seen in Fig. 26-2 that the resting potential of an axon is relatively insensitive to small increases in $[K^+]_o$ when compared to that of glia. Except in cases of synchronous repetitive impulses in a nonmyelinated nervous pathway, the accumulation of K+ will affect very little conduction of the nervous impulse. On the other hand, at synapses even small changes in [K+] can have important effects on the spontaneous release of transmitter as well as the release following a nerve impulse [13, 34]. Thus, fluctuations of $[K^+]_o$ around nerve terminals and cell bodies in the nervous system could exert an influence on the integrative activity at synapses. The effects are, however, quite complicated, and it is difficult to assess their functional significance. For example, a small increase in $[K^+]_o$ around a neuron would tend to depolarize the cell toward threshold, thus increasing the chances of an excitatory influence producing an action potential. On the other hand, release of excitatory and inhibitory transmitters will be changed by depolarization of the presynaptic terminal.

The overall result on the impulse activity of the cell is difficult to predict. In addition, it is necessary to consider effects of [K+] on pacemaker activity, sensitivity of postsynaptic receptors to transmitters, and on the production and time course of afterpotentials in both presynaptic and postsynaptic cells [26]. Another consideration is the effect of changes in $[K^+]_o$ on the longer term functions of the synapse; for example, facilitation and posttetanic potentiation [24].

GLIAL CONTRIBUTION TO EXTERNAL POTENTIALS

Current will flow between parts of the glial syncytium depolarized by activity in adjacent neurons and parts near inactive neurons due to the difference in membrane potential at the two points. These currents apparently can be recorded from the surface of the structures [28]. Figure 26-6B shows a simultaneous recording of extracellular action potential and glial membrane potential during repetitive stimulation of a frog optic nerve. It can be seen that the time course of the rise and decay of the whole nerve negative afterpotential is similar to the change in glial membrane potential. What is the contribution of changes in glial membrane potential to the extracellular record? This question has been quantitatively studied by Cohen and Kuffler (personal communication) in the *Necturus*

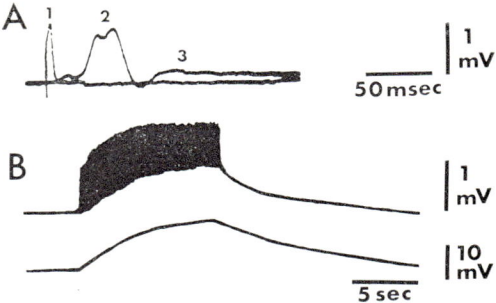

FIG. 26-6. Intracellular and extracellular recordings from frog optic nerve. (*A*) Extracellular *monophasic* record of compound action potential set up by a single maximal nerve stimulus; short-latency deflection (1) is due to medullated axons and is followed by more slowly conducting, nonmedullated fibers (2). Last is small negative afterpotential (3). (*B*) Upper record: Same recording conditions as in (*A*), but stimulation at 10 sec and displayed at a slower sweep speed. Summation of negative afterpotentials. Lower record: Simultaneous recording with an intracellular electrode in a glial cell. Note similar time course of rising phase of glial depolarization with potential recorded with surface leads. Calibrations: (*A*) and (*B*), upper trace, same amplification, different time base; (*B*) both records, same time base, different amplification [27].

optic nerve. In these experiments the extracellular potential was recorded from the whole nerve across a sucrose gap and the glial membrane potential near the gap. A second current-passing electrode was inserted in a glial cell to depolarize the glial cells but not the axons. Under these conditions 22–46 percent of the change in glial membrane potential could be recorded from the whole nerve with the extracellular leads. In other experiments, the axons were subjected to repetitive stimulation, and a posttetanic hyperpolarization was recorded extracellularly at a time when the glial cells were still depolarized. During these stages the axons are apparently greatly hyperpolarized due to activity in an electrogenic pump, while the external [K+] is still elevated and causing depolarization of the glial cells.

These experiments point out the great difficulty in trying to interpret potential changes recorded from the surface of the nervous system. Glial cells become depolarized following activity in either excitatory or inhibitory axons. At the same time, the neurons may be hyperpolarized or depolarized due to transmitter effects or afterpotentials. Therefore, external currents resulting from potential changes in neurons and glia might be in the same or opposite direction. The magnitude and sign of the potential recorded from the surface will depend on magnitude and direction of the potential change in each type of cell, as well as the relative volumes of underlying neurons and glia.

REFERENCES

1. Ames, A., III, Higashi, K., and Nesbett, F. B. Relation of potassium concentration in choroid-plexus fluid to that in the plasma. *J. Physiol.* (London) 181:506, 1965.
2. Bennett, M. V. L., Aljure, E., Nakajima, Y., and Pappas, G. D. Electrotonic junctions between teleost spinal neurons: Electrophysiology and ultrastructure. *Science* 141:262, 1963.
3. Brightman, M. W. The distribution within the brain of ferritin injected into cerebrospinal fluid compartments. II. Parenchymal distribution. *Amer. J. Anat.* 117:193, 1965.
4. Brightman, M. W., and Reese, T. S. Junctions between intimately apposed cell membranes in the vertebrate brain. *J. Cell Biol.* 40:648, 1969.
5. Bradbury, M. W. B., and Davson, H. The transport of potassium between blood, cerebrospinal fluid and brain. *J. Physiol.* (London) 181:151, 1965.
6. Bradbury, M. W. B., and Kleeman, C. R. Stability of the potassium content of cerebrospinal fluid and brain. *Amer. J. Physiol.* 213:519, 1967.
7. Cohen, M. W., Gerschenfeld, H. M., and Kuffler, S. W. Ionic environment of neurones and glial cells in the brain of an amphibian. *J. Physiol.* (London) 197:363, 1968.
8. Cooper, E. S., Lechner, E., and Bellet, S. Relations between serum and cerebrospinal fluid electrolytes under normal and abnormal conditions. *Amer. J. Med.* 18:613, 1955.
9. Davson, H. *Physiology of the Cerebrospinal Fluid*. London: Churchill, 1967.
10. Fencl, V., Miller, T. B., and Pappenheimer, J. R. Studies on the respiratory response to disturbances of acid-base balance, with deductions concerning the ionic composition of cerebral interstitial fluid. *Amer. J. Physiol.* 210:459, 1966.
11. Frankenhaeuser, B., and Hodgkin, A. L. The after-effects of impulses in the giant nerve fibres of *Loligo*. *J. Physiol.* (London) 131:341, 1956.
12. Furshpan, E. J. "Electrical transmission" at an excitatory synapse in a vertebrate brain. *Science* 144:878, 1964.
13. Gage, P. W., and Quastel, D. M. J. Dual effect of potassium on transmitter release. *Nature* (London) 206:625, 1965.
14. Golgi, C. *Opera Omnia*. Milano: U. Hoepli, 1903, vol. 2.
15. Horstman, E., and Meves, H. Die Feinstruktur des molekularen Rindengraues und ihre physiologische Bedeutung. *Z. Zellforsch.* 49:569, 1959.
16. Huxley, A. F., and Stämpfli, R. Effect of potassium and sodium on resting and action potentials of single myelinated nerve fibres. *J. Physiol.* (London) 112:496, 1951.
17. Karahashi, Y., and Goldring, S. Intracellular potentials from "idle" cells in cerebral cortex of cat. *Electroenceph. Clin. Neurophysiol.* 20:600, 1966.
18. Katzman, R., Graziani, L., Kaplan, R., and Escriva, A. Exchange of cerebrospinal fluid potassium with blood and brain: Study in normal and ouabain perfused cats. *Arch. Neurol.* (Chicago) 13:513, 1965.
19. Kuffler, S. W. Neuroglial cells: Physiological properties and a potassium mediated effect of neuronal activity on the glial membrane potential. *Proc. Roy. Soc.* [Biol.] 168:1, 1967.
20. Kuffler, S. W., and Nicholls, J. G. The physiology of neuroglial cells. *Ergebn. Physiol.* 57:1, 1966.
21. Kuffler, S. W., Nicholls, J. G., and Orkand, R. K. Physiological properties of glial

cells in the central nervous system of amphibia. *J. Neurophysiol.* 29:768, 1966.

22. Kuffler, S. W., and Potter, D. D. Glia in the leech central nervous system. Physiological properties and neuron-glia relationship. *J. Neurophysiol.* 27:290, 1964.

23. Leusen, I. The influence of calcium, potassium and magnesium ions in cerebrospinal fluid on vasomotor system. *J. Physiol.* (London) 110:319, 1950.

24. Liley, A. W., and North, K. A. K. An electrical investigation of effects of repetitive stimulation on mammalian neuromuscular junction. *J. Neurophysiol.* 16:509, 1953.

25. Maturana, H. R. The fine anatomy of the optic nerve of *Anurans*—an electron microscope study. *J. Biophys. Biochem. Cytol.* 7:107, 1960.

26. Nicholls, J. G., and Baylor, D. A. The after effects of nerve impulses on glial cells and integrative processes in leech ganglia. *Proc. I.U.P.S.* 6:117, 1968.

27. Nicholls, J. G., and Kuffler, S. W. Extracellular space as a pathway for exchange between blood and neurons in central nervous system of leech: The ionic composition of glial cells and neurons. *J. Neurophysiol.* 27:645, 1964.

28. Orkand, R. K., Nicholls, J. G., and Kuffler, S. W. The effect of nerve impulses on the membrane potential of glial cells in the central nervous system of amphibia. *J. Neurophysiol.* 29:788, 1966.

29. Palay, S. L. The morphology of synapses in the central nervous system. *Exp. Cell. Res.* Suppl., 5:275, 1958.

30. Pappenheimer, J. R. The Ionic Composition of Cerebral Extracellular Fluid and Its Relation to Control of Breathing. *Harvey Lect.* 61:71, 1967.

31. Peters, A. The formation and structure of myelin sheath in the central nervous system. *J. Biophys. Biochem. Cytol.* 8:431, 1960.

32. Reed, D. J., Woodbury, D. M., Jacobs, L., and Squires, R. Factors affecting distribution of iodide in brain and cerebrospinal fluid. *Amer. J. Physiol.* 209:757, 1965.

33. Reese, T. S., and Karnovsky, M. J. Fine structural localization of a blood brain barrier to exogenous peroxidase. *J. Cell Biol.* 34:207, 1967.

34. Takeuchi, A., and Takeuchi, N. Changes in potassium concentration around motor nerve terminals produced by current flow, and their effects on neuromuscular transmission. *J. Physiol.* (London) 155:46, 1961.

35. Voeller, K., Pappas, G. D., and Purpura, D. P. Electron microscope study of development of cat superficial neocortex. *Exp. Neurol.* 7:107, 1963.

36. Wardell, W. M. Electrical and pharmacological properties of mammalian neuroglial cells in tissue culture. *Proc. Roy. Soc.* [*Biol.*] 165:326, 1966.

37. Windle, W. F. *Biology of Neuroglia.* Springfield, Ill.: Thomas, 1958.

Discussion

MORPHOLOGY OF NEUROGLIAL CELLS*

SANFORD L. PALAY

The relation between neurons and neuroglial cells in the central nervous system has long puzzled anatomists and physiologists. Aside from the production of the myelin sheath, no function has been agreed upon for the neuroglia, although a number of hypotheses have been put forward (see discussion in [5]). Most of these proposals are variations on one or more of the following ideas: (1) Neuroglial cells provide physical support for nerve cells and their processes. (2) Neuroglial cells provide pathways for nutrients and metabolic products to pass between blood vessels and nerve cells. (3) Neuroglial cells insulate nerve cells and their processes from one another. (4) Neuroglial cells are concerned with the more complex and persistent phenomena of brain activity such as memory and learning. (5) Neuroglial cells are reserve cells activated by injury to the nervous system and are concerned with filling in defects and repair. There is no compelling evidence for any of these ideas except for the insulation and repair hypotheses, which are strongly supported in regard to oligodendroglia by the existence of myelin and in regard to astrocytes by certain kinds of scars and plaques. But modern electrophysiological data have not as yet provided any definite evidence that neuroglial cells do anything at all; modern biochemical data have been extremely difficult to obtain and are largely controversial not only with respect to their significance but also to their pertinence. Consequently, neuroglial research remains hazardous and anyone who ventures to support an old hypothesis or propose a new one does so at his peril.

As Orkand has pointed out, the processes of neuroglial cells encapsulate nerve cells and segregate them from the non-nervous tissue and to some extent from one another. This property is best exemplified by the myelin sheath, the most regular and elaborate structure produced by neuroglial cells. It consists of the surface membrane of a glial cell wrapped helically around an axon and compacted into a paracrystalline array. In the peripheral nervous system the myelin-producing cell is the Schwann cell; in the central nervous system it is the oligodendrocyte.

Astrocytic Lamellar Processes

This tendency to form membranous expansions is not, however, confined to the Schwann cells and oligodendrocytes; it is also displayed by astrocytes. As Fig. D26-1 shows, slender astrocytic processes are inserted between neural elements in the neuropil. These processes are actually extremely thin lamellae given off from the cell body and main processes of protoplasmic astrocytes. They can be so thin that their opposite surfaces are only a few Ångstrom units apart (arrows in Fig. D26-1). Sometimes these lamellae are piled up into two or three layers, but they never become compact as the myelin sheath does.

Certain nerve cells are characteristically encapsulated in one or two astrocytic lamellae, which cover the cell body and all of the processes, except for small openings where preterminal axons slip through and come into synaptic contact with the neuronal surface. One of these neurons is shown in Fig. D26-2, which is an electron micrograph of a Purkinje cell in the rat's cerebellum. This entire cell is ensheathed in astrocytic layers, including the dendritic tree and the axon, shown here as it leaves

---

* The original work reported in this discussion was supported by PHS Research Grant NB03659 from the National Institute of Neurological Diseases and Stroke.

the cell body. Other cells with similar capsules are pyramidal cells in the cerebral cortex and small cells in the substantia gelatinosa. There are also numerous cells that do not have an astrocytic sheath, for example, granule cells and basket cells in the cerebellar cortex. These apparently are not isolated by any intervening cellular structure. Thus, for example, hundreds of granule cell axons can be found traveling together in parallel array without any glial investment and therefore in even closer contact with one another than are axons in unmyelinated nerve. This arrangement is encountered quite frequently in the central nervous system.

THREE KINDS OF GLIA-NEURONAL RELATIONSHIPS IN THE CENTRAL NERVOUS SYSTEM. (a) Nerve cells can be entirely naked, that is, directly apposed one to another without any intervening neuroglial cell, as in the granule cell layer of the cerebellar cortex.

(b) Nerve cells can be surrounded completely or partially by an oligodendrocyte, as in the myelinated fibers of the white matter or in the anterior horn of the spinal cord and the cerebral cortex, where oligodendrocytes are often satellites to the large neuronal perikarya.

(c) Nerve cells can be surrounded completely or partially by astrocytes, as in the cerebellar cortex or the lateral vestibular nucleus, where Purkinje cells and Deiters' giant cells, respectively, are typical examples.

The last type of arrangement is extremely common. Astrocytes, not oligodendrocytes, are generally the true satellites of the neuron throughout the gray matter of the central nervous system. In some places where, at the light microscope level, the neuronal perikarya appear to have oligodendrocyte satellites, examination in the electron microscope may reveal that neighboring astrocytes are insinuating their tenuous laminar processes between the oligodendrocytes and the neuron. A good example of this arrangement is seen in the lateral vestibular nucleus [6]. Even where the oligodendrocyte does come into direct apposition with the neuronal perikaryon it usually occupies only a small part of the neuronal surface, the rest being preempted by astrocytic processes and synaptic terminals.

The important point here is not, however, precise identification of the perineuronal satellite cell, but recognition of the coherence of the central nervous tissue. All available space is occupied by cellular elements separated only by shallow intercellular clefts. As Orkand reported in this chapter, these clefts are quite sufficient for the transport of nutrients, metabolic products, and ions between blood vessels and cells residing in the central nervous system. Because the spaces are so narrow, it is likely that their content is readily susceptible to modification by the cells on their borders and that the cells in turn are sensitive to the microenvironment provided by extracellular fluid. Orkand has given an example of this reciprocal relationship in his description of the results of potassium ion accumulation. Studies of this type may eventually elucidate the significance of lamellar astrocytic processes that everywhere fill the interstices between the neurons.

Astrocytic Lamellar Processes, Capillaries, and Synapses

The importance of neuroglia and especially astrocytic lamellar processes in regulating the microenvironment of central nervous tissue is indicated by their morphological relation to the blood vessels. As illustrated in Fig. D26-3, astrocytic lamellae surround the capillaries and separate them

FIG. D26-1. Gray matter in anterior horn of cervical spinal cord from rat. Figure shows small field of neuropil between perikarya of motor neurons. Dendrites (D) of several sizes are seen in transverse and oblique section. Seated upon them are axonal terminals (t) containing synaptic vesicles and mitochondria. Thin astrocytic lamellae (A) are disposed in spaces intervening between neural elements. Some of these are so attenuated that they consist of little more than cell membrane (arrows). Small unmyelinated axons (ax) and one myelinated fiber (max) also lie within this field. $\times 38,000$

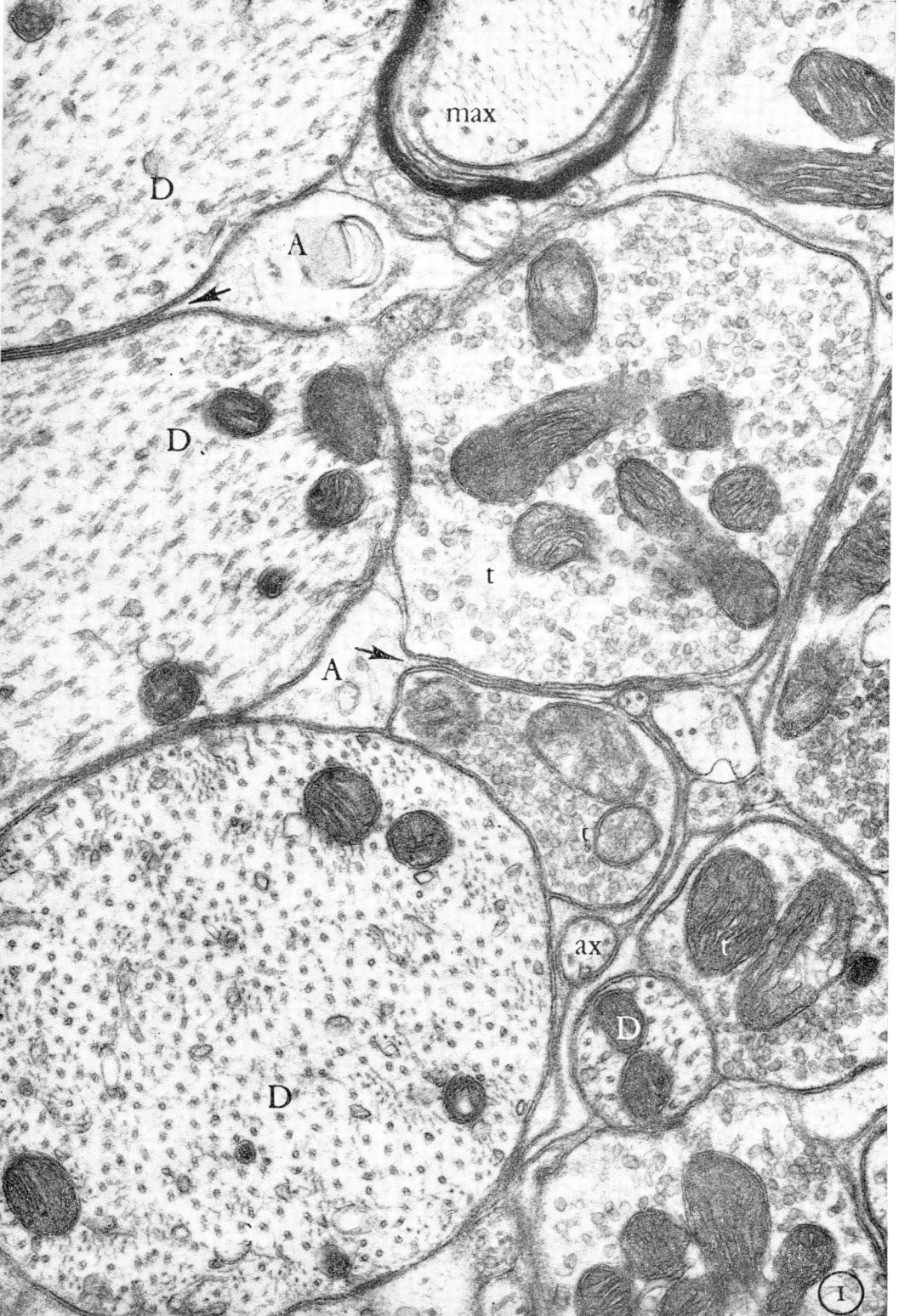

Fig. D26-2. Cerebellar cortex of rat. Figure shows base of a Purkinje cell at point where its axon exits from perikaryon. Both perikaryon (P) and initial segment of axon (ax) are ensheathed in astrocytic lamellae (A), which separate them from terminal branches of basket fibers in the neighborhood. ×34,000.

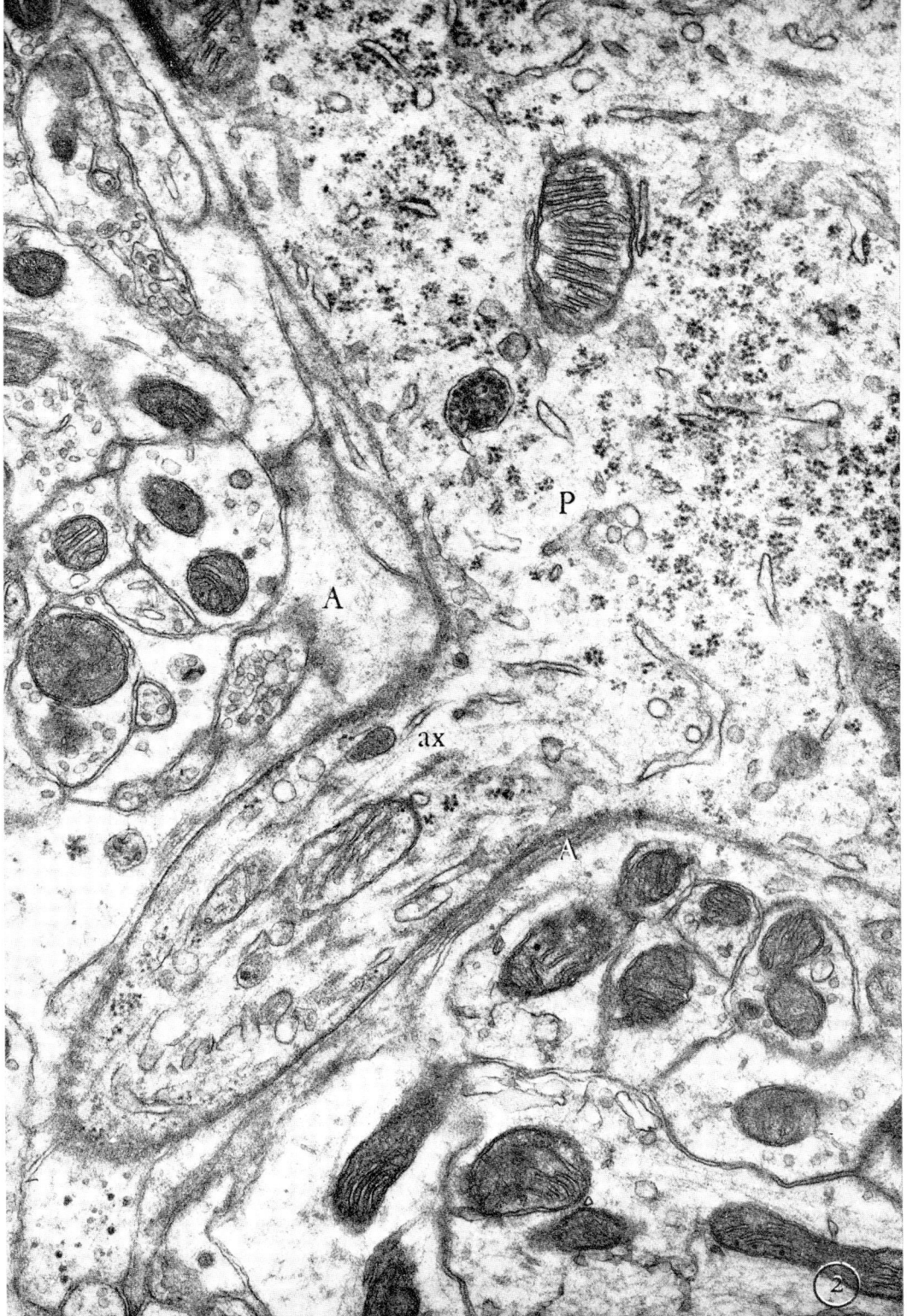

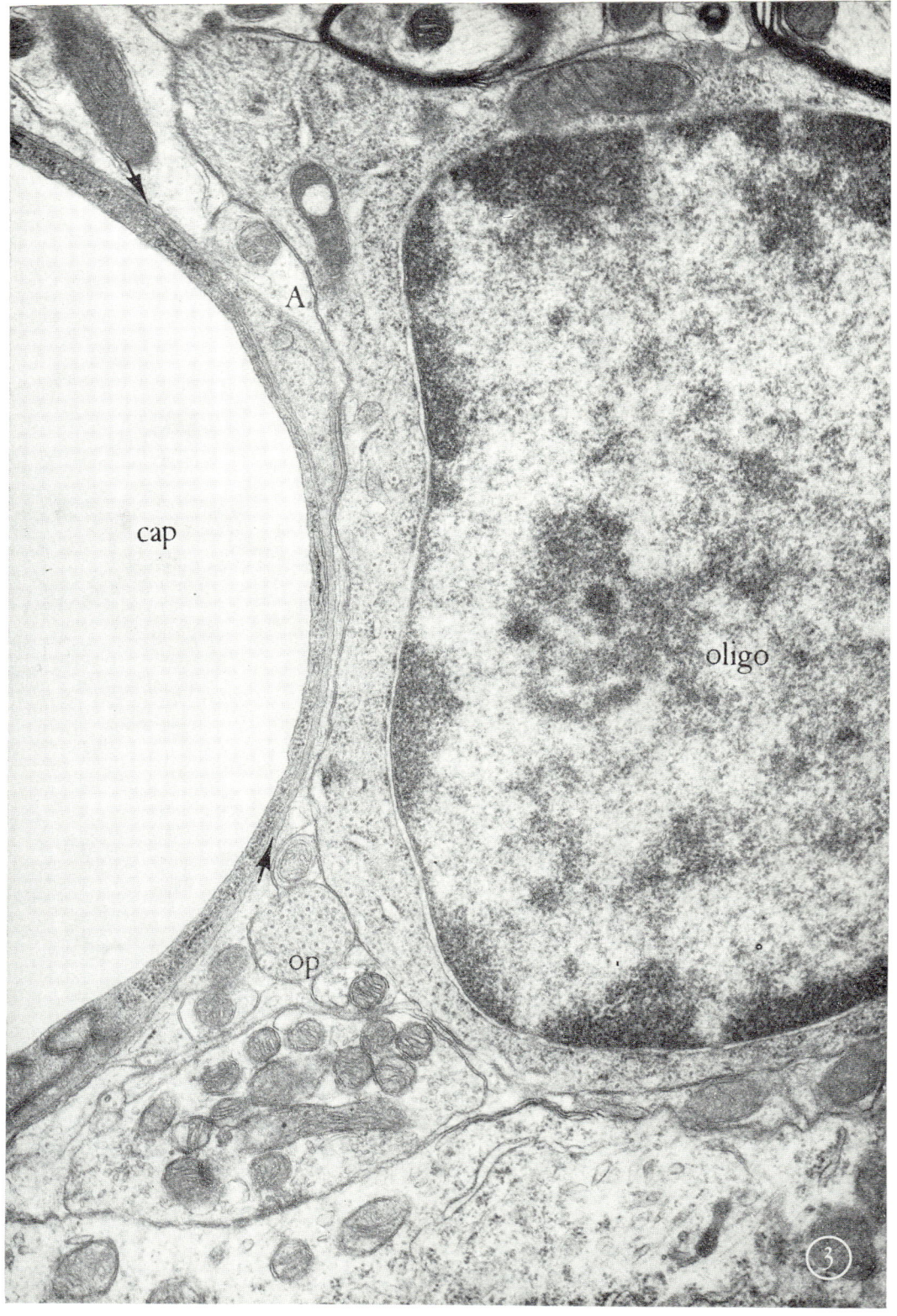

from the brain tissue proper. Although it is now generally conceded [1] that this glial investment does not constitute a blood-brain barrier, such an arrangement means that all substances passing between the blood vessel and the neural tissue must pass over or through an astrocytic process and consequently may be subject to modification by this cell.

Some 70 years ago Ramón y Cajal [2] proposed that neuroglial cells, especially those we now call astrocytes, served an insulating function, leading nerve fibers to their proper destinations and confining nervous currents to their proper territories. Several years ago, Peters and Palay [3, 4] suggested a refinement of this concept, derived from a study of distribution of astrocytic processes in various parts of the central nervous system. It was hypothesized that neuroglial cells served to insulate receptive surfaces of the nerve cell from nonspecific or extraneous synaptic influences, either in the form of transmitter chemicals or local imbalance of ions. The studies described by Orkand lend some slight support to this as yet untested idea. Whether or not these concepts are correct, it seems clear from recent physiological work that neuroglial cells are not just stuffing, space fillers created to maintain the plump shape of the brain.

REFERENCES

1. Brightman, M. W., and Reese, T. S. Junctions between intimately apposed cell membranes in the vertebrate brain. *J. Cell Biol.* 40:648, 1969.
2. Cajal, S. R. *Histologie du système nerveux de l'homme et des vertébrés.* Paris: Maloine, 1909, vol. 1. Reprinted, Madrid: Consejo Superior de Investigaciones Científicas, 1952.
3. Palay, S. L. The Role of Neuroglia in the Organization of the Central Nervous System. In Rodahl, K., and Issekutz, B. (Eds.), *Nerve as a Tissue.* New York: Hoeber Med. Div., Harper & Row, 1966, pp. 3–10.
4. Peters, A., and Palay, S. L. An electron microscope study of the distribution and patterns of astroglial processes in the central nervous system. *J. Anat.* 99:419, 1965.
5. Peters, A., Palay, S. L., and Webster, H. de F. *The Fine Structure of the Nervous System.* New York: Hoeber Med. Div., Harper & Row, in press.
6. Sotelo, C., and Palay, S. L. The fine structure of the lateral vestibular nucleus in the rat. *J. Cell Biol.* 36:151, 1968.

FIG. D26-3. Anterior horn of cervical spinal cord of rat. Small capillary (cap) lies at the left side of figure with oligodendrocyte (oligo) beside it and perikaryon of motor neuron at bottom. Capillary endothelium varies in thickness but is smooth and shows little sign of pinocytosis. Surrounding it is a thin basal lamina (arrows) consisting of condensed extracellular matrix. Next layer is formed by astrocytic lamellae (A) which everywhere separate neural tissue, in strict sense, from other tissues. In this figure a highly attenuated astrocytic lamella intervenes between capillary wall and oligodendrocyte. The latter cell gives off a process from its upper pole, and a smaller process (op) can be seen in transverse section beside lower end of cell. ×29,000.

27

Theoretical Concepts of Synchrony

MARVIN MINSKY

WHAT CAN CAUSE a collection of normally independent units suddenly to act simultaneously? One way is to have a central control system, with lines radiating out to each of the units. At the other extreme, an attempt could be made to imagine a distributed system in which negotiations circulate between nearby units, culminating in global agreement about action at some future moment. When a great many neurons fire at once, or periodically, there must be *some* synchronizing mechanism. It could be as simple as a rapid chain reaction originating from some center. Or it might be a complex and sudden *constructive interference* effect of propagating wave patterns.

This article makes no pretense of concern with any specific theory of epilepsy or, for that matter, of neurons. It is an attempt to collect a variety of ideas about synchrony from the huge range of activities in modern mathematics.

SYNCHRONIZATION OF REFRACTORY CONDUCTION NETWORKS

Our first model is concerned with the kinds of synchronous activity that can be maintained in a pulse-conduction medium with all-or-none excitation and refractory period. The surprisingly simple and general conclusions described here were established by Selfridge [17] in developing some of the suspicions of Wiener and Rosenblueth [19] about the mechanisms of cardiac flutter. The theorems (for this is a mathematical rather than a physiological theory) appear to apply equally well to waves in uniform sheets, volumes, or mixed reticula of volumes, sheets, and networks of conducting fibers. The theory does *not* attempt to represent the behavior of networks containing unilateral elements, like synapses, that do not propagate activity equally in all directions.

Consider first an annular disc of a conduction medium that (1) is all or none, (2) has constant conduction velocity in all directions, and (3) has a definite refractory time. Then if any point is excited, a wave will spread out from that center.

Figure 27-1 shows the advancing wave front as a solid line, the refractory area as shaded, and the trailing recovery wave as a dotted line. Eventually, the wave dies out completely, partly by reaching the region's edge and partly by mutual annihilation of colliding fronts (Fig. 27-2).

It can be shown that *no matter what the geometry of the medium and the choice of the stimulus points, the activity from a single volley will disappear; no circulating loops can arise.*

But it is possible, with a two-volley stimulus, to start perpetual cycles in which a wave circulates around a boundary. To do this, start a pair of waves, as in Fig. 27-1, and then stimulate a region that completely covers one of the recovery fronts, as in Fig. 27-3. This produces a third wave (its mate does not propagate because it is in the refractory region) that persists forever after the original pair is annihilated.

Now imagine that a number of such unpaired wavefronts have been created somehow in a medium with the same local properties but with an arbitrarily complicated geometry (Fig. 27-4). Selfridge's main theorem shows that: *if all external stimulation is stopped, the entire activity will even-*

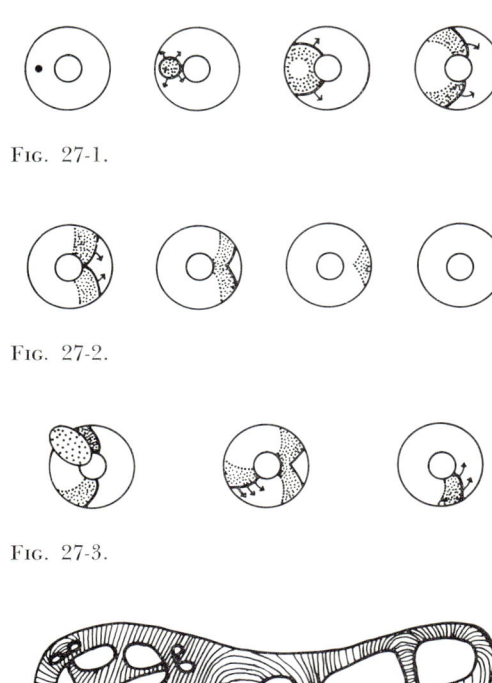

FIG. 27-1.

FIG. 27-2.

FIG. 27-3.

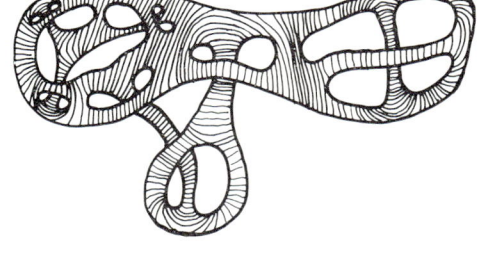

FIG. 27-4.

tually take on a single repetitive rhythm. That is, all points will fire at the same frequency or, more precisely, with the same exactly repeating rhythm—although not in the same phase. Thus, two basically different cyclic activities cannot be maintained, such as might be expected if waves were to circulate around two boundaries of different length. Although we cannot here give all details of the complicated proof, we can show, in the case of two wave cycles, why both cannot persist indefinitely. Figure 27-5A shows a two-loop system. The closer wave spacing in the right-hand loop means that its points are excited with a higher mean frequency than those of the left-hand loop. If there were no *bridge* between the loops, the two frequencies could persist forever. But the time diagram (Fig. 27-5B) shows how the higher frequency pulses invade relentlessly the low-frequency domain.

With each pulse, the higher frequencies occupy a little more territory. Eventually this progression will invade the left-hand loop and destroy its native rhythm, with the final result as shown in Fig. 27-5C.

Mathematical proof shows that this is typical of what happens in more complicated networks: the pulses from some one circular path eventually dominate all others. Selfridge's proof uses a mathematical argument based on the numbers of intersections of wavefronts with closed paths; this is based in part on some ideas of H. Poincaré. The proof is complicated by the fact that there can exist *active boundaries* dynamically maintained in the interiors of uniform regions. Such a boundary can arise by stimulating a region containing a refractory recovery front, as shown in Fig. 27-6: this leads to a spiral wavefront originating from a point that oscillates back and forth along a line in the region's interior. In some computer-simulation experiments upon a somewhat different model, Farley and Clark [7] and Farley [6] report spiral phenomena that are presumably related to this.

Such an interior wave source, once started, persists in place even though there is no anatomically distinctive site there. It is basically unstable, however, because each turn of the spiral comes into contact with the refractory recovery front of the previous wave, so that an infinitesimal increase in refractory time could snuff it out. Other minor fluctuations could make its locus drift about. A possible stabilizing influence will be mentioned in the following section.

To summarize: a uniform propagation medium with refractory period, of any shape and connection structure, will become entirely dominated by a single rhythm. This rhythm could originate from a parasitic interior disturbance with no *anatomic* locus. All of these arguments assume that the network is isolated from external stimuli.

THEORETICAL CONCEPTS OF SYNCHRONY 757

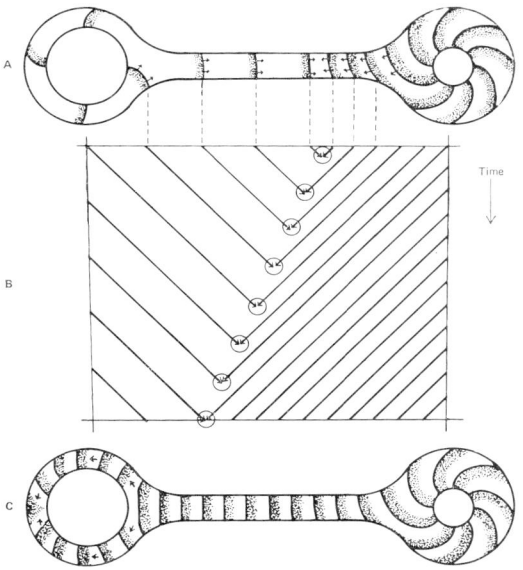

FIG. 27-5.

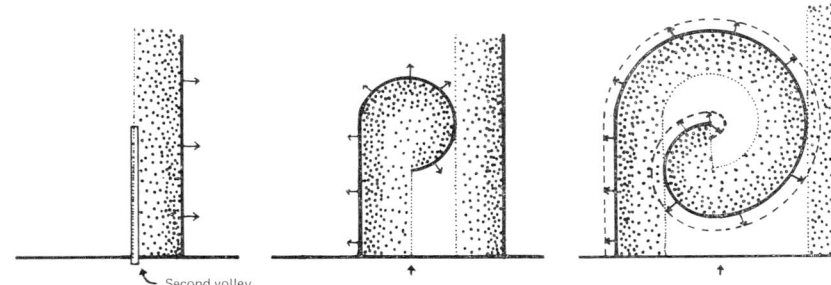

FIG. 27-6.

SYNAPTIC DELAY AND REGULARIZATION OF RHYTHMS

In the early computers, information was stored in *circulating delay lines* as patterns of pulses. Because in any real medium there are always velocity fluctuations, frequency dispersions (different frequencies propagating at different velocities), and other disturbances, one cannot depend on a circulating pattern to persist unchanged indefinitely; always included in computers are synchronization and pulse-reshaping devices in the loop. There is one kind of propagation disturbance that is particularly interesting in that it tends to smooth out irregular rhythms, and it is a condition to be expected in most neural activity. It is discussed here because of suspicion that it would stabilize the *interior wave sources* mentioned in the previous section, which would otherwise be too transient to be of serious concern.

Consider a closed circular ring of wave-conducting material, in which several unequally spaced pulses are circulating (Fig. 27-7). The ring may be thought of either as composed of chained neurons and synapses, in which case the pulses' velocities will depend mainly upon the synaptic delays, or

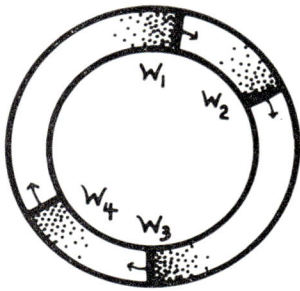

Fig. 27-7.

as a continuous band, in which case the velocities will depend upon the membrane's recovery and excitation properties. Consider the case in which *the conduction speed at any point is a decreasing function of the time since the last previous excitation of that point.*

In the discrete model (the one with cells and synapses) this supposes that the delay between excitation and firing increases when pulses come closer together. In Fig. 27-8, we show two regions in which this is true and one where it is not.

Observing the pattern in Fig. 27-7, note that the waves w_1 and w_3 are following their predecessors w_2 and w_4 rather closely. Therefore, assuming intervals for which $(dD)/(dT)$ is negative, w_1 and w_3 are in regions of relatively slow conductions, as compared with w_2 and w_4. Then w_1 and w_3 will become retarded and w_2 and w_4 advanced, relative to one another. Thus, they will tend to become more equally spaced.

In fact, if the time intervals involved all lie in the region in which the slope $(dD)/(dT)$ *of the delay curve is negative, then the waves will approach exactly equal spacing.* The equilibrium will be approached with the exponential-decay rapidity. (In the discrete case of separate neurons, it is required that $0 > \dfrac{dD}{dT} > -1$ for otherwise the *correction* would be larger than the *error* and equal spacing would not be a stable configuration.) This theorem can be proved by solving the differential or difference equations that describe the deviations of present pulse positions from the limiting configuration of the same number of equally spaced pulses. Incidentally, the speed at which the rhythm becomes perfectly regular warns away from models of memory, even of very short-term memory, in which information is stored in loops by *pulse-interval modulation,* for information in this form is swiftly destroyed. This theorem was discussed, although not very thoroughly, by Minsky [15].

Here again we observe a phenomenon in which an assembly of many parts comes to oscillate, with each part at the same frequency and without any *global* synchronization mechanism. The situation is *not* like the mechanics of a spring-and-mass ring system (Fig. 27-9) because its forces act only in one direction and because there are no *inertial* effects. It *does* behave rather like such a system in which the springs are highly *damped,* for example, by immersion in a highly viscous liquid. In such a system, the equal-spacing result is intuitively obvious.

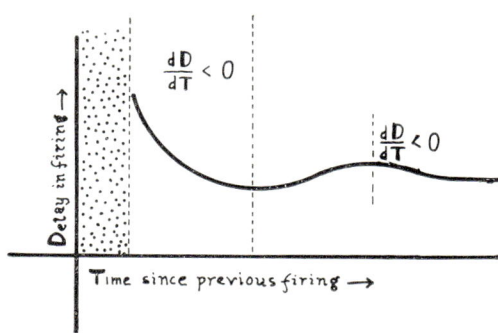

Fig. 27-8.

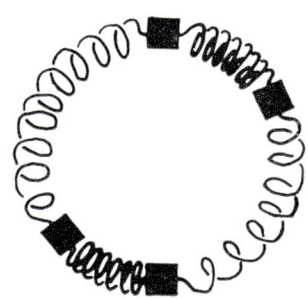

Fig. 27-9.

Finally, going back to the last remarks in the previous section concerning possible *interior foci* of oscillation, it can be seen how such parasitic activity might well be more stable in a network whose refractory periods and conduction velocities share some of the properties of Fig. 27-8. For now each advancing wave could remain a safe, stable, distance in back of the refractory rear of its predecessor. However, this author has not studied this mathematically.

SOME PSEUDOEXPLOSIVE MECHANISMS

There is little to be said about networks of interconnected elements in general. But by suitable choice of excitatory and inhibitory connections and of time constants of refractoriness and recovery, networks can be designed that maintain various levels of activity, with various degrees of stability. The general level of activity will usually increase with facilitation and decrease with enhancement of inhibition and refractoriness. A network can be designed to maintain a moderate and stable steady state when suitably initialized, yet to be hypersynchronously explosive under different initial conditions. An excessive burst might leave a net very quiet, so that after recovery it is ripe for another epidemic of firing, and so on: the same net in its normal state could maintain a stable inhibition-excitation balance. Models of such systems will not be made, simply because there are so many ways of proceeding.

Instead, some highly synthetic models will be discussed in which explosive activities can be seen that are not in the family of those just mentioned. As models for neural activity, even epileptic, they are probably quite absurd. Instead, they are presented to build a sort of museum of exotic phenomena that could be helpful when older ideas fail and new ones must be sought.

Our first model was suggested by E. Fredkin [unpublished, c. 1962] in discussing the theory of self-reproducing machines. Consider a linear array of cells in which each can affect only its two neighbors (Fig. 27-10). The peculiar constraint is imposed that a cell will be excited if, and only if, *exactly one* of its two neighbors fire. Conceivably, the cells might respond only to gradients and hence not to balanced symmetrical stimulation. Then if a single cell is initially fired, the sequence of states results as depicted in Fig. 27-11. The numbers of excited cells, as time proceeds, is the sequence 1, 2, 2 4, 2 4 4 8, 2 4 4 8 4 8 8 16, ... If b_n is the number of ones in the binary numeral for n, the nth term in this sequence is 2^{b_n}. It is not the rate of growth that is impressive (since $2^{b_n} \leq n$), but the explosive *drops* to just two firing cells, at the $\{2, 4, 8, 16, 32, . . .\}$th moments. And, despite its apparent triviality, the network has an astounding property of "self-replication of an arbitrary pattern," as shown in Fig. 27-12.

Note how the whole of Fig. 27-11 is replicated within the alternating lattice positions descending from one of the initially stimulated points. It can be seen in the figure how the initial pattern becomes diffused but emerges again as two copies at the $\{2, 4, 8, 16, 32, . . .\}$th moments. In the intervening periods, the pattern's information is distributed in a convoluted manner different from, but reminiscent of, holographic images. Similar phenomena occur in the corresponding two-dimensional and three-dimensional versions of the model, with 4 and 8 copies in those cases. Again, a functional model is not proposed (in this case, it might be tempting to think of memory concepts), but a conceptual entity is proposed, to be thought about. The Fredkin pattern copier requires a too-critical temporal matching of the elements' parameters to work reliably on large arrays without some sort of external global pacemaker to keep the units in temporal synchrony.

Proceeding to another idea of how a simultaneous explosion might occur in a large network, first recall a rather silly model: that which children call *counting off*. In a long line of soldiers, each can talk

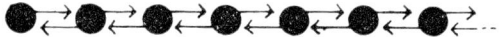

Fig. 27-10.

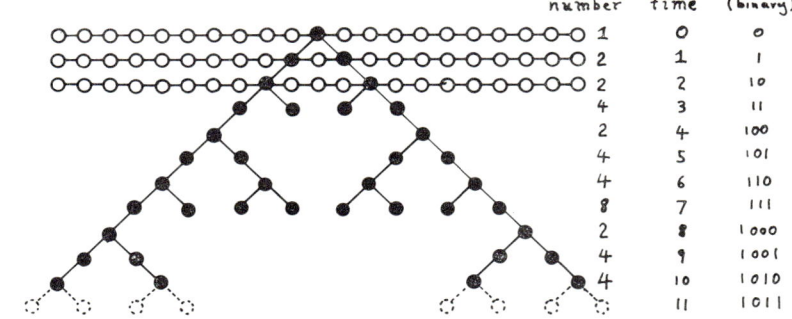

FIG. 27-11.

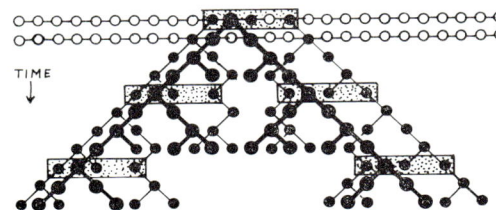

FIG. 27-12.

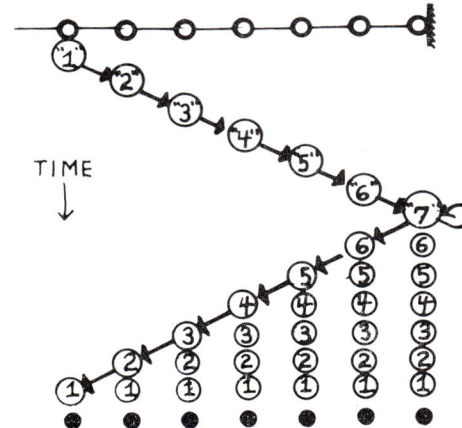

FIG. 27-13.

only to his two neighbors. How can it be arranged that the whole line (which might be many miles long) will all step forward at the same time? Figure 27-13 shows the time graph of one simple way to arrange this.

After the "General" at the left starts the sequence, the first soldier shouts "one." When any soldier hears his left-hand neighbor's number, he adds one to it and, after a one-second delay, tells it to his neighbor on the right. When the wave reaches the farthest right soldier, he starts to count *down* and informs his neighbor on the *left*. As the counting-down wave proceeds back to the beginning, each soldier counts down, and (if they all count at the same rate) they will all step forward together at the count of "one"! An objection can be raised to the requirement that all can count at exactly the same rate, but to some extent this can be synchronized locally. A more urgent objection is to the supposed ability of the units *to remember arbitrarily large numbers* while counting. (The problem is not interesting for any *fixed* small number of units.) Therefore, we proceed to another model that places no memory load on the units.

In the next model, it is convenient to replace the line of discrete, individual men by a uniform, continuous-propagation fiber. We shall make the usual stipulation that *the fiber can maintain two different wave types with two different speeds!* (This is not really unprecedented, for a glass rod can support three independent mechanical waves, to say nothing of an optical wave, of grossly different velocities. But in the neurological context it might be easier simply to imagine two different but parallel fibers.) In fact, we shall require the F (for Fast) wave to travel with three times the velocity of the S (for Slow) wave. The significance of the number 3 is seen in Fig. 27-14. At an initial moment, both an S wave and an F

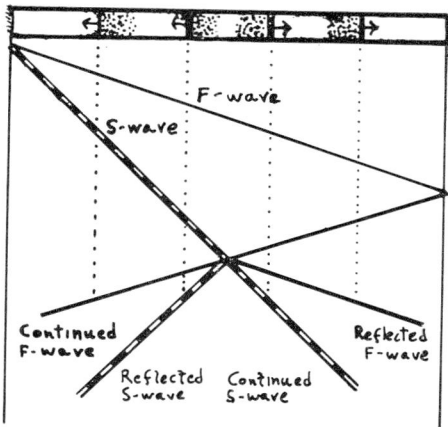

FIG. 27-14.

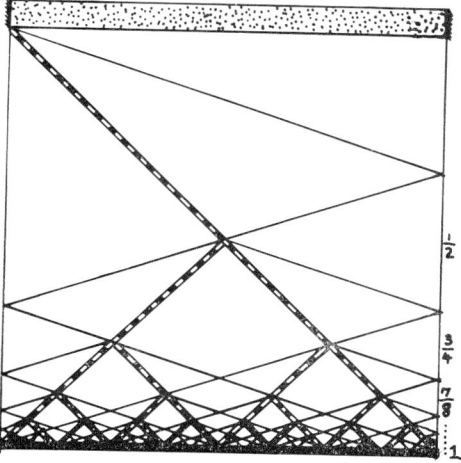

FIG. 27-15.

wave are started from one end of the fiber; we assume that an *F* wave will be *reflected* when it reaches the end of the fiber. Reflection is, of course, incompatible with nerve impulse because of refractoriness. Neurophysiologists who at this point must be becoming quite angry (and justifiably so) can imagine another pair of fibers for conducting pulses in the other direction.

Note, in Fig. 27-14, how the 3:1 velocity ratio causes the two waves to meet at the exact midpoint of the fiber. This event, occurring at the *global* center, at a point that is *locally* without any anatomic distinction whatever, is the key idea. Two more postulates can now be made:

(1) *When two F waves meet, they pass through one another (or reflect, which has the same effect).*

(2) *When an F wave meets an S wave, they both reflect and continue. That is, four waves result, as shown in the lower part of Fig. 27-14.*

The complete time course of the resulting events is depicted in Fig. 27-15. A truly explosive burst of activity occurs at just the moment when the initial *S* wave reaches the distal end of the fiber. The number of pulses doubles and redoubles; that the activity grows exponentially in time would be an understatement: in fact, it would become infinite at the terminal moment in a finite time. Returning to the image of the individual soldiers, the postulate is added that:

(3) *When two S waves meet near a soldier, he shall step forward.*

We now have a no-memory solution to the synchronization problem. Various other properties of this kind of *linear-array* computer have been studied extensively: in Hennie [12], in Blum and Hewitt [3], and in Minsky and Papert [16]; the above model is developed in detail in Fischer [9]. There are analogous solutions for two-dimensional and three-dimensional arrays.

The 3:1 model is sensitive to nonuniformity along the fiber; this could prevent a synchronous explosion. Another model, discovered by Balzer [1] appears to be better in this respect: it has only one kind of wave and explodes even more quickly (two-thirds as soon), but its soldiers are more complicated; they each contain a two-state *flip-flop*. Figure 27-16 (supplied by M. Paterson, who discovered it independently) only suggests how the soldiers work, but, since the details are not important to our discussion, they will be left as a sort of puzzle to the reader who can spare the time. It is amazing that the mechanism works perfectly even when the number of soldiers is not exactly a number like 2, 4, 8, 16, and so on.

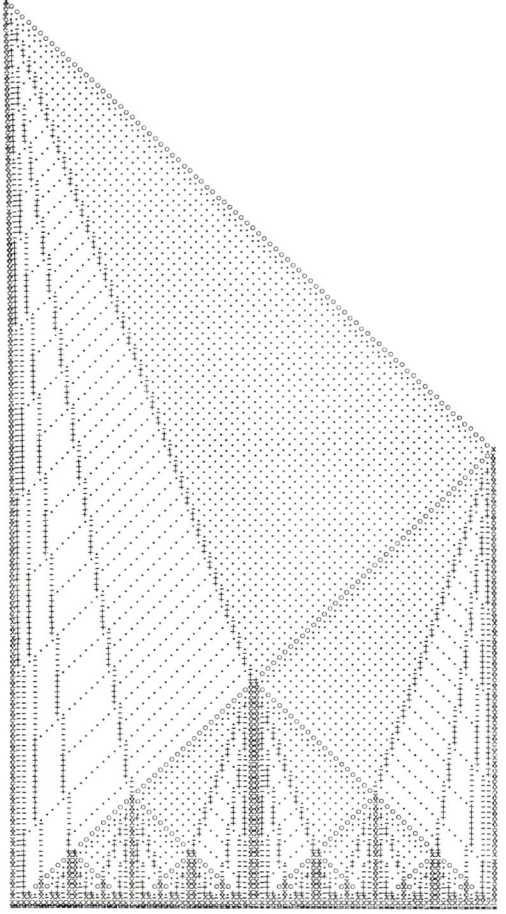

Fig. 27-16.

ACTIVITY OF LINEARLY COUPLED OSCILLATORS

A false appearance of synchrony can come about if there is an assortment of independent oscillators vibrating at different, but only slightly different, frequencies. Consider, for example, three oscillators whose periods are 7, 8, and 9 seconds. If started together in phase, they will come back into phase in $504 = 7 \cdot 8 \cdot 9$ seconds; at that time, the *sum* of their amplitudes will be larger than at any intervening time. With closer frequencies the phase interval will be even larger and it will also be larger with a larger number of independent oscillators. The phase interval is the least common multiple of the separate periods, that is, the shortest interval that is exactly divisible by each.

When a group of oscillators have identical frequencies, this will not happen, of course; they will remain in whatever mutual phase relation they are started. But this is a treacherous mathematical abstraction because, physically, there is usually some small amount of *coupling*. Some extremely elementary, but seldom understood facts about the behavior of coupled oscillator systems should be pointed out.

The first observation is: when identical oscillators, or nearly identical oscillators, are coupled by the purest and simplest interaction—a weak linear coupling (explained below)—then they are *not*, usually, brought into phase; instead the system actually behaves as though it had two not quite equal frequencies, hence shows a very long interval between apparent synchronies. And for a large number of oscillators, the phase duration can become extremely large. (For nonlinear coupling, quite different effects are obtained, as will be seen in a subsequent section.)

It is best to think of a mechanical system in which vibration is due to the relation between an elastic force and an inertial force, as shown in Fig. 27-17. Two identical mass-and-spring devices are shown, with displacement-indicator scales. The physics of such a system will be reviewed briefly.

The *force* exerted by a *linear* spring S upon its associated mass M is proportional to its compression Δ, that is, it obeys Hooke's law, $F = K\Delta$, relating force and displacement. Since the acceleration of M obeys Newton's law

$$F = Ma = M \frac{d^2 \Delta}{dt^2}$$

we have the "harmonic oscillator" equation

$$\frac{d^2 \Delta}{dt^2} = \frac{K}{M} \Delta$$

whose solutions have the form

$$A \sin \{\sqrt{(K/M)} \, [t + phase]\}$$

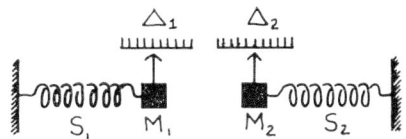

FIG. 27-17.

where A is an arbitrary amplitude and *phase* is an arbitrary time phase. The frequency formula $\sqrt{(K/M)}$ shows how the frequency increases with the spring stiffness K and decreases with the mass M.

To *couple* our two oscillators with a third linear spring, as shown in Fig. 27-18, let the new spring have Hooke's constant K^*. The great discovery of classical analysis is that such a system can be analyzed into *normal modes,* and, in this case, we can think of the two kinds of vibration shown in Fig. 27-19.

In the upper part of Fig. 27-19, the two

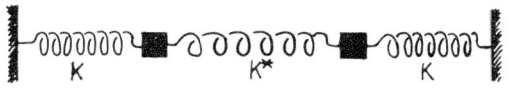

FIG. 27-18.

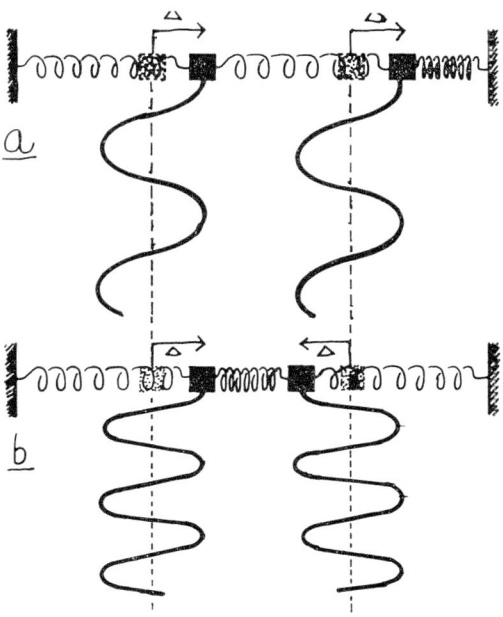

FIG. 27-19.

masses are started together with equal displacements. *Since the coupling spring is never compressed,* it may be ignored, and both halves of the system vibrate as before with the old frequency $\sqrt{(K/M)}$.

In the lower half of Fig. 27-19, the two masses move oppositely. Here the coupling spring is really engaged and, observing the symmetry about the center, it can be seen that each mass *sees* a spring whose Hooke's constant is $(K + 2K^*)$. This is a stiffer spring, so this *mode* has a higher frequency, as suggested in the drawing. It is a mathematical fact, deriving from the linear equation

$$\frac{d^n(u+v)}{dt^n} = \frac{d^n u}{dt^n} + \frac{d^n v}{dt^n}$$

about derivatives in general, that superimposed vibrations in these two modes proceed with absolute independence. If the system is started with equal amounts of each mode of Fig. 27-19, this is equivalent to beginning with the displacement of just one of the masses. The resulting vibration is depicted in Fig. 27-20.

The familar phenomenon is now seen in which all the energy seems to begin in the vibration of one excited mass, but after a while seems all transferred to the other mass and periodically to shift from one to the other. The time for this transfer is longer when the spring K^* is weaker—indeed, the time is determined by approximating the least common multiple of $\sqrt{K}$ and $\sqrt{(K + 2K^*)}$, which will be huge when K^* is very small. (Ignore the fact that there may not be any *exact* common multiple.)

The "trained intuition" of the physicist is not deceived by the "illusion" that the energy is shifting. He has learned to think in terms of the energies as residing in the A and B modes (and not, naively, in the masses). In this frame of reference, there are two independent oscillations, and the energy in each is separately conserved; the *exchange* is only in the mind of the observer who is unduly impressed by the *amplitudes,* which in fact play no direct role in the system's analysis. (In *nonlinear* systems, the amplitudes do have a fundamental role and the analysis is drastically different.)

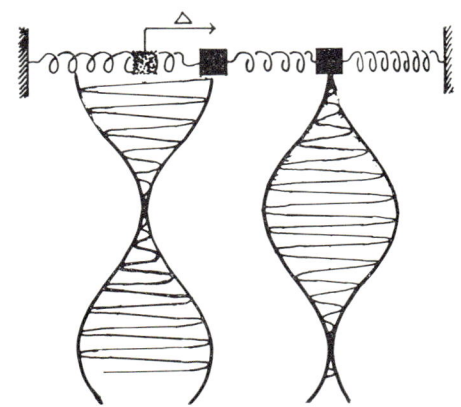

Fig. 27-20.

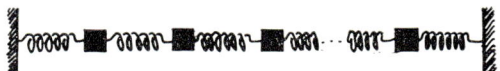

Fig. 27-21.

The basic observation, then, is that upon introducing linear coupling between identical oscillators, new modes and frequencies of oscillations are usually created. Then, because weak coupling makes *small* frequency changes, it produces *long* phase-synchrony intervals. If there were n independent oscillators, or (the same thing) a system with n normal modes (subconfigurations that have simple sinusoidal motion), the *sum* of their displacements (amplitudes) would usually be expected to be of the order of $\sqrt{n}$ times the average individual displacement. (Regard this either as a *statistical* fact about adding numbers from independent sources or as a consequence of the fact that the *energies* really add, and amplitudes are square roots of energies.) But, at great intervals, be prepared for amplitudes of the order of n. For large values of n this becomes extremely rare, and in any realistic model the least-common-multiple effect will be dominated by even extremely small nonlinearities of the system, to be discussed in the next section. Neuronal circuits are bound to be so nonlinear that the classical linear theory above could be, at best, misleading.

NONLINEAR COUPLING

Figure 27-21 shows a well-understood system in the classic analysis of wave motion: a series of N identical masses and $N + 1$ identical springs. This system has N normal modes, all of which have different frequencies. Consider now the effect of *nonlinear* springs; springs will be used that violate Hooke's law. Thus, instead of $F = K\Delta$,

$$F = K(\Delta + c\Delta^2)$$

might be used for each spring. A square-law term with a coefficient c has been added to make the spring nonlinear, this being a method mathematicians often find helpful: a quadratic system is usually the simplest to exhibit the nonlinear phenomenon in question.

Mathematical analysis of nonlinear vibration systems, even as simple as this one, is astoundingly difficult; it is often necessary to resort to computers for numerical calculation. This was done by Fermi, Pasta, and Ulam [8] for the system being discussed. Suppose, in analogy to what happens in classical statistical mechanics, that in the system of Fig. 27-21 the nonlinear interactions would cause energy to flow from any one "pure" mode to all other modes until they all share it equally—at least when averaged over time. (The energy of the system is still conserved, because while the nonlinearity changes the exact way potential energy is stored in the springs, it does not introduce any dissipation or frictionlike effects.) In classic theories used to model the mechanics of gases as systems of many degrees of freedom with nonlinear coupling, an *equipartition* phenomenon is discovered in which the energy eventually is dispersed equally among all degrees of freedom or modes, as a statistical time average. But this does not happen here, at least within any reasonable time interval. Instead, the investigators were surprised to find that the system, when initially excited in its lowest frequency mode (the concept of *normal mode* can still be defined in nonlinear systems in terms of very small displace-

THEORETICAL CONCEPTS OF SYNCHRONY 765

ments), seems to return after rather a long time to very nearly its initial configuration, as shown in Fig. 27-22. In other words, the system does not behave as though it were decaying toward a *thermal equilibrium*.

According to Zabusky [20], this phenomenon is now at least partially understood. In a series of analyses by Kruskal and Zabusky on some analogous situations, it was found that even though the system is *dispersive* (different frequencies have different wave velocities), the system tends to support certain kinds of physically localized pulses, which the investigators called *solitons*, that propagate with persistent individual characteristics. For example, in some cases they can collide and pass through one another with little effect except for a transient acceleration, which is illustrated in Fig. 27-23.

The recurrence phenomenon indicated in Fig. 27-22 can then be explained by the fact that in the intervening period, energy is packaged in the form of a collection of traveling solitons, which do not get thermally fragmented in a random or quasi random fashion. The soliton phenomena can be seen in a motion picture by Zabusky et al. [21]. Again a kind of system is seen in which relatively dispersed activity can rather suddenly recombine to put all its energy into one distinct mode.

Returning to the general topic of coupled nonlinear oscillators, a very broad general-

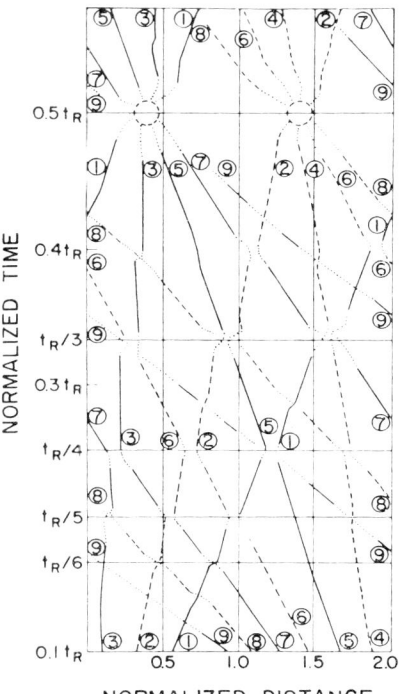

FIG. 27-23. From Zabusky [20].

ization can be made that probably is usually true in the limiting case of very weak coupling. At the beginning of the previous section it was mentioned that independent oscillators whose periods have whole-number ratios will come *into phase* at intervals exactly divisible by all the oscillators' periods. When frequencies do not have whole-number ratios, for example if there is a ratio of $\sqrt{2}:1$, the rhythm of the group will never be exactly repeated in the independent case. But this is physically unrealistic fiction, because all physical systems have *some* nonlinear coupling. And whenever two (or more) oscillators are coupled nonlinearly, they will usually approach (as a limit) a stable periodic rhythm. (All of this assumes that the effects of noise can be neglected.)

If the coupling is weak, that is, if relatively little energy (or its equivalent) is being transformed between the systems, then each oscillator will behave very much as it did before coupling. The natural frequencies will be affected only slightly, but they must

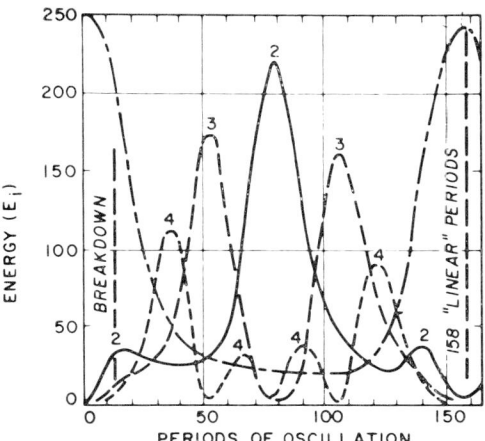

FIG. 27-22. From Zabusky [20].

change so that there are only whole-number ratios. Mathematically, this can be done with arbitrarily small changes: for example, $1:\sqrt{2}$ could change to $1000/1414$ or to any rational approximation to $\sqrt{2}$. (Two oscillators with frequency ratios of $1000/1414$ will not repeat their rhythm exactly until 707 periods of the faster one, for this gives the smallest interval divisible by both periods.) The stronger the coupling, the larger the changes that can be forced upon the oscillators, hence the shorter can become the period of repetition. Harmon and Lewis [10] cite a variety of examples of such frequency division effects, both in models and in physiological preparations. When the coupling is extremely strong, of course, both systems will lock together with the same period.

Unfortunately, the mathematical theory of coupled nonlinear oscillators is difficult, even in its qualitative aspects. Sources of information are, for example, Bogolubov and Mitropolsky [4], Cole [5], as well as other works on nonlinear partial differential equations.

OTHER TOPICS

NEURAL MODELS. There is a large literature of theories about how neurons perform various functions. The review of Harmon and Lewis [10] provides a good introduction to many theories at many levels of organization.

BRANCHING PROCESSES. Hypersynchrony can come about when the level of inhibition (or other activity regulator) is reduced: this will tend toward chain-reaction explosions. A great deal is known about chain reactions both from classic population genetics and from modern nuclear reactor theory; Harris [11] and Birkhoff [2] are good sources.

CONNECTEDNESS. If there is a general change in the levels of thresholds in a network, this changes the functional density of connections between elements. There are many questions for which an answer might be wanted about average densities of connections. For example, if there are n cells and P is the probability that any two are directly connected, what is the probability that there is an indirect path between two cells? A variety of such questions are discussed in Jacobs [13] and Solomonoff [18]. Kaufman [14] gives some interesting results on the number of different dynamic cycles in random McCulloch-Pitts networks with certain interconnection probabilities.

CONCLUDING REMARKS

A variety of formal treatments of some of the properties of neural nets is available which may be useful in thinking about the problems of epilepsy. In addition, modern mathematics is now moving in several directions that may be helpful in formulating hypotheses regarding mechanisms which may be operating to produce neurosynchrony such as occurs in epilepsy.

REFERENCES

1. Balzer, R. M. Studies Concerning Minimal Time Solutions to the Firing Squad Synchronization Problem. Carnegie Institute of Technology (Dissertation, 1966.)
2. Birkhoff, G., and Wigner, E., (Eds.). *Nuclear Reactor Theory, Symposia in Applied Mathematics.* American Mathematic Society, 1961, vol. 11.
3. Blum, M., and Hewitt, C. Automata on a Two-Dimensional Tape. In *Eighth Annual Symposium on Switching and Automata Theory.* New York: I.E.E.E., 1967.
4. Bogolubov, N., and Mitropolsky, Y. *Asymptotic Methods in the Theory of Nonlinear Oscillations.* New York: Gordon and Breach, 1961.
5. Cole, J. D. *Perturbation Methods in Applied Mathematics.* Waltham, Mass.: Blaisdell, 1968.
6. Farley, B. G. Some Similarities between the Behavior of a Neural Network Model and Electrophysiological Experiments. In *Self-Organizing Systems.* Washington: Spartan Books, 1962.

7. Farley, B. G., and Clark, W. A. Activity in Networks of Neuron-like Elements. In *Information Theory (Fourth London Symposium)*. London: Butterworth, 1961.

8. Fermi, E., Pasta, J. R., and Ulam, S. M. Studies of Nonlinear Problems. I. *Los Alamos Rep.* LA–1940 (May), 1955. Also in *Collected Works of E. Fermi*. Chicago: University of Chicago Press, 1965, vol. II, pp. 978–988.

9. Fischer, P. C. Generation of primes by a one-dimensional real-time iterative array. *J. Ass. for Computing Machinery (J.A.C.M.)* 12:388, 1965.

10. Harmon, L. D., and Lewis, E. R. Neural modeling. *Physiol. Rev.* 46:513, 1966.

11. Harris, T. E. *Theory of Branching Processes*. Berlin: Springer, 1963.

12. Hennie, F. C. *Iterative Arrays of Logical Circuits*. Cambridge, Mass.: M.I.T. Press, 1962.

13. Jacobs, I. M. *Connectivity in Probabilistic Graphs*, Tech Rep. 356. Cambridge, Mass.: Research Lab. of Electronics, M.I.T., Sept. 1959.

14. Kaufman, S. A., and McCulloch, W. S. Random nets of formal genes. *Quart. Progr. Rep.* 88:340, 1968. (Cambridge, Mass.: Res. Lab. of Electronics, M.I.T.)

15. Minsky, M. *Neural Nets and the Brain-Model Problem*. Princeton University (Dissertation, 1954.)

16. Minsky, M., and Papert, S. *Perceptrons*. Cambridge, Mass.: M. I. T. Press, 1969.

17. Selfridge, O. G. Some notes on the theory of flutter. *Arch. Inst. Cardiol. Mex.* 18:177, 1948.

18. Solomonoff, R. J., and Rapaport, A. Connectivity of random nets. *Bull. Math. Biophys.* 13:107, 1951.

19. Wiener, N., and Rosenblueth, A. Conduction of impulses in cardiac muscle. *Arch. Inst. Cardiol. Mex.* 16:205, 1946.

20. Zabusky, N. J. Synergetic Approach to Nonlinear Wave Problems. In Ames, W. F. (Ed.), *Nonlinear Partial Differential Equations*. New York: Academic, 1967, pp. 223–258.

21. Zabusky, N. J., Kruskal, M. D., and Deem, G. S. *Formation, Propagation, and Interaction of Solitons* (16 mm silent motion picture, 1965). Available on loan: Film Library, Bell Telephone Labs., Murray Hill, N. J.

Discussion

MODELS OF BRAIN FUNCTION
VALENTINO BRAITENBERG

This discussion was prepared without benefit of having seen Minsky's presentation in this chapter. Hence it will be limited to a few points which can be considered basic to how well a model reflects known data about brain.

First, the discussion will center on two aspects related to the question of what position the brain occupies between the two extremes of the purely digital and the purely analog machine.

The brain has a fibrous structure whose fibers (in the human brain), if placed end to end, would reach from here to the moon. Most of the information handled within the brain, if not all of it, is transmitted on the basis of messages traveling along these fibers. Occasional cross-talk occurs in the form of electrical or chemical interactions, whether as part of the normal function or as a disturbance, we do not know, but on the whole messages are not broadcast like waves in a continuous medium. A most disturbing feature about Hoyle's Black Cloud, which in its conversation with scientists on earth proved not only to be able to think but to learn as well, was the fact that it lacked the filamentous structure which appears to be in the brain an essential prerequisite of ordered interaction and of stability of the kind that memory would imply. For the contrary to be convincing, a theoretician must prove that specificity of frequencies (in the world system of radio broadcasting for instance), or some other form of temporal rather than spatial tag, may easily replace the specificity of point-to-point connections, but this proof would be desirable in a quantitative form. A network of elongated conductors remains the most efficient means of obtaining the specificity of connections which, with reason, is called in technical application the *wiring*.

Having established the spatially discrete nature of animal brains, which up to the present is not a distinguishing characteristic in regard to any of the artificial computing devices, consider next (a) whether information about intensity is also compressed in a limited number of discrete states, and (b) whether information about time of occurrence is also given in terms of a discrete succession of instants. The two questions are best discussed together since both are related to a well-known description of nervous activity in terms of propositional calculus [3]. Here, all that occurs in a nerve network is represented essentially by indicating, for a discrete succession of times, which of a limited number of neurons is in one of the two possible states: activity or rest. This implies that many different degrees of excitation, for example, all superthreshold ones, will elicit the same response in a neuron; in other words, information on how much the excitation was above threshold will be irretrievably lost at the next stage. This is probably not so on the basis of all that is known about synaptic transmission; the time of spike occurrence under certain conditions may depend on intensity of the excitation which produced it; hence not only is information about intensity preserved and coded in time beyond the synapse, but it will also determine if the spike will interfere at the next junction with other concurrent spikes. To put this another way, the intensity of the excitation at one point will reflect itself in the logical structure of the network.

Further experimental evidence leads to the supposition that in many instances when nerve fibers transmit spikes, what they communicate are graded quantities such as intensity of sensory stimulation coded as (average) frequency of a random spike-generating process. Also, some of the models characterized by very faithful representation of the experimental reality, such as Reichardt's model of the optomotor reactions in the beetle [4] or Hartline and Ratliff's model of lateral inhibition in the eye of *Limulus* [1], are expressed in terms of continuous quantities.

There has been no final word on the significance of individual spikes on the question of whether they may be understood as *symbols*, for example, in an abstract representation of quantities such as numbers in a digital computer, or always only as *signs*, as they obviously are in the aforementioned instance of representation of sensory excitation as spike frequency (to use Susanne Langer's distinction of signs of symbols [2]). The brain may yet have surprises in store for us, even in such fundamental aspects as the kind of language in which it encodes its own internal rumblings.

POINTS IN NEUROANATOMY

The role of the internal spatial coordinates of the brain is only imperfectly understood. It is still an open question why the right brain perceives the left half of the world, and even the naive question, why we don't see things upside down as they appear on our retina, is only superficially ridiculous. The brain itself seems to take very seriously the projection of its own internal spatial coordinates onto the external coordinates of the world. Putting aside the puzzle of the inverted projection of the world onto the brain, stop to consider the fact that once the orientation of the internal coordinates of a segment of brain with regard to the outside coordinates is established for one sensory modality, the same orientation can be found valid for other sensory modalities as well, even for the internal coordinates of the motor apparatus. Thus in the cortex, *right cortex* clearly means *to the left of my nose, up* in the cortex means *down* for vision, for the tactile sense, and even for the representation of the motor output.

In the chain of insects' visual ganglia, projection of the visual field can be strictly followed through from level to level. Everywhere the brain seems to take advantage of the fact that objects in the sensory spaces have certain properties (such as continuity of outline, sharp margin, continuity of motion and of velocity, and certain correlations between mechanical, optical, acoustical, and dynamic properties of these objects) which are best discovered if the representation of objects within the brain is in the form of images that retain some of these properties, and move in spaces which in some primitive sense conform to the outside space.

Space within the brain does not always represent space in the outside world. It may represent something as simple as frequency in one of the coordinates of the auditory cortex, or something probably quite complicated, or at least quite abstract in the cerebellar cortex; the unresolved ambiguous situation regarding the cerebellar *homunculus* would seem to indicate this.

One important point should be added lest these coordinates within the brain be taken in too literal a Cartesian sense. A straight line of the outside world will be represented within the brain as a continuous line, but generally not as a straight line. The spaces in which these coordinates are embedded are freely distorted in various ways: bent, stretched, or folded; the familiar example is, of course, the cerebral cortex whose surface in the case of larger animals increases more than proportionally to the square of the linear dimensions of the animal. In larger animals it will be folded or wrinkled in the familiar manner, almost as a handkerchief on which the various homunculi and sensory coordinates had been previously painted. Apparently in this folding process, what is preserved with respect to the unfolded cortex are the neighborhood relations of the elements, not the metrics of the representation.

Of even greater interest, we find examples occasionally where distances are preserved. The cerebellum also has a folded cortex in some species and not in others. As in the case of the telencephalic cortex, it is partly a question of body size and of some proportionality of the cerebellum's surface with a higher power than the second of the linear dimension. However, richly folded cerebellums occur, for example, in some electric fishes, where such an explanation cannot be applied. The interesting observation is that in fishes, in man, or in birds, whenever the cerebellar cortex is enlarged to an extent that it must be folded in order to be tucked into the cranial cavity, folds running in one of two directions (anteroposterior) in which elements of the cortical sheet are organized seem to be strictly avoided. Such folds would distort distances in the arrangement of elements in the laterolateral direction, and it is justifiable, therefore, to interpret these distances as having importance for some type of analog calculation that is performed in the cerebellum.

Properties of Neurons in Brain

Finally, to be pointed out, are those properties of neurons which will give an edge to natural brains over artificial brains for quite some time to come.

In physiological properties, the decisive trick is certainly conduction along axons without decrement. The distributed amplification along the line, which frees the signal from the chore of carrying along its own energy and allows signals to be multiplied at the branching points practically without any limit, frees the constructor from bothersome energetic considerations, when he is actually planning a network for the elaboration of information. This is certainly important for plastic networks which, when made of neurons, make automatic adjustment of the energy supply along with any change of logical structure.

In morphological properties, neurons are surprisingly macroscopical objects. Their dendrites alone, with which they absorb excitation (or inhibition) from the diffuse gas of axonal terminations, may extend over several millimeters. If these dendritic fields are described either as solids (by indicating the boundaries which contain all the dendrites of a given neuron), or as densities of dendrites around the cell body according to Sholl [5], their macroscopical shape is seen as quite characteristic for different neuron types, therefore presumably important functionally. Each neuron is affected by distribution of excitation within the brain at any one moment through its own characteristic weighting function, represented by its dendritic tree. If neurons are observed as such functions of space, it is discovered that the most amazing of their properties is that they can freely compenetrate one another. They can make any intersection imaginable, and one may be even completely contained in the other. The outlines of these dendritic fields (and analogously the regions of the axonal terminations) may be interpreted as Venn diagrams in logic. Here will be found any possible situation truly represented in such complex nerve networks as the cerebral cortex, where neurons, possessing in this macroscopical sense diameters of hundreds and even thousands of microns, are packed together so closely that their average separation is no more than 20 μ.

If this scheme of neurons as densely packed Venn diagrams reflects a basic property of the nervous system, technology will be hard put to imitate it, since it can scarcely be imagined how objects such as the dendritic trees of neurons in the cerebral cortex could be so densely packed without encountering insurmountable mechanical difficulties. A condition would be to learn to use the trick fundamental in creation of the cortex: to put neurons together initially as ball-shaped objects and let them grow their cell processes once they are in place.

REFERENCES

1. Hartline, H. K., and Ratliff, F. Inhibitory interaction of receptor units in the eye of *Limulus*. *J. Gen. Physiol.* 40:357, 1957.
2. Langer, S. *Philosophy in a New Key*. New York: New American Library, 1961.
3. McCulloch, W. S., and Pitts, W. A. A logical calculus of the ideas imminent in

nervous activity. *Bull. Math. Biophys.* 5: 115, 1943.

4. Reichardt, W., and Varju, D. Übertragungseigenschaften im Auswertesystem für das Bewegungssehen. *Z. Naturforsch.* 14b: 447, 1959.

5. Sholl, D. A. *The Organization of the Cerebral Cortex*. London: Methuen, 1956.

28
Perspectives in Neuropathology

ALFRED POPE

IF, AS SEEMS LIKELY at this writing, most human epilepsy is the result of brain damage, then as part of an overview of basic science potentialities for this clinical problem it is appropriate to examine the present state and future role of neuropathology in the study of seizures. In general keeping with the spirit of this volume, the discussion will be projective rather than retrospective and primarily concerned with assessment of those aspects of contemporary neurobiology pertinent for reevaluation of classical writings on the morbid anatomy of epilepsy, and for suggesting lines of investigation with particular promise for achieving insights into its ultrastructural, physiological, and biochemical pathology.

For present purposes, the neuropathology of epilepsy will be construed as broadly defined to comprise identification and analysis of morphological and biochemical characteristics complementary to the altered temporal sequences in brain action that specify the abnormal physiology of the epilepsies. So defined, it signifies the search for, and consideration of, changes in *structure* in the geometrical sense at all levels of tissue analysis, from molecular architecture to neuronal connectivity, that are necessary and sufficient for the epileptic state in individual units or cell assemblies. An ancillary aspect must be consideration of the metabolic machinery essential for maintenance of cellular fine structure and the function of excitable membranes.

Given the definitions of epileptogenicity employed throughout this volume, identification of scientific questions in the sphere of neuropathology is relatively easy in terms of current neurobiological sophistication. Answers to the questions, however, are for the most part nonexistent; the treatment must necessarily be mainly speculative. Nevertheless, the issues are provocative, and it is very much within the spirit of this treatise to juxtapose the scholarly assessments of basic mechanisms that comprise the contents of the volume with the pathophysiological challenges of human epilepsy, in the hope that this will lead to fruitful consequences. Some of the wealth of material in earlier chapters of this volume must of necessity be referred to in the discussion that follows.

PATHOLOGY OF HUMAN EPILEPSY

From the beginning of its history, neuropathology addressed itself to a search for the "lesion of epilepsy." This resulted in a large but inconclusive literature which has been repeatedly reviewed [21, 29] and which it would be inappropriate to reexamine in any detail here.

Many authors have reported that in idiopathic epilepsy (defined as seizures without identifiable focal origins, though undoubtedly in many instances these were simply not recognized) there are generalized, usually symmetrical, pathological changes in the cerebrum. Particular emphasis has been upon neuron outfall and gliosis in the hippocampus, especially in Sommer's sector (Rose's field H1). Ammon's horn sclerosis of this type should not be confused with the phenomenon of localized incisural sclerosis often associated with temporal lobe seizures [24].

In the isocortex, bizarre nerve cells, marginal gliosis, affecting primarily the plexiform layer, and laminar or pseudolaminar lesions in the supragranular layers (II–III) have also frequently been described. Most current opinion would consider these changes to be nonspecific, in all probability the result of repeated convulsions rather than in any sense causative, and probably mainly due to attendant cerebral hypoxia, the lesions of which they resemble both in nature and distribution [30]. Not infrequently, the brains of epileptics fail to reveal any clear-cut neuropathological changes at the level of light microscopy.

By contrast, epileptogenic foci in human cerebral cortex may be one consequence of many kinds of pathological processes directly affecting the cortex. Most important, undoubtedly, is craniocerebral trauma including perinatal injury. Other common neuropathological processes frequently resulting in the development of symptomatic seizures include: infection (especially subacute or chronic localized sepsis leading to encapsulated abscesses of the hemisphere); neoplasia (either involving cortical invasion by intrinsic or metastatic lesions or encroachment upon cortex by extracerebral tumors); healed cerebral infarction with scarring of cortex; and spontaneous cortical degenerations of many types (Alzheimer's, Pick's diseases, Huntington's chorea, neuronal storage diseases, and others). Certain diffuse processes such as the cerebral lipidoses and Creutzfeldt-Jakob disease are commonly associated with the phenomenon of myoclonus. Evidently there is something relatively peculiar and specific about the neuronal circuitry of the cortex that, in contrast to most CNS gray matter, makes it prone to episodic hyperactivity as a result of slowly developing, destructive lesions.

In all of the processes associated with development of focal epilepsy, the lesion is, in a crude sense, causative. More precisely, it is altered cortex at the border of the primary abnormality that is the epileptogenic zone. However, the morbid biological properties of epileptogenic cortex and the special intrinsic characteristics that produce an irritative environment and/or alterations in the structure or connectivity of the affected neurons, that in turn confer upon them their epileptogenicity in susceptible individuals, are poorly understood. The inspiration of experimental steps directed towards revelation of these factors represents the primary challenge of this volume.

For all forms of epilepsy, with or without recognizable foci of origin, the phrase "in susceptible individuals" must be emphasized. The role of heredity in the genesis of major and minor forms of attacks in man appears established, as brought out by Metrakos (Chap. 24). However, the mode of participation of genetic information and the nature of the coding error remain wholly obscure. It is important to stress once more that a still remote but major challenge for future students of the molecular biology and genetic engineering of the nervous system will be to provide insights concerning the biochemical genetics and pathways to ultimate control of the epilepsies.

The Meningocerebral Cicatrix. This is the prototype pathological lesion of posttraumatic epilepsy in man. The classical neuropathological descriptions of human cortical epileptogenic scars (including localized atrophic lesions) by Penfield and associates [23, 24] and his hypothesis concerning their development remain the most imaginative and provocative attempt to explain and understand the pathogenesis of a discharging focus.

Figure 28-1 reproduces Penfield's well-known diagrammatic representation of the basic pathological features of a meningo-

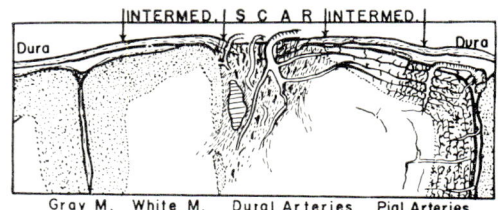

FIG. 28-1. Schematic representation of meningocerebral cicatrix and adjacent cortex. Central aganglionic scar is bordered by intermediate zone of partially damaged brain shown in terms of nerve cells (left) and blood vessels (right). (From Penfield and Jasper [24, chap. VII, fig. 15], by permission of the authors and publisher.)

cortical scar. The primary lesion is characteristically the consequence of a depressed skull fracture with inadequate reduction and debridement. The result is an area of traumatic necrosis in the subjacent cortex with ultimate repair producing a central aganglionic, relatively avascular, collagenous, fibrous tissue scar adherent to the overlying dura and immediately surrounded by a mixed fibroastrocytic type of encapsulation. At the frontier between the scar and surrounding cortex there is a zone of partial destruction of gray matter, resulting in islands of preserved neurons embedded in regions of replacement astrogliosis. In this intermediate zone between scar and normal brain the vascularization may be of a dual nature, arising partly in the usual way from pial blood vessels and partly from neovascularization by vessels of dural origin that penetrate from the central fibrous tissue mass.

There is abundant clinical and physiological evidence showing the abnormal border containing partially isolated (?deafferented) neurons to be the epileptogenic region [24]. It is from this frontier zone that electrocorticographic recordings demonstrate localization of spontaneous random spikes and sharp waves, and occasionally overt seizure discharges. It is also from this region that during craniotomy, electrical stimulation can provoke electrographic seizure activity and often reproduce the patient's habitual seizure pattern or his characteristic aura or both. Finally, surgical extirpation of the identified focus may abolish or significantly modify the clinical attacks.

Penfield's hypothesis states that continuing destructive changes within the frontier zone somehow induce its epileptogenic properties. He has provided pathological evidence strongly suggesting that chronic, progressive, destructive changes do indeed continue sometimes for years following the initial injury. This is evidenced by the continuing presence in the epileptogenic frontier zone of hypertrophied degenerating astrocytes, acutely swollen oligodendrocytes, and activated microglia including macrophages containing phagocyted neutral lipid. These changes have been attributed to recurrent episodes of hypoxic damage as a result of abnormal vasoconstriction (for brain) because of the presence of those arterioles derived from the dura (hence from the external carotid artery) which normally display greater vasomotor responsivity than do those derived from the pial circulation. Increased numbers of nerve fibers can, in fact, be demonstrated on some of the vessels in the partially damaged cortex at the frontier of a meningocerebral cicatrix [23].

The foregoing hypothesis would be compatible (in part) with some of the other processes affecting cortex that may produce epileptogenic lesions (tumors, abcesses, infarcts, and the like). However, while consistent with neuropathological evidence in the case of a meningocortical scar, proof is lacking with respect to specificity for the induction of an epileptogenic state [22], and the hypothesis still leaves unexplained the misbehavior of neurons in the actual epileptogenic site. The hypothesis seems clearly inadequate to account for focal epilepsy associated with the primary, spontaneous, neuronal degenerations or with the occasional establishment of autonomous mirror foci due to transcommissural bombardment. Indeed, the latter phenomenon indicates that a lesion identifiable by light microscopy is not essential for the development of localized epileptogenicity.

Unfortunately, few details are known concerning the microphysiology and molecular pathology of epileptogenic cortical lesions in man. Unit electrical recordings have been obtained by Ward (Chap. 10; see also Rayport [27]) and both gross and semimicro biochemical data have been reported in human spike foci [4, 26, 31]. It should now be possible to study the microcirculation in situ by means of polarographic and radiographic techniques. In view of the evidence for prolonged necrobiosis at the frontier of cortical scars, studies on cellular catabolic mechanisms, especially the proteolytic and lipolytic capabilities of constituent lysosomes, might be of significance. Explorations in the spheres of ultrastructure and microchemistry of the kinds outlined below should, in principle, be exceedingly illuminating. However, technical and logistical difficulties inherent in all such investigations are only magnified in the case of human material. Therefore, experimental models must also be employed for advancement of knowledge on the pathophysiology of epileptogenic lesions.

EXPERIMENTAL MODELS

Experimental epilepsies have been referred to throughout this volume, and the epileptologist is indeed fortunate that models are available that closely mimic the neurological properties of focal epilepsy in man. For the most part, as in human focal epilepsy, these result from chronic irritation due to foreign body reaction in gray matter, the most effective agents being certain specific chemical compounds (aluminum hydroxide, penicillin, cobalt, and others). Histopathologically, these experimental lesions (especially the alumina cream induced foci) resemble in certain respects the human prototype [2, 20] but they also show important differences; no common pattern at this level of analysis has been identified. Furthermore, repetitive and continuing physiological stimulation appears to be a sufficient condition for establishment of epileptogenic neuron assemblies, as in the case of independently firing autonomous mirror foci. Together with the human epileptogenic lesions considered above, these experimental paradigms constitute the main neuropathological states resulting in the appearance of *epileptic neurons* as defined by Ward [32]. Can ultrastructural, macromolecular, metabolic or environmental common denominators be established for neurons located in such diverse lesions but sharing unrestrained hypersynchronous discharge characteristics?

Figure 28-2 is an elementary depiction of a neuron as a physical-chemical system including distribution of its metabolic machinery in relation to cytological structure. The schematic details should be self-evident and will be described only in relation to the considerations that follow.

What factors are associated with conversion of such a cell to an epileptic neuron as operationally defined by Ward, Ajmone-Marsan, and others in earlier chapters in terms of unit pathophysiology? Such questions may be appropriately discussed in relation to: (a) surface membrane structure

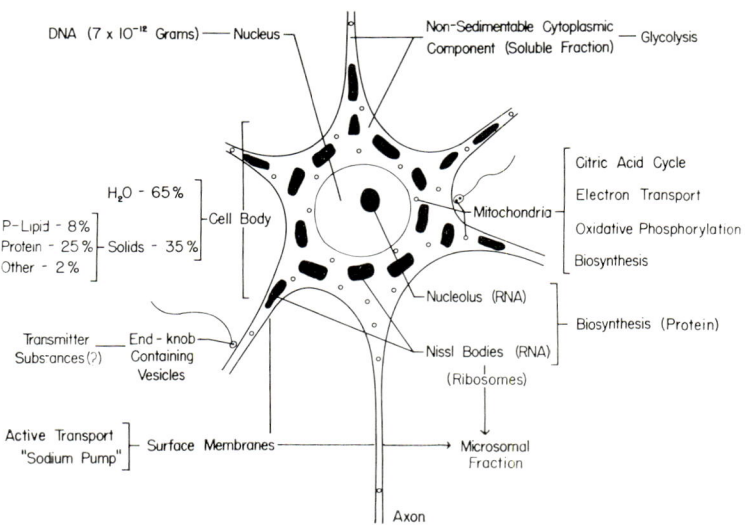

Fig. 28-2. Schematic representation of nerve cell body and proximal portions of its processes displaying elementary chemical composition and distribution of major metabolic systems in relation to cytological substructure.

and function; (b) intracellular metabolic systems responsible for maintaining structural integrity of the cell including its membrane; (c) status of the cell's milieu interne including the neuroglial sheath; and (d) relationship of the single epileptic cell to others in its component network. Contemporary methodologies theoretically appropriate for comparative analyses at the cellular and subcellular levels in relation to microphysiological properties include: (a) techniques of ultrastructure research (electron microscopy, polarization optics, x-ray diffraction, and others); (b) microscopic cytochemistry including fluorescence microscopy and electron histochemistry; (c) quantitative microchemistry suitable for single cell analyses as developed and applied to the nervous system, especially by Lowry [17], Hydén [11, 12], and Giacobini [8, 9]. With further refinement and increased versatility enabling sophisticated structural and metabolic chemistry on samples of cellular and subcellular dimensions, these direct microchemical techniques would appear to this author to be those of choice for eventually establishing a definitive comparative chemical pathology of single epileptic neurons.

Surface Membranes. It is virtually axiomatic that comparative analyses of the presynaptic and postsynaptic membranes will be all important for full understanding of the epileptic state. Indeed, unit neurophysiology can almost be equated with membrane dynamics, and discernible disturbances in the latter are potentially of central significance for the pathophysiology of seizures. Ion fluxes correlatable with membrane polarization depend upon the action of metabolic systems for active transport, and these in turn upon the molecular architecture and conformational states of constituent protein-lipid macromolecular complexes. This critically important role of the membrane fine structure is emphasized and elaborated upon by a number of contributors to this volume, notably McIlwain (Chap. 4), De Robertis (Chap. 6), Tower (Chap. 22), and Wolfe (Chap. 28).

The principles and techniques of unit-level neurobiology are logically applicable to the epileptic neuron in the search for changes in several aspects of membrane structure and function. Thus, correlative data on alterations in the molecular architecture of axonal and dendritic membranes and on the status of the monovalent cation transport system could provide crucial information regarding the genesis of pathological polarization. In this regard, the suggestive experiments reported by Lewin and McCrimmon [15], showing elevation of sodium and potassium stimulated adenosinetriphosphatase (membrane or transport ATPase) in epileptogenic rat cortex (freezing lesions), demand exploitation at the subcellular level. Similarly, simultaneous examinations of the ultrastructural characteristics of both somatic and dendritic axon terminals (including their vesicles) and of the concentrations and turnover rates of excitatory and inhibitory neurotransmitters should be potentially illuminating. Is there evidence at the unit level for increased production and/or release or for decreased catabolism of excitatory biogenic amines? Conversely, is there evidence for decreased production and/or release or for increased catabolism of inhibitory substances?

Alterations in the activities of enzymes concerned with the metabolism of neurotransmitters may be indicative in this regard. Data obtained some years ago revealed elevation of acetylcholinesterase (AChE) activity in both monkey (alumina cream) and human epileptic foci, presumably reflecting elevated acetylcholine turnover corresponding with observed increased rates of neuronal discharge [26, 31]. Possible imbalances in the metabolism of neurogenic amines either leading to, or the consequence of, chronic neuronal hyperactivity, require exact and refined analysis in terms of the known cytological loci of such events. If enzyme activities are employed as indices of altered turnover rates, it is important to evaluate the results in terms of the principles of induced, adaptive enzyme changes. Thus, such apparent discrepancies as the increased AChE activity in focal discharging lesions and its decreased activity in isolated cortical slabs [28] are easily reconciled if the changes are assumed to be indicative in the first instance of chronic hyperactivity of cholinergic neuron systems and in the second of their relative quiescence due to (partial) deafferentation. In general, the relative activities of enzymes involved in the molecular equivalents of neuronal firing patterns, especially in chronic epileptogenic lesions, will reflect rates of discharge of the constituent neuron assemblies. The results, therefore, must be interpreted with great caution with respect to possible etiological significance.

Cell Metabolism. Intracytoplasmic organelles and membrane systems are the sites for metabolic transformations that convert nutrient energy into molecular forms (the high-energy phosphate bonds of ATP and analogous nucleotides), utilizable for cellular work, including sustenance of surface membrane dynamics and maintenance of cytoplasmic structure throughout the protoplasmic and axonal expansions of neurons. The complex metabolic machinery for protein and lipid turnover involved in these events has not been examined in detail in epileptic foci. In view of established high rates of protein turnover during neuronal activity, the importance of axonal protein transport, and the critical requirement for maintenance of molecular membrane structure, it would appear vital to examine the comparative states of the polynucleotide (RNA)-mediated metabolic systems for protein synthesis in epileptic neurons. The histochemical findings described by Morrell (Chap. 13), indicating increased RNA concentrations in the neurons of experimental mirror foci, provide an intriguing further stimulus for this line of attack.

Relationships of energy metabolism to epilepsy for whole brain and for in vitro preparations have been presented by McIlwain and Passonneau (Chap. 4), and Sokoloff (Chap. 22); their relevance is critical and clear. It is also apparent that comparative analysis at the level of neuron units and small assemblies could be of major significance. Experimentally, this is approachable (in principle) by adequate miniaturization of such existing methods as those of Lowry [18, 19] and Chance [3] and their associates, for monitoring steady-state concentrations of key substrates and metabolites and levels of enzymatic catalysis in relation to ongoing functional activity.

Environment. Three types of observations suggest themselves in the search for local changes in the milieu interne surrounding the epileptic neuron that might be conducive to, or associated with its abnormal polarization and rate of discharge. They are: (a) changes in composition of the extracellular fluid adjacent to the neuronal membrane; (b) factors producing interference with exchanges of blood gases, substrates, and ionic species between vascular compartment and nerve cell (such as local alterations in the blood-brain barrier or the astroglial sheath or both); and (c) changes in the enigmatic neuron-oligodendrocyte satellite relationship.

The importance and feasibility (in part) of the environmental approach have been brought out in the articles of Orkand and Palay (Chap. 26). Comparative ultrastructural analysis of neuron-glial relationships in epileptic foci is realistic and practical. Refined electrolyte measurements at subcellular loci are also theoretically practicable by means of electron-probe analyses [10] or microflame photometry [14]. Similarly, single-cell microchemistry, especially as developed for fresh tissue samples by Hydén and associates [12, 13], Giacobini [8], and Epstein and O'Connor [5], has already led to suggestive information on the chemical interdependency of single nerve cells, their satellite oligodendroglia, and other elements of the neuropil. Techniques such as the foregoing are suitable and available for immediate application to problems of altered homeostasis in experimental and human epileptogenic cortex; the results of their utilization might have considerable impact. A further potential development might be the use of polarographic techniques for demonstrating local changes in gas tensions, or other homeostatic displacements in the micro-environment of epileptic foci, which could be correlated with the observable dc potential shifts described by Caspers (Chap. 14).

Cell Assemblies. Alterations in neuron connectivity and synaptology are obviously not determinable at the unit level alone, but require composite study of exact and total three-dimensional morphology and macromolecular substructure in tissue samples of gross anatomical dimensions. (In terms of fresh weight, sample sizes might vary from a few milligrams to the order of magnitude of grams.) As pointed out by Szentágothai (Chap. 2) for ultrastructural definitions alone, such an undertaking is of a degree of complexity that almost defies analysis. For the molecular level of emergence, the magnitude of the task for full descriptive evaluation is several times greater, and the problem is compounded by current deficiencies in requisite analytical methods. Nevertheless, first approximations of several neurobiological parameters are feasible and might establish significant leads in this sphere.

Comparative morphological studies using combined Golgi and electron microscopic techniques, as exemplified by the contributions of Szentágothai and Colonnier (Chap. 2), are clearly well suited for ultimate determination of the comparative, anatomical fine structure of epileptogenous tissue. The pioneer observations described by Ward (Chap. 10) showing decreased dendritic branching and reduction of dendritic spines of epileptic neurons with apparently correlated deafferentation are highly significant steps in this direction. Since dendritic spines apparently serve to increase the membrane surface for synaptic contacts primarily of an inhibitory nature, their selective disappearance would be consistent with a relative increase in excitatory input to the affected ganglion cell.

If, as suggested by Szentágothai (Chap. 2), intracortical star cells and Golgi type II cells are mainly inhibitory in their actions, is there evidence for a relatively specific outfall of such neurons in partially damaged areas of cortex with epileptogenic properties? Is it possible that differential counts of synaptic morphological types and analyses of their contained vesicles, prepared according to the procedures of De Robertis (Chap. 6), might provide complementary histological or biochemical evidence indicative of imbalances between excitatory and inhibitory synapses and/or the production and content of excitatory and inhibitory transmitter agents in such cortex?

Potentialities for the qualitative and quantitative histochemical analyses of tissues and cells, operationally definable by low- and high-power light microscopy, are now considerable; a wealth of baseline information on the histochemistry and cytochemistry of the nervous system is currently available [1, 7]. The obvious applicability of classic microscopic histochemistry for study of the histological components of epileptogenic lesions is particularly well exemplified by fluorescence microscopy for in situ localization of biogenic amines [6], as described in full by Dahlström (Chap. 8).

Architectonic cell assemblies can now also be systematically analyzed by means of a wide and versatile repertoire of microchemical techniques for quantitative analysis of microgram-sized tissue samples. For cerebral cortex, this enables description of its chemoarchitectonic fine structure, and establishment of normative data permitting detection of subtle changes in microchemical properties before the appearance of histopathological lesions [25]. In the case of epilepsy, an example of this approach is extension by Lewin and McCrimmon of their studies on Na-K ATPase in freezing lesions of rat cortex, demonstrating the elevation of activity to be limited to the middle cortical layers [16]. Analysis by the methods and principles of structural and enzymatic microchemistry would seem a particularly feasible and appropriate means for achieving a relatively refined biochemical description of epileptogenic cortical foci.

CONCLUSION

Table 28-1 provides a recapitulation of the experimental armentarium available to the contemporary neuropathologist and suitable for quantitative analysis of structural and metabolic properties of epileptogenic cortical lesions. The basic premise for such investigations must be that in the discharging focus, changes in the geometrical conformations of tissue components and in the metabolic events responsible for normal maintenance and function of the macromolecular substructure are part of

TABLE 28-1. Levels for Study of Biochemical Neuropathology

Anatomical Resolution	Observation and Identification	Neurobiological Samples	Biochemical and Biophysical Methods
Gross	Unaided eye	Brain, spinal cord, peripheral nerves, regional subdivisions	Standard structural and metabolic neurochemistry (gm and mg samples)
Histological	Microscope, low power	Nuclei, tracts, architectonic cell assemblies	Quantitative histochemistry (μg samples)
Cytological	Microscope, high power	Single cells, nuclei, processes, organelles	Quantitative histochemistry (mμg and $\mu\mu$g samples)
Ultrastructural	Electron microscope	Cytological fine structure, macromolecules	Biophysical optics

the causal sequence for epileptogenicity. If valid, neurochemistry and neuropathology have a significant role to play in further elucidation of the exact pathologic physiology of the epilepsies. However, meaningful information within biochemical and neuropathological frames of reference can only be achieved through investigations that also include immediate, sophisticated, correlative observations on the part of neurophysiology and neuropharmacology.

Together, current knowledge and microtechnology of the neurosciences applied to comparative analyses of the cellular constituents of epileptogenic cortex should yield highly significant information regarding its inherent pathological properties that result in or are associated with its abnormal physiology. It is to be hoped that one of the consequences of this volume will be multidisciplinary efforts in this sphere, especially those directed at new knowledge concerning the pathogenesis of focal epilepsy in man.

REFERENCES

1. Adams, C. W. M. (Ed.). *Neurohistochemistry*. Amsterdam: Elsevier, 1965.
2. Barrera, S. E., Kopeloff, L. M., and Kopeloff, N. Brain lesions associated with experimental epileptiform seizures in the monkey. *Amer. J. Psychiat.* 100:727, 1944.
3. Chance, B. Spectrophotometry of intracellular respiratory pigments. *Science* 120:767, 1954.
4. Elliott, K. A. C., and Penfield, W. Respiration and glycolysis of focal epileptogenic human brain tissue. *J. Neurophysiol.* 11:485, 1948.
5. Epstein, M. H., and O'Connor, J. S. Respiration of single cortical neurons and of surrounding neuropile. *J. Neurochem.* 12:389, 1965.
6. Falck, B., Hillarp, N.-Å., Thieme, G., and Torp, A. Fluorescence of catechol amines and related compounds condensed with formaldehyde. *J. Histochem. Cytochem.* 10:348, 1962.
7. Friede, R. L. *Topographic Brain Chemistry*. New York: Academic, 1966.
8. Giacobini, E. Metabolic Relations between Glia and Neurons Studied in Single Cells. In Cohen, M. M., and Snider, R. S. (Eds.), *Morphological and Biochemical Correlates of Neural Activity*. New York: Hoeber Med. Div., Harper & Row, 1964.
9. Giacobini, E. The intracellular localization of cholinesterase. *J. Histochem. Cytochem.* 8:419, 1960.
10. Hale, A. J. Electron Probe Microanalysis as a Quantitative Cytochemical Method.

In Wied, G. L. (Ed.), *Introduction to Quantitative Cytochemistry*. New York: Academic, 1966.

11. Hydén, H. Cytophysiological Aspects of the Nucleic Acids and Proteins of Nervous Tissues. In Elliott, K. A. C., Page, I. H., and Quastel, J. H. (Eds.), *Neurochemistry* (2d ed.). Springfield, Ill.: Thomas, 1962.

12. Hydén, H. Dynamic Aspects of the Neuron-Glia Relationships. A Study with Microchemical Methods. In Hydén, H. (Ed.), *The Neuron*. Amsterdam: Elsevier, 1967.

13. Hydén, H., and Pigon, A. A. A cytophysiological study of the functional relationships between oligodendroglial cells and nerve cells of Deiters' nucleus. *J. Neurochem.* 6:57, 1960.

14. Keesey, J. C. Flame photometric analysis of sodium and potassium in nanogram samples of mammalian nervous tissue. *J. Neurochem.* 15:547, 1968.

15. Lewin, E., and McCrimmon, A. ATPase activity in discharging cortical lesions induced by freezing. *Arch. Neurol.* (Chicago) 16:321, 1967.

16. Lewin, E., and McCrimmon, A. The intralaminar distribution of sodium-potassium activated ATPase activity in discharging cortical lesions induced by freezing. *Brain Res.* 8:291, 1968.

17. Lowry, O. H. The Chemical Study of Single Neurons. *Harvey Lect.* 58:1, 1962–63.

18. Lowry, O. H., Passonneau, J. V., Hasselberger, F. X., and Schulz, D. W. Effect of ischemia on known substrates and cofactors of the glycolytic pathway in brain. *J. Biol. Chem.* 239:18, 1964.

19. Lowry, O. H., and Passonneau, J. V. The relationships between substrates and enzymes of glycolysis in brain. *J. Biol. Chem.* 239:31, 1964.

20. Mayman, C. I., Manlapaz, J. S., Ballantine, H. T., and Richardson, E. P., Jr. A neuropathological study of experimental epileptogenic lesions in the cat. *J. Neuropath. Exp. Neurol.* 24:502, 1965.

21. Meyer, A. Epilepsy. In *Greenfield's Neuropathology* (2d ed.). Baltimore: Williams & Wilkins, 1963.

22. Penfield, W., and Bridgers, W. H. Progressive tissue destruction in epileptogenic lesions of the brain. *Trans. Amer. Neurol. Ass.* 68:158, 1942.

23. Penfield, W., and Humphreys, S. Epileptogenic lesions of the brain. A histological study. *Arch. Neurol. Psychiat.* 43:240, 1940.

24. Penfield, W., and Jasper, H. H. *Epilepsy and the Functional Anatomy of the Human Brain*. Boston: Little, Brown, 1954.

25. Pope, A. Structural and Enzymatic Microchemistry of Human Cerebral Cortex. In Bailey, O. T., and Smith, D. E. (Eds.), *The Central Nervous System* (International Academy of Pathology Monograph). Baltimore: Williams & Wilkins, 1968.

26. Pope, A., Morris, A. A., Jasper, H. H., Elliott, K. A. C., and Penfield, W. Histochemical and action potential studies on epileptogenic areas of cerebral cortex in man and the monkey. *Res. Publ. Ass. Res. Nerv. Ment. Dis.* 26:218, 1946.

27. Rayport, M. The Jacksonian hypothesis: A reappraisal in the light of single unit recording in focal epileptogenic gray matter of man. *Electroenceph. Clin. Neurophysiol.* 24:287, 1968.

28. Rosenberg, P., and Echlin, F. A. Cholinesterase activity of chronic partially isolated cortex. *Trans. Amer. Neurol. Ass.* 90:195, 1965.

29. Scholz, W. Epilepsie. In Bumke, O. (Ed.), *Handbuch der Geisteskrankheiten* XI. Berlin: Julius Springer, 1930.

30. Scholz, W. The contribution of pathoanatomical research to the problem of epilepsy. *Epilepsia* (Amst.) 1:36, 1959, series 4.

31. Tower, D. B., and Elliott, K. A. C. Activity of acetylcholine system in human epileptogenic focus. *J. Appl. Physiol.* 4:669, 1952.

32. Ward, A. A., Jr. The epileptic neurone. *Epilepsia* (Amst.) 2:70, 1961, series 4.

Discussion

FEATURES OF CHEMICAL STRUCTURE OF SYNAPTIC MEMBRANES*

LEONHARD S. WOLFE

A rereading of Penfield and Jasper, *Epilepsy and the Functional Anatomy of the Human Brain* [31], in the hope that 15 years later something really new could be added to their discussion of pathogenetic processes of local seizure initiation in man, proved presumptuous. Still unknown are the significant chemical changes associated with partial damage in brain which predispose to epileptic discharge; how local instability of oxygen tension or relative ischemia seem to be just the conditions favoring epileptic discharge; what biochemical changes in the border zones separate obvious pathology from normal tissue; what metabolic links are lost between neurons and glial cells in an epileptogenic focus; and what constitutes, in molecular detail, postsynaptic membrane instability or submaximal depolarization.

The difficulty is deciding which questions and projects are accessible by techniques now available and would lead to the smallest number of interpretations of possible results. Eight years ago, with Elliott [52], chemical studies in relation to convulsive conditions were reviewed; it was felt that in human epilepsy, particular attention should be given to the possibility that abnormal behavior of epileptogenic tissue is due to response of normal neurons to an abnormal, chemical environment. Discussion here will be restricted to three topics: concept of the greater cell membrane, the gangliosides, and the prostaglandins. The latter two groups of acidic lipids may be of considerable importance in structure and function of membranes of synaptic complexes and receptor surfaces. Detailed knowledge of the chemistry of presynaptic and postsynaptic membranes is clearly needed before pathological changes in membrane excitability can be fully understood.

CONCEPT OF THE GREATER CELL MEMBRANE

The greater cell membrane consists of the plasma membrane and the polysaccharide-rich cell coat. A variety of membrane models have been proposed for the organization of lipid and protein within the plasma membrane which can be broadly classified into two types: bilayer models, and globular or subunit models. Bilayer membrane models are based on the well-known lipid-bilayer membrane model of Davson and Danielli [14] in which a bimolecular leaflet of lipid is sandwiched between monolayers of hydrophilic protein and penetrated by polar pores. General applicability of the bimolecular leaflet concept has been questioned; the widely varied functional properties of different biological membranes do not seem compatible with the simple bilayer structure. Existence of differentiated globular substructures within cell membranes is now widely accepted; evidence for or against these membrane models has been discussed in detail [20, 24, 29]. A general feeling is that reversible transitions between globular arrangements and various types of bimolecular leaflet structures may be very important in physiological events. Several types of plasma membrane models are summarized in Fig. D28-1.

The role of carbohydrate-containing materials at the surface of cell membranes is now receiving much greater attention. Rambourg and Leblond [34] by periodic acid

---

* Research supported by Medical Research Council of Canada and Multiple Sclerosis Society of Canada.

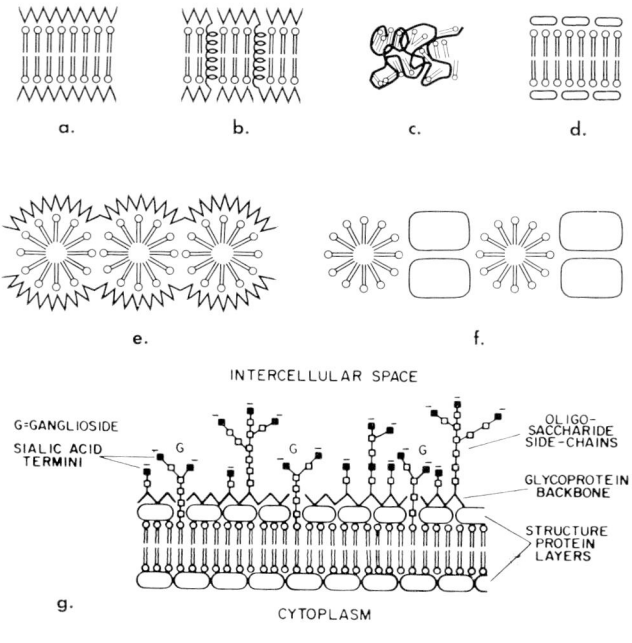

Fig. D28-1. Several types of membrane models based on lipid bilayer, globular, and subunit concepts of structure. (a) Classical Davson-Danielli model of lipid bilayer between layers of protein. (b) Model of Lenard and Singer has protein forming cross links through the membrane. (c) Benson model has protein within the lipid as a lipoprotein complex. (d) Protein subunits on surface of lipid bilayer. (e), (f) Lipid micellar models of Lucy. (g) Lehninger model of greater cell membrane of neurons. See [24, 29] for further details.

silver methenamine and colloidal thorium-staining procedures followed by electron microscopy have recently shown that a carbohydrate-rich cell coat is a common and likely universal feature of cells. The glycoproteins of the outer surface of membranes which have been studied in any detail show chemical characteristics quite distinct from secreted glycoproteins (low mannose content, high galactosamine ratio, and predominance of serine and threonine linked covalently to carbohydrate, see [29]).

It is important to appreciate that the dividing line between the cell surface and the immediate environment of cells is really arbitrary. In addition to the glycoprotein surface coat, acidic mucopolysaccharides of the extracellular space may also become associated by adsorption [33]. Properties of these surface constituents must be considered in any discussion of the environment of neuronal membranes, particularly at synapses, since they are of profound importance in the control of monovalent and divalent cation-binding properties. In brain, the acidic mucopolysaccharides in the extracellular spaces are mainly hyaluronic acid and chondroitin sulfates unassociated with collagen. The shape of these polymers depends upon their charge density and the adsorption of counterions that shield the mutually repulsive anionic charges [23, 33].

In the presence of counterions such as Na^+ and Ca^{2+}, these polymers undergo profound changes in viscosity and space-filling properties and tend to become more compact and spherical in shape. The selectivity of acidic mucopolysaccharides and glycoproteins for various cations depends upon the polarizability of the anionic groups and the valence, hydrated radii, and relative concentrations of the counterions. At equal concentrations the carboxylate anion of hyaluronic acid prefers Ca^{2+} to either Na+ or K+ and this property is specific over all other divalent cations. However, sodium can displace calcium if the local concentration is sufficiently high. The complex polymers of the intercellular space between neurons and glial cells are dynamic constituents and likely undergo rapid changes in their conformation during neuronal activity.

One of the most distinctive features of the chemical composition of neuronal membranes, particularly at the synapse, is their high content of complex glycoproteins and glycolipids [24]. Both these classes of compounds contain many terminal residues of the nine-carbon sugar N-acetylneuraminic acid (one of the sialic acids) which are negatively charged at neutral pH and appear to be mainly responsible for surface negative charge. The Lehninger membrane model (Fig. D28-1) conceptualizes particularly well the neuronal membrane and the carbohydrate-rich surface which is often completely overlooked in most membrane models.

The neuronal sialoglycoproteins or sialomucopolysaccharides are an extraordinarily complex group of molecules which may contain up to 50 percent carbohydrate [8, 9]. The chemical problems involved in their isolation and complete structural determination are at present quite formidable and the study of these molecules has only begun. Nothing is known about their tertiary structure or conformational changes in different environments but their properties undoubtedly contribute in an important way to the specificities of synapses and the local environment. Preliminary studies suggest active metabolic turnover [2] and there is great interest at the moment in the immunological properties and specificities of their carbohydrate sequences. In considering pathological changes in membrane excitability, the role of these surface-coat constituents and the adsorbed glycosaminoglycan polymers must not be overlooked. For example, loss of the calcium-binding sites at the surface of cells is now considered a primary factor in the ability of cells to metastasize. Are changes in the calcium-binding sites a factor in the development of epilepsy? It is not known if there are changes in the acidic mucopolysaccharides or membrane glycoproteins in epileptogenic brain.

Gangliosides—Glycolipids of Synaptic Membranes

Gangliosides are a family of sialoglycolipids mainly localized to the nervous tissue of vertebrates [25, 40–42, 48, 49]. Although certain gangliosides of simpler carbohydrate structure, for example, hematoside or GM_3 ganglioside by the Svennerholm nomenclature [41], occur along with neutral glycosphingolipids as minor lipid components localized in the plasma membranes of many tissues [18], the lipids of the neuronal plasma membrane are the richest source of the more complex gangliosides. Four types predominate in normal human brain [39] (Table D28-1).

The parent ganglioside of this glycolipid series is the monosialoganglioside, GM_1, from which the other types are derived by further attachment of from one to three sialic acid groups to the terminal galactose or to another sialic acid. The sialic acid of brain is exclusively N-acetylneuraminic acid. The GM_1 monosialoganglioside has the structure shown in Fig. D28-2. Monosialogangliosides occur predominantly in

Table D28-1. Major Gangliosides of Adult Human Brain

Type	Nomenclature	Distribution of Types. Mean % Lipid NANA	
		Cerebral Cortex	Cerebellum
Major Monosialoganglioside	GM_1	10 (6–12)	7
Disialoganglioside I	GD_{1a}	21 (17–24)	15
Disialoganglioside II	GD_{1b}	31 (28–35)	26
Trisialoganglioside I	GT_1	31 (29–32)	43
Totals		93	91

NANA = N-acetylneuraminic acid. Data summarized from Suzuki [39].

Galactosyl-(β,1→3)-N-acetylgalactosaminyl-(β,1→4)-galactosyl-(β,1→4)-glucosylceramide
|
N-acetylneuraminyl (2→3)

Fig. D28-2. Structure of the monosialoganglioside.

the axon whereas the polysialogangliosides are concentrated in the nerve endings [40, 42]. These gangliosides do not occur in glial cells or the myelin sheath [16, 19]. In development, the increase in polysialoganglioside content of the brain parallels very closely the maturation of neurons and establishment of axodendritic and axosomatic synapses [38]. Gangliosides are not uniformly distributed throughout the brain, but their occurrence is concentrated in regions densely supplied with synaptic endings [24]. A number of studies have been made on the distribution of these lipids in subcellular fractions of developing and adult brain of a number of mammalian species including man [15, 22, 50].

A cholinergic nerve-ending particle fraction contains the highest concentration of gangliosides relative to protein [22]. They do not occur in free mitochondria, synaptic vesicles, or a noncholinergic nerve-ending fraction rich in glutamic decarboxylase (possibly the endings containing γ-aminobutyric acid). The gangliosides in isolated nerve-ending fractions from adult or immature brain are concentrated in the outer membranes [22, 38, 46]. De Robertis and co-workers [15, 22] have shown that these membranes are also enriched in acetylcholinesterase, adenyl cyclase, a particulate phosphodiesterase, and the ($Na^+ + K^+$) stimulated oubain-sensitive adenosinetriphosphatase. Since nerve-ending particle fractions often seen in the electron microscope have pieces of the postsynaptic membrane still attached, it is not as yet completely clear whether gangliosides occur in both presynaptic and postsynaptic membranes or only in presynaptic membrane.

Our studies on ganglioside localization within neurons, adjacent neuropil, and glial-enriched samples isolated from the lateral vestibular nucleus of the ox strongly suggest a concentration of these lipids in the axon terminals on dendrites and cell bodies [16]. We also isolated from newborn rat brain a subcellular membrane fraction which appeared to be derived from the nerve endings [38]. These membranes contained 7–9 percent gangliosides mainly as polysialogangliosides based on membrane dry weight or 13–16 percent of the total membrane lipids. This is a 4-to-5-times greater concentration than in total gray matter lipids and agrees well with the calculations by Salganicoff and Koeppe [37] that nerve endings represent 15 percent of the brain volume. Technical limitations taken into consideration, the evidence is fairly good that polysialogangliosides are concentrated in the presynaptic terminal membrane. However, there is no precise understanding of their function at these sites; suggestions of their role in cation transport are still highly speculative [26]. The strong negative charge of the ionized carboxyl group of sialic acid may be important in influencing physiological properties such as the transport of monovalent cations. There is good evidence that gangliosides are the specific membrane constituents which bind tetanus toxin and perhaps other toxins; this might suggest a role in neurotransmitter release [27, 43].

Isolation of clean cholinergic and noncholinergic nerve-ending particle fractions (synaptosomes of Whittaker) [46, 47] by well-controlled subcellular fractionation techniques permits much more direct biochemical investigation of synaptic metabolism, as well as the structure and composition of its various membrane components. Recent calculations show that 15 percent of the brain volume in the rat can be ascribed to nerve endings; within this space, 50 percent of the total brain Krebs-cycle turnover goes on, together with a high percentage of γ-aminobutyric acid synthesis and carbon dioxide fixation. [37].

It has generally been assumed that non-membrane-bound proteins of the axon terminals were supplied by somatoaxonal flow. Ribosomes are not seen under the electron microscope in synaptic regions of neurons [30]. However, recent studies on the ribonucleic acid content and protein-synthetic capacity of isolated synaptosomes, in which ribosomal contamination was well controlled, have shown that these preparations do indeed contain significant amounts of membrane-bound ribonucleic acid and exhibit protein-synthesizing activity for membrane-bound mitochondrial as well as soluble proteins [1, 28]. Thus the synaptic region appears to be a part of the neuron in which there is intense metabolic turnover and which may be autonomous from the perikaryon to a much greater extent than previously realized. Interference in the microenvironment of axon terminals might be reflected very rapidly in altered energy metabolism in this local neuronal compartment, and provide just the appropriate local conditions for membrane instability and seizure initiation.

Prostaglandins—Lipids Formed in Postsynaptic Membranes?

The story of prostaglandins goes back to the independent findings of Goldblatt and von Euler in the early thirties, that seminal plasma of man and the seminal vesicles of sheep contained active principles with the properties of lipid acids which contracted the uterus and intestinal smooth muscle, and lowered the blood pressure. Isolation, separation, and crystallization of several different types of prostaglandins in milligram amounts led to their complete chemical characterization in the last ten years through the superb chemical investigations of Bergström, Ryhage, Samuelsson, Sjövall, and co-workers at the Karolinska Institute [4, 5, 6, 7, 32, 45]. The natural prostaglandins are a new and unique class of unsaturated hydroxy- or hydroxyketo-long-chain fatty acids with potent and exceedingly diverse pharmacological properties. They occur in very small quantities in many tissues including the central nervous system. The major prostaglandin isolated from brain is PGF_{2a} which has the chemical structure shown in Fig. D28-3.

Soon after the chemical structures of the prostaglandins were determined, it was shown that these lipids originate from free all-*cis* polyunsaturated eicosenoic acids of the so-called essential fatty acid type. The conversion of these fatty acids into prostaglandins is initiated by an enzymatic stereospecific removal of a hydrogen atom followed by the addition of molecular oxygen and specific molecular rearrangements. Prostaglandin synthetase, as the reaction sequence is called, is a tightly membrane-bound enzyme system. In the brain, the commonest essential polyunsaturated fatty acid is arachidonic acid from which the most abundant brain prostaglandin, PGF_{2a}, is derived.

The discovery of this relationship between prostaglandins and essential fatty acids has stimulated reexamination of the very old problem of what it is that makes essential fatty acids essential. There is growing appreciation that it might be their ability to act as precursors to the prosta-

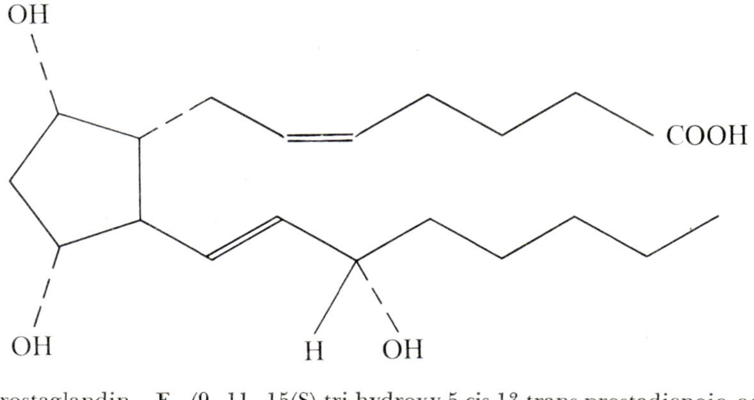

Fig. D28-3. Prostaglandin $F_{2a}(9_a,11_a,15(S)$-tri-hydroxy-5-cis,13-trans-prostadienoic acid).

glandins since only those fatty acids which have the right chemical structure and can be converted into biologically active prostaglandins are active in reversing essential fatty acid deficiency in animals [3]. All the evidence at present indicates that prostaglandins are formed locally in tissues and may be released into venous effluents or superfusing fluids. Prostaglandins are cleared very rapidly from the blood stream by metabolism in the lung and liver to biologically inactive metabolites which appear in the urine. Arachidonic acid, the fatty acid precursor of the brain prostaglandins, does not occur as the free acid but is esterified in the membrane phospholipids. Prostaglandins, however, do not occur in tissues esterified to phospholipids or other lipids [21].

Since triglycerides or cholesterol esters do not occur normally in brain, it appears that the source of the precursors for brain prostaglandins is likely from arachidonic acid, cleaved from certain membrane phospholipids through the activity of specific, membrane-bound phospholipases, known to occur in brain. A relationship exists between the activity of phospholipase A_2 and the amounts of prostaglandins formed in tissues, but the details will not be discussed here [12, 44]. Prostaglandin formation may originate from a sequence of linked enzymatic reactions initiated in membrane phospholipids. What initiates or controls prostaglandin formation?

Very recently, a number of independent studies have shown that prostaglandin release from tissues is accelerated in a stimulus-dependent fashion following stimulation of central or certain types of peripheral autonomic neural pathways [5, 6, 12, 13, 32, 35]. The investigations of Ramwell and Shaw [35] have shown that direct electrical stimulation of the somatosensory cortex of the cat, transcallosal stimulation, or stimulation of the contralateral radial nerve increases prostaglandin release into fluids superfusing the cortex. Following these studies, it was suggested that prostaglandins might represent a new class of transmitter substances. Our own work indicates that prostaglandins arise from postsynaptic sites, most likely the postsynaptic membrane itself, or receptor regions of the cell membrane [11, 12].

These studies were performed on an isolated rat-stomach preparation in which the effect of both sympathetic and vagal nerve stimulation could be studied independently. This preparation was chosen since the cholinergic receptors are of the muscarinic type similar to those in the cerebral cortex. The increased release of prostaglandins E_2 and F_{2a} from the serosal surface of the rat stomach when the vagal nerves were stimulated was completely inhibited by hyoscine. Furthermore, the prostaglandins did not arise from a preformed store but were formed de novo during the period of nerve stimulation. With Coceani, a simple model was proposed which relates prostaglandin formation to membrane function [11]. We are aware that this might be premature, but it has been very useful for our experimental designs. Our concept is that prostaglandin formation within membranes is initiated by activation of a specific phospholipase, which cleaves off arachidonic acid as the free acid. This fatty acid comes into contact with the membrane prostaglandin synthetase, which converts it into PGE_2 and PGF_{2a}, depending on the particular local concentration of sulfhydryl-containing cofactors. This sequence is greatly accelerated by stimulation of receptor sites or the postsynaptic membrane. The prostaglandins formed within the membrane structure would then control excitability through effects on calcium binding and availability associated with metabolism (for example, membrane-bound ATP and possibly the formation of cyclic 3,′5′adenosinemonophosphate).

Thus we regard prostaglandins as modulators of transmitter action at the receptor level [11]. Prostaglandin formation will occur only within discrete regions of the effector cell membrane which may well have phospholipids of unique properties. The reaction sequence by which prostaglandins are formed is thought to represent a basic response of specific regions of many cell membranes to a wide variety of challenges.

Although knowledge of the prostaglandins is rapidly expanding and a wealth of new data, particularly on pharmacological actions, is appearing in the literature, the physiological role and mechanism of action of these lipids is obscure. Two general hypotheses of the primary site of action of prostaglandins have been advanced: (1) prostaglandins modulate membrane-bound adenyl cyclase activity by feedback inhibition of hormonally stimulated cyclic 3',5'-adenosinemonophosphate formation [4]; (2) prostaglandins regulate the calcium distribution and fixation in cellular compartments after stimulation of receptor sites by neurohormones [10, 11].

In conclusion, brief mention should be made of our most recent experiments which suggest that prostaglandins may affect calcium distribution in effector cells. We investigated the effect of a prostaglandin (PGE_1) on the exchange of radioactive calcium in the smooth muscle of the rat-stomach fundus strip and taenia coli under strict isometric conditions. Our previous investigation and those of Clegg, Hall, and Pickles [10, 51] had revealed that the smooth-muscle contracting action of these lipids was due to a direct action on the smooth muscle cells and was dependent upon the presence of calcium in the perfusion medium. When the effect of prostaglandins on calcium exchange was studied, some unique and highly interesting effects were obtained with concentrations of prostaglandins as low as 10 picograms per ml (approximately $3 \times 10^{-11}M$); such doses do not cause contraction.

It was found that prostaglandin E_1 significantly decreased calcium efflux during an efflux phase of half-time of about 5 min at 38°C, but had no effect on calcium influx. Furthermore, total calcium content was significantly increased by 0.2–0.3M and this excess calcium had accumulated in a slowly exchangeable fraction. These results provide a possible explanation for the greatly increased sensitivity (*enhancement effect*) to all agonists caused by previous exposure to low noncontractile doses of prostaglandins in smooth muscle.

Calcium is a known essential in order for physiological stimuli to lead to normal effector responses. If it is assumed that the properties of muscarinic receptors are similar in smooth muscle and on neuronal membranes, then the brain prostaglandins formed and released upon stimulation may control neuronal responses by their action on distribution of calcium between membrane and cytoplasmic phases. If this is true, then the prostaglandins would have particular pertinence in the pathogenesis of epilepsy. For example, in the presence of a compromised oxygenation of the local environment of neurons, or if widespread deafferentation has taken place, the formation of prostaglandins may be greatly decreased in certain neurons in response to normal stimuli. Although calcium uptake following stimulation might occur normally, its distribution in membrane and metabolic compartments may be uncontrolled and lead to marked changes in membrane stability and in the depolarization-repolarization cycles of the neuronal membrane.

Acknowledgments. I thank Dr. A. L. Lehninger and the National Academy of Sciences for permission to reproduce part of Fig. D28-1.

REFERENCES

1. Austin, L., and Morgan, I. G. Incorporation of ^{14}C-labelled leucine into synaptosomes from rat cerebral cortex in vitro. *J. Neurochem.* 14:377, 1967.
2. Barondes, S. Incorporation of radioactive glucosamine into macromolecules at nerve endings. *J. Neurochem.* 15:699, 1968.
3. Beerthuis, R. K., Nugteren, D. H., Pabon, H. J. J., and Van Dorp, D. A. Biologically active prostaglandins from some new odd-numbered essential fatty acids. *Rec. Trav. Chim. Pays-Bas* 87:461, 1968.
4. Bergström, S. The prostaglandins: Members of a new hormonal class. *Science* 157:382, 1967.
5. Bergström, S., Carlson, L. A., and Weeks, J. R. The prostaglandins: A family of

biologically active lipids. *Pharmacol. Rev.* 20:1, 1968.

6. Bergström, S., and Samuelsson, B. (Eds.). *Prostaglandins,* Proc. II Nobel Symposium. Uppsala: Almqvist and Wiksell, 1967.

7. Bergström, S., and Samuelsson, B. The prostaglandins. *Endeavour* 27:109, 1968.

8. Brunngraber, E. G., and Brown, B. D. Preparation and properties of sialomucopolysaccharides obtained from rat brain. *Biochem. J.* 103:65, 1967.

9. Brunngraber, E. G., Dekirmenjian, H., and Brown, B. D. The distribution of protein-bound N-acetylneuraminic acid in subcellular fractions of rat brain. *Biochem. J.* 103:73, 1967.

10. Clegg, P. C., Hall, W. J., and Pickles, V. R. The action of ketonic prostaglandins on the guinea-pig myometrium. *J. Physiol.* (London) 183:123, 1966.

11. Coceani, F., Dreifuss, J. J., Puglisi, L., and Wolfe, L. S. Prostaglandins and Membrane Function. In Mantegazza, P. (Ed.), *Peptides, Amines and Prostaglandins.* New York: Academic, 1968, in press.

12. Coceani, F., Pace-Asciak, C., Volta, F., and Wolfe, L. S. Effect of nerve stimulation on prostaglandin formation and release from the rat stomach. *Amer. J. Physiol.* 213:1056, 1967.

13. Davies, B. N., Horton, E. W., and Withrington, P. G. The occurrence of prostaglandin E_2 in splenic venous blood of the dog following splenic nerve stimulation. *Brit. J. Pharmacol.* 32:127, 1968.

14. Davson, H., and Danielli, J. F. *The Permeability of Natural Membranes.* London: Cambridge University Press, 1943.

15. De Robertis, E. Ultrastructure and cytochemistry of the synaptic region. *Science* 156:907, 1967.

16. Derry, D. M., and Wolfe, L. S. Gangliosides in isolated neurons and glial cells. *Science* 158:1450, 1967.

17. Derry, D. M., and Wolfe, L. S. Ganglioside analyses of serial cryostat sections through Ammon's horn and cerebellar folia. *Exp. Brain Res.* 5:32, 1968.

18. Dod, B. J., and Gray, G. M. The lipid composition of rat liver plasma membranes. *Biochim. Biophys. Acta* 150:397, 1968.

19. Eichberg, J., Whittaker, V. P., and Dawson, R. M. C. Distribution of lipids in subcellular particles of guinea-pig brain. *Biochem. J.* 92:91, 1964.

20. Korn, E. D. The structure of biological membranes. *Science* 153:1491, 1966.

21. Lands, W. E. M., and Samuelsson, B. Phospholipid precursors of prostaglandins. *Biochim. Biophys. Acta* 164:426, 1968.

22. Lapetina, E. G., Soto, E. F., and De Robertis, E. Gangliosides and acetylcholinesterase in isolated membranes of the rat brain cortex. *Biochim. Biophys. Acta* 135:33, 1967.

23. Laurent, T. C. Physicochemical characteristics of the acid glycosaminoglycans. *Fed. Proc.* 25:1037, 1966.

24. Lehninger, A. L. The neuronal membrane. *Proc. Nat. Acad. Sci. USA* 60:1069, 1968.

25. Lowden, J. A., and Wolfe, L. S. Studies on brain gangliosides. *Canad. J. Biochem.* 42:1587, 1964.

26. McIlwain, H. *Chemical Exploration of the Brain.* Amsterdam: Elsevier, 1963.

27. Mellanby, J., Van Heyningen, W. E., and Whittaker, V. P. Fixation of tetanus toxin by subcellular fractions of brain. *J. Neurochem.* 12:77, 1965.

28. Morgan, I. G., and Austin, L. Synaptosomal protein synthesis in a cell-free system. *J. Neurochem.* 15:41, 1968.

29. Northcote, D. H. Structure and function of plant-cell membranes. *Brit. Med. Bull.* 24:107, 1968.

30. Palay, S. L., and Palade, G. E. Fine structures of neurones. *J. Biophys. Biochem. Cytol.* 1:69, 1955.

31. Penfield, W., and Jasper, H. *Epilepsy and the Functional Anatomy of the Human Brain.* Boston: Little, Brown, 1954.

32. Pickles, V. R. The prostaglandins. *Biol. Rev.* 42:614, 1967.

33. Quintarelli, G. (Ed.). *Chemical Physiology of Mucopolysaccharides.* Boston: Little, Brown, 1967.

34. Rambourg, A., and Leblond, C. P. Electron microscope observations on the carbohydrate-rich cell coat present at the surface of cells in the rat. *J. Cell Biol.* 32:27, 1967.

35. Ramwell, P., and Shaw, J. E. Spontaneous and evoked release of prostaglandins from cerebral cortex of anesthetized cats. *Amer. J. Physiol.* 211:125, 1966.

36. Ramwell, P. W., Shaw, J. E., Clarke, G. B., Grostic, M. F., Kaiser, D. G., and Pike, J. E. Prostaglandins. In Holman, R. (Ed.), *Progress in the Chemistry of Fats and Other Lipids.* New York: Pergamon, 1968, pp. 9, 75.

37. Salganicoff, L., and Koeppe, R. E. Subcellular distribution of pyruvate, carboxylase, diphosphopyridine nucleotide and triphosphopyridine nucleotide isocitrate dehydrogenases and malate enzyme in rat brain. *J. Biol. Chem.* 243:3416, 1968.

38. Spence, M. W., and Wolfe, L. S. Gangliosides in developing rat brain. *Canad. J. Biochem.* 45:671, 1967.

39. Suzuki, K. The pattern of mammalian brain gangliosides. *J. Neurochem.* 12:969, 1965.

40. Suzuki, K. Gangliosides in myelin fractions of developing rat brain. *Biochim. Biophys. Acta* 144:375, 1967.

41. Svennerholm, L. Chromatographic separation of human brain gangliosides. *J. Neurochem.* 10:613, 1963.

42. Svennerholm, L. The gangliosides. *J. Lipid Res.* 5:145, 1964.

43. Van Heyningen, W. E. The fixation of tetanus toxin, strychnine, serotonin and other substances by ganglioside. *J. Gen. Microbiol.* 31:375, 1963.

44. Vogt, W., Suzuki, T., and Babilli, S. Prostaglandins in SRS-C and in a Darmstoff preparation from frog intestinal dialysates. *Mem. Soc. Endocrinol.* 137, 1966.

45. Von Euler, U. S., and Eliasson, R. *Prostaglandins.* New York: Academic, 1968.

46. Whittaker, V. P. Synaptic transmission. *Proc. Nat. Acad. Sci. USA* 60:1081, 1968.

47. Whittaker, V. P., Michaelson, I. A., and Kirkland, R. J. A. The separation of synaptic vesicles from disrupted nerve-ending particles ("synaptosomes"). *Biochem. J.* 90:293, 1963.

48. Wiegandt, H. Ganglioside. *Ergebn. Physiol.* 57:190, 1966.

49. Wiegandt, H. The structure and function of gangliosides. *Angew. Chem.* [Eng.] 7:87, 1968.

50. Wolfe, L. S. The distribution of gangliosides in subcellular fractions of guinea-pig cerebral cortex. *Biochem. J.* 79:348, 1961.

51. Wolfe, L. S., Coceani, F., and Pace-Asciak, C. Brain Prostaglandins and Studies of the Action of Prostaglandins on the Isolated Rat Stomach. In Bergström, S., and Samuelsson, B. (Eds.), *Prostaglandins*, Nobel Symp. 2:265. New York: Interscience, 1967.

52. Wolfe, L. S., and Elliott, K. A. C. Chemical Studies in Relation to Convulsive Conditions. In Elliott, K. A. C., Page, I. H., and Quastel, J. H. (Eds.), *Neurochemistry* (2d ed.). Springfield, Ill.: Thomas, 1962.

29

Epilepsy, Neurophysiology, and Some Brain Mechanisms Related to Consciousness

WILDER PENFIELD

IT WAS MY PURPOSE in undertaking this study to reconsider a long experience with epilepsy and with the associated electrical exploration of the human cerebral cortex, hoping that a late overall analysis would lead to new interpretations. I am happy to say it has brought me a clearer view of brain function. I hope it may be of some service to others.

John Hughlings Jackson saw that epilepsy could be his guide to an understanding of brain function: "Epilepsy," he said, "is the name for occasional sudden excessive, rapid and local discharges of grey matter."

By means of this hypothesis and the concept of spread of discharge from point to point in the cortex, Jackson made two forward steps: (1) He explained the mechanism of an epileptic seizure, and (2) he came on a clue to the delimitation of areas of cortex and the localization of function in the brain.

He proposed the following hypothesis: There was, he argued, in any case of epilepsy, an area of gray matter so abnormally nourished that it reached a high tension and exploded from time to time. The discharge was followed by local fatigue of the nerve cells in the gray matter, and thus there was interference with the normal function of that part of the cortex during and immediately following the attack.

Ictal Discharge and Surgeon's Electrode

As far as surgery is concerned, it may be said that a thoughtful approach to radical treatment of epilepsy began in the neurosurgical clinic of Otfried Foerster in Germany just over forty years ago. Theodore Rasmussen has made a critical assessment of the present-day surgical treatment, its methods, and its successes [13]. I shall not refer to this, but pass instead to some functional deductions.

Experience has shown us that any effect an epileptogenic lesion may have on the brain can be reproduced by electrical stimulation if strength of stimulus is carefully modulated. We may conclude then that the Jacksonian explosive discharge, produced by what he called "high tension," is, at least in part, an electrical phenomenon.

Neurophysiology of Epilepsy

Unlike most human ailments, there are, in each epileptic seizure, certain invariable characteristics. A statement of them should formulate the neurophysiology of epilepsy. If we bear this in mind, the epilepsies throw much light on mechanisms of the brain.

Interference with local function is the effect of ictal discharge or electrical stimulation in any epileptogenic area of gray matter. Active responses result, as I concluded in a study of the excitable cortex of conscious man in 1958 [5], only when that gray matter provides axonal conduction along functional tracts to a secondary ganglionic station at a distance. The gray matter in the secondary station, since it is not subjected to the disturbance of the unphysiological electrical discharge, can act, so to speak, in a physiological manner.

Thus, as shown in Fig. 29-1, stimulation of motor cortex produces active responses from gray matter in medulla or spinal cord; stimulation of sensory cortex produces active responses in related nuclei of diencephalic gray matter; stimulation of interpretive cortex produces two types of response. There are then two different secondary ganglionic stations to be discovered.

If we would learn about brain function, we must look beyond the local areas of stimulation and discover the mechanisms involved. Each local cortical seizure provides a glimpse of a partially separable mechanism within the total function of man's master organ.

Sensory and Motor Areas

Let us consider for a moment the familiar motor and sensory areas of the cortex (Fig. 29-2). The motor stream of impulses from the higher brain stem makes a detour to motor cortex on the way out to the muscles, and the incoming stream of impulses makes a detour to the various sensory areas, on the way in (Fig. 29-3). If some functional addition is made in each of these sensory and motor way-stations, it gives these cortical detours purpose. But the interference effect prevents cortical stimulation from throwing any light on that addition. It may well be that the way of making this addition must be acquired by each individual early in life and the convolutions programmed. There is evidence that the animal kept in the dark during the first weeks that follow birth is functionally blind when he opens his eyes on a world that is seen too late.

Hubel and Wiesel have used single-cell recording techniques and natural stimuli to study the function of visual sensory cortex. They conclude, in recent work, that unless the striate cortex is trained early for binocular vision, there develops a cortical defect as compared with normal. Exposing the retina of a kitten to light alone serves to prevent atrophy of the geniculate ganglia. But only the eyes, working together under the direction of the kitten's own interest, can train the cortex to receive binocular vision. If the cortex is not trained early, a cortical defect results [3].

If the visual cortex must be programmed during kittenhood, one may well surmise that the other sensory areas must also be programmed during the earliest learning period.

It is likely too that similar programming is necessary in the motor cortex before the stream of outflowing voluntary impulse can receive the local functional addition which would give this cortical detour a purpose of its own (Figs. 29-3 and 29-7). Thus it may

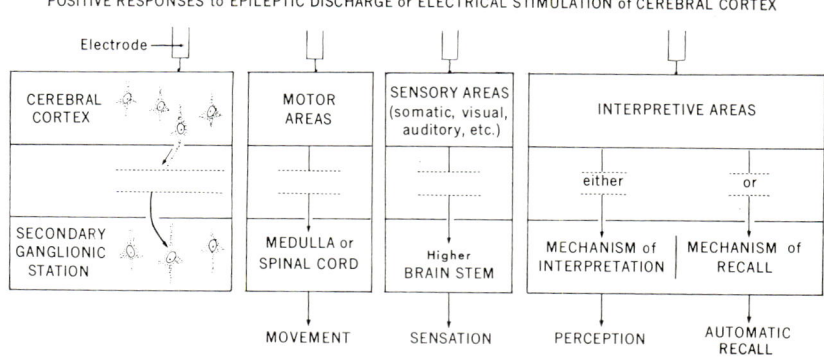

FIG. 29-1. Positive responses: Stimulation (or epileptic discharge) interferes with function of gray matter locally. It produces active response only in those areas of cerebral cortex from which axonal conduction along a functional tract activates some *distant* ganglionic station. Cortical responses are of four types: muscular movement, sensation, interpretive perception, or recall of conscious experience. (Drawn by Eleanor Sweezey.)

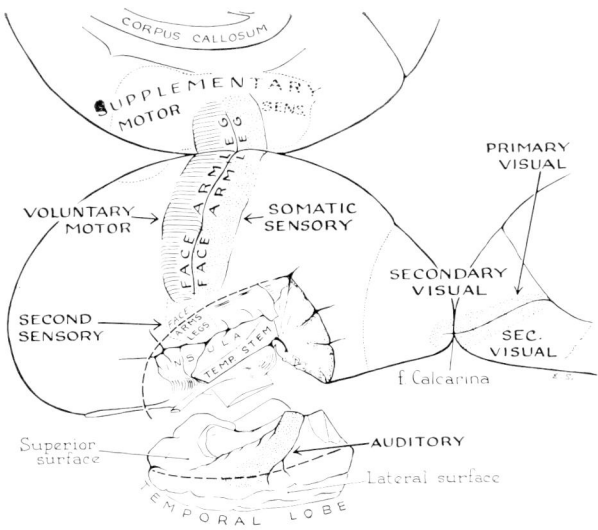

Fig. 29-2. Primary transmitting areas (sensory, stippled; motor, lined) and some secondary sensory and motor areas in the cortex of the left hemisphere as outlined by electrical stimulation. Parts of the mesial surfaces are shown. The temporal lobe is cut and turned down to expose its superior surface. Note the primary auditory sensation area on the transverse gyrus of Heschl. Stimulation of the normally buried insular cortex produces sensory and motor responses from the alimentary system, mouth to rectum. (From Penfield and Roberts [12].)

well be that cells should begin to function and axons to conduct according to a normal functional timetable.

Cerebral Cortex

Man's brain differs from that of other mammals chiefly because of the large amount of uncommitted cortex that has appeared behind the sensorimotor strip and because of the added frontal cortex anterior to it. Man's sensory and motor areas are crowded from the surface down into deep fissures and sulci.

Figures 29-4 and 29-5 show how man makes use of some of the new cortex that is not committed to sensory or motor function. Accidental destruction of the temporal (and neighboring parietal) speech area of Wernicke, in childhood, produces aphasia. But after a time, speech is reestablished on the other side and the child develops a normal command of language [12]. The same complete lesion in adult life (after age 12) would result in permanent aphasia.

In adult life, the homologous area of temporoparietal cortex in the nondominant hemisphere has developed a function of its own. It is part of the interpretive cortex. Its complete removal results in spatial disorientation, *apractognosia* [2].

This means that the patient has lost the awareness of orientation in space. The astonishing fact is that, although the initial structure of the cortex is the same on the two sides, the individual establishes the mechanism of speech in one side and the mechanism of space orientation in the other during childhood. The one gives no active responses to stimulation. The other does.

To Learn Is to Program

Electrical discharge in the temporal speech area of an adult produces aphasia. This is the interference-effect. The patient is aware of it only when called upon to speak or to read or to understand speech. There is no active response to the discharge. Stimulation of the homologous area in the minor hemisphere and the interpretive cortex elsewhere produces an active response which may be (a) the recall of an

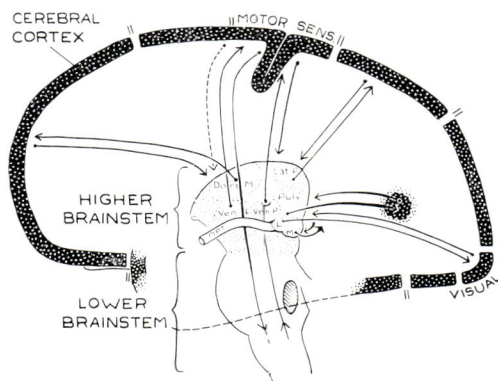

FIG. 29-3. Cerebral cortex and higher brain stem. The somatic sensory inflow is shown from periphery to thalamus and its detour out to cortex (SENS) and back to higher brain stem, shown by lines and arrows. The inflow of the other forms of discriminative sensation is shown similarly. The voluntary motor outflow originates in higher brain stem, as suggested in Fig. 29-7, is interrupted in the motor cortex, and then passes down to medulla and spinal cord. (From Penfield and Jasper [9].)

auditory or visual experience [11], or (b) a sudden interpretation of present experience [4].

Teaching an infant the mother tongue can be carried out when he is paying attention. The voluntary, or the involuntary, act of paying attention precedes and accompanies all learning. While paying attention to speech, the infant begins to program his cerebral cortex on one side only. This seems to bring about a considerable degree of specialization of function in the minor hemisphere as well. But it may well be concomitant rather than secondary. Who can say? As the infant begins to perceive the meaning of nonverbal experience, he is evidently programming the remainder of the uncommitted cortex.

Speech, too, is, in a very real sense, an interpretation, and thus it may be said that the uncommitted cortex is programmed by the child for the interpretation of verbal and nonverbal material separately. The data used by man in speaking, reading, and writing are predominantly visual and auditory, and the same is true of nonverbal perception. In other species, smell and taste, balance and touch, play a more important role.

One may surmise that a child who had never heard the spoken word would, in time, come to use the uncommitted cortex on the two sides as interpretive cortex and devote it all to nonverbal perception. This may well be the case among the other animals since they do not speak. Unfortunately, even the most cooperative dog cannot inform the surgeon what comes to his mind when an electrode is applied to the cortex! His behavior, however, during sleep, when he seems to dream of action, shows that he, too, must have a record of past experience. My own canine companion often runs and yelps in pantomime of what I've seen him do in waking life.

The motor and the sensory mechanisms constitute the brain's output and input. It is not surprising, perhaps, that an electric discharge of one volt, regularly repeated at 60 cycles per second, should cause sensory or motor cells to send out a stream of neuronal impulses and thus activate their distant nerve cell-stations. But it did come as

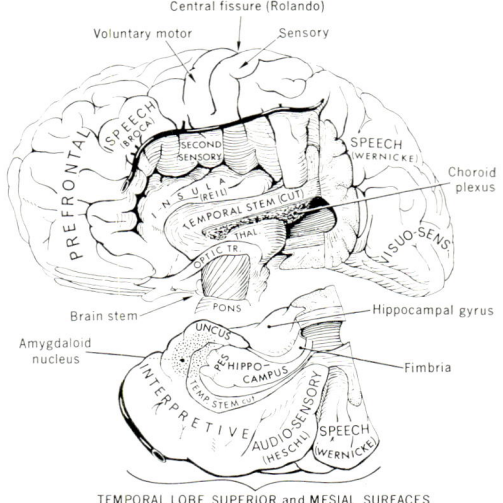

FIG. 29-4. Left cerebral hemisphere. The temporal lobe has been cut across and turned down to show the *superior* and *mesial temporal surfaces*. Note that the audiosensory cortex of Heschl's gyrus is bounded by speech posteriorly and interpretive cortex anteriorly. (Drawn by Eleanor Sweezey.)

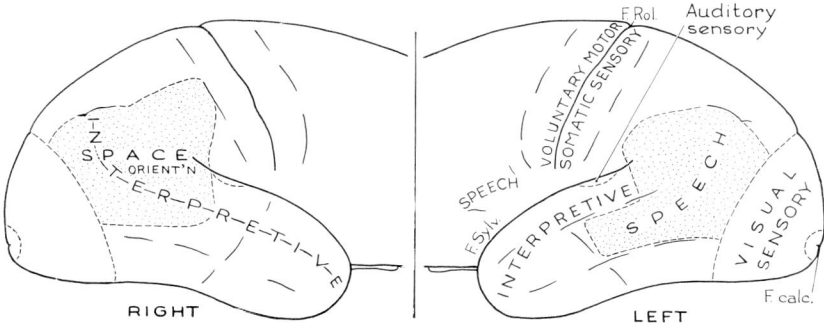

Fig. 29-5. Lateral surfaces of the posterior parts of both hemispheres of a human adult. On the dominant side interference aphasia is produced by stimulating in the area marked speech. Experiential and interpretive responses are produced in the interpretive cortex. The area marked *space orientation* on the nondominant side (right) was outlined by study of the results of cortical excision. Complete removal produces spatial disorientation without aphasia. (From Penfield [7].)

a great surprise when an electrode applied to what we now call the interpretive cortex produced active responses. Perhaps if we had listened to the teaching of epilepsy and had understood the significance of what Jackson called "psychical seizures," we would have expected these responses to the electrode.

I shall now discuss the meaning of these responses in terms of mechanisms of normal function.

The Interpretive Cortex

There are two related mechanisms revealed by stimulation of the interpretive cortex. (a) There is a brain mechanism whose function is to send neuronal signals that interpret the relationship of the individual to his immediate environment. The action is automatic and subconscious, but the signal appears in consciousness. One segment of the circuitry that produces the signal has been demonstrated, that is, the flow of axonal potentials from cells in the interpretive cortex to a ganglionic station somewhere in the subcortex. (The perception that things are familiar, and perhaps the feeling of fear, would certainly seem to call for some access to the mechanism of recall. But perception of position in space and of movement toward an individual, or away, would not seem to require the scanning of past records after the child had learned that enlargement in size with increase in sound means approach, while the reverse means departure.) There is no clue, as yet, to where the secondary (the subcortical) station is located.

(b) Second, there is a brain mechanism capable of setting in motion the patterned movement of electrical potentials that once accompanied the state of mind and the succession of thoughts that made consciousness what it was during certain moments of this man's distant past. One link in the mechanism that switches on this replay has been demonstrated: A cellular station in the interpretive cortex of one temporal lobe, by means of its conducting axons, activates a distant area of gray matter. This distant area, being activated physiologically, switches on, as its active response, the replay of experience and keeps it going.

How often do *psychical* responses (interpretive or experiential) occur? Perhaps it would serve a useful purpose to insert, here and there, an answer to questions that come up repeatedly in discussion of this work. It has been my own habit, in every exploration, to obtain a somatic motor or a sensory response in order to identify the fissure of Rolando and to determine the strength of stimulus to be used in any attempt to reproduce the initial phenomenon in the attacks of that particular patient. But, as a rule, no effort was made to produce psychical responses unless psychical phenomena had occurred in the patient's habitual minor seizures. In about 50 cases, there were psychical responses of varying content from different points. To obtain temporal lobe responses, in any case, the stimulus usually had to be increased by one volt, or occasionally two (see [9]).

My associate, Phanor Perot, and I made a final summary of the initial Montreal experience [11]. Out of 1288 such operations, there were 520 with electric stimulation of the cortex of one temporal lobe. In 40 of these there were positive experiential responses; there were none as the result of stimulation of other areas. These responses were not epileptic in any of the 40 cases. The response ceased when the electrode was withdrawn or the current shut off. Fifty-three of the patients, suffering from temporal-lobe epilepsy, complained, in advance, of experiential seizures. This analysis was up to 1961. According to Rasmussen, about 20 percent of the published experiential and interpretive responses were obtained while he or one of my other associates was carrying out the operation.

Neurosurgeons who rely on electrocorticography for guidance during cortical excision are not apt to take time to stimulate the cortex. On the other hand, I had used stimulation as a guide in temporal excisions before the art of electroencephalography was highly developed. I have continued to use it, when there is time and opportunity, since that time.

Opportunity-to-learn walks into the operating room with any surgeon who has unanswered questions in his mind. The good of the patient is his first consideration. But as he works on the exposed brain, he should talk to reassure an alert and understanding subject. Opportunity stands at his elbow then. Like an unseen Puck, it whispers to him from time to time: "This chance may never come again. Stop for just a moment. Consider. Apply the electrode. Listen to what the patient says. Control and verify his response critically while you still can."

The recall of a man's past awarenesses, when it is evoked, is complete and detailed. There are none of the fanciful elaborations that occur in a man's dreaming. Music repeated over and over again varies not at all. Intelligent patients assert it must have happened that way.

Are we to conclude, then, that the whole of a man's conscious experience is recorded thus? My reply is "No." One should not go beyond the evidence. It may be.

It is clear that, at least when an individual's attention is focused on auditory and visual phenomena, a complete engram is left behind in the brain. When I say "a complete engram," I mean that what the individual paid attention to was recorded leaving out all else—leaving out all incoming sensory information that was ignored at the moment.

To illustrate from our published experience, here is an experiential response that was largely auditory: The patient, J.T., exclaimed with astonishment, when a point on the superior surface of the right temporal lobe was stimulated just anterior to the auditory convolution, "Yes, Doctor, yes, Doctor! Now I hear people laughing—my friends in South Africa." When asked, after the current was shut off, he said they were his "two cousins Bessie and Ann Wheliaw." He did not know why they were laughing. Some days after the operation I discussed the matter with him. He remembered it all and said he was standing with his cousins and that they were all laughing together at something. This was only a brief flashback. It began too late to include the joke that had gone before. While lying on the operating table, he perceived who his companions were and where they were and what they were doing. But he could not recall the awareness that had been his a few moments before. Only the sound and the awareness of his cousins had come to him.

On the other hand, such flashbacks may be largely visual. H. P., a fifteen-year-old girl, said, when the electrode was applied briefly to her right second temporal convolution anteriorly, "I am seeing somebody." After an interval the electrode was reapplied to the same point without warning her. She was silent. Then she said, "It is coming again." I asked her if she saw somebody and she replied, "Sure, a boy." Sometime later, the electrode was applied a centimeter distant on the first temporal convolution. "A dream is starting," she said. "There are a lot of people . . . in the living room. I think one of them is my mother." When asked if they were speaking, she said she did not know.

In another case, stimulation of a point on the superior surface of the left first temporal convolution, deep in the fissure of Sylvius, caused her (D.F.) to hear a song. Fifteen minutes later, the point was stimulated again without the patient's knowledge. She heard it again, the same song. After that, I took time out to stimulate the point again and again at intervals [6].

Each time, she heard the same song played by an orchestra. She described it and hummed an accompaniment to it. She thought we were turning on a phonograph in the operating room. No one explained to her otherwise. Other points in the temporal cortex were stimulated but only one produced an active response, a feeling of fear. (I have considered fear to be a type of interpretive response.)

Almost a year after her return home, I wrote to her, explaining as best I could, what had happened during the operation. She was a very intelligent young woman, and I shall quote from her reply:

"Today is a year that [since] you operated on me, and I suppose you are wondering how I am coming along. . . .

"Now to your questions: I heard the song right from the beginning and, you know, I could remember much more of it right in the operating room. . . .

"There were musical instruments. . . . It was as though it were being played by an orchestra. Definitely it *was not* as though I were imagining the tune to myself. I actually heard it. . . . I finally got hold of a copy of this piece and played it on the piano the other Sunday.

"Thanks again for better health."

The anterior portion of the left temporal lobe was removed at the operation. There was an atrophic, epileptogenic lesion within it. She was right-handed.

LOCALIZATION IN THE INTERPRETATIVE CORTEX

We may now consider the localization of experiential and interpretive responses taken together: In Fig. 29-6 I have made a map of the posterior portions of the right and left hemispheres. The major (temporal) speech area is shown by stippling in the left hemisphere and the spatial-orientation area in the right. A rough idea of the distribution of all the psychical responses may be given by reference to it, and a few remarks are in order about the meaning of the map.

When either an experiential response or an interpretive response has a strongly auditory content or when it is both auditory and visual, it comes from the first temporal convolution of one side or the other. There, it is near the auditory sensory gyrus (Fig. 29-4). If either type of response is strongly visual, it comes from the nondominant side reasonably near the visual sensory cortex, and only rarely from the dominant side. See Fig. 29-6, a map drawn to show both interpretive and experiential responses.

This argues for some interrelationship between the mechanism of interpretation and that of recall. And yet the electrode never activated both—an experience from the past and an interpretation of the present—at the same time.

The perception of *familiarity* calls for special consideration. It is produced almost exclusively by stimulation of the minor interpretive cortex but in an area more anterior, as shown in Fig. 29-6. Feelings of fear, unreality, lonesomeness, or of being somewhere else were produced in either temporal region, but they were too infrequent in our series to allow conclusion as to special localization.

In ordinary life, the automatic signal, which informs a conscious individual that present experience is familiar, comes to everyone, I suppose. If it is accurate, and it usually is, one must be using an automatic mechanism that can scan a record of the past, a past that has *not* faded. This perception of familiarity is not limited to auditory or visual experience at all, but apparently applies to all that enters consciousness. A person seen may be labeled as "seen before (déjà vu)," a bar of music as "heard before," a sequence of events as "happened before."

Such perceptions must depend upon a scanning mechanism somewhere in the

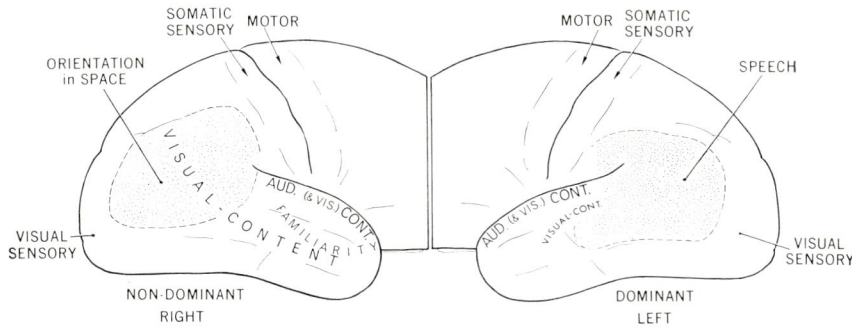

Fig. 29-6. Location of stimulation points producing *psychical responses,* analyzed according to *content.* Recall of strongly visual experience was produced, in the great majority of cases, from interpretive cortex on the nondominant side, rarely on the other side (visual-content). The same was true of interpretive signals that had to do with things seen. They were rare on the dominant side.

On the first temporal convolution of both sides [marked: AUD. (& VIS.) CONT.] purely auditory, or mixed auditory and visual, experiential responses and interpretive responses were produced. The interpretive response of familiarity appears, as a result of stimulation, only on the nondominant side as far as our experience goes. (Drawn by Eleanor Sweezey.)

brain as well as upon the record of consciousness. This is further justification for the point of view that the recall mechanism, demonstrated in this body of evidence, somehow plays a part in the *automatic* and subconscious process of interpretation of present experience.

Voluntary Recall

One may assume that when any individual turns his attention to a selected moment in the very recent past he makes use of the record that was described above. But whether he makes use of the interpretive cortex to activate that record is not at all clear. Certainly, the details of one's conscious experience fade progressively and are soon beyond the reach of voluntary recollection. If they did not do so, it would be difficult to distinguish events of today from those of yesterday. Thus an awareness of overvivid memories might well confuse the present.

The hippocampal formations certainly play an essential role in the voluntary or conscious recall of past experience: Bilateral removal of these formations puts an end to the voluntary recall at least of recent events. The hippocampi may, as well, play an essential role in the laying down of the engram that makes voluntary recall of sequential experience possible. But the absence of these structures produces little interference with the memory and use of speech, no loss of the perception of orientation in space. The learned skills and the perception of concepts are preserved.

Thus it is clear that an engram of memory is to be recognized in many of the brain's mechanisms. An engram is the *lasting trace* or the *permanent impression* left behind in the nervous system by psychical experience. I have discussed engrams elsewhere to the best of my ability quite recently [7].

The recall mechanism that is demonstrated by epileptic discharge or electrical stimulation in the interpretive cortex seems to be part of a perception and interpretation system that is automatic. What is its relationship to voluntary recall?

ICTAL DISCHARGE IN THE DIENCEPHALON

I asked myself that question at the beginning of this review—and do so again now. We may apply the physiological principles of an epileptic fit to the higher brain stem as well as the cortex. What more can epilepsy teach us?

There is another phenomenon we have

not considered. When local discharge, occurring in the cortex, is severe enough, the discharging state is communicated by *projection* along neuron pathways to gray matter lying at a distance [9]. Thus, a secondary discharging state is produced. If this secondary discharge occurs in gray matter of the higher brain stem, it produces loss of consciousness during (a) generalized convulsion or (b) automatism.

Men, in olden times, looked on a generalized convulsive attack as a *seizure* of the mind and the body by a spirit. Frightened, they watched the poor fellow fall and froth at the mouth perhaps, and soil himself. The Greeks, meanwhile, opened their cloaks and spat on themselves to keep the evil spirit away. In later centuries, Christians crossed themselves. What men did in the Orient I do not know. Perhaps someone will tell me.

There is an invariable loss of consciousness during a general convulsion. The patient will have a subsequent amnesia for the period of the discharge and the period of neuronal fatigue that follows it.

But there is another epileptic state in which consciousness is lost, or is seriously disturbed, without generalized convulsion. Amnesia for the period always follows. This is *automatism*. At such times the body carries on as though it had become an automaton, doing things (sometimes crude, sometimes complicated) that it might well have carried out "subconsciously" in normal life.

It is my good fortune to have restudied, from time to time, the patterns of epileptic seizures with one brilliant, hard-working associate after another [8, 9, 10]. Spread of discharge is local or by axonal projection to secondary ganglionic areas.

There are significant differences in the results of spread-by-projection (it may also be called spread-by-bombardment) depending on where, in the cerebral cortex, the epileptogenic lesion is located:

(1) Sensory and motor area discharge may lead, by projection, to a generalized convulsion and with it loss of consciousness, but never simple automatism.

(2) Temporal discharge may produce either one (convulsion or automatism). If it produces automatism, that may or may not be followed in turn by a generalized seizure.

(3) Anterior frontal (prefrontal) discharge may also produce either. That is to say, it may precipitate a generalized convulsion. Or, it may produce automatism, which in turn may or may not be followed by a major convulsion.

We were first aware of these differences in the effect of projection when Kristiansen, after examining 95 cases in our clinic, pointed out that there were 29 examples of local motor seizures, 55 somatic sensory, and 11 visual sensory seizures. None developed automatism during the evolution of attacks. Many, however, went from localized manifestation directly to generalized seizures.

AUTOMATISM

Automatism Following Temporal Lobe Discharge. This form is frequent. Feindel found that, in a series of 155 patients who suffered from seizures arising in one temporal lobe, the majority (78 percent) exhibited behavioral automatism at one time or another. They did this occasionally at the outset of the attack, more often after preliminary psychical, sensory, or brief motor phenomena. He and I discovered that automatism could be produced by stimulation, during operation. It could be produced only deep in the periamygdaloid region beneath the uncus (Fig. 29-4). But it never appeared as a simple response to the electrode's stimulus. Instead, it developed only when stimulation was followed by epileptic afterdischarge. We concluded that the automatism was associated with extension of discharge into gray matter centrally placed in higher brain stem [1].

Automatism Following Prefrontal Discharge. This form of automatism may be distinguished, by experienced clinicians, from that which appears in temporal lobe cases. The difference is not, however, in the automatism itself so much as in the associated phenomena produced by discharge in neighboring areas of cortex, usually before projection to subcortical gray matter.

Thus, in temporal cases, there may easily

be added phenomena from discharge in the interpretive cortex, or the insular cortex, and the second-sensory cortex at the bottom of the fissure of Sylvius (Figs. 29-2 and 29-4).

The prefrontal area is separated from the Rolandic motor gyrus by a zone of cortex that is devoted (from above down) to the supplementary motor area, the adversive-turning area and, on the dominant side, the speech area of Broca. Thus frontal automatism may well be preceded by turning of the body or the gaze. Otherwise frontal automatism resembles a petit mal attack.

Stimulation of the prefrontal cortex produces no active simple responses, and neither the patient nor an observer is aware of any outward manifestation. Even an epileptic discharge passes unobserved in the prefrontal area, unless an electrographic recording is in process. After recording electrodes had been applied to the exposed cortex (electrocorticography), we have produced a local discharge by stimulating the prefrontal cortex and followed its transition to subcortical discharge, observing, meanwhile, that the patient changed from normal behavior to automatism [9].

When a prefrontal epileptogenic lesion that is giving rise to recurring attacks of automatism is located deep in a fissure or sulcus, and thus is at a distance from the scalp, the electroencephalograph is apt to miss the initial one-sided discharges and to pick up only the bilaterally synchronous wave-and-spike abnormality so characteristic of petit mal seizures. Thus the automatic behavior and the electrographic abnormality produced in petit mal attacks and frontal automatism may be quite similar.

Petit Mal Automatism. A petit mal attack has its focus of irritation in the higher brain stem. If it is like other fits, the originating discharge takes place in an area of gray matter. This, we may then assume, lies in the higher brain stem.

In each attack, the loss of consciousness is initial. Sometimes there is also a sudden pallor or a fluttering of the eyelids, sometimes a brief bilateral jerk of muscles, sometimes a sudden nod or a fall that signals momentary interference with the midbrain's maintenance of erect posture. But there are no continuing generalized convulsive spasms. The patient may continue to walk or even to play the piano or to drive an automobile for a time.

The clinician recognizes, in a petit mal seizure, the sudden lapse of consciousness without initial one-sided phenomena. If there is movement, it is symmetrical and fleeting. The electroencephalographer recognizes in it a brain-wave change that is symmetrical. It presents the typical spike and slow wave sequences. It is obvious that the discharge must take place in central gray matter that has equal access of communication to both hemispheres. Jackson concluded simply that the discharge producing these fits occurred at the "highest level" of brain function.

Following his line of thought, the fact that there are such fits proves the existence of an area of gray matter which forms an essential part of a mechanism of the mind. The hypothesis, then, is an obvious one, that this gray matter normally plays a role in the neuronal action that *corresponds* to each successive state of consciousness. During automatism, ictal discharge interferes with the action of that mechanism so selectively that the sensory and the motor mechanisms, and the conditioned reflexes of human skills, may still operate for a time. This is, in a sense, a first step in the direction of localization. It attracts attention to diencephalon and to mesencephalon, that is, the higher brain stem. Compression or injury in this region also extinguishes awareness and is followed by amnesia.

Discharge during a petit mal seizure produces no active response. It interferes with function in the area of discharge just as a fit in the speech cortex interferes with the function of the speech mechanism. In the one case, interference produces unconsciousness; in the other, aphasia. One may conclude, then, that there is, largely in the higher brain stem (Figs. 29-3 and 29-7), a mechanism whose action corresponds with conscious activity.

In passing, let me say that it would be wrong to jump to philosophical conclusions —to assume that neuronal activity here produces the conscious state in the first

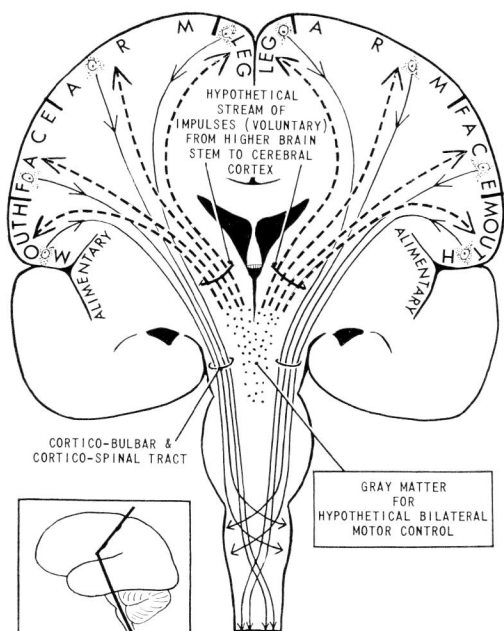

FIG. 29-7. Bilateral motor-control system. The angulated vertical section passes through the human brain as shown in the inset. Motor areas of cortex from leg to mouth are shown in the precentral gyrus. The ganglionic area in which epileptogenic discharge produces (grand mal) generalized convulsion is suggested by the dotted zone. The exact localization of this gray matter is yet to be discovered.

place. It would be equally premature to assume that the mental state produces the neuronal activity and determines its pattern. A critical scientist can only establish the fact that the two sequences do correspond, the mental and the physical. So much is clear.

GENERALIZED CONVULSION

For the purpose of discussion, consider a patient who has an attack of petit mal. If the discharge that produces automatism, instead of subsiding, increases in violence, the picture changes suddenly. The patient has a grand mal generalized convulsion. The sudden change means there has been spread of the ictal (epileptic) ganglionic discharge from an area of gray matter, in which only interference was produced, to an area capable of active response. The interference, with the mechanism related to consciousness alone, has been followed by discharge in gray matter that has for its function bilateral motor control. There are two mechanisms then. One has to do with consciousness alone and a second with bilateral motor control as well as consciousness.

On the basis of this hypothesis, generalized convulsion does not signify global discharge of cerebral gray matter. It would be enough if ictal discharge occurred in the gray matter of the higher brain stem that conducts to both hemispheres. It is assumed that discharge there interferes with the cerebral mechanism related to consciousness. The discharge in the higher brain stem may be primary, as in grand mal cases. It may be secondary when cortical epileptogenic lesions are present.

All generalized convulsions as studied by a clinician, or by an electrophysiologist, vary little from case to case. The patterns at the beginning may differ, depending on the place of initial discharge, but the end result is much the same.

After the muscular spasms cease, the loss of consciousness continues through the postictal period of ganglionic fatigue and electrographic silence. Only the automatic control of respiration, located in the medulla oblongata, has escaped the dreadful command of this diencephalic gray matter. At onset, there may be a very brief period of unconsciousness before convulsion begins. If so, the electroencephalogram, in that brief period, often has, I am told, the form characteristic of petit mal automatism.

On the assumption that all epileptic seizures are caused by a discharge in gray matter, we conclude that there are in the higher brain stem two areas of gray matter symmetrically placed. The one produces automatism when subjected to discharge. The other produces unconsciousness and convulsion.

During an attack of automatism, one sees the patient at times carry out sequences of purposeful acts like those a normal individual might well carry out when he is focusing his attention on something else.

It is sometimes obvious that the automaton, in addition to his preservation of motor skills, may preserve a short-term purpose, with which his automatic mechanism was somehow endowed shortly before the onset of the attack.

Thus, the central motor mechanism can, it seems, accept a purpose and carry it out. This throws light on the automatic integration of motor activity that is normally carried out by this central *motor mechanism*. Other patients follow a purpose established as a habit—like the man who, during his attacks of automatism, would put on his hat and coat and then set off for the bus terminal.

It is a common experience that one can program his own motor mechanism. In my own case, on leaving the house in the morning and stepping into my automobile, prepared to drive, I find it necessary to stop and plan what streets to follow according to that morning's purpose. After that, it is possible to think of other things and yet to arrive at the planned destination. But if I omit this moment of preliminary street planning, I automatically deliver myself to the Neurological Institute, even when I wanted to arrive at another rendezvous. Thus, we may all of us recognize the potential automaton within ourselves.

A Mechanism That Corresponds with the Mind

The behavior of the patient during an attack of automatism throws a revealing light on a neuronal mechanism that must be related to consciousness. It can be neatly and selectively *switched off* by the interference of discharge. What the automaton lacks is what this mechanism makes possible.

Under normal conditions, it is the neuronal action in this mind mechanism that makes the conscious elaboration of new purposes and of conscious control possible. There is a corresponding parallelism, one may assume, between the changing content of a man's mind and the progressive action of this mechanism. Assuming this, however, does not enable one to explain the nature of thought or of thought control.

Engram

The switching off of the mechanism that corresponds with and makes possible the action of the mind tells us something about the mechanism and the mind, much as aphasic interference tells us about the speech mechanism and the verbal processes of mind.

Can this mechanism that corresponds with awareness be switched on as well as off? What is an experiential response if it is not a switching on of that mechanism? When an electrode is placed on the interpretive cortex of one temporal lobe and a strip of past experience is brought to mind, is it this mechanism that is activated? Yes, I think it must be. At all events, since no other hypothesis presents itself, let us assume that it is.

This means that the ictal discharge (or electrical stimulation) in the interpretive cortex causes the mind's mechanism to repeat its previous action. On this basis, automatism is the result of interference with the mind mechanism and experiential response is the result of activation of the same mechanism.

If true, we face a startling opportunity to draw a conclusion: The mechanism that corresponds with mind must lay down its own permanent record within itself. There must be a thread of *permanent facilitation* that runs through its own neuronal action during each man's waking hours.

The engram of the stream of consciousness is evidently formed by the single passage of impulses while the individual's attention is focused. Attention, then, by some selective effect, must determine what is to be recorded. How is this brought about? Whatever the answer to that question may be, it is a fact that the things of which the subject is aware are recorded. Ten years later, a stream of axonal impulses from the interpretive cortex can revive the whole state of consciousness and cause it to flow from one awareness to succeeding ones. One must conclude that the imprinting of the engram takes place while the individual is still paying attention.

Facilitation for a second passage of impulses along a path of neuronal connections is well known to physiologists. Elsewhere in the nervous system, it is largely a temporary phenomenon. But here the facilitation is permanent.

Temporary facilitation of active response to stimulation of the motor cortex of the mammalian brain, for example, was studied by Sherrington and his pupils. For a time after the first application of the electrode to a cortical point, they found the threshold to be reduced for subsequent stimulations.

This temporary facilitation applies similarly to stimulation of the human motor cortex in our experience and also to the sensory cortex. When we began to stimulate the interpretive cortex, we found the same evidences of temporary facilitation. Thus a second and third stimulation may produce the same response, and there is enough facilitation so that if the later electrode applications are at a distance, say of a centimeter, the same response may still be obtained. The same song comes back or the same familiar scene. But these are all effects due to temporary change in the cortex, or perhaps in the secondarily activated ganglionic station.

While the cortical electrode is recalling the past, the patient has what Jackson called a "doubling of consciousness."

DISCUSSION

Finally, to summarize, it is evident that all mechanisms that play a role in the integrated neuronal action of the brain are related to consciousness. Certainly the speech mechanism, interpretive perception, and the automatic recall of past experience are intimately involved in what one might consider psychical processes. The localized epileptic seizure and cortical stimulation have thrown light on these mechanisms as well as on the more familiar sensory and motor mechanisms.

Thus, when we turn from the cerebral cortex to the fits that are produced by discharge within the higher brain stem, two types of attack emerge. And two neuronal mechanisms begin to emerge from the brain's central integrating and coordinating activity.

Automatism. There is first, evidently, an area of gray matter within the higher brain stem in which discharge produces ictal automatism. During discharge (and in the period of subsequent cellular fatigue) the neuronal mechanism that corresponds with mental activity is paralyzed. When ictal discharge originates in that gray matter, the automatism has all the features of the petit mal variety of seizures. But the same neuronal mechanism may be paralyzed secondarily by bombardment from an epileptogenic focus in frontal or temporal areas. The beginning is different, the eventual automatism much the same.

Convulsion. Secondly, there is an area of gray matter in the brain stem in which discharge produces active response in the motor systems of both hemispheres. This precipitates a generalized convulsion. It is the grand mal seizure produced by initial local discharge. But an identical major seizure is produced secondarily when bombardment from one of the various areas of the cerebral cortex touches it off.

The central motor control mechanism (Fig. 29-7), is, one may assume, what carries on in normal life when a man turns his thought and attention to matters unrelated to his own behavior. From the point of view of function, it is apparent that during an attack of automatism the central motor mechanism continues to function. The behavior of an epileptic automaton, deprived of conscious control, throws a startling light on that mechanism.

Thus, discharge in the *automatism-producing* gray matter allows one to see that the central control mechanism can still call on the skills and perceptions established by previous conditioning of the various specialized areas of the cortex. On the other hand, discharge in the *convulsion-producing* gray matter of the higher brain stem tells us nothing of all that. It shows only that the gray matter now discharging is part of the bilateral motor mechanism of the brain.

The second mechanism that emerges has, in it, an area of gray matter in the higher brain stem that produces automatism when it becomes the site of epileptic discharge. This interferes with the action of a neuronal mechanism related to consciousness, a mechanism that corresponds to, and accompanies, the current transactions of the mind.

What, then, of the sequential record of

consciousness that we know exists? The hypothesis presents itself that the neuronal record of conscious experience is, in fact, a thread of permanent facilitation formed within the ganglionic circuitry of that same mechanism which corresponds with mind. Recall of past conscious experience would then be possible when a continuing stream of neuron impulses finds its way to the engram thread.

Thus the recall of past experience could be an activation of the engram, a reactivation. And the secondary ganglionic station which produces experiential recall may be the same as the gray matter which produces automatism when subject to primary discharge. If not the same, then there must be another available ganglionic station in the mechanism.

As far as higher brain-stem localization is concerned, it may be said that the central motor-control mechanism has a major area of gray matter located somewhere there. But the mechanism itself cannot be so delimited. It extends far beyond the limits of brain stem. The same is true of the mechanism that corresponds with the sequences of the mind—the gray matter in which ictal discharge produces petit mal automatism is in the higher brain stem. But the mind's mechanism (if I may call it that) must constantly reach out to, and involve, other mechanisms of the brain.

The diencephalon of man has its bulging thalamic nuclei from which the various areas of cerebral cortex are outgrowths. The brain is like a tree. Neither trunk nor branch can function alone.

Once I pointed out the evidence of the existence of "neuronal circuits which are most intimately associated with the initiation of voluntary activity and with the sensory summation prerequisite to it." They were to be sought, I suggested, within the "old brain. . . . All regions of the brain may well be involved in normal conscious processes but the indispensable substratum of consciousness lies outside the cerebral cortex, probably in the diencephalon" (Penfield, 1938).

It seemed better to refer to higher brain stem, including thus the midbrain and perhaps upper pons with the diencephalon.

Later, I began to use the expression centrencephalic coordinating and integrating system (Penfield, 1952) and referred to the petit mal and grand mal attacks that arise in the gray matter of the higher brain stem as centrencephalic seizures. Unfortunately some workers, who misunderstood my meaning, thought of a separate area and coined the term "centrencephalon" as though there were a new anatomical subdivision.

Function, I suppose, is never localized in gray matter, whether it has been mapped thus on the cerebral cortex or in a nucleus. Function may only be localized in a wider ranging mechanism. All these mechanisms are only partly separable for our examination, since they play a coordinated role in overall brain function.

Finally, the evidence derived from the study of the epilepsies suggests that, within the coordinating activity we have described as centrencephalic, there are two brain mechanisms. One has to do with the mind, the other with central control of the motor system. During automatism, the former mechanism is out of action while the latter carries on by virtue of the programming that has already come to it.

Epilogue

There are obvious analogies between a computer and the brain. Conditioning the brain is somewhat like programming a computer. To learn is to program. Learning, it seems, whether it has to do with skills, or words or concepts or sequences of behavior, takes place within the focused limits of conscious attention.

The mind and its corresponding mechanism controls attention. It is, in a sense, the mind with its mechanisms that programs the brain. Thus, the mind seems to program the central motor mechanism, establishing its skills, as well as the short-term purposes that an automaton exhibits during some attacks of automatism.

The sequential engram that we have discussed is not the only engram. Engrams are laid down in the mechanisms of motor skill, speech, perception, and memorization. Finally, it is evident that man learns while paying attention, and perhaps only then,

When he focuses his attention, he is always programming his brain. This is a reasonable hypothesis and one of great importance to those who would teach.

REFERENCES

1. Feindel, W., and Penfield, W. Localization of discharge in temporal lobe automatism. *A.M.A. Arch. Neurol. Psychiat.* 72:605, 1954.
2. Hécaen, H., Penfield, W., Bertrand, C., and Malmo, R. The syndrome of apractognosia due to lesions of the minor cerebral hemisphere. *A.M.A. Arch. Neurol. Psychiat.* 75:400, 1956.
3. Hubel, D. Eleventh Bowditch Lecture. Effects of distortion of sensory input on the visual system of kittens. *Physiologist* 10:17, 1967.
4. Mullan, S., and Penfield, W. Illusions of comparative interpretation and emotion. Production by epileptic discharge and electrical stimulation of the temporal cortex. *A.M.A. Arch. Neurol. Psychiat.* 81:269, 1959.
5. Penfield, W. *The Excitable Cortex in Conscious Man.* Liverpool: Liverpool University Press, 1958; Springfield, Ill.: Thomas, 1958.
6. Penfield, W. Some mechanisms of consciousness discovered during electrical stimulation of the brain. *Proc. Nat. Acad. Sci. USA* 44:51, 1958.
7. Penfield, W. Engrams in the human brain. *Proc. Roy. Soc. Med.* 61:831, 1968.
8. Penfield, W., and Gage, L. Cerebral localization of epileptic manifestations. *A.M.A. Arch. Neurol. Psychiat.* 30:709, 1933.
9. Penfield, W., and Jasper, H. *Epilepsy and the Functional Anatomy of the Human Brain.* Boston: Little, Brown, 1954.
10. Penfield, W., and Kristiansen, K. *Epileptic Seizure Patterns.* Springfield, Ill.: Thomas, 1950.
11. Penfield, W., and Perot, P. The brain's record of auditory and visual experience. *Brain* 86:595, 1963.
12. Penfield, W., and Roberts, L. *Speech and Brain-Mechanisms.* Princeton, N.J.: Princeton University Press, 1959.
13. Rasmussen, T. Neurosurgical Treatment of Focal Epilepsy. In Niedermeyer, E. (Ed.), *Modern Aspects of Neurology.* Basel and New York: Karger, to be published.

30

A Prospectus

A. EARL WALKER

ADVANCES in medicine rarely develop at an even pace but tend to occur in spurts, followed by periods in which, although gains are consolidated, relatively little new is added. This has been the case with the epilepsies. Toward the end of the last century, the clinical manifestations of the various epilepsies were described in precise terms. However, no insight into basic mechanisms occurred until electrical current was used to stimulate the nervous system. The demonstration that such excitation produced motor responses that resembled epileptic seizures seen in the clinic stimulated thinking neurologists to consider epileptic manifestations in terms of electrical theories of nervous function. Accordingly Hughlings Jackson, although not personally involved in the physiological studies that were being carried out in laboratories of continental Europe and England in the latter part of the nineteenth century, deduced hypotheses for mechanisms of epileptic attacks on the basis of astute clinical observations. It was almost fifty years before the next advance came with the introduction of electrical recording techniques. Development of thermionic valves for amplification of minute currents made it possible for physiologists to study electrical potentials developed by cells of the nervous system and to record them both indirectly through scalp and directly by means of electrodes placed upon or within individual cells. Pioneering work by Berger [2], Adrian and Matthews [1], and Rosenbleuth and Cannon [7] served as the foundation for new conceptualization of epileptic mechanisms. Working with this precise instrumentation in the last thirty years, investigators both in the clinic and in the laboratory have been revealing new concepts of brain function. In epilepsies, particularly important clinical observations and experimental findings have been reported over the years by the Montreal group. This monograph is a fitting tribute to physiological studies carried out by Dr. Jasper in the laboratory and by Dr. Penfield in the operating room. Certainly much research presented in this volume has been stimulated by their ideas of the mechanisms of epilepsy.

This book is not only a compendium of current knowledge of epilepsy, but will serve as the foundation for further advances in this field. In what direction and with what instruments will these new advances develop? Obviously it is impossible to imagine what new techniques might be developed in the next few years by which new concepts of epileptic mechanisms might be constructed. The comments that will be expressed should not be construed as criticisms of current endeavors, but merely as flights of imagination into the future.

GENETIC CONSIDERATIONS

Genetic factors that might be operative in the epilepsies should be explored in the future. Unfortunately we are not quite sure which functional or structural criteria to use in looking for genetic factors.

One could examine the chromosomes for morphological or immunochemical abnormalities that might be associated with a primary or secondary epileptic trait. A primary genetic factor would decrease the inherent threshold of brain to epileptic seizures. A secondary trait would produce a local cerebral or systemic disorder predisposing to epilepsy. For some of the latter disorders, such as phenylketonuria and maple syrup disease, discussed in this volume, a specific enzyme defect has been identified. However, the mechanism by which retained degradation products induce the epileptic state is not yet clarified. Models that might be induced by simple overloading with a known breakdown product or by blocking by an antienzyme should afford promising leads for investigation of the basic epileptic state.

Further study of chromosomal characteristics of individuals with hereditary defects associated with epilepsy might be quite revealing. Granted that light microscopic examination cannot show a specific epileptic gene, there is the chance that the ultrastructure revealed by electron microscopy or x-ray diffraction might disclose an *epileptic configuration* in the deoxyribonucleic acid (DNA) of the chromosome; if so, it could be searched for in persons with various types of epilepsy and in siblings of epileptics, thus establishing the hereditary factor.

Demographic explorations are handicapped by the lack of definition of the condition. It is not clear as to whether one should look for individuals who have had overt clinical seizures or for those who have only abnormalities in the electroencephalogram. If it is the latter, should one consider only the abnormalities present under resting conditions or those that may be induced by various activating procedures? And what type of EEG pattern should be considered epileptic? Or should all so-called dysrhythmic patterns be considered? Then the question arises if the electroencephalographic study should be confined to individuals of certain ages, such as preadolescence or adolescence, when the percentage of positives might be at its peak. These considerations have made the study of the genetic factors in epilepsy difficult. In the future, if, as seems possible, all citizens of the country will have their medical history from birth put on magnetic tape, it may not be difficult to carry out a meaningful epidemiological study. With detailed medical records of pregnancy, birth, infancy, and childhood of each person, a significant study should be feasible that would define genetic factors in various epilepsies and establish the role of such predispositions in acquired seizure states associated with organic brain disease.

FUNCTION AND STRUCTURE

With the development of instruments to examine the ultrastructure of cells, it became possible to define the structural substrate of certain conditions which were thought previously to be functional derangements. Since it is now possible to produce epilepsies by various physical and chemical means, which presumably generate fits by different mechanisms, a comparative examination of the ultrastructure of neurons, glia, and even blood vessels, after induction of such seizures, would be of considerable interest. An epileptogenic agent that affects an enzyme system that is impeding utilization of glucose would probably induce different changes in cell structures than one which modified permeability of the cell membrane to ion transfer, thus effecting a state of cerebral edema. This approach to the basic mechanisms of an epilepsy is quite feasible with techniques at hand, although careful controls will be essential to avoid complicating artifacts. Because manifestations of convulsions induced by various agents have such different clinical patterns, neuronal response as determined by microelectrodes and ultrastructural changes may reflect more systemic alterations secondary to seizure than primary neural epileptogenic mechanisms. Structural adaptive phenomena to continuous epileptic discharge might well be discernible by electron microscopic examination for some days after a barrage.

One might look at this problem from a different standpoint and explore the effects of known structural alterations of the cell. The elimination of some boutons from soma and dendrites of cells in the precentral convolution by lesions of thalamus, corpus callosum, and prefrontal and parietal cortex would allow one to examine the remaining structure and function of partially denuded cortical neurons. The correlation of physiological activity of such deafferented neurons with their ultrastructural characteristics and enzyme systems might clarify some of the confusion regarding the hypersensitivity of the isolated neuron.

Finally, the fine morphological changes that occur at or in the cell membrane as the result of generalized or localized trauma to the head, which may be associated with neuronal discharge, should give some insight into the structural derangements of one type of epileptic activity.

FUTURE BIOCHEMICAL TRENDS

Tower has presented strong evidence that epileptogenic agents can act by interference with the integrated enzyme chain between glucose and oxygen. Their common effect is an inhibition of enzyme action at some point in this cycle. Since drugs that affect a specific stage in the development of energy can now be synthesized, the biochemist has an ideal opportunity to study the specific effects of modifying cell activity by interruption of energy cycles at various levels, thus allowing the buildup of degradation products that must interfere with energy-dependent enzyme systems of the membrane which regulate the ionic environment of the cell. If systematically studied, this aspect of cellular metabolism, which has only been sporadically explored in the past, should yield fascinating information regarding many mechanisms that cause a cell to discharge repetitively.

Perhaps the analysis of the biochemical changes might be simplified if the unit is considered a system including blood vessel, glia, neuron, and finally ependyma somewhat comparable to the glomerular system of the kidney. In brain, energy-dependent enzymal systems are responsible for the transport of ions and molecules along these channels. Interference with this mechanism at any point may result in changes producing repetitive cellular discharge. Such a system concept offers a dynamic approach to metabolic problems of brain. Within this framework, the acid-base regulation of brain requires further consideration, for both its local and general homeostasis relates to seizure induction.

The majority of acquired epilepsies are associated with organic lesions of the brain characterized by connective tissue and glial scars with blood vessel proliferation. Except for morphological descriptions of these areas, little attention has been paid to their dynamic and chemical properties. Yet, if they behave as other scars, their presence in the brain should produce marked alterations in the energy-dependent transport systems. Little is known of the enzyme activity of new vessels and of their ability to pass oxygen, glucose, and electrolytes in a form available to the cells either in early or late stages of cicatrization. One might assume that as the scar contracted such vessels would be unable to transport molecules and ions across their endothelium. In addition, decreased flow might impair thermoregulation of the area. Thermistor determinations of the progressively scarring area may indicate that tissue temperatures vary sufficiently to interfere with activities of thermosensitive enzymes. Under normal circumstances even augmented blood flow, as a cortical seizure develops, is unable to carry off heat developed by energy systems so that local temperature rises $0.3°C$ or more. With impaired vascular responses, this hyperpyrexia may be greatly increased.

The progressive gliosis in the scarred area may well modify local metabolism and, in fact, may be an adaptive response to a decreasing amount of available energy sources. Metabolic properties of such glia, which may be quite unlike those of the normal astrocytes of the cortex, are demonstrable by such techniques as Cartesian diver microrespirometry and enzyme assays of submicrogram samples (Lowry [4]). These metabolic studies may indicate the adequacy of the local circulation; if insufficient, the hypoxia is known to predispose to epileptic neuronal activity. The great variation in number of mitochrondria seen in reactive glia would suggest a considerable range in energy requirements.

The few electron microscopic observations of reparative processes on neuronal membrane suggest that following injury there is complete disruption of the terminating boutons with replacement of many by glial, probably astrocytic, processes. The effect of such changes on the enzyme systems related to membrane permeability is unknown. A study of enzyme changes as a cerebral scar develops and matures might give considerable insight into the basic processes that predispose a neuron to hyperactivity. Such an investigation should include not only the enzymes required for energy but the turnover of the more permanent constituents of the cells. For genesis of an epilepsy, changes in the latter might be particularly important. One would be especially interested in the activity of cells that at the site of traumatically disrupted axons had developed terminal balls. Do such cells maintain functional connections in cortex or subcortical structures?

Finally, normal transport of degradation products and water to capillaries and to the ependyma may well be severely impeded by the scar. Both electron microscopic and biochemical studies would be valuable to demonstrate such changes.

With increasing evidence that repetitive stimulation to discharge of a cell is associated in some cases at least, with a buildup of protein substances resembling ribonucleic acid (RNA), the identification of such materials becomes of paramount importance. Several techniques that have been developed recently should aid in this problem.

X-ray diffraction of macromolecules has given great insight into the chemical structure and arrangement of many biological substances, particularly proteins. Analysis of the crystal structure of protein is impressive for its unique information. Although computers have made it possible to process the great amount of data needed in these studies, protein crystallography remains an area for team research. The structures of ribonucleic acid and deoxyribonucleic acid have been studied by these techniques. The structure of DNA has reached a stage where the helix dimensions have been defined under a number of conditions. The study of RNA- and DNA-like substances, particularly in neurons that have been stimulated for some period of time to give rise to autonomous discharge as in a mirror focus, would be of great interest and importance in understanding biochemical adaptive mechanisms involved in the storage of data.

The principles of fluorescent immunebody reaction might be applied to identification of protein or lipoprotein molecules even if their structure and chemical composition is not known. Macromolecules within the cell such as RNA or DNA may act as potent antigens (Parker and Halloran [5]). Their identification by fluorescent antibody techniques would open new pathways for exploration of mechanisms related to storage of data within the cell. Studies of immunochemistry of enzymes such as lactic dehydrogenase, which might be modified under epileptic conditions, indicate that replacement of a single amino acid in the enzyme may be detected by microcomplement fixation techniques. Although time consuming, a systematic study of the state of enzyme systems in the epilepsies could yield essential information. Use of antibody-to-enzyme reactions might be fruitful in tracing the compound relationships of many enzyme systems.

FUTURE PHYSIOLOGICAL ADVANCES

Physiological studies of properties of neurons and their environment using electronic instrumentation, so well documented in this volume, have given much insight into characteristics of cell membranes and their appendages which relate to epileptic discharge. In those discussions, problems relating to membrane polarization, inhibitory and excitatory presynaptic and postsynaptic potentials, and paroxysmal depolarization and hyperpolarization shifts have been defined and need no further elaboration in this chapter. These mechanisms relate to the individual neuron and occur in the interictal state without overt manifestations of epilepsy. The essence of epileptic discharge is the synchronization of firing of neurons. Both release of inhibitory influences tending to confine discharges and facilitation of excitatory elements have been considered to produce this synchrony. Structural connections at cellular levels have been implicated. It might be advisable, however, to examine the possibility that unison in this type of rapid firing occurs between axons of a tract. There is evidence that field effects modify the thresholds of excitability in peripheral nerves; such effects may be equally operative in the brain where many fibers are poorly myelinated or unmyelinated. Further study of the mode of transmission of impulses in pyramidal and extrapyramidal fiber systems during generalized epileptic discharge might explain the stereotyped pattern of muscular contractions during the seizure. The relationship of fast and slow conducting fibers to this phenomenon has yet to be elucidated.

Unison firing begins at the focus and propagates to secondary sites, which discharge in time with the primary focus. As secondary and tertiary points join in synchronous discharge, the pacemaker shifts from the original focus to secondary or tertiary points, where it continues to regulate spiking until termination of the seizure. Mechanisms involved not only in pacemaking but also in transfer are poorly understood. This shifting interrelationship of primary, secondary, and tertiary foci is of particular relevance to the more general control of cerebral activity by the reticular system.

The steady potentials of the cerebral cortex have been shown to exert a potent effect upon epileptic neuronal activity. Although inhibitory actions of cortical neurons are ineffective in eliminating epileptic discharge, shifts of potential, particularly that of spreading depression, are quite capable of arresting discharge. Local factors such as pH or CO_2 and O_2 tension, modulating steady potentials, are well known, but much less information is available regarding modification of these polarities by cortical and subcortical activity. During cortical epilepsy, marked shifts in direct current have been demonstrated at or near the focus, but what shifts occur in different parts of the hemispheres as the attack progresses? Perhaps even more important would be knowledge of slow potential changes in subcortical ganglia as the convulsion passes through its cycles. Instrumentation is sufficiently developed to permit such studies.

With the increasing use of computers, the complicated interrelationships of systems should be subject to analysis. Thus, by the use of implanted microsensors for telemetering data, the extracellular and intracellular records of unit activity, the pH, the local blood flow, the temperature, the O_2 tension and O_2 consumption, the steady potentials and effects of various inputs (such as physiological and pharmacological) to the focus should be capable of correlation. Such dynamic concepts of epileptic discharge should give better insight in basic mechanisms.

CHRONOLOGICAL ASPECTS OF EPILEPSY

In a subject such as epilepsy in which the phenomena are periodic, the timing of events becomes particularly important. This dimension of biology termed *chronobiology* offers a means of displaying quantitative estimates of rhythmic parameters in terms of their levels, amplitude, and various phase relations at each of a number of frequencies. Rhythm, a statistically validated physiological change recurring with a reproducible waveform that may be synchronized by primary or secondary environmental factors, in biology (biorhythm) is amenable to frequency synchronization that persists after elimination of the primary synchronizing effect. Obviously these rhythms are, to some extent, obscured by biological noise stemming from unidentified sources and interfering with the signal. However, because such noise has no relationship to a given event, when transformed into frequency spectrum, the variants of energy corresponding to biological noise are spread out more or less uniformly, in contrast to rhythmic phenomena that occur in a narrow spectral band. The spectrum of rhythms is quite wide, varying from circa annual to circa sigma. While many rhythms may be recognized by inspection of phenomena, some require electronic computers for macroscopic or microscopic display of the rhythm and for the subsequent estimation of their parameters.

Rhythms that have received the most attention in recent years have been of the circadian range and relate to such phenomena as rest, activity, sleep, wakefulness, and body temperature. Higher frequency rhythms seen in electroencephalograms or electrocardiograms, although well recognized from the standpoint of chronobiology, have been studied to a lesser extent.

Of obvious importance to the discharge frequency of neurons are such factors as body temperature, pH of the blood, and steady potential of the brain. It is apparent that these parameters, having cycles of varying length, may make for increased membrane excitability at certain times, as when individual peaks coincide and summate.

The circadian nature of epileptic attacks has been demonstrated by Griffiths and Fox [3], who reviewed almost 40,000 fits in 110 males in the Litchfield Epileptic Colony in England and found that many patients tended to have their daily fits between 6 and 7 A.M. or between 10 P.M. and midnight. The relationship of these attacks to the stages of sleep—a secondary rhythm —and particularly to REM, might be not only of scientific but of therapeutic value. A longer periodicity in terms of weeks or months, especially related to the menstrual periods, may characterize epileptic rhythm.

Only a beginning has been made in assessment of clinical rhythms that may modulate the course of epileptic processes. Further studies along this line may give not only insight into basic mechanisms involved in epilepsy but a rational basis for therapeusis.

ALLERGIC PHENOMENA AS BASIC MECHANISM IN EPILEPSY

Concepts involved in allergy may be of considerable importance in epileptic events. These relate to the neutralization of or the aggravated reaction (hypersensitivity) to certain toxic properties of an antigen. The idea that allergic phenomena may play a role in epilepsy stems from the possibility of developing autoantigens of neural material. At the present time, two types of autoantigen have been demonstrated in the nervous system, those related to experimental allergic neuritis and those to experimental allergic encephalomyelitis. Many epileptic manifestations arise within the brain as the result of organic disease, which result in the breakdown of neurons, white matter, and glia, all liberating proteins and lipids theoretically capable of antigenicity. The blood-brain barrier provides a mechanism by which specific neural substances may be isolated from the rest of the body indefinitely. The breakdown of this barrier in conditions such as trauma or infection might be associated with a release of cerebral antigens to stimulate the lymphocytic system. A second insult may well be responsible for both acute and chronic manifestations of cerebral sensitivity. Although this idea has been expressed previously, no serious attempt has been made to test the hypothesis. Such an autoimmune reaction has been suggested as the explanation of the late epileptic manifestations of electric shock injuries of the brain. Both acute traumatic cerebral edema, sometimes associated with convulsions, and late developing posttraumatic epilepsy could be related to allergic phenomena.

UNRESOLVED CLINICAL PROBLEMS

Perhaps it is appropriate to conclude a prospectus by an inquiry into clinical questions that future investigations into basic mechanisms of epilepsy might be expected to answer. The clinician has difficulty in explaining a number of phenomena associated with seizures. The first is why one patient suffering from a certain condition has a seizure whereas another with the same disorder does not. The second concerns the periodicity or intermittency of attacks. The third relates to the seizure pattern, be it focal or generalized, and as a corollary, why is it different in neonatal and adult life? The fourth phenomenon is the factors that initiate seizures after a head injury and those responsible for recession of seizures some years later. Finally, clinicians would like to know the teleological significance of seizures. These are some questions to which future investigation might be directed.

Let us examine these points. The first relates to the susceptibility to epilepsy as illustrated by the observation that only a certain percentage of patients with parasagittal meningiomas develop seizures. Genetic factors have been suggested, but no well-documented genealogical study has been presented to indicate that heredity plays a significant role. Such random factors as the anatomical relationship of the lesion to inhibitory cortical zones, the interruption of cortical blood supply by the tumor either as the result of vascular occlusion or steal, and local humoral agents, perhaps derived from the tumor, do not seem, when considered independently, sufficiently epileptogenic to have a causal relationship. The sorting of these jigsaw pieces into a plausible epileptogenic matrix remains for future workers.

The second issue relates to the intermittent character of the attacks. Although much has been written of the sequences, both electrical and chemical, that accompany the transformation of an aggregate of cells into a convulsing unit, rather little has been said of the factors, other than sensory input, that precipitate the discharge. There is no convincing evidence that hormones, electrolytes, pH, or water imbalance are the primary initiators of the attack. Interictal discharges become self-propagating if the cortical chemical milieu favors a positive potential shift, but the cortical and subcortical determinants of such shifts are poorly understood. The factors that arrest the attack are also inadequately defined. Although cortical exhaustion has been suggested, available evidence indicates that neither lack of pO_2 nor ATP is responsible. Perhaps a subcortical pacemaker using a chemical pendulum may modify the cortical potentials sufficiently to cause an arrest of neurons which have little reserve energy mechanism.

The factors that fashion the pattern of a seizure seem to be related to cortical sites of epileptic susceptibility and to well-established anatomical pathways. However, it is yet to be resolved why one of several available pathways is favored and the means by which this preferential pathway of discharge becomes a deep rut for later seizure discharges to follow. There is no doubt that the mechanism is complex and involves both facilitatory and inhibitory elements, perhaps in varying proportions.

The pathogenesis of seizures which begin days, weeks, or even years after a cerebral injury and their subsequent spontaneous recession has been speculated upon many times. In neonatal isolated cortex, the transformation of pyramidal to internuncial cells, which predisposes to a localized discharge, may be a factor, but in adult brain this metamorphosis does not occur. Denervation hypersensitivity has been suggested as a possible factor; perhaps akin to this is the hypersensitivity of the immune response. Chronic anoxemia of partially damaged neurons at the margin of a scar has been proposed, but a more attractive hypothesis suggests that the blood vessel wall itself may be altered by the scarring to prevent the transport of the high-energy metabolites. However, no theory has stood the test of either science or time.

Finally, the purpose of the seizure in the economy of the organism remains to be resolved. One may consider the cellular discharges as only a pathological response, but there is the possibility that such repetitive discharges of the neuron serve to preserve the cell or organism from irreparable damage. The constant discharge of a group of neurons might preempt certain functional systems so that they are either physiologically unavailable or overstimulated. The paroxysmal elimination of such discharges might restore these systems to their physiological state. The personality alterations, loss of memory, or impairment of libido in patients with psychomotor epilepsy may be examples of this principle. Certainly some epileptics believe that they feel better and think clearer after a seizure; attendants have noted personality disturbances the day or so before a patient has a seizure.

FINALE

Obviously, in a brief discussion of the future studies of basic mechanisms in epilepsy, it is impossible to explore all the available avenues for progress. Many other techniques, such as polarography and radioautography, might have been used to illustrate future advances. However, the fact seems obvious that in this field, as in the world of Ulysses, "though much is taken, much abides."

REFERENCES

1. Adrian, E. D., and Matthews, B. H. C. The Berger rhythm. Potential changes from the occipital lobes in man. *Brain* 57:355, 1934.
2. Berger, H. Ueber das Elektrenkephalogram des Menschen. I. Mitteilung. *Arch. Psychiat. Nervenkr.* 87:527, 1929.
3. Griffiths, G. M., and Fox, J. T. Rhythm in epilepsy. *Lancet* 2:409, 1938.
4. Lowry, O. H. Quantitative Analysis of Single Nerve Cell Bodies. In Waelsch, H. (Ed.), *Ultrastructural and Cellular Chemistry of Neural Tissue.* New York: Harper and Row, 1962, p. 69.
5. Parker, C. W., and Halloran, M. J. The Production of Antibodies to Mononucleotides, Oligonucleotides, and DNA. In Plescia, O. J., and Braun, W. (Eds.), *Nucleic Acids in Immunology.* New York: Springer, 1968, p. 724.
6. Richter, C. P. *Biological Clocks in Medicine and Psychiatry.* Springfield, Ill.: Thomas, 1965.
7. Rosenblueth, A., and Cannon, W. B. Cortical responses to electrical stimulation. *Amer. J. Physiol.* 135:690, 1943.
8. Tower, D. B. *Neurochemistry of Epilepsy.* Springfield, Ill.: Thomas, 1960.

Index

Accommodation and block, 65–66
Acetazolamide, 670
  petit mal and, 714
Acetoxycycloheximide, protein synthesis and memory, 372
Acetylcholine, 105–111
  brain decreases during convulsion, 186
  cerebellum and, 111
  cerebral cortex and, 106–109
  direct postsynaptic action of, 335
  discharges after, paroxysmal repetitive, 513
  exciting long-isolated cerebral cortical tissue, 160–161
  ganglia and, basal, 109–110
  -induced paroxysms in isolated cortex, in cat, 424
  presynaptic function of, 201
  release, 201–203
    compared with monoamines, 221–222
    cortical, 109
  rhinencephalon and, 106–109
  role of
    anticholinesterases and, 612–614
    in releasing inhibitory transmitters, 204
  spinal cord and, 110–111
  supersensitivity of denervated ganglion cells to, 335–338
  thalamus and, 110
Acetylcholinesterase, 105
  electron microscopy and, 200
ACh. *See* Acetylcholine
AChE. *See* Acetylcholinesterase
Acid-base
  balance, and petit mal, 713
  changes
    in epilepsy, 714–715
    seizures and, 713–714
  mechanisms in epilepsy, 713–715
  metabolism
    didione effects on, 670–671
    diphenylhydantoin effects on, 657–661
    in petit mal, 714
    trimethadione effects on, 670–671
Action potential. *See* Potential
Activation
  processes, 79–80
  Schaffer collateral, 243
Active transport, 53
Adenosinephosphates after electroshock, in rat, 87
Adenosinetriphosphatase
  cation transport by, 91
  pentylenetetrazol and, 151
  properties of, 91
Adenotriphosphate, 86–87
  as central transmitter, 119
  lack of, 620
ADP, 254
Adrenal-pituitary imbalance and seizures, 717–719
Adrenergic transmissions, 197–199
Afferents, 13–18
  fibers
    course and distribution in cerebral cortex, 14
    feedback, 436
Afterdepolarization, 254
Afterdischarge
  activities, examples of, 367
  hippocampal, inhibitory and excitatory actions in, 588
  neocortical, inhibitory and excitatory actions in, 588
  oscillatory, enhancement in cerebral explant, 512
  projection and, 430
    corticofugal, in monkey, 431
  repetitive, in CNS explants, 510
  seizure, and inhibition, 581–588
  self-sustained, after epicortical stimulation, 404–405
Afterhyperpolarization, 254
Age and spike-wave EEG traits, 705
Aging and pyridoxal-5′-phosphate pool size, 620
AHP, 254
Allergic phenomena as mechanism in epilepsy, 812
Allocortex, cerebral, 29
Allylglycine
  amino acids and, free, 146–147
  cerebellar cortex changes due to, 147–148
  convulsions and, possible mechanism, 148–151
  convulsive states and, experimental, 146–151
  enzymes and, 146–148
  GABA and, 146
  GAD inhibition by, 147
  nerve ending changes due to, 147
Amine(s)
  biogenic
    content in synaptic vesicles, 141
    diphenylhydantoin and, 667
    distribution of, 138
    MSO and, 145
  storage granules, 221
Aminergic nerve endings, 137–138
Amino acid(s), 113–119
  actions, 115–117
  diphenylhydantoin effects on, 667–668
  disorders
    complicated by seizures, 715
    in epilepsy, etiologic significance of, 716–717
  distributions, 114
  free, and allylglycine, 146–147
  inactivation, 117–118
  ketogenic diet and, 712
  mechanisms in epilepsy, 715–717
  metabolism
    diphenylhydantoin effects on, 662–666
    in epilepsy, 715–716
  methobarbital and, 712
  release of, 118
  seizures and, 185–186
  transmitter function of, 118–119
  trimethadione and, 712
Aminoaciduria in petit mal, 716
Ammonia
  levels, and MSO, 101
  seizures and, 185–186

815

INDEX

Ammonium chloride, 192
  inducing conditions predisposing to seizures, 188
Amphetamine, 220
Amygdala and localized seizure threshold curves, in rat, 729
Analysis, voltage clamp, of repetitively firing neuron, 76
Anesthetics and acetylcholine, 108–109
Animal
  behavior, diphenylhydantoin actions on, 686–687
  model, baboon as, 566
Anions, monovalent, 672–675
Anodal block, 66
Anomalous rectification, 80
Anoxia, 101–103
  energy reserves and, in mice, 102
Anticholinesterases
  acetylcholine role and, 612–614
  excitatory effects of, 191–192
  functional, 199–201
  reserve, 199–201
Anticonvulsants
  action mechanisms, 647–681
  REM sleep and, 464–467
  responses to, 539
Antiepileptic mechanisms, membrane, 72–73
Apoenzyme and pyridoxal-5′-phosphate pool size, 620
Apomorphine, 220
Apractognosia, 793
Architecture of cerebral cortex, 13–28
Arecoline blocking postsynaptic inhibition, 172–174
L-Aspartic acid, actions, 115–116
Association systems in brain and hormones, 730
Astrocytic lamellar processes, 747–753
Astroglial swelling after pentylenetetrazol, 151
  interpretation of, 153–154
ATP. See Adenosinetriphosphate
ATPase. See Adenosinetriphosphatase
Atropine, 612
  effects of, 107–108
Audiogenic epilepsy, 565
Audiogenic stimulation, energy expenditure changes after, 100
Audiosensitive epilepsy, 565
Aura and focal seizure, 4
Automaticity and diphenylhydantoin, 654
Automatism, 799–801, 803
  afterdischarge
    prefrontal, 799–800
    temporal lobe, 799
  petit mal, 800–801
  -producing gray matter, 803
Autonomic effectors, and disuse supersensitivity, 334–335
Autoradiography
  dense cells, 364
  mirror focus and, 363
  RNA turnover in secondary epileptogenic foci cells, 360–368
Awakening epilepsies, 454
Axodendritic synapse, 354
  in newborn kitten, 483
Axon
  -collaterals, and cultures, 511–512
  giant, voltage clamping of, in squid, 59
  radiating from neuron, drawing of, 230
  stimuli, epileptic neurons, 281–282
Axosomatic synapse, 354, 490–492
  hippocampus, in kitten, 489

Barbiturates, convulsant, 179–180
Basket cells, features of, 16, 245–247
Behavior, diphenylhydantoin actions on
  animal, 686–687
  human, 685–686
Biochemical lesion and epilepsy, 113
Biochemical processes
  didione effects on, 670–672
  diphenylhydantoin effects on, 657–668
  trimethadione effects on, 670–672
Biochemical trends, future, 809–810
Biogenic amines. See Amines
Biologic models of trigger epilepsy, 557–558
Biophysics of nerve membrane, 41–75
Block
  accommodation and, 65–66
  anodal, 66
  cathodal, 65
  depolarization, 66
  hyperpolarization, 66
  inactivation, 66
Blockade, cholinergic, central neuron supersensitivity after, 339–340
Blood
  -brain barrier, 163, 738
  flow, cerebral
    during convulsions, drug-induced, 640–642
    during convulsions, pentylenetetrazol-induced, 640
    during convulsions, pyridoxine deficiency, 644
  energy metabolism and, 639–646
  pressure, and diphenylhydantoin, 654
  vessels, in epileptic brain, 639–640
Border cells, 30
Brain
  association systems in, and hormones, 730
  -blood barrier, 163, 738
  epileptic, vessels in, 639–640
  function, models of, 768–771
  immature
    seizure susceptibility of, 481–505
    seizure susceptibility of, enhancement and maturation patterns, 497–501
    stability of, 481–505
  mechanisms
    excitatory, 229–252
    inhibitory, 229–252
    related to consciousness, 791–805
  metabolites, and pentylenetetrazol, 99
  nature of, spatially discrete, 768
  neural, of kitten, 482
  glial, 482
  neurons, properties of, 770
  normal
    morphology of, synaptic region, 137–144
    neurochemistry of, 159–163
    neurochemistry of, synaptic region, 137–144
  proteins from, electrophoresis of, 693
  research, and epilepsies, 10–11
  stem transection, and diphenylhydantoin, 683–684
  tissue, electrical activity of, in culture, 506–516
Branching processes, 766
Bromide, 672–675
  anticonvulsant action of, 73
Buffers, spatial, 154, 743
Bursts
  firing. See Firing burst
  spike, recorded from cell bodies, 324
  spindle, and secondary current generators, 417
  strychnine, after depolarization inactivation, 412

Cable properties, 55
  experimental measurement in muscle fiber, 56
Calcium concentration and Na+ and K+ conductance, 68
Calculation of waves, 414
Callosal fibers, termination sites of, 35
Cannon's law, status of today, 329–335
Capacitors, 48–49
Capillaries and astrocytic lamellar processes, 748–753
Carbohydrate metabolism
  didione effects on, 671–672
  diphenylhydantoin effects on, 661–662
  trimethadione effects on, 671–672
Carbon dioxide and seizure discharge inhibition, 384
Cartridges, synaptic, 15, 20, 36
Catamenial epilepsy, 721–722
Cataplexy, 465
Catecholamines, 111–113
  cerebral cortex and, 112
  rhinencephalon and, 112
  spinal cord and, 113
  subcortical structures and, 112–113
Cathodal block, 66
Cation, transport, active, 90–93
Cell(s)
  assemblies, 778–779
  basket-type, 16
    features of, 245–247
  bodies, spike bursts recorded from, 324
  border, 30
  cellular relations in vertebrate nervous system, 739
  cerebral cortex
    semidiagrammatic drawing of, 25
    types, 13
  dense, 363
    autoradiography of, 364
  elongated, cable properties of, 55–58
  explosive, 8
  follower, synchronization of population, 581
  fractionation techniques, 139
  ganglion, denervated, 335–338
  giant, 30
  glial
    depolarization of, 742
    physiologic properties of, 741–742
    secondary current generators and, 417–418
  idle, 294, 742
    secondary current generators and, 417

inhibitory, 249
intracellular energy-yielding processes, 10
intracellular studies of propagation mechanisms, 441–451
membrane
  capacitance, 49
  charge, 49
  greater cell membrane, 782–788
  potentials, 90
metabolism, experimental models, 778
molluscan, 76–80
nerves, body of, schematic representation, 776
neuroglial, morphology of, 747–753
PT. See Pyramidal tract cells
Purkinje. See Purkinje cells
pyramidal tract. See Pyramidal tracts cells
Renshaw, 204
  pathway through, 240
  responses in precruciate gyrus after electrical stimulation, 398
stellate. See Stellate cells
Cellule à double bouquet dendritique, 20
Central nervous system. See Nervous system
Centrencephalic EEG trait, 701–702
Centrencephalic epilepsy, 565, 701, 703–704
Centrencephalic structures and spike-wave complex, 402
Centrencephalic system, 536
  of neurons, 433–434
Cerebellar excitatory factor, 119
Cerebellum
  acetylcholine and, 111
  cortex. See also Cortex
    changes due to allylglycine, 147–148
    light microscopy of, in rat, 148–150
    glomerular synapse of, electron microscopy of, in rat, 152
  homunculus, 769
  irradiated, Purkinje cell characteristics in, 501
Cerebrospinal fluid, regulation of, 740
Cerebrum
  blood flow. See Blood flow
  cortex. See also Cortex
    acetylcholine and, 106–109
    afferent fibers in, course and distribution of, 14

application of metals to, 264–265
architecture of, 13–28
area 17, degenerating fibers in, 32
catecholamines and, 112
cells, semidiagrammatic drawing of, 25
cells, types of, 13
effects of neostigmine on, in cat, 423
electron microscopy, in rat, 153
epileptic. See Epileptic cerebral cortex
heterogeneity of, 29–40
5-hydroxytryptamine and, 112
immature, stability of, 486–487
immature, supersensitivity and, 349
isolated, disuse supersensitivity and, 342–345
isolated, epileptiform activity in, 343
isolated and normal, neurotransmitters in, 159–165
isolated, partially, supersensitivity and, 350–354
isolated, stimulation and, 349–355
lamination, 13
mature, supersensitivity and, 349
models of, 29
modified Golgi-Cox preparations, in cats, 351
neurophysiology and, 793
undercut, procedures, 351–354
energy metabolism, 83–97
hemispheres
  electrical stimulation, in mice, 85
  left, 794
peduncle
  potentials evoked by stimulation, 258
  responses evoked by stimulation, 254
respiration, 83–84
ChAc, 105
CHEB, 179
  motoneurons and, 180
Chemical induction, 556–557
Chemical receptor, isolation of, 144
Chloralose and microreflex, 560
Chloride
  estradiol and, 733
  ions, 51–52
  post-DS hyperpolarization and, 321

INDEX

Chlorimipramine, 220
p-Chloro-phenylalanine, 220
Chlorpromazine, 89–90, 220
Choline acetyltransferase, 105
Cholinergic blockade
   central neuron supersensitivity after, 339–340
   of postsynaptic inhibition, 171
Cholinergic nerve-ending membranes, isolation of, 141
Cholinergic propagation mechanisms, 423–426
Cholinergic transmissions, 197–199, 204–205
Chronobiology, 811
Cicatrix, meningocerebral, 774–776
   schematic representation of, 774
Circuit
   local
      action potential propagation and, 43
      current flow, 65
      propagation of impulse, 65
   neuron, basic, 24–26
Circulation and diphenylhydantoin, 654
Clamp. See Voltage clamp
Clamping. See Voltage clamping
Clarke's column region, electron microscopy of, in cat, 134
Clonic spasms and diphenylhydantoin, 685
CNS. See Nervous system, central
Collosal pathway, integrity of, in rabbit, 359
Commissural section and propagation of seizures, 439
Compensatory processes and stimulation effects on isolated cortex, 349–350
Compulsory nervous control, 332
Computer models, 560–561
   of trigger epilepsy, 557–558
Concentration gradient, 47
Concentration potential, energy difference, 51
Concepts in epilepsy, historical development of, 2–3
Conductance
   inactivation of, 61
   IPSPs, 576
      properties in hippocampus and neocortex, 577
   membrane ionic, 52
   potassium, 61, 64
   sodium, 61, 64
Conduction
   phenomena, 41–44
   refractory networks, synchronization of, 755–756
   velocity, and diphenylhydantoin, 654

Conductivity of intracortical pathways, 345
Confusional phase, in baboon, 567
Confusional state, in baboon, 567
Coniine blocking postsynaptic inhibition, 171
Connectedness, 766
Consciousness, brain mechanisms related to, 791–805
Constructive interference, 755
Contact
   excitatory type, 37
   inhibitory type, 37
Contractility and diphenylhydantoin, 653–654
Convulsants
   acetylcholine and, 108–109
   actions
      direct stimulation, 175–180
      mechanisms, 167–183
      mechanisms, general, 167–180
      neurochemistry, 184–193
   barbiturates, 179–180
   electrogenic pumps and, 175
   energy metabolites and, 99–101
   excitation enhancement by, 167–169
   induction by, 557
   inhibition block by, 167
      postsynaptic, 169–171
      presynaptic inhibition and, 174–175
   responses to, 537–538
Convulsion(s), 803
   allylglycine and, possible mechanism, 148–151
   drug-induced, cerebral blood flow and metabolic rate in, 640–642
      pentylenetetrazol, 640
   electroshock, hyperglycemic effects of, 720
   energy metabolism during, 642
   febrile, 705
   generalized, 801–802
   -producing gray matter, 803
   pyridoxine deficiency and, 642–644
   spinal cord, development of, 536
Convulsive activity and REM sleep, 463–464
Convulsive discharges, 161
   neurochemical correlates of, 185–186
Convulsive states
   experimental, ultrastructural and neurochemical studies, 144–154
   neurotransmitters and, 160
Convulsive tendency, 705

Convulsive threshold and REM sleep deprivation, 463
Corneal reflexes, inhibition of, 477
Cortex. See also Cerebrum, cortex
   electrogenic, ictal activity in, 405–406
   elements, 397
   inducing inhibition of reflexes, 478
   interpretive, 795–798
      localization in, 797–798
   intracortical propagation mechanism, 422–427
   isoelectric region, recording from, 413
   neurons. See Neurons
   precruciate, surface activity and dc recording of intracellular activity, in cat, 412
   responses, superficial, in kitten, 498
   thalamocortical interrelationships, 429–433
Corticofugal influences by PT cells, 258–259
Counseling, genetic, 703–704
Coupling, 762
   linearly coupled oscillators, 762–764
   nonlinear, 764–766
   springs, 763
Cranial nerves and forebrain inhibition, 474–477
P-creatine and electrical stimulation, in mice, 99
Creutzfeldt's disease, myoclonus latency in, 549
Critical electrodes, 390
Cross dependence, patterns of, 340
Current
   densities, transcortical, 411
   depolarizing, 65
   electric, 49–50
   generator
      primary, 411–416
      secondary, 417–418
   membrane ionic, 52
   synaptic
      EPSP and, 132
      time course of, 131–132
Cystic tumor of right hemisphere, 434

DA (dopamine), 111, 216, 220
Daughter-foci, 443
Davson-Danielli model, 783
DC potential shifts. See Potentials, dc shifts
Deafferentation, 270–279
   dendritic changes, 272–273
   spinal neurons, 273–275

INDEX 819

trigeminal spinal complex, 275–276
Degeneration hypothesis and isolated cortex stimulation, 350
Dendrites
  apical, 353
    axonal neuropil and, 22
    terminal twigs of, 353
  basal, 352
  deafferentation and, 272–273
  immature cortical neurons, spike generation in, 492–495
  impulse initiation in
    in kitten, 495
    suppression of, 494
  potential, 682
  propagation in, in kitten, 495
  Purkinje cell
    in immature brain, 499–501
    retardation of, 499
  radiating from neuron, drawing of, 230
  synapse-studded, 31
Denervation
  compensation for, mechanisms of, 332–333
  ganglion cells, 335–338
  hypersensitivity, 498
  law of, 329
  meaning of, 329–331
  neurons, 335–338
    epileptic, 282–284
  supersensitivity, 162, 330
Deoxyribonucleic acid transformation into protein structure, 690
Dependence
  cross, patterns of, 340
  physical
    depression and, 340
    disuse theory of, 340–341
  SEL and, 357
Depolarization, 43, 63
  block, 66
  glial cells, 742
  ictal EEG phenomena and, 405
  inactivation, strychnine burst after, 412
  paroxysmal depolarization shifts, 300, 358
    clonic phase, 310
    epileptic neurons and, 320–324
    generation, intracellular current pulses and, 321
    generation, mechanisms of, 322–324
    penicillin and, 400
    penicillin focus, in cat, 401
    penicillin inducing, 300
    synaptic activity and spike potentials in generating neurons, 321
    synaptic mechanisms, 301–305
    tonic phase, 310
    triggering of, 302–303
    typical, development of, 314
  soma, absence of, 243
  steady state, in epileptic neuronal aggregate, 322
Depolarizing potentials. See Potentials
Depressant drugs, 340
Depression
  disuse supersensitivity and, 342
  physical dependence and, 340
  postconvulsive, 641
  postictal, and diphenylhydantoin, 685
  spreading, 293–296
    complete, segments from, 295
    potential changes measured during, 295
Desmethylimipramine, 220
Didione, 668–672
  effects
    biochemical processes, 670–672
    nervous system, 668–670
    neurotransmitters, 672
  structure of, 648
Dielectric, 49
Diencephalon, ictal discharge in, 798–799
Diffuse epilepsies, 454
Diffuser effect, 545
Diffusion, 47
  constant, 47
  spread by, 426–427
  through intercellular clefts, 737–738
Dimethadione. See Didione
Dimethyl-14C-D-tubocurarine, binding capacity, 143
Diphenylhydantoin, 647–668, 682–688
  acetylcholine and, 666–667
  actions
    anticonvulsant, 72–73
    on behavior, animal, 686–687
    on behavior, human, 685–686
    dc and ac responses and, 379
    on heart, 685
    on peripheral nerve, 684–685
    on polynucleotide systems, 687
    at various CNS levels, 682–684
  CNS development and, 539
  distribution in cerebral cortex, in rat, 665
  effects, 720
    acetylcholine, 666–667
    acid-base metabolism, 657–661
    amino acid, 667–668
    amino acid metabolism, 662–666
    biochemical processes, 657–668
    biogenic amines, 667
    carbohydrate metabolism, 661–662
    electrolytes, 657–661
    energy metabolism, 661–662
    excitable tissues, 647–657
    ileum, 656
    lipid metabolism, 662–666
    muscle, cardiac, 653–655
    muscle, skeletal, 655–656
    muscle, smooth, 656–657
    muscle, smooth, vascular, 653–655
    nervous system, 647–653
    neurotransmitters, 666–668
    nucleic acid metabolism, 662–666
    protein metabolism, 662–666
  induced seizures and
    chemically, 539
    electrically, 539
  petit mal and, 619
  structure of, 648
Discharge
  afterdischarge. See Afterdischarge
  basic rhythm of, 443
  convulsive, 161
    neurochemical correlates of, 185–186
  electrographic, evoked by light stimulation, 548–549
  epileptic
    focal, and sleep, 456–458
    generalized, and sleep, 455–456
  epileptiform
    nonepileptic neuronal aggregates and, 324–327
    projected, synaptic activities during, 326–327
  epileptogenic
    inhibitory, 327
    synaptic influences on, 446–450
  evoked, in long-term culture, 509
  focal repetitive, and focal seizure ontogeny study, 532
  frequencies, 78–79

Discharge—*Continued*
  ictal
    in diencephalon, 798–799
    surgeon's electrode and, 791
  interneuron, 596
  limited afterdischarge technique, 432
  multiple
    factor responsible for, 132–133
    transmitter action and, 130–135
  prefrontal, automatism after, 799–800
  pyramidal
    during REM of desynchronized sleep, 459
    focal, independence of, in epileptogenic lesion, 442
    ILS inducing, in photosensitive baboon, 568
    interictal, 400–404
    repetitive, after acetylcholine, 513
    repetitive, after eserine, 513
  seizure
    immature cortical neurons and, in neonate, 482–487
    inhibition, and CO_2, 384
  spike
    light stimulus producing, 544
    strychnine waves and, 402
  spontaneous oscillatory, in long-term cultures, 509
  stimuli-evoked, in cultures, 509–511
  temporal lobe, automatism after, 799
  wave, light stimulus producing, 544
Disinhibition theories and inhibitory connections, 579–581
Disuse
  compensation for, mechanisms of, 332–333
  hypothesis, and isolated cortex stimulation, 350
  neurons, 335–338
  potentiation, 331
  in sympathetic nerve endings, 336
  sensitization, 331
  supersensitivity. *See* Supersensitivity
  theory of physical dependence, 340–341
DMO. *See* Didione
^{14}C-DMTC, binding capacity, 143
DNA transformation into protein structure, 690
Dopamine (DA), 111, 216, 220
Dorsal spinocerebellar tract neuron response to electrodes, 132
DPH. *See* Diphenylhydantoin
Drugs
  action by direct stimulation, 175–180
  anticonvulsant. *See* Anticonvulsants
  blocking postsynaptic inhibition, 169–174
  convulsant. *See* Convulsants
  depressant, 340
  effects on CNS, 197–205
  electrogenic pumps and, 175
  inducing conditions predisposing to seizures, 186–191
  inducing convulsions. *See* Convulsions
  neurons and, action site, 220
  presynaptic inhibition, 174–175
  stimulant, 340
DSCT neuron response to electrodes, 132
DSs. *See* Depolarization
Dual recurrent system hypothesis, 593–596
Dysrhythmia, paroxysmal, 3

Echelon processing, 26–27
Edema, astroglial, after pentylenetetrazol, 151
  interpretation of, 153–154
Effectors, autonomic, and disuse supersensitivity, 334–335
Efflux, 54
Electrical activity
  of brain tissue in culture, 506–516
  of heart, 654–655
Electrical properties of membranes, 48–50
Electrical stimulation
  cerebral hemispheres, in mice, 85
  changes after, 98–103
    energy expenditure, 99–100
  P-creatine and, in mice, 99
  induction, 557
  K movements after, 88
  Na movements after, 88
  precruciate gyrus after, 398
  sleep and, 455
Electric current, 49–50
Electrochemical equilibrium, 45
Electrochemical potential, 50–52
  difference, 50–51
Electrode(s)
  critical, 390
  reference, 390
    indifferent, 411
  surgeon's, and ictal discharge, 791
Electrodecremental seizures, 84
Electrodiffusion, 50–52
Electroencephalography
  abnormalities
    febrile convulsions, 705
    focal epilepsy, 706
  centrencephalic EEG traits, 701–702
  changes during apnea after ventilation with oxygen, 385
  ethyl chloride lesion, in rabbit, 358
  focal seizure ontogeny study, in monkey
    adult, 529–531
    newborn, 520–522
    puberty, 525–526
  ictal phenomena, 404–407
  neuronal mechanisms underlying, 397–410
  probands with focal EEG, 705–706
  pyridoxine dependency, 643
  spike-wave abnormality, bilaterally synchronous, 435
  spike-wave EEG trait, 704, 707
    age and, 705
  spike-wave electrical disturbances, 422
  vitamin B_6 dependency, 616–618
  waves, spontaneous, in animals without epileptic lesions, 397–400
Electrogenic cortex, ictal activity in, 405–406
Electrogenic pumps
  drugs affecting, 175
  IPSP, 576–579
  spike and synaptic activation of, 578
Electrographic discharges evoked by light stimulation, 548–549
Electrographic effects in experimental model, 558–559
Electrolyte(s)
  balance, in petit mal, 711, 713
  CNS development and, 537
  didione and, 670–671
  diphenylhydantoin effects on, 657–661
  disorders predisposing to seizures, 709–710
  imbalance in epilepsy, 711–713
  ketogenic diet and, 712
  mechanisms, in epilepsy, 709–713
  mephobarbital and, 712
  metabolism
    in epilepsy, 710–711
    ouabain and, 625–628
  trimethadione and, 670–671, 712
Electron micrograph of neuropil, 21

Electron microscopy
  acetylcholinesterase, 200
  cells
    pyramidal, 16–18
    stellate, 18
  cerebellum, glomerular synapse of, in rat, 152
  cerebral cortex, in rat, 153
  Clarke's column region, in cat, 134
  MSO effects in brain, 145–146
  Purkinje cells, basal region, in rat, 151
  synapses, 15–18
Electrophoresis of proteins from brain, 693
Electroshock
  adenosinephosphates and phosphocreatine after, in rat, 87
  convulsions, hyperglycemic effects of, 720
  seizure patterns, development of
    maximal, 536
    minimal, 535–536
Electrotonus, 55
Emotional induction, 555–556
Endocrine function, CNS biochemical development and seizure activity, 731–734
Energetics of seizure and chemical changes, 185
Energy
  -consuming reactions, 90–93
  expenditure
    changes after audiogenic stimulation, 100
    changes after electrical stimulation, 99–100
  metabolism
    cerebral, 83–97
    cerebral blood flow and, 639–646
    didione effects on, 671–672
    diphenylhydantoin effects on, 661–662
    during convulsions, 642
    hypoxia and, 623–625
    trimethadione effects on, 671–672
  metabolites in experimental seizures, 98–103
  reserves, and anoxia, in mice, 102
  -stores and, intermediated, 85–90
  -yielding processes, 83–85
  intracellular, 10
Enervation, 330
Enzymes
  allylglycine and, 146–147
  defects, and abnormal neural function, 693–697
  distribution of, 138, 143

  membrane-bound, 142
  MSO and, 145
"Ephaptic" excitation and potential fields, 427
Ephaptic mechanisms
  hippocampus and, 443–446
  in local seizure spread, 441–446
Epicortical stimulation, self-sustained afterdischarge after, 404–405
Epilepsy
  acid-base changes in, 714–715
  acid-base mechanisms in, 713–715
  allergic phenomena as mechanism in, 812
  amino acid disorders in, etiologic significance of, 716–717
  amino acid mechanisms in, 715–717
  amino acid metabolism in, 715–716
  audiogenic, 565
  audiosensitive, 565
  awakening, 454
  biochemical lesion and, 113
  biochemical trends, future, 809–810
  brain research and, 10–11
  catamenial, 721–722
  centrencephalic, 565, 701, 703–704
  chronological aspects of, 811–812
  clinical challenges of, 1–12
  clinical, genetic studies in, 700–708
    animal studies, 702–703
  clinical problems, unresolved, 812–814
  concepts, historical development of, 2–3
  diffuse, 454
  definitions, early, 1
  derivation of term, 1
  electrolyte imbalance in, 711–713
  electrolyte mechanisms in, 709–713
  electrolyte metabolism in, 710–711
  essential, 4
  excitable membranes in, 41
  experimental challenges of, 1–12
  familial, 701–702
  focal, surgery of, 706–707
  function and, 808–809
  genetic, 701–702
    inheritance mode, 701
  genetics and, 807–808
  idiopathic, 2, 4
  induction mechanisms in patients, 545–558

  learning curve for, 366–367
  lesion of, and neuropathology, 10
  models of, experimental, 263–279
  neurobiology and, 10–11
  neuroendocrine mechanisms in, 717–722
  neurophysiology of, 791–793
  partialis continua, 8
  pathology of, 773–776
  petit mal. See Petit mal
  photoepilepsy. See Photoepilepsy
  photogenic, 565
  photosensitive, 565
  physiological advance, future, 810–811
  prospectus, 807–814
  psychomotor, 5
  reading, 555
  reflex, 308
  reflex, in baboon, 566–571
    clinical signs continuing after ILS, self-sustained, 567
    clinical signs during ILS, 566–567
    electrical sign variations, 570
    electrographic signs after ILS, 569–570
    electrographic signs during ILS, 567–568
    evoked potentials, 570–571
  sensory precipitation of, 458
  sex hormones in, 721
  sleep and, 453–467
  spike-wave, 704–705
  startle, model, 554–557
  stimulus-sensitive, 544, 565
  structure and, 808–809
  of subcortical origin, 704
  sympathetic, 2
  trigger, models, 557–558
  vessels of brain in, 639–640
Epileptic cerebral cortex, in monkey
  Golgi-Cox preparations, 272
  interictal spontaneous activity of single unit, 266
  rhythmic repetitive bursts of unit potentials, 267
  spontaneous action potentials in, 280
Epileptic configuration, 808
Epileptic discharges. See Discharges
Epileptic focus, 324
Epileptic mechanisms, membrane, 72–73
Epileptic nerve tissue
  primary, 422
  projected, 422
  secondary, 422
Epileptic neuron. See Neuron

Epileptic spike, 265, 279
Epileptic triggers, internal, 555
Epileptiform activity in chronically isolated cortex, 343
Epileptiform discharge
　nonepileptic neuronal aggregates and, 324–327
　projected, synaptic activities during, 326–327
Epileptogenic agents, topical effects of, acute, 299–319
　ictal episode development, 309–311
　in penicillin focus, 309
　ictal phase, 300, 308–311
　interictal phase, 299–308
Epileptogenic discharge
　inhibitory, 327
　synaptic influences on, 446–450
Epileptogenic focus
　neuron in, 268–270
　secondary, RNA turnover in cells of, 360–368
　in sigmoid gyrus, 598
Epileptogenic lesions
　secondary
　　dependence and, 357
　　development of, 357–359
　　independence and, 357
　　split, independence of focal paroxysmal discharges in, 442
EPSP(s), 230
　changes in amplitude and duration, graphic display of, 307
　giant, 358
　　recurrent, 591
　in motoneuron, 231, 236
　prolonged, in immature brain, in kitten, 485
　synaptic current and, 132
Equations
　Hodgkin-Huxley, 64, 81
　Nernst, 51
Equilibrium
　electrochemical, 45
　potential, 50
　　potassium, 51
　thermal, 765
Equipartition phenomenon, 764
Ergothioneine as central transmitter, 119
Eserine, paroxysmal repetitive discharges after, 513
Estradiol
　chloride and, 733
　dipropionate, and seizures, in rat, 729–730
Ethyl chloride lesion, electroencephalography of, in rabbit, 358
Evoked responses, transition from central to complex, in explants, 507–515

Evoked seizures, 544
Excitability, 55–66
　hippocampus, immature, 495–497
　molecular mechanisms of, 66–70
　neocortex, immature, 495–497
　prerequisites for, 44–55
Excitable membranes
　in epilepsy, 41
　intrinsic properties of, 58–63
Excitation
　diphenylhydantoin and, 647–653
　enhancement by convulsants, 167–169
　"ephaptic," and potential fields, 427
　phenomena, 41–44
Excitatory impingement and ictal episode, 310–311
Excitatory mechanisms in brain, 229–252
Excitatory phenomena and epileptogenic agents, 308
Excitatory postsynaptic potentials. See EPSPs
Excitatory seizure. See Seizure
Experimental models, 558–561, 776–780
Explosive cells, 8
Expressive phenomena, 556

Facial nerve, 477
Facilitation, permanent, 802
Familiarity, 797
Fast prepotential
　activation of, 492
　induction of, in kitten, 494
Fatty acids, fluoro-, inducing conditions predisposing to seizures, 188–189
Febrile convulsions, 705
Feedback afferent fibers, 436
Feed-forward inhibition, 575
Fever and pyridoxal-5'-phosphate pool size, 620
Fibers
　afferent
　　course and distribution in cerebral cortex, 14
　　feedback, 436
　callosal, termination sites of, 35
　dorsal-root, tracing action potential recorded from, 42
　nerve, method for studying electrical activity of, 42
Fields, potential, and "ephaptic" excitation, 427
Filter, low pass, 416
Firing
　burst
　　epileptic neurons, analysis of patterns, 276–279

　　epileptic neurons, long first-interval, 278
　　normal neurons, 276
　neuron, epileptic, 267–269, 276–279
Fluid
　cerebrospinal, regulation of, 740
　environment of neurons and glia, 738–740
Fluorescence histochemistry of monoamines in CNS, 212–227
Fluro-fatty acids inducing conditions predisposing to seizures, 188–189
Flux, 47
　membrane ionic, 52
Focal seizure ontogeny study, in monkey, 517–534
　adult, 527–532
　　anatomical substrate, 531–532
　　clinical expression, 527–529
　　electroencephalographic expression, 529–531
　discharge, repetitive focal, 532
　discussion, 532–534
　material of, 517–519
　method of, 519
　newborn, 519–524
　　clinical expression, 519–520
　　electroencephalographic expression, 520–522
　　histology, 522–524
　propagation, 532
　puberty, 524–527
　　anatomical substrate, 526–527
　　clinical expression, 524–525
　　electroencephalographic expression, 525–526
　results of, 519–532
Foci, 289–292
　chronic
　　alumina, 292
　　epileptic neuron, 263–289
　daughter-foci, 443
　epileptic, 324
　epileptogenic. See Epileptogenic foci
　mirror. See Mirror focus
　penicillin. See Penicillin focus
Follower cell population, synchronization of, 581
Follower neurons, 270, 587
Forebrain, basal, inhibition, 474–479
Fornix
　deafferented, 492
　inhibition and penicillin, 589
　intact, 492
　recurrent connections in, 583
　seizure in
　　excitatory, 585–586

inhibitory, 586–587
  mechanisms of, 587–588
FPP. See Fast prepotentials
Fractionation techniques, 139
Frequency potentiation, 605–607
Frequency sensitivity, 607–608
F wave, 761

GABA, 113
  actions, 116–117
  allylglycine and, 146
  discussion of, 114–115
  inducing conditions predisposing to seizures, 187–188
  as inhibitory transmitter, 140
  long-isolated cerebral cortical tissue and, 161
  role of, and vitamin B_6 dependency, 614–620
GAD inhibition by allylglycine, 147
Gamma-aminobutyric acid. See GABA
Ganglia
  basal, and acetylcholine, 109–110
  cells, denervated, 335–338
  sympathetic denervated, and collateral growth, 336–337
Gangliosides, 694–696, 784–786
  major, of adult human brain, 784
Gangliosidosis, 696
Gap junction, 737
Gene(s)
  action
    mechanism of, 689–690
    mode, 702
  associations, 702
  frequency, 701
  linkage, 702
  regulation, 702
  switch, 702
Generators. See Current generators
Genetic counseling, 703–704
Genetic defects and abnormal neural function, 691–692
Genetic deletion of apoenzyme, 620
Genetic epilepsy, 701–702
  inheritance mode, 701
Genetic heterogeneity, 700–701
Genetics, 807–808
  model systems and, 690–692
  molecular, 9
  of seizure susceptibility, 689–699
Genetic studies in clinical epilepsy, 700–708
  animal studies, 702–703

Geometry, neuropil, tentative, 23–24
Giant cells, 30
Giant synaptic contacts, 133
Glia
  cells
    depolarization of, 742
    physiologic properties of, 741–742
    secondary current generators and, 417–418
    contribution to external potentials, 744–745
    density of, 163
    fluid environment of, 738–740
    membrane potential, 742
    potassium concentration and, 740
  -neuronal relationships in CNS, 748
L-Glutamate and long-isolated cerebral cortical tissue, 160
Glutamate and MSO, 101, 145
Glutamic acid, 89
L-Glutamic acid, 114
  actions, 115–116
Glutamine and MSO, 145
Glycine
  actions, 116–117
  discussion of, 115
Glycolipids of synaptic membranes, 784–786
Glycolysis, 84–85
Golgi complex, in kitten, 488
Golgi technique, neuron prepared by, 77
Gradient, concentration, 47
Grand mal and focal seizures, 4
Granules, amine storage, 221
Gray matter
  automatism-producing, 803
  convulsion-producing, 803
  spinal cord, in rat, 748–749
Gyrus
  Heschl's, 794
  precruciate, electrical stimulation of, 398
  sigmoid, epileptogenic focus in, 598

Hallucinations, hypnagogic, 465–467
Haloperidol, 89, 220
Heart
  diphenylhydantoin and, 653–655, 685
  electrical activity of, 654–655
  output, and diphenylhydantoin, 654
Hemisphere(s)
  cerebral, left, 794
  lateral surfaces of posterior parts, 795
  right, cystic tumor of, 434

Hemoglobinopathy, 691
Hemoglobin Yakima, 691
Heschl's gyrus, 794
Heterogeneity
  cerebral cortex, 29–40
  clinical, 700–701
  genetic, 700–701
Hippocampus
  afterdischarge, inhibitory and excitatory actions in, 588
  axosomatic synapses of, in kitten, 489
  conductance IPSPs in, 577
  ephaptic mechanisms and, 443–446
  excitatory mechanisms in, 241–244
  excitatory pathways in, 240–247
    recurrent, 593
  formation, in rabbit, schematic drawings, 605
  immature
    excitability of, 495–497
    inhibition in, 487–492
  inhibition, 487–492
    frequency dependence of, 604–609
    interictal spike, 590
    organization of, 604–609
    postsynaptic, postulated pathways, 246
  inhibitory mechanisms in, 244–247
  inhibitory pathways in, 240–247
  neurons
    busy appearance of, 496
    Golgi complex of, in kitten, 488
    IPSPs and, in kitten, 491
    in kitten, 488–491, 493
    pyramidal, membrane potential in, in kitten, 493
    pyramidal, spike potential of, 445
    spike potentials from, in kitten, 493
    synchronization, 445
  pyramidal cells, impulse initiation during seizure, 585
  responses evoked by stimulation, 244
  seizure activity in
    initiation of, 446
    transition from interictal spike, 599
  seizure threshold curves, localized, in rat, 729
  spikes in, interictal, 591
    penicillin, 597
Histamine as central transmitter, 119

824 INDEX

Histochemistry
  fluorescence, of monoamines in CNS, 212–227
  mirror focus, 357–370
  neurotransmitters, 162
Histology
  focal seizure ontogeny study, newborn, 522–524
  neurotransmitters, 162
Hodgkin cycle, 43, 63
Hodgkin-Huxley equations, 64, 81
Homunculus, cerebellar, 769
Hormones
  seizure development and, 727–736
  sex
    in epilepsy, 721
    in seizures, 720–722
5-HT. See 5-Hydroxytryptamine
Human behavior and diphenylhydantoin, 685–686
Hydrazides, 620
  convulsant
    inducing conditions predisposing to seizures, 187–188
    pyridoxal phosphate and, 192
Hydrazones, pyridoxal, 620
5-Hydroxytryptamine, 111–113, 216, 220
  cerebral cortex and, 112
  rhinencephalon and, 112
  spinal cord and, 113
  subcortical structures and, 112–113
Hyperexcitability, 322
Hyperglycemic effect of seizures, 720
Hypernatremia and seizures, 710
Hyperpolarization, 43
  block, 66
  excitatory seizure termination by, 584
  PDSs and, 307
  post-DS, and chloride, 321
Hyperpolarizing potentials. See Potentials
Hypersensitivity, denervation, 498
Hypersynchronous nature of spike, in immature brain, 484
Hypersynchrony, 3
Hypnagogic hallucinations, 465–467
Hypocalcemia and seizures, 710
Hypoglycemia, 189–190
  complex wave pattern during, in cat, 401
  insulin-induced, in cat, 398–399
  seizures and, 719–720

sharp waves recorded during, 400
Hyponatremia and seizures, 709–710
Hypothesis, dual recurrent system, 593–596
Hypothyroidism, 732
Hypoxia, 101–103
  energy metabolism, 623–625

Ictal activity in electrogenic cortex, 405–406
Ictal discharge. See Discharge
Ictal EEG phenomena, 404–407
Ictal episode
  excitatory impingement and, 310–311
  spontaneous, in penicillin focus, in cat, 406
  topical epileptogenic agents and, 309–311
Ictal phase and epileptogenic agents, 300, 308–311
Idle cells, 294, 742
  secondary current generators and, 417
Ileum, effects of diphenylhydantoin on, 656
Imipramine, 220
Immature brain, stability and seizure susceptibility of, 481–505
Immature nervous system, 652
Impulse, 55
  excitatory, 37
  initiation in cells during seizure, 585
  nerve, 41–44
  propagation of, local circuits, 65
Inactivation
  amino acids, 117–118
  of conductance, 61
  potassium, 81
  processes, 79–80
  transmitter, changes affecting, 332
Independence
  focal paroxysmal discharges in epileptogenic lesion and, 442
  SEL and, 357
Indifferent reference electrode, 411
In-file behavior, 48
Influx, 54
Inhibition
  afferent collateral, 249–250
  block by convulsants, 167
  evoked by surface shock, 161
  feed-forward, 575
  forebrain, basal, 474–479
  fornix and penicillin, 589
  hippocampal, 246

frequency dependence of, 604–609
  immature, 487–492
  organization of, 604–609
  integrative actions of, 579–581
  mechanisms, 162
  postsynaptic, 233–238
    drugs blocking, 169–174
    hippocampus, postulated pathways, 246
    potentials, ionic mechanisms of, 576–579
  presynaptic, 237–238
    drugs affecting, 174–175
    generalizations about, 237–238
    pharmacological, 673
  reciprocal, 575
  recurrent, 249–250, 575
    frequency sensitivity of, 607-608
  reflexes, corneal, 477
  RNA and, 365
  seizure afterdischarge and, 581–588
  spikes and, interictal, 588–598
    in neocortex and hippocampus, 590
  surround, 324–326, 575
Inhibitory cells, 249
Inhibitory connections
  mutually
    in interneurons, 583
    in neurons, 581
  parallel, 581–582
  series, 579–581
Inhibitory mechanisms in brain, 229–252
Inhibitory pathways, two types of, 249
Inhibitory postsynaptic potentials. See IPSPs
Input forcing techniques, 561
Insulin
  excess, and seizures, 719–720
  induced hypoglycemia, in cat, 398–399
Intellectual induction, 555–556
Interference, constructive, 755
Interictal paroxysmal activity after penicillin poisoning, 400–402
Interictal paroxysmal discharges, 400–404
Interictal phase and epileptogenic agents, 299–308
Interictal spikes. See Spikes
Intermediates and energy-stores, 85–90
Interneuron
  discharge, 596
  inhibitory, 511

mutually inhibitory connections and, 583
spinal cord, reflex responses of, 462
Interpretive cortex, 795-798
localization in, 797-798
Ion(s)
chloride, 51-52
concentrations
in cells, and electric potentials, 44
maintenance of, 54
conductance, 52
potassium, 61
sodium, 61
current, 52
potassium, 60-61
sodium, 60
exchange, during activity, 66
flux, 52
through membranes, factors determining, 46
major, typical concentrations of, 45
mechanisms of inhibitory postsynaptic potentials, 576-579
membrane permeability, increased, 72
metabolism, 731-733
movements through membranes, 44-48
active transport, 45-47
diffusion, 47-48
passive forces, 44-45
permeation, and membrane structure, 48
potassium, 51, 60-61
sodium, 52, 60-61
Iontophoretic application of strychnine to PT cells, 305
Iproniazide, 220
IPSP(s), 233
antidromic, 413
attenuation, in immature brain, 488
conductance, 576
properties in hippocampus and neocortex, 577
direct disynaptic, 576
electrogenic pump, 576-579
hippocampal neuron, in kitten, 487, 491
immature brain and, 488, 491-492
ionic mechanisms of, 576-579
in motoneuron, 236
prolonged, in neuron, in kitten, 487
Isocortex, cerebral, 29

Isoelectric region of cortex, recording from, 413
"Jacksonian march," 83
Jacksonian seizures, 517
Jakob-Creutzfeldt disease, myoclonus latency in, 549
K
cation transport by, 91
movements after electrical stimulation, 88
properties of, 91
K+
active transport of, 44
channels
distinctive characteristics of, 67-68
selectivity of, 68
special characteristics of, 68
conductance
calcium concentration and, 68
temperature dependence of, 68
regulation of Na+-K+ pumping rate, 71-72
role of, 71
separability of Na+ and K+ channels, 67
voltage dependence of, 61
Ketogenic diet
electrolytes and amino acids, 712
petit mal and, 714
Kindling phenomenon, 366-368
Kinetics, potassium conductance changes, 62-63

Labilization, 168
Lamellar processes, astrocytic, 747-753
Lamina 3, neuropil geometry in, 24
Lamination of cerebral cortex, 13
Lasting trace, 798
Latency, 42
Law
Cannon's, status of today, 329-335
of denervation, 329
L-DOPA, 220
Learning
curve for epilepsy, 366-367
programming and, 793-795
Lehninger model, 783
Lenard and Singer model, 783
Light
microscopy, of cerebellar cortex, in rat, 148-150
periodic variation in response to, 550
stimulation. See Stimulation

Lipid(s)
components of membranes, 695-696
formed in postsynaptic membranes, 786-788
metabolism, 733
didione effects on, 671-672
diphenylhydantoin effects on, 662-666
trimethadione effects on, 671-672
model, 783
status epilepticus and, 186
Locus ceruleus, in rat, 213-215
Low pass filter, 416
LSD, 220
Lucy model, 783

Magnesium depletion and seizures, 710
Masseteric reflex, 475
Maturational factors in seizures, 535-541
Maturation patterns, neuronal, and seizure susceptibility of immature brain, 497-501
Membrane(s)
antiepileptic mechanisms, 72-73
-bound enzymes, 142
cells. See Cells
electrical properties of, 48-50
epileptic mechanism, 72-73
excitable. See Excitable membranes
greater cell, 782-788
ionic flux, current, and conductance, 52
lipid components of, 695-696
models, 777-778, 783
nerve
biophysics of, 41-75
-ending. See Nerves, endings
phenomena, and cerebral energy metabolism, 83-97
postsynaptic abnormalities, 322
potentials. See Potentials
pyramidal tract cells, electrical parameters of, 254-255
response to voltage steps, 78
structure, and ion permeation, 48
subsynaptic, 229
surface, experimental models, 777-778
synaptic. See Synaptic membranes
voltage change, 64

Memory
    acetoxycycloheximide and, 372
    -enhancer, 686
    storage, long-term
        mirror focus and, 371–374
        occurrence of, 371–373
Meningocerebral cicatrix, 774–776
    schematic representation of, 774
Mephobarbital, electrolytes and amino acids, 712
Metabolic rates in drug-induced convulsions, 640–642
Metabolism
    acid-base. See Acid-base
    amino acid. See Amino acid
    carbohydrate. See Carbohydrate
    cell, experimental models, 778
    changes, in denervated ganglion cells, 337–338
    during convulsions
        pentylenetetrazol, 640
        pyridoxine deficiency, 644
    electrolyte
        in epilepsy, 710–711
        ouabain and, 625–628
    energy. See Energy
    factors in pyridoxal-5′-phosphate pool size, 620
    ionic, 731–733
    lipid. See Lipid
    nucleic acid. See Nucleic acid
    protein. See Protein
    pyridoxine, 621–622, 644
Metabolites
    brain, and pentylenetetrazol, 99
    cerebral cortex, and MSO, in mice, 100
    energy, and experimental seizures, 98–103
Metals, application to cerebral cortex, 264–265
Methionine sulfoximine
    actions
        on biogenic amines, 145
        on enzymes, 145
        possible mechanism, 146
    ammonia levels and, 101
    cerebral cortex metabolites and, in mice, 100
    convulsive states and, experimental, 144–146
    effect in brain, electron microscopy of, 145–146
    glutamate and, 101, 145
    glutamine and, 145
    inducing conditions predisposing to seizures, 190–191

α-Methyl-p-tyrosine, 221
Microelectrode studies of penicillin focus, 320–328
Microreflexes, 548
    chloralose and, 560
Microscopy
    electron. See Electron microscopy
    light, of cerebellar cortex, in rat, 148–150
Microspectrophotometry of mirror focus, 359–360
Mind, mechanism that corresponds with, 802–803
Mirror focus
    establishment of, 371
    histochemistry of, 357–370
    independent intracellular microelectrode record, in frog, 358
    memory storage and, long-term, 371–374
    microspectrophotometry of, 359–360
    physiology of, 357–370
Mode(s), normal, 763–764
Model(s)
    animal, baboon as, 566
    brain function, 768–771
    cerebral cortex, 29
    computer, 560–561
    Davson-Danielli, 783
    epilepsy
        experimental, 263–279
        startle, 554–557
        trigger, 557–558
    epileptic neuron, 279–284
    experimental, 263–279, 558–561
    in neuropathology, 776–780
    Lehninger, 783
    of Lenard and Singer, 783
    lipid, 783
    of Lucy, 783
    membrane, 783
    myoclonus, 559–560
    neural, 766
    neurochemical mechanisms, selected, 612–628
    photoepilepsy, quantitative, 551–552
    proteins, 783
    seizures, photoepileptic, 551
    spikes, interictal, 595
    systems, and genetics, 690–692
Modulation, pulse-interval, 758
Molecular genetics, 9
Molecular mechanisms of excitability, 66–70
Molluscan cells, 76–80
Monoamines
    CNS, fluorescence histochemistry of, 212–227

    intraneuronal distribution of, 213–214
    neurons. See Neurons
    release of, 221–222
        compared with ACh, 221–222
Monosialaganglioside, structure of, 785
Monosynaptic reflexes during REM sleep, 461
Monovalent anions, 672–675
Morphology
    neuroglial cells, 747–753
    synaptic region of normal brain, 137
Motoneuron(s)
    CHEB and, 180
    decentralized, 330
    EPSPs in, 231, 236
    inhibitory pathways to, 240
    IPSPs in, 236
    pentylenetetrazol and, 177–178
    trigeminal motor nucleus, 476
Motor
    areas, and neurophysiology, 792–793
    -control system, bilateral, 801
    function, paradoxical improvement of, 5
Movement, evolving, 26
MSO. See Methionine sulfoximine
Muscarinic cholinoceptive site, 335
Muscle, diphenylhydantoin effects on, 653–657
Mutation rate, 701
Mutually inhibitory connections, 581
    in interneurons, 583
Myelination and CNS development, 537
Myocardium and diphenylhydantoin, 653–654
Myoclonus
    latency in Jakob-Creutzfeldt disease, 549
    models, 559–560
    twitches during desynchronized sleep, 459

Na
    cation transport by, 91
    movement after electrical stimulation, 88
    properties of, 91
Na+
    active transport of, 44, 53
    channels
        distinctive characteristics of, 67–68
        model of, 68–69

selectivity of, 68
voltage-induced confirmation change in, 69–70
conductance
activation of, 61–62
calcium concentration and, 68
inactivation of, 61–62
temperature dependence of, 68
inactivation, model of, 62
pump, 53
regulation of Na+-K+ pumping rate, 71–72
role of, 71
separability of Na+ and K+ channels, 67
voltage dependence of, 61
NE. *See* Norepinephrine
Negativity, surface, 413–414
Neocortex. *See also* Cerebral cortex
afterdischarge, inhibitory and excitatory actions in, 588
conductance IPSPs in, 577
immature, excitability of, 495–497
interictal spikes in, 592
inhibition, 590
potentials, generation of, 411–420
pyramidal neurons, in newborn kitten, 482
Neostigmine, effects on cerebral cortex, in cat, 423
Nernst equation, 51
Nerve(s)
abnormal function
enzymatic defects resulting in, 693–697
genetic defects and, 691–692
activity, and neuroglia, 742–744
cell body, schematic representation of, 776
cranial, and forebrain inhibition, 474–477
endings
aminergic, 137–138
changes due to allylglycine, 147
membranes, cholinergic, isolation of, 141–142
membranes, noncholinergic, isolation of, 141–142
membranes, receptor properties of, 142–144
nonaminergic, 137–138
nonaminergic, inhibitory synapses and, 138–140
sympathetic, disuse potentiation in, 336
epileptic tissue
primary, 422
projected, 422

secondary, 422
facial, 477
fibers, method for studying electrical activity of, 42
growth factor, 696
impulse, 41–44
membrane, biophysics of, 41–75
models, 766
networks activated in CNS tissues developing in culture, 506–515
oculomotor, evoked potentials, in cat, 475
optic, recordings from, 744
peripheral, diphenylhydantoin actions on, 684–685
spinal, and forebrain inhibition, 477–478
systems, development of, 537–539
Nervous control, compulsory, 332
Nervous system
central
biochemical development, seizure activity, and endocrine function, 731–734
development and growth, 535–537
diphenylhydantoin and, 539, 682–684
excitatory pathways in, 239–250
explants, repetitive afterdischarges in, 510
glia-neuronal relationships in, 748
inhibitory pathways in, 239–250
inhibitory transmission in, 203–205
intrinsic capacity to organize neural networks, 506
monoamines in, fluorescence histochemistry of, 212–227
strychnine effects on, 304–305
tissues developing in culture, neural networks activated in, 506–515
didione effects on, 668–670
diphenylhydantoin effects on, 647–653
peripheral, strychnine effects on, 313
proteins of, 692–693
trimethadione effects on, 668–670
vertebrate, cellular relations in, 739
Neural brain, of kitten, 482
glial, 482

Neuroanatomy, 769–770
Neurobiology and epilepsies, 10–11
Neurochemical correlates of convulsive discharge, 185–186
Neurochemical mechanisms, 611–638
Neurochemistry
brain, normal, 159–163
synaptic region, 137
challenge to, 9–10
convulsants, 184–193
convulsive states, experimental, 144–154
ultrastructural, 137–158
Neuroendocrine mechanisms in epilepsy, 717–722
Neuroglia
cells, morphology of, 747–753
nerve activity and, 742–744
-neuronal interactions, 737–746
diffusion through intercellular clefts, 737–738
Neurohumoral transmitters, 196–197
Neuromorphology, challenge to, 10
Neuropathology, perspectives in, 773–781
Neuron(s)
action site of drugs, 220
antagonistic motoneuronal pools during desynchronized sleep, 466
brain, properties of, 770
central, supersensitivity after cholinergic blockade, 339–340
circuit, basic 24–26
cortical, immature
seizure discharges in neonate and, 482–487
spike generation in dendrites of, 492–495
deafferented, 270–279, 329–348
dendrites and axons radiating from, drawing of, 230
denervated, 282–284, 335–338
disused, 335–338
DS generating, synaptic activity and spike potentials in, 321
DSCT, responses to electrodes, 132
epileptic, 10, 263–288, 776
aggregate, steady state depolarization in, 322
axon stimuli, 281–282
chronic foci, 321–322
as chronic foci, 263–288
chronic foci, alumina, 292
deafferentation, 270–279

Neuron(s), epileptic—*Continued*
  denervation and, 282–284
  depolarization shift and, 320–324
  electrophysiological characteristics of, 320–324
  firing, 267–269
  firing, burst, analysis of patterns, 276–279
  firing, burst, long first-interval, 278
  interictal activity of, 265–270
  models of, 279–284
  raster displays of, 277
  spike densities of, 277
  in epileptogenic focus, 268–270
  excitatory, PT cells as, 256–270
  firing, 267–269, 276–279
    burst, normal neurons, 276
    repetitively, voltage clamp analysis of, 76
    spontaneous, 70–72
    spontaneous, consequences of repetitive firing, 71
    spontaneous, mechanism of, 70
  fluid environment of, 738–740
  follower, 270, 587
  glia-neuronal relationships in CNS, 748
  hippocampal. *See* Hippocampus, neurons
  isolated, 329–348
  long-isolated cerebral cortex tissue and, 160
  maturation patterns, and seizure susceptibility of immature brain, 497–501
  mechanisms underlying EEG, 397–410
  membrane potentials, 385
  monoamine
    central, pharmacology of, 218–222
    distribution of, 215
    function of, 222–223
    main systems, schematic drawing, 218
    mapping out of central systems, 217–218
    morphology of, 212–213
  mutually inhibitory connections in, 581
  neuroglial-neuronal interactions, 737–746
    diffusion through intercellular clefts, 737–738
  nonepileptic aggregates, and epileptiform discharge, 324–327
  nucleus, dorsal lateral geniculate, axonal projections of, 31
  oscillator, 535
  pacemaker, 587
  polarization of. *See* Polarization
  prepared by rapid Golgi technique, 77
  projected epileptiform activity during projected discharge, 326
  pyramidal, in kitten
    arciform, 499
    hippocampal, membrane potential in, 493
    hippocampal, spike potentials from, 493
    neocortex, 482
  spinal, deafferentation, 273–275
  surround inhibition and, 325
  synchronization, 398
    hippocampal, 445
  system, 241
    centrencephalic, 433–434
Neuropathology, 773–781
  biochemical, levels for study, 780
  models in, experimental, 776–780
Neurophysiology, 791–805
  challenge to, 8–9
Neuropil
  axonal, and apical dendrites, 22
  cortical, 18–27
  electron micrograph of, 21
  geometry, tentative, 23–24
Neurotransmission and CNS development, 537
Neurotransmitters. *See also* Transmitters
  in cerebral cortex, normal and isolated, 159–165
  didione effects on, 672
  diphenylhydantoin effects on, 666–668
  trimethadione effects on, 672
Newborn
  focal seizure ontogeny study, in monkey. *See* Focal seizure ontogeny study, in monkey
  immature cortical neurons and seizure discharges of, 482–487
NGF, 696
Nialamide, 216, 220
Nicotinic cholinoceptive sites, 335
Nitrogen balance and petit mal, 713
Noncholinergic transmission, 204–205
Nonlinear coupling, 764–766

Nonlinear springs, 764
Norepinephrine, 111, 220
  modification of synthesis, uptake, and release by drugs, 198
Normal modes, 763–764
NSD-1015, 220
Nucleic acid metabolism
  didione effects on, 671–672
  diphenylhydantoin effects on, 662–666
  trimethadione effects on, 671–672
Nucleus
  geniculate, lateral
    polarization of, 389–393
    polarization of, transcortical, 392–393
    records from, in cat, 390
  thalamic, and spike-wave complex, 404
  trigeminal
    mesencephalic, 475
    motor, motoneuron of, 476

Oligodendrocyte, 751–753
Ontogeny. *See* Focal seizure ontogeny study
Operon, 702
Optic nerve, recordings from, 744
Oscillator(s)
  linearly coupled, 762–764
  neurons, 535
Ouabain, 91
  electrolyte metabolism and, 625–628

Pacemaker neurons, 587
Pacemaker potential, 70, 76
Pacemaker systems, subcortical, 447–449
Paradoxical improvement of motor function, 5
Parallel inhibitory connections, 581, 582
Paralysis, sleep, 465
Parathyroid deficiency and seizures, 719
Paroxysm, ACh-induced, in isolated cortex, in cat, 424
Paroxysmal depolarization shifts. *See* Depolarization
Paroxysmal discharge. *See* Discharge
Paroxysmal states, DC potential shifts in, 375–388
Passive transport, 53
Pathology of epilepsy, 773–776
pCO_2
  changes during apnea after ventilation with oxygen, 385
  dc shifts and, seizure type, 380–382

P-creatine and electrical stimulation, in mice, 99
PDSs. See Depolarization
Peduncle, cerebral
  potentials evoked by stimulation, 258
  responses evoked by stimulation, 254
Penicillin
  effects of, 305–308
  focal seizure ontogeny study and, 517, 532
  focus
    epileptiform activity in, 300
    epileptogenic, and surround inhibition, 325
    ictal episode in, 309
    ictal episode in, spontaneous, in cat, 406
    microelectrode studies of, 320–328
    PDSs in, in cat, 401
  fornix and inhibition, 589
  hippocampal interictal spike, 597
  PDSs and, 30, 400–401
  poisoning, interictal paroxysmal activity during, 400–402
Pentylenetetrazol
  astroglial swelling after, 151
    interpretation of, 153–154
  ATPase and, 151
  brain metabolites and, 99
  convulsive states and, experimental, 151–154
  dc potential shifts and, 384
  direct stimulation by, 175–179
  -induced convulsive potentials, in cat, 403
  inducing convulsions, blood flow and metabolism during, 640
  motoneuron and, 177–178
  phosphohydrolases and, 151, 153
  potentials, 402
  seizure, clonic phase, in cat, 407
Perikaryon, 750–753
Permanent facilitation, 802
Permanent impression, 798
Permeability, 48
Persisting elements method, 16
Petit mal, 547
  absence, 6
  acetazolamide in, 714
  acid-base balance and, 713
  acid-base metabolism in, 714
  aminoaciduria in, 716
  automatism and, 800–801
  classical attack, 422
  diphenylhydantoin in, 619
  electrolyte balance and, 713

idiopathic, 7
ketogenic diet in, 712, 714
mephobarbital in, 712
nitrogen balance and, 713
seizures, centrencephalic, 6
status, 435
trimethadione in, 619, 712
pH and seizure type dc shifts, 380–382
Pharmacogenetics, 703
Pharmacological presynaptic inhibition, 673
Pharmacology
  of monoamine neurons, 218–222
  of synaptic transmitters, 195–211
Pheniprazine, 220
Phenobarbital, 89, 675
  structure of, 648
Phenocopy, 701
Phenoxybenzamine, 220
Phosphocreatine, 86–87
  after electroshock, in rat, 87
Phosphohydrolases and pentylenetetrazol, 151, 153
Phosphorylation and pyridoxal-5'-phosphate pool size, 620
Photoepilepsy, 545–548
  central mechanisms in, 549–550
  models, quantitative, 551–552
Photoepileptic seizures, models, 551
Photogenic epilepsy, 565
Photogenic seizures, in baboon, 565–573
Photomotor microreflex, 548
Photosensitive epilepsy, 565
Physical dependence
  depression and, 340
  disuse theory of, 340–341
Physiological advances, future, 810–811
Physiology of mirror focus, 357–370
Pilocarpine blocking postsynaptic inhibition, 171–172
Pituitary-adrenal imbalance and seizures, 717–719
pO_2
  changes during apnea after ventilation with oxygen, 385
  dc shifts and, 383
  seizure type, 380–382
Poisoning, penicillin, interictal paroxysmal activity after, 400–402
Polarization
  anatomical arrangements basic to studies of, 390
  ictal episode and, 310–311
  neurons

cortical, 389–395
geniculate, 389–395
nucleus, geniculate lateral, 389–393
applied polarization, 391–392
transcortical polarization, 392–393
primary visual response and, 392
surface anodal, in kitten, 494
Polymorphism, balanced, 702
Polynucleotide systems, diphenylhydantoin actions on, 687
Polysynaptic reflexes during REM sleep, 461
Pore protein, 67
Positivity, surface, and ictal EEG phenomena, 405
Postictal depression and diphenylhydantoin, 685
Postjunctional elements, sensitivity of, 332
Postsynaptic inhibition. See Inhibition
Postsynaptic membrane
  abnormalities, 322
  lipids formed in, 786–788
Postsynaptic potentials. See Potentials
Posttetanic potentiation and diphenylhydantoin, 682
Potassium, 87–90
  accumulation, consequences of, 743–744
  concentration, and membrane potential, 741
  glial, 740
  conductance, 61–64
    changes, kinetics of, 62–63
  equilibrium potential, 51
  inactivation, 81
  ions, 51, 237
    conductance, 61
    current, 60–61
  -sodium exchange, active, 53–54
Potency of prejunctional elements, 332
Potential(s)
  action, 42, 55
    generation, 43–44
    prediction from voltage-clamp data, 63–66
    primary current generators and, 416–417
    propagated, calculated from Hodgkin-Huxley equations, 64
    propagation, 43–44
  PT cells, 253–254
  spontaneous, in epileptic cerebral cortex, in monkey, 280

Potential(s), action—*Continued*
tracing, dorsal-root fiber, 42
changes measured during spreading depression, 295
concentration, energy difference, 51
convulsive, pentylenetetrazol-induced, in cat, 403
cuneate surface, of cerebral peduncle, 258
dc shifts, 375–388
  cortical, types of, 377
  delayed clonic phase type, 377
  main types associated with seizure activity, 376–377
  origin and functional significance of shifts, 383–385
  in paroxysmal states, 375–388
  pentylenetetrazol and, 384
  pO_2 and, 380–383
dc shifts, seizure type, 377–382
  diphenylhydantoin action and, 379
  distribution, 377–378
  EEG waves and, 378–380
  pCO_2 and, 380–382
  pH and, 380–382
  pO_2 and, 380–382
  polarity, 377–378
  time course, 377–378
dc shifts, spreading depression type, 377, 382–383
dendritic, 682
depolarizing
  cellular mechanisms of, 589–590
  pathways mediating, 590–593
electric
  energy difference, 51
  ion concentration in cells and, 44
electrochemical, 50–52
  difference, 50–51
equilibrium, 50
  potassium, 51
evoked
  enhancement, in immature brain, 512–513
  oculomotor nerve, in cat, 475
  in photosensitive baboons, 570–571
  in precruciate gyrus after electrical stimulation, 398
  prolongation, in immature brain, 512–513
  in ventrobasal thalamus, 247

excitatory postsynaptic. *See* EPSPs
extracellular, to entorhinal stimulation, 242
fields, and "ephaptic" excitation, 427
gial contribution to, 744–745
hyperpolarizing
  cellular mechanisms of, 589–590
  pathways mediating, 590–593
inhibitory postsynaptic. *See* IPSPs
maintenance of, 54–55
membrane
  cellular, 90
  glial, 742
  glial, and potassium concentration, 740
  immature brain and, 484
  neuron, 385
  neuron, hippocampal pyramidal, in kitten, 493
  potassium concentration, and, 741
  traces, two superimposed, 79
neocortical, generation of, 411–420
neuronal membrane, 385
pacemaker, 70, 76
pentylenetetrazol, 402
postsynaptic
  excitatory. *See* EPSPs
  inhibitory. *See* IPSPs
  primary current generators and, 411–416
resting, 42
PT cells, 253–254
slow hump, 682
spike
  antidromic, in kitten, 486
  DS generating neurons and, 321
  hippocampal pyramidal neuron, 445
  hippocampal pyramidal neuron, in kitten, 493
steady, 375
  changes during apnea after ventilation with oxygen, 385
strychnine, 402
synaptic
  giant, DS as, 320
  time course of, 130–131
transmembrane, 50
  steady-state, 54–55
unit, rhythmic repetitive bursts in epileptic cortex, in monkey, 267

Potentiation
  disuse, 331
  in sympathetic nerve endings, 336
  frequency, 605–607
  posttetanic, and diphenylhydantoin, 682
Precruciate gyrus, electrical stimulation of, 398
Prefrontal discharge, automatism after, 799–800
Pregnancy and pyridoxal-5′-phosphate pool size, 620
Prejunctional elements, potency of, 332
Prepotentials. *See* Fast prepotentials
Presynaptic abnormalities, 322–324
Presynaptic function of acetylcholine, 201
Presynaptic inhibition. *See* Inhibition
Presynaptic terminal, 239
Probands
  with focal EEG, 705–706
  treated surgically for focal epilepsy, 706–707
Programming and learning, 793–795
Projection, 799
  afterdischarge and, 430
  corticofugal projection, in monkey, 431
  over long conducting pathways, 427–433
  strychnine spikes, in cat, 429
  type of spontaneous activity and acetylcholine, 107
Propagation
  in dendrites, in kitten, 495
  distinguished from spread, 422
  extracellular studies, 421–440
  focal seizure ontogeny study and, 532
  of impulse, local circuits, 65
  mechanisms of, 421–440
    cholinergic, 423–426
    intracellular studies, 441–451
    intracortical, 422–427
    over long conducting pathways, 427–433
  of seizures, and commissural section, 439
  spike, interictal, 596–598
Proprioceptive induction, 555
Prospectus, 807–814
Prostaglandins, 786–788
  as central transmitters, 119
  structure, 786

Protein(s)
  from brain, electrophoresis of, 693
  DNA transformation into structure of, 690
  metabolism, 733–734
    didione effects on, 671–672
    diphenylhydantoin effects on, 662–666
    trimethadione effects on, 671–672
  model, 783
  of nervous system, 692–693
  pore, 67
  synthesis
    acetoxycycloheximide and, 372
    inhibitors of, 93
Protriptyline, 220
Pseudoexplosive mechanisms, 759–761
PST characteristics, defining in immature brain, 484–485
Psychical responses, 798
PT cells. See Pyramidal tract cells
PTZ. See Pentylenetetrazol
Pulse-interval modulations, 758
Pump, 47
  electrogenic. See Electrogenic pump
  inhibition, 72
  Na+, 53
Purkinje cells, 750
  characteristics in irradiated cerebellum, 501
  dendrites
    immature brain, 499–501
    retardation of, 499
  electron microscopy of, 16–18
    basal region, in rat, 151
  microphotographs of, 500
Pyramidal tract cells, 253–261
  axonal conduction velocity, 253
  biophysical properties, 253–256
  classification, 253–256
  corticofugal influences by, 258–259
  as excitatory neurons, 256–257
  frequency potentiation of, 606
  hippocampal, impulse initiation during seizure, 585
  intracortical synaptic mechanism, 257–258
  iontophoretic application of strychnine to, 305
  membranes, electrical parameters of, 254–255
  potential
    action, 253–254
    resting, 253–254
  studies of, 253–261

  synaptically activated, 243
  synaptic organization of, 256–259
  vesicular
    flattened, 16
    spheric, 16
Pyridoxal phosphate and convulsant hydrazides, 192
Pyridoxal-5′-phosphate pool size, 620–622
  apoenzyme and, 620
  metabolism factors, 620
  supply factors, 620
Pyridoxine
  deficiency, and convulsions, 642–644
  dependency, electroencephalography of, 643
  metabolism of, 621–622

Raster displays of epileptic neurons, 277
Reading epilepsy, 555
Rebound
  character of withdrawal symptoms, 340–341
  effect, 339
Recall, voluntary, 798
Receptor
  chemical, isolation of, 144
  -properties of nerve-ending membranes, 142–144
Reciprocal inhibition, 575
Rectification, anomalous, 80
Recurrent inhibition, 575
Reeler mouse, 697
Reference electrodes, 390
  indifferent, 411
Reflex(es)
  corneal, inhibition of, 477
  cortically induced inhibition of, 478
  discussion of term, 565
  epilepsy. See Epilepsy
  masseteric, 475
  mechanisms, and sensory precipitation, 543–564
  microreflexes, 548
    chloralose and, 560
  monosynaptic
    during REM sleep, 461
    spinal, effects of tenotomy on, 338–339
  polysynaptic, during REM sleep, 461
  responses of interneurons in spinal cord, 462
  seizures, 544
Refractory period, 65
REM sleep. See Sleep
Renshaw cells, 204
  pathway through, 240
Repetitive activity, capacity for, 332

Repolarization, 63–65
Reserpine, 220
Respiration, cerebral, 83–84
Resting potential, 42
Rhinencephalon
  acetylcholine and, 106–109
  catecholamines and, 112
  5-hydroxytryptamine and, 112
Rhythm(s)
  of discharge, basic, 443
  regularization of, and synaptic delay, 757–759
Ribonucleic acid
  concentration, hypotheses about, 365–368
  inhibition and, 365
  synthesis, cerebral, 373–374
  turnover in secondary epileptogenic foci cells, 360–368
RNA. See Ribonucleic acid
Rubral activity during REM sleep, 459

Schaffer collateral activation, 243
SCRs, in kitten, 498
Secondary bilateral synchrony, 555
Seizure(s)
  acid-base changes and, 713–714
  activity
    associative, and hormones, 730–731
    CNS biochemical development and endocrine function, 731–734
    generalized, and hormones, 727–728
    in hippocampus, initiation of, 446
    localized, and hormones, 727–730
  adrenal imbalance and, 717–719
  afterdischarge, and inhibition, 581–588
  amino acid disorders complicated, 715
  amino acids and, 185–186
  ammonia and, 185–186
  centrencephalic, 6–7
    petit mal, 6
    simple absence, 6
  cerebral
    generalized, 7
    unlocalized, 7
  chemically induced, 537–538
    diphenylhydantoin and, 539
  classification, 3–7
  dc potential shifts associated with, 376–377
    origin and functional significance of, 383–385
  definition, early, 1

832   INDEX

Seizure(s)—Continued
  development
    associative activity, and hormones, 730–731
    at cellular level, 629
    electroshock patterns, maximal, 536
    electroshock patterns, minimal, 535–536
    generalized activity, and hormones, 727–728
    hormones and, 727–736
    localized activity, and hormones, 728–730
  discharges. See Discharge
  drug-induced conditions predisposing to, 186–191
  electrically induced, and diphenylhydantoin, 539
  electrodecremental, 84
  electrolyte disorders predisposing to, 709–710
  estradiol dipropionate and, in rat, 729–730
  evoked, 544
  excitatory
    in fornix, 585–586
    termination by hyperpolarization, 584
  experimental
    energy metabolites in, 98–103
    mechanisms, 289–298
  focal, 4–6
    aura and, 4
    cortical, diphenylhydantoin and, 682–683
    distribution of initial phenomena in, 5
    ontogeny study. See Focal seizure ontogeny study
  generalized, of sudden bilateral onset, 433–436
  in hippocampus, transitions of interictal spike, 599
  hyperglycemic effects of, 720
  hypernatremia and, 710
  hypocalcemia and, 710
  hypoglycemia and, 719–720
  hyponatremia and, 709–710
  impulse initiation in pyramidal cells, 585
  induction, and experimental models, 559
  inhibitory, in fornix, 586–587
  insulin excess and, 719–720
  Jacksonian, 517
  light stimulation inducing, 558
  local, spread, ephaptic mechanisms in, 441–446
  magnesium depletion and, 710
  maturational factors in, 535–541
  mechanisms of, 7–10
  experimental, 289–298
    in fornix, 587–588
  parathyroid deficiency and, 719
  pattern, after brain stem transection, and diphenylhydantoin, 683–684
  pentylenetetrazol, clonic phase, in cat, 407
  photoepileptic, models, 551
  photogenic, in baboon, 565–573
  pituitary imbalance and, 717–719
  precipitated, 544
  propagation, and commissural section, 439
  psychomotor, 6
  psychoparetic, 6
  recording, in monkey, 265
  reflex, 544
  sex hormones and, 720–722
  somesthetic induced, 554–555
  sound-induced, 552–554
  spatial spread of, limiting, 601
  stimulus-sensitive, 544
  strychnine, and diphenylhydantoin, 684
  susceptibility
    genetics of, 689–699
    of immature brain, 481–505
    of immature brain, enhancement and maturation patterns, 497–501
    regional variability in, 608
  synaptic inhibition in, 575–603
  thyroid imbalance and, 719
  tonic, and diphenylhydantoin, 685
  transition to, 596–598
  triggers of. See Triggers
  withdrawal, and disuse supersensitivity, 341–342
SEL. See Epileptogenic lesions
Semantic information, 548
Sensitivity
  frequency, 607–608
  of postjunctional elements, 332
Sensitization, disuse, 331
Sensitizing factor, 330
Sensorimotor cortex, in normal monkey, 271
Sensory areas and neurophysiology, 792–793
Sensory precipitation
  of epilepsy, 458
  reflex mechanisms and, 543–564
Series inhibitory connections, 579–581
Sex hormone
  in epilepsy, 721
  seizures and, 720–722
Shock, surface, inhibition evoked by, 161
Sigmoid gyrus, epileptogenic focus in, 598
Sleep, 453–473
  deprivation, 458–464
    epilepsy and, 458–464
  desynchronized, 453
    antagonistic motoneuronal pools during, 466
    myoclonic twitches during, 459
    REM of, monosynaptic and polysynaptic reflexes during, 461
    REM of, pyramidal discharge during, 459
    REM of, rubral activity increase during, 459
  electrical stimulation during, 455
  epilepsy and, 453–467
  epileptic discharges and
    focal, 456–458
    generalized, 455–456
  mechanisms of, 453–473
  paralysis, 465
  REM, 459
    anticonvulsant experiments, 464–467
    convulsive activity and, 463–464
    deprivation, convulsive threshold and, 463
    interruption of, 460–463
  sleep epilepsies, 454
  synchronized, 453
Slow hump potential, 682
Sodium, 87–90
  conductance, 61, 64
  diethyldithiocarbamate, 220
  ion, 52
    conductance, 61
    current, 60
    -potassium exchange, active, 53–54
  transport, active, 52–54
    energy requirements for, 53
Solitons, 765
Soma, depolarization absence, 243
Somesthetic induced seizures, 554–555
Sound-induced seizures, 552–554
Spasms, clonic, and diphenylhydantoin, 685
Spatial buffers, 154, 743
Spike(s), 289–292
  activation of electrogenic Na+ pump, 578
  bursts, recorded from cell bodies, 324
  densities of epileptic neurons, 277
  discharges. See Discharge

EEG intervals, and cortical dc shifts, 378
epileptic, 265, 279
epileptiform focal, in immature brain, 482
  hypersynchronous major, 484
epileptogenic agents and, topical, 300
generation in dendrites of immature cortical neurons, 492–495
ILS inducing, in photosensitive baboon, 567
induction, in kitten, 494
interictal
  cortical, 293
  hippocampal, 590–591, 599
  hippocampal penicillin, 597
  inhibition and, 588–598
  inhibition in neocortex and hippocampus, 590
  mechanisms in generation of, 593–596
  model of, 595
  in neocortex, 590–592
  propagation of, 596–598
  restriction of, 596–598
  transition to seizure in hippocampus, 599
intracellular, initiation of, 444
negative field, 445
potentials. See Potentials
responses, and transcortical current densities, 411
strychnine, projection of, in cat, 429
-wave
  abnormality, bilaterally synchronous, 435
  complex, 402–404
  EEG trait, 704, 707
  EEG trait, age and, 705
  electrical disturbances in EEG, 422
  epilepsy, 704–705
Spindle
  activity and diphenylhydantoin, 682
  bursts, and secondary current generators, 417
Spine
  cord
    acetylcholine and, 110–111
    anterior horn of, in rat, 751–753
    catecholamines and, 113
    convulsions, development of, 536
    disuse supersensitivity in, 338–339
    gray matter of, in rat, 748–749
    5-hydroxytryptamine and, 113
    interneurons, reflex responses of, 462
    spontaneous activity in, in cat, 274
    stimulation of, 535–537
    strychnine effects on, 306–307
  nerves, and forebrain inhibition, 477–478
  neurons, deafferentation, 273–275
  reflexes, monosynaptic, effects of tenotomy of, 338–339
  trigeminal spinal complex
    deafferentation of, 275–276
    spontaneous activity in, 275
Spread
  by diffusion, 426–427
  distinguished from propagation, 422
  local seizure, ephaptic mechanisms in, 441–446
Spreading depression, 293–296
  complete, segments from, 295
  potential changes measured during, 295
Spring(s)
  coupling, 763
  nonlinear, 764
Stability of immature brain, 481–505
Status epilepticus and lipids, 186
Steady potential. See Potential
Steady state
  concentration, maintenance of, 54–55
  definition, 54
  transmembrane potential, 54–55
Stellate cells, 18–19
  degenerating terminals of, 34
  electron microscopy of, 18
  giant, 30
Stimulant drugs, 340
Stimulation
  audiogenic, energy expenditure changes after, 100
  cerebral cortex and, isolated, 349–355
  electrical. See Electrical stimulation
  epicortical, self-sustained afterdischarge after, 404–405
  light
    electrographic discharges evoked by, 548–549
    seizure due to, 558
    spike and wave discharges produced by, 544
    photic, comparison of normal and epileptic responses to, 550
  spinal cord, 535–537
  surface folial, in irradiated kittens, 501
  thalamus, 292–296
Stimulus, 55
  -sensitive
    epilepsy, 544, 565
    seizures, 544
Strychnine
  action of, 117
  blocking postsynaptic inhibition, 169–171
  burst after depolarization inactivation, 412
  effects of, 305–308
    on CNS, 304–305
    excitatory, 600
    on peripheral nervous system, 313
    on spinal cord, 306–307
  iontophoretic application to PT cells, 305
  potentials, 402
  seizures, and diphenylhydantoin, 684
  spikes, projection of, in cat, 429
Subcortical pacemaker systems, 447–449
Substance P as central transmitter, 119
Subsynaptic membrane, 229
Subthreshold, 42
Supersensitivity
  central neurons after cholinergic blockade, 339–340
  cerebral cortex and, partially isolated, 350–354
  of denervated ganglion cells to acetylcholine, 335–338
  denervation, 162, 330
    differentiated from disuse supersensitivity, 331
  disuse, 329–348
    development during depression, 342
    differentiated from denervation supersensitivity, 331
    properties, in autonomic effectors, 334–335
    spinal cord, 338–339
    withdrawal seizures and, 341–342
    withdrawal symptoms as, 339–342
  meaning of, 330–332
  nonspecific, 334
Suprathreshold, 42
Surgeon's electrode and ictal discharge, 791
Surgery of focal epilepsy, 706–707
Surround inhibition, 324–326, 575

S wave, 761
Swelling. *See* Edema
Switch genes, 702
Synapse(s)
    astrocytic lamellar processes and, 748–753
    axodendritic, 354
        in newborn kitten, 483
    axosomatic, 354, 490–492
        in hippocampus, in kitten, 489
    connections, and cultures, 511–512
    degenerating, in cat, 33
    electron microscopy of, 15–18
    excitatory, 229–239
        action, 230–233
        frequency potentiation of, 605–607
    glomerular, of cerebellum, electron microscopy of, in rat, 152
    inhibitory, 37, 229–239, 575–603
        nonaminergic nerve endings and, 138–140
    structural features of, 229–230
    -studded dendrites, 31
    trophic change mediated by, 495
Synaptic activation of electrogenic Na+ pump, 578
Synaptic activity
    in DS generating neurons, 321
    during projected epileptiform discharges, 326–327
Synaptic cartridges, 15, 20, 36
Synaptic cleft, 239
Synaptic contacts, giant, 133
Synaptic current
    EPSP and, 132
    time course of, 131–132
Synaptic delay and rhythm regularization, 757–759
Synaptic influences on epileptogenic discharges of neocortex, 446–450
Synaptic inhibition in seizures, 575–603
Synaptic knob, 229
    excitatory activated, 235
Synaptic mechanisms of PDSs, 301–305
Synaptic membranes
    chemical structure of, 782–790
    glycolipids of, 784–786
Synaptic organization of PT cells, 256–259
Synaptic potentials. *See* Potentials
Synaptic region of brain, normal
    morphology of, 137–144
    neurochemistry of, 137–144

Synaptic transmitters
    central, 105–129
    pharmacology of, 195–211
Synaptic vesicles, 229, 239
    amines of, biogenic, 141
    elliptical, 141
    flattened, 141
    isolation of, 141
    neurotransmitters and, 160
    quantal release of transmitter and, 140–141
Synaptology, 229
Synaptosomes, 159
Synchronization
    of follower cell population, 581
    mechanism, global, 758
    of neurons, 398
        hippocampal, 445
    of refractory conduction networks, 755–756
Synchrony, 755–767
    secondary bilateral, 555
    theoretical concepts of, 755–767

Tay-Sachs disease, 694–695
Temporal lobe discharge, automatism after, 799
Tenotomy, effects on monosynaptic spinal reflexes, 338–339
TEPP, 612–613
    inducing conditions predisposing to seizures, 187
Terminals
    degenerating, 34
    presynaptic, 239
Termination sites, of callosal fibers, 35
Terminology and reflex mechanisms, 543–545
Tetrabenazine, 220
Tetraethylpyrophosphate, 612–613
    inducing conditions predisposing to seizures, 187
Tetrodotoxin, 89
Thalamocortical interrelationships, 429–433
Thalamus
    acetylcholine and, 110
    activity, 449–450
    excitatory mechanisms in, 247–249
    inhibitory mechanisms in, 247–249
    nucleus, and spike-wave complex, 404
    stimulation, 292–296
    ventrobasal, electrical potentials evoked in, 247

Thebaine blocking postsynaptic inhibition, 171
Theory, disuse, of physical dependence, 340–341
Thermal equilibrium, 765
Threshold, 42, 65
    -all-or-nothing, 42
    decrease, 72
Thyroid imbalance and seizures, 719
Time course
    synaptic current, 131–132
    synaptic potential, 130–131
Tonic seizure and diphenylhydantoin, 685
Transmissions
    adrenergic, 197–199
    cholinergic, 197–199, 204–205
    inhibitory, in CNS, 203–205
    noncholinergic, 204–205
Transmitter(s). *See also* Neurotransmitters
    action, and multiple discharge, 130–135
    amino acid transmitter function, 118–119
    inactivation, changes affecting, 332
    inhibitory, role of acetylcholine in releasing, 204
    neurohumoral, 196–197
    quantal release, and synaptic vesicles, 140–141
    removal, changes affecting, 332
    synaptic. *See* Synaptic transmitters
Transmitting areas, primary, 793
Transport
    active, 53
    passive, 53
Tranylcypromine, 220
Trigeminal
    nucleus
        mesencephalic, 475
        motor, motoneuron of, 476
    spinal complex
        deafferentation of, 275–276
        spontaneous activity in, 275
Trigger(s)
    epileptic, internal, 555
    multisensory, 565–566
Triggered seizures, 544
Triggering phenomenon, 302
Trimethadione, 668–672
    effects
        biochemical processes, 670–672
        nervous system, 668–670
        neurotransmitters, 672
    electrolytes and amino acids, 712
    petit mal and, 619
    structure of, 648

INDEX 835

Tumor, cystic, of right hemisphere, 434

Ultrastructural neurochemistry, 137–158
Ultrastructure, experimental convulsive states, 144–154
Use hypothesis and isolated cortex stimulation, 350

Vesicles. *See* Synaptic vesicles
Vessels
    diphenylhydantoin and, 653–655
    epileptic brain, 639–640
Visual response, primary, and polarization, 392
Vitamin B_6
    deficiency, in rat, 621
    -dependency, 622
        electroencephalography of, 616, 618
        gamma-aminobutyric acid and, 614–620

Voltage
    clamp
        analysis, repetitively firing neuron, 76–82
        data, prediction of action potential from, 63–66
    clamping, 58
        in giant axon, in squid, 59
        technique, 77–78
    dependence, 61
    steps, response of membrane to, 78
Voluntary recall, 798

Wave(s) 289–292
    calculation of, 414
    clonic phase, 405
    complex pattern during hypoglycemia, in cat, 401
    dc potential shifts and, seizure type, 378–380
    discharges, light stimulus producing, 544
    EEG, spontaneous, in animals without epileptic lesions, 397–400
    F, 761
    ILS inducing, in photosensitive baboon, 567
    interior wave sources, 757
    responses, and transcortical current densities, 411
    S, 761
    sharp, 399–400
        hypoglycemia and, 400
    slower, 399
    -spike. *See* Spike-wave
    spindle, 397–399
    strychnine, and spike discharges, 402
    tonic phase, 405
Wiring, 768
Withdrawal seizures and disuse supersensitivity, 341–342
Withdrawal symptoms
    as disuse supersensitivity, 339–342
    rebound character of, 340–341